Core Curriculum for
Maternal-Newborn Nursing

Core Curriculum for
Maternal-Newborn Nursing

Third Edition

Susan Mattson, PhD, RNC, CTN
Professor and Chairperson, College of Nursing
Adult Health/Parent Child Division
Arizona State University
Tempe, Arizona

Judy E. Smith, PhD, RN, WHNP-C
Professor
Director of Graduate Nursing Program
California State University—Long Beach
Long Beach, California

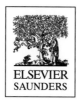

ELSEVIER
SAUNDERS

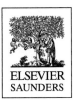

ELSEVIER
SAUNDERS

11830 Westline Industrial Drive
St. Louis, MO 63146

Notice

Nursing is an ever-changing field. Standard safety precautions must be followed, but as new
research and clinical experience broaden our knowledge, changes in treatment and drug therapy
may become necessary or appropriate. Readers are advised to check the most current product
information provided by the manufacturer of each drug to be administered to verify the
recommended dose, the method and duration of administration, and contraindications. It is the
responsibility of the licensed prescriber, relying on experience and knowledge of the patient, to
determine dosages and the best treatment for each individual patient. Neither the publisher nor
the author assumes any liability for any injury and/or damage to persons or property arising
from this publication.

Previous editions copyrighted 2000, 1993

Library of Congress Cataloging-in-Publication Data
Core curriculum for maternal-newborn nursing/edited by Susan Mattson, Judy E.
  Smith.–3rd ed.
      p. ; cm.
   Includes bibliographical references and index.
   ISBN-13: 978-0-7216-0322-3 ISBN-10: 0-7216-0322-X
     1. Maternity nursing–Outlines, syllabi, etc. I. Mattson, Susan. II. Smith, Judy E.
   [DNLM: 1. Maternal-Child Nursing–Outlines. 2. Curriculum–Outlines. WY 18.2
C7965 2004]
RG951.N33 2004
618.2'0231–dc22   2004047368

Executive Editor: Michael S. Ledbetter
Senior Developmental Editor: Laurie K. Gower
Publishing Services Manager: Catherine Jackson
Project Manager: Clay S. Brocker
Design Manager: Amy Buxton

ISBN-13: 978-0-7216-0322-3
ISBN-10: 0-7216-0322-X

Printed in the United States of America

Last digit is the print number: 9 8 7 6 5

Contributors

Linda Bond, PhD, RNC
Professor Emerita, Kirkhof School
of Nursing
Grand Valley State University
Allendale, Michigan
Physiology of Pregnancy

Linda Callahan, CRNA, PhD
Associate Professor, Department
of Nursing
California State University
Long Beach, California
*Genetics; Fetal and Placental
Development and Functioning;
Surgery in Pregnancy*

**Natalie Diane Cheffer, RN, CPNP,
PhD**
Assistant Professor, Department
of Nursing
California State University
Long Beach, California
*Adaptation to Extrauterine Life and
Immediate Nursing Care;
Newborn Biologic/Behavioral
Characteristics and Psychosocial
Adaptations*

Diana E. Clokey, MS, RD, RPh, CDE
Diabetes in Pregnancy Program
Coordinator, School of Medicine
University of New Mexico
Albuquerque, New Mexico
Endocrine and Metabolic Disorders

Catherine R. Coverston, PhD, RNC
Assistant Professor, College
of Nursing
Brigham Young University
Provo, Utah
Psychology of Pregnancy

**Sandra L. Gardner, RN, MS, CNS,
PNP**
Neonatal/Perinatal/Pediatric
Consultant
Director, Professional Outreach
Consultation
Aurora, Colorado
Ethics

Elizabeth Gilbert, RNC, MS, CFNP
Family Nurse Practitioner in Private
Practice
Associate Dean and Associate
Professor, College of Nursing
Grand Canyon University
Phoenix, Arizona
Labor and Birth at Risk

**Starre Haney, RN, MS, TNCC-I,
ENPC**
Emergency Department Clinical
Educator
Scottsdale Healthcare Osborn
Scottsdale, Arizona
Trauma in Pregnancy

**Patricia Grant Higgins, PhD, RN,
BSHEd, BSN, MN**
Professor Emerita, College
of Nursing
The University of New Mexico Health
Sciences Center
Albuquerque, New Mexico
Postpartum Complications

Marcia Liden Jasper, BSN, MS, RNC
Clinical Associate Professor, College of
Nursing
Arizona State University
Tempe, Arizona
Antepartum Fetal Assessment

Denise G. Link, RNC, DNSc
Women's Health Nurse Practitioner
Clinical Associate Professor, College
  of Nursing
Arizona State University
Tempe, Arizona
  Reproductive Anatomy, Physiology,
  and the Menstrual Cycle; Family
  Planning

Susan Mattson, PhD, RNC, CTN
Professor and Chairperson, College
  of Nursing
Adult Health/Parent Child Division
Arizona State University
Tempe, Arizona
  Ethnocultural Considerations in the
  Childbearing Period; Intimate Partner
  Violence

Jacqueline M. McGrath, PhD, RN,
  NNP, CCNS
Assistant Professor, College of Nursing
Arizona State University
Tempe, Arizona
  Identification of the Sick Newborn

Barbara A. Moran, MS, MPH, CNM
Certified Nurse Midwife
Andersen & Maanavi, Ltd.
Fairfax, Virginia
  Maternal Infections; Substance Abuse in
  Pregnancy

Susan Saffer Orr, PT, CLC, IBCLC
Lactation Consultant
Torrance Memorial Medical Center
Torrance, California;
Columbia Pediatrics
Long Beach, California
  Breastfeeding

Judith H. Poole, PhD, BSN, BA, MN
Perinatal Clinical Nurse Specialist
Presbyterian Healthcare System
Charlotte, North Carolina
  Hypertensive Disorders in Pregnancy;
  Hemorrhagic Disorders

Margaret A. Putman, RN, MS, NNP
Neonatal Nurse Practitioner
Neonatology Associates, Ltd.
Phoenix, Arizona
  Risks Associated with Gestational Age
  and Birth Weight

Debra Ann Rannalli, RN, PNP, MSN
Pediatric Nurse Practitioner
ABC Pediatrics
Los Alamitos, California
  Newborn Biologic/Behavioral
  Characteristics and Psychosocial
  Adaptations

Janet Scoggin, PhD, CNM
Certified Nurse Midwife
Life Choices Women's Clinic
Phoenix, Arizona
  Physical and Psychologic Changes

Judy E. Smith, PhD, RN, WHNP-C
Professor, Department of Nursing
California State University
Long Beach, California
  Age-Related Changes

Kathleen V. Smith, RNC,
  BSN, MSN
Assistant Professor
Clarkson College
Omaha, Nebraska;
Casual Staff Nurse
Beautiful Beginnings, Alegent Mercy
  Hospital
Council Bluffs, Iowa
  Normal Childbirth

Keiko L. Torgersen, BSN, MS, RNC
Colonel, United States Air Force
Commander 319th Medical Group
Grand Forks Air Force Base
Grand Forks, North Dakota
  Intrapartum Fetal Assessment

Gail M. Turley, RNC, MSN,
  CNAA
Director of Nursing, Clinical Practice,
  and Research
Crozer-Chester Medical Center
Upland, Pennsylvania
  Essential Forces and Factors in Labor

Cheryl Wallerstedt, MS, RNC, IBLCE,
  FACCE
Perinatal Outreach Educator/Program
  Manager
School of Medicine, Department of
  Obstetrics & Gynecology
University of New Mexico
Albuquerque, New Mexico
  Endocrine and Metabolic Disorders

Contributors **vii**

Roxena Wotring, RN, MS
Clinical Assistant Professor, College
of Nursing
Arizona State University
Phoenix, Arizona
Environmental Hazards

**Margaret Yancy, RN, MS, WHNP,
ANP-C**
Faculty, College of Nursing
Arizona State University
Tempe, Arizona;
Women's Health Nurse Practitioner
Maternal Outreach Mobile
(MOMmobile)
St. Joseph's Hospital & Medical Center
Phoenix, Arizona
Other Medical Complications

Preface

This book is intended to be used by practicing nurses for several purposes. First, it can be a study guide for those wishing to sit for certification examinations in maternal-newborn nursing. Basic and complex information is presented and accompanied by an extensive reference list to augment the knowledge base.

Second, the text may be used by development personnel and educators as an orientation for new staff, a source of information for nurses entering or returning to maternal-newborn nursing, and a reference for nurses on those units.

Third, this book can be a classroom text, particularly for students requiring a resource or reference. It is not designed to be a primary text for undergraduate students, but it could be a resource for those graduate students in women's health nurse practitioner programs who want to review some of the material relating to pregnancy that will be needed for their practice.

This edition has several significant changes that should make the book more usable for a wider audience yet keep the content directed toward the original audience. There is no longer a section on "complications of the newborn"; instead, most of the content has been integrated into those chapters dealing with maternal complications, with reference to how the condition affects the fetus or neonate. This will make it easier for the maternal-newborn or LDR nurse to identify the high-risk infant and the care required until the baby stabilizes or can be transferred (if necessary). Theoretical information about the continued care of high-risk neonates with selected conditions is briefly presented. The information is included to provide a basis from which the maternal-newborn nurse may give answers to parents' questions and provide anticipatory guidance to new parents of sick neonates.

Although nursing diagnoses have been used throughout the book, we do wish to remind the reader that all nursing diagnoses are fluid, designed to be tested in practice and refined. Thus wording may differ from some NANDA publications or other authorities in the field. This approach is not to imply that one is right and another wrong, but simply that certain terminology fits more appropriately in some settings than in others and is used to express the need of a particular client at that time. We also gave the contributors the option of using clinical pathways rather than nursing diagnoses if this terminology seemed more appropriate for the material in that chapter.

We hope this text will be helpful to those of you using it for all purposes. Its editing has been an educational and a character-building experience for us both.

Susan Mattson
Judy E. Smith

Acknowledgments

We would like to acknowledge the contributors to the previous edition:

Dorothy A. Austin, CNM, MS
Labor and Delivery at Risk

Hector Balcazar, MS, PhD
Nutrition

Arlene Blix, DrPH, RN
Environmental Hazards

Linda Bond, PhD, RN
Physiology of Pregnancy

Gail Brown, RNC, WHNP
Trauma in Pregnancy

Linda Callahan, CRNA, PhD
Surgery in Pregnancy

Kevin Copeland, RN, CNNP
Congenital Abnormalities

Michelle Copeland, MSN, CPNP
Congenital Abnormalities

Kathryn V. Deitch, PhD, RNC
Reproductive Anatomy, Physiology, and the Menstrual Cycle; Age-Related Concerns; Family Planning

Nancy Byram Del Mar, MPH, RN, CHES
Trauma in Pregnancy

Melodee J. Deutsch, MS, MPH, RNC, CPHQ
Ethics

Maureen Heaman, BN, MN, RN
Other Medical Complications

Patricia Grant Higgins, PhD, RN
Postpartum Complications

Lucy Hosmer, CNM, MS
Trauma in Pregnancy

Linda Howard-Glenn, MN, RNC
Adaptation to Extrauterine Life and Immediate Nursing Care; Newborn Biological/Behavioral Characteristics and Psychosocial Adaptations

Marcia Liden Jasper, BSN, MS, RNC
Antepartum Fetal Assessment

Wendee L. Johnson, MSN, RN
Infant of a Diabetic Mother

Kathleen A. Kalb, PhD, RNC
Endocrine and Metabolic Disorders

Bonnie Kellogg, DrPH, RN
Genetics; Fetal Development; Placental Development and Functioning

Susan Mattson, PhD, RNC, CTN
Ethnocultural Considerations in the Childbearing Period; Nutrition; Domestic Violence

Barbara A. Moran, MS, MPH, CNM
Maternal Infections; Substance Abuse in Pregnancy

Phyllis Muchmore, BSN, MHA
Respiratory Distress; Sepsis in the Newborn

Leith Merrow Mullaly, MSN, RNC, ACCE, IBCLC
Psychology of Pregnancy

Margaret Putman, BS, MS
Risks Associated with Gestational Age and Birth Weight; The Drug-Dependent Neonate

Susan Saffer Orr, BS, RPT, CLC
Breastfeeding

Judy Schmidt, MSN, MA, EdD
Intrapartum Fetal Assessment;
Hemorrhagic Disorders

Janet Scoggin, CNM, PhD
Physical and Psychological Changes

Diane Shannon, MSN, RN
Hypertension in Pregnancy

Mary E. Sheridan, CNM, MN
Labor and Delivery at Risk

Judy E. Smith, PhD, RNP-C
Domestic Violence; Hyperbilirubinemia;
The Drug-Dependent Neonate

Kathleen V. Smith, BSN, MSN, RNC
Normal Childbirth

**Gail M. Turley, BSN, BSN, RNC,
CNAA**
Essential Forces and Factors in Labor

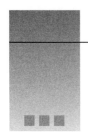

Contents

SECTION ONE

REPRODUCTION: FETAL AND PLACENTAL DEVELOPMENT, 1

1 Reproductive Anatomy, Physiology, and the Menstrual Cycle, 3
DENISE G. LINK

2 Genetics, 23
LINDA CALLAHAN

3 Fetal and Placental Development and Functioning, 41
LINDA CALLAHAN

SECTION TWO

NORMAL PREGNANCY, 73

4 Ethnocultural Considerations in the Childbearing Period, 75
SUSAN MATTSON

5 Physiology of Pregnancy, 96
LINDA BOND

6 Psychology of Pregnancy, 124
CATHERINE R. COVERSTON

SECTION THREE

MATERNAL-FETAL WELL-BEING, 145

7 Age-Related Concerns, 147
JUDY E. SMITH

8 Antepartum Fetal Assessment, 161
MARCIA LIDEN JASPER

9 Environmental Hazards, 201
ROXENA WOTRING

SECTION FOUR

INTRAPARTUM PERIOD, 225

10 Essential Forces and Factors in Labor, 227
GAIL M. TURLEY

11 Normal Childbirth, 271
KATHLEEN V. SMITH

12 Intrapartum Fetal Assessment, 303
KEIKO L. TORGERSEN

SECTION FIVE

POSTPARTUM PERIOD, 369

13 Physical and Psychologic Changes, 371
JANET SCOGGIN

14 Breastfeeding, 387
SUSAN SAFFER ORR

15 Family Planning, 409
DENISE G. LINK

SECTION SIX

THE NEWBORN, 419

16 Adaptation to Extrauterine Life and Immediate Nursing Care, 421
NATALIE DIANE CHEFFER

17   Newborn Biologic/Behavioral Characteristics and Psychosocial Adaptations, *437*
NATALIE DIANE CHEFFER AND DEBRA ANN RANNALLI

18   Risks Associated with Gestational Age and Birth Weight, *465*
MARGARET A. PUTMAN

19   Identification of the Sick Newborn, *497*
JACQUELINE M. MCGRATH

SECTION SEVEN

COMPLICATIONS OF CHILDBEARING, *535*

20   Intimate Partner Violence, *537*
SUSAN MATTSON

21   Hypertensive Disorders in Pregnancy, *554*
JUDITH H. POOLE

22   Maternal Infections, *592*
BARBARA A. MORAN

23   Hemorrhagic Disorders, *630*
JUDITH H. POOLE

24   Endocrine and Metabolic Disorders, *660*
CHERYL WALLERSTEDT AND DIANA E. CLOKEY

25   Trauma in Pregnancy, *703*
STARRE HANEY

26   Surgery in Pregnancy, *727*
LINDA CALLAHAN

27   Substance Abuse in Pregnancy, *750*
BARBARA A. MORAN

28   Other Medical Complications, *771*
MARGARET YANCY

29   Labor and Delivery at Risk, *818*
ELIZABETH GILBERT

30   Postpartum Complications, *850*
PATRICIA GRANT HIGGINS

SECTION EIGHT

ETHICS AND ISSUES, *871*

31   Ethics, *873*
SANDRA L. GARDNER

Index, *895*

REPRODUCTION: FETAL AND PLACENTAL DEVELOPMENT

1 Reproductive Anatomy, Physiology, and the Menstrual Cycle

DENISE G. LINK

OBJECTIVES

1. Identify and locate the female organs of reproduction.
2. Describe the physiologic functioning of the female reproductive system.
3. Identify the parameters of normal menstruation, including cycle interval, duration of menstrual flow, and age for menarche and menopause.
4. Describe the physiologic changes in the ovaries, uterus, and cervix that occur during the menstrual cycle.
5. Explain the physiologic pathways of the hypothalamic-pituitary-ovarian axis and their relationship to the normal menstrual cycle.
6. Describe deviations from normal anatomy that affect reproduction.
7. Describe deviations from normal physiology that affect reproduction.
8. Identify the common deviations from normal parameters in the menstrual cycle.
9. Analyze the data from a reproductive history and physical examination to determine overt and covert anatomical and physiologic factors that could affect pregnancy.
10. Prepare a set of nursing interventions for teaching pertinent concepts of anatomy and physiology to clients.

INTRODUCTION
Female Organs of Reproduction
A. **External genitals:** Vulva (Figure 1-1)
    1. Mons pubis (or mons veneris)
        a. A rounded pad of subcutaneous fatty tissue over the symphysis pubis; covered with pubic hair
        b. Function is the protection of the symphysis pubis during intercourse.
    2. Labia majora
        a. Two rounded folds of fatty and connective tissues, covered with pubic hair, that extend from the mons pubis to the perineum
        b. Function is the protection of the vaginal introitus.
    3. Labia minora
        a. Narrow folds of hairless skin located within the labia majora; begin beneath the clitoris and extend to the fourchette.
        b. Highly vascular and rich in nerve supply; glands lubricate the vulva.
        c. Function is erotic; swell in response to stimulation and are highly sensitive.

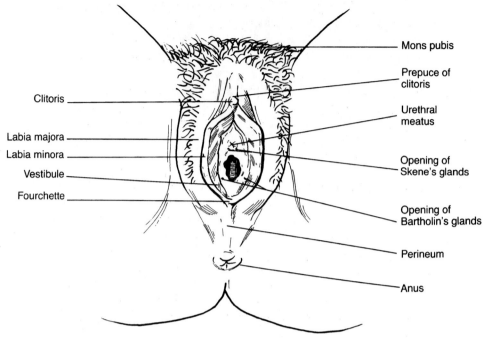

Clitoris

Labia majora

Labia minora

Vestibule

Fourchette

Mons pubis

Prepuce of clitoris

Urethral meatus

Opening of Skene's glands

Opening of Bartholin's glands

Perineum

Anus

FIGURE 1-1 ■ Female external genitals.

4. Prepuce of clitoris is a hood-like covering over the clitoris
5. Clitoris
   a. An erectile organ located beneath the pubic arch that consists of shaft and glans
   b. Secretes smegma, a pheromone (olfactory erotic stimulant).
   c. Extremely sensitive to touch, pressure, and temperature
   d. Function is sexual stimulation.
6. Vestibule
   a. An oval-shaped area whose boundaries are the clitoris, fourchette, and labia minora; contains the following:
      (1) Urethral meatus
         (a) The terminal portion of the urethra, with puckered or slit appearance
         (b) Located 2.5 cm (1 in) below the clitoris.
      (2) Skene's glands
         (a) Located inside the urethral meatus.
         (b) Produce mucus for lubrication.
      (3) Hymen
         (a) Tough, elastic, perforated, mucosa-covered tissue across the vaginal introitus
         (b) Hymenal opening might be absent or small, impeding menstrual flow and intercourse.
         (c) Characteristics of the hymen vary widely among women; the presence or absence of the hymen can neither confirm nor rule out sexual experience.
      (4) Bartholin's glands
         (a) Located at the base of each of the labia minora, just inside the vaginal orifice.
         (b) During coitus, secrete mucus that is hospitable to sperm.

7. Fourchette is a point located midline below the vaginal opening where the labia majora and labia minora merge.
8. Perineum
   a. Skin-covered muscular tissue located between the vaginal opening and the anus
   b. The area of a midline episiotomy
   c. Might be lacerated during childbirth.
B. **Internal organs** (Figure 1-2)
   1. Vagina
      a. A tubular structure located behind the bladder and in front of the rectum; extends from the introitus to the cervix.
      b. Thin-walled; composed of smooth muscle; capable of great distension as well as collapse.
      c. Lined with a glandular mucous membrane that is arranged in folds called rugae.
      d. Highly vascular and relatively insensitive; adds little sensation for the female during coitus.
      e. Functions as the outflow track for menstrual fluid and for vaginal and cervical secretions, the birth canal, and the organ for coitus.
   2. Uterus
      a. Located behind the symphysis pubis between the bladder and the rectum.
      b. Muscular, hollow, smooth, mobile, nontender, firm, and symmetric
      c. In a woman who has not been pregnant, uterine size ranges from 5.5 to 8 cm (2.2 to 3.2 in) in length, 3.5 to 4 cm (1.4 to 1.6 in) in

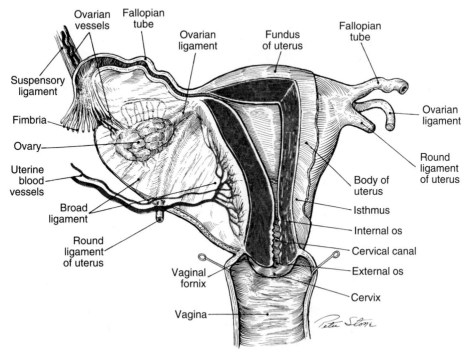

FIGURE 1-2 ■ Female reproductive organs. Front uterine wall has been removed so that the fallopian tube, uterus, cervical canal, and vagina are seen as a continuous channel. (From Langley, L.L., Telford, I.R., & Christensen, J.B. [1980]. *Dynamic anatomy and physiology*. New York: McGraw-Hill. Copyright Mosby.)

width, and 2 to 2.5 cm (0.8 to 1 in) in depth; size increases after childbirth.
  d. Is similar in shape to a light bulb or pear.
  e. Comprises four parts:
  (1) Fundus
    (a) The upper, rounded portion above the insertion of the fallopian tubes
    (b) Beginning at the 20th week of pregnancy, uterine size is measured in centimeters from the height of the fundus to the top of the symphysis pubis.
  (2) Corpus (or body) is the main portion of the uterus, located between the cervix and the fundus.
  (3) Isthmus
    (a) Also called the lower uterine segment during pregnancy.
    (b) Joins the corpus to the cervix.
  (4) Cervix (or neck of the uterus)
    (a) Divided into two portions: the portion above the site of attachment of the cervix to the vaginal vault is called the supravaginal portion; the portion below the attachment site that protrudes into the vagina is called the vaginal portion.
    (b) Composed of fibrous connective tissue.
    (c) Diameter varies from 2 to 5 cm (0.8 to 2 in), depending on childbearing history.
    (d) Length is usually 2.5 to 3 cm (1 to 1.2 in) in the nonpregnant woman.
    (e) Vaginal portion is smooth, firm, and doughnut shaped, with visible central opening called the external os.
    (f) Internal os is the opening of the cervix inside the uterine cavity.
    (g) Cervical canal forms the passageway between the vagina and the uterine cavity; major feature is the ability to stretch to a diameter large enough to allow passage of an infant's head and then to return to a closed position.
    (h) Produces mucus in response to cyclic hormones; thickened cervical mucus can block the passage of sperm and bacteria; thin cervical mucus facilitates the movement of sperm and prolongs sperm life; observation of changes in cervical mucus is important in fertility awareness methods of family planning.
    (i) At maturity, the cervical vaginal surface is covered with squamous epithelium; cervical canal is lined with columnar epithelium.
      (i) Area where two types of epithelium meet is called the squamocolumnar junction (s-c junction; also called the transformation zone or T-zone).
      (ii) Prior to puberty, the cervix is covered with columnar epithelium, and the s-c junction is located on the outer surface of the cervix.
      (iii) Beginning at puberty, under the influence of estrogen, the s-c junction gradually recedes back toward the external os, with squamous epithelium replacing the columnar epithelium.
      (iv) The s-c junction is the most frequent site of changes associated with the development of cervical cancer; cells from the s-c junction and other areas of the cervix are assessed via the Papanicolaou (Pap) test.

     f. Uterine position (Figure 1-3)
        (1) Five positions are possible:
           (a) Anteflexed
           (b) Anterior (anteverted)
           (c) Midposition
           (d) Posterior (retroverted)
           (e) Retroflexed
     g. Uterine support (see Figure 1-2)
        (1) Anterior ligament extends from the anterior cervix to the bladder.
        (2) Cardinal (transverse) ligaments
           (a) Portion of the broad ligaments
           (b) Contain uterine blood vessels and ureters.
           (c) Connected to the lateral margins of the uterus.
        (3) Posterior ligament extends from the posterior cervix to the rectum.
        (4) Uterosacral ligaments
           (a) Extend from the cervix over the rectum to the sacral vertebrae.
           (b) Maintain traction on the cervix to hold the uterus in position.
     h. Uterine wall
        (1) Composed of three layers:
           (a) Endometrium is a highly vascular mucous membrane that responds to hormone stimulation first by hypertrophy and then by secretion to prepare to receive the developing ovum; sloughs if pregnancy does not occur, resulting in menstruation; if pregnancy occurs, sloughs after delivery.
           (b) Myometrium is composed of smooth muscle in layers.
              (i) Outer layer is composed of longitudinal fibers, which predominate in the fundus and provide power to expel the fetus.
              (ii) Middle layer is composed of fibers interlaced with blood vessels in a figure-eight pattern; contraction following childbirth helps control blood loss.
              (iii) Inner layer is composed of circular fibers concentrated around the internal cervical os; provides sphincter action to help keep the cervix closed during pregnancy.
           (c) Parietal peritoneum covers most of the uterus, except for the cervix and a portion of the anterior corpus.
3. Fallopian tubes or oviducts (see Figure 1-2)
     a. Attached to the uterine fundus and curve around each ovary.
     b. Provide a passageway for the ovum into the uterus.
     c. 10 cm (4 in) in length and 0.6 cm (0.25 in) in diameter

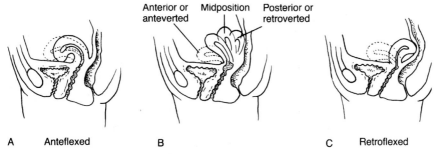

FIGURE 1-3 ■ Uterine positions.

        d. Comprises four parts:
- (1) Infundibulum: the most distal portion; funnel-shaped; covered with fimbriae that pull the ovum into the tube by creating a wavelike motion
- (2) Ampulla: next most distal portion and site of fertilization
- (3) Isthmus: narrowed part of the tube; closer to the uterus
- (4) Interstitial: narrowest portion, which passes through the uterine myometrium and opens into the uterine cavity

        e. Functions include:
- (1) Capture of the ovum
- (2) Transport of the ovum into the uterus via peristaltic activity and wavelike motion of the cilia
- (3) Secretion of nutrients to support the ovum during transport

   4. Ovaries (female gonads) (see Figure 1-2)
- **a.** Comparable with the testes in the male.
- **b.** Located on either side of the uterus, below and behind the fimbriated ends of the oviducts.
- **c.** Supported by the ovarian ligaments and the mesovarian portion of the broad ligament.
- **d.** Similar to almonds in size and shape; smooth, mobile, slightly tender, and firm.
- **e.** Functions include ovulation and production of hormones (estrogen, progesterone, and androgens).

C. Support for organs of reproduction
   1. Circulation
- **a.** Blood is supplied to the pelvis by arteries branching from the hypogastric artery (which branches from the iliac artery, a division of the aorta).
- **b.** Major pelvic arteries include the uterine, vaginal, pudendal, and perineal arteries.
- **c.** Ovarian arteries branch directly from the aorta.
- **d.** Lymphatic drainage is accomplished from the uterus, ovaries, and fallopian tubes to nodes around the aorta, with some use of the femoral, iliac, and hypogastric nodes.

   2. Pelvic floor and perineum
- **a.** Functions include:
  - (1) Support of the suspended internal organs of reproduction
  - (2) Support for sphincter control, allowing for expansion of the vagina with expulsion of the fetus, and closure of the vagina after delivery
- **b.** Pelvic diaphragm (Figure 1-4)
  - (1) Levator ani muscles
    - (a) Puborectalis
    - (b) Iliococcygeus
    - (c) Pubococcygeus
  - (2) Coccygeal muscles
- **c.** Urogenital diaphragm (see Figure 1-4): transverse perineal muscles
- **d.** Perineum (see Figure 1-4)
  - (1) Bulbocavernous muscle
  - (2) Ischiocavernous muscle
  - (3) Anal sphincter muscles
  - (4) Perineal strength can be increased through pelvic floor (Kegel) exercises.
- **e.** Perineal body
  - (1) Wedge-shaped area between the vagina and the rectum
  - (2) Anchor point for muscles, ligaments, and fascia of the pelvis

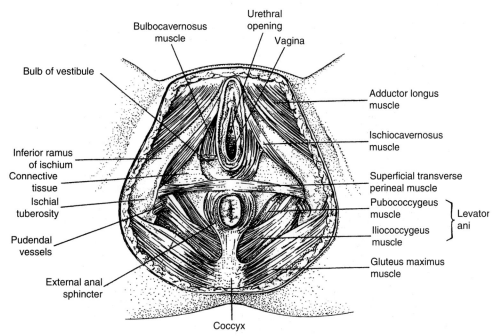

FIGURE 1-4 ■ Muscles of the pelvic floor, from below. (From Sloane, E. [2002]. *Biology of women* [4th ed.]. Albany, NY: Delmar.)

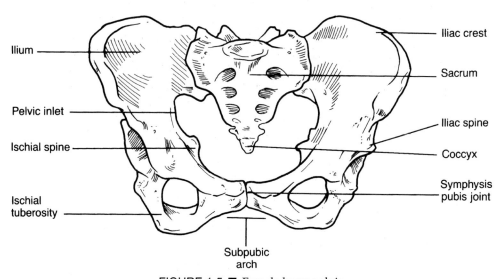

FIGURE 1-5 ■ Female bony pelvis.

3. Bony pelvis (Figure 1-5)
   a. Functions include support and protection of pelvic structures, and support for a growing fetus during gestation.
   b. Components include:
      (1) Ilium
         (a) Iliac crests
         (b) Anterior, superior iliac spines

(2) Ischium
  (a) Ischial spines
  (b) Ischial tuberosities
(3) Pubic bone
  (a) Symphysis pubis joint
  (b) Subpubic arch
(4) Sacrum; sacral promontory
(5) Coccyx
c. Ilium, ischium, and pubic bones fuse after puberty; the pelvic bone then is called the right or left innominate bone.
d. False pelvis (Figure 1-6)
  (1) Area of the pelvis above the anterior, superior iliac spines
  (2) Provides no useful data for estimating the size of the birth canal.
e. True pelvis (see Figure 1-6)
  (1) Comprises three pelvic planes.
    (a) Pelvic inlet is bordered by anterior, superior iliac spines and the sacral promontory.
    (b) Midpelvis is the area between the inlet and the outlet.
    (c) Pelvic outlet is bordered by ischial tuberosities and the coccyx.
4. Nervous innervation
  a. Motor nerves
    (1) Parasympathetic fibers from the sacral nerves stimulate pelvic vasodilation and inhibit uterine contractions.
    (2) Sympathetic motor nerves from ganglia between T-5 and T-10 stimulate pelvic vasoconstriction and uterine contractions.
  b. Sensory nerves
    (1) Fibers from ovaries and uterus transmit pain sensations to the spinal cord at T-11 to L-1.
    (2) Pain in ovaries, oviducts, and uterus is difficult to differentiate; might be felt in flank, inguinal, vulvar, or suprapubic area.

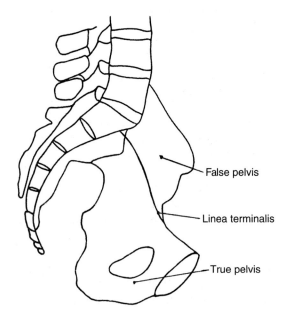

False pelvis

Linea terminalis

True pelvis

FIGURE 1-6 ■ True pelvis and false pelvis divided by the linea terminalis. (From Ross Laboratories. *Clinical Education Aid No. 18*, Columbus, OH 43216.)

D. Menstruation

1. Menarche (onset of the first menstrual period) normally occurs between the ages of 9 and 16 years, with a mean age of 12.8 years in the United States.

2. Menstrual cycles in the first 2 years postmenarche tend to be irregular; irregular menstrual cycles are associated with irregular ovulation.

3. Menstrual cycles are timed from the first day of menstrual bleeding; the first day of bleeding is marked as day 1 of the cycle.

4. Menstrual cycle length ranges normally from 21 to 36 days; 95% of women have a cycle length between 25 and 32 days.

5. Duration of bleeding ranges from 1 to 8 days; most women report a menstrual flow that lasts from 3 to 5 days.

6. Amount of blood lost averages 30 ml (1 oz) per menstrual period; a normal range is between 20 and 80 ml (⅔ and 2 ⅔ oz).

7. Cessation of menses (menopause) occurs between the ages of 35 and 60 years, with an average age of 51 years in the United States.

8. The menstrual cycle is divided into two phases:
   a. Follicular phase
      (1) Starts with day 1 of menses.
      (2) Multiple follicles are maturing in the ovary; the term primary is given to the follicle selected for maturation during this cycle.
      (3) Maturing follicle is called a graafian follicle.
      (4) Estrogen is produced in the follicles.
      (5) Follicular phase ends with the release of the egg from the mature follicle (ovulation).
      (6) Normal variation in length of this phase is 7 to 22 days (e.g., it would be 14 days in a 28-day cycle).
      (7) The endometrium is in the proliferative phase and thickens during this period of rapid growth.
      (8) At the end of this phase, the external cervical os dilates slightly to admit sperm; the cervix becomes softer.
      (9) Cervix produces mucus that is thin, clear, slippery, stretchy, copious in quantity, and designed to aid sperm in passage through the cervix; the stretching property is called spinnbarkeit.
      (10) Ovulation usually occurs within 24 hours before, during, or after the last day of this slippery, copious discharge.
   b. Luteal phase
      (1) Starts with ovulation.
      (2) Follicle that releases the ovum becomes the corpus luteum.
      (3) Corpus luteum produces both estrogen and progesterone.
      (4) Lasts 14 days if conception does not occur.
      (5) Endometrium is in the secretory phase; increasingly vascular and filled with glandular secretions, ready to support a fertilized ovum.
      (6) If no conception occurs, the corpus luteum deteriorates, and levels of estrogen and progesterone decrease.
      (7) Menstruation begins, signaling the start of a new cycle.

9. Common deviations from normal in the menstrual cycle
   a. Amenorrhea: defined as an absence of menstrual periods; pregnancy is a common cause.
      (1) Primary amenorrhea
         (a) Is failure of the onset of menstruation:
            (i) By age 14 in the absence of secondary sex characteristics
            (ii) By age 16 in the presence of secondary sex characteristics

(b) Might be due to chromosomal defects.
  (i) Congenital agenesis of the ovaries or uterus
  (ii) "Streak" ovaries: non-functional; will not produce ova or the hormones necessary to initiate puberty

(2) Secondary amenorrhea
  (a) Cessation of menses prior to age 40 in a previously menstruating woman
  (b) Defined as absence of menses for 6 months or the equivalent of three cycles in a woman who does not menstruate every month.

(3) Menarche usually requires a minimum height of 152.4 cm (5 ft) and a minimum weight of 47.5 kg (105 lb), with a fat-to-lean ratio of 1:3; females with body fat levels below 16% seldom menstruate.

(4) Menarche delay is common in girls who are competitive athletes, have eating disorders such as anorexia nervosa, or participate in activities in which extreme thinness is valued, such as ballet and gymnastics; might lead to the development of osteoporosis if estrogen levels are consistently low.

b. Anovulatory cycles
  (1) Common in both the early years following menarche and the years close to menopause
  (2) A graafian follicle matures, and estrogen is produced, but ovulation does not occur.
    (a) Corpus luteum does not form and progesterone is not available.
    (b) Uterine lining thickens in response to estrogen.
    (c) Progesterone-induced signal to start and stop the menstrual flow is absent.
  (3) Might result in light, irregular menses, and difficulty in conceiving, or might result in frequent, prolonged, heavy menstrual flow.

c. Inadequate (short) luteal phase
  (1) Corpus luteum stops producing hormones prematurely or produces inadequate levels of estrogen and progesterone.
  (2) Can lead to infertility.
  (3) Can cause early pregnancy losses when progesterone levels are too low to support the pregnancy until the placental formation is complete.
  (4) Diagnosed by analysis of serum progesterone levels and treated with progesterone.

E. **The hypothalamic-pituitary-ovarian axis**
  1. Responsible for the control of the hormones that affect reproduction.
  2. Sphenoidal sinus in the brain houses the pituitary gland, and the hypothalamus is located directly above the pituitary gland.
  3. Pituitary gland is divided into two parts: the anterior and the posterior; function/control of the two sections are separate and distinct.
  4. Hypothalamus releases hormones (called releasing factors) into the hypophysial portal system that supplies the anterior pituitary; these hormones provide instructions to the anterior pituitary.
  5. Releasing factors signal the anterior pituitary to produce hormones, which in turn stimulate certain target organs to produce hormones.
  6. Releasing factors are produced by the hypothalamus in response to the decreasing levels of hormones being produced by the target organs; when the levels of hormones from the target organs increase, the hypothalamus responds by decreasing the releasing factor hormones sent to the anterior pituitary.

7. This type of system is called a feedback loop; when rising levels of target organ hormones result in a decrease in the releasing factor and stimulating hormones, the system is called a negative feedback loop.
8. Target organs include the ovaries, the thyroid, and the adrenal cortex.
9. Feedback loop functioning for the ovary
    a. During menstruation, a message is sent through the central nervous system to the hypothalamus that circulating levels of estrogen are low.
    b. Hypothalamus responds by sending gonadotropin-releasing hormone to the anterior pituitary.
    c. Anterior pituitary responds by sending first follicle-stimulating hormone (FSH) and then luteinizing hormone (LH) to the ovary.
    d. Ovary responds to FSH by selecting a follicle for maturation and choosing from among several follicles that are undergoing early development and producing estrogen; the chosen follicle that begins to mature is called the graafian follicle.
    e. LH stimulates the graafian follicle to release the egg, and ovulation occurs; the graafian follicle becomes a corpus luteum, which produces both estrogen and progesterone.
    f. There are now high circulating levels of both estrogen and progesterone.
        (1) If conception does not occur, circulating levels of both estrogen and progesterone gradually decrease as the corpus luteum disintegrates.
        (2) When estrogen levels are again low, menstruation begins, another message is sent to the hypothalamus, and the cycle begins again.

CLINICAL PRACTICE

A. **Assessment**
   1. Subjective assessment (health interview or history)
      a. Health history, including previous or current disorders that might affect reproductive function or impact on pregnancy
          (1) Endocrine disorders
              (a) Hypothyroidism or hyperthyroidism
              (b) Hypertension
              (c) Diabetes mellitus (types 1 and 2 gestational diabetes)
              (d) Parathyroidism
              (e) Adrenal disorders
          (2) Pelvic infection
              (a) Interferes with conception through the formation of scar tissue in response to inflammation.
              (b) Can be asymptomatic.
              (c) Infection and resultant scarring of the fallopian tubes, which leaves the oviducts blocked, is a major cause of infertility.
          (3) Endometriosis
              (a) Causes significant pain with menstruation and interferes with conception.
              (b) Scar tissue is formed in response to inflammation or bleeding from ectopic endometrial implants (functioning endometrial tissue that has migrated outside of the uterus).
          (4) Uterine fibroids
              (a) Benign tumors that alter the shape of the uterus and its ability to expand
              (b) Might cause excessive menstrual bleeding.
              (c) Common in women older than 35 years

b. Surgical history
  (1) Pelvic surgery (i.e., ovarian cystectomy or uterine myomectomy) increases risk of formation of adhesions that interfere with conception or maintenance of a pregnancy.
  (2) Repetitive dilatation and curettage procedures for diagnosis or pregnancy termination; might result in the following:
    (a) Asherman syndrome
        (i) Uterine scar tissue forms, usually as a result of aggressive curettage.
        (ii) Scar tissue interferes with the normal cyclic changes in the endometrium (uterine lining).
    (b) Incompetent cervix
        (i) Due to repetitive, forced dilation of the cervix
        (ii) Cervix is unable to remain closed during pregnancy, which leads to spontaneous abortion or preterm labor (see Chapter 26 for discussion of surgery as treatment for incompetent cervix).
  (3) A cone biopsy/cryosurgery, laser surgery to cervix, and LEEP (loop electrosurgical excision procedure)
    (a) Risk of scarring, which prevents conception
    (b) Risk of incompetent cervix
c. Reproductive history
  (1) Puberty is characterized by developmental milestones that provide evidence that ovaries and uterus are present and functioning, such as the following:
    (a) Secondary sex characteristics, including breast development and the appearance of axillary and pubic hair (Tanner scale)
    (b) Menarche occurring before the age of 16 years
  (2) Menstrual history
    (a) Age at menarche
    (b) Date of the last menstrual period and determination of whether or not the last menstrual period was a normal one for the woman
    (c) The usual cycle length and the cycle length for this period
    (d) The usual duration of bleeding and the duration of bleeding for this cycle
    (e) The usual amount of bleeding and the amount of bleeding for this cycle
    (f) Cramps
        (i) Present or absent
        (ii) Degree of interference with normal activities
    (g) Clots
        (i) Present or absent
        (ii) Number and size
    (h) Molimina symptoms
        (i) Are defined as cyclic symptoms associated with menses.
        (ii) Examples include premenstrual bloating, breast tenderness, and irritability.
        (iii) Presence is due to estrogen and progesterone.
        (iv) Molimina symptoms plus regular and normal menses imply a pattern of normal ovulation.
  (3) Reproductive functioning
    (a) Pregnancy history
        (i) Number of confirmed pregnancies: gravida

(ii) Number of term pregnancies (pregnancies that lasted at least 37 weeks)

(iii) Number of preterm pregnancies (confirmed pregnancies that ended between 20 and 37 weeks' gestation)

(iv) Number of confirmed pregnancies that ended before 20 weeks' gestation: spontaneous and induced abortions

(v) Number of children who are currently living

(vi) Difficulty in conceiving

(vii) Causes of pregnancy losses

(viii) Problems in perinatal period

(ix) Labor: preterm or prolonged

(x) Delivery: type of anesthesia, episiotomy, vacuum extraction, or forceps used; cesarean birth

(xi) Postpartum period: hemorrhage, infection, difficulty with healing of lacerations or episiotomy (e.g., fistula formation)

d. Sociocultural history

(1) Attitudes and values toward menstruation

(a) Common cultural attitudes include menstruation as illness, as a state of uncleanliness, as a time of decreased competence, and as causing fear of contamination.

(b) Some American Indian cultures isolate the menstruating woman.

(c) Orthodox Judaism requires a ritual bath after menstruation.

(d) In post–World War II Japan, a policy of menstrual leave for "incapacitated" women was enacted.

(e) In the United States and the United Kingdom, criminal court cases have been tried with defenses of diminished capacity from premenstrual syndrome pleaded for women accused of acts of violence.

(2) Sexual practices that can lead to increased risk of pelvic infection and affect fertility

(a) Multiple partners

(b) Recent change in sexual partners

(c) Failure to use a condom when indicated

2. Objective assessment (physical examination)

a. General survey

(1) Secondary sex characteristics: Tanner Stages of Development (Figure 1-7)

(2) Pelvic examination

(a) External genitalia

(i) Structural abnormalities (i.e., evidence of female circumcision procedure common in some cultures)

(ii) Evidence of infection, as signaled by discharge from glands

(iii) Hymenal opening

(b) Internal organs

(i) Vagina

■ Color, integrity, and presence of discharge

■ Rectocele or cystocele is the herniation of the vaginal wall with the rectum or the bladder protruding into the vagina.

■ Uterine prolapse is the relaxation of vaginal support, with the uterus in the vagina.

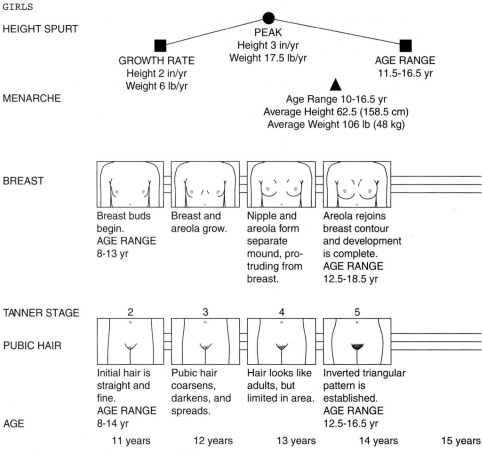

FIGURE 1-7 ■ Tanner Maturity Rating Scale (Female). (From Tanner, J.M. [1962]. *Growth at adolescence* [2nd ed.]. Oxford, UK: Blackwell Scientific Publications.)

       (ii) Cervix: parity and appearance
- Structural abnormalities
- Patency
- Evidence of infection

      (iii) Uterus
- Size, shape, consistency, and mobility
- Position

      (iv) Adnexa
- Size, shape, consistency, and mobility of ovaries
- Oviducts usually not palpable.

  (c) Bony pelvis
      (i) Estimate of anterior-posterior diameter of the pelvic inlet (i.e., the distance between sacral promontory and subpubic arch [12.5 to 13 cm])
      (ii) Prominence of ischial spines and bispinous diameter (11 cm)
      (iii) Prominence of coccyx (see Chapter 10 for a complete discussion of pelvic measurements)

3. Diagnostic procedures
  a. Menstrual calendar
  b. Blood chemistry, including lipid levels

      c. Hemoglobin and hematocrit
         (1) Anemia might result from excessive menstrual blood loss.
         (2) Anemia is usually when hemoglobin levels are below 12 g/dl and hematocrit levels are below 37%.
      d. FSH and LH levels
         (1) Elevated when ovaries are not functioning normally with cyclic ovulation.
         (2) FSH levels higher than 40 mIU/ml and LH levels higher than 25 mIU/ml are diagnostic for anovulation.
         (3) Normal levels of FSH are 5 to 30 mIU/ml and normal LH levels are 5 to 20 mIU/ml in women.
         (4) FSH level is a better indicator of ovarian function than gonadal hormone levels.
      e. Prolactin
         (1) Elevated levels block the action of estrogen.
         (2) Normal levels are 0 to 23 mg/dl.
      f. Thyroid function tests
         (1) Identify hyperthyroidism and hypothyroidism.
         (2) Normal nonpregnant values are:
            (a) Serum thyroxine (T_4), 5 to 12 µg/dl
            (b) Serum triiodothyronine (T_3), 80 to 200 mg/dl
            (c) Thyroid-stimulating hormone, 2 to 5.4 mIU/ml
      g. Progesterone
         (1) Level is tested on menstrual cycle days 21 to 23 (28-day cycle).
         (2) Provides evidence of ovulation.
         (3) Low levels after conception might lead to a spontaneous abortion.
      h. Testosterone and dehydroepiandrosterone sulfate (DHEAS)
         (1) Androgens are produced by the normal ovary and the adrenal gland.
         (2) High levels usually are associated with anovulation and amenorrhea.
      i. Endometrial biopsy
         (1) Evaluates the influences of hormones on the uterine lining.
         (2) Is performed on days 21 to 23 of a 28-day cycle.
         (3) Estrogen and progesterone, which are present after ovulation, produce the characteristic changes in the microscopic lining of the uterus.
   4. Potential psychosocial responses to the reproductive assessment
      a. Concerns
         (1) Modesty
         (2) Feelings of invasion of privacy
         (3) Strangers invading privacy
         (4) Gender of examiner; same or different
      b. Meaning of examination for the woman
      c. Desire for assurances that all structures appear normal

B. Nursing Diagnoses
   1. Deficient knowledge related to normal anatomy and physiology of the female reproductive system
   2. Altered functioning related to deviation from normal anatomical or physiologic status of the female reproductive system
   3. Deficient knowledge related to a lack of understanding of the physical changes that occur during the normal menstrual cycle

C. Interventions/Outcomes
   1. Deficient knowledge related to normal anatomy and physiology of the female reproductive system

    a. Interventions
      (1) Assess current level of understanding.
      (2) Identify inaccuracies or gaps in knowledge.
      (3) Identify the woman's interest in increasing her knowledge.
      (4) Formulate a teaching plan.
      (5) Evaluate the effectiveness of the implemented plan.
    b. Outcomes
      (1) The woman will be able to explain anatomic or physiologic functioning in the areas in which previous inaccuracies or gaps were identified.
      (2) The woman will state that her learning needs were met.

2. Altered functioning related to deviation from normal anatomic or physiologic status of the female reproductive system
    a. Interventions
      (1) Identify the specific alteration in function.
      (2) Identify the physiologic basis for the alteration in function.
      (3) Formulate a management plan with the woman.
      (4) Assess the woman's level of understanding of both the problem and plan of management.
      (5) Formulate a teaching plan to increase understanding.
      (6) Implement the management plan and the teaching plan.
      (7) Evaluate the effectiveness of the implemented plans.
      (8) Communicate the effectiveness to other members of the health care team.
    b. Outcomes
      (1) The woman will repeat an accurate description of the specific problem of alteration in functioning.
      (2) The woman will describe the proposed management plan accurately.
      (3) The woman will state that her health care needs were met.

3. Deficient knowledge related to a lack of understanding of the physical changes that occur during the normal menstrual cycle
    a. Interventions
      (1) Assess the current level of knowledge of the cyclic physical changes that occur in a normal menstrual cycle.
      (2) Provide necessary instruction for learning gaps that have been identified.
      (3) Reassess the level of knowledge of physical changes attributed to the menstrual cycle after instruction.
    b. Outcomes
      (1) The woman will describe the timing of the physical changes that commonly occur during her own menstrual cycle.
      (2) The woman will identify whether or not those changes are within the normal range.
      (3) The woman will identify potential changes in her menstrual cycle that require the attention of a health care professional.

HEALTH EDUCATION

Appropriate, age-specific, individualized instruction regarding reproductive anatomy and physiology should be presented by the health care provider. Health education about the menstrual cycle should also be provided according to an assessment of the current level of knowledge of the woman as well as her current level of understanding of the subject. The teaching plan should use the particular concerns of the woman or the particular details of her diagnosis to help her understand both her own situation and the parameters of normal functioning.

A. **Identify the purpose of the instruction.**
B. **Identify the characteristics of the learner.**
   1. Assess the current level of understanding.
   2. Identify the learning needs.
   3. Identify the level of comfort with the subject matter.
   4. Identify the level of comfort of members of the group with each other.
C. **Choose an instructional method appropriate to the learning needs and comfort level of the participants.**
D. **Develop a teaching plan.**
E. **Implement the teaching plan.**
F. **Evaluate the effectiveness of the teaching plan in terms of meeting the learning needs of the participants.**
G. **Alter the teaching plan.**
H. **Implement the alterations.**
I. **Reevaluate the teaching plan.**

CASE STUDIES AND STUDY QUESTIONS

An 18-year-old girl has decided to see a health care provider to find out "why I'm so slow in developing." Her last physical examination was 5 years ago; she reports no serious illnesses and no operations. Her chief complaints are lack of breast development and delayed onset of menstruation. She is 156 cm (5 ft, 1 in) tall and weighs 48 kg (105 lb). She states that she has never had a menstrual period, does not have to shave her underarms and legs, and has never had acne. Pertinent physical findings include an absence of secondary sex characteristics, including a lack of breast development and of axillary hair and pubic hair. A vaginal examination was attempted but not completed because of an imperforate hymen. The primary diagnosis is delayed puberty.

1. Further assessment and intervention for this client:
   a. Should be delayed because there is a wide variation in the onset of menses and breast development among young girls.
   b. Are necessary because the development of secondary sex characteristics and the onset of menstruation normally occur by the age of 16 years.
   c. Are not essential because breast development normally precedes menstruation by several years.
   d. Should focus on treatment of her imperforate hymen.

2. Further studies reveal a chromosomal karyotype of XX, the presence of a very small uterus, and "streak" ovaries. Exogenous sources of estrogen and progesterone are recommended to trigger the onset of puberty for this young woman. She will need to take these hormones:
   a. Only until her own ovaries are stimulated to begin producing hormones.
   b. Only until she decides to become pregnant.
   c. Until well past the normal time for menopause because "streak" ovaries are nonfunctioning and will never produce the necessary hormones.
   d. She will not need to take these hormones because her ovaries will begin functioning soon.

3. The imperforate hymen:
   a. Must be treated because menstrual flow started by the use of hormone therapy can be trapped and prevented from exiting the vagina.
   b. Should be treated when she decides to become sexually active.
   c. Should be treated when she decides to become pregnant.
   d. Does not require treatment because it will be broken when she has sexual intercourse.

4. This girl wants to know about her childbearing capabilities. She will:
   a. Be able to have as many children as she wishes as long as she takes the necessary hormones.
   b. Need to use birth control to prevent unwanted pregnancies.
   c. Not be able to become pregnant without donor eggs because "streak" ovaries are nonfunctioning and do not contain ova.
   d. Not be able to become pregnant because of her imperforate hymen.

Mrs. A, 25 years old and married, wants to use the techniques of natural family planning to help her to conceive. She had her first menstrual period at the age of 12 years. Her periods are regular, occur every 28 days, and last 4 to 5 days. She has no trouble with cramping or excessive flow. She has noticed breast tenderness, feelings of heaviness and bloating, and irritability in the few days before each period. She also notices an increase in her vaginal discharge in the middle of her cycle; the discharge is thin, slippery, stretchy, and clear.

5. She is probably experiencing:
   a. Regular ovulation because her periods are regular and she is experiencing normal moliminal symptoms.
   b. A vaginal infection because of the repetitive discharge.
   c. Anovulatory cycles because she is not having trouble with cramps or clots.
   d. Some anovulatory cycles because her cycle length varies by a few days and is not always consistent.

6. The breast tenderness, bloating, and irritability are due to:
   a. The effects of falling levels of estrogen during this phase of the cycle.
   b. The effects of progesterone produced by the corpus luteum after ovulation occurs.
   c. The effects of rising levels of testosterone during this phase of the cycle.
   d. These symptoms have no relationship to the levels of hormones in the body.

7. Clear, slippery cervical mucus that occurs at midcycle has a quality of stretchiness called spinnbarkeit. This quality is associated with cervical changes, including:
   a. The opening of the cervical os to aid the sperm in moving into the uterus.
   b. The closing of the cervical os to become more hostile to sperm.
   c. The shortening of the cervix to prepare for cervical dilation in labor.
   d. A maturation of the cervix that occurs after puberty.

ADDITIONAL STUDY QUESTIONS

8. All of the following are components of the external female genitalia except the:
   a. Vulva
   b. Vestibule
   c. Fourchette
   d. Vagina

9. The middle layer of the uterine myometrium is composed of smooth muscle fibers in figure-eight patterns around major blood vessels. This is called a living ligature because:
   a. Contraction of these fibers after childbirth or an abortion helps prevent massive blood loss.
   b. These fibers provide support for the major blood vessels that innervate the uterus.
   c. These fibers contract before the placenta detaches from the uterine wall, thus preventing blood loss from the umbilical cord.

10. Which of the following statements is untrue for the ovaries?
    a. Normally are the size of almonds in women during the reproductive years.
    b. Are comparable to the testes in the male.
    c. On examination, should be fixed and nonmobile.
    d. Are responsible for the production of estrogen, progesterone, and the androgens.

11. Which of the following uterine positions is considered abnormal?
    a. Anteflexed
    b. Anterior
    c. Posterior
    d. Retroflexed
    e. None of the above.

12. Blocked oviducts are a major cause of infertility. They are most often the result of:
    a. Pelvic inflammatory disease
    b. Congenital abnormality
    c. Exposure to diethylstilbestrol (DES)
    d. Cone biopsy

13. Which of the following describes a menstrual cycle that is within the normal parameters?
    a. Age at menarche: 11 years; cycle length: 42 days; duration of menses: 3 days; blood loss: light.
    b. Age at menarche: 8 years; cycle length: 28 days; duration of menses: 4 days; blood loss: heavy.
    c. Age at menarche: 12 years; cycle length: 26 to 28 days; duration of menses: 5 days; blood loss: moderate.
    d. Age at menarche: 12 years; cycle length: 14 days; duration of menses: 8 days; blood loss: heavy.

14. During the menstrual cycle, the hormone progesterone is produced:
    a. Throughout the cycle
    b. From days 1 to 14 by the graafian follicle
    c. From days 14 to 28 by the graafian follicle
    d. Beginning just after ovulation by the corpus luteum

ANSWERS TO STUDY QUESTIONS

1. b	5. a	9. a	13. c
2. c	6. b	10. c	14. d
3. a	7. a	11. e	
4. c	8. d	12. a	

REFERENCES

Bickley, L.S., & Szilagyi, P.G. (2003). *Bates's guide to physical examination and history taking* (8th ed.). Philadelphia: Lippincott, Williams & Wilkins.

Guyton, A.C., & Hall, J.E. (2001). *Textbook of medical physiology* (10th ed.). Philadelphia: W.B. Saunders.

Lowdermilk, D.L., & Perry, S.E. (2004). *Maternity & women's health care* (8th ed.). St. Louis: Mosby.

Novak, E., Hilliard, P., & Berak, J. (Eds.). (2002). *Novak's gynecology* (13th ed.). Philadelphia: Lippincott, Williams & Wilkins.

Speroff, L., Glass, R., & Kase, N. (1999). *Clinical gynecologic endocrinology and infertility* (6th ed.). Philadelphia: Lippincott, Williams & Wilkins.

Thibodeau, G.A, & Patton, K. (2003). *Anthony's textbook of anatomy and physiology* (17th ed.). St. Louis: Mosby.

2 Genetics

LINDA CALLAHAN

OBJECTIVES

1. Discuss the potential importance of the National Human Genome Project on patient care.
2. Define the terms commonly used in genetic conditions.
3. Describe the implications of an increased amount of chromosomal material, the deletion of genetic material, and the translocation process in chromosomal disorders.
4. Explain the basic mendelian modes of inheritance.
5. Identify client situations that indicate the need for a chromosomal analysis.
6. Assess the emotional impact on couples of the birth of an infant with a genetic disorder.
7. Discuss the responsibility and needed competencies of the nurse in initial counseling and referral of patients for further genetic testing and counseling.

INTRODUCTION

A. **The National Human Genome Project** (Lorentz et al., 2002)
   1. First discussed in the 1980s; officially launched in 1990
   2. Goals include sequencing the entire human genome (achieved in April, 2003), identifying human DNA sequence variations, identifying and determining the function of individual genes, and studying the ethical, legal, and social implications of information and technologic outcomes of the Human Genome Project on human beings and society.
   3. Increased understanding of the genotype will allow:
      a. Development of targeted health promotion strategies
      b. Potential disease prevention
      c. Genotype-tailored drugs to optimize therapeutic effects while minimizing negative drug interactions and side effects
      d. Eventual correction of disease states by development of gene transfer technology (gene therapy)
B. **Definition:** Genetics is a medical science concerned with the transmission of characteristics from parent to child (Horowitz, 2000; Guttmacher & Collins, 2002).
   1. Gene: the basic hereditary unit; a DNA sequence required for production of a functional product, usually a protein
   2. Genotype: an individual's genetic makeup
   3. Phenotype: the outward appearance or expression of the genes
   4. Allele: an alternative form of a gene; the wild type allele is the most common form of a gene found within a population
   5. Mutation: a rare alternative form of an allele; occurs in less than 1% of the population
   6. Polymorphism: a common alternative form of an allele; occurs in more than 1% of the population
   7. Genome: complete DNA sequence containing all of the genetic information for an individual

C. Foundation of inheritance

   1. Cell division: all beings begin life as a single cell (zygote). The single cell continues to reproduce itself by the process of either mitosis or meiosis.

     a. Mitosis is the process of cell division in which new cells are made. The new cells have the same number and pattern of chromosomes as the parent cell (46 chromosomes comprising 44 autosomes and 2 sex chromosomes); mitosis occurs in five stages (Figure 2-1).

       (1) Interphase: before cell division, the DNA replicates itself.

       (2) Prophase: the strands of chromatin shorten and thicken; the chromosomes reproduce; spindles appear, and the centrioles migrate to the opposite poles of the cell; the membrane separating the nucleus from the cytoplasm disappears.

       (3) Metaphase: the chromosomes line up along the poles of the spindle.

       (4) Anaphase: the two chromatids separate and move to the opposite ends of the spindle.

       (5) Telophase: a nuclear membrane forms, the spindles disappear, and the centrioles relocate to the outside of the new nucleus; toward the end of this phase, the cells divide into two new cells, each with its own nucleus and each having the same number of chromosomes as the parent cell.

     b. Meiosis is a process of cell division that occurs in the sperm and ova and is known as gametogenesis; this process decreases the number of chromosomes by 50% (from 46 to 23 per cell) and occurs in two successive cell divisions (Figure 2-2).

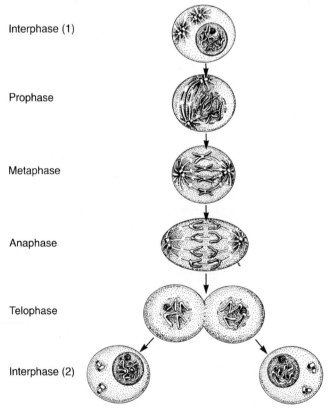

Interphase (1)

Prophase

Metaphase

Anaphase

Telophase

Interphase (2)

FIGURE 2-1 ■ The process of mitosis.

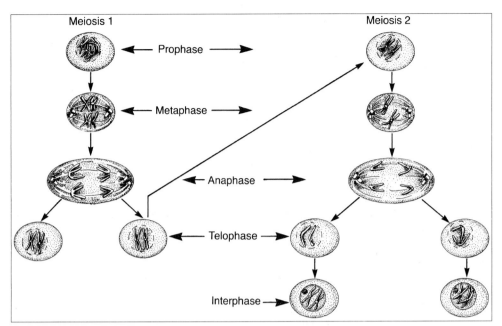

FIGURE 2-2 ■ The process of meiosis.

(1) The first division consists of four phases.
    (a) Prophase: the chromosomes move close together.
       (i) Crossover of genetic material can take place at this time.
      (ii) Crossover accounts for the wide variation of features seen within same-parent siblings.
    (b) Metaphase: spindle fibers attach to separate chromosomes.
    (c) Anaphase: intact chromosome pairs migrate to opposite ends of the cell (the distribution of maternal and paternal chromosomes is random).
    (d) Telophase: the cell divides into two cells, each with 50% (23) of the usual number of chromosomes (22 autosomes and 1 sex chromosome).
(2) Second division
    (a) The chromatids of each chromosome separate and move to the opposite poles of each of the daughter cells.
    (b) This is followed by each of the cells dividing into two cells, which results in four cells (spermatogenesis and oogenesis).
       (i) Spermatogenesis is continuous from puberty to senescence.
      (ii) Oogenesis is noncontinuous.
         ■ Begins in utero, and by the fifth intrauterine month, a full complement of primary oocytes has been produced.
         ■ Primary oocytes are dormant until puberty, at which time one or two will complete the meiotic cycle each month during a woman's reproductive years.
    (c) During the meiotic division, two of the chromatics might not move apart when the cell divides; this lack of separation is called autosomal nondisjunction; this is also the stage at which breakage can occur, resulting in abnormalities of chromosomal structure such as that producing cri du chat syndrome.

    2. Genetic information is present on the chromosomes (Tefferi et al., 2002).

      a. Chromosomes are composed of DNA, a complex protein that carries the genetic information.

      b. DNA occurs as a double-stranded helix found in the cell nucleus.

        (1) Two long strands of DNA molecules are wound around each other.

        (2) The strands are linked by chemical bonds.

        (3) The strands are complementary.

        (4) The chains comprise sequences of four nitrogen base subunits (adenine, guanine, thymine, and cytosine).

      c. Genes are the smallest known unit of heredity.

        (1) Genes are present on the chromosomes.

        (2) Each gene codes for a particular cellular function.

        (3) Genes occur in pairs (alleles) derived from the mother and father during reproduction.

        (4) Each gene has a specific location on the chromosomes.

        (5) Genetic errors can occur when there are changes in the location of the gene.

    3. Chromosomes form a genetic blueprint that comprises tightly coiled structures of DNA.

      a. Chromosomes are threadlike structures within the nucleus of the cell that carry the genes.

      b. Humans have 46 chromosomes in each body cell (22 pairs of autosomes and 1 pair of sex chromosomes [diploid]).

      c. The sex cells contain 23 chromosomes (haploid).

      d. Abnormalities of chromosome number are as follows (Lashley, 1998; Guttmacher & Collins, 2002).

        (1) Paired chromosomes fail to separate during cell division (nondisjunction).

        (2) If nondisjunction occurs during meiosis (before fertilization), the fetus usually will have abnormal chromosomes in every cell (trisomy or monosomy).

          (a) Trisomy is a product of the union between a normal gamete (egg or sperm) and a gamete that contains an extra chromosome.

            (i) The individual will have 47 chromosomes; one "pair" will have three chromosomes instead of two.

            (ii) Examples of trisomies are Down syndrome (47, XY, +21 [the extra chromosome is in the 21st pair]); trisomy 18 (47, XX, +18); and trisomy 13 (47, XY, +13).

          (b) Monosomy is the product of a union between a normal gamete and a gamete with a missing chromosome.

            (i) The individual will have 45 chromosomes instead of 46.

            (ii) Monosomy of an entire autosome is incompatible with life.

            (iii) Complete monosomy of a sex chromosome is compatible with life; an example is a female with only one X chromosome (45, XO); known as Turner syndrome.

        (3) If nondisjunction occurs after fertilization, the fetus might have two or more chromosomes that evolve into more than one cell line (mosaicism), each with a different number of chromosomes (Lashley, 1998).

          (a) Different body tissues might have different chromosome numbers or a mixture of cells, depending on when the nondisjunction occurred.

(b) Clinical signs and symptoms vary in mosaicism; they can be severe or inapparent, depending on the number and location of the abnormal cell line.

e. Abnormalities in chromosome structure are as follows:

(1) Abnormalities of the chromosomes involving only a part of the chromosome.

(2) Chromosomes have a primary constriction called the centromere (Figure 2-3).

(a) The short arm of the chromosome is designated by the letter p.

(b) The long arm of the chromosome is designated by the letter q.

(3) Abnormalities can occur by translocation, by deletions, or by additions (Lashley, 1998).

(a) Translocation occurs when the individual has 45 chromosomes, with one of the chromosomes fused to another chromosome (usually number 21 fused to number 14) (see Figure 2-3).

(i) The person has the correct amount of chromosomal material (45, t[14q21q]), but it has been rearranged; this individual is known as a balanced translocation carrier.

(ii) When such an individual and a structurally normal mate have a child, there is a possibility that the offspring:

■ Will receive the carrier parent's abnormal 21/14 chromosome and a normal 14 and 21 from the other parent; thus, the child will be a carrier.

■ Will receive the abnormal chromosome, plus a normal 21 from the carrier parent; this will result in an extra amount of chromosomal material for the 21 pair (unbalanced translocation), and the child will have Down syndrome (46,14,t[14q21q]).

(b) Additions and/or deletions: a portion of a chromosome can be added or lost, which will result in adverse effects on the infant.

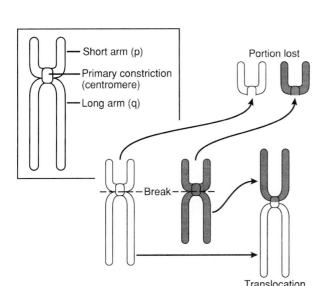

FIGURE 2-3 ■ The process of translocation. Detail shows chromosomal representation. (Adapted from Genetics Screening and Counseling Service, Texas Department of Mental Health and Mental Retardation.)

(i) Deletions and additions result from a small breakage in the chromosomal structure during early cell division.

(ii) An example of the consequences of a deletion is the cri du chat syndrome, in which a small amount of chromosomal material is missing from the short arm of chromosome 5 (5p–).

D. Modes of inheritance (mendelian)

1. Many diseases are caused by an abnormality of a single gene or a pair of genes.

2. Autosomal dominant inheritance: autosomal dominant disorders occur when an individual has a gene that produces an effect whenever it is present (homozygous or heterozygous); this gene overshadows the other gene of the pair.

   a. Mode of transmission (Figure 2-4)

   b. Characteristics

      (1) Affected individuals generally have an affected parent; the family tree (genogram) might show several generations of individuals with the condition.

      (2) The affected individual has a one in two (50%) chance with each pregnancy of passing the abnormal gene on to his or her child.

      (3) Males and females are equally affected.

      (4) An unaffected individual cannot transmit the disorder to his or her children.

      (5) A mutation (a gene that has been spontaneously altered) can result in a new case.

      (6) Autosomal dominant disorders vary greatly in the degree of characteristics that are seen within a family (e.g., in Marfan syndrome, the parent might have only elongated extremities but the child might have a more involved condition, including dislocation of the lens of the eye and severe cardiovascular abnormalities).

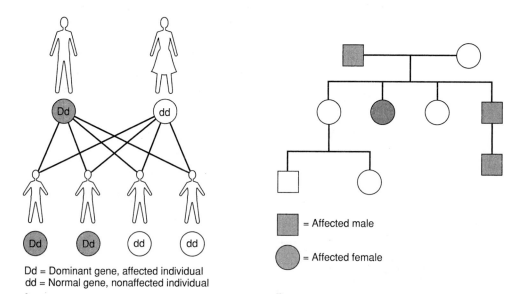

Dd = Dominant gene, affected individual
dd = Normal gene, nonaffected individual

A

B

= Affected male

= Affected female

FIGURE 2-4 ■ Dominant inheritance. **A,** Autosomal dominant inheritance. One parent is affected. Statistically, the offspring have a one in two chance of being affected, regardless of gender. **B,** Autosomal dominant genogram.

3. Autosomal recessive inheritance: an individual has an autosomal recessive disorder if he or she has a gene that produces its effects only when there are two genes on the same chromosome pair (homozygous trait).

    a. A carrier state can occur (heterozygote).

        (1) An individual with the abnormal gene does not manifest obvious symptoms.

        (2) When two carriers pass on the same abnormal gene, the condition might appear.

    b. Mode of transmission (Figure 2-5).

    c. Characteristics

        (1) An affected individual has clinically normal parents, but the parents are both carriers for the abnormal gene.

        (2) The carrier parents have a one in four (25%) chance with each pregnancy of passing the abnormal gene on to their offspring; in this case, when a recessive gene is received from each parent, the child will have the disorder.

        (3) If the offspring of two carrier parents is clinically normal, there is a one in two (50%) chance that he or she will be a carrier, like the parents.

        (4) Males and females are affected equally.

        (5) The family genogram usually shows siblings affected in a horizontal pattern.

        (6) There is an increased risk if intermarriage occurs (consanguineous matings); individuals who are closely related are more likely to have the same genes in common.

        (7) Recessive disorders tend to be more severe in their clinical manifestations.

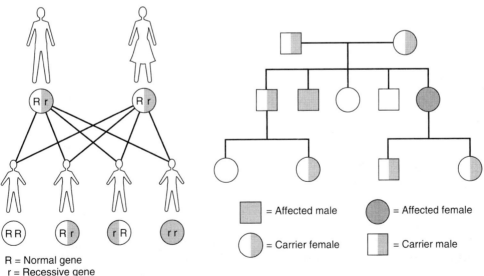

R = Normal gene
r = Recessive gene
Rr = Carrier, nonaffected individual
rr = Affected individual

A   B

FIGURE 2-5 ■ Recessive inheritance. **A,** Autosomal recessive inheritance. Both parents are the carriers. Statistically, the offspring have a one in four chance of being affected, regardless of gender. **B,** Autosomal recessive genogram.

(8) The presence of certain autosomal recessive genes can be detected in the normal carrier parent; examples of diseases for which carrier screening is available are sickle cell anemia, Tay-Sachs disease, and cystic fibrosis.

4. Sex-linked dominant inheritance
   a. The gene is located on the X chromosome of either the mother or the father.
   b. The gene only needs to be present on one X chromosome for symptoms to be manifested.
   c. Mode of transmission—similar to dominant inheritance (see Figure 2-4), but the gene in question is carried only on the X chromosome.
   d. Characteristics
      (1) All individuals with the gene exhibit the disorder.
      (2) It appears in every generation.
      (3) There is a one in two chance of the female child being affected if the mother is affected.
      (4) All the female children are affected if the father has the affected gene.
      (5) None of the male children is affected if the father has the affected gene.
   e. Examples of sex-linked dominant conditions are: vitamin D–resistant rickets, polydactyly, polycystic renal disease (adult).

5. Sex-linked recessive inheritance
   a. Sex-linked or X-linked disorders are those for which the gene is carried on the X chromosome.
   b. A female might be heterozygous or homozygous for a trait carried on the X chromosome because she has two X chromosomes.
   c. A male has only one X chromosome, and there are some traits for which no comparable genes are located on the Y chromosome; in this case, the gene will be expressed.
   d. The X-linked recessive disorders are manifested only in the male who carries the gene.
   e. Mode of transmission (Figure 2-6).
   f. Characteristics
      (1) There is no male-to-male transmission; fathers pass on their Y chromosome to their sons and their X chromosome to their daughters.
      (2) Affected males are related through the female line.
      (3) There is a one in two (50%) chance with each pregnancy that a carrier mother will pass the abnormal gene on to her son, who will then be affected.
      (4) There is a one in two (50%) chance with each pregnancy that a mother will pass the abnormal gene to her daughter, who will then be a carrier like herself.
      (5) A father affected with an X-linked condition cannot pass the disorder on to his sons, but all of his daughters will be carriers.
      (6) Occasionally, a female carrier demonstrates the symptoms of an X-linked disorder; this situation is probably due to the random inactivation of the second X chromosome.
   g. Examples of X-linked recessive disorders are color blindness (red-green), Duchenne's muscular dystrophy, and hemophilia A and B.

E. **Polygenic or multifactorial disorders**
   1. Many common congenital malformations are caused by the interaction of many genes and environmental factors, such as health status, age of the parents, and/or exposure to pollutants and viruses.

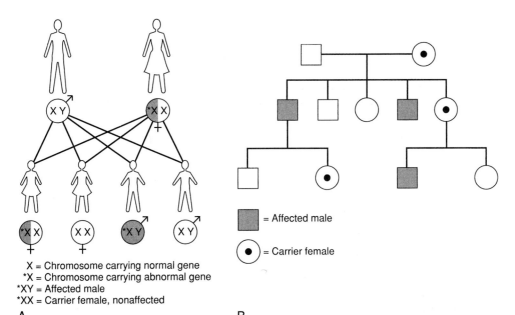

X = Chromosome carrying normal gene
*X = Chromosome carrying abnormal gene
*XY = Affected male
*XX = Carrier female, nonaffected

A   B

FIGURE 2-6 ■ Recessive inheritance. **A,** X-linked recessive inheritance. The mother is the carrier. Statistically, the male offspring have a one in two chance of being affected, and none of the females will be affected. The female offspring have a one in two chance of being carriers. **B,** X-linked genogram.

2. Characteristics
  a. Malformations vary from mild to severe.
  b. The more severe the defect, the greater the number of genes involved.
  c. There is often a gender bias in occurrence rates for specific malformations.
    (1) Congenital hip dysplasia occurs more frequently in females.
    (2) Pyloric stenosis occurs more frequently in males.
    (3) When a member of the less commonly affected gender manifests the condition, more genes must be present to cause the defect.
  d. In the presence of environmental influences, it might take fewer genes to manifest the disease.
  e. In contrast with gene disorders, in multifactorial inheritance an additive effect occurs:
    (1) When more than one family member is affected.
    (2) In proportion to the severity of the condition in the child.
  f. Risk factors are determined by the distribution of cases found in the general population.
  g. The risk of occurrence is usually 2% to 5% for all first-degree relatives but is higher (10% to 15%) if more than one member is affected.
F. **Complex disorders occur when:**
  1. Multiple genes specify proteins whose effects, when expressed, combine to produce a particular phenotype.
  2. Expression of these specific proteins is environmentally influenced to variable degrees throughout individual development, maturation, and aging.
  3. Some examples of complex disorders include hypercholesterolemia, depression, schizophrenia, essential hypertension, and type 2 diabetes mellitus.
  4. The prevalence of such disorders is generally high in the population.

5. Individual disease occurrence is not easily traced through the pedigree; there might not be a clear path of inheritance or segregation.
6. The age at disease onset is often during adult years when reproduction has already occurred.
7. The threshold for disease expression can be affected by a number of different variables; such variables are often controlled to decrease risk of disease expression (e.g., weight control to decrease the incidence of type 2 diabetes mellitus onset).

CLINICAL PRACTICE

A. **The health care professional, at a minimum, should:**
   1. Appreciate his/her personal limitations of genetic expertise;
   2. Understand the social and psychological implications of genetic services;
   3. Know how and when to make a referral to a genetics professional; and,
   4. Strive to meet the knowledge, skills, and attitudes competencies as outlined by National Coalition for Health Professional Education in Genetics (NCHPEG) in 2001. (Competencies are available at *www.nchpeg.org*.)

B. **Assessment**
   1. Family history: take a thorough family history going back at least three generations (genogram) (Figure 2-7) (Harris & Verp, 2001).
   2. Information to be gathered about all three generations should include:
      a. Legal names, including maiden names of all family members
      b. Racial, ethnic background, and country of origin
      c. Place and date of birth
      d. Occupation
      e. Current and past health status
      f. Age and cause of death
      g. Presence of birth defects, retardation, or repetitive family traits
      h. Any miscarriages, stillbirths, or severe childhood illnesses/deaths
      i. Environmental, occupational exposures, and social history
      j. Medication and drug use history
   3. Physical findings: evaluate all systems; chromosomal disorders affect multiple body systems, and many gene disorders have subtle signs that will be detected only through careful assessment of, for example, skin pigmentation, color of sclera, fingernail patterns, texture of hair, and neurologic responses.
   4. Diagnostic tests that might be performed are:
      a. Maternal serum alpha-fetoprotein (AFP) to screen for neural tube defects (elevated) or Down syndrome (low) in the fetus.
         (1) AFP alone detects only 20% of Down syndrome fetuses.
         (2) AFP in combination with human chorionic gonadotropin (hCG) levels and assessing for levels of unconjugated estriol can improve the rate of detection.
         (3) If AFP, hCG, and unconjugated estriol levels are indicative, the mother can be counseled to undergo chromosome analysis to verify the diagnosis.
      b. Chromosomal and biochemical analyses via chorionic villi sampling or amniocentesis.
      c. DNA analysis can be performed on the fetus.
      d. Developmental assessment of parents or siblings as indicated by possible risk status established by a family history (such as Fragile X syndrome).

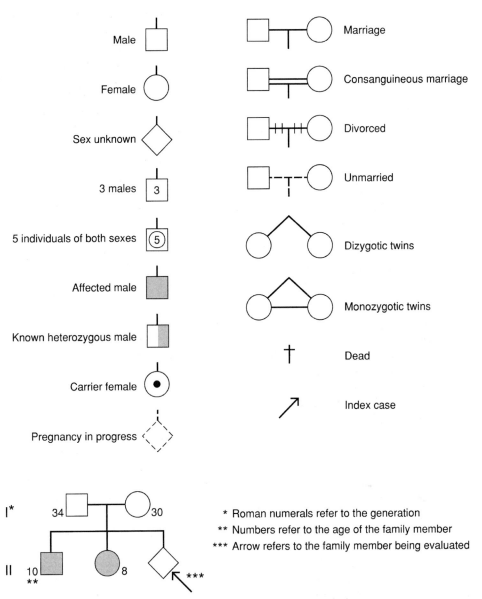

* Roman numerals refer to the generation
** Numbers refer to the age of the family member
*** Arrow refers to the family member being evaluated

FIGURE 2-7 ■ Common genogram symbols.

  e. Fetal ultrasonography for suspected structural disorders (e.g., omphaloceles, renal agenesis).
  f. Newborn screening tests (phenylketonuria [PKU], galactosemia, hypothyroidism).
  g. Other laboratory tests as indicated by physical signs and symptoms.
5. Some indications for prenatal diagnostic testing include the following (Lashley, 1998; Burke, 2002):
  a. Pregnancy at risk for chromosomal aberration
    (1) Maternal age over 35
    (2) Known chromosomal abnormality in the parent
    (3) Previous pregnancy with recognized chromosomal abnormality or observable malformation

      (4) Previous stillbirth or perinatal death in which the cause is unknown
      (5) History of infertility in either parent
      (6) Diagnostic tools—amniocentesis, chorionic villus sampling. Obvious malformations might be observed utilizing ultrasound.
   b. Pregnancy at risk for neural tube defects
      (1) High maternal blood levels of AFP
      (2) Previous child with neural tube defect
      (3) Presence of neural tube defect in either parent or a close relative
      (4) Diagnostic tools—amniocentesis, ultrasound (See Chapter 26 for information on intrauterine fetal surgery for neural tube defect repair.)
   c. Pregnancy at risk for X-linked inherited disorder
      (1) Mother known to be a carrier
      (2) Presence of a close maternal male relative who is affected
      (3) Diagnostic tools—amniocentesis, chorionic villus sampling
   d. Pregnancy at risk for detectable, inherited, biochemical disorders
      (1) Parents are known carriers or are affected
      (2) Previous children born with a biochemical disorder
      (3) Close family members with a known inherited biochemical disorder
      (4) Diagnostic tools—amniocentesis, chorionic villus sampling
   e. Miscellaneous
      (1) Extreme parental anxiety
      (2) Significant exposure to radiation, infection, drugs, or chemicals
      (3) Presence of diabetes mellitus in the mother
      (4) Birth of a previous child with a structural abnormality
      (5) Family history of structural abnormality
      (6) Diagnostic tools—amniocentesis, chorionic villus sampling, ultrasound (Exception: chorionic villus sampling is not indicated in mothers with diabetes mellitus.)
 6. Social, legal, and ethical implications associated with prenatal diagnosis
   a. Option of pregnancy termination/selective reduction for certain conditions
   b. Right of individual to refuse prenatal diagnostic procedures
   c. Right to privacy and ownership of sample taken
   d. Possibility of an ambiguous finding with a resultant dilemma regarding the proper course of action to be taken
C. Nursing Diagnoses
 1. Deficient knowledge related to factors of heredity, infant potential, and community resources
 2. Risk for ineffective family coping related to physical and/or mental handicap of a family member
 3. Risk for interrupted family processes related to diagnosis of a genetic disorder in the fetus or newborn
 4. Risk for impaired parenting related to the diagnosis of a genetic disorder in the fetus or newborn
 5. Grieving related to loss of a normal child
 6. Risk for social isolation of the family and the infant related to embarrassment about child's appearance and/or behavior and lack of knowledge
D. Interventions/Outcomes
 1. Deficient knowledge related to factors of heredity, infant potential, and community resources
   a. Interventions
      (1) Explain appropriate genetic information to the family.

(2) Discuss implications of the condition for the parent, the infant, and the siblings.

(3) Provide written educational material or refer the family to the appropriate agency (such as the March of Dimes National Foundation) for educational materials.

(4) Refer the family to a genetics center for a complete evaluation with appropriate genetic counseling.

(5) Maintain a supportive attitude toward the family's questions, need for clarification, and final decision about actions to be taken.

(6) Explain diagnostic procedures and emphasize the purpose, anticipated findings, and possible side effects.

b. Outcomes

(1) The family demonstrates an understanding of the information provided through feedback and appropriate questions.

(2) The family has obtained the appropriate diagnostic tests.

2. Risk for ineffective family coping related to physical and/or mental handicap of a family member

a. Interventions

(1) Assure family members that they do not need to rush into a decision.

(2) Provide the necessary information and resources for the family to make an informed decision.

(3) Encourage family members to verbalize their feelings.

(4) Interact with family members to encourage individual feelings of self-worth.

(5) Recognize that grief is appropriate during a difficult decision-making process.

b. Outcomes

(1) The family is able to make appropriate decisions.

3. Risk for interrupted family processes related to diagnosis of a genetic disorder in the fetus or newborn

a. Interventions

(1) Explain that grief is appropriate during a difficult decision-making process.

(2) Encourage family members to verbalize their feelings.

(3) Interact with family members to encourage individual feelings of self-worth.

(4) Refer family members to appropriate resources to deal with current crises.

b. Outcomes

(1) The family is able to make appropriate decisions.

(2) Family members are able to provide each other with the necessary emotional and physical support and care.

4. Risk for impaired parenting related to diagnosis of a genetic disorder in the fetus or newborn

a. Interventions

(1) Explain appropriate genetic information to the family.

(2) Discuss implications of the condition.

(3) Interact with the family to encourage feelings of self-worth.

(4) Explain that grief is appropriate during a difficult decision-making process.

(5) Refer the family to the appropriate agency to assist in the parenting of an affected child.

    b. Outcomes

        (1) Family members have obtained needed services.

        (2) Family members are able to make appropriate decisions.

  5. Grieving related to the loss of a normal child

    a. Interventions

        (1) Assure family members that they do not need to rush into a decision.

        (2) Provide privacy and encourage family members to verbalize their feelings.

        (3) Explain that grief is a normal response.

        (4) Provide the necessary information and resources.

    b. Outcomes

        (1) Family members verbalize grief and feelings of loss.

        (2) Family members make the appropriate decisions.

  6. Risk for social isolation of the family and the infant related to embarrassment about the child's appearance and/or behavior and lack of knowledge

    a. Interventions

        (1) Explain appropriate genetic information to the family.

        (2) Discuss the implications of the condition and the resources available to the family.

        (3) Maintain a supportive attitude toward the family.

        (4) Encourage family members to verbalize their feelings.

        (5) Refer family members to appropriate agencies to deal with their concerns.

    b. Outcomes

        (1) The family is able to provide necessary care for the affected infant.

        (2) The family has obtained services from referral agencies.

        (3) The family is able to make the appropriate decisions.

HEALTH EDUCATION

A. **Explain the known causes for the condition (the genetics of the disorder).**

B. **Describe the referral agencies that are available for the follow-up and support.**

C. **Explain the reproductive options and recurrence risks.**

D. **Discuss available treatment options.**

E. **Discuss the prognosis of the condition.**

F. **Discuss the measures to be taken to prevent the condition in future offspring.**

CASE STUDIES AND STUDY QUESTIONS

Mrs. C, 43 years old, gravida 3, para 2 (G3, P2) is at 16 weeks' gestation. She underwent a prenatal diagnostic test for chromosomal abnormalities. She received the result of the test, which was 47,XY,+21 (male with Down syndrome). Otherwise, the pregnancy has been normal with no complications to date.

  1. What information would you need to know to assist Mr. and Mrs. C in understanding the cause of chromosomal abnormalities?

    a. A history of maternal substance use during pregnancy

    b. The level and quality of prenatal care received to date

    c. The family history of chromosomal abnormalities

    d. The delivery history of previous children

2. Mr. and Mrs. C do not understand what 47,XY, 21 means. What is the correct interpretation?
   a. The 47th chromosome has 21 extra genes and XY refers to gender.
   b. There is an extra chromosome in the 21st pair and XY refers to gender.
   c. The 21st chromosome has additional genetic material and XY refers to location on the gene.
   d. The number 47 refers to the type of test and 21 refers to the number of abnormal cells identified.

3. Mr. and Mrs. C believe that they must have done something that caused this abnormality in their fetus. You can tell them:
   a. They are not responsible because this was an accident that occurred in early cell division before fertilization.
   b. Mrs. C might have had a viral infection in the first few days after conception.
   c. Mr. C might have been exposed to an environmental toxin during adolescence, thus altering his ability to produce normal sperm.
   d. Mrs. C might have exposed the embryo to an environmental toxin that altered the basic cell structure.

4. Mr. and Mrs. C are concerned about the potential risks to their future grandchildren. What is an appropriate response?
   a. With each occurrence of a chromosomal abnormality, there is an increased risk of recurrence of 2% to 5%.
   b. Recommend that their children undergo regular chromosomal monitoring to rule out a future translocation.
   c. Recommend that only male children should consider future pregnancies because they would not be at risk.
   d. The recurrence risk should not be higher than that for the general population.

Mrs. K is a 29-year-old white woman. She is a G1, P1 and has delivered an infant boy. The child was diagnosed as having achondroplasia (a type of dwarfism that is inherited via the autosomal dominant mode [Figure 2-8]). The child weighs 2722 g (6 lb) and is in no apparent distress. Upon further questioning, you learn that Mr. K is 45 years old and has achondroplasia. Mrs. K has three sisters with no health problems, and her parents are living and well. Mr. K has one brother and one sister; both are normal. Mr. K's mother is living and well; Mr. K's father is dead and he, too, had achondroplasia. Both Mr. and Mrs. K are interested in future pregnancies.

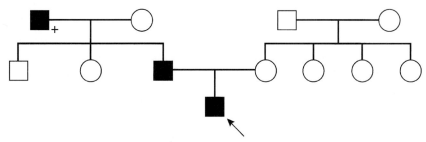

FIGURE 2-8 ■ Mr. and Mrs. K.

5. The couple does not understand what autosomal dominant means. You tell the couple that an autosomal dominant condition is:
   a. A disorder that is caused by a single gene that overshadows a gene that is at the same location on the other chromosome pair
   b. A condition that occurs when each parent contributes a gene for the particular disorder
   c. A condition that produces a result that is severe and usually is not correctable
   d. A condition that is caused by a combination of many genes and an environmental factor

6. Because they would like to have other children, they are interested in knowing the recurrence risk for this condition. The estimated risk is:
   a. Quite small
   b. 10% to 15%
   c. 25%
   d. 50%

7. Mr. and Mrs. K note that two individuals with achondroplasia in their family were males, and they would like to know if boys are at a greater risk. You advise them that this dominant condition:

   a. Has a 25% increased risk for males.
   b. Occurs in both males and females.
   c. Occurs more frequently when the woman is older than 35 years old.
   d. Has a 50% increased risk for males.

Mr. and Mrs. Y were contacted by their pediatrician because their newborn son's screening PKU test results were abnormal (the PKU level was elevated). The infant is now 5 days old and appears normal, although a little colicky. Further testing verified the diagnosis of PKU. Mr. and Mrs. Y are in their late 20s; they have three normal daughters, and Mr. Y is convinced that if their next child is a girl, she will be normal. Mrs. Y has one sister who has three normal children. Her parents died in an automobile accident when she was small. Mr. Y is an only child, and his parents died when he was a young child (Figure 2-9).

8. The couple does not understand what autosomal recessive means. You could tell them that an autosomal recessive condition is:
   a. A disorder that is caused by a single gene that overshadows a gene that is at the same location on the other chromosome pair.
   b. A condition that occurs when each parent contributes a

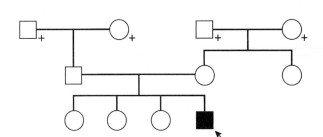

FIGURE 2-9 ■ Mr. and Mrs. Y.

gene for the particular disorder.

c. A condition that produces a result that is not severe and usually is correctable.

9. Because they would like to have other children, they are interested in knowing that the recurrence risk for this condition is:
   a. Extremely small
   b. 10% to 15%
   c. 25%
   d. 50%

10. Mr. and Mrs. Y do not understand why the girls were normal and the boy was not; they would like to know if only a boy would be at risk. You advise them that this recessive condition:
    a. Has a 25% increased risk for males.
    b. Occurs in both males and females

c. Occurs more frequently in women older than 35 years old.
d. Has a 50% increased risk for males.

11. The couple has difficulty believing that the condition is inheritable in their family, because no one else has a similar problem. You can explain to them that recessive disorders:
    a. Occur among siblings versus occurring from generation to generation.
    b. Occur in a random pattern in the first two or three generations.
    c. Have a high frequency of mutations in the original case.
    d. Usually skip a generation before they manifest themselves.

ANSWERS TO STUDY QUESTIONS

1. c	4. d	7. b	10. b
2. b	5. a	8. b	11. a
3. a	6. d	9. c	

REFERENCES

Bennett, R.L. (1999). *The practical guide to the genetic family history*. New York: Wiley-Liss.

Burke, W. (2002). Genetic testing. *New England Journal of Medicine, 347*(23), 1867-1875.

Guttmacher, A.E. & Collins, F.S. (2002). Genomic medicine: A primer. *New England Journal of Medicine, 347*(19), 1512-1520.

Harris, C.M. & Verp, M.S. (2001). Prenatal testing and interventions. In Mahowald M.B., Scheuerle, A.S., McKusick, V.A., & Aspinwall, T.J. (Eds.). *Genetics in the clinic:* *Clinical, ethical, and social implications for primary care* (pp. 59-74). St. Louis: Mosby.

Horowitz, M. (2000). *Basic concepts in medical genetics: A student's survival guide*. New York: McGraw-Hill.

Lashley, F.R. (1998). *Clinical genetics in nursing practice* (2nd ed.). New York: Springer.

Lorentz, C.P., Wieben, E.D., Tefferi, A., Whiteman, D.A.H., & Dewald, G. (2002). Primer on medical genomics, part I: History of genetics and sequencing the human genome. *Mayo Clinic Proceedings, 77*(8), 773-782.

Tefferi, A., Wieben, E.D., Dewald, G.W., Whiteman, A.H., Bernard, M.E., & Spelsberg, T.C. (2002). Primer on medical genomics, part II: Background principles and methods in molecular genetics. *Mayo Clinic Proceedings*, 77(8), 785-808.

3 Fetal and Placental Development and Functioning

LINDA CALLAHAN

OBJECTIVES

1. Describe the process of fertilization.
2. Discuss the stages of placental development.
3. Describe the functions of the placenta.
4. Explain the implications of ineffective placental development on fetal development.
5. Describe the functions of the amniotic fluid.
6. Identify the important milestones for the development of fetal organs, such as the heart, lungs, kidney, and brain.
7. Identify the periods when the developing body systems of the fetus are most susceptible to teratogenic influences.

INTRODUCTION

A. **Pregenesis**
  1. Encompasses the time after formation of the germ cells and before union of sperm and egg.
  2. Begins with differentiation and migration of primitive germ cells to the genital ridge and ends with the formation of the gametes (karyogamy).
  3. Aneuploidies (abnormal numbers of chromosomes) might occur as a consequence of abnormal meiotic division of chromosomes during gamete formation.
B. **Conception**
  1. Fertilization usually occurs in the ampulla of the fallopian tube.
  2. Estrogen levels increase during ovulation, aiding fertilization and easing transit of the ovum down the fallopian tube.
  3. The ovum membrane is surrounded by two layers of tissue.
    a. An inner layer called the zona pellucida
    b. An outer layer called the corona radiata (Figure 3-1)
  4. In a single ejaculation, 400 million spermatozoa are deposited in the vagina, reaching the fallopian tubes within 5 minutes by frantic movement of their flagellar tails.
    a. A sperm undergoes two processes before it is able to penetrate the ovum.
      (1) Capacitation: structural changes occur once in the female genital tract.

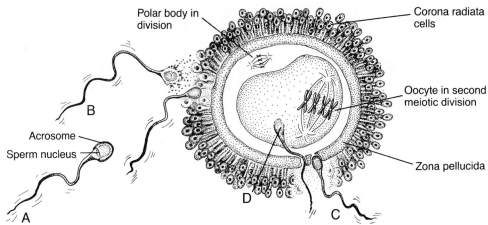

FIGURE 3-1 ■ Process of fertilization. **A,** Sperm moves toward ovum using movement of the flagellum. **B,** Acrosomal reaction. **C,** Sperm penetrates corona radiata and zona. **D,** Once sperm penetrates the ovum, fusion of the oocyte and sperm cell membranes occurs.

        (2) Acrosomal reaction: the sperm releases enzymes (see Figure 3-1).
          (a) Hyaluronidase causes separation of the corona radiata.
          (b) Acrosin and neuraminidase allow the sperm to enter the zona pellucida.
     b. Ova are considered fertile for approximately 24 hours after ovulation, whereas sperm, although viable for 72 hours, are believed to be fertile for only 24 hours.
     c. At the moment of penetration, the oocyte completes the second meiotic division (see Figure 3-1) whereas cellular changes prevent other sperm from entering the ovum (zona reaction).
  5. With fertilization, the diploid number (46) of chromosomes is restored, and cell division begins.
     a. Within the cell, the nuclei of the spermatozoon and oocyte unite, and their nuclear membranes disappear.
     b. The chromosomes pair up, and a new cell, the zygote, which contains a new combination of genetic material, is formed.
C. Pre-embryonic stage: the first 2 weeks after fertilization; the blastogenetic period is the first 4 weeks of human development.
  1. This stage is characterized by rapid cell division, cell differentiation, and the development of embryonic membranes and germ layers.
     a. First week (Figure 3-2)
       (1) Division of the zygote occurs within the first 30 hours.
       (2) The zygote continues to divide into a solid ball of cells (the morula).
       (3) The morula floats inside of the uterus for 2 or 3 days obtaining nourishment from the mucous lining of the uterus and the fluid in the uterine cavity.
       (4) Two distinct layers of cells develop as the morula hollows out.
         (a) The inner cell mass (blastocyst), which will form the embryo, the amnion, and the yolk sac membrane
         (b) The outer cell layer (trophoblast), which becomes the fetal side of the placenta and chorion

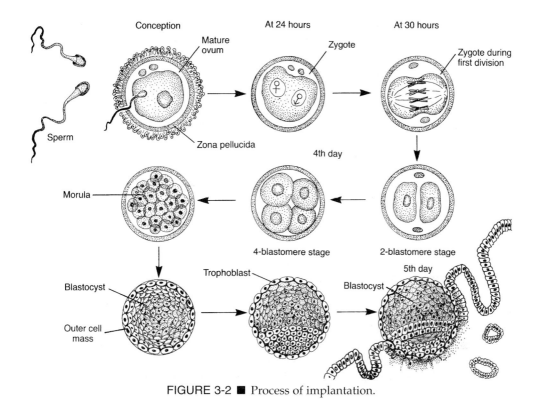

FIGURE 3-2 ■ Process of implantation.

    (5) Zona pellucida disappears at about 5 days.
        (a) The blastocyst enlarges.
        (b) The trophoblast attaches to the endometrial epithelium and begins
            the process of implantation.
    (6) The attached portion of the trophoblast develops into two layers.
        (a) The internal cellular layer is called the cytotrophoblast.
        (b) The outer layer is called the syncytiotrophoblast, which invades
            the endometrial epithelium by the end of the seventh day.
        (c) Embedding is completed by the 11th day, with the site of
            attachment usually being the upper part of the posterior uterine
            wall. Attachment can occur anywhere, even extrauterine.
  b. Second week
    (1) The inner cell mass differentiates into two cell layers: the endoderm
        (the inside of the embryo) and the ectoderm (the outside of the
        embryo).
        (a) The amniotic cavity appears as a space between the inner cell
            mass and the trophoblast.
        (b) When the embryo becomes a cylinder, the amnion surrounds it
            and forms the amniotic sac.
    (2) By the end of the second week, the embryonic cells and the amniotic
        and yolk sacs are attached to the chorionic sac by a slender band,
        which becomes the umbilical cord.
    (3) Malformations that occur during the pre-embryonic stage seldom
        result in a viable fetus.

   c. Placental development
- (1) Description: the placenta is a temporary disc-shaped organ that connects the fetus to the uterine wall and provides for fetal respiration and metabolic and nutrient exchanges between the maternal and fetal circulations.
- (2) Approximately 5 to 6 days after fertilization, the blastocyst adheres to the endometrium.
- (3) Blastocyst penetrates toward the maternal capillaries by eroding the uterine epithelium; this erosion process continues until the blastocyst is completely embedded in the uterine wall.

   d. Decidua: the portion of the endometrium enveloping the developing fertilized ovum (Figure 3-3)
- (1) On approximately the 14th day, the endometrium changes at the site of implantation and becomes the decidua.
- (2) Implantation causes the adjacent decidual cells to engorge with glycogen and lipids (decidual reaction).
- (3) The swollen decidual cells release their contents during the erosion process to provide nourishment to the embryo.
- (4) The decidua divides into three layers:
  - (a) Decidua capsularis—covers the embryoblast.
  - (b) Decidua basalis—maternal portion of the placenta that supplies vessels to nourish the intervillous spaces.
  - (c) Decidua parietalis—lines the remainder of the uterine cavity.

   e. Placenta
- (1) When the embryoblast is partially embedded in the decidua, two distinct layers of cells can be seen in the trophoblast.
  - (a) Inner layer (cytotrophoblast) is made of mononuclear cells.
  - (b) Outer layer (syncytiotrophoblast) consists of multinucleated cells and is responsible for the erosive ability of the trophoblast.
- (2) The cytotrophoblast and the syncytiotrophoblast separate the maternal and fetal circulations and are called the placental barrier.

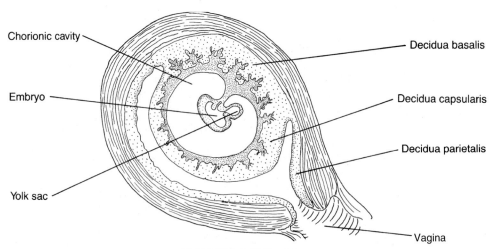

FIGURE 3-3 ■ Decidua.

(3) On approximately the ninth day, spaces (vacuoles) appear in the syncytium; these fuse together to form lacunae (intervillous spaces), which develop into an interconnecting system.

(4) On approximately the 11th day:
   (a) Invading syncytium encounters the congested capillaries of the decidua.
   (b) Syncytium enzymes break down the vessel walls, releasing blood into the lacunae.
   (c) Eventually, the syncytium encounters the larger arteries and veins and establishes a directional flow of blood.
   (d) Blood enters the lacunae.
      (i) The embryo experiences rapid growth because of a high concentration of nutrients.
      (ii) This growth results in an increase in the distance that nutrients must travel by diffusion to reach the embryo.

(5) Chorionic villi develop between the 9th and 25th days (Figure 3-4).
   (a) The chorion (trophoblastic cells) is the first placental membrane to form, enclosing the embryo, amnion, and yolk sac and growing outward, forming finger-like projections called villi within which blood vessels develop.
   (b) Initially, the chorion covers the whole chorionic surface but with fetal growth the intraluminal villi become compressed and degenerate.
   (c) Villi located below the embryo continue to grow, forming a large surface for exchange with villi that contact the decidua basalis to become anchoring villi.
      (i) Decidual septa form between anchoring villi, which results in 15 to 20 lobes (cotyledons).
      (ii) Exchange of gases and nutrients occurs in this vascular system.
   (d) Other villi float free and conduct most of the exchange between mother and developing fetus.
   (e) No further villi are formed after the 12th week.

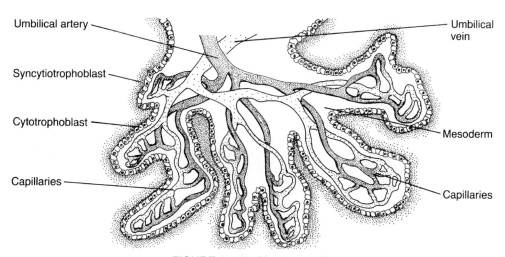

FIGURE 3-4 ■ Chorionic villi.

    D. Embryonic stage: begins with the folding of the disk in week two of
       development.
      1. Third week
         a. Gastrulation
           (1) The embryonic disc converts into a trilaminar embryonic disc
               comprising three germ layers: ectoderm (to become the epidermis and
               the nervous system); mesoderm (to become the smooth muscle); and
               endoderm (to become the epithelial lining of the respiratory and
               digestive tracts).
           (2) The process is completed in the third week with the formation of
               intraembryonic mesoderm by the primitive streak.
         b. Proliferation and migration of cells from the primitive streak give rise to
           mesenchyme (Figure 3-5, *A*).
           (1) Cells spread cranially and caudally.
           (2) Cells begin to form the embryonic endoderm, which give rise to the
               lining of the digestive and respiratory tracts.
           (3) The cells that remain on the surface of the embryonic disc form
               the layer of cells called the embryonic ectoderm, which develop into
               the nervous system (i.e., the sensory epithelium of the eye, ear, and
               nose).
         c. The mesenchymal cells migrate cephalid under the embryonic ectoderm
           and form the notochordal process (Figure 3-5, *B*).

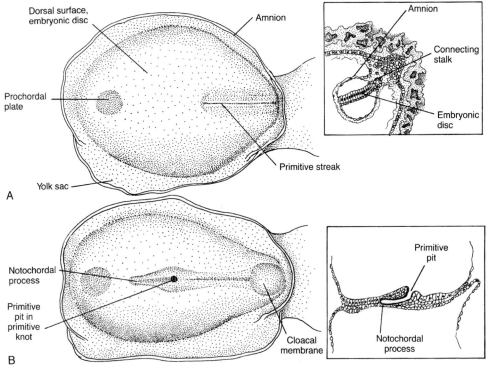

FIGURE 3-5 ■ Schematic of embryonic disc and extraembryonic membranes. **A,** Embryonic
disc. **B,** Extraembryonic membranes.

(1) These cells grow until they reach the prochordal plate, the future site of the mouth.
(2) Caudal to the primitive streak is a circular area called the cloacal membrane, which becomes the anus.
(3) The primitive streak continues to form mesoderm until the end of the fourth week.
(4) The notochord develops by transformation of the notochordal process by the end of the third week of gestation.
  d. Neurulation is the process of developing the neural plate, neural folds, and neural tube.
(1) Neural plate (Figure 3-6)
  (a) Embryonic ectoderm lying over the notochord thickens to form the neural plate.
  (b) It first appears near the primitive knot and enlarges to form a neural groove, which becomes bounded by the neural folds on each side.
(2) Neural tube
  (a) By the third week, the neural folds begin to fuse, forming the neural tube.
  (b) This occurs near the middle of the embryo and progresses toward the cranial and caudal ends.
(3) Neural crest (Figure 3-7)
  (a) Cells lying along the neural fold migrate ventrolaterally on each side of the neural tube forming an irregular mass called the neural crest.
  (b) These cells migrate throughout the embryo and give rise to the spinal ganglia.
  (c) The neural crest cells also form the meninges of the brain and spinal cord, the adrenal medulla, and several components of the skeletal and muscular parts of the head.
  e. Somite development (Figure 3-8, *A*)
(1) Some of the mesoderm form columns that divide into paired cuboidal bodies (somites).

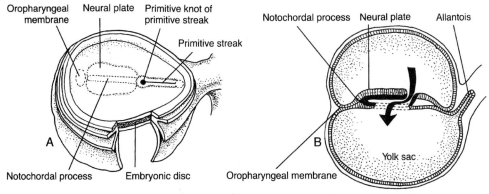

FIGURE 3-6 ■ Embryonic disc at approximately 3 weeks. Neural plate. **A,** Horizontal section showing notochordal process and associated mesenchyme stimulating ectoderm to form the neural plate. **B,** Vertical section showing the notochordal process beginning to degenerate. (Adapted from Moore, K.L. [1988]. *Essentials of human embryology* [p. 19]. Philadelphia: B.C. Decker.)

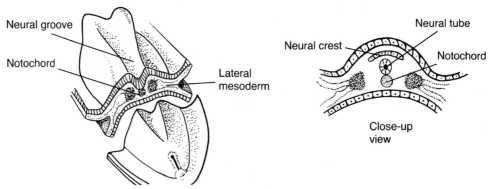

FIGURE 3-7 ■ Transverse section of developing embryo at 3 weeks. (Adapted from Moore, K.L. [1988]. *Essentials of human embryology* [p. 20]. Philadelphia: B.C. Decker.)

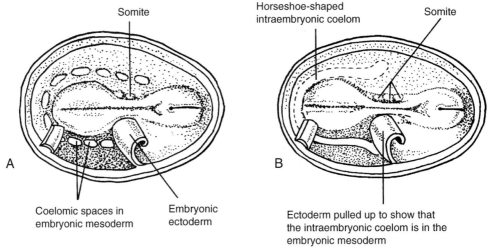

FIGURE 3-8 ■ Dorsal view of the developing embryo. (Adapted from Moore, K.L. [1988]. *Essentials of human embryology* [p. 23]. Philadelphia: B.C. Decker.)

    (2) Mesenchymal cells from the somites will become the vertebral column, the ribs, the sternum, the skull, and associated muscles.

  f. Intraembryonic coelom

    (1) Cavities in the lateral mesoderm form a horseshoe-shaped cavity called the intraembryonic coelom (Figure 3-8, *B*).

    (2) The intraembryonic coelom divides the lateral mesoderm into two layers.

      (a) Somatic layer is continuous with the extraembryonic mesoderm covering the amnion.

      (b) Visceral layer is continuous with the extraembryonic mesoderm covering the yolk sac.

    (3) During the second month, the intraembryonic coelom will become the pericardial, the pleural, and the peritoneal cavities.

  g. Primitive cardiovascular system (Figure 3-9)

    (1) Blood vessels start forming in the extraembryonic mesoderm of the yolk sac, connecting stalk and chorion at the end of the third week.

    (2) Mesenchymal cells (angioblasts) aggregate to form blood islands.

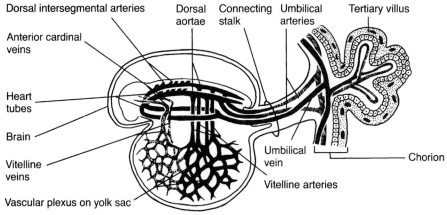

FIGURE 3-9 ■ Primitive cardiovascular system (at about 20 days). (Adapted from Moore, K.L. [1988]. *Essentials of human embryology* [p. 61]. Philadelphia: B.C. Decker.)

    (3) Mesenchymal cells arrange around cavities in the blood islands to form the endothelium of primitive blood vessels, which go on to develop into a series of vascular networks.

    (4) Primitive blood cells develop from the endothelial cells of the vessels in the walls of the yolk sac; blood formation does not begin in the embryo until the fifth week.

    (5) The primitive heart is a tubular structure formed from the mesenchymal cells in the cardiogenic area.

        (a) Paired endocardial heart tubes develop and fuse to form a primitive heart.

        (b) The heart tubes join blood vessels in the embryo, connective stalk, chorion, and yolk sac, forming a primitive cardiovascular system.

        (c) The primitive blood cells begin to circulate at the end of the third week as the tubular heart begins to beat.

  h. Malformations that might occur during this stage:

    (1) Anencephaly, as a result of a defect in the closure of the anterior neural tube, which results in the degeneration of the forebrain

    (2) Cyclopia, as a result of an alteration in the prechordal mesodermal development, and producing secondary defects of the midface and forebrain

    (3) Ectromelia (congenital absence of a limb)

    (4) Ectopia cordis (heart remains outside of the thoracic cavity)

2. Fourth week

  a. The neural tube is open at the rostral and caudal neuropores, and the embryo is almost straight (Figure 3-10, *A* and *B*).

  b. The first and second pairs of the branchial arches (future head and neck) are visible.

  c. The otic placodes (primordia of the internal ears) are developed.

  d. By the middle of the fourth week, the embryo is cylindric and curved because of the folding of the median and horizontal planes.

    (1) The rostral neuropore closes.

    (2) The upper limb buds appear as small swellings on the lateral wall (Figure 3-10, *C*).

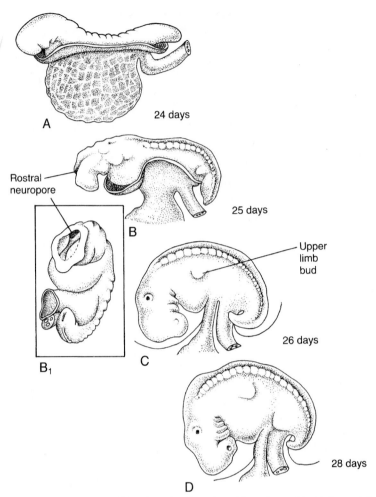

A 24 days

Rostral neuropore

B 25 days

B₁

C 26 days

Upper limb bud

D 28 days

FIGURE 3-10 ■ Development of head and tail regions (fourth week). (Adapted from Moore, K.L. [1988]. *Essentials of human embryology* [p. 29]. Philadelphia: B.C. Decker.)

    (3) The heart is a distinct prominence on the surface of the embryo.
    (4) The otic pits are formed.
  e. By the end of the fourth week, the embryo is C-shaped.
    (1) The oral cavity begins while the esophagotracheal septum begins to divide into the esophagus and the trachea.
    (2) The stomach, the pancreas, and the liver begin to form.
    (3) Upper limb buds have a flipper shape (Figure 3-10, *D*).
    (4) Lower limb buds appear as small swellings (Figure 3-11, *A*).
    (5) Four pairs of branchial arches and lens placodes (the lens of the eye) have developed.
    (6) A tail is prominent at this time.
  f. Malformations that might occur during this stage of development:
    (1) Meningomyelocele results from a defect in the closure of the posterior neural tube.
    (2) Esophageal atresia and tracheoesophageal fistulas can occur as a result of the lateral septation of the foregut.

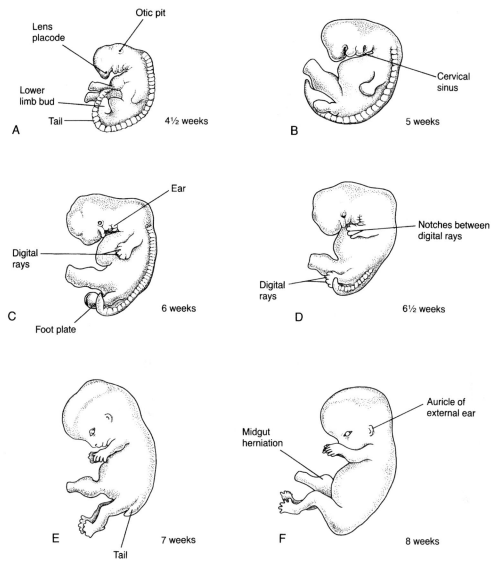

FIGURE 3-11 ■ Embryo from 4 weeks to 8 weeks. (Adapted from Moore, K.L. [1988]. *Essentials of human embryology* [p. 37]. Philadelphia: B.C. Decker.)

      (3) Extravasation of the bladder occurs if the infraumbilical mesenchyme does not migrate effectively.

  3. Fifth week (Figure 3-11, *B*)

    a. The embryo is approximately 8 mm (⅜ in) in length.

    b. The head grows because of the rapid development and differentiation of the brain.

    c. The cranial nerves have developed.

    d. Atrial division in the heart begins.

    e. Upper limbs become paddle-shaped.

    f. Malformations that can occur during this stage:

      (1) Cleft lip and other facial clefts result from a defect in the closure of the lip.

      (2) Transposition of the great vessels can occur if the aorticopulmonary septum fails to spiral.

      (3) Nuclear cataracts.

      (4) Microphthalmia (small eyeballs).

      (5) Carpal and pedal ablation.

4. Sixth week (Figure 3-11, C and D)

   a. The embryo is 12 mm (½ in) long.

   b. The fissures of the brain are obvious.

   c. The heart begins to divide into chambers, and the liver begins to form red blood cells.

   d. The trachea and lung buds appear, and the oral and nasal cavities are formed.

   e. The upper and lower jaw begin to form; upper lip and palate development also occur.

   f. Embryonic sex glands appear.

   g. Skeletal and muscular systems.

      (1) Ossification of the jaw and skull begins.

      (2) The wrist and elbow are identifiable.

      (3) Ridges called digital rays (future fingers and thumb) form on the paddle-shaped hands.

      (4) Muscle begins to develop.

   h. The primordia of the external acoustic meatus and external ear are present; the external, middle, and inner ears continue to form.

   i. Malformations that can occur during this period:

      (1) Rectal atresia with fistula occurs if there is a defect in the lateral septation of the cloaca into the rectum and urogenital sinuses.

      (2) Diaphragmatic hernia occurs when there is a defect in the closure of the pleuroperitoneal canal.

      (3) Ventricular septal defect results during the closure of the ventricular septum.

5. Seventh week (Figure 3-11, E)

   a. The embryo is approximately 18 mm (¾ in) in length.

   b. Fetal heartbeat can be heard and fetal circulation begins.

   c. Gastrointestinal system

      (1) The tongue separates, and the palate begins to fold inward.

      (2) The stomach assumes its final shape.

      (3) The diaphragm separates the abdominal and thoracic cavities.

   d. Genitourinary system

      (1) The bladder and the urethra separate from the rectum.

      (2) The sex glands begin to differentiate into testes or ovaries.

   e. Skeletal and muscular systems

      (1) Notches develop between the digital rays of the hand.

      (2) Digital rays appear in the developing feet.

   f. The optic nerve forms, the eyelids appear, and the eye lenses begin to thicken.

   g. Malformations that can occur during this period:

      (1) Duodenal atresia resulting from an error in the recanalization of the duodenum

      (2) Pulmonary stenosis

      (3) Brachycephalism (shortening of the head)

      (4) Alteration in sexual characteristics

      (5) Cleft palate

6. Eighth week (Figure 3-11, *F*)
   a. The embryo is 2.5 to 3 cm (1 in) in length and weighs 8 g (0.25 oz).
   b. Sensory and motor neurons have functional connections, and the embryo is able to contract large muscles.
   c. Development of the heart is complete, and the circulatory system through the umbilical cord is formed.
   d. Gastrointestinal system
      (1) Abdomen protrudes because the intestines are in the proximal part of the umbilical cord.
      (2) Anal membrane perforates, and rectal passage opens.
      (3) Lips are fused.
   e. External genitalia begin to differentiate.
   f. Skeletal and muscular systems
      (1) Distinct notches are present between the toes.
      (2) The fingers and toes are distinct and separated.
      (3) Differentiation of the cells occurs in the primitive skeleton.
      (4) Cartilaginous bones begin to ossify.
      (5) Muscle development begins in the trunk, limbs, and head.
   g. The eyes are open but fuse at the end of the eighth week while the auricles of the external ear assume their final appearance.
   h. Malformations that can occur during this period:
      (1) Persistent opening of the atrial septum
      (2) Digital stunting
E. **Fetal stage:** every organ system and external structure is present, and the remainder of gestation is devoted to refining the function of the organs.
   1. Placental growth continues until the 20th week; beyond 20 weeks the placenta increases only in thickness.
      a. At term
         (1) Placenta is round and flat; approximately 15 to 20 cm (6 to 8 in) in diameter and 2.5 cm (1 in) thick.
         (2) Placenta weighs approximately one-sixth of the weight of the infant.
         (3) Maternal surface (red and blue in color):
            (a) Arises from the decidua basalis.
            (b) Has multiple lobules (cotyledons).
         (4) Fetal surface (smooth, white, and shiny in appearance):
            (a) Develops from the chorionic villi.
            (b) Contains branches of umbilical veins and arteries.
            (c) Is covered with the chorionic and the amniochorionic membranes.
      b. Circulation (Figure 3-12)
         (1) Maternal placental circulation
            (a) Oxygenated blood enters the intervillous spaces from the decidua basalis.
            (b) Maternal blood pressure directs the blood toward the chorionic villi.
            (c) Deoxygenated blood leaves the intervillous spaces through openings in the cytotrophoblast and enters the endometrial veins.
            (d) Uterine contractions compress intervillous spaces, forcing the blood into the uterine veins.

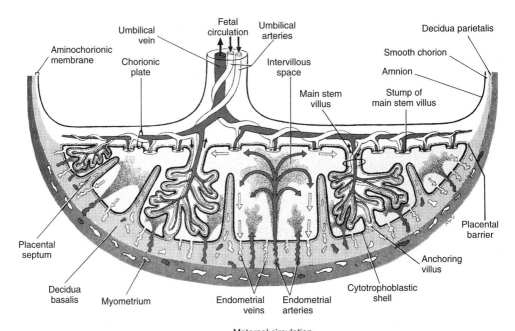

Maternal circulation

FIGURE 3-12 ■ Placental circulation. Arrangement of the placental blood vessels. Blood of the fetus flows through the umbilical arteries into the fetal capillaries in the villi and then back to the fetal circulation through the umbilical vein. Maternal blood is transported by the uterine arteries to the intervillous space and leaves by the uterine veins to go back to the maternal circulation. (From Moore, K.L. [1988]. *The developing human* [p. 109]. Philadelphia: W.B. Saunders.)

(2) Fetal placental circulation
    (a) Deoxygenated blood leaves the fetus through the two umbilical arteries.
    (b) Umbilical arteries divide into multiple branches as they enter the chorionic villi.
    (c) Oxygenated blood returns via venules and veins in the chorionic villi.
    (d) The veins in the chorionic villi join to form the umbilical vein.
2. Mechanism of placental transfer (Table 3-1)
    a. The passage of substances from mother to fetus against a concentration gradient (active transport) requires expenditure of energy by the cells and can be inhibited by substances that interfere with energy production.
        (1) Amino acids, iron, calcium, iodine, and water-soluble vitamins are transported by this process.
    b. Defects or breaks in the placental membrane allow for the transfer of large cells, such as red blood cells.
        (1) This process is responsible for Rh sensitization.
        (2) This can only occur when the mother is Rh negative and the fetus is Rh positive.
        (3) Rh-positive fetal cells enter the maternal system through a break or defect in the placenta.

■ TABLE 3-1
■ ■ **Placental Transfer**

Type of Transfer	Products Transferred
Active transport	Amino acids
	Iron
	Calcium
	Iodine
	Water-soluble vitamins
Breaks in membrane	Rh factors that result in isoimmunization
Bulk flow	Water
Diffusion	Oxygen
	Carbon dioxide
	Electrolytes
	Lipid-soluble vitamins
Facilitated diffusion	D-Glucose
Pinocytosis	Some immunoglobulins

  (4) Maternal system develops antibodies to the Rh-positive fetal cells.
  (5) Process occurs most frequently during delivery.
  c. Bulk flow.
  (1) Transfers substances by osmosis through micropores in the membrane.
  (2) This process maintains the maternal-fetal exchange of water.
  d. Diffusion
  (1) The process by which molecules that present at higher levels of concentration move more rapidly toward areas of lower concentrations across a membrane.
  (2) Molecular size determines rate of movement; also, the higher the temperature, the greater the activity.
  (3) Provides the mechanism for the transfer of respiratory gases (oxygen and carbon dioxide), electrolytes, and some lipid-soluble vitamins.
  (4) Limitations in diffusion are a major factor in placental failure.
  e. Facilitated diffusion
  (1) Occurs on a maternal to fetal concentration gradient without an expenditure of energy.
  (2) Occurs at a rate greater than that of simple diffusion.
  (3) D-Glucose, galactose, and some oxygen are transported.
  (4) Substances that are highly fat soluble cross the placenta at a faster rate.
  f. Pinocytosis
  (1) Is the transfer by invagination into the cell membrane of a molecule, which then crosses to the opposite side. Examples include:.
   (a) Microdrops of plasma are taken up by the trophoblasts.
   (b) Trophoblasts transport immunoglobulins from the plasma to the fetus.
3. Transfer disorders
  a. Separation of the placenta from the uterine wall
  (1) Placenta previa
  (2) Placental infarcts
  (3) Abruptio placentae

    b. Intervillous coagulation and ischemic necrosis

    c. Alterations in the membrane as a result of calcifications, thickening, and degeneration can alter permeability.

    d. Usually result from a problem in maternal circulation.

      (1) Hypertensive disorders in pregnancy.

      (2) Diabetes mellitus.

      (3) Severe maternal malnutrition.

    e. For placental insufficiency to occur, a major portion of the placenta must be involved.

4. Placental function

    a. Respiration

      (1) Oxygen in the maternal blood crosses the placental membrane and enters the fetal blood supply by diffusion.

      (2) Carbon dioxide returns to the maternal system across the placental membrane.

      (3) Actual fetal pulmonary respiration does not take place in utero.

    b. Nutrition

      (1) Water, inorganic salts, carbohydrates, fats, proteins, and vitamins pass from the maternal blood through the placental membrane into the fetal system via enzymatic carriers.

      (2) The placenta metabolizes glucose and stores it in the form of glycogen until the fetal liver is able to function.

    c. Excretion

      (1) Waste products cross the placental membrane and enter the maternal blood.

      (2) Waste products produced by the fetus are minimal due to the dominance of anabolic (building rather than breaking down activities) metabolism.

    d. Protection

      (1) Placental barrier prevents the transfer of many harmful substances from the maternal blood system.

      (2) Maternal immunity is transferred to the fetus across the placenta.

    e. Storage: placenta stores carbohydrates, proteins, calcium, and iron.

    f. Hormonal production

      (1) The placenta secretes and synthesizes hormones necessary for the maintenance of the pregnancy and for fetal development.

      (2) These hormones are the steroid hormones, estrogen and progesterone; the protein hormones, human chorionic gonadotropin, and human chorionic somatomammotropin (also known as human placental lactogen); and thyrotropin.

5. At 9 to 12 weeks

    a. By 12 weeks, the fetus is 8 cm (3 in) in length and weighs about 45 g (1.6 oz).

    b. Brain and neurologic system

      (1) Divisions of the brain begin to develop.

      (2) The head is large and constitutes almost half of the fetus's size.

      (3) The neck is distinct from the head and body.

      (4) Neurons appear at the caudal end of the spinal cord.

      (5) By the 12th week, spontaneous movements of the fetus occur; lip movements indicate the development of the sucking reflex.

    c. Heart and circulatory system

      (1) Red blood cells are produced in the liver by the ninth week.

      (2) By the 12th week, the spleen begins to produce red blood cells.

    d. Gastrointestinal system
      (1) The buccopharyngeal and anal membranes open (the intestinal system from mouth to anus is patent).
      (2) Intestinal loops are visible in the proximal end of the umbilical cord and re-enter the abdomen during the 11th week.
      (3) By the 12th week, the face is well formed and broad.
        (a) The nose begins to protrude.
        (b) The chin is small and receding.
        (c) Tooth buds appear.
        (d) The palate is complete.
      (4) Bile secretions begin.
    e. Genitourinary system
      (1) The kidneys begin to produce urine (amniotic fluid volume increases).
      (2) Well-differentiated genitals appear.
      (3) Urogenital tract is developed.
    f. Skeletal and muscular systems
      (1) The limbs are long and slender.
      (2) The digits are well formed, and the fetus can curl the fingers and make a tiny fist.
      (3) The legs are still shorter and less developed than the arms.
      (4) Primary ossification centers appear, and ossification begins in the skull and long bones.
      (5) Involuntary muscles in the viscera begin to appear.
    g. Eyes and ears
      (1) Eyes are widely spaced and fused.
      (2) Ears are set low and beginning to acquire an adult shape.
    h. Endocrine and immunologic systems
      (1) The thyroid begins to secrete hormones.
      (2) Lymphoid tissue develops in the fetal thymus.
    i. Malformations that can occur during this period:
      (1) Cleft palate
      (2) Malrotation of the gut
      (3) Omphalocele
      (4) Meckel's diverticulum
6. Between 13 and 16 weeks, there is a period of rapid growth.
    a. At 13 weeks, the fetus is about 9 cm (3.6 in) in length and weighs between 55 and 60 g (2 oz).
    b. Brain and neurologic system
      (1) Fetal movements are present.
      (2) Thumb sucking can be detected by ultrasonography.
    c. Respiratory system
      (1) Bronchial tubes are branching out in the primitive lungs.
      (2) Lungs are fully shaped.
    d. Gastrointestinal system
      (1) Hard and soft palates are developed.
      (2) Fetus begins to swallow amniotic fluid.
      (3) Fetus is able to produce meconium in the intestinal tract.
      (4) Liver and pancreas begin to produce secretions.
      (5) Gastric and intestinal glands begin to form.
    e. Genitourinary system
      (1) The ovaries have differentiated.
      (2) Primordial follicles containing primitive oocytes and ova (oogonia) are visible.

        (3) External genitalia are formed.

        (4) Kidneys assume the normal shape.

   f. Skeletal and muscular systems

        (1) More muscle tissue develops.

        (2) Ossification of the skeleton occurs.

        (3) By the 16th week, skeletal structure is identifiable.

        (4) Lower limbs are longer than the upper limbs.

        (5) Hard tissue in the jaw begins to form.

   g. Eyes, ears, skin, and hair

        (1) Downy lanugo hair begins to develop.

        (2) Fetal skin is transparent and the blood vessels are visible.

        (3) Eyes move to the front of the face.

        (4) Ears migrate upward and are fully formed.

7. At 17 to 20 weeks

   a. At 20 weeks, the fetus measures 19 cm (8 in) and weighs between 435 and 465 g (1 lb, 0.5 oz).

   b. Myelination of the spinal cord begins.

   c. Heart tones are audible with a fetoscope.

   d. Respiratory system

        (1) Lung development continues.

        (2) Gas exchange does not occur at this stage, although primitive respiratory-type movements begin.

        (3) Bronchial branching is complete, and pulmonary capillary beds are forming.

        (4) Terminal sacs (alveoli) are developing.

   e. Gastrointestinal system

        (1) Fetus is able to suck and swallow amniotic fluid.

        (2) Peristaltic movements begin.

   f. Skin and hair

        (1) Subcutaneous deposits of brown fat make the skin less transparent.

        (2) Nipples begin to develop over the mammary glands.

        (3) The head has wool-like hair; the eyebrows and eyelashes form.

        (4) Nails are present on both fingers and toes.

        (5) Muscles develop and fetal movements are felt by the mother.

        (6) The sebaceous glands become active and produce a greasy substance called vernix caseosa, which covers and protects the fetus from the effects of the amniotic fluid by preventing the skin from becoming chapped and hardened.

   g. Endocrine and immunologic systems

        (1) Detectable levels of fetal antibodies are present.

        (2) The fetus stores iron, and the bone marrow begins to function.

8. At 21 to 24 weeks

   a. At 24 weeks, the fetus is 28 cm (11.2 in) long and weighs approximately 780 g (1 lb, 10 oz).

   b. Brain and neurologic system

        (1) The fetus has a reflex hand grip.

        (2) By the sixth month, the fetus will exhibit a startle reflex.

        (3) The brain structure is mature.

c. Heart and circulatory system
   (1) The fetal heartbeat is audible through a stethoscope.
   (2) The blood in the capillaries is visible.
d. Respiratory system
   (1) The alveoli of the lungs are beginning to form.
   (2) Secretory epithelial cells in the interalveolar walls begin to secrete surfactant.
      (a) Surfactant facilitates expansion of the alveoli, but not in a quantity sufficient to prevent respiratory distress syndrome (RDS).
      (b) A fetus born at this stage might survive.
   (3) Lecithin can be detected in the amniotic fluid.
   (4) Respiratory movements might occur, and gas exchange is possible.
   (5) The nostrils reopen.
e. Genitourinary system: the testes descend to the inguinal ring.
f. Skeletal and muscular systems: the muscles are developed and the fetus is more active.
g. Eyes, ears, skin, and hair
   (1) The eyes are fully developed and will open.
   (2) The hair is growing longer.
   (3) Eyebrows and eyelashes have formed.
   (4) The ears are flat and shapeless, but the fetus can hear.
   (5) The skin is red and wrinkled, with little subcutaneous fat.
   (6) Skin ridges on the palms and soles of the feet are forming.
   (7) The skin is less transparent because of deposits of brown fat.
   (8) Vernix caseosa covers the entire body.
   (9) Fingernails are well developed.
h. Endocrine and immunologic systems: immunoglobulin G (IgG) levels in the fetus reach maternal levels.

9. At 25 to 29 weeks
   a. The fetus is now between 35 and 38 cm (14 to 15 in) in length and weighs about 1200 g (2 lb, 10.5 oz).
   b. Brain and neurologic system
      (1) The brain continues to mature and grow in size.
      (2) The nervous system is complete enough to provide some regulation of the body functions and body temperature.
   c. Heart and circulatory system: erythropoiesis ends in the spleen and begins in the bone marrow.
   d. Respiratory system
      (1) Respiratory system is developed enough to provide gaseous exchange.
      (2) Lungs are capable of breathing air, but the fetus will need intensive care to survive.
      (3) Surfactant forms on the alveolar surfaces.
   e. Genitourinary system
      (1) In the male, the testes descend into the scrotal sac.
      (2) In the female, the clitoris is prominent, and the labia majora are small and do not cover the labia minora.
   f. Skin and hair
      (1) Adipose tissue begins to accumulate.
      (2) Eyebrows and eyelashes develop.

10. At 30 to 34 weeks
    a. The fetus is gaining weight from an increase in muscle and fat.
    b. The fetus will grow from about 1200 g (2 lb, 10.5 oz) and a length of about 38 cm (14-15 in) to 2000 g (4 lb, 6.5 oz) and a length of 40 cm (16 in).
    c. Brain and neurologic system
        (1) The central nervous system has matured enough to direct breathing movements and partially control body temperature.
        (2) Reflexes are present.
    d. Respiratory system
        (1) The lungs are not fully developed, but the fetus can survive if born at this stage.
        (2) The lecithin/sphingomyelin (L/S) ratio is approximately 1.2:1 at 30 weeks increasing to greater than 2:1 by 38 weeks.
    e. Genitourinary system
        (1) The testes descend into the scrotum; scrotum is small and rugae are present anteriorly.
        (2) Clitoris is covered and labia majora increase in size.
    f. Skeletal and muscular systems: distal femoral ossification centers develop.
    g. Eyes, ears, skin, and hair
        (1) Pinna is still folded and soft.
        (2) Skin is less wrinkled, and the fetus is more filled out.
        (3) Fingernails extend to the ends of the finger tips.
11. At 35 to 38 weeks
    a. The fetus is 46 cm (17.5 in) in length and weighs 2600 g (6 lb).
    b. A fetus born at this time has a fairly good chance of surviving.
    c. Respiratory system: the L/S ratio is greater than 2:1 by 38 weeks.
    d. Genitourinary system
        (1) Scrotum is small, and rugae are present anteriorly.
        (2) Clitoris is covered, and labia majora increase in size.
    e. Skeletal and muscular systems: distal femoral ossification centers develop.
    f. Eyes, ears, skin, and hair
        (1) The body and extremities are filling out.
        (2) The fetus is less wrinkled.
        (3) Lanugo is disappearing.
        (4) The fetus has a firm grasp and begins to orient to light.
12. At 39 to 40 weeks, the fetus is considered full-term.
    a. The fetus is approximately 50 cm (20 in) in length and weighs between 3000 and 3600 g (6 lb, 10 oz and 7 lb, 15 oz).
    b. Genitourinary system
        (1) The testes should be palpable in the inguinal canals.
        (2) The labia majora are well developed.
    c. Ears, skin, and hair
        (1) The skin is smooth and has a polished look.
        (2) Vernix caseosa is present, with the heaviest deposits in the creases and folds of the skin.
        (3) The chest is prominent and slightly smaller than the head.
        (4) The mammary glands protrude in both sexes.
        (5) The fetal body fills most of the uterine cavity, and the amniotic fluid volume diminishes to about 500 ml.
        (6) Lanugo remains on shoulders and upper back only.
        (7) Ear lobes become firm as the cartilage thickens.

     d. Malformations that might occur during this period

       (1) Patent ductus arteriosus

       (2) Cryptorchidism (failure of the testes to descend into the scrotum)

13. Postterm (42 weeks and beyond).

     a. Fetuses might gain weight, thus increasing the difficulty of labor or might lose weight because parts of the placenta fail to function.

     b. Fetus might pass meconium due to hypoxia from placental insufficiency.

     c. Nails and hair continue to grow.

14. Congenital malformations

     a. Approximately 3% to 4% of all live-born infants have obvious malformations.

     b. Genetic factors are involved in more than 33% of all congenital malformations.

     c. Environmental factors cause approximately 7% of malformations.

       (1) Organs and parts of the embryo affected will be determined by the time of ingestion or exposure to teratogens (an environmental agent that causes malformations) (Figure 3-13). (See Chapter 9 for a complete discussion of environmental hazards.)

       (2) The organs and fetal system are most sensitive to teratogens during periods of rapid growth in the first trimester.

F. Placental abnormalities

1. Extrachorial placentas: situation in which the membrane is 1 cm or more central to the chorionic plate

     a. Causes

       (1) Might be the result of lateral placental growth or implantation that was too deep, causing an undermining of the membranes.

       (2) Hemorrhage and separation with resealing

     b. Are common in the placentas of extramembranous pregnancies.

       (1) Associated rare occurrence: amniotic fluid might leak throughout the pregnancy because of rupture of the membranes.

       (2) The ruptured membrane might retract to such an extent that the pregnancy is extramembranous and the fetus is no longer contained within the amniotic sac.

       (3) The newborn can have pulmonary hypoplasia because of a lack of amniotic fluid and a resultant inability to inspire in utero.

     c. Possibly exists in 20% of placentas.

       (1) Are more common in multigravid pregnancies.

       (2) Familial occurrence has been noted.

       (3) Are not related to maternal age.

     d. Are usually of no major fetal consequence but, if severe, can cause:

       (1) Prematurity

       (2) Hemorrhage

       (3) Fetal growth retardation

2. Amniotic bands (Table 3-2)

     a. Believed to arise from ruptures in the amnion, resulting in floating strands and cords of the amnion.

     b. Etiology is unknown, but ruptures usually occur near the cord insertion site.

       (1) Inflammation and trauma are possible causes.

       (2) Amnionic bands have occurred in some pregnancies after amniocentesis has been performed.

       (3) Oligohydramnios might be present.

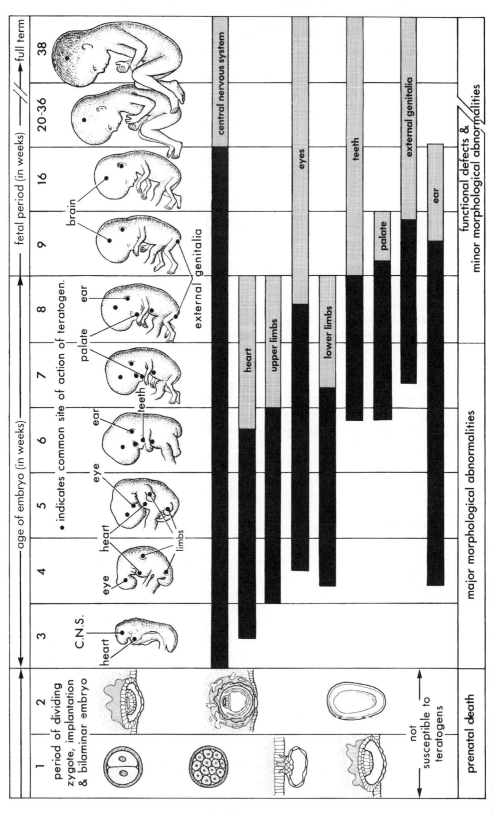

FIGURE 3-13 ■ Schematic illustration of the critical periods in human development. (From Moore, K.L. [1988]. *The developing human: Clinically oriented embryology* [4th ed.; p. 143]. Philadelphia: W.B. Saunders.)

■ TABLE 3-2
■ ■ **Abnormalities Resulting from Amnionic Bands**

Fetal Age	Abnormality Most Likely Seen
3 weeks	Anencephaly
	Facial distortions
	Facial clefting
	Encephaloceles
5 weeks	Cleft lip
	Choanal atresia
	Limb reduction
	Syndactyly
	Abdominal wall defects
	Thoracic wall defects
	Scoliosis
7 weeks and after	Ear deformities
	Amputations
	Distal lymphedema
	Foot deformities
	Omphaloceles

Adapted from Smith, D.W. (1982). *Recognizable patterns of human malformation: Genetic, embryologic, and clinical aspects* (3rd ed.). Philadelphia: W.B. Saunders.

   c. The floating amnionic strands are sticky and can adhere to the fetus.
      (1) The bands might restrict embryonic development; facial defects, such as clefts and encephaloceles, and thoracic and abdominal defects, such as gastroschisis, can result.
      (2) If the bands constrict the extremities, amputation and constriction bands on limbs and digits can result.
G. Cord
   1. Description: the cord is the connecting link between the fetus and the placenta; it usually contains one large vein and two smaller arteries.
   2. Development
      a. Formed from the union of the amnion, yolk, and connecting stalk
      b. First trimester
         (1) The body stalk, which attaches the embryo to the yolk sac, contains blood vessels that extend into the chorionic villi.
         (2) The body sac fuses with the embryonic portion of the placenta to provide a circulatory pathway from the chorionic villi to the embryo.
         (3) The body stalk elongates and becomes the umbilical cord.
            (a) The vessels of the cord decrease to one large vein and two smaller arteries.
               (i) The umbilical vein contains placental oxygenated blood that returns to the fetus.
               (ii) The arteries carry unoxygenated blood to the placenta.
            (b) Approximately 1% of umbilical cords have only two vessels—an artery and a vein; this condition is frequently associated with congenital malformations.
               (i) Sirenomelia, in which the lower limbs are fused, giving the infant a "mermaid" appearance

(ii) VATERS syndrome, which can comprise any or all of the following.
- Vertebral and ventricular septal defects
- Anal atresia
- Tracheoesophageal fistula
- Esophageal atresia
- Radial and renal dysplasia
- Single umbilical artery

(iii) Trisomies 13 and 18

(c) The cord has no nerves.

(4) Specialized gelatinous connective tissue, called Wharton jelly, surrounds the blood vessels and prevents compression of the cord.

(5) At term, the average cord is about 55 cm (22 in) long.
  (a) A cord shorter than 32 cm (13 in) might indicate problems with the fetus.
    (i) There can be renal agenesis.
    (ii) A short cord is often associated with pulmonary hypoplasia.
    (iii) May predispose to abruptio placentae or cord rupture.
  (b) An unusually long cord is associated with cord prolapse and fetal entrapment.

(6) The cord can attach itself to the placenta at various sites, but central insertion into the placenta is considered normal; abnormalities include:
  (a) Velamentous insertion, in which the cord is implanted at the edge of the placenta, and fetal vessels separate in the membranes before reaching the placenta.
    (i) Increased incidence of structural defects in the fetus occurs.
- Congenital hip dislocation
- Asymmetric head shape

    (ii) Can increase risk for intrauterine growth restriction and preterm birth.
  (b) Vasa praevia is associated with velamentous insertion of the cord, in which the vessels lie over the internal cervical os in front of the fetus.
    (i) The vessels might be compressed, compromising oxygen exchange in the fetus.
    (ii) If the vessels rupture, the fetus might experience severe blood loss, which can occur when membranes rupture.
  (c) Marginal insertion (battledore)
    (i) Occurs in 2% to 15% of gestations.
    (ii) Is associated with a higher-than-normal frequency of preterm labor and birth

(7) The cord can appear twisted or spiraled.
  (a) This is most likely caused by fetal movement.
  (b) A true knot in the cord rarely occurs; when there is a true knot in the cord, the cord is usually longer than normal, allowing the fetus to pass through a loop in the cord.
  (c) So-called false knots are more common.
    (i) False knots are caused by the folding of the cord vessel.
    (ii) False knots are not usually a problem for the developing fetus.

(8) When the umbilical cord is around the neck of the fetus, it is called a nuchal cord.

H. Amniotic fluid: the pale, straw-colored fluid in which the fetus floats.
   1. Development
      a. Early pregnancy
         (1) Shortly after fertilization, a cleft forms in the morula.
         (2) As the cleft enlarges, it becomes fused with the surrounding amnion, creating the amniotic sac.
         (3) The sac then fills with colorless fluid, which increases in volume to 50 ml at 12 weeks' gestation.
         (4) The fluid is produced by the amnionic membrane.
      b. Second trimester to delivery (Figure 3-14)
         (1) Fetus modifies amniotic fluid through the processes of swallowing and urinating.
         (2) The volume can also be modified through movement of fluid through the fetal respiratory tract.
   2. Volume
      a. There is a wide range of amniotic fluid volume during pregnancy.
      b. Normal approximations of volume.
         (1) At 12 weeks, there is approximately 50 ml.
         (2) At 20 weeks, there is approximately 400 ml.
         (3) At 36 to 38 weeks, there is approximately 1 L.
         (4) Volume decreases after 38 weeks.
   3. Function
      a. Provides a medium for fetal movement.
      b. Protects the fetus against injury from external causes.
      c. Assists in maintaining temperature.
      d. Provides nourishment to fetus.
      e. Might be an important factor in dilating the cervical canal.
      f. Prevents the amnion from adhering to the developing fetus.
   4. Composition
      a. Consists of approximately 98% water.
      b. Is alkaline in reaction (pH is 7.0 to 7.25).
      c. Early pregnancy
         (1) Is similar in composition to maternal plasma.

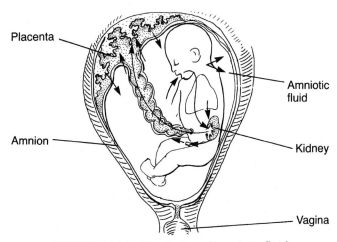

FIGURE 3-14 ■ Circulation of amniotic fluid.

(2) Contains a lower protein concentration than maternal plasma.

(3) Is nearly devoid of particulate matter.

d. Second trimester to delivery (see Figure 3-14).

(1) As pregnancy progresses, phospholipids (from the lung) accumulate.

(2) Variable amounts of particulate matter occur from the shedding of fetal cells, lanugo, scalp hair, and vernix caseosa into the fluid.

(3) Osmolality decreases.

(4) Fluid becomes hypotonic as a result of fetal urination.

(5) Fluid contains higher levels of urea, creatinine, and uric acid than the plasma.

5. Abnormalities in volume

a. Oligohydramnios (decreased amounts of amniotic fluid).

(1) Less than 500 ml; between 32 and 36 weeks

(2) Common causes

(a) Amniotic leakage

(b) Abnormalities of the fetal kidneys (e.g., renal agenesis)

(3) Primary oligohydramnios associated with fetal abnormalities

(a) Renal agenesis

(b) Polycystic kidneys

(c) Urinary tract obstructions

(4) Oligohydramnios that occurs during or before the second trimester; usually associated with a poor pregnancy outcome

(a) Compression of the fetus

(b) Fetal death due to respiratory insufficiency and a lack of lung development

b. Hydramnios (increased amounts of amniotic fluid)

(1) Exceeds 2 L of fluid between 32 and 36 weeks.

(2) Is often associated with poor fetal outcomes because of tendency toward:

(a) Preterm delivery

(b) Fetal malpresentation

(c) Cord prolapse

(3) Hydramnios that occurs during or before second trimester spontaneously resolves in 45% of the cases, resulting in normal outcomes.

(4) Pathogenesis is usually unclear.

(a) Is possibly caused by defective regulation of fluid transfer across the amniochorion

(b) Occurs more frequently with Rh-sensitized pregnancies, monozygotic multiple pregnancy, and gestational or insulin-dependent diabetes mellitus

(c) Occurs frequently with fetal gastrointestinal obstructions or atresias

CLINICAL PRACTICE

A. Assessment

1. History

a. Ascertain the date of day 1 of the last menstrual period to monitor fetal development.

b. It is important to ascertain the dates of maternal immunizations for rubella, rubeola, and mumps.

      c. Knowledge of any infections during pregnancy is important because viruses are known to cross the placental barrier and the timing of viral infections might determine the type and extent of fetal injury.

      d. A thorough family history is needed to detect potential inheritable diseases.

      e. A complete medical history can identify maternal high-risk conditions, such as diabetes mellitus, that might adversely affect fetal development.

      f. A comprehensive assessment of drug intake should include prescription, over-the-counter, and illicit drugs, alcohol, and nicotine; teratogenic effects of chemical substances will be determined by the stage of fetal development at the time of drug consumption.

      g. Previous pregnancies and outcomes

      h. Known uterine infections

      i. Episodes of bleeding, hypertension, and trauma

  2. Physical findings.

      a. Excessive weight gain or lack of weight gain during pregnancy

      b. Delayed or accelerated uterine growth related to gestational age might indicate problems with fetal development.

      c. Physical signs of placental risk

        (1) Bleeding

        (2) Sudden and severe abdominal pain

        (3) Uterine rigidity

        (4) Fundal height not appropriate for gestational age

  3. Diagnostic procedures

      a. Monitoring of uterine growth by measuring fundal heights

      b. Ultrasonography

        (1) Monitors fetal growth and development.

        (2) Can identify major congenital malformations such as hydrocephalus, renal agenesis, and anencephaly.

        (3) Location of the placenta

        (4) Placental grading

        (5) Amniotic volume

      c. Maternal serum alpha-fetoprotein (msAFP).

        (1) Lower-than-normal results might indicate a chromosomal abnormality such as trisomy 21 (Down syndrome).

        (2) Elevated maternal AFP level might indicate a neural tube defect but is also normally associated with multiple pregnancy.

      d. Amniocentesis is the withdrawal of fluid from the amniotic cavity.

        (1) Identifies chromosomal abnormalities.

        (2) Assesses the fluid for AFP levels to rule out open-neural tube defects.

      e. Chorionic villi sampling is performed for chromosome analysis and selected metabolic tests on the fetus (see Chapter 8 for a complete discussion of antenatal testing).

      f. Kleihauer-Betke test is used to determine if vaginal bleeding is of maternal or fetal origin.

B. Nursing Diagnoses

  1. Risk for congenital malformation related to exposure to teratogens

  2. Risk for delayed growth and development related to inadequate maternal nutrition

   3. Risk for altered development related to genetic disorder
   4. Risk for deficient or excess fluid volume related to impaired placental transport
   5. Risk for altered fetal growth related to impaired placental transport of nutrients
   6. Risk for impaired fetal gas exchange related to impaired placental transport

C. **Interventions/Outcomes**
   1. Risk for congenital malformation related to exposure to teratogens
      a. Interventions
         (1) Assess for exposure to infection, chemicals, or environmental factors.
         (2) Identify the stage of fetal development at which exposure occurred.
         (3) Provide parents with the information they need to understand risks and make appropriate medical and health decisions about the pregnancy.
         (4) Refer parents to appropriate resources to assess the effects of exposure (e.g., to a genetic center or tertiary high-risk obstetric services).
         (5) Maintain an accepting and supportive approach toward the parents.
         (6) Listen to their fears and concerns, and provide health information that is appropriate to their level of understanding.
      b. Outcomes
         (1) Parents are able to express an understanding of the risks from exposure.
         (2) Parents have obtained appropriate services from referral agencies.
         (3) Parents have made an appropriate decision regarding the outcome of the pregnancy that is based on their values and needs.
   2. Risk for delayed growth and development related to inadequate maternal nutrition
      a. Interventions
         (1) Assess maternal nutritional intake to identify deficiencies.
         (2) Assess maternal understanding of nutritional needs for fetal development.
         (3) Educate the mother about healthy nutritional intake.
         (4) Provide supplements for nutritional deficiencies, as indicated.
            (a) Supplement the mother's diet with vitamins and iron.
            (b) Refer the parents to a nutritionist for further counseling or to Women, Infants, and Children (WIC) nutritional supplement program, if eligible .
      b. Outcomes
         (1) Maternal nutritional intake improves.
         (2) Fetus continues to grow.
         (3) Mother obtains services from referral sources.
   3. Risk for altered development related to genetic disorder
      a. Interventions
         (1) Assess parents for a genetic history.
         (2) Interpret risks, as indicated.

      (3) Refer the parents for genetic counseling, as indicated.

      (4) Provide appropriate information to assist the couple in making decisions about the outcome of pregnancy.

      (5) Maintain a nonjudgmental attitude toward the couple, and allow the couple to discuss fears and concerns.

   b. Outcomes

      (1) Parents have made an appropriate decision about the outcome of the pregnancy, based on their values and needs.

      (2) Parents have obtained the necessary services from referral sources.

4. Risk for deficient or excess fluid volume related to impaired placental transport

   a. Interventions

      (1) Explain diagnostic tests (ultrasonography and amniocentesis) to the pregnant woman and her family.

      (2) Remain with the pregnant woman during procedure, if possible.

      (3) Clarify misconceptions and allow the pregnant woman and her family to discuss fears and concerns.

      (4) Ensure that the pregnant woman and her family understand the test results and the test's implications.

   b. Outcomes

      (1) The pregnant woman and her family can explain the reason for the diagnostic procedure.

      (2) The pregnant woman reports an understanding of test results.

      (3) The pregnant woman and her family report decreased fear and anxiety.

5. Risk for altered fetal growth related to impaired placental transport of nutrients

   a. Interventions

      (1) Explain the importance of adequate nutritional intake.

      (2) Discuss the possible consequences of poor nutritional intake.

      (3) Evaluate maternal nutritional intake.

   b. Outcomes

      (1) The pregnant woman complies with proposed nutritional program.

      (2) The pregnant woman can explain the possible negative consequences to the fetus resulting from poor maternal nutritional intake.

6. Risk for impaired fetal gas exchange related to impaired placental transport

   a. Interventions

      (1) Explain the possible outcome of poor fetal gas exchange.

      (2) Explain the importance of compliance with the testing regimen.

      (3) Reinforce the need for lateral position to improve uteroplacental circulation when the client is recumbent.

   b. Outcomes

      (1) The pregnant woman can explain the possible outcome to fetus of poor gas exchange.

      (2) The pregnant woman agrees to comply with recommended antepartal testing.

      (3) The pregnant woman agrees to lie in the lateral position when recumbent during the remainder of the pregnancy.

HEALTH EDUCATION

A. **Nutritional needs for adequate fetal development**
   1. Calories: 2300 to 2400 per day.
   2. Protein: 74 to 76 g/day.
   3. Carbohydrates: increased requirement to allow for protein uptake for fetal development.
   4. Fat: provides energy, and fat deposits increase in the fetus from 2% at midpregnancy to 12% at term.
   5. Vitamins and minerals: a slight increase in intake is needed to provide for the growth of new tissue in the fetus.
B. **Effects of chemical use (smoking, alcohol, and drugs) on the fetus**
   1. Timing of ingestion and amount of chemical consumed
   2. Effect on fetus (teratogenic)
      a. Intrauterine growth restriction
      b. Premature birth
      c. Congenital malformations, determined by the effects on developing systems
      d. Newborn withdrawal
   3. Importance of eliminating chemical use during pregnancy
C. **Reasons for and the procedures used in ultrasonography and amniocentesis**
D. **Importance of prenatal visits for assessing fetal well-being**
E. **Importance of relating any unusual symptoms to health care provider**
F. **Implications of any symptoms**
G. **Review of the stages of fetal development and the role of the placenta and amniotic fluid**

STUDY QUESTIONS

1. The most critical stage of physical development for the unborn child occurs:
   a. During the pre-embryonic stage
   b. From the 3rd to the 8th week of development
   c. From the 9th to the 20th week of development
   d. From the 20th week to delivery

2. The major function of vernix caseosa is to:
   a. Protect fetal skin from the amniotic fluid.
   b. Prevent adhesions to the amniotic sac.
   c. Enhance the nutrient balance of the amniotic fluid.
   d. Prevent the excessive shedding of fetal tissue.

3. During which weeks of development is the fetus first able to provide some regulation of its own body functions and body temperature?
   a. At 17 to 20 weeks
   b. At 21 to 24 weeks
   c. At 25 to 29 weeks
   d. At 30 to 34 weeks

4. The main function of the placenta is to:
   a. Provide a nutrient exchange between maternal and fetal circulations.
   b. Ensure that the fetus is protected from trauma.
   c. Provide a mechanism for the direct exchange of oxygen and carbon dioxide.
   d. Allow for the elimination of excess fetal hormones.

5. Which of the following statements best describes placental development?
   a. It develops rapidly, with limited changes after the first month.
   b. It continues to develop and grow throughout pregnancy.
   c. Major growth and development occur in the first trimester.
   d. There are two major stages of development; these are in the first and third trimesters.

6. What is the major reason for monitoring placental growth and function?
   a. To predict fetal positioning at time of birth.
   b. To evaluate fetal well-being.
   c. To predict gestational age at delivery.
   d. To indicate risk factors for chromosomal abnormalities.

7. Which of the following are the major functions of amniotic fluid?
   a. Provides respiratory and nutritional exchange between fetal and maternal circulation.
   b. Is a major component of fetal blood circulation and hormone production.
   c. Protects the fetus from injury by cushioning it from trauma, and maintains a constant temperature.
   d. Is an important component in monitoring and altering fetal biochemical status.

ANSWERS TO STUDY QUESTIONS

1. b   5. c
2. a   6. b
3. c   7. c
4. a

REFERENCES

Buster, J.E., & Carson, S.A. (2002). Endocrinology and diagnosis of pregnancy. In S.G. Gabbe, J.R. Niebyl, & J.L. Simpson, (Eds.), *Obstetrics: Normal and problem pregnancies* (4th ed.; pp. 3-25). London: Churchill Livingstone.

Collins-Nakai, R., & McLaughlin, P. (2002). How congenital heart disease originates in fetal life. *Cardiology Clinics, 20*(3), 367–383.

Craven, C., & Ward, K. (1999). Embryology, fetus, and placenta. In J.R. Scott, P.J. Di Saia, C.B. Hammond, & W.N. Spellacy (Eds.), *Danforth's obstetrics and gynecology* (8th ed.; pp. 29-46). Philadelphia: Lippincott, Williams & Wilkins.

Hirschi, K.K., & Keen, C.L. (2000). Nutrition in embryologic fetal development. *Nutrition, 16*(7-8), 495-499.

Moore, K.L., & Persaud, T.V. (1998). *Before we are born: Essentials of human embryology and birth defects* (5th ed.). Philadelphia: W.B. Saunders.

Opitz, I.M., & Clark, E.B. (2000). Heart development: An introduction. *American Journal of Medical Genetics, 97*(4), 238-247.

Pahal, G.S., Jauniaux, E., & Kinnon, C. (2000). Normal development of human fetal hematopoiesis between 8th and 17th week gestation. *American Journal of Obstetrics and Gynecology, 183*(4), 1029-1034.

Ross, M.G., Ervin, M.G., & Novak, D. (2002). Placental and fetal physiology. In S.G. Gabbe, J.R. Niebyl, & J.L. Simpson (Eds.). *Obstetrics: Normal and problem pregnancies.* (4th ed.; pp. 37-54). London: Churchill Livingstone.

Schmidt, J.V., & McCartney, P.R. (2000). History and development of fetal heart assessment: a composite. *Journal of Obstetric, Gynecologic, and Neonatal Nursing, 29*(3), 295-305.

Utiger, R.D. (1999). Maternal hypothyroid and fetal development. *New England Journal of Medicine, 341*(8), 601-602.

NORMAL PREGNANCY

4 Ethnocultural Considerations in the Childbearing Period

SUSAN MATTSON

OBJECTIVES

1. State the need for a cultural assessment of the childbearing family.
2. Describe data to be collected through a cultural assessment.
3. Perform a cultural assessment of a childbearing family.
4. Use data obtained to formulate a care plan for the childbearing family.
5. Analyze data obtained from a cultural assessment for potential problem areas.
6. Formulate nursing interventions to prevent anticipated problems identified from the assessment.
7. Identify barriers to care that are frequently encountered by the culturally diverse client.
8. Identify ways to decrease barriers to care encountered by the culturally diverse client.

INTRODUCTION

A. **Transcultural nursing is concerned with the provision of nursing care in a manner that is sensitive to the needs of individuals, families, and groups.**
   1. A major aim of transcultural nursing is to understand and assist members of diverse cultural groups with their nursing and health care needs.
   2. Nursing interventions that are culturally relevant to the needs of the client decrease the possibility of conflict or misunderstanding arising from people from different backgrounds (Andrews, 1995).
   3. The goal of transcultural nursing is "to develop a scientific and humanistic body of knowledge to provide culture-specific and culture-universal nursing care practices" (Andrews, 2003, p. 4).
      a. Culture-specific refers to particular values, beliefs, and patterns of behavior that tend to be special or unique to a group and that do not tend to be shared with members of other cultures.
      b. Culture-universal refers to the commonly shared values, norms of behavior, and life patterns that are similarly held among cultures about human behavior and lifestyles (Leininger & McFarland, 2002).
   4. Applying transcultural concepts to nursing practice includes:
      a. Identifying cultural needs
      b. Understanding the cultural context of the client and family
      c. Using culturally sensitive strategies to meet mutually satisfying goals

5. A common problem faced by nurses who want to use cultural data is knowing what data to collect and how to use the data effectively.
   a. A major purpose of collecting cultural data is to give the nurse greater insight into and understanding of:
      (1) The nature and behavior of clients
      (2) The problems that clients encounter in health promotion and maintenance
      (3) Clients' ways of coping with illness
   b. These data should be relevant to potential or actual nursing problems.
   c. Transcultural knowledge is used to augment, clarify, explain, or assist in attaining client-centered goals.
B. **The overall goal is to develop and sustain cultural (and linguistic) competence among health care professionals.**
   1. The concept refers to a complex integration of knowledge, attitudes, and skills that enhance cross-cultural communication and appropriate/effective interactions with others (American Academy of Nursing, 1992, 1993).
   2. Cultural competence has been defined as a process, as opposed to an end point, in which the nurse continuously strives to work effectively within the cultural context of individuals, families, or communities from diverse cultural backgrounds (Andrews & Boyle, 1997; Meleis, 1999; Purnell & Paulanka, 2003; Wells, 2000).
   3. Cultural and linguistic competence have been defined and issued as standards from the Office of Minority Health at the U.S. Department of Health & Human Services (1999) as the ability of health care providers and organizations to understand and effectively respond to the cultural and linguistic needs brought by the clients to the health care encounter.
C. **Childbearing is a time of transition and social celebration of great importance in any society (Lauderdale, 2003).**
   1. Many cultures have particular customs and beliefs that dictate activities and behavior during this time.
      a. Some might be considered *prescriptive* in nature: phrased positively, and describing expectations of behavior.
         (1) Might involve wearing special articles of clothing
         (2) Might involve ceremonies
         (3) Might be recommendations for physical activity and/or diet
      b. Others are *restrictive:* phrased negatively, and limiting choices or behaviors; usually directed toward:
         (1) Activity—physical and sexual
         (2) Work and environment
         (3) Emotions
      c. A third area of beliefs is the *taboo*—restrictions with serious supernatural consequences.
         (1) Often involve exposure to moon and sun at certain times of the day
         (2) Might refer to witchcraft as a mechanism, or avoidance of some types of people (widows, people in mourning)
         (3) Often refer to food choices (Lauderdale, 2003)
   2. The labor and delivery and postpartum periods might also be governed by unique customs
      a. Cultural factors influencing labor and delivery center on a general attitude toward:
         (1) Birth
         (2) Methods of dealing with the pain of labor

(3) Preferred positions during delivery

(4) The role of support persons and health practitioners

   b. Many cultures consider the postpartum period to be one of increased vulnerability for both mother and infant.

     (1) Dietary and activity prescriptions are common at this time and might be in conflict with the usual Western methods of obstetric care.

     (2) Infant care also varies from culture to culture in regard to:

       (a) Bathing

       (b) Swaddling

       (c) Feeding

       (d) Care of the umbilical cord

       (e) Circumcision

D. The different ways in which a particular society views this transitional period and manages childbirth depend on the culture's beliefs about health, medical care, reproduction, and the role and status of women (Figure 4-1).

   1. Pregnancy and childbirth practices in Western society have changed dramatically during the past two decades. A few of the trends that

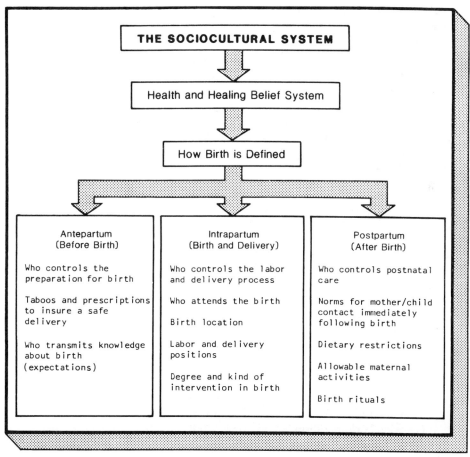

FIGURE 4-1 ■ Components of the childbearing system. A culturally diverse woman, familiar with her own ethnic group's childbearing system, might feel estranged by the dominant culture's birth practices. (From Mattson, S., Galanti, G., Lettieri, C., & Kellogg, J. [1986]. *Culture and health module 2: The family and life cycle in transcultural perspective* [p. 60]. Long Beach, CA: Statewide Nursing Program, Consortium of the California State University.)

require nurses to examine and rethink how we can better care for our clients include:

  a. An increase in the number of women in the workforce
  b. Advances in reproductive technology
  c. Self-care
  d. Alternative therapies
  e. Increase in health information available to consumers on the Internet
  f. The large influx of refugees and immigrants (Tiedje, 2000)

2. Subcultures within the United States and Canada have very different practices, values, and beliefs about childbirth and the roles of men, women, social support networks, and health care practitioners.

3. Additionally, religious background, regional variations, age, urban or rural background, sexual preferences, and other individual characteristics all contribute to cultural differences surrounding the childbearing period.

4. Great variations exist in the social class, ethnic origin, family structure, and social support networks of women and their families. One must keep in mind the individual differences that are present within cultures as well as those found between cultures.

5. Culturally competent care for ethnic minority women requires a delicate balance in assumptions that drive the assessment process and the resultant care plans.

  a. One must balance the assumption that those women who immigrated from a similar region share similar values and beliefs that influence how they will respond to the childbirth experience with the assumption of diversity among women from the same area (Meleis, 2003).

  b. Women's experiences that profoundly influence their childbirth experience include all of the individual characteristics described above; therefore the descriptions of the various "populations" in this chapter must be viewed within the context of diversity within each group.

CLINICAL PRACTICE

A. Assessment

  1. Introduction

    a. Cultural assessment is defined as assessment of:
      (1) Shared beliefs
      (2) Values
      (3) Customs that have relevance to health behaviors (Tripp-Reimer & Brink, 1984)

    b. It is performed to identify patterns that might assist or interfere with a nursing intervention or planned treatment regimen.

    c. To understand why birth is managed in a particular way, it is necessary to view the process in terms of the society's:
      (1) Social organization
      (2) Political and economic system
      (3) Medical theory

    d. In addition, Kay (1982) delineated specific cultural data for the four periods during childbearing: antepartum, intrapartum, postpartum, and newborn period. In this chapter, assessment needs during each of these four periods are discussed. (For specific details about particular cultural groups, see the material referenced in appropriate chapters and sections; see also the appendix at the end of this chapter.)

2. History
   a. Antepartum period
      (1) Determinants of the society's acceptance of the pregnancy
         (a) Acceptable age
         (b) Marriage requirements
         (c) Acceptable father
         (d) Pregnancy frequency
      (2) Consideration of pregnancy as a state of illness or of health
      (3) Behavioral expectations
         (a) Dietary prescriptions or restrictions
            (i) Adherence to the hot or cold theory of health and diet (especially with Hispanic and Asian clients)
               ■ This theory describes the intrinsic properties of foods, beverages, medicines, and their effects on the body.
               ■ Health is maintained through a balance of these forces.
               ■ If an imbalance occurs, illness results.
               ■ To produce balance (and restore or maintain health), illness and conditions such as pregnancy are treated with substances having the opposite property of the illness (i.e., pregnancy is considered to be a hot state; thus, any treatments must be of a cold nature).
                  — Temperature and spiciness do not determine classification, however, this varies among cultural groups.
                  — Generally, warm or hot foods are believed to be easier to digest than cold or cool foods.
               ■ These properties of hot and cold are also part of the yin-yang belief system prevalent among Asian approaches to health and diet (Andrews, 1989).
            (ii) Another unfamiliar practice that nurses might encounter is that of pica, or the ingestion of nonfood substances, especially clay or starch.
               ■ Pica is often practiced by black women, usually in the rural southern United States.
               ■ There are many explanations for why this occurs.
                  — A result of an iron deficiency that leads to the craving
                  — A carryover from behaviors practiced in Africa
         (b) Activity restrictions or prescriptions, including the use of massage as a treatment for the various ills experienced during pregnancy
         (c) Expression of emotions, including anger, fear, and anxiety
      (4) People from whom to seek advice, and the appropriate time to do so
         (a) Women from many cultures might refuse to seek early prenatal care because they consider pregnancy a normal and healthy state.
         (b) Fear, modesty, and a wish to avoid a physical examination by a male care provider might also prevent some women from seeking care from Western providers (Andrews, 1989).
   b. Intrapartum period
      (1) Appropriate setting for labor and delivery to occur

(2) Appropriate attendants for support and as a "practitioner"
  (a) Most non-Western cultures see childbearing as being within the woman's domain.
    (i) Support during labor and assistance after delivery are usually provided by women relatives or friends.
    (ii) It is unusual, and should not be expected, for a father from a non-Western culture to provide this support and caretaking.
  (b) Male caregivers might be refused.
(3) Expectations of pain control, including what expressions of discomfort are permitted and expected
(4) Restrictions and prescriptions for activity, including ambulation and massage
(5) Dietary recommendations, including the continuation of intake of food and drink; possible preference for herbal teas
(6) Expected length of labor
  (a) Behaviors that are necessary to ensure the appropriate length, including diet and activity
  (b) Expected interventions if the time is prolonged
(7) Expected and ideal positions for facilitating pushing and delivery
  (a) Squatting
  (b) Sitting
  (c) Side-lying
(8) Appropriate disposition of placenta and umbilical cord after delivery
  (a) Some cultural groups believe that burying the placenta, the umbilical cord, or both in a particular place will bring good fortune to the child and family.
  (b) Others wish to preserve the cord through drying to use it medicinally at a later time.
c. Postpartum period
  (1) Activity restrictions and prescriptions
    (a) The postpartum period is viewed by many as one that is fraught with dangers for both mother and infant.
      (i) One way to protect against danger is for the mother to remain quietly in bed, with little activity to disturb her.
      (ii) This includes a restriction on:
        ■ Ambulating
        ■ Bathing (especially showering)
        ■ Infant caretaking
        ■ Other activities seen as normal from a Western medical perspective
    (b) In some cultures, women are considered to be in a state of impurity during the puerperium, which often coincides with the period of lochial flow. Common behaviors include:
      (i) Seclusion and avoidance of contact with others
      (ii) Avoidance of sexual relations
  (2) Dietary restrictions and prescriptions
    (a) Many of the same requirements that are based on a theory of hot and cold also affect postpartum guides.
    (b) The puerperium is a cold time, so foods should be hot in nature; women will avoid fruits and vegetables that are considered cold.

(3) Appropriateness of therapeutic heat and cold
   (a) Western practitioners often use cold packs or sitz baths for perineal comfort and healing.
   (b) These practices are not acceptable to women from many cultures.
      (i) Cold air and water are frequently believed to be harmful.
      (ii) They are believed to cause uterine problems and even infertility when they enter the uterus through the vagina (Greener, 1989).

d. Newborn period
   (1) Feeding of the infant, including the method and timing of the first feeding
      (a) A society's advocacy of breastfeeding varies, and many influences must be considered.
      (b) Although American women are choosing to breastfeed in increasing numbers, immigrants from developing and poorer countries see bottle-feeding as the modern way to provide nourishment to their infants.
      (c) Several cultural groups, including Hispanic and Arab women, in particular, believe that colostrum is bad for the infant and prefer to bottle-feed until their milk comes in.
   (2) Bathing of the infant, including:
      (a) Time of the first bath
      (b) Appropriate person to perform the bath
      (c) Measures used to protect the infant during the procedure
         (i) Traditional Hispanics believe that both the head and feet should be wet.
         (ii) Water will be placed on the head at the same time that the body is immersed in the bath (Clark, 1978).
   (3) Sleeping arrangement provided for the infant and what is done to promote sleeping
      (a) Women often keep the infant physically as close as possible, often sharing the same bed.
      (b) This is particularly true if ritual seclusion and limited activity are enforced.
   (4) Swaddling practices
   (5) Circumcision
      (a) Cultures vary greatly in their beliefs about this practice.
      (b) Ritual circumcision is frequently practiced in traditional Judaism and among followers of Islam.
   (6) Caretaking of the infant at home
      (a) Appropriate person to do so
      (b) Length of time that the infant is allowed to cry before being attended to
         (i) Some cultures expect that infants will be picked up and attended to (usually breastfed) immediately.
         (ii) Others believe that the infant should be allowed to cry for a certain period.
      (c) Care of the umbilical cord
         (i) Hispanic, Filipino, and black women might use an abdominal binder or "belly band" to protect the umbilical area against dirt, injury, or hernia.

           (ii) These binders are usually not seen by the Western care provider because they are removed before office or clinic visits.

           (iii) Oils might also be applied to the umbilical cord stump (Greener, 1989).

    (7) Ritual beautification varies according to cultural interpretation and might be done to avoid the evil eye. Navajo infants undergo piercing of their ears and insertion of turquoise earrings to provide protection from evil forces (Kay, 1982).

    (8) Attachment behaviors toward the infant

        (a) Asian and Middle Eastern women, in particular, might be erroneously assessed as demonstrating maladaptive attachment behaviors.

        (b) Asian women maintain a distance and do not praise their infants because of a fear of evil influences harming the infant if he or she were seen to be joyfully received.

        (c) Middle Eastern women believe that the mother is the one deserving of praise for her great work in producing the infant (Meleis & Sorrell, 1981).

  3. Physical findings

    a. Differences in pelvic shape and size related to race (see Chapter 10 for further discussion)

    b. Differences in infant size related to ethnic influences (see Chapter 17 for further discussion)

  4. Psychosocial findings

    a. Refusal to accept or use Western medical services

    b. Distress occurs when care is provided without cultural competency; for example, when:

      (1) Modesty is not acknowledged and protected.

      (2) Male caretakers are provided.

      (3) There are inappropriate expectations of participation by the expectant father or husband and restrictions on other family members' presence.

      (4) There are inappropriate expectations of caretaking activities of the client in regard to herself and her infant.

B. Nursing Diagnoses

The North American Nursing Diagnosis Association (NANDA) has attempted to define the phenomenon of nursing and identify those health care problems that are within the scope of nursing practice; there are, however, objections to the use of NANDA diagnostic categories and defining characteristics in international or transcultural contexts (Andrews, 1995).

  1. The nursing diagnoses are focused primarily on biophysical and psychologic "disturbances," "alterations," "impairments," or some deficit states that have been developed by North American nurses.

  2. The diagnoses are also based, to a large extent, on Anglo-American Western cultural values, norms, and standards, which have questionable relevance and usefulness with non-Anglo cultures and subcultures.

  3. Selection from the current list of nursing diagnoses might result in the nurse imposing culturally inaccurate and inappropriate labels on clients from diverse backgrounds (Geissler, 1991, 1992).

4. Positive health descriptors, caring modalities, and assets or strengths of cultures in dealing with human conditions need to be added to the more pathologic and medically oriented negative conditions currently emphasized (Leininger, 1990).
5. Transcultural nursing diagnoses can be adopted that will expand the scope of practice to include the specific cultural needs of clients and reflect cultural sensitivity rather than bias; for example:
   a. Adherence to traditional beliefs about hot and cold
   b. Impaired verbal communication related to language barrier
   c. Adherence to the traditional cultural group's dietary beliefs
   d. Adherence to the traditional cultural group's activity practices
   In addition, more familiar diagnoses are also appropriate.
   e. Fear secondary to an unknown environment
   f. Anxiety related to culturally unusual expectations for behavior and treatment
C. **Interventions/Outcomes**
   1. Adherence to traditional beliefs about hot and cold
      a. Interventions
         (1) Offer warm drinks immediately postpartum.
         (2) Offer heat lamps or hot packs rather than sitz baths or ice application to the perineum.
         (3) Provide extra blankets for warmth.
         (4) Provide a balance between the hot and cold forces by offering medications with warm liquids, if requested by client.
      b. Outcomes
         (1) Client successfully balances hot and cold elements in diet, medication, and treatment regimens, as evidenced by her expression of satisfaction.
   2. Impaired verbal communication related to language barrier
      a. Interventions
         (1) Provide and use an interpreter, when necessary.
         (2) Use the interpreter appropriately.
            (a) Most women prefer another woman when discussing intimate matters.
            (b) The interpreter should not be a child.
               (i) It is not appropriate for a child to have knowledge of childbearing.
               (ii) The child will have unusual power over the parent because of the knowledge gained.
            (c) Refrain from using slang or medical jargon that might be difficult for the interpreter to translate.
         (3) Assess the client's ability to read and write before providing written information in the native language.
      b. Outcomes
         (1) Client experiences an increase in communication with the nurse through the appropriate use of an interpreter.
   3. Adherence to the traditional cultural group's dietary practices
      a. Interventions
         (1) Assess what foods the client prefers to eat or not to eat.
         (2) Encourage preferred dietary practices if they are not shown to cause harm to the mother or fetus.

(3) Permit and encourage family members to bring foods into the hospital if necessary.

   b. Outcomes

      (1) Client expresses satisfaction with dietary provisions.

4. Adherence to traditional cultural group's practices

  a. Interventions

    (1) Assess what practices the mother wishes to follow related to

      (a) Bathing

      (b) Ambulation

      (c) Infant caretaking

      (d) Support persons

      (e) Dietary practices (for mother and infant)

    (2) Modify usual hospital practices to accommodate client preferences.

      (a) Explain the rationale for early ambulation.

      (b) Encourage the mother to move frequently in bed and perhaps to sit by the bedside rather than to completely ambulate.

      (c) Provide an opportunity for bathing in bed with warm water, rather than showering.

      (d) Encourage family members or the other support person to assume care of the infant.

  b. Outcomes

    (1) Client expresses satisfaction with activity level and caretaking responsibilities.

5. Fear secondary to an unknown environment

  a. Interventions

    (1) Encourage family members to remain with the client if so desired.

    (2) Explain procedures and reinforce the explanations given by others.

      (a) Use terminology that is understood.

      (b) Avoid taboo or inappropriate language or terminology.

    (3) Include family members in decision making, particularly the expectant father or husband.

    (4) Incorporate traditional practices as expressed by the client into the care plan when possible.

    (5) Avoid practices in conflict with cultural traditions, when possible.

  b. Outcomes

    (1) Client experiences a decrease in fear of the unknown environment:

      (a) By describing expected behaviors or treatment

      (b) Through use of a family member for support and decision making

      (c) By using traditional elements of care

      (d) By avoiding practices that conflict with cultural traditions

6. Anxiety related to culturally unusual expectations for behavior and treatment

  a. Interventions

    (1) Assess the level of anxiety through overt and covert manifestations.

    (2) Assess the client's expectations for behavior and treatment.

(3) Incorporate culturally traditional expectations into the care plan.
   (a) Allow the activity and position of choice during labor and delivery.
   (b) Allow the family member of choice to provide support.
   (c) Alter Western expectations for activity and hygiene during the postpartum period to allow comfort for the new mother.
   (d) Observe mother-infant interactions in the context of cultural expectations.
b. Outcomes
   (1) Client experiences less anxiety about unexpected behaviors and treatment:
      (a) By sharing with the nurse culturally expected behaviors
      (b) By using usual behaviors, when possible
      (c) By expressing an understanding of the need to use unfamiliar behaviors, when necessary

HEALTH EDUCATION

A. **Before education can begin with culturally diverse clients, the assessment just described must be performed to establish a valid data base.**
   1. Strategies that are based on cultural knowledge are more likely to be successful than those not based on such data.
   2. Unless based on cultural information, nursing interventions might be inappropriate or incomplete, rather than allowing modification to meet the client's cultural needs.
B. **Approaches might:**
   1. Integrate scientific knowledge and folk practices, if necessary.
   2. Affect the client's behavior.
   3. Result in understanding on the nurse's part about why change cannot occur.
C. **Educational strategies**
   1. Explain the rationale for a scientific approach to care if it is significantly different from that proposed by the client.
   2. If proposed practices are not harmful to the mother or fetus, allow them to continue.
   3. If proposed practices are harmful, attempt to alter behaviors to include more beneficial ones.
   4. Elicit assistance and support from the established caretaker in the family (e.g., a grandmother or an aunt).
   5. Obtain approval and consent for treatment from the proper person (e.g., the husband or father).
   6. Demonstrate how scientific and folk practices can be combined to provide optimal care for the mother and infant.
   7. Recognize when compromise is not possible without destroying the family's entire cultural belief system.

CASE STUDIES AND STUDY QUESTIONS

Mrs. G, a Mexican-American, has come to your antepartum clinic for the first time. She is a gravida 3, para 2 (G3, P2) and is at 32 weeks' gestation. Through an interpreter, she tells you that she is feeling fine, had no problems with her previous pregnancies, and has come for prenatal care only at the urging of the nurse in the well-child clinic where her two children receive immunizations. She believes it is important to balance the hot and cold humors and eats according to the prescriptions for accomplishing this during pregnancy; she avoids "hot" foods, iron preparations, and milk (because of lactose intolerance). She is kept active caring for her family (her children are ages 2 and 5 years) and believes that this will ensure a small infant and an easy delivery; she also believes that sleeping flat on her back protects the fetus from harm.

1. Who is the best person to serve as an interpreter for this woman?
   a. A woman 20 to 30 years old
   b. A man 20 to 30 years old
   c. A young girl in her early teens
   d. A young boy 8 to 10 years old

2. What is an appropriate approach to discussing her possible dietary deficiencies?
   a. Tell her the beliefs in a balance of hot and cold are superstition.
   b. Tell her that it is important that she include milk and an iron preparation in her diet.
   c. Explore with her acceptable alternatives to milk and iron preparations that she can ingest.
   d. Refer her to a nutritionist who will construct a specific diet for her.

3. What is an appropriate question to ask this woman?
   a. "Will your husband be with you during labor and delivery?"
   b. "Who will you want to be with you during labor and delivery?"
   c. "Are you attending any childbirth preparation classes?"
   d. "Do you know that sleeping on your back is actually bad for the infant?"

4. What is a good approach for the nurse in caring for this woman?
   a. Instruct her in the components of a balanced diet.
   b. Tell her the benefits of regular and early prenatal care.
   c. Enroll her and her husband in a childbirth preparation class.
   d. Ensure female care providers as often as possible.

You are assigned to care for Mrs. T, a Vietnamese woman who gave birth 12 hours previously. When you enter the room, she is lying in bed with the infant in the bassinet beside her. There is a full bottle in the crib. She has not had a shower, and most of her food remains on her breakfast tray. She has had only the tea and toast. When you exclaim over the infant, she merely turns her head away and does not comment.

5. What is an appropriate comment or question for her regarding her food intake?
   a. "If you don't eat more, you won't have the strength to care for your infant."
   b. "Why didn't you eat your cereal, juice, and fruit?"
   c. "Do you have special food requirements during this time that I could help with or that your family could bring in?"
   d. "Don't you like our food?"

6. What should you assess about her activity and bathing?
   a. Whether there are cultural restrictions on her activity that prohibit her from showering at this time
   b. When she will take a shower
   c. When she will get out of bed and ambulate
   d. Whether she is going to feed the infant soon

7. How would you expect this mother to behave toward her infant?
   a. Expresses great joy about the birth of the infant.

b. Appreciates compliments about the infant by the staff.
c. Willing to take complete charge of caring for the infant.
d. Remains distant toward the infant during the first few days, with caretaking done by others.

8. Who would you expect to be at her bedside helping her to take care of herself and the infant?
   a. No one
   b. Her mother or grandmother
   c. Her husband
   d. Her neighbors

You are interviewing Ms. G, a 17-year-old gravida 2, para 1 (G2, P1) black woman originally from Georgia, who, at 28 weeks' gestation, is now attending your prenatal clinic for the first time.

9. Which of the following questions are appropriate for you to ask when taking her history?
   a. "Do you have any special food requirement or cravings that you need to follow during pregnancy?"
   b. "Do you believe any special restrictions on your activity are necessary for a safe pregnancy?"
   c. "Do you consider pregnancy an illness?"
   d. "Why haven't you come in for prenatal care before? You know you should have done so."
   e. "Aren't you a little young to be pregnant for the second time?"
   (1) a, c, e
   (2) a, b, c
   (3) b, c, e
   (4) a, b

Mrs. C, a Laotian, her husband, and her mother come into the labor and delivery area. She is a 20-year-old gravida 1, para 0 (G1, P0) at term. When being examined, she frequently pulls the sheet over herself and looks away from her husband, who appears uncomfortable. She is found to be 7 cm dilated, completely effaced, and at 0 station. She sits upright in the bed, only grimacing with contractions. Her mother asks if her daughter may have a cup of hot tea to drink.

10. What are important components of a care plan for this family?
    a. Determine which family member(s) the patient would prefer to support her during labor.
    b. Make sure that the patient has ice chips at the bedside at all times.
    c. Assess the patient frequently for signs and behavior indicative of increasing discomfort.
    d. Provide for as much privacy and modesty as possible.
    e. Insist that the patient lie on one side or the other during the rest of her labor.
    (1) All of the above
    (2) a, c, d
    (3) a, c
    (4) b, c, e

11. Which of the following are essential to providing effective perinatal care to families of different cultures?
    a. Including cultural and family assessments as part of the routine history
    b. Insisting that the family adhere to scientific and medical principles of care at all times
    c. Assessing all culturally different beliefs as harmful
    d. Providing the services of an interpreter if a language barrier exists
    e. Fostering an attitude of respect for alternative healing practices
    (1) a, c, e
    (2) b, c, e
    (3) a, d, e
    (4) All of the above

12. Which of the following might prevent culturally diverse families from seeking maternity care in health care institutions in the United States?

a. The presence of interpreters to assist with language differences

b. Culturally competent care provided by health care practitioners

c. Clinics that are easily accessible and in local neighborhoods

d. Long clinic waits in urban centers that are structured to accommodate clients as a group, not as individuals

ANSWERS TO STUDY QUESTIONS

1. a	4. d	7. d	10. 2
2. c	5. c	8. b	11. 3
3. b	6. a	9. 2	12. d

REFERENCES

American Academy of Nursing. (1992). AAN expert panel report: Culturally competent health care. *Nursing Outlook, 40*(6), 277-283.

American Academy of Nursing. (1993). *Promoting cultural competence in and through nursing education.* Subpanel on Cultural Competence in Nursing education. New York: American Academy of Nursing.

Andrews, M. (1989). Culture and nutrition. In J. Boyle, & M. Andrews (Eds.), *Transcultural concepts in nursing care* (pp. 333-355). Glenview, IL: Scott, Foresman/Little, Brown College.

Andrews, M. (1995). Transcultural nursing care. In M. Andrews, & J. Boyle (Eds.), *Transcultural concepts in nursing care* (2nd ed.; pp. 49-96). Philadelphia: Lippincott.

Andrews, M. (2003). Culturally competent nursing care. In *Transcultural concepts in nursing care* (4th ed.). M. Andrews, & J. Boyle (Eds.), (pp. 15-35). Philadelphia: Lippincott, Williams & Wilkins.

Andrews, M., & Boyle, J. (1997). Competence in transcultural nursing care. *American Journal of Nursing, 98*(8), 16AAA-16DDD.

Clark, A. (1978). *Culture, childbearing, health professionals.* Philadelphia: F.A. Davis.

Geissler, E. (1991). Transcultural nursing and nursing diagnoses. *Nursing and Health Care, 12*(4), 190-192.

Geissler, E. (1992). Nursing diagnoses: A study of cultural relevance. *Journal of Professional Nursing, 8*(5), 301-307.

Greener, D. (1989). Transcultural nursing care of the childbearing woman and her family. In J. Boyle, & M. Andrews (Eds.), *Transcultural concepts in nursing care* (pp. 95-119). Glenview, IL: Scott, Foresman/ Little, Brown College.

Kay, M. (1982). *Anthropology of human birth.* Philadelphia: F.A. Davis.

Lauderdale, J. (2003). Transcultural perspectives in childbearing. In M. Andrews, & J. Boyle (Eds.), *Transcultural concepts in nursing care* (4th ed). Philadelphia: Lippincott, Williams & Wilkins.

Leininger, M. (1990). Issues, questions, and concerns related to the nursing diagnosis cultural movement from a transcultural nursing perspective. *Journal of Transcultural Nursing, 2*(1), 23-32.

Leininger, M., & McFarland, M. (2002). *Transcultural nursing: Concepts, theories, research & practice.* New York; McGraw-Hill.

Meleis, A. (1999). Culturally competent care. *Journal of Transcultural Nursing, 10*(1), 12.

Meleis, A. (2003) Theoretical consideration of health care for immigrant and minority women. In P. Hill, J. Lipson, & A. Meleis (Eds.), *Caring for women crossculturally* (pp. 1-10). Philadelphia: F.A. Davis

Meleis, A., & Sorrell, L. (1981, May–June). Bridging cultures. Arab-American women and their birth experiences. *American Journal of Maternal-Child Nursing, 6*(3), 171-176.

Miller-Karas, E. (1990, Summer). Ethnicity and perinatal patient care. *Mid-Coastal California Perinatal Outreach Program Newsletter*, 1-3.

Office of Minority Health. (1999). *Assuring cultural competence in health care: Recommendations for national standards and an outcomes-focused research agenda.* Washington, DC: Department of Health & Human Services, U.S. Public Health Service. Available online at *www.omhrc.gov/clas/ds.htm.*

Purnell, L., & Paulanka, B. (2003). *Transcultural health care: A culturally competent approach.* Philadelphia: F.A. Davis.

Tiedje, L. (2000). Returning to our roots: 25 years of maternal/child nursing in the community. *MCN The American Journal of Maternal Child Nursing, 25*(6), 315-317.

Tripp-Reimer, T., & Brink, P. (1984). Cultural brokerage. In G. Bulechek & J. McCloskey (Eds.), *Nursing interventions: Treatment for nursing diagnoses.* Philadelphia: W.B. Saunders.

Tripp-Reimer, T., Brink, P., & Saunders, J. (1984). Cultural assessment: Content and process. *Nursing Outlook, 32*(2), 78-82.

Wells, M. (2000). Beyond cultural competence: A model for individual and institutional cultural development. *Journal of Community Health Nursing, 17*(4), 189-199.

ADDITIONAL RESOURCES

Alexander, G., Mor, J., Kogan, M., Leland, N., & Kieffer, E. (1996). Pregnancy outcomes of U.S.-born and foreign-born Japanese Americans. *American Journal of Public Health, 86*(6), 820-824.

Al-Shahri, M. (2002). Culturally sensitive caring for Saudi patients. *Journal of Transcultural Nursing, 13*(2), 133-138.

Andrews, M., & Boyle, J. (2003). *Transcultural concepts in nursing care* (4th ed). Philadelphia: Lippincott, Williams & Wilkins.

Berry, A. (1999). Mexican American womens' expressions of the meaning of culturally congruent prenatal care. *Journal of Transcultural Nursing, 10*(3), 203-212.

Callister, L., Semenic, S., & Foster, J. (1999). Cultural and spiritual meanings of childbirth: Orthodox Jewish and Mormon women. *Journal of Holistic Nursing, 17*(3), 280-295.

Callister, L., & Vega, R. (1998). Giving birth: Guatemala women's voices. *Journal of Obstetric, Gynecologic and Neonatal Nursing, 27*(3), 289-295.

Choi, E. (1995). A contrast of mothering behaviors in women from Korea and the United States. *Journal of Obstetric, Gynecologic and Neonatal Nursing, 24*(4), 363-369.

Edwards, N., & Boivin, J. (1997). Ethnocultural predictors of postpartum infant-care behaviours among immigrants in Canada. *Ethnicity and Health, 2*(3), 163-176.

Hill, P., Lipson, J., & Meleis, A. (2003). *Caring for women cross-culturally.* Philadelphia: F.A.Davis.

Hyman, I., & Dussault, G. (2000). Negative consequences of acculturation on health behaviour, social support and stress among pregnant Southeast Asian immigrant women in Montreal: An exploratory study. *Canadian Journal of Public Health, 91*(5), 357-360.

Kridli, S. (2002). Health beliefs and practices among Arab women. *MCN The American Journal of Maternal child Nursing, 27*(3), 178-182.

Mattson, S., & Lew, L. (1992). Culturally sensitive prenatal care for Southeast Asians. *Journal of Obstetric, Gynecologic and Neonatal Nursing, 21*(1), 48-54.

Morgan, M. (1996). Prenatal care of African American women in selected USA urban and rural cultural contexts. *Journal of Transcultural Nursing, 7*(2), 3-9.

Office on Women's Health. Available online at *www.4woman.gov*.

Pritham, U., & Sammons, L. (1993). Korean women's attitudes toward pregnancy and prenatal care. *Health Care for Women International, 14*(2), 145-153.

Purnell, L., & Paulanka, B. (2003). *Transcultural health care: A culturally competent approach* (2nd ed). Philadelphia: F.A. Davis.

Spector, R. (2000). *Cultural diversity in health and illness* (5th ed). Upper Saddle River, NJ: Prentice Hall Health.

Spring, M., Ross, P., Etkin, N., & Deinard, A. (1995). Sociocultural factors in the use of prenatal care by Hmong women, Minneapolis. *American Journal of Public Health, 85*(7), 1015-1017.

Weber, S. (1996). Cultural aspects of pain in childbearing women. *Journal of Obstetric, Gynecologic, and Neonatal Nursing, 25*(1), 67-72.

4-1 Quick Reference Guide to Ethnocultural Differences

■ TABLE 4-1
■ ■ **Antepartum Variations**

	Native American	Black	Asian	Hispanic	Arab Heritage
Pregnancy normal	Yes	Yes	Yes (must maintain balance between yin/yang)	Yes	Yes (but seek care)
Prefer female attendants	Yes	No	Yes	Yes	Yes
Diet	Often have lactose intolerance (especially Eskimos, who are used to high protein and low carbohydrates)	Pica; eat salty (soul) foods; avoid acids; use sassafras tea; are at risk for overeating of fats and carbohydrates	Often are vegetarian; use herbal teas; often have lactose intolerance (tofu is a good alternative; also	Are clay eaters; use herbal teas and remedies; use much fat in cooking; may not consider greens to be vegetables use fish bones for calcium); may not eat eggs; may refuse iron (believe it causes a difficult recovery)	If Moslem, eat no pork or pork products, caffeine, or alcohol
Activity	Should be active	Should continue sexual activity	Remain moderately active; avoid sexual activity in third trimester	Are active; use massage	Have no restrictions
Emotions	Should be happy	Avoid stress	Should be serene, calm, and not sad	Do not quarrel with husband	Have no special needs

■ TABLE 4-2
■ **Intrapartum Variations**

	Native American	Black	Asian	Hispanic	Arab Heritage
Prefer female attendants	Yes; some want the whole family (Navajo)	Yes (especially mother or grandmother)	Yes	Yes	Yes
Pain	Endure quietly	Usually are taught not to show weakness or call attention to themselves	Should not show pain; shameful to scream; often avoid verbal expression; use no medication (Samoan)	Endure pain with patience, but consider it acceptable to cry out	Are verbally expressive; cry and scream loudly; refuse medication
Positions	Choose various positions; often use birth chair	Choose various positions	Like to move around, but must stay warm to not lose heat; come to hospital in advanced labor; squatting (Laotian, Hmong)	Use massage; will use birth chair; like to move around and walk; come to hospital in advanced labor	Choose various positions
Food and drink	Have no special needs	Have no special needs	Drink herbal teas	Drink manzanilla tea (makes uterine contractions stronger)	Have no special needs

TABLE 4-3
■ Postpartum Variations

	Native American	Black	Asian	Hispanic	Arab Heritage
Hot and cold beliefs	Not applicable	Prevent cold air from entering uterus; wear pad and use abdominal binder	Believe that exposure to cold may cause arthritis or asthma; avoid showers, ice packs, and ice water; use hot blankets; avoid drafts	Believe that exposure to cold may cause sterility; use abdominal binder	Have no special needs
Diet	Drink hot herbal teas	Use sassafras tea; avoid eggplant, okra, tomatoes, cold drinks, and milk (Haitians); avoid chitterlings, liver, and onions (southern Blacks believe that these will affect breast milk)	Drink ginseng tea; eat only "hot" foods (chicken every day, plus other meats and fish for 30 days; may eat warm, dry, salty foods with little liquid [Korean, Vietnamese]; avoid fruits and green vegetables)	Eat cold food for 1 to 2 months; corn gruel is good; avoid acidic foods (citrus fruits, vegetables, chili, pork)	Have no special needs
Activity	Have no special needs	See themselves as sick; avoid bathing, washing hair, and heavy work	Need to rest; relatives do all work, including care of the infant; avoid contact with others and going out into the sun	Remain indoors, stay in bed up to 1 month; avoid strenuous work and bathing; avoid sexual contact for 40 days	Expect a lot of visitors; often request pain medications
Purification	Take a ritual batch on the fourth postpartum day (Navajo)	Not applicable	Avoid sexual contact for 3 to 4 months	Take a ritual batch 2 weeks postpartum	Not applicable

TABLE 4-4
■ Variations in Newborn Care

	Native American	Black	Asian	Hispanic	Arab Heritage
Breastfeeding	Yes; urban dwellers may use bottle	Yes; urban dwellers may use bottle	Yes	Yes (after milk comes in); consider colostrum bad for the infant; use bottle	Varies
Special clothes	Use cradle boards in urban areas	Use belly bands to prevent hernias	Wear old, ragged clothes (southeast Asians)	Swaddle tightly; abdominal binder is common (infant is susceptible to "bad air")	Do not plan ahead for the infant, which would tempt the evil eye; often have no layette ready
Activity	Consider infants important to the family; keep infant close and handle often	Not applicable	Keep infant close continuously; have no circumcision performed	Believe that the infant is vulnerable to the evil eye (if a stranger admires the infant, believe should touch the infant to dispel harm); no circumcision performed	Believe that the infant is vulnerable to the evil eye and needs protection
Praise of infant	Not applicable	Not applicable	No; believe that praise will call the attention of the gods to the vulnerable newborn	Yes	No; praise mother instead; if do praise the infant, touch wood or mention God's blessing

TABLE 4-5
Biologic Variations to Consider

	Native American	Black	Asian	Hispanic	Arab Heritage
Sickle cell trait	Yes	Yes	No	No	Yes
Diabetes	Yes (especially Pima and Papago of Arizona)	No	No	No	No
Abnormal hemoglobin (other than sickle cell)	No	No	Yes (especially Thais and Cambodians)	No	No
Tuberculosis	No	No	Yes (especially recent refugees)	No	No

5 Physiology of Pregnancy

LINDA BOND

OBJECTIVES

1. Describe systemic changes occurring in the woman's body during pregnancy.
2. Describe changes in the uterus, cervix, vagina, and vulva during pregnancy.
3. Identify the presumptive, probable, and positively diagnostic signs and symptoms of pregnancy.
4. Differentiate between normal and abnormal laboratory findings observed during pregnancy.
5. Define optimal nutritional adequacy based on pregnancy outcome indicators.
6. Identify specific changes in nutrient requirements during pregnancy.
7. Examine patterns of weight gain recommendations during pregnancy for different women.
8. Design an individualized patient education plan based on data from the history.
9. Detect potential complications of pregnancy based on data from a history, a physical examination, and laboratory test results.
10. Formulate nursing interventions to prevent anticipated problems identified from the nursing assessment.

INTRODUCTION

A. **Conception and the 40 weeks of gestation constitute a time of numerous changes within a woman's body, often unbeknown to the woman**
   1. Regular health care supervision is necessary to ensure that subtle and untoward changes will not go undetected, ensuring a positive outcome for mother, infant, and the entire family.
   2. The course of pregnancy and the outcome are directly related to the nutritional status of the mother.
   3. The health care team is responsible for monitoring expected physiologic and psychologic changes and for providing health teaching for greater understanding of the events of pregnancy as well as preparation for the post-pregnancy events.
B. **Maternal system changes**
   1. Reproductive system
      a. Uterus
         (1) Size increases to 20 times that of nonpregnant size.
            (a) Hyperplasia and hypertrophy of myometrial cells, including muscle fibers, occur.
            (b) Increases are related to estrogen and progesterone, with mechanical factors of stretching related to the developing fetus.
         (2) Wall thins to 1.5 cm (0.6 in) or less (changes from almost a solid globe to a hollow vessel).

(3) Weight increases from 70 g to 1100 g (1.8 oz to 2.2 lb).
(4) Volume (capacity) increases from less than 10 ml to 5 L (2 tsp to 1 gal).
(5) Uterine contractility (Braxton Hicks contractions)
    (a) Irregular, painless contractions due to structural and functional changes in myometrium resulting from estrogen increases in pregnancy.
    (b) As pregnancy advances, these contractions become more intense, frequent, and easily felt.
    (c) Braxton Hicks contractions do not typically lead to cervical changes.
(6) Shape changes from that of an inverted pear to that of a soft globe that enlarges, rising out of the pelvis by the end of the first trimester.
(7) Endometrium is called the decidua after implantation.
    (a) Decidua vera: all of the uterine lining that is not in contact with the fetus
    (b) Decidua basalis: uterine lining beneath implantation
    (c) Decidua capsularis: portion of the decidua that covers the embryo

b. Cervix
(1) Softening related to increased vascularity, edema, slight hypertrophy, and hyperplasia (Goodell's sign).
(2) Cervical glands occupy approximately half of the cervical mass near term.
(3) Mucus plug (operculum) fills the cervical canal soon after conception.
    (a) Formed from the thick mucus produced by endocervical glands
    (b) Function is to prevent ascending infections

c. Ovaries and fallopian tubes
(1) Anovulation results from the suppression of follicle-stimulating hormone (FSH) and luteinizing hormone (LH) related to high levels of estrogen and progesterone.
(2) Corpus luteum remains active for 6 to 7 weeks into pregnancy, producing progesterone and estrogen to maintain pregnancy; after 6 to 7 weeks' gestation, the placenta will produce the progesterone to maintain pregnancy.

d. Vagina
(1) Increased vascularity results in bluish, violet discoloration (Chadwick's sign)
(2) Hypertrophy and hyperplasia of epithelium and elastic tissues
(3) Leukorrhea, with an acid pH of 3.5 to 6.0, functions to control the growth of pathogens.

e. Vulva
(1) Increased vasculature
(2) External structures enlarged due to hypertrophy of structures, along with fat deposits

f. Breasts
(1) Changes begin soon after conception.
(2) External changes
    (a) Size increases; weight increases by about 400 g (12 oz).
    (b) Breasts become nodular.
    (c) Skin appears thinner.
    (d) Blood vessels become more prominent with a twofold increase in blood flow.

(e) Areola and nipples
  (i) Pigmentation darkens, beginning during the first trimester.
  (ii) Montgomery's tubercles become more prominent.
  (iii) Secondary pinkish areola might develop.
  (iv) Nipples enlarge and become more erect (second trimester).
(3) Internal changes
  (a) Proliferation of glandular tissue and lactiferous ducts begins in first trimester (influenced by estrogen and progesterone).
  (b) Alveoli begin producing colostrum.
    (i) Pre-colostrum, which is a thin, clear liquid, can be found in acini cells in early second trimester.
    (ii) Colostrum is the creamy, white to yellowish pre-milk secreted as early as 16 weeks' gestation.

2. Cardiovascular system
  a. Heart
    (1) Slight enlargement (hypertrophy) (approximately 12%)
    (2) Auscultatory changes
      (a) Exaggerated split heard in first sound.
      (b) Second and third sounds are more obvious.
      (c) Systolic and diastolic murmurs are common.
    (3) Shift in chest contents: heart is displaced upward and to the left in late pregnancy.
  b. Hemodynamic changes
    (1) Heart rate increases by 15 to 20 beats/min (20% increase).
    (2) Cardiac output increases by 30% to 50% during first two trimesters and then declines to about 20% near term.
    (3) Blood volume increases by 1500 ml or 40% to 50% (might be even greater with multiple births) over prepregnancy level.
    (4) Stroke volume increases by as much as 30% over prepregnancy level.
    (5) Vasodilation occurs because of progesterone.
    (6) Arterial blood pressure
      (a) Readings, positional variations (Lowdermilk & Perry, 2004; Walsh, 2001)
        (i) Supine hypotension results from uterine pressure on inferior vena cava (supine hypotensive syndrome).
        (ii) Left lateral recumbent position is optimal for cardiac output and uterine perfusion.
        (iii) Brachial artery pressure is highest when woman is sitting.
      (b) Systolic and diastolic pressures begin to fall in the first trimester; they decrease until midpregnancy and then slowly rise back to the 1st trimester level.
    (7) Venous pressure does not change despite the increase in blood volume.
      (a) Increased vascular capacity influenced by hormonal changes.
      (b) Pressure below the uterus is increased related to large pelvic veins and those distal to the uterus.
        (i) Venous pooling might occur late in pregnancy after long periods in the upright position.
        (ii) Late in pregnancy, the enlarged uterus might also contribute to slowed venous return, pooling, and dependent edema.

  c. Hematologic changes
    (1) Red blood cell (RBC) production escalates.
        (a) Total RBC volume increases approximately 33% (450 ml) with iron supplementation.
        (b) Blood iron levels in RBC volume increase only approximately 18% (250 ml).
    (2) White blood cell (WBC) count increases 5000 to 12,000/mm; might normally increase to 20,000/mm during parturition without infection.
        (a) WBCs in pregnant women are less effective in fighting infection and disease than they are in nonpregnant women.
        (b) History and physical examination must confirm diagnosis of infection.
    (3) Blood volume expansion is made up of increased volume of plasma and increased numbers of RBCs (plasma volume increases more rapidly than RBC production and causes hemodilution or physiologic anemia of pregnancy).
        (a) Primary function is to offset blood loss at delivery.
        (b) Supplies the hypertrophied vascular system during pregnancy.
    (4) Clotting factors increase
        (a) Plasma fibrin levels increase by approximately 40%.
        (b) Fibrinogen levels increase by approximately 50%.
        (c) Pregnancy is a hypercoagulable state, placing the woman at risk for thrombosis and alterations in coagulation (e.g., disseminated intravascular coagulation).
    (5) Hemoglobin and hematocrit decrease (in relation to plasma volume).
        (a) Hemoglobin of less than 11 g/dl indicates anemia.
        (b) Hematocrit lower than 35% indicates anemia.
3. Respiratory system
  a. Respiratory rate and maximal breathing capacity remain unchanged while vital capacity might increase slightly.
  b. Tidal volume, minute ventilatory volume, and minute oxygen uptake increase as pregnancy advances, as evidenced by deeper breathing.
  c. Carbon dioxide output increases.
  d. Increased vascularity of the upper respiratory tract is influenced by increased estrogen levels.
  e. Thoracic circumference increases by 5 to 7 cm (2 to 3 in), and the diaphragm elevates approximately 4 cm (1.5 in).
  f. Basal metabolic rate increases and oxygen requirement increases by 30 to 40 ml/min.
  g. Acid-base balance: arterial blood is slightly more alkaline.
4. Urinary system
  a. Renal structure changes.
    (1) Influenced by
        (a) Hormone effects, particularly the influence of progesterone on smooth muscle
        (b) Uterine pressure
        (c) Alterations in the cardiovascular system, including increased cardiac output and increased blood volume
    (2) Collection system changes (physiologic hydronephrosis)
        (a) Renal pelvis dilates.
        (b) Ureters elongate and become tortuous; the upper one third of the ureters might dilate (particularly the right ureter).

(c) Urinary stasis or stagnation occurs and increases the danger of pyelonephritis.
(3) Increased urinary frequency is related to the increasing size of the uterus and its pressure on the bladder.
(4) Bladder is pulled up into the abdominal cavity by the growing uterus, and the bladder tone is decreased.
  b. Renal function changes
(1) Changes in kidney function occur to accommodate a heavier workload while maintaining stable electrolyte balance and blood pressure.
  (a) Increased glomerular filtration rate
  (b) Increased renal plasma flow
(2) Urine output is 25% higher during pregnancy.
(3) Laboratory values (Cunningham, Gant, Leveno, Gilstrap, Hauth, & Wenstrom, 2001; Walsh, 2001)
  (a) Glucosuria might occur (might not be abnormal; warrants further evaluation and monitoring).
  (b) Proteinuria is abnormal, except in very concentrated urine or in the first-voided specimen on arising (total urine protein of 250 to 300 mg in 24 hours is a warning of impaired kidney function and/or pregnancy-induced hypertension).
5. Gastrointestinal system
  a. Mouth and teeth
(1) Gums become hyperemic, swollen, and soft (friable) and have a tendency to bleed (estrogen influence).
(2) Saliva becomes more acidic.
  (a) Production remains unchanged. (Ptyalism occurs in a few women.)
  (b) Some women experience a sense of increased saliva production due to decreased swallowing associated with nausea and vomiting.
(3) Teeth remain unchanged.
  b. Gastrointestinal tract
(1) Smooth muscle relaxation and decreased peristalsis occur related to the progesterone influence; this can lead to:
  (a) Decreased motility, resulting in fluids and nutrients remaining in the intestine longer, facilitating greater absorption but also resulting in constipation.
  (b) Hemorrhoids: associated with constipation, increased venous pressure, and pressure of the gravid uterus.
  (c) Heartburn, slowed gastric emptying, and esophageal regurgitation (reflux).
(2) Positional changes of organs occur because of uterine enlargement.
  (a) Upward displacement of the stomach
  (b) Colon shifted and compressed
  c. Liver function undergoes insignificant, minor changes.
  d. Gallbladder
(1) Volume is increased, muscle tone decreased.
(2) Emptying time is prolonged, which could lead to formation of gallstones.
(3) Retained bile salts can lead to pruritus.

6. Musculoskeletal system
   a. Distension of the abdomen and a shift in the center of gravity can result in lordosis.
   b. Relaxation and increased mobility of joints occur because of the hormones relaxin and progesterone, and lead to a characteristic "waddle gait."
   c. Diastasis recti, a separation of the rectus muscles of the abdominal wall, is associated with the enlarging uterus in some women.
7. Integumentary system
   a. Skin undergoes hyperpigmentation (primarily due to estrogen influence).
      (1) Melasma (also called chloasma) is the blotchy, brownish "mask of pregnancy."
      (2) Linea alba can darken and become linea nigra (abdomen).
      (3) Nipples, areolae, axillae, vulva, and perineum all darken.
      (4) Moles (nevi), freckles, and recent scars might darken.
   b. Hair: some women may note increased growth.
   c. Connective tissue fragility can cause striae gravidarum (breasts, abdomen, thighs, and inguinal area).
   d. Blood vessels have increased permeability, causing:
      (1) Edema
      (2) Spider nevi or angiomas
      (3) Palmar erythema
   e. Skin disorders and skin problems associated with pregnancy include non-inflammatory pruritus and acne vulgaris (especially in the first trimester).
8. Endocrine system
   a. Pituitary gland
      (1) Anterior lobe: slight increase in size
         (a) FSH and LH production is suppressed.
         (b) Thyrotropin and adrenocorticotropic hormones might increase slightly.
         (c) Melanotropin production is increased.
         (d) Human placental lactogen (HPL) (human chorionic gonadotropin [HCS]) production is suppressed.
         (e) Prolactin production is increased.
      (2) Posterior lobe: oxytocin production gradually increases as the fetus matures.
   b. Thyroid gland activity and hormone production increases.
      (1) Gland enlarges (related to increased vascularity and growth of glandular tissue).
      (2) Thyroxine (T_4) level, unbound to plasma proteins, remains unchanged (triiodothyronine [T_3] and T_4 increase but are bound to thyroxine-binding globulin [TBG]).
      (3) Basal metabolic rate (BMR) increases up to 15% to 20% by term.
   c. Parathyroid gland activity increases, and blood levels of parathyroid hormone are elevated to meet the demands for growth of the fetal skeleton.
   d. Adrenal glands: little change in function
   e. Pancreas: insulin production increased throughout pregnancy to compensate for placental hormone insulin antagonism
      (1) Insulin antagonists (HPL [HCS], estrogen, progesterone, and adrenal cortisol) decrease tissue sensitivity or the ability to use insulin.
      (2) Normal beta cells can meet the increased demand for insulin.

    (3) Women with poor pancreatic function might develop true diabetes during pregnancy. (See Chapter 24 for a complete discussion of diabetes in pregnancy.)

  f. Ovaries

    (1) Estrogen (also from adrenal cortex and later the placenta) is responsible for:

      (a) Enlargement of breasts, uterus, and genitals

      (b) Fat deposit changes

      (c) Alterations in thyroid function and nutrient metabolism

      (d) Changes in sodium and water retention

      (e) Hematologic changes

      (f) Vascular changes

      (g) Stimulation of melanin-stimulating hormones, hyperpigmentation

    (2) Progesterone from the corpus luteum (later, the placenta) is responsible for:

      (a) Facilitating implantation

      (b) Decreasing uterine contractility

      (c) Development of secretory ducts and the lobular-alveolar system of the breasts

      (d) Fat deposit changes

      (e) Reducing smooth muscle tone

      (f) Increasing sensitivity of respiratory system to carbon dioxide

      (g) Reducing gastric motility

    (3) Relaxin from the corpus luteum (later, the placenta) is thought to be responsible for musculoskeletal changes.

9. Immunologic system

  a. Resistance to infection is decreased due to depressed leukocyte function, which can also lead to improvement in certain autoimmune diseases.

  b. Immunoglobulin (Ig) levels

    (1) Maternal IgG levels are decreased because of cross-placental transfer to the fetus starting at about 16 weeks' gestation; increased transfer occurs near term.

    (2) Maternal IgA and IgM levels remain relatively stable (Cunningham et al., 2001).

C. Pregnancy signs and symptoms

  1. Presumptive evidence of pregnancy

    a. Signs

      (1) Amenorrhea

      (2) Breast changes: increase in size, tenderness

      (3) Vaginal mucosa discoloration (Chadwick's sign)

      (4) Skin pigmentation changes (melasma/chloasma, linea nigra, and linea alba)

    b. Symptoms

      (1) Nausea with or without vomiting

      (2) Urinary frequency

      (3) Weight gain

      (4) Constipation

      (5) Fatigue

      (6) Perception of fetal movement (quickening)

      (7) Maternal perception of pregnancy

2. Probable evidence of pregnancy
    a. Signs
        (1) Abdominal enlargement and striae
        (2) Uterine changes: softening of isthmus (Hegar's sign); Cervical softening (Goodell's sign)
        (3) Braxton Hicks contractions
        (4) Ballottement of the fetus
        (5) Endocrine tests positive for human chorionic gonadotropin (hCG) levels
    b. Symptoms are the same as presumptive symptoms.
3. Positive evidence of pregnancy
    a. Fetal heartbeat (distinct from the heart sounds of the mother) heard by the examiner
    b. Fetal outline confirmation by sonography
    c. Fetal movement detected by examiner
D. **Nutritional consideration during pregnancy:** although attitudes have varied over the years and within cultures about desirable weight gain, much of the recent scientific body of knowledge allows some general observations.
    1. Prepregnancy weight and weight gain
        a. Weight before pregnancy and weight gain during pregnancy are directly related to the birth weight of the infant and the incidence of morbidity and mortality.
        b. Prepregnancy weight and height along with stores of micronutrients affect health and size of the newborn (Kaiser & Allen, 2002).
        c. Body mass index (BMI) is commonly used to evaluate weight for height.
            (1) BMI is expressed as weight/height^2 in which weight is in kilograms (kg) and height is in meters (m)
            (2) BMI classifications are used to categorize nutritional status based on prepregnancy measurements (Cesario, 2003).
                (a) Underweight: BMI less than 18.5
                (b) Healthy/normal weight: BMI 18.6 to 24.9
                (c) Overweight: BMI greater than 25.0 to 29.9
                (d) Obese: BMI greater than 30.0
        d. A weight gain of between 11.5 and 16 kg (25 and 35 lb) is recommended for healthy pregnant women (Reifsnider & Gill, 2000).
            (1) Weight gain should be steady throughout the pregnancy and depends upon the stage of pregnancy.
                (a) Progressive weight gain during pregnancy is essential to ensure normal fetal growth and development and the deposition of maternal stores.
                (b) Recommended weight gain during pregnancy is determined largely by prepregnancy weight for height (Lowdermilk & Perry, 2004).
            (2) Approximately 200 to 450 g/wk (½ to 1 lb/wk) should be adequate during the second and third trimesters.
        e. Weight gain for overweight women is recommended at between 7 and 11.5 kg (15 and 25 lb), depending on nutritional status and degree of obesity (Cesario, 2003).
            (1) Women must be aware of the adverse effects of maternal malnutrition on infant growth and development.
            (2) All pregnant women should gain at least enough weight to equal the weight of the products of conception.

(3) Dietary restriction can result in inadequate intake of essential nutrients and in catabolism of fat stores.
  (a) This process augments the production of ketones leading to ketonuria, which has been found to be correlated with pre-term labor.
  (b) Long-term effects of mild ketonemia during pregnancy are not known. (See Chapter 24 for discussion of endocrine disorders.)
(4) Ideally, obese women should address weight management issues before conception.
  f. If prepregnancy weight is estimated at 10% to 20% below ideal body weight, the mother is considered to have poor nutritional status.
    (1) This might also indicate an inability to attain proper weight or the presence of poor or unusual dietary habits.
    (2) It is recommended that gains for pregnant, underweight women be 12.5 to 18 kg (28 to 40 lb).
    (3) Emphasis should be placed on the quality of food intake.
2. Nutritional needs during pregnancy
  a. Energy and calorie requirements are increased during pregnancy due to deposition of new tissue, increased metabolic expenditure, and increased energy needed to move the pregnant body.
  b. Optimal weight gain from a nutritionally sound diet contributes to a successful pregnancy (Lederman, 2001).
  c. Nutrients needed during pregnancy can be obtained with a diet that provides all essential nutrients, fiber, and energy in adequate amounts.
    (1) Dietary supplementation is justified when there is concern that adequate nutrition or a well-balanced diet is compromised.
      (a) Indicators of nutritional risk include:
        (i) Adolescence
        (ii) Short interval between pregnancies
        (iii) Obesity or low prepregnancy weight
        (iv) Use of alcohol, drugs, or tobacco
        (v) Poor dietary habits
        (vi) Poverty; lack of access to food-distribution programs
        (vii) Multiple gestation pregnancy
        (viii) Medical conditions (e.g., diabetes, heart disease, errors in metabolism)
        (ix) Social conditions (e.g., homelessness, battering)
    (2) Vegetarian diets have many variations; however, almost all contain vegetables, fruits, legumes, nuts, seed, and grains (Lowdermilk & Perry, 2004) (Figure 5-1).
      (a) For strict vegetarians (vegans), vitamin B_{12} supplement or fortified foods are recommended.
      (b) Vitamin B_6, iron, calcium, zinc intake might also be low, so intake must be assessed and supplements added as needed.
    (3) To meet the increased need for iron during the second and third trimesters, a low-dose iron supplement is recommended (60 mg ferrous iron daily).
  d. To meet the energy needs of pregnancy, the recommended dietary allowance (RDA) states that pregnant women need 300 kcal/day over prepregnancy intake.

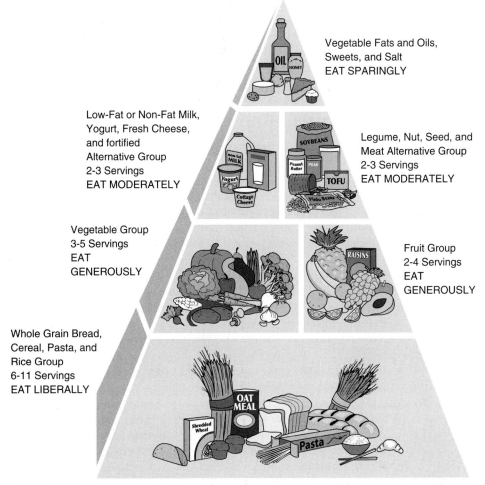

FIGURE 5-1 ■ Vegetarian food guide pyramid. (Adapted from U.S. Department of Agriculture, Washington, DC.)

    e. These additional kilocalories can be adequately met by the following recommended increases:
        (1) Milk intake from 480 ml (2 cups) prepregnancy to the recommended 720 to 960 ml (3 to 4 cups)
        (2) Protein intake by 1 serving
        (3) Fruits and vegetables by 2 servings
        (4) Breads and cereals by 1 to 2 servings
  3. Achieving nutritional adequacy during pregnancy is closely associated with meeting the nutrient requirements based on the RDAs.
    a. Protein requirements are increased for the development of new tissue; currently, the RDA for pregnant women includes an additional 10 to 12 g per day for a daily total of 60 g of protein.
    b. Vitamins and mineral requirements are usually increased during pregnancy.
        (1) Folic acid
            (a) Should be increased from 400 to 600 fg/day to support increase in RBC production, cell division, and DNA synthesis.

      (b) This need can be met by an increased intake of leafy green vegetables, citrus fruits, and fortified ready-to-eat cereals.

   (2) B vitamin requirements are increased because of energy metabolism.

      (a) Adequate intake of protein foods and grains should meet this requirement.

      (b) The RDA for the B vitamins is as follows:

         (i) Riboflavin: 1.4 mg

         (ii) Thiamin: 1.4 mg

         (iii) Pyridoxine (B_6): 1.9 mg

         (iv) Niacin: 18 mg/NE

         (v) B_{12}: 2.6 fg

   (3) Vitamin C

      (a) The RDA during pregnancy is 70 mg/day or 10 mg/day more than the prepregnancy intake.

      (b) This need is easily met by a minimal increase of foods rich in vitamin C (e.g., citrus fruits, certain melons, peppers, leafy green vegetables).

   (4) Vitamin A

      (a) The RDA is not different during pregnancy.

      (b) Adequate vitamin A can be obtained from consuming, at least every other day, a yellow, orange, or red vegetable or fruit or a leafy green vegetable, and/or fortified butter or margarine.

   (5) Vitamin K

      (a) Essential for assisting in the normal process of blood clotting.

      (b) Maternal dietary deficiency is rare.

   (6) Calcium

      (a) Requirement remains at 1000 to 1300 mg/day to ensure adequate calcium for changes in bone metabolism during pregnancy and for development of the fetal skeleton and deciduous teeth.

      (b) Phosphorus and vitamin D are also involved in bone and calcium metabolism, and imbalances of either might affect calcium requirements.

   (7) Iron requirements are greatly increased during pregnancy because of increased maternal blood volume and fetal demands.

      (a) The current RDA for iron is 30 mg/day.

         (i) It is difficult to get adequate iron intake from food sources during pregnancy; therefore, iron supplements (simple ferrous salts) are prescribed.

         (ii) Food sources include deep green leafy vegetables, enriched breads and cereals, legumes, liver, and dried fruits.

      (b) Pica, or consumption of nonfood substances, might displace more nutritious foods and interfere with absorption of nutrients, especially iron.

         (i) Either pica or iron deficiency anemia should lead to the investigation for the other problem.

         (ii) Women at highest risk for pica are from rural or inner-city areas, black, or those who have a family or childhood history of pica (Kaiser & Allen, 2002).

   (8) Sodium

      (a) Is currently not restricted unless a medical condition so warrants.

      (b) No fewer than 2 to 3 g of sodium should be consumed daily during a normal pregnancy.

(9) Other requirements can be met by a well-balanced diet and include
    (a) Vitamin E (10 mg/day)
    (b) Zinc (15 mg/day)
    (c) Iodine (175 fg/day)

4. Nutrition for optimal fetal health
  a. The fetus is dependent on the maternal host for nutrients.
  b. Because the fetus is in a state of growth and development, deprivation of essential nutrients can lead to stunted growth, various birth abnormalities, or spontaneous abortions.
  c. Nutritional knowledge in this area is not yet complete. Human research is based on observation and epidemiologic data (Worthington-Roberts & Williams, 1997).
  d. The following evidence is based on animal studies and is not conclusive or extensive (Worthington-Roberts & Williams, 1997).
    (1) Riboflavin (vitamin B_2) deficiency has been associated with poor skeletal formation.
    (2) Pyridoxine (vitamin B_6) deficiency has been associated with neuromotor problems.
    (3) Vitamin B_{12} deficiency has been associated with hydrocephalus.
    (4) Folic acid deficiencies are associated with neural tube defects.
    (5) The fetal growth stage known as hyperplasia, the time during the first trimester when the cells are rapidly dividing and multiplying, requires folic acid and vitamin B_{12}, which play a role in the synthesis of nucleic acids and prevention of neural tube defects.
    (6) The next fetal growth stage, known as hypertrophy, occurs during the second and third trimesters of pregnancy when the cells increase in size, and require amino acids and vitamin B_{12} for protein synthesis.
    (7) Iron is essential to maintain the maternal hemoglobin levels, which, in turn, supply oxygen to the developing fetus.
    (8) Inadequate caloric intake increases the risk of delivering an infant with intrauterine growth restriction (IUGR).
    (9) Excessive caloric intake (preexisting obesity or obesity that develops during pregnancy) increases the likelihood of macrosomia and the associated increases in operative births, birth trauma, and infant mortality.

CLINICAL PRACTICE

A. Assessment (comprehensive general health examination at first prenatal visit)
  1. History
    a. Current pregnancy
      (1) Menstrual history
        (a) Last menstrual period
        (b) Previous menstrual period
        (c) Last normal menstrual period
        (d) Menarche, age of onset
    b. Signs and symptoms (See earlier discussion of pregnancy signs and symptoms.)
    c. Risk assessment (at risk for a problem pregnancy)
      (1) Younger than 16 years, older than 35 years (See Chapter 7 for a complete discussion.)

    (2) History of induced abortions

    (3) Previous stillbirth or neonatal loss

    (4) Infant born prematurely, large for gestational age (LGA), with isoimmunization, or with congenital anomaly

    (5) History of maternal malignancy, genital tract anomaly, or medical indication for termination of previous pregnancy

    (6) Substance use or abuse: tobacco products, alcohol, or illicit or prescription drugs (See Chapter 27 for a complete discussion.)

    (7) Environmental factors: exposure to high levels of noise; radiation; or pollution of air, food, and water

    (8) Occupational hazards: anesthetic gases, lead, or paternal exposure to toxic agents (can transfer to female partner during intercourse) (See Chapter 9 for complete discussion of environmental effects.)

    (9) Abuse assessment; research suggests that intimate partner violence might increase during pregnancy. Screening should be instituted for women with unusual bruising, injury, or depression (Barash & Weinstein, 2002) (Refer to Chapter 20 for a complete discussion.)

2. Obstetric and gynecologic history
   a. Gravida/para system or gravidity, term, preterm, abortions, living children (G/TPAL) system
   b. Sexual history, including sexually transmitted diseases: syphilis, gonorrhea, herpes genitalia, trichomoniasis, condylomata acuminata (genital human papillomavirus [HPV] infection or genital warts), hepatitis B, chlamydial infection, and human immunodeficiency virus (HIV) infection (See Chapter 22 for a complete discussion.)
   c. Contraceptive history and use
   d. Infertility problems
   e. Description of previous pregnancies and their outcomes (length of gestations, type of delivery, and fetal outcome, including birth weight and maternal complications)

3. Cultural assessment including racial or ethnic background (refer to Chapter 4 for complete discussion)

4. Medical history
   a. Childhood diseases (especially infectious diseases)
   b. Other diseases (e.g., diabetes, asthma, urinary tract infections, varicosities, seizures)
   c. Surgery (blood transfusions)
   d. Injuries (especially to the pelvic region)
   e. Allergies (especially to drugs)
   f. Immunizations (especially rubella and chicken pox)
   g. Alcohol, caffeine, tobacco, and other drug use, including prescription, over-the-counter, and recreational drugs
   h. Exercise patterns
   i. Elimination patterns
   j. Sleep patterns
   k. Any significant stress
   l. Relationships with significant others, including potential for abuse

5. Nutrition history
   a. Overall factors to consider
      (1) Parity, in addition to the time intervals between each pregnancy, has an effect on nutrition reserves and the outcome of pregnancy, and it might generate increased nutritional needs.

       (a) Primigravidas usually gain more weight during pregnancy than multigravidas.

       (b) Short time intervals between pregnancies increase the challenge for nutrient repletion and maintenance of adequate nutrient stores.

       (c) A woman who had a previous low birth weight, IUGR, or preterm delivery needs to be identified in subsequent pregnancies for early counseling and assessment.

    (2) Age is an important consideration.

       (a) Adolescent pregnancy adds important considerations to clinical assessment.

          (i) Pregnant adolescents who, at the time of conception, are less mature gynecologically and undernourished have the greatest risks.

          (ii) Infants born to teenagers suffer a higher incidence of prematurity (fewer than 37 weeks), stillbirth, and low birth weight (fewer than 2500 g).

       (b) At the other range of the age spectrum, older women (40+) might incur more health risks during pregnancy than younger women (this effect is confounded with parity and might be associated with concurrent chronic illnesses). (See Chapter 7 for further considerations of age.)

    (3) Women of very low socioeconomic status are at risk for undernutrition, which leads to inadequate nutrient and energy intake, poor weight gain, and increased pregnancy complications and poor pregnancy outcomes.

    (4) A more careful dietary assessment is needed for women with chronic diseases, such as pregnancy-induced hypertension, diabetes, and cardiovascular disease, to prevent nutrition-related complications. (See Chapters 21, 24, and 28, respectively, for further discussion.)

    (5) Ethnic/cultural and religious background may determine which foods are customarily desirable and those that are not consumed.

    (6) Allergies might determine the need for dietary substitutions or supplements.

    (7) Women with multiple fetuses are advised to consult a dietician or nutritionist to ensure optimal nutrition and weight gain.

  b. A 24-hour recall, a verbal or written recollection of all foods, meals, and snacks eaten within the last 24-hour period can be helpful.

    (1) Food frequency analysis: the number of times each week a basic food is eaten

    (2) Additional factors to be considered

       (a) Where food is eaten

       (b) How much is eaten

       (c) How food is prepared (e.g., fried with a bread coating)

       (d) Which foods or odors seem to precipitate discomfort?

       (e) Which foods are limited and for what reasons

    (3) Compare data with the daily food guide recommendations for pregnancy and lactation (Figure 5-2) (it is not necessary to compute the RDA because it has been calculated into the guide).

6. Family medical history

  a. Health status of parents and siblings

  b. Family incidence of diabetes, cardiovascular disease, and hypertension

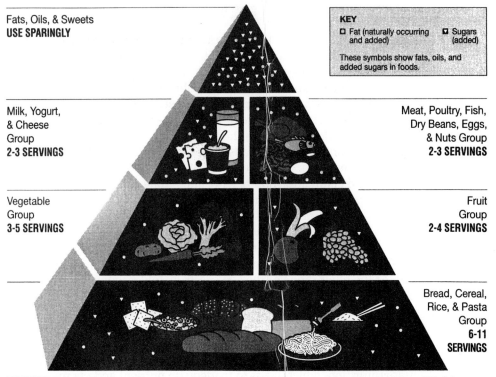

FIGURE 5-2 ■ Food guide pyramid. (Courtesy U.S. Department of Agriculture, Washington, DC.)

    c. Genetic and congenital diseases, abnormalities, or unexplained stillbirths
    d. Multiple births
  7. Father's health history
    a. Current health status, including health problems
    b. Blood type and rhesus (Rh) factor
    c. Family medical history
    d. Alcohol and drug use and abuse
  8. Social, family, and emotional history
  9. Review of physical systems
    a. General: weight change, fatigue, night sweats, chills or fever
    b. Skin, hair, and nails
    c. Head, ears, eyes, nose, and throat
    d. Mouth and teeth
    e. Breasts
    f. Respiratory
    g. Cardiovascular
    h. Gastrointestinal
    i. Genitourinary
    j. Musculoskeletal
    k. Neurologic (especially history of seizure activity)
    l. Hematologic
    m. Endocrine
    n. Psychiatric (mental disorders, especially depression)

B. **Physical examination**
  1. Initial visit
     a. Temperature, pulse, and respiration; blood pressure; height; and weight
     b. Breasts (changes consistent with early pregnancy)
     c. Abdomen (changes consistent with pregnancy)
     d. Pelvis (external genitalia, vagina, uterus, cervix, and adnexa) (See Chapter 1 for a complete discussion of anatomy and Chapter 10 for pelvic sizes and shapes.)
        (1) Bony pelvis, internal
           (a) Diagonal conjugate measurement: 12.5 cm
           (b) Sacral curve and shape (concave)
           (c) Ischial spines (prominence or bluntness)
           (d) Coccyx (moveable)
        (2) Pelvic outlet
           (a) Subpubic arch 4-to-5 cm wide and rounded
           (b) Distance between ischial tuberosities (biischial diameter) more than 11 cm
  2. Calculation of expected delivery date (EDD), expected confinement date (ECD), expected date of birth (EDB)
     a. Nägele's rule: 1st day of last menstrual period – 3 months + 7 days + 1 year (Littleton & Engebretson, 2002)
     b. Ultrasonic examination: measurement of crown-to-rump length; most accurate in first trimester to date the gestation.
  3. Physical assessment of nutritional status (Table 5-1)
     a. Blood pressure readings above 140/90 mmHg or an increase of 30 mmHg systolic or 15 mmHg diastolic over baseline blood pressure might indicate pregnancy-induced hypertension, if combined with other signs.
     b. Temperature readings above 37° C (98.6° F) might indicate infection, which might increase basal metabolic rate and protein requirements.
     c. Weight and height; calculation of BMI

■ TABLE 5-1
■ ■ **Physical Assessment of Nutritional Status**

Signs of Good Nutrition	Signs of Poor Nutrition
GENERAL APPEARANCE	
Alert, responsive, energetic, good endurance	Listless, apathetic, cachectic, easily fatigued, looks tired
WEIGHT	
Normal for height, age, body build	Overweight or underweight
POSTURE	
Erect, arms and legs straight	Sagging shoulders, sunken chest, humped back
MUSCLES	
Well developed, firm, good tone, some fat under skin	Flaccid, poor tone, undeveloped, tender, "wasted" appearance

Continued

■ TABLE 5-1
■ ■ Physical Assessment of Nutritional Status—cont'd

Signs of Good Nutrition	Signs of Poor Nutrition
NERVOUS CONTROL	
Good attention span, not irritable or restless, normal reflexes, psychological stability	Inattentive, irritable, confused, burning and tingling of hands and feet, loss of position and vibratory sense, weakness and tenderness of muscles, decrease or loss of ankle and knee reflexes
GASTROINTESTINAL FUNCTION	
Good appetite and digestion, normal regular elimination, no palpable organs or masses	Anorexia, indigestion, constipation or diarrhea, liver or spleen enlargement
CARDIOVASCULAR FUNCTION	
Normal heart rate and rhythm, no murmurs, normal blood pressure for age	Rapid heart rate, enlarged heart, abnormal rhythm, elevated blood pressure
HAIR	
Shiny, lustrous, firm, not easily plucked, healthy scalp	Stringy, dull, brittle, dry, thin and sparse, depigmented, can be easily plucked
SKIN (GENERAL)	
Smooth, slightly moist, good color	Rough, dry, scaly, pale, pigmented, irritated, easily bruised, petechiae
FACE AND NECK	
Skin color uniform smooth, pink, healthy appearance; no enlargement of thyroid gland; lips not chapped or swollen	Scaly, swollen, skin dark over cheeks and under eyes, lumpiness or flakiness of skin around nose and mouth; thyroid enlarged; lips swollen, angular lesions or fissures at corners of mouth
ORAL CAVITY	
Reddish pink mucous membranes and gums; no swelling or bleeding of gums; tongue healthy pink or deep reddish in appearance, not swollen or smooth, surface papillae present; teeth bright and clean, no cavities, no pain, no discoloration	Gums spongy, bleed easily, inflamed or receding; tongue swollen, scarlet and raw, magenta color, beefy, hyperemic and hypertrophic papillae, atrophic papillae; teeth with unfilled caries, absent teeth, worn surfaces, mottled
EYES	
Bright, clear, shiny, no sores at corners of eyelids, membranes moist and healthy pink color, no prominent blood vessels or mound of tissue (Bitot's spots) on sclera, no fatigue circles beneath	Eye membranes pale, redness of membrane, dryness, signs of infection, Bilot's spots, redness and fissuring of eyelid corners, dryness of eye membrane, dull appearance of cornea, soft cornea, blue sclerae
EXTREMITIES	
No tenderness, weakness, or swelling; nails firm and pink	Edema, tender calves, tingling, weakness; nails spoon-shaped, brittle
SKELETON	
No malformations	Bowlegs, knock-knees, chest deformity at diaphragm, beaded ribs, prominent scapulas

From Lowdermilk, D., Perry, S., & Bobak, I. (1997). *Maternity & women's health care* (6th ed.). St. Louis: Mosby.

d. Special nutritional consideration/problems
   (1) A vegetarian diet needs special consideration (Fisher, 1999).
      (a) Generally, a vegetarian diet is practiced because of physiologic, philosophic, or religious commitments.
      (b) Ensuring adequate protein and vitamin intake is an important consideration (Mangels, 2000).
      (c) Foods are usually combined to ensure enough protein in the diet (examples: legumes and grains; legumes and seeds; seeds and grains).
         (i) Only animal proteins are complete.
         (ii) By combining particular vegetable proteins, a complete source of essential amino acids can be achieved.
      (d) Vegetarianism classifications are
         (i) Ovolacto: excludes all animal protein but includes eggs and dairy products and all plant foods.
         (ii) Lacto: excludes all animal protein and eggs but includes dairy products and all plant foods.
         (iii) Vegan: excludes all animal products, including eggs and dairy products; diet consists of plant foods only.
   (2) Obesity: recent research has confirmed that obese pregnant women have a higher incidence of obstetric complications.
      (a) These women are at an increased risk for developing pregnancy-induced hypertension, diabetes, wound complications, thromboembolism, urinary tract infections, prolonged labor, and postpartum hemorrhage.
      (b) Obese women are at a greater risk to deliver macrosomic infants.
      (c) Newborns of obese mothers might also become obese infants.
      (d) Weight loss is not recommended during pregnancy; low-carbohydrate or low-calorie diets are ketogenic and can cause glucose deprivation to the fetal brain.
   (3) Pica is the compulsive ingestion of nonfood substances that have little or no nutritive value; one suggested reason for pica is that the body is lacking in some essential nutrient (Littleton & Engebretson, 2002).
      (a) The most commonly ingested substances are:
         (i) Dirt
         (ii) Clay
         (iii) Dry laundry starch
         (iv) A variety of other substances have also been known to be eaten, however, such as:
            ■ Ice
            ■ Hair
            ■ Gravel
            ■ Charcoal
            ■ Antacid tablets
            ■ Baking soda
            ■ Coffee grounds
            ■ Inner tubes
      (b) Pica is neither a new phenomenon nor one that is solely correlated to a geographic area, race, creed, culture, gender, or socioeconomic status.
      (c) Etiology and medical implications are not well understood, but the practice can lead to:

      (i) Inadequate intake of essential nutrients

      (ii) Intake of substances that might contain toxic compounds

      (iii) Interference with the absorption of certain minerals (e.g., iron)

      (iv) Lactose intolerance should not hinder the pregnant woman's ingestion of calcium-fortified foods during pregnancy.
- Suggested substitutions for milk or dairy products that are fairly well tolerated are:
  — Calcium-fortified tofu
  — Soy milk
  — Canned salmon with bones
  — Naturally aged hard cheese
  — Milk products (e.g., yogurt, sweet acidophilus milk, buttermilk, chocolate milk, cocoa)
  — Fortified orange juice
  — Commercial products that contain lactase (e.g., Lactaid)
- Although leafy green vegetables are high in calcium, the bioavailability of calcium may be inhibited by phytates.

4. Diagnostic procedures
  a. Pregnancy test (hCG levels in serum or urine) (Cunningham et al., 2001; Walsh, 2001)
    (1) Radioimmunoassay (RIA)
      (a) Based on antibodies against beta subunit hCG, radioimmunoassay is accurate as early as 1 week postovulation.
      (b) Other bioassay tests are prone to false-positive and false-negative results because of cross-reaction with LH.
      (c) Test time 1 to 5 hours, viewed as a disadvantage
    (2) Enzyme-linked immunosorbent assay (ELISA) most popular test
      (a) Monoclonal antibody binds with hCG (levels as low as 5 mIU/ml) in serum
      (b) Positive test indicated by color change in as little as 5 minutes
      (c) Home pregnancy tests (based on ELISA technology) are sensitive and accurate as early as day 1 of the expected menstrual cycle (provided the directions have been carefully followed).
  b. Blood
    (1) Complete blood count with differential smear
    (2) Hemoglobin, 12 to 16 g/dl (less than 11 g/dl might indicate iron-deficiency anemia)
    (3) Hematocrit, 38% to 47% (less than 35% may indicate iron-deficiency anemia)
    (4) Type and Rh factor
    (5) Antibody screen (Rh, D [Rho], rubeola, varicella, and toxoplasmosis)
    (6) Rubella titer more than 1:10 to confirm immunity
    (7) Screening for genetic diseases based on family history, ethnic or racial background (e.g., Tay-Sachs disease, thalassemia, sickle cell anemia)
    (8) Syphilis tests (serologic test for syphilis or Venereal Disease Research Laboratory [test] [VDRL])
    (9) Hepatitis B screen
    (10) Additional testing might be indicated based on the woman's history: HIV, alpha-fetoprotein, *Chlamydia,* rubeola, tuberculosis or group B streptococcus.

    c. Urinalysis: urine screening for glucose, protein, RBCs, WBCs, and bacteria
      (1) Ketone and glucose: elevated levels might indicate gestational or overt diabetes mellitus; low intake or absorption of ketones might indicate starvation ketosis.
      (2) Protein (albumin): increased levels after 20 weeks in the presence of hypertension might indicate preeclampsia.
    d. Cervical smears
      (1) Papanicolaou
      (2) Gonorrhea culture
      (3) *Chlamydia* culture
      (4) Herpes simplex (types 1 and 2), if indicated by history or observation
    e. Periodic revisits: normal pregnancy (National Guideline Clearinghouse [NGC], 2002; Walker, McCully, & Vest, 2001; Wilkinson, 2000)
      (1) Schedule is usually
        (a) Monthly until 28 weeks' gestation
        (b) Biweekly from 28 to 36 weeks' gestation
        (c) Weekly from 36 weeks until delivery
        (d) Healthy women might be placed on a reduced number or visits (9 vs the traditional 14) (Walker, McCully, & Vest, 2001).
      (2) Interval history: physical symptoms and maternal well-being, including emotional adjustment
      (3) Blood pressure and weight
      (4) Urinalysis: glucose and protein (dipstick, first morning voided specimen) (evidence suggests that this practice should be phased out as routine) (NGC, 2002)
      (5) Fetal well-being
        (a) Fundal height (Figure 5-3)
          (i) Fundus elevates out of pelvic area and can be palpated just above the symphysis pubis at about 12 weeks.
          (ii) Fundus rises to the level of the umbilicus at about 20 weeks and to the xiphoid process near term.
        (b) Value of symphysis-fundal height measurement called into question as a valid measure of fetal size and weight (Neilson, 2002)
        (c) Fetal heart rate
        (d) Fetal position determination: Leopold's maneuvers (See Chapter 10 for complete discussion of Leopold's maneuvers.)
        (e) Other possible tests: chorionic villus sampling, fetal movements determined by examiner, nonstress test (See Chapter 8 for complete discussion of antepartum fetal testing.)
        (f) Ultrasonography considered optional by some providers (Barash & Weinstein, 2002; Bickler & Neilson, 2003; NCG, 2002)
          (i) Controversy over value of routine screening in second trimester (Barash & Weinstein, 2002)
          (ii) Routine early screening is related to a decrease in induction rate for postterm infants.
          (iii) Routine late screening has not been shown to decrease morbidity or mortality.
      (6) Pelvic examination if indicated
      (7) Repeated or additional laboratory examinations
        (a) Maternal serum alpha-fetoprotein concentration at 15 to 20 weeks (elevated levels associated with neural tube defects)

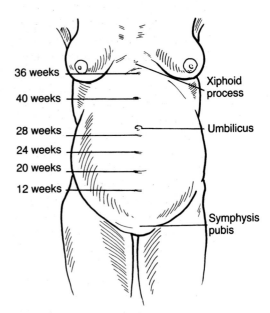

36 weeks

40 weeks

Xiphoid process

28 weeks

24 weeks

20 weeks

Umbilicus

12 weeks

FIGURE 5-3 ■ Fundal height.

Symphysis pubis

    (b) Hemoglobin or hematocrit at 26 to 28 weeks

    (c) Glucose screen at 24 to 28 weeks

    (d) Antibody screen (D [Rho]) at 28 weeks

    (e) Group B streptococci at 35 to 37 weeks (American College of Obstetricians and Gynecologists [ACOG], 2003)

    (f) Triple screen or multiple marker (must offer, but remains the client's choice) at 16 to 18 weeks (Barash & Weinstein, 2002; Cunningham et al., 2001) (See Chapter 8 for further discussion.)

        (i) Maternal serum alpha-fetoprotein (MSAFP), hCG, and unconjugated estriol examined (expanded MSAFP test)

        (ii) Low levels might be associated with Down syndrome and other chromosomal abnormalities

        (iii) High levels might be associated with poor pregnancy outcomes

    (g) Tests for sexually transmitted diseases, if indicated (e.g., gonorrhea)

C. Nursing Diagnoses

    1. Deficient knowledge related to normal physical responses to pregnancy

    2. Constipation related to changes in gastrointestinal tract normally occurring in pregnancy

    3. Imbalanced nutrition: more than body requirements related to excessive intake of calories

    4. Imbalanced nutrition: less than body requirements related to inadequate information about nutritional needs during pregnancy

    5. Activity intolerance related to fatigue related to physiologic changes of pregnancy

D. Interventions/Outcomes (Johnson, Maas, & Moorhead, 2000; McCloskey & Bulechek, 2000)

    1. Deficient knowledge related to normal physical responses to pregnancy

        a. Interventions

        (1) Instruct client on importance of regular prenatal care throughout entire pregnancy.

        (2) Encourage parents to attend prenatal classes.

   (3) Instruct client on danger signs that warrant immediate reporting.
      (a) Vaginal bleeding
      (b) Leaking of fluid from the vagina
      (c) Sudden swelling of the face or fingers
      (d) Headache not relieved by normal measures
      (e) Blurred vision
      (f) Abdominal pain
      (g) Chills or fever
      (h) Severe or prolonged vomiting
   (4) Give client anticipatory guidance about physiologic changes accompanying pregnancy.
   (5) Assist client in managing changes associated with pregnancy.
   (6) Refer client to childbirth preparation class.
   b. Outcomes
   (1) Client can provide description of physical and psychologic changes of pregnancy.
   (2) Client can identify warning signs of pregnancy complications.
   (3) Client acknowledges importance of prenatal education.
   (4) Client acknowledges importance of prenatal care.
2. Constipation related to changes in gastrointestinal tract normally occurring in pregnancy
   a. Interventions
   (1) Instruct client/family on the relationship of diet, exercise, and fluid intake to constipation.
   (2) Explain etiology of problem and rationale for actions to client.
   (3) Encourage increased fluid intake, unless contraindicated.
   (4) Instruct on high-fiber diet.
   (5) Instruct on the appropriate use of laxatives.
   (6) Teach client how to keep a food diary.
   (7) Evaluate recorded intake for nutritional content.
   b. Outcomes
   (1) Client's elimination pattern is within expected range.
   (2) Client's stool is soft and formed.
   (3) Client ingests adequate fluids.
   (4) Client ingests adequate fiber.
3. Imbalanced nutrition: more than body requirements related to excessive intake of calories
   a. Interventions
   (1) Determine client's food intake and eating habits.
   (2) Facilitate identification of eating behaviors to be changed.
   (3) Discuss nutritional requirements and client's perception of recommended diet.
   (4) Discuss client's food likes and dislikes.
   (5) Assist client in recording what is usually eaten in a 24-hour period.
   (6) Discuss the meaning of food.
   (7) Increase physical activity (e.g., walking).
   (8) Use accepted dietary standards to assist client in evaluating adequacy of dietary intake.
   (9) Evaluate progress of dietary modification goals at regular intervals.
   b. Outcomes
   (1) Oral food intake adequate
   (2) Oral fluid intake adequate

4. Imbalanced nutrition: less than body requirements related to inadequate information about nutritional needs during pregnancy
   a. Interventions
      (1) Teach client and family meal planning and how to increase caloric intake.
         (a) A balanced diet is composed of 55% to 60% carbohydrate calories, 12% to 15% protein calories, and 25% to 30% fat calories.
         (b) The food selection should incorporate highly nutrient-dense foods.
         (c) Selection of foods should fit the person's lifestyle, cultural norms/traditions, and budget.
         (d) Recommend eating small meals frequently to obtain adequate kilocalories for weight gain and protein conservation.
      (2) Teach client about the balance between excessive exercise and rest; might need to eliminate if maternal weight is too low.
      (3) Provide education about the higher risk of adverse birth outcomes.
         (a) Weight gain of at least 12.5 to 18 kg (28 to 40 lb).
         (b) Limit foods that have empty calories.
         (c) Recommend eating between meals.
      (4) Refer to community agencies as appropriate.
         (a) Consider referral to WIC program (Special Supplemental Program for Women, Infants & Children) for those who fulfill eligibility requirements.
         (b) Encourage participation in support groups as appropriate.
         (c) Provide referral/consultation with other health-team members as appropriate.
      (5) Chart weight-gain progress.
   b. Outcomes
      (1) Nutrient intake adequate
      (2) Food and fluid intake adequate
      (3) Energy level acceptable
      (4) Weight at acceptable level
5. Activity intolerance related to fatigue caused by the physiologic changes of pregnancy
   a. Interventions
      (1) Determine client's health beliefs concerning physical exercise.
      (2) Inform client about health benefits and physiologic effects of exercise.
      (3) Instruct client about appropriate type of exercise for pregnancy.
      (4) Instruct client about conditions warranting cessation of or alteration in the exercise program.
      (5) Instruct client on proper warm-up and cool-down exercises.
      (6) Assist client in developing appropriate exercise program to avoid fatigue.
   b. Outcomes
      (1) Perceived importance of taking action
      (2) Perceived threat from inaction
      (3) Perceived benefits of action
      (4) Perceived control of health outcome

HEALTH EDUCATION

A. **First trimester**
   1. Physiologic changes of pregnancy with resulting discomforts
      a. Pain and tingling in breasts

   b. Nausea and vomiting (morning sickness)
   c. Urinary frequency
   d. Fatigue
   e. Mood swings
  2. Danger signs that should be reported
   a. Vaginal bleeding
   b. Abdominal cramping
   c. Severe and prolonged vomiting
  3. Health teaching (use principles of teaching and learning)
   a. Schedule of return visits for routine prenatal care
   b. General hygiene
   c. Comfort measures for trimester-related discomforts
   d. Anticipatory guidance regarding duration of current discomforts
   e. Sexual activity
   f. Physical activities, exercise, and rest
    (1) Exercise is safe in uncomplicated pregnancies (Lively, 2002).
    (2) Mild to moderate exercise is encouraged.
    (3) Athletes should avoid sports that carry a risk of abdominal trauma.
    (4) Recommend adequate hydration and nutrition essential for well-being of client and fetus (Dundas & Taylor, 2002).
   g. Nutritional guidance, weight gain, and diet
    (1) Multiple pregnancy
     (a) Theoretically, the nutritional needs of a woman carrying more than one fetus should be greater to support extra blood volume and placental/fetal tissue.
     (b) There has been no formal evaluation of needs, however, and specific guidelines have not been developed (Reifsnider & Gill, 2000).
     (c) Total weight gain recommendations are between 40 and 45 lb (18.2 to 20.5 kg) for twins and 45 to 50 lb (20.5 to 22.7 kg) for triplets.
     (d) General dietary recommendations include the following:
      (i) Follow all dietary recommendations of non-risk pregnancy (see earlier).
      (ii) Eat nutrient-dense foods.
      (iii) Increase protein and calcium intake as necessary.
      (iv) Eat small, frequent meals.
    (2) For women who are vegetarians, the assumption of malnutrition is not supported by nutrition research, although supplements may be recommended to meet nutritional needs.
   h. Encourage avoidance of alcohol (leading cause of mental retardation; fetal alcohol syndrome).
   i. Educate on smoking cessation (if indicated).
B. Second trimester
  1. Physiologic changes with resulting discomforts
   a. Enlargement of abdomen
   b. Skin pigmentation
   c. Striae gravidarum
   d. Vascular spiders

        e. Constipation

        f. Heartburn

        g. Leg cramps

        h. Groin pain from round ligament stretching

        i. Leukorrhea

   2. Danger signs that should be reported

        a. Vaginal bleeding

        b. Burning or painful urination

        c. Signs of fever

        d. Reduction in or absence of fetal movements

        e. Nausea and vomiting

        f. Abdominal pain or cramping

        g. Swelling of face or fingers, headaches, visual disturbances, or epigastric pain

   3. Health teaching

        a. Reinforcement and reiteration of previous teaching

        b. Comfort measures specific to trimester-related discomforts

        c. Anticipatory guidance regarding duration of current discomforts

        d. Choices of prenatal education classes

        e. Signs and symptoms of preterm labor

C. Third trimester

   1. Physiologic changes with resulting discomforts

        a. Dyspnea

        b. Leg and feet cramps

        c. Constipation

        d. Indigestion, heartburn

        e. Pedal edema

        f. Fatigue

        g. Vaginal discharge

        h. Urinary frequency

        i. Braxton Hicks contractions

   2. Danger signs that should be reported

        a. Visual disturbance

        b. Headache

        c. Hand and facial edema

        d. Fever

        e. Vaginal bleeding

        f. Abdominal pain; uterine contractions

        g. Premature rupture of membranes

        h. Decreased or lack of fetal movement

   3. Health teaching

        a. Signs and symptoms of labor/preterm labor

        b. When to call the health care provider, when to go to the hospital or birthing place

        c. Comfort measures for trimester-related discomforts

        d. Anticipatory guidance regarding duration of present discomforts

        e. Reinforcement and reiteration of previous teaching

CASE STUDIES AND STUDY QUESTIONS

Ms. L is a 26-year-old woman who has registered at the clinic for prenatal care. She reports fatigue, nausea, and constipation. Her last normal menstrual period was 8 weeks ago, and the home pregnancy test result was positive. This is her first pregnancy.

1. Presumptive signs of pregnancy include:
   a. Ballottement
   b. Braxton Hicks contractions
   c. Breast changes
   d. Positive pregnancy test results

2. The bluish discoloration of the vagina is known as:
   a. Chadwick's sign
   b. Hegar's sign
   c. Goodell's sign
   d. Braxton's sign

3. A normal physiologic change associated with the first trimester of pregnancy is:
   a. Increased respirations
   b. Increased peristalsis
   c. Increased resistance to infection
   d. Increased cardiac output

4. Health teaching of particular importance at this early stage of pregnancy includes:
   a. Comfort measures for trimester-related discomforts
   b. Choices of prenatal education classes
   c. Signs and symptoms of labor
   d. Infant feeding techniques

Ms. T, at 27 weeks' gestation, comes to the clinic for a routine prenatal visit. This is her fourth pregnancy, and she has four living children (with one set of twins).

5. How would her obstetric history be recorded?

6. Routine laboratory tests that should be repeated at this visit include:

   a. hCG level
   b. Rubella titer
   c. Antibody screen
   d. Complete blood count with differential smear

7. She reports feeling fatigued and is bothered by constipation. These symptoms are related to the hormone:
   a. Estrogen
   b. hCG
   c. Thyroxine
   d. Relaxin

8. Her hemoglobin value is 11.7 g/dl. Which factor explains this finding?
   a. The trimester of pregnancy
   b. Hemodilution of pregnancy
   c. The presence of iron-deficiency anemia
   d. Greater-than-expected weight gain

Ms. S, age 16, is a finicky eater. She is very weight conscious and has tried several fad diets in the past. Ms. S rarely eats breakfast; when she does, it consists of a glass of orange juice and a piece of toast. At noon, she usually eats an apple or an orange. After school, she is famished and snacks on cookies, soda, and ice cream. Frequently, her evening meal consists of pizza, or a milk shake and a hamburger. She has just learned that she is pregnant, and she is horrified that she might become fat. Her medical history includes anemia. Present weight is 112 lb (50.9 kg) and height is 5 ft, 7 in (1.86 m).

9. How much weight should she gain to ensure a healthy pregnancy?
   a. 28 to 40+ lb
   b. 25 to 35 lb
   c. More than 55 lb
   d. 15 to 22 lb

10. The RDAs for energy include an extra _____ kilocalories to support needs associated with the second

and third trimesters of pregnancy.
a. 200
b. 250
c. 300
d. 350

11. When assessing the nutritional status of Ms. S, one of the best methods for obtaining dietary information is to:
a. Consult with family members.
b. Ask her where she usually eats.
c. Ask her how many meals she eats.
d. Obtain a verbal and written 24-dietary recall.

12. Which of the following factors is not a nutritional risk at the onset of pregnancy or during pregnancy?
a. Low hemoglobin or hematocrit
b. BMI within 90% to 110% of standard prepregnancy BMI
c. Inadequate weight gain
d. Poverty

ADDITIONAL STUDY QUESTIONS

13. The increase in uterine size during pregnancy is primarily the result of which of the following factors?
a. Growth of the fetus
b. Formation of new muscle fibers
c. Increase in blood circulation to the uterus
d. Stretching of existing muscle fibers

14. The primary source of the hormones estrogen and progesterone during early pregnancy is the:
a. Placenta
b. Anterior lobe of the pituitary gland
c. Corpus luteum
d. Adrenal cortex

15. The expected height of the fundus at 20 weeks' gestation is:

a. At the xiphoid process
b. At the umbilicus
c. Halfway between the symphysis pubis and umbilicus
d. At the symphysis pubis

16. A pregnant woman should immediately report which of the following symptoms to her health care provider?
a. Leg cramps
b. Abdominal pain
c. Dyspnea
d. Heartburn

17. Normal physiologic responses to pregnancy include:
a. Increased cardiac output
b. Increased peristalsis
c. Increased respirations
d. Increased blood pressure

ANSWERS TO STUDY QUESTIONS

1. c
2. a
3. d
4. a
5. G4, P3
6. c
7. d
8. b
9. a
10. c
11. d
12. b
13. d
14. c
15. b
16. b
17. a

REFERENCES

American College of Obstetricians and Gynecologists. (2003). *ACOG Advises Screening All Pregnant Women for Group B Strep*. Washington, DC: Author. Retrieved February 13, 2003 from *www.acog.org/from_home/publications/press_releases/nr11-29-02-1.cfm*.

Barash, J.H., & Weinstein, L.C. (2002). Preconception and prenatal care. *Primary Care Clinical Office Practice, 29*, 519-542.

Bickler, L., & Neilson, J.P. (2003). Routine Doppler ultrasound in pregnancy. In *The Cochrane Library*, Vol 1. Oxford: Update Software.

Cesario, S.K. (2003). Obesity in pregnancy: What every nurse should know. *AWHONN Lifelines 7*, 119-125.

Cunningham, F.G., Gant, N.F., Leveno, K.J., Gilstrap, L.C. III, Hauth, J.C. & Wenstrom, K.D. (2001). *Williams obstetrics* (21st ed.). New York: McGraw-Hill.

Dundas, M.L., & Taylor, S. (2002). Perinatal factors, motivation, and attitudes concerning pregnancy affect dietary intake. *Topics in Clinical Nutrition, 17,* 71-79.

Fisher, M. (Winter 1999). Vegan pregnancy. Retrieved March 11, 2003 from *www.midwiferytoday.com*.

Johnson, M., Maas, M., & Moorhead, S. (2000). *Nursing Outcomes Classification (NOC)* (2nd ed.). St. Louis: Mosby.

Kaiser, L.L., & Allen, L. (2002). Position of the American Dietetic Association: Nutrition and lifestyle for a healthy pregnancy outcome. *Journal of the American Dietetic Association, 102*(10), 1479-1490.

Lederman, S.A. (2001). Pregnancy weight gain and postpartum loss: Avoiding obesity while optimizing the growth and development of the fetus. *Journal of the American Medical Women's Association, 56*(2), 53-58.

Littleton, L.Y, & Engebretson, J.C. (2002). *Maternal, neonatal, and women's health nursing*. Albany, NY: Delmar-Thompson Learning.

Lively, M.W. (2002). Sport participation and pregnancy. *Athletic Therapy Today, 7,* 11-15.

Lowdermilk, D.L., Perry, S. E. (2004). *Maternity & women's health care* (8th ed.). St. Louis: Mosby.

Mangels, R. (2000). Protein in the vegan diet. The Vegetarian Resource Group. Retrieved March 11, 2003, from *www.vrg.org/nutrition/protein.htm*.

McCloskey, J.C., & Bulechek, G.M. (2000). *Nursing interventions classification (NIC)* (3rd ed.). St. Louis: Mosby.

National Guideline Clearinghouse (NGC). (August 2002). Routine prenatal care. Retrieved March 11, 2003 from *www.Guideline.gov/VIEWS/*.

Neilson, J.P. (2002). Symphysis-fundal height measurement in pregnancy. In *The Cochrane Library*, Vol 4. Oxford: Update Software.

Reifsnider, E., & Gill, S.L. (2000). Nutrition for the childbearing years. *Journal of Obstetric, Gynecologic, and Neonatal Nursing, 29*(1), 43-55.

Walker, D.S., McCully, L., & Vest, V. (2001). Evidence-based prenatal care visits: When less is more. *Journal of Midwifery and Women's Health, 46*(3), 146-151.

Walsh, L.V. (2001). *Midwifery: Community-based care during the childbearing year*. Philadelphia: W.B. Saunders.

Wilkinson, L.D. (2000). Care and counseling by trimester. *Family Practice Recertification, 22*, 61-76.

Worthington-Roberts, B.S., & Williams, S.R. (1997). *Nutrition in pregnancy and lactation* (6th ed.). Boston: McGraw-Hill.

6 Psychology of Pregnancy

CATHERINE R. COVERSTON

OBJECTIVES

1. Describe two stages of family development pertinent to pregnancy.
2. List the developmental tasks of pregnancy.
3. List the general concepts in Rubin's tasks of pregnancy.
4. Discuss two psychosocial findings in normal pregnancy.
5. Discuss strategies to minimize self-concept disturbances during pregnancy.
6. Discuss risks related to eating disorders during pregnancy.
7. Discuss the effects of increased technology in America on a woman's psychological experience of pregnancy.
8. Describe three needs of fathers during labor and delivery.
9. Identify two reactions of fathers to pregnancy.
10. Describe changes in sexual feelings and behaviors in pregnancy.
11. Discuss the concept of developmental crises in pregnancy.
12. Describe how to assist families in developing a birth plan and selecting childbirth education.
13. Enumerate maternal behaviors exhibited during pregnancy validation.
14. Describe maternal behaviors exhibited during fetal embodiment.
15. Differentiate maternal behaviors seen during fetal distinction.
16. List the most common maternal behaviors observed in role transition.
17. Identify maternal behaviors indicative of Rubin's task of safe passage as it relates to the last trimester of pregnancy.
18. Describe issues seen in the last trimester involving acceptance of the child by others.

INTRODUCTION

Pregnancy is a time of increased susceptibility to psychologic stress for expectant mothers and fathers. Pregnancy and childbearing are developmental phases in family life that are often characterized by ambivalence and conflicting emotions, as expectant parents face significant role and lifestyle changes.

CLINICAL PRACTICE

A. Assessment
    1. History
        a. Family background
            (1) Economic status

(2) Marital status
(3) Age
(4) Support system
(5) Self-esteem
(6) Role models
(7) Culture
(8) Religion
(9) Stability of living conditions
   b. Obstetric experience
(1) Previous pregnancies
(2) Prior pregnancy outcomes
(3) Pregnancy experiences of extended family and friends
(4) Previous experience with infants and neonates
(5) Unresolved grief or anger related to previous experiences
   c. Current pregnancy
(1) Wanted or unwanted
(2) Planned or unplanned
(3) Mother's health: healthy or unhealthy before and during this pregnancy
(4) The woman's and partner's learning capabilities and/or limitations
(5) Whether the woman has healthy or unhealthy personal relationships
(6) The status of her pregnancy: low risk or high risk
2. Duvall's stages of family development
   a. Married couple beginning a family
(1) Attainment of a satisfying relationship
(2) The dyad is the easiest and first relationship of family development
   b. Expectant family: role preparation
(1) Reorganization of the household for the infant
(2) Development of new patterns of making and spending money
(3) Realignment of tasks and responsibilities
(4) Adaptation of sexual relationship to the pregnancy
(5) Reorientation of relationships with relatives
(6) Adaptation of relationships with friends and associates
(7) Increase in knowledge about pregnancy, birth, and parenting
(8) Adaptation to accelerated emotional changes
   c. Childbearing family (from the time of the first birth to the time when the last child attains the age of 30 months)
(1) Adjust to a changing relationship (i.e., dyad to triad).
(2) Encourage the development of the new infant.
(3) Introduce each new infant to the existing siblings.
3. Psychosocial findings
   a. Thoughts and desires
(1) Food cravings might occur during pregnancy.
(2) Sexual behaviors, desires, and thoughts vary throughout pregnancy.
      (a) Might decrease in late pregnancy for some.
      (b) Might remain unchanged for others.
(3) Dream life is very active in pregnancy.

        (4) Chronic fatigue, especially during the first and third trimesters, might influence desires and thoughts.

    b. Mood swings

        (1) Ambivalence about becoming a mother appears in early pregnancy in most women.

        (2) Irritability might increase throughout pregnancy and might peak in the ninth month, when fatigue is the greatest.

        (3) Increased sensitivity might exist throughout the entire pregnancy.

        (4) A sense of vulnerability tends to peak during the seventh month.

        (5) The woman might experience frustration with her own indecisiveness throughout the pregnancy.

        (6) Normal fears might exist (e.g., about the health of the infant and about her ability to give birth safely).

  4. Pregnancy as a developmental (maturational) crisis

    a. Danger of increased psychologic vulnerability at this time

    b. Increased opportunity for personal growth

    c. Increased susceptibility to stress because of potential for changes in areas such as work, housing needs, and access to care

    d. Alteration in role and identity for each parent and for each member of the family

  5. Developmental tasks of pregnancy progressive over time

    a. Pregnancy validation

        (1) Most women have an initial ambivalence about being pregnant.

        (2) Many women experience fantasies and dreams about themselves and how pregnancy will change their lives.

    b. Fetal embodiment

        (1) The woman incorporates the fetus into her body image.

        (2) She becomes dependent on her partner or on significant others.

        (3) She is typically introspective and calm.

    c. Fetal distinction

        (1) The woman conceptualizes her fetus as a separate individual.

        (2) She accepts her new body image and might characterize it as being full of life.

        (3) She typically becomes more dependent on her mother or feels closer to her mother at this time.

    d. Role transition

        (1) She prepares to separate from and give up the physical, symbiotic attachment with her fetus.

        (2) She becomes anxious about impending labor and delivery.

        (3) She exhibits "nesting" behaviors or a need to get all the supplies needed for the infant (preterm labor is a major disruption of the need to nest).

        (4) She becomes impatient with her awkward body and is anxious for pregnancy to end; she states frequently that she is tired of being pregnant.

        (5) She feels prepared to mother the infant.

  6. Rubin's tasks of pregnancy occur concurrently with each other.

    a. General principles

        (1) Pregnancy progressively becomes a part of the woman's total identity.

(2) The woman is able to share relatively little of her sensory experience with others, which makes her feel unique.

(3) The woman's focus turns progressively inward as the pregnancy advances.

(4) The woman generally becomes overly sensitive.

(5) She seeks the company of other women, especially other pregnant women.

(6) The absence of a female support system during pregnancy is a singular index of a high-risk pregnancy.

b. Acceptance of pregnancy and incorporating the reality of pregnancy into her self-concept is called "binding-in."

(1) First trimester: she accepts the idea of pregnancy, but not of the child.

(2) Second trimester: there is a dramatic change, with the sensation of fetal movement (quickening); she becomes aware of the child as a separate entity within her.

(3) Third trimester: she wants the child and is tired of being pregnant.

c. Acceptance of the child

(1) First trimester: acceptance of the pregnancy by herself and others.

(2) Acceptance of the child by others is the keystone of a successful adjustment to pregnancy.

(3) Second trimester: the family needs to relate to the infant (e.g., as a son or brother).

(4) Third trimester: the critical issue is the unconditional acceptance of the child; conditional acceptance implies rejection.

d. Reordering of relationships and learning to give of herself

(1) First trimester: examines what needs to be given up.

(a) Trade-offs for having the infant

(b) Might grieve the loss of a carefree life

(2) Second trimester: identifies with the child.

(3) Third trimester: has decreased confidence in her ability to become a good mother to her child.

e. Safe passage: Rubin suggests that this task usually receives most of the woman's attention.

(1) First trimester: focuses on herself, not on her infant.

(2) Second trimester: develops an attachment of great value to her infant.

(3) Third trimester: has concern for herself and her infant as a unit.

(a) At the seventh month, she is in a state of high vulnerability.

(b) She sees labor and delivery as deliverance and as a hope, not as a threat.

7. Expectant fathers

a. Psychosocial findings during pregnancy

(1) Couvade: some men actually experience symptoms of pregnancy.

(a) Weight gain

(b) Nausea

(c) Other common physical symptoms of pregnancy

(2) Expectant fathers vary widely in their reactions to pregnancy as well as to the psychologic and physical changes in the woman.

(a) Some enjoy the role of nurturer.

(b) Some experience alienation, which might lead to extramarital affairs.

       (c) Some view the pregnancy as a proof of masculinity and assume a dominant role.

       (d) Some believe pregnancy has no meaning and carries no particular responsibility to the mother or child.

b. Paternal tasks of pregnancy

  (1) First trimester: announcement phase

       (a) Must cope with ambivalence about becoming a father.

       (b) Strives to accept the biologic fact of pregnancy.

       (c) Attempts to take on the expectant father role.

  (2) Second trimester: moratorium phase

       (a) Often has a delay of "binding-in" to the pregnancy compared with the woman.

       (b) Accepts the woman's changing body.

       (c) Accepts the reality of the fetus, particularly when fetal movement is felt.

       (d) Adapts to the changes in their sexual relationship.

         (i) Frequently has fears about harming the fetus during sexual intercourse.

         (ii) Might experience a potential rivalry with a male obstetrician.

       (e) Experiences confusion when dealing with the woman's intense introspection.

       (f) Fantasizes about the father-child relationship (with the child not as an infant but as an older child—playing ball, for example).

  (3) Third trimester: focusing phase

       (a) Negotiates what his role will be during labor and delivery.

       (b) Prepares for the reality of parenthood.

       (c) Might change his self-concept and image (e.g., might shave his beard and buy new clothes).

       (d) Engages in preparing the nursery.

       (e) Copes with fears about the mutilation or the death of his partner and child.

c. Fathers at labor and birth

  (1) Benefits

       (a) Might dispel his feelings of alienation.

       (b) Might increase his sense of significance and importance.

       (c) Might increase his sense of control.

       (d) Might increase his appreciation for his laboring woman/partner.

       (e) Might develop a closer attachment to his newborn earlier in the father-child relationship.

  (2) Roles of fathers during labor and birth

       (a) A *coach* is very involved and needs a high level of control.

       (b) A *teammate* needs less control but provides emotional and physical support.

       (c) A *witness* is there as a companion, provides support, but looks to others for instruction and support; needs very little control.

  (3) There is a need for sensitivity to a father's unfamiliarity with such things as:

       (a) Unfamiliar sights; for example:

         (i) His wife/girlfriend in pain and grimacing

         (ii) Bulging perineum

　　　　(iii) Blood and fluids
　　　　(iv) Others touching his partner in intimate ways
　　　(b) Unfamiliar sounds; for example:
　　　　(i) Moans, grunts
　　　　(ii) Hospital noises
　　　(c) Unfamiliar smells; for example:
　　　　(i) Vaginal discharge, amniotic fluid
　　　　(ii) Cleaning solutions and medications
　　　(d) The father has his own needs
　　　　(i) Fatigue
　　　　(ii) Hunger
　　　　(iii) Fears and concerns
　　(4) Other considerations about expectant fathers at labor and birth
　　　(a) Some cultures bar men from labor and birth (e.g., certain Middle Eastern cultures).
　　　(b) Some men do not want to be present for labor and/or birth.
　　　(c) Some women do not want the father to see them "like that."
8. Other family members' psychosocial reactions to pregnancy and childbirth
　a. Expectant siblings
　　(1) Reaction to pregnancy is age dependent.
　　(2) Siblings might express excitement and anticipation.
　　(3) Siblings might verbalize negative reactions.
　　(4) Siblings might be unaware or noncommittal.
　　(5) Siblings who are present at birth need a caretaker whose major focus is meeting the needs of the sibling (i.e., involvement or withdrawal from the process).
　　(6) Siblings might exhibit ambivalent reactions to a newborn in the home.
　　　(a) Show affection and excitement
　　　(b) Might vacillate, with regressive behavior, anger, or both.
　b. Expectant grandparents
　　(1) Often express excitement and anticipation.
　　(2) Might express resentment (e.g., "I'm too young to be someone's grandmother!").
　　(3) Might verbalize anger if the pregnancy was unplanned or if the mother is a teenager or is unwed.
　　(4) Often express anxiety about the health and well-being of the expectant mother (daughter or daughter-in-law) and fetus.
　　(5) Might be concerned about the expectant parents' age, income, and emotional stability to have a child.
9. Single expectant mother's psychosocial needs
　a. Reason for single status needs to be assessed to better understand the meaning of pregnancy
　　(1) Single by choice: pregnancy might have been by artificial insemination.
　　(2) Single by accident; for example, a woman became a widow after conception or became pregnant through rape.
　　(3) Single by divorce or separation after conception.
　　(4) Single and pregnant by a casual acquaintance (unplanned or planned).

    b. Presence or absence of strong support persons can significantly influence the woman's adaptation to pregnancy.

    c. Future plans for the child are an important factor influencing the mother's psychologic needs (i.e., is she planning to keep and raise the child or planning to place the child for adoption? Is she a surrogate parent?).

  10. Ethnocultural considerations

    a. In the United States, there are mixed cultural messages about behavior during pregnancy and birth.

    b. Technologic culture is dominant in U.S. health care.

      (1) Use of technology creates a potential to increase stress and anxiety in the pregnant woman.

        (a) Moral and ethical dilemmas frequently are associated with diagnostic tests.

        (b) The woman's interpersonal and emotional needs and feelings might be missed or ignored in favor of technologic information.

      (2) There is an increased chance of caregivers' shifting their focus from the woman to the equipment.

      (3) The concept of "tentative pregnancy" involves the inability or unwillingness to fully accept or embrace one's pregnancy until all prenatal diagnostic test results have been received.

      (4) Technology might prevent women from viewing pregnancy with the "ignorant bliss" of earlier generations.

      (5) The woman might feel that she must trust technology more than her own instincts and inner self.

    c. General principles regarding pregnancy among varying cultures

      (1) Pregnancy is considered to be normal, not a state of illness in many cultures (e.g., some American Indian tribes, most Latin cultures).

      (2) Women of some cultures might only seek care if they believe there is something wrong or for technology, such as ultrasound.

      (3) Pregnancy often has many rigid taboos (e.g., some African nations).

      (4) Pregnancy might be viewed as only woman's work (e.g., Middle Eastern cultures).

      (5) Yin-yang: everything in nature is balanced; for example, hot/cold (e.g., Korean cultures).

      (6) Some cultures stress pregnancy behaviors that are protective, whereas others do not (avoidance of substance abuse, improved diet).

      (7) Protective behaviors might be compromised as immigrants become more acculturated and give up protective behaviors (e.g., use of tobacco, less healthy food such as fast food).

  11. Psychosocial alterations affecting perinatal adaptation and outcomes

    a. Postpartum mood disorders

    b. Eating disorders

      (1) Three types in the *Diagnostic and Statistical Manual of Mental Disorders* (fourth edition) (DSM-IV):

        (a) Anorexia nervosa

          (i) Intentional loss of body weight 15% below recommended weight

            ■ Body image distortion and amenorrhea common

            ■ Preoccupation with weight and eating

        (ii) Achieved by severe food restriction, exercise, fasting, as well as purging through vomiting; laxative and diuretic abuse; and diet pills

        (iii) Affects about 0.3% to 1% of the population.

        (iv) Very difficult to treat; often chronic and concurrent with other psychiatric disorders

    (b) Bulimia nervosa

        (i) Binge eating with purging; excessive exercise

        (ii) Usually normal weight

        (iii) Undue focus on body image

    (c) Eating disorders not otherwise specified

        (i) Do not meet criteria for anorexia or bulimia but might binge eat.

        (ii) Pregnancy might push a woman into full-blown anorexia or bulimia.

(2) Effects on pregnancy

    (a) Anorexia nervosa

        (i) Fertility: contrary to popular belief, women with anorexia do not seem to have decreased fertility, even with amenorrhea.

        (ii) Complications

           ■ Higher cesarean rates

           ■ Higher rate of miscarriages

           ■ Low infant birth weight

           ■ Higher incidence of congenital malformation

    (b) Bulimia nervosa

        (i) Symptoms increase in pregnancy.

        (ii) Might smoke or restrict eating to control weight.

        (iii) Complications

           ■ Higher miscarriage rate

           ■ Hypertension more common

    (c) Complications associated with all eating disorders

        (i) Infant

           ■ Low birthweight infants

           ■ Low APGAR scores

           ■ Higher occurrence of breech presentation

           ■ Higher incidence of cleft palate

           ■ Higher incidence of stillbirth

        (ii) Mother

           ■ Higher incidence of bleeding during pregnancy

           ■ Delay in wound healing

           ■ Complications no more prevalent in women with eating disorders than in any other pregnancy if normal pregnancy weight gain is maintained

(3) Detection of eating disorders

    (a) Evaluate feelings about being weighed.

    (b) Evaluate history of amenorrhea, unexplained pregnancy loss, or infants with difficulties.

    (c) Evaluate for history of sexual or physical abuse as well as other psychiatric disorders.

    (d) Determine if cosmetic surgery has been obtained to alter the body.

(e) Evaluate history, which is likely to indicate many weight gains and losses in the past.

(f) Evaluate exercise and caffeine patterns, food allergies or phobias, restrictions such as vegetarianism.

(g) Look for failure to gain weight in two consecutive visits during the second trimester.

c. Grief and loss in the perinatal period

  (1) Grief and loss might be triggered by several events related to pregnancy.

    (a) Spontaneous abortion

      (i) Loss of various roles and privileges associated with pregnancy

      (ii) Loss of trust in one's body; feelings of inadequacy as a woman

      (iii) Might feel guilt if she had been ambivalent about the pregnancy.

      (iv) Father of the infant might not have the same sense of the reality of the pregnancy as the mother.

      (v) The lack of any "rituals" related to spontaneous abortion might leave the woman feeling alone and unsupported.

      (vi) Each member of a couple or family will likely grieve differently and might be perceived as unsupportive or unfeeling by the others.

    (b) Relinquishing child for adoption

    (c) Loss of the perfect child

      (i) Preterm or ill child

      (ii) Child of a gender other than that wanted

  (2) Parental reaction

    (a) Parents will likely experience a grief response that includes shock, denial, depression, equilibrium, and acceptance and reorganization of the family (Klaus & Kennell, 1982).

    (b) Might separate from the preterm or ill child, which can delay attachment.

    (c) Might anticipate grief of potential loss of ill infant.

    (d) Might acknowledge failure to produce a healthy infant.

    (e) Might change ways of relating to the infant in face of the threat of disability or death.

    (f) Might strive to learn to live with the special needs of their infant.

12. Childbirth preparation education: the goal of childbirth education is to assist individuals and family members to make informed decisions about pregnancy and birth based on knowledge of their options and choices; the goal is operationalized via the provision of specific information about the components of a healthy pregnancy and the process of labor and birth; necessary tools and skills to deal with pregnancy, labor, and birth are acquired.

a. Basic underlying principles of childbirth education are:

  (1) Partner or support person participation is important.

  (2) Relaxation and breathing strategies can be learned and practiced as a conditioned response to the stimulus of a uterine contraction.

        (3) Relaxation and breathing patterns are aids to cope with labor pain and enhance labor effectiveness.

        (4) Knowledge of choices, options, and alternatives can empower a laboring woman and her support person.

        (5) Confidence in one's ability to accomplish unmedicated birth is the most important predictor of success.

    b. Various approaches are available; the two most common are:

        (1) Lamaze

           (a) Active relaxation strategies to deal with pain of labor (e.g., touch, imagery, music, hydrotherapy)

           (b) Basic breathing awareness and breathing strategies

        (2) Bradley

           (a) Diaphragmatic breathing (i.e., from the abdomen) is believed to be most efficient for relaxation during labor.

           (b) Women are taught to become aware of their own breathing to determine the rate and depth of breath to take in labor.

        (3) Others

           (a) Many childbirth educators have taken what they believe are the best of several approaches and created a hybrid approach.

           (b) Many childbirth educators will tailor a program that is right for the couple.

        (4) Women and their partners should be encouraged to explore broadly the many options available for childbirth through books, articles, classes, and films.

        (5) Women who are unable to attend prenatal classes due to bedrest or other situations might find an educator willing to work with them individually.

B. Nursing Diagnoses

  1. Risk for disturbed body image related to bodily changes, eating disorders

  2. Ineffective role performance related to taking on new roles; changes in roles related to pregnancy

  3. Risk for situational low self-esteem related to pregnancy complications, changes in body image, roles

  4. Ineffective sexuality patterns related to changes in libido during pregnancy

  5. Interrupted family processes related to developmental stressors of pregnancy or loss

  6. Anxiety related to fear of the unknown

  7. Readiness for enhanced family coping related to opportunity for growth/mastery

  8. Risk for impaired parenting related to lack of knowledge and skills

  9. Impaired adjustment related to mood disorder, eating disorder, or loss

  10. Anticipatory grieving related to ill or preterm newborn

  11. Dysfunctional grieving related to stillbirth, ill or preterm newborn, loss of perfect child, loss of pregnancy, or loss of desired labor or birth experience

C. Interventions/Outcomes

  1. Risk for disturbed body image related to bodily changes, eating disorders

  2. Ineffective role performance related to taking on new roles; changes in roles related to pregnancy

  3. Risk for situational low self-esteem related to pregnancy complications, changes in body image, roles

    a. Interventions

        (1) Use effective listening and nonjudgmental communication skills.

        (2) Encourage woman to seek early and continuous prenatal care.

        (3) Provide resources—books, magazines, videos, and support groups—to assist in role changes of pregnant woman to a new mother.

        (4) Encourage childbirth and child care classes.

        (5) Encourage family to provide material symbols of role changes.

           (a) Maternity clothes

           (b) Infant equipment

        (6) Explain normal, expected emotional ramifications of pregnancy and role changes.

        (7) Help couple to set realistic goals and expectations for themselves.

        (8) Explore expectations for labor.

           (a) Birth plans

           (b) Choice of support persons

           (c) Options and opportunities for decision making to increase self-esteem

        (9) Offer realistic concepts of early parent-infant attachment process.

           (a) Provide early infant contact.

           (b) Explain normal newborn behaviors.

      (10) Evaluate weight gain and other possible signs of eating disorders.

    b. Outcomes

        (1) Woman has received prenatal care.

        (2) Couple has attended childbirth and/or child care classes.

        (3) Woman exhibits acceptance of role (e.g., can be concerned about being a good mother but not ambivalent about becoming a mother).

        (4) Woman gains appropriate weight in the pregnancy.

        (5) Woman has determined how she will feed her child (by breast or bottle).

        (6) Couple has chosen the possibilities for the infant's name.

        (7) Couple has prepared the home for the infant.

        (8) Couple negotiates options and desires for labor and birth.

        (9) Parents demonstrate an active interest in the newborn at birth.

4. Ineffective sexuality patterns related to changes in libido during pregnancy

    a. Interventions

        (1) Explain wide variety of sexual feelings and behaviors

           (a) Couple might enjoy sexual activity more because there is:

               (i) No fear of pregnancy

               (i) No need for contraceptive use (which, depending on the method, could have disrupted spontaneity)

               (iii) Increased pelvic congestion with fulminating orgasm (Some women experience their first orgasm during pregnancy.)

               (iv) Increased vaginal lubrication

               (v) Perception of the pregnancy as very sensuous

           (b) Couple might have decreased desires and responses because of:

               (i) Negative body image (might be experienced by the man, the woman, or both)

      (ii) A belief in myths about harming the fetus by intercourse

      (iii) Physical symptoms such as fatigue, nausea, and vomiting, which might influence desire and response

      (iv) Psychologic restriction some couples feel toward sexual intercourse during pregnancy

      (v) Taboos that some cultural and social groups have against sexual intercourse during pregnancy

  (2) Determine and fulfill informational needs

    (a) There are many ways of expressing affection and intimacy beyond intercourse alone (e.g., kissing, massage, and romantic dinner).

    (b) Positions for intercourse might need to change as the uterus grows (e.g., to side-lying or female superior).

    (c) Masturbation or manual stimulation might cause a more intense orgasm than intercourse (needs to be avoided if intercourse is contraindicated for preterm labor risk).

    (d) Provide accurate information about the safety of intercourse throughout a normal pregnancy.

    (e) Pregnancy is a time of vulnerability, and couples need to be encouraged to be sensitive to one another's needs for affection and intimacy.

    (f) Orgasm causes harmless contractions and does not cause any problems in normal pregnancy.

    (g) Blowing into the vagina is contraindicated because of the potential of causing an air embolus.

  (3) Contraindications to intercourse

    (a) Ruptured membranes: contraindicated because of potential for infection

    (b) Incompetent cervix: contraindicated because of potential to cause preterm labor

    (c) Spotting or bleeding: contraindicated, especially with a placenta previa

    (d) Preterm labor history in current pregnancy: contraindicated because of potential to start premature labor

b. Outcomes

  (1) Comfort level is established for open dialogue with health care provider about sexual questions and concerns.

  (2) Couple maintains intimacy during pregnancy.

  (3) Couple can discuss satisfaction with options for expressing affection.

5. Interrupted family processes related to developmental stressors of pregnancy or loss

  a. Interventions

    (1) Offer anticipatory guidance about normal developmental stressors of pregnancy, such as:

      (a) Ambivalence during early pregnancy

      (b) Vulnerability

      (c) Impatience, irritability

      (d) Active dream/fantasy life

    (2) Encourage couple to ask questions.

    (3) Help couple appreciate the normal and universal nature of the emotional changes in pregnancy and identify areas of stress.

      (4) Acknowledge ethical dilemmas and emotional stress of some prenatal diagnostic testing procedures.

      (5) Discuss common phases through which men progress during pregnancy.

        (a) Announcement phase: when diagnosis is made

        (b) Moratorium phase: occurring during early pregnancy, when there is often little overt interest on the expectant father's part

        (c) Focusing phase: related to new role as father, which occurs during late pregnancy

      (6) Provide encouragement that couple's adaptive coping strategies are effective (or help the couple alter them if the strategies are not working).

      (7) Help couple to identify and use support systems.

  b. Outcomes

      (1) Couple can verbalize feelings and concerns to each other and to the health care provider.

      (2) Couple discusses available support systems and uses them (family, friends, and other expectant families).

      (3) Couple attends childbirth or child care classes together.

      (4) Couple demonstrates mutual support.

      (5) Couple seeks help with emotional concerns about prenatal testing.

6. Anxiety related to fear of the unknown

  a. Interventions

      (1) Offer education and information on individual basis and encourage attendance at childbirth classes.

      (2) Explain all procedures and rationales before implementing them and keep parents informed of progress.

      (3) Help couple verbalize fears and determine the level of anxiety (from mild anxiety to panic).

      (4) If anxiety is related to a specific maternal or fetal complication, refer the couple to an appropriate resource.

      (5) Avoid overburdening couple with too much information at one time.

      (6) Assist family to develop a realistic birth plan to better focus on concerns and to gain a sense of control for themselves.

        (a) Primigravida: help to focus on alternatives and to transform dreams and fantasies into real choices.

        (b) Multigravida: assess what went well in the last labor and birth and what she would like to change this time.

  b. Outcomes

      (1) Couple develops a realistic birth plan with several different alternatives and options.

      (2) Couple seeks appropriate resources for specific problems.

      (3) Couple can verbalize fears to health care providers and to each other.

      (4) Couple demonstrates a calm demeanor with relaxed voices and body language.

      (5) Couple states a feeling of less anxiety and fearfulness.

7. Readiness for enhanced family coping related to opportunity for growth/mastery

  a. Interventions

(1) Offer couple the necessary information for decision making.
(2) Encourage couple to make decisions based on realistic alternatives.
(3) Praise couple each time the couple demonstrates effective coping (e.g., a birth plan, breathing in synchrony, and mutual support).
(4) If couple is not coping effectively, actively help them regain control.
(5) Offer oneself as role model to demonstrate skills the couple can learn (e.g., relaxation strategies, breathing techniques, breastfeeding guidance).
(6) Help couple to envision changes in plans (e.g., undergoing an unplanned epidural procedure) as an appropriate coping mechanism within context of a particular situation and not as a failure.
  b. Outcomes
(1) Couple verbalizes a sense of pride of accomplishment.
(2) Couple discusses resources and support systems used during pregnancy and childbirth.
(3) Couple seeks to understand any events during labor and birth that were unclear or misinterpreted and to put them into an appropriate context.
(4) Couple expresses realistic uncertainties about infant care while expressing confidence in the ability to learn.
8. Risk for impaired parenting related to lack of knowledge and skills
  a. Interventions
(1) Help parents to develop realistic expectations of themselves as parents.
    (a) Primigravida: help to shift the focus from the common myth of blissful newborn parenting to a more realistic view of initial sleep deprivation and disorganization.
    (b) Multigravida: help to identify how a new infant will change her present family constellation and assess family plans to incorporate the new infant into the family's daily life.
(2) Offer hands-on demonstration/return demonstration opportunities for infant care (e.g., bathing or cord care) to increase practical parenting skills.
(3) Give parents community resources to solicit assistance and support, as needed.
(4) Send parents home from hospital with written materials to reinforce hospital staff teaching about infant care and parenting.
  b. Outcomes
(1) Couple demonstrates basic infant care skills with confidence.
(2) Couple verbalizes a plan for meeting early parenting demands.
(3) Couple identifies appropriate resources to offer assistance.
9. Impaired adjustment related to mood disorder, eating disorder, or loss
  a. Interventions
(1) Assess frequently.
(2) Provide motivational stimulation for health-directed behavior.
(3) Use praise to affirm weight gain, coping abilities, and adjustment.
(4) Provide consultation with appropriate health care providers.
(5) Provide support group information and encouragement.

       (6) Evaluate grief response of father and mother of ill or preterm infants separately as well as together.
- **b.** Evaluation
  - (1) Women with eating disorders will gain adequate weight during pregnancy and transit through the postpartum period without additional difficulties.
  - (2) Women with mood disorders will demonstrate appropriate care of self and infant.
  - (3) Couples experiencing loss of the perfect child will experience an appropriate adjustment.
- **10.** Anticipatory grieving related to ill or preterm newborn
  - **a.** Interventions
    - (1) Provide information and support.
    - (2) Allow parents to participate in care as much as they desire and as is possible.
    - (3) Encourage couple to talk about their feelings and concerns.
  - **b.** Outcomes
    - (1) Couple will verbalize their feelings and concerns; ask appropriate questions.
    - (2) Couple will verbalize realistic expectations.
- **11.** Dysfunctional grieving related to stillbirth, ill or preterm newborn, loss of perfect child, loss of pregnancy, or loss of desired labor or birth experience
  - **a.** Interventions
    - (1) Provide information and support.
    - (2) Allow venting of feelings and concerns.
    - (3) Encourage parental participation in care.
    - (4) Assess parental grief responses; provide validation of their experience and feelings.
    - (5) Provide "tokens" of stillborn or expired infant with pictures, hair clippings, handprints and footprints, etc.
    - (6) Maintain continuity in caregivers as possible.
    - (7) Refer to support groups.
  - **b.** Outcomes
    - (1) Couple will demonstrate both individual and family progress in the grieving process.
    - (2) Parents of ill or preterm infants will participate in infant care.

HEALTH EDUCATION

A. Early pregnancy
1. Developmental tasks of pregnancy
   - **a.** Mother: acceptance of pregnancy integration into her self-system
   - **b.** Father: announcement and realization of the pregnancy
   - **c.** Couple: realignment of relationships and roles
2. Psychosocial changes of pregnancy
   - **a.** Ambivalence about pregnancy
   - **b.** Introversion
   - **c.** Passivity and difficulty with decision making
   - **d.** Sexual and emotional changes
   - **e.** Changing self-image
   - **f.** Ethical dilemmas of prenatal testing

B. Second trimester
   1. Developmental tasks of pregnancy
      a. Mother: binding-in to the pregnancy, ensuring safe passage, and differentiating the fetus from herself
      b. Father: anticipation of adapting to the role of fatherhood
      c. Couple: realignment of roles and division of tasks
   2. Psychosocial changes
      a. Active dream and fantasy life
      b. Concerns with body image
      c. Nesting behaviors
      d. Sexual behavior adjustment
      e. Expanding to a variety of methods of expressing affection and intimacy

C. Third trimester
   1. Developmental tasks of pregnancy
      a. Mother: separating herself from the pregnancy and the fetus; trying various caregiving methods
      b. Father: role adaptation; preparation for labor and birth
      c. Couple: preparation of the nursery
   2. Psychosocial changes
      a. Dislikes being pregnant but loves the child.
      b. Although anxious about childbirth, the mother also sees labor and delivery as a deliverance.
      c. The couple experiments with various mothering or fathering roles.
      d. Mother is introspective.

D. Evaluation
   1. Couple can verbalize the educational content.
   2. Couple seeks assistance and support with psychologic concerns.
   3. Couple demonstrates insight into psychologic processes (e.g., increasing introspection and isolation during labor).

CASE STUDY AND STUDY QUESTIONS

Mrs. L is a 30-year-old primigravida and the last of her friends to become pregnant. Although she and her husband wanted a child, they had not expected it to happen so quickly after stopping birth control pills. She confided to the nurse that she was not sure she really wanted to be pregnant. When her ultrasound and alpha-fetoprotein tests were normal, she began to really embrace pregnancy. She frequently spent time with her friends and family who had children to learn about their experiences.

Mr. L was very excited about the pregnancy and had nausea when his wife did and even gained more weight than she did in the first trimester. However, Mrs. L was experiencing strange dreams and fantasies and was beginning to think she was crazy until her friends told her they had also had strange dreams. Her mother, who is a labor nurse, bought them almost every book about pregnancy and birth that was available at the local bookstore. Some of the ideas the couple read sounded really strange and "far-out." However, as they continued to read, they found ideas that were comfortable for them. Mr. L was enthusiastic about learning to be a good support person for Mrs. L, but wanted Mrs. L to have the most say about the experience, because it was she who would actually experience labor. They learned that the hospital in which they would deliver had a very high induction and epidural rate, and wished that they had known more before they chose their care provider and hospital. They were concerned about their ability to accomplish their dreams of an unmedicated birth in such an environment. Their childbirth educator helped them to develop a birth plan and coached them in assertiveness techniques while encouraging them to explore alternatives just in case not all went according to the ideal. They arrived in the labor suite feeling confident and able.

1. When a woman desires to have a child and learns that she is pregnant, her emotions might include:
   a. Ambivalence
   b. Joy
   c. Surprise
   d. All of the above

2. Men whose partners are pregnant sometimes experience sympathetic feelings and symptoms called:
   a. Pseudopregnancy
   b. Male pregnancy
   c. Couvade
   d. Pseudogestation

3. Pregnant women who tell the nurse about strange dreams should be:
   a. Referred to a psychiatrist.
   b. Assured that such dreams are common and normal in pregnancy.
   c. Offered a psychosocial interpretation.
   d. Told to ignore them.

4. The concept of developing a birth plan:
   a. Should upset nurses who are the real experts about labor and birth.
   b. Is illegal in some states.
   c. Is acceptable only in home births.
   d. Increases a couple's sense of control and mastery.

5. Many Native American women do not seek prenatal care because:
   a. They see tribal healers instead.
   b. They remain in bed throughout pregnancy.
   c. They believe that pregnancy is normal, and it is, therefore, unnecessary to see a doctor.
   d. None of the above.

6. The critical third-trimester issue in acceptance of the child is that:
   a. The nursery is ready.
   b. The family describes the fetus as a real person.
   c. Acceptance is unconditional.
   d. The father is concerned about the infant's well being.

7. Nesting behaviors are disrupted by:
   a. Baby showers
   b. Preterm labor
   c. Father's business plans
   d. Anxiety about labor

8. Two third-trimester developmental tasks of expectant fathers include:
   a. His changing image and negotiation of his role during labor and delivery
   b. Taking on the expectant father role and preparing the nursery
   c. Preparing for parenthood and accepting the woman's changing body
   d. Dealing with the woman's introspection and accepting the biologic fact of pregnancy

9. A common principle found among many ethnic cultures is that:

a. Pregnant women are sick.
b. Everything in nature is balanced (e.g., yin/yang)
c. A pregnant woman must wear a gold necklace in labor.
d. A pregnant woman's mother must be barred from the birth.

10. If expectant parents tell the labor nurse that they have taken childbirth classes, have chosen a possible name for their infant, have decided to breastfeed, and have prepared their home for the newborn, the nurse can surmise they are successfully coping with changes in:

a. The expectant couple role
b. Self-concept as a couple
c. The developmental stressors of pregnancy
d. Anxiety

ANSWERS TO STUDY QUESTIONS

1. d	4. d	7. b	10. b
2. c	5. c	8. a	
3. b	6. c	9. b	

REFERENCES

Aguilera, D.C., & Messick, J.M. (1986). *Crisis intervention: Theory and methodology* (5th ed.). St. Louis: Mosby.

Altender, R.R., Kenner, C., Greene, D., & Pohorecki, S. (1998). The lived experience of women who undergo prenatal diagnostic testing due to elevated maternal serum alpha-fetoprotein screening. *MCN The American Journal of Maternal Child Nursing, 23*(4), 180-186.

Ayers, S., & Pickering, A.D. (2001). Do women get posttraumatic stress disorder as a result of childbirth? A prospective study of incidence. *Birth, 28*(2), 111-118.

Bartels, R. (1999). Experience of childbirth from the father's perspective. *British Journal of Midwifery, 7,* 681-683.

Callister, L.C., & Birkhead, A. (2002). Acculturation and perinatal outcomes in Mexican immigrant childbearing women: A literature review. *Journal of Perinatal and Neonatal Nursing, 16*(3), 22-38.

Bloom, K.C. (1998). Perceived relationship with the father of the baby and maternal attachment in adolescents. *Journal of Obstetric, Gynecologic, and Neonatal Nursing, 27*(4), 420-430.

Draper, J. (2002). "It's the first scientific evidence": Men's experience of pregnancy confirmation. *Journal of Advanced Nursing, 39*(6), 563-570.

Duvall, E. (1985). *Marriage and family development.* New York: Harper & Row.

Elek, S.M. (2002). Couples' experiences with fatigue during the transition to parenthood. *Journal of Family Nursing, 8,* 221-240.

Franko, D.L., Blais, M.A., Becker, A.E., Delinsky, B.A., Flores, A.T., Ekeblad, E.R., et al. (2001). Pregnancy complications and neonatal outcomes in women with eating disorders. *American Journal of Psychiatry, 158*(9), 1461-1466.

Freeman, A. (2000). The influences of ultrasound-stimulated paternal-fetal bonding and gender identification. *Journal of Diagnostic Medicine and Sonography, 16,* 237-241.

Gennaro, S., Kamvendo, L.A., Mbwaza. E., & Kershbaumer, R. (1998). Childbearing in Malawi, Africa. *Journal of Obstetric, Gynecologic, and Neonatal Nursing, 27*(2), 191-196.

Graham, J.E., Lobel, M., & DeLuca, R.S. (2002). Anger after childbirth: An overlooked reaction to postpartum stressors.

Psychology of Women Quarterly, 26, 222-233.

Howard, J.Y., & Berbiglia, V.A. (1997). Caring for childbearing Korean women. *Journal of Obstetric, Gynecologic, and Neonatal Nursing, 26*(6), 665-671.

Johnson, M.P. (2002). The implications of unfulfilled expectations and perceived pressure to attend the birth on men's stress levels following birth attendance: A longitudinal study. *Journal of Psychosomatic Obstetrics and Gynecology, 23*(3), 173-182.

Kitson, C. (2002). Fathers experienced stillbirth as a waste of life and needed to protect their partners and express grief in their own way. *Evidence-Based Nursing, 5*(2), 61.

Klaus, M.H., & Kennell, J.H. (1982). Maternal-infant bonding (2nd ed.). St. Louis: Mosby.

Koniak-Griffin, D., & Turner-Pluta, C. (2001). Health risks and psychosocial outcomes of early childbearing: A review of the literature. *Journal of Perinatal and Neonatal Nursing, 15*(2), 1-17.

Korenman, S., Kaestner, R., & Joyce, T. (2002). Consequences for infants of parental disagreement in pregnancy intention. *Perspectives on Sexual and Reproductive Health, 34*(4), 198-205.

Kridli, S.A. (2002). Health beliefs and practices among Arab women. *MCN The American Journal of Maternal Child Nursing, 27*(3), 178-182.

Lindgren, K. (2001). Relationships among maternal-fetal attachment, prenatal depression, and health practices in pregnancy. *Research in Nursing and Health, 24*(3), 203-217.

Lothian, J.A. (2000). The birth plan revisited. *Journal of Perinatal Education, 9,* 8-12.

Lothian, J.A. (2001). Back to the future: Trusting birth. *Journal of Perinatal and Neonatal Nursing, 15*(3), 13-22.

Lynch, M. (2001). Being there: Kids on hand at siblings' birth. *Nursing Spectrum, 11*(6), 18.

Matthey, S. (2002). Postpartum issues for expectant mothers and fathers. *Journal of Obstetric, Gynecologic, and Neonatal Nursing, 3*(4), 428-435.

Meighan, M. (1999). Living with postpartum depression: The father's experience. *MCN The American Journal of Maternal Child Nursing, 24*(4), 202-208.

Mercer, R.T. (1990). *Parents at risk.* New York: Springer.

Mitchell-Gieleghem, A., Mittelstaedt, M.E., & Bulik, C.M. (2002). Eating disorders and childbearing: Concealment and consequences. *Birth, 29*(3), 182-191.

Molina, J.W. (2001). Traditional Native American practices in obstetrics. *Clinical Obstetrics and Gynecology, 44*(4), 661-670.

Moore, S. (2001). Question of the quarter: How can midwives best facilitate the bonding process between mother/baby in pregnancy, birth, and postpartum? *Midwifery Today, 58,* 68.

Moyer, A. (1999). Decisions about prenatal testing for chromosomal disorders: Perceptions of a diverse group of pregnant women. *Journal of Women's Health and Gender Based Medicine, 8*(4), 521-531.

Orr, S.T., & Miller, C.A. (1997). Unintended pregnancy and the psychosocial well-being of pregnant women. *Women's Health Issues, 7*(1), 38-146.

Perla, L.J. (2002). Patient compliance and satisfaction with nursing care during delivery and recovery. *Journal of Nursing Care Quality, 16*(2), 60-66.

Polomeno, V. (1999). Sex and babies: Pregnant couples' postnatal sexual concerns. *Journal of Perinatal Education, 8,* 9-18.

Rubin, R. (1984). *Maternal identity and the maternal experience.* New York: Springer.

Sagrestano, L.M., Feldman, P., Rini, C.K., Woo, G., & Dunkel-Schetter, C. (1999). Ethnicity and social support during pregnancy. *American Journal of Community Psychology, 27*(6), 869-898.

Sandelowski, M. (2000). *Devices and desires: Gender, technology, and American nursing.* Chapel Hill, NC: The University of North Carolina Press.

Smith-Battle, L.(1997). Change and continuity in family caregiving practices with young mothers and their children. *Image The Journal of Nursing Scholarship, 29,* 125-129.

Sobey, W.S. (2002). Barriers to postpartum depression prevention and treatment: A policy analysis. *Journal of Midwifery and Women's Health, 47*(5), 331-336.

Strong, T.H. (2000). *Expecting trouble: What expectant parents should know about prenatal care in America.* New York: New York University Press.

Terycyak, A.P., Johnson, S.B., Roberts, S.F., & Cruz, A.C.(2001). Psychological response to prenatal genetic counseling and amniocentesis. *Patient Education and Counseling, 43*(1), 73-84.

Wagner, T. (1997). Perinatal death: How fathers grieve. *Journal of Perinatal Education, 6,* 9-16.

MATERNAL-FETAL WELL-BEING

7 Age-Related Concerns

JUDY E. SMITH

OBJECTIVES

1. Identify the risks of childbearing that are related to adolescents.
2. Identify the risks of childbearing that are related to advanced maternal age.
3. Distinguish between the risks that can be attributed solely to biologic age factors and the risks that can be attributed to sociocultural and economic factors.
4. Select nursing interventions that correspond to the developmental level of a pregnant adolescent.
5. Design and implement health education that reflects a sensitivity to the specialized needs of younger expectant parents and older expectant parents

INTRODUCTION

Pregnancy that occurs at the two age extremes (younger than 19 years and older than 35 years) of a woman's childbearing years places the expectant mother and the fetus at risk for age-related complications. However, the increased risks of age extremes might be related more to sociocultural and economic factors than to the biologic factors of age. Many of these risks can be minimized through the use of current technology, education, and consistent prenatal care. Certainly, preexisting biologic conditions might require management by a high-risk team, regardless of the age of the woman. The maternal mortality risk for adolescents younger than 15 years has been reported to be two to five times that of pregnant women aged 20 to 24 (Nichols & Zwelling, 1997).

Pregnancy in women 35 years and older who deliver in settings in which current technology is available might be at no higher risk for an adverse outcome than pregnancy in younger women. The trend toward high technology to treat infertility has led to the possibility of childbirth in women of any age (Nichols & Zwelling, 1997). Using surrogacy or egg donors, women well into the menopausal years can have children.

More than 900,000 adolescents become pregnant each year in the United States (American Medical Association [AMA], 2001). Although teen pregnancies have been decreasing steadily during the past decade, the United States still has the highest teen pregnancy rate among all developed countries (Elfenbein & Felice, 2003). With early and thorough prenatal care, adolescents older than the age of 15 years experience no greater risks than those of the general pregnant population. Although the incidence of certain complications might be higher because of age extremes, the nursing diagnoses, interventions, and evaluations remain relatively unchanged from those for the general pregnant population with the same complications.

CLINICAL PRACTICE

Adolescence

A. Assessment
   1. History (specifics to add related to the adolescent's age)

   a. Age at menarche

     (1) Several of the first menstrual cycles are anovulatory and irregular, making gestational dating difficult.

     (2) Long bone growth is incomplete until approximately 2 years after menarche, and the pelvis does not reach adult size until 1 to 3 years after menarche; there is an increased risk of cephalopelvic disproportion (CPD) among young adolescents because of lack of pelvic maturity (Olds, London, Ladewig, & Davidson, 2004).

   b. Number of sexual partners

     (1) Having multiple sexual partners increases the risk of concurrent sexually transmitted diseases; adolescents will frequently have serial monogamous relationships (i.e., one short-term, monogamous relationship that is followed by another, and then another).

     (2) Each year, adolescents who are 15 to 19 years old account for 25% of all reported cases of sexually transmitted diseases in the United States (Nichols & Zwelling, 1997).

   c. Knowledge about how conception occurs

   d. Planned or unplanned pregnancy: most teen pregnancies are unintentional (Raines, 2004; Sherwen, Scoloveno, & Weingarten, 1999).

   e. Previous pregnancies

     (1) Term or preterm

     (2) Spontaneous abortions

     (3) Therapeutic abortions

   f. Contraceptive use: only approximately 40% of teens seek contraceptive services within 1 year of becoming sexually active (Sherwen et al., 1999).

     (1) Type

     (2) Frequency of use

     (3) Last time used

     (4) Non-use

   g. Dietary intake

     (1) Is frequently inadequate in adolescents; there is a high incidence of pregnancy-related, iron-deficient anemia in pregnant adolescents who are younger than 17 (Raines, 2004; Olds et al., 2004).

     (2) Caloric restriction can occur when the pregnant adolescent attempts to "not get fat," to control abdominal protrusion, or to deny the pregnancy to herself and others (Olds et al., 2004).

     (3) Overeating might occur to mask the bodily changes of pregnancy.

     (4) The incidence of eating disorders might be high among adolescents as a group.

     (5) Good maternal weight gain during an adolescent pregnancy improves fetal growth and reduces mortality (Olds et al., 2004).

       (a) Young, pregnant adolescents should strive for a weight gain at the upper end of the range for an adult pregnant woman.

       (b) Young, pregnant adolescents should consume as much as 50 kcal/kg of nutrition per day, if active.

   h. Prenatal care

     (1) Some adolescents have no prenatal care, might not have known they were pregnant, or continue to deny their pregnancy.

     (2) Prenatal care is frequently started in middle-to-late pregnancy (Raines, 2004).

     (3) Sporadic prenatal care and missed appointments are prevalent.

(4) Adolescents who lack adequate and early prenatal care have an increased incidence of spontaneous abortions, placental disorders, and prolonged labors (National Center for Health Statistics, 2001).
  i. Alcohol, tobacco, and illicit drug use
  j. Support system
   (1) Financial
   (2) Emotional: father of child
   (3) Marital status
   (4) Parents' awareness of and attitude toward their teen-aged daughter's pregnancy
  k. Attendance at prenatal classes
2. Developmental assessment
  a. The overall developmental tasks of an adolescent are:
   (1) Acceptance of and comfort with one's body image
   (2) Internalization of a sexual identity and role
   (3) Development of a personal value system
   (4) Development of a sense of productivity
   (5) Identification of a life's work
   (6) Achievement of a sense of independence
   (7) Development of an adult identity
  b. The early-adolescent girl (younger than 15 years):
   (1) Is a concrete thinker.
   (2) Usually has some degree of discomfort with normal body changes and body image.
   (3) Usually has only a minimal ability to foresee the consequences of her behavior and see herself in the future.
   (4) Usually has an external locus of control.
  c. The middle-adolescent girl (15 to 17 years):
   (1) Is prone to experimentation and challenges.
    (a) Drugs and alcohol
    (b) Sex
    (c) Feeling invulnerable
   (2) Seeks independence and frequently turns to her peer group for support, information, and advice; pregnancy at this age can force a parental dependency and interfere with her striving for independence.
   (3) Is capable of formal operational thought and abstract thinking, but might have difficulty anticipating the long-term implications of her actions.
  d. The late-adolescent girl (17 to 19 years):
   (1) Is developing individuality.
   (2) Is capable of thinking abstractly and anticipating consequences.
   (3) Is capable of problem solving and decision making.
   (4) Can picture herself in control.
3. Physical findings (specifics related to the adolescent girl's age)
  a. Bone growth is still incomplete in early adolescence.
   (1) If pregnancy occurs before bone growth is complete, it can interfere with or arrest further bone growth.
    (a) The first 2 to 4 years after menarche carry the highest risk (Raines, 2004; Olds et al., 2004).
    (b) An increase of estrogen during this time, caused by pregnancy, can lead to the early closure of the epiphysis.

(2) Pelvic bones have not reached adult female dimensions: the incidence of cephalopelvic disproportion, leading to cesarean section, is increased (Raines, 2004).

b. Signs of pregnancy-induced hypertension (See Chapter 21 for a complete discussion of pregnancy-induced hypertension.)

(1) Pregnancy-induced hypertension is one of the most prevalent medical complications in young, pregnant adolescents (Raines, 2004).

(2) Higher incidence might be due to:

(a) Suboptimal uterine vascular development.

(b) Poor nutrition practices by adolescents.

(3) Blood pressure elevations might be missed because of low baseline values.

c. Signs of intrauterine growth restriction (See Chapter 18 for a complete discussion of intrauterine growth restriction.)

(1) Morbidity in babies of adolescents might be attributed to two common causes: prematurity and low birth weight.

(2) Adolescents have a higher incidence of low-birthweight infants, especially very young girls aged 16 or younger (Kirchengast & Hartmann, 2003).

(3) Fundal height and gestational age discrepancy might be noted.

(4) Inadequate nutritional status might be evidenced by low weight gain; nutritional needs include:

(a) Additional amounts of protein, iron, and calcium needed to support the adolescent's growth and fetal development (Raines, 2004; Olds et al., 2004).

(b) Folic acid supplementation (Raines, 2004).

(5) Signs of infection (See Chapter 22 for a complete discussion of intrauterine infection and Chapter 19 for a discussion of congenital infections of the neonate.)

B. **Nursing Diagnoses**

1. Delayed growth and development of the adolescent related to pregnancy

2. Interrupted family processes related to the adolescent's denial of pregnancy

3. Deficient knowledge related to adequate nutrition during pregnancy

4. Noncompliance with prenatal care and instructions related to a lack of understanding of the value of prenatal care to pregnancy outcome

C. **Interventions/Outcomes**

1. Delayed growth and development of the adolescent related to pregnancy

a. Interventions

(1) Adapt the nutritional requirements of pregnancy to the individual adolescent's likes, cultural influences, economic resources, and peer-group habits.

(a) Instruct the adolescent about how to make the most nutritious selections from fast-food menus without attracting peer attention.

(b) Instruct the adolescent about how to select and plan for healthy snacks when she is both away from home and at home.

(2) Adapt all interventions to correspond with the adolescent's developmental level.

(a) Help her to develop and use decision-making skills that are appropriate to her developmental level; because teens tend to be self-centered, consider ways to motivate her to participate in health care and health education.

   (b) Help her to develop and use problem-solving skills that are appropriate to her developmental level; focus on those areas that are of most concern to her; present information in terms of how it will make life easier for her (Nichols & Zwelling, 1997).
   (c) Actively involve her in her own care.
    (i) Have her listen to fetal heart tones.
    (ii) Have her place her hands on palpable fetal parts in late pregnancy and help her to visualize the fetal position.
    (iii) Help her to see how good nutrition benefits her skin and hair texture and how it prevents her from gaining excess weight.
 b. Outcomes
  (1) Pregnant adolescent will be able to select and consume a nutritious diet without feeling conspicuous among her peers.
  (2) Pregnant adolescent will show an active involvement in her own care.
  (3) Pregnant adolescent will seek information and make decisions that are appropriate for her developmental level.
2. Interrupted family processes related to the adolescent's denial of pregnancy
 a. Interventions
  (1) Develop a trusting relationship with the adolescent.
   (a) Listen attentively.
   (b) Maintain a nonjudgmental approach.
   (c) Avoid sounding like a parent to the adolescent (i.e., avoid using the word *should,* giving unwanted advice, making decisions for her).
   (d) Recognize the unique problems of the adolescent as they relate to her individual situation.
   (e) Determine her individual strengths, and compliment her on these strengths.
  (2) Assist her in developing and using decision-making and problem-solving skills related to her developmental level.
   (a) Encourage her to include her family as a resource, if appropriate, in decision making and problem solving.
   (b) If inappropriate to include her family in the decision-making process, encourage the adolescent to communicate to her family the thoughts and resources she used to arrive at her decisions.
   (c) Support and encourage her well-thought-out decisions; praise her abilities and her approximations toward thoughtful decisions.
  (3) Seek involvement of the adolescent's mother, older sister, or other close female relative, if appropriate.
 b. Outcomes
  (1) Pregnant adolescent will develop a trusting relationship with the nurse.
  (2) Pregnant adolescent will be able to include her parents or another relative in the problem-solving process, if at all possible, and seek the support of her family, if appropriate.
3. Deficient knowledge related to adequate nutrition during pregnancy
 a. Interventions
  (1) Adapt nutritional requirements of pregnancy to the individual adolescent's likes, cultural influences, economic resources, and peer-group habits.
  (2) Instruct adolescent about how to make the most nutritious selections from fast-food menus without attracting peer attention.

(3) Instruct adolescent about how to select and plan for healthy snacks when she is both away from home and at home.

(4) Describe to her how good nutrition benefits her skin and hair texture and how it prevents her from gaining excess weight.

b. Outcomes

(1) Pregnant adolescent will select and consume all nutrients necessary for continued individual growth and fetal development.

4. Noncompliance with prenatal care and instructions related to a lack of understanding of the value of prenatal care to pregnancy outcome

a. Interventions

(1) Give specific information about the effect or purpose of each procedure that is conducted during a prenatal visit.

(a) Explanations must be appropriate to the adolescent's developmental level.

(b) Provide attractive drawings of the fetus at the current gestational stage, and inform the client of the appearance and capabilities of the fetus at every visit.

(c) Adolescents have a tendency to be egocentric.

(i) Effects of maternal health and habits on the fetus might not be regarded as important by the adolescent.

(ii) Emphasize the effects of health maintenance and practices on her own individual well-being (see previous discussion under alteration in growth and development).

(2) Adapt prenatal instructions to the adolescent's lifestyle as much as possible.

b. Outcomes

(1) Adolescent will seek prenatal care within the first trimester of her pregnancy.

(2) Adolescent will receive consistent prenatal care throughout her pregnancy.

(3) Pregnant adolescent will demonstrate an adequate knowledge of the value of prenatal care and demonstrate compliance with instructions.

Advanced Maternal Age

In 2001 the U.S. birth rates for women; in the age range of 35 to 39 years rose 30%; in the age range of 40 to 44 years old, 47%; and in the age range of 45 to 49 years of age, 190% when compared with the rates of 1990 (Blickstein, 2003). Clearly, pregnancy at or beyond what was commonly thought of as the far end of a woman's reproductive age has become more prevalent. With implementation of infertility technologies, the boundaries of reproductive age have been challenged.

A. Assessment

1. History

a. Conception problems: can occur in up to 25% of women in the age range of 35 to 39 years old and in up to 50% of women in their 40s (Bradley, Horan, & Molloy, 2004)

(1) Any tests, treatments, or procedures that were used to facilitate conception

(a) Diagnostic tests

(i) Ovarian function

(ii) Semen analysis

(iii) Uterine assessment

         (iv) Hormonal function tests

         (v) Endometrial assessment

         (vi) Tubal patency assessment

     (b) Treatments/procedures

         (i) Fertility drugs to induce ovulation

         (ii) Artificial insemination

     (c) Assisted reproductive technologies (Gardella, 2004)

         (i) In vitro fertilization (IVF): oocyte fertilized in the laboratory; resulting embryo transferred to uterus

         (ii) Gamete intrafallopian transfer (GIFT): gametes (oocyte and sperm) transferred to fallopian tubes; (zygote transfer = ZIFT)

         (iii) Intracytoplasmic sperm injection (ICSI): one sperm injected into the cytoplasm of the oocyte

         (iv) Assisted hatching: hole made in zona pellucida with microinjection needle or laser to enhance embryo hatching (used with frozen embryos)

         (v) Donor oocytes: oocytes retrieved from donor, inseminated, and resulting embryo transferred to recipient using IVF

         (vi) Gestational carrier: IVF with resulting embryos transferred to the uterus of another woman who will carry the pregnancy

         (vii) Embryo cryopreservation: pregnancy can be achieved by using previously frozen embryos from IVF, GIFT, or ZIFT

         (viii) Embryo donation: previously cryopreserved embryos are donated to be transferred to the uterus of a recipient woman who has been prepared for implantation with estrogen and progesterone

  (2) Duration of the conception problem

  (3) Gynecologic conditions predisposing to fertility problems

     (a) Uterine fibroids

     (b) Endometriosis

     (c) Pelvic inflammatory disease (PID)

b. Previous pregnancies

  (1) Problems conceiving

  (2) Complications during the pregnancy

c. Planned or unplanned pregnancy

d. Occupation or career

  (1) Women older than 35 years might have advanced in their careers to a level of high responsibility and high stress. They:

     (a) Frequently are college educated.

     (b) Frequently have high achievement needs.

     (c) Usually have a deep psychologic investment in their careers.

  (2) Career women older than 35 years might have difficulty balancing a career with the physical and psychologic demands of pregnancy.

  (3) Women older than 35 years might have difficulty with or feel an increased ambivalence about changing their roles.

     (a) During the postpartum period, women must make decisions about whether to return to work and, if they plan to, when they will return.

        (b) They must make decisions about obtaining adequate child care if they will return to work and must deal with the feelings of combining motherhood and a career.

    e. Chronic diseases, which are more common in women older than 35 years, might affect the pregnancy (e.g., arthritis, hypertension, diabetes).

  2. Physical assessment (specific to advanced maternal age)

    a. Genetic testing (See Chapter 2 for a complete discussion of genetics.)
        (1) Incidence of chromosomal abnormalities increases with age.
        (2) Chorionic villi sampling or amniocentesis is performed for the detection of chromosomal abnormalities.

    b. Signs of diabetes (See Chapter 24 for a complete discussion of diabetes in pregnancy.)
        (1) Blood glucose tolerance screening, if not performed as a routine screening in all pregnant women, is usually performed in pregnant women older than 35 years.
        (2) Incidence of gestational diabetes is increased in women older than 35 years (Jolly, Sebire, Harris, Robinson, & Regan, 2000)

    c. Signs of hypertension or pregnancy-induced hypertension (See Chapter 21 for a complete discussion of hypertensive disorders in pregnancy.)
        (1) Incidence of pregnancy-induced hypertension is increased in women older than 35 years (Heffner, 2002; Olds et al., 2004; Dulitzki, Soriano, Schiff, Chetrit, Mashiach, & Seidman, 1998).
        (2) Women with chronic hypertension have an increased incidence of superimposed pregnancy-induced hypertension.

    d. Presence of uterine fibroids
        (1) Increased incidence in women older than 35 years (Seoud, Nassar, Usta, Melhem, Kazma, & Khalil, 2002)
        (2) Can cause pregnancy and labor complications

    e. Fundal height and due-date discrepancy
        (1) Women older than 35 years are at higher risk for low birth weight, term infants (birth weight below the 5th percentile); breech presentations; preterm delivery prior to 32 weeks, and stillbirths (Sheiner, Shoham-Vardi, Hershkovitz, Katz, & Mazor, 2001; Jolly et al., 2000).
        (2) There is an increased incidence of multiple gestation in women older than 35 years; however, there is a better perinatal outcome of twins and triplets (Blickstein, 2003).

    f. Vaginal bleeding: there is an increased incidence of gestational bleeding in women older than 35 years (see Chapter 23 on hemorrhagic disorders in pregnancy for a complete discussion of bleeding during pregnancy).
        (1) Increased incidence of abruptio placentae (Jolly et al., 2000)
        (2) Increased incidence of placenta previa (Jolly et al., 2000)
        (3) Increased incidence of trophoblastic disease, particularly in women who are older than 40 years (Poole, 1997)

    g. For pregnant women over the age of 35, and particularly those who have had infertility treatment/assisted reproduction, there is an increased incidence of cesarean section, both elective and emergency (Seoud et al., 2002; Sheiner et al., 2001; Jolly et al., 2000; Dulitzki et al., 1998).

B. Nursing Diagnoses

  1. Anxiety and fear related to possible complications of pregnancy

2. Anxiety and fear related to possible chromosomal abnormalities in the fetus

3. Risk for impaired parenting related to late childbearing

C. Interventions/Outcomes

1. Anxiety and fear related to possible complications of pregnancy

   a. Interventions

   (1) Treat the pregnancy as normal unless specific complications are identified.

   (2) Reassure client that good nutrition, health habits, and consistent prenatal care significantly reduce the risks associated with advanced maternal age.

   (3) Stress importance of consistent prenatal care to detect any complications early, when treatment is most effective.

   (4) Review danger signs in pregnancy, and rehearse the appropriate responses to them so that the client feels confident about what to do.

   b. Outcomes

   (1) Client of an advanced maternal age will feel that her pregnancy is normal, unless specific complications are identified.

   (2) Pregnant client of an advanced maternal age who has identified risks and complications will feel confident in the care and treatment she receives to minimize her risks and complications.

   (3) Client of an advanced maternal age will seek and receive early prenatal care.

2. Anxiety and fear related to possible chromosomal abnormality in the fetus

   a. Interventions

   (1) Encourage genetic counseling to identify risks, and discuss implications of testing to enhance decision making.

   (2) Decision to undergo amniocentesis or a chorionic villi sampling might be related to beliefs and attitudes about abortion; therefore, the nurse must respect the client's decision.

   (3) Support client and encourage her to ventilate her anxiety during days of waiting for amniocentesis or chorionic villi sampling results.

   b. Outcomes

   (1) Pregnant client of an advanced maternal age will make an informed choice about whether she will undergo genetic studies and will feel confident about her decision.

   (2) Pregnant client of an advanced maternal age and her partner will understand what is taking place on a technical level during the waiting period after amniocentesis for a chromosomal study and will verbalize their frustration and anxiety associated with delayed results.

3. Risk for impaired parenting related to late childbearing

   a. Interventions

   (1) Encourage expectant parents' attendance at parenting classes before the infant's birth.

   (2) Identify and promote individual strengths and the advantages related to late childbearing.

       (a) Financial security has usually been achieved.

       (b) Education has usually been completed.

       (c) Expectant mother usually is secure in a career or occupation.

       (d) Marriage or relationship has had opportunity to stabilize.

    (e) Woman has had a child-free period for personal development before childbearing.
    (f) Personal maturity will generally result in mothers who are more accepting and feel less conflict in their parenting role.
  (3) Anticipate the informational needs of older couples.
    (a) Handling feelings of social isolation that might occur because peers have children who are already teenagers
    (b) Coping with increased energy required to care for newborn and developing strategies to meet the added energy demands
      (i) Getting help in the house, if finances permit
      (ii) Sharing care of newborn with partner
      (iii) Planning naps
      (iv) Preparing and eating simple, nutritious meals
  b. Outcomes
   (1) Pregnant client of an advanced maternal age and her partner will feel confident in their ability to parent their newborn.
   (2) Expectant couple of an advanced age will develop a plan to meet the high-energy demands of newborn care and tailor it to their individual lifestyle.

HEALTH EDUCATION

A. Adolescence
  1. Preparation for childbirth classes focused on pregnant adolescents' special concerns
   a. Lack of knowledge about conception and pregnancy, as well as labor and delivery
   b. Alteration in body image issues
   c. Isolation from peer groups
   d. Alteration in education and career goals and plans
  2. Female anatomy and physiology: before, during, and after pregnancy
  3. Conception and contraception
  4. Information about pregnancy alternatives to assist in decision making
   a. Abortion
   b. Adoption: public and private
   c. Single parenting
  5. Parenting classes for adolescents
   a. Child development
   b. Child safety
   c. Discipline
   d. Child-care arrangements
  6. Setting realistic short-term and long-term goals
   a. Returning to school or continuing educational plans
   b. Career or life plans
   c. Adequate child care
   d. Financial considerations
   e. Social relationships
B. Advanced maternal age
  1. Preparation for childbirth and parenting skill classes developed to accommodate the special concerns and needs of older expectant parents
  2. Alteration in lifestyles and habits to adapt to a child
  3. Combining career and quality parenting

CASE STUDIES AND STUDY QUESTIONS

Ms. C is a 14½-year-old high-school student, gravida 1, para 0 (GI, P0). Her last menstrual period was approximately 5 months ago, as best she remembers. She has had unprotected intercourse sporadically during the past year. She has had three sexual partners since she became sexually active and one steady boyfriend for the past 6 months. She states that her parents are unaware that she is sexually active and would never suspect that she might be pregnant. In fact, she is surprised that her pregnancy test result is positive and stated that she "doesn't do it that often." She says that her periods have always been irregular since the beginning. (Menarche was at age 12). Skipping a few months was not unusual, and she did not think much about it. She states that recently it has been difficult to control her weight, that she has had to be stringent about what she eats, and that some days she does not eat at all, just to stay at her present weight. She complains that, despite all this effort, her clothes are uncomfortably tight and she feels fat. She denies tobacco or other drug use and states that she drinks beer only at parties. She has come to the clinic for birth control. The results of a physical examination are as follows: blood pressure, 118/60; height, 162.6 cm (5 ft, 4 in); weight 52.6 kg (116 lb) (prepregnant weight, 52.6 kg); urine, trace protein, no sugar; fundal height , 14 cm; ultrasound test results, intrauterine pregnancy at 16 weeks' gestation.

1. Ms. C states that she cannot believe she is pregnant and that maybe a mistake has been made in the tests. This remark is not unusual because, appropriate to her age, she:
    a. Has the ability to foresee the consequences of her behavior but will not admit it to herself or to anybody else.
    b. Is a concrete thinker and has difficulty believing something she cannot see, such as a 16-week pregnancy.
    c. Really does know she is pregnant because she is capable of thinking abstractly but cannot deal with the thought of her parents' finding out that she is sexually active and now pregnant.

2. From the physical findings and her history, she is at greatest risk for and already showing signs of:
    a. Intrauterine growth restriction
    b. Pregnancy-induced hypertension
    c. Gestational diabetes
    d. Sexually transmitted disease because of her multiple sexual partners

3. She proudly states that she has not gained any weight but complains that her clothes are fitting tighter and that she feels fat. The most appropriate intervention would be to:
    a. Reinforce the fact that she is pregnant and needs to eat more to support her own growth and the growth of her fetus.
    b. Tell her not to worry about gaining weight, and explain to her that after she has had the child, she will return to her normal weight.
    c. Review her food intake during the past 24 hours, determine her likes and dislikes, and adapt a nutritious diet to her needs.
    d. Encourage her to wear looser clothing so that she will not feel so constricted.

Ms. C explains that it was difficult for her to get to the clinic. She had to make an excuse to her mother and had to get an older friend to give her a ride. When given the schedule for prenatal clinic visits, she states that the appointments are too frequent and, in her opinion, nothing much is done at each visit. She says she will come as often as she can, but she does not know how often that will be.

4. Her anticipated missed appointments represent the largest problem in the management of adolescent pregnancy, which is:
   a. An adolescent seeks independence; however, the clinic represents authority and has rules.
   b. The pregnant adolescent pictures herself in control and resents being told what she has to do.
   c. Late and inconsistent prenatal care is the cause of most of the complications associated with adolescent pregnancy.

Mrs. M, 42, is an accountant with a prestigious firm in a large metropolitan area. She typically works long hours and must travel on occasion. She enjoys the responsibilities of her career as well as the authority of her position. She has been married to her husband, 43, for 10 years. They had always planned to have a family, but Mrs. M wanted time to develop her career. She is now pregnant for the first time. She has a history of uterine fibroids, one of which measures 3 cm. Physical findings are as follows: blood pressure, 130/82; height, 167.6 cm (5 ft, 6 in); weight, 64.9 kg (143 lb), prepregnant weight, 59 kg (130 lb); urine, no protein/no sugar; fundal height, 26 cm; ultrasound results show an intrauterine pregnancy at 25 weeks' gestation and marginal placenta previa.

At 16½ weeks' gestation, Mr. and Mrs. M elected to have amniocentesis performed for genetic testing. They had to wait nearly 2 weeks (10 business days) for the results, making Mrs. M. 18½ weeks into gestation before any information was available.

5. Mr. and Mrs. M were undecided about what their actions would be if the fetus had chromosomal abnormalities. An important intervention with them would be:
   a. To assist them in clarifying and deciding what their decision is before getting the results so that their emotions will not confuse their decision.
   b. To encourage them to talk about their anxieties and concerns about the upcoming results and to delay their final decision making until the results are known.
   c. To have them put their worry about the test results aside because there is nothing that they can do about it during the waiting period, and they will just make themselves more anxious by worrying.

6. Because of the marginal placenta previa, Mrs. M is instructed to immediately report any vaginal bleeding, no matter how slight. There is a possibility that the birth will have to be by cesarean section. She cries and wonders aloud why she just cannot be normal, like any other pregnant woman. She states she feels so out of control. The best intervention for her is one based on the concept that:
   a. This is a normal feeling for all pregnant mothers, and she will just have to work through it psychologically.
   b. Because of her age, her fears are heightened related to the fact that she might not have another chance to have a child.
   c. She is exaggerating her situation and creating her own anxiety.
   d. Her career and lifestyle have elements of personal control in them to which she has become accustomed; feeling out of control is distressing for her.

7. Pregnant women older than 35 years have a higher incidence of all of the following except:
   a. Neural tube defects
   b. Gestational diabetes
   c. Multiple gestation
   d. Pregnancy-induced hypertension

8. Women older than 35 years have a higher incidence of gestational bleeding related to:
   a. An incompetent cervix
   b. Clotting abnormalities
   c. Abruptio placentae
   d. Anemia

ANSWERS TO STUDY QUESTIONS

1. b   5. b
2. a   6. d
3. c   7. a
4. c   8. c

REFERENCES

American Medical Association (AMA). (2001). *Healthy Youth 2010.* Chicago: Author.

Blickstein, L. (2003). Motherhood at or beyond the edge of reproductive age. *International Journal of Fertility in Women's Medicine, 48*(1), 17-24.

Bradley, L., Horan, M., & Molloy, P. (2004). Pregnancy and childbearing. In M. Condon (Ed.), *Women's health*, (p. 467). Upper Saddle River, New Jersey: Pearson Prentice Hall.

Dulitski, M., Soriano, D., Schiff, E., Chetrit, A., Mashiach, S., and Seidman, D. (1998). Effects of very advanced maternal age on pregnancy outcome and rate of cesarean delivery. *Obstetrics and Gynecology, 92*(6), 935-939.

Elfenbein, D., & Felice, M. (2003). Adolescent pregnancy. *Pediatric Clinics of North America, 50*(4), 781-800, viii.

Gardella, J. (2004). Infertility. In E. Youngkin, & M. Davis (Eds.). *Women's health: A primary care clinical guide* (3rd ed.; p. 254). Upper Saddle River, New Jersey: Pearson Prentice Hall.

Heffner, L. (2002). Pregnancy in the older woman. In K. Carlson, S. Eisenstat, F. Frigoletto, & I. Schiff (Eds.). *Primary care of women* (2nd ed.). St. Louis: Mosby.

Jolly, M., Sebire, N., Harris, J., Robinson, S., & Regan, L. (2000). The risks associated with with pregnancy in women aged 35 years or older. *Human Reproduction, 15*(11), 2433-2437.

Kirchengast, S., & Hartmann, B. (2003). Impact of maternal age and maternal somatic characteristics on newborn size. *American Journal of Human Biology, 15*(2), 220-228.

National Center for Health Statistics. (2001). National survey of family growth. Retrieved June 15, 2002 from *www.cdc. gov/nchs/nsfg.htm.*

Nichols, R., & Zwelling, E. (1997). *Maternal newborn nursing: Theory and practice.* Philadelphia: W.B. Saunders.

Olds, S., London, M., Ladewig, P., & Davidson, M. (2004). *Maternal-newborn nursing* (7th ed.; pp. 391-430). Upper Saddle River, New Jersey: Pearson Prentice Hall.

Poole, J. (1997). Maternal hemorrhagic disorders. In D.L. Lowdermilk, S.E. Perry, & I.M. Bobak (Eds.), *Maternity & women's health care* (6th ed.; pp. 761-793). St. Louis: Mosby.

Raines, D. (2004). Assessing adolescent women's health. In E. Youngkin, & M. Davis (Eds.), *Women's health: A primary care clinical guide* (3rd ed.; pp. 39-52). Upper Saddle River, New Jersey: Pearson Prentice Hall.

Seoud, M., Nassar, A., Usta, I., Melhem, Z., Kazma, A., & Khalil, A. (2002). Impact of advanced maternal age on pregnancy outcome. *American Journal of Perinatology, 19*(1), 1-8.

Sheiner, E., Shoham-Vardi, I., Hershkovitz, R., Katz, M., & Mazor, M. (2001). Infertility is an independent risk factor for cesarean section among nulliparous women aged 40 and above. *American Journal of Obstetrics and Gynecology, 185*(4), 888-892.

Sherwen, L., Scoloveno, M., & Weingarten, C. (1999). *Maternity nursing* (3rd ed.; pp. 228-289). Stamford, Connecticut: Appleton & Lange.

8 Antepartum Fetal Assessment

▪▪▪

MARCIA LIDEN JASPER

OBJECTIVES

1. Describe the various fetal diagnostic tests performed to evaluate fetal development and well being.
2. Explain the risks and benefits of the various fetal diagnostic tests.
3. Identify high-risk pregnancy conditions that require fetal surveillance, and discuss appropriate tests for each condition.
4. List the steps in performing each test.
5. Explain the sensitivity of testing parameters for fetal well being.
6. Describe client needs for high-risk pregnant clients undergoing a fetal diagnostic testing program and the interventions that might be helpful.

INTRODUCTION

A basic understanding of the physiologic principles of fetal life is required to understand how the various diagnostic tests determine fetal well being and identify abnormal development (see Chapter 3 for additional information on fetal development).

In every pregnancy, basic fetal assessment is conducted at every prenatal visit by assessing for fundal height, presence of fetal movement, and auscultation of the fetal heart rate. In the high-risk pregnancy, fetal assessment becomes more specialized. The information gleaned from these tests and procedures allows the health care provider to manage the pregnancy better, weighing the risks versus the benefits of uterine environment versus the external or neonatal intensive care unit (NICU).

The American Academy of Pediatrics and American College of Obstetricians and Gynecologists (AAP/ACOG, 2002) and ACOG (1999) list some of the more common high risk conditions of pregnancy that include (but are not limited to) the following:
1. Maternal conditions
   a. Hypertensive disorders
   b. Antiphospholipid syndrome
   c. Hyperthyroidism
   d. Hemoglobinopathies
   e. Cyanotic heart disease
   f. Systemic lupus erythematosus
   g. Chronic renal disease
   h. Insulin treated diabetes mellitus
2. Pregnancy-related conditions
   a. Pregnancy-induced hypertension
   b. Decreased fetal movement
   c. Oligohydramnios
   d. Intrauterine growth restriction
   e. Postterm pregnancy
   f. Isoimmunization

    g. Previous fetal anomalies
    h. Multiple gestation
    i. Polyhydramnios
3. Genetic assessment may be done for clients of certain ethnic origins or with a personal or family history of genetic defect.

    Initiation of fetal surveillance for most at-risk clients begins about 32 to 34 weeks' gestation but may begin as early as 26 to 28 weeks with some high-risk conditions (ACOG, 1999). For genetic concerns, assessment can begin in the first trimester.

    In summary, "the goal of antepartum fetal surveillance is to prevent fetal death" (ACOG, 1999, p. 1).

ROLE OF THE NURSE

For each test, the role of the nurse will vary. For some tests, the nurse will provide direct assistance to the physician or health care provider. In others, the nurse conducts the test him or herself. In all cases, the nurse must be able to explain the procedure to the client, as well as to understand the results so that these may be either interpreted and reinforced to the client, providing appropriate nursing interventions or education when required.

A. Fetal growth and development
  1. The normal length of gestation for full fetal development is 280 days (40 weeks) from the first day of the mother's last menstrual period (LMP) or 266 days (38 weeks) from actual conception; because the conception date is usually not known, the delivery date given to the mother is the estimated date of confinement (EDC), with a range of plus or minus 2 weeks to account for variations in time of ovulation from LMP.
  2. With unknown LMP, an estimation of gestational age (EGA) can be determined by estimating fetal size; one method is to measure the distance from the upper aspect of the maternal symphysis pubis to the top of the uterus (fundal height).
    a. Given a normal uterus, normal amniotic fluid volume, and a nondiabetic singleton gestation, a 20-week fetus usually causes a fundal height of 20 cm, with a normal growth rate of 1 cm per week until 36 weeks, after which engagement of the presenting part may occur.
    b. If a discrepancy is found in the size-for-dates estimate, ultrasonography can be performed, preferably in the first or second trimesters, a time that demonstrates the most steady growth rates.
      (1) First trimester
        (a) The gestational sac can be measured and visualized during the first 13 weeks; measurements provide an estimated gestational age with plus or minus 9 days' accuracy (Robinson, 1980).
        (b) Crown rump length (CRL) can also be evaluated and has been accurate in 95% of cases within plus or minus 4.7 days.
      (2) Second trimester
        (a) Biparietal diameter is a fairly accurate method of determining fetal age between 13 and 30 weeks' gestation, providing accuracy of plus or minus 10 days (Robinson, 1980); after 30 weeks, a significant difference to the altered growth rates may be found in the small-for-gestational-age (SGA), average-for-gestational-age (AGA), and large-for-gestational-age (LGA) fetuses seen in the graphs demonstrating intrauterine growth curves of weight, head growth, and length developed by Lubchenko in 1963 (Robinson, 1980).

(b) Femur length

(c) Ratios between fetal head and abdominal circumference

c. Human intrauterine growth charts have been developed that are clinically useful in assessing adequate serial fetal growth; the normal fetus grows from a weight of 2 to 4 g (0.1 to 0.12 oz) and less than 2 to 3 cm (1 in) at the onset of the fetal period (the beginning of the ninth week), up to an average weight of 3000 to 3600 g (6 lb, 10 oz to 7 lb, 15 oz) and a length of 48 to 53 cm (19 to 21 in) at term.

3. Fetal organ growth is not synchronous; fetal systems grow in staggered periods.

a. Because all body organ systems are present at least in rudimentary form by the end of the embryonic stage (8 weeks), the fetal period involves tissue and organ specialization and growth accompanied by changes in body proportions.

b. Depending on their level of development, the systems have a varying degree of susceptibility to malformations caused by environmental agents and maternal conditions.

c. The fetal heart is usually large enough at 18 to 20 weeks' gestation to be audible with a DeLee stethoscope; this finding is another confirmation of gestational age and, if not found at 20 weeks, can mean the fetus is not as old as expected.

4. Viability can be defined in terms of ability or capacity of a product of conception to survive for a finite time in a defined environment.

a. Most authorities believe that 23 weeks (menstrual dating) is the time of earliest survival (Little, 1990). Cooper, Goldenberg, Creasy, DuBard, Davis, Entman, et al. (1993) report the survival at 23 weeks to be 1.8%, increasing to 97.9% by 33 weeks.

b. Some systems are more immediately critical than others for survival; the respiratory system is critical because gas exchange must occur even if assisted ventilation is used.

(1) Pulmonary maturity generally is not achieved until approximately 37 weeks' gestation.

(2) Surfactant—the substance that prevents the collapse of the alveoli—increases significantly at the 34th week; the absence of surfactant contributes to respiratory distress, a common condition of prematurity.

(3) Surfactant is stored in lamellar bodies, discharged into the alveoli, and carried into the amniotic cavity and pulmonary fluid (Druzin, Gabbe, & Reed, 2002).

(4) Phospholipids make up most of surfactant, the most common being lecithin and the second most common being phosphatidylglycerol (PG).

(5) The presence of lecithin increases significantly at about the 35th week of gestation.

(6) PG appears at 35 weeks' gestation and increases rapidly between 37 and 40 weeks.

B. **Fetal physiologic responses**

1. Adequate tissue oxygenation in the fetus is accomplished by an umbilical vein PO_2 level of 28.9 ± 7 mmHg (Silverman, Suidan, Wasserman, Antoine, & Young, 1985), the critical level of hypoxia that triggers an adaptive response being 17 to 18 mmHg (Freeman & Lagrew, 1990).

2. Without adequate oxygen, the metabolism of glucose is incomplete, causing a buildup of lactic acid, a potent acid capable of rupturing brain cells; the level of lactic acid (metabolic acidosis) is measured by:

      a. The pH of the blood: by fetal scalp sample
        (1) Reassuring: greater than 7.25
        (2) Borderline: 7.2 to 7.25
        (3) Acidosis: less than 7.2; critical
        (4) Potentially damaging: less than 7.0 (McDuffie & Haverkamp, 1991)
      b. The amount of base (HCO_3) used by the body to buffer the acid present (base deficit greater than 8)

3. A diminished oxygen reserve has numerous causes.
      a. Uteroplacental insufficiency (refer to Chapter 3 for additional discussion of placental function)
      b. Umbilical cord compression
      c. Fetal complications (e.g., sepsis, hemorrhage, anemia)

4. The fetus's attempt to adapt to a diminished oxygen supply involves a complex array of responses.
      a. These biophysical responses vary according to certain factors present in each situation.
        (1) Severity and acuteness of onset of hypoxemia
        (2) Preexisting fetal condition
        (3) Presence of compounding factors (e.g., hyperglycemia)
        (4) Level of maturity of reflexes and endocrine systems
      b. In the healthy fetus, adaptations facilitate transport of oxygen (Meschia, 1999).
        (1) Fetal hemoglobin has a higher affinity for oxygen than does adult hemoglobin.
        (2) Cardiac output is high for body size and metabolism.

5. According to Manning and Harman (1990), asphyxia is the presence of both hypoxia and acidemia; the fetal biophysical responses to asphyxia may be divided into two categories:
      a. Acute, or immediate, responses such as changes in central nervous system (CNS) function
      b. Chronic responses, such as reduction in amniotic fluid production, impaired fetal growth, and increased probability of ischemic neonatal complications

6. Porto (1987) and others believe that there is usually a progressive response to asphyxia, following the CNS embryologic developmental phases, with the area developed last being the most sensitive to hypoxia.
      a. The medulla, which controls heart reactivity, is the last area to develop; thus, a loss of fetal ability to accelerate (a nonreactive nonstress test) should be the first CNS response to asphyxia.
      b. Prolonged exposure is needed to lose the CNS responses of fetal movement, breathing, and then tone, which are responses regulated by neurologic areas with earlier embryologic development.
      c. This understanding of progressive fetal biophysical response to asphyxia is useful clinically in ruling out false-positive findings; with a maternal complaint of decreased fetal movement, if testing shows presence of fetal heart accelerations (reactive nonstress test), the mother can be reassured of fetal well being.
      d. In a true case of asphyxia, the CNS would already have lost the ability to stimulate fetal heart acceleration before the loss of the ability to stimulate movement.

7. With a decrease in oxygen, decreased fetal movement occurs, a measurement used in fetal movement counting, as well as with the biophysical profile, and indirectly with the nonstress test in regard to the association of fetal movement with increased fetal heart rate accelerations (Richardson & Gagnon, 1999).

C. **Comparison of fetal surveillance tests:** sensitivity of testing parameters (see Chapter 12 for a complete discussion of fetal assessment)
   1. Reflex late deceleration
      a. The most sensitive indicator of fetal hypoxia is a late deceleration of the fetal heart rate, which is triggered by chemoreceptors sensing a PO_2 of less than 20 mmHg (Caldeyro-Barcia, Casacuberta, & Bustos, 1968; Cibils, 1981).
      b. This response occurs before changes in pH, baseline fetal heart rate (FHR), variability, or reactivity (Martin, de Haan, van der Wildt, Jongsma, Dilleman, & Arts, 1979; Porto, 1987).
      c. Early work by Adamsons and Myers (1977) in monkeys showed that when late decelerations lasted for less than an hour, no neurologic damage occurred; a degree of hypoxia is demonstrated without CNS depression during this clinical experience, making it an excellent time for intervention for the term or fully developed fetus to prevent neurological damage (Freeman & Lagrew, 1990).
   2. Accelerations
      a. When hypoxia lasts long enough for anaerobic metabolism of glucose to cause lactic acid buildup, the pH falls below 7.22, and FHR accelerations disappear (Murata, Martin, Ikenoue, Hashimoto, Taira, Sagawa, et al., 1982).
      b. The foundation work by Myers, Beard, and Adamson (1969) demonstrated that lactic acid is a potent acid and that severe asphyxia can cause swelling in the brain and eventually rupture the cells.
   3. Variability
      a. Variability decreases as the degree of hypoxia and acidosis increase (Parer, 1999).
      b. When moderate (also called normal or average) FHR variability (6 to 25 beats per minute) (Parer, 1999) was present 30 minutes before delivery, only 2% of newborns had Apgar scores below 7 at 5 minutes (Krebs, Petres, Dunn, Jordaan, & Segreti, 1979).
      c. This gives a 98% accuracy in predicting fetal well being, regardless of the presence of periodic decelerations, making the presence of variability the most reassuring aspect of FHR monitoring.
   4. Biophysical profile
      a. Prolonged hypoxia is needed to lose the CNS response of breathing, fetal movement, and then tone (Vintzileos, Campbell, Ingardia, & Nochimson, 1983).
      b. Chronic hypoxia can also cause a protective redistribution of cardiac output away from organ systems not vital to fetal life (lung, kidney, and gut) and toward vital organs (heart, brain, adrenals, and placenta).
      c. With decreased placental, renal, and pulmonary perfusion, urine production and lung fluid flow are decreased, which results in decreased amniotic fluid.

CLINICAL PRACTICE
Fetal Movement Assessment by Client
A. Introduction
In all pregnancies, fetal movement is a sign of fetal well being. In high-risk pregnancies, the fetus may be at increased risk for altered perfusion. Fetal movement is a

noninvasive method of screening that should be taught to all high-risk pregnant women. In low-risk pregnancies, perception of fetal movement is discussed at every prenatal visit, and women are told to inform their health care provider if a decrease occurs. Daily fetal movement counting is included for high-risk pregnant women.

B. Assessment
1. History: physiologic basis
   a. Fetal activity expresses fetal condition in utero, and daily evaluation of fetal movements provides an inexpensive, noninvasive way of assessing fetal well being.
   b. Decreased activity in a previously active fetus may reflect disturbance of placental function and may be a clue to impending demise (Sadovsky, 1985a).
   c. Many variables (e.g., fetal resting state, maternal glucose load, medications, exercise), however, make the interpretation of fetal movement (FM) patterns confusing (Queenan, 1985).
2. Physical findings
   a. According to Sadovsky (1990), the mean daily FM recording (DFMR) rises from about 200 in the 20th week to a maximum of 575 in the 32nd week of gestation and then decreases gradually thereafter until delivery, with a mean of 282 daily FMs.
   b. The periods of decreased activity at term may be related to fetal sleep states, which increase with maturity (Richardson & Gagnon, 1999).
   c. Except for very low DFMRs, and especially when a definite trend toward decreasing motion is noted, the clinical value of the absolute number of FMs has not been established; the only exception is when FMs cease entirely for 12 hours.
   d. Interpretation is complicated because every pregnancy has its own rhythm, and a woman's perception is subjective; when compared with an FM-sensing device, however, there was an 80% to 90% correlation with maternal perception of FM (Sadovsky, 1990).
   e. Many women report that fetal activity during the day is not constant; therefore it would be incorrect to evaluate FM only once a day for a short period.
3. Interpretation: practitioners use various protocols to identify FM (ACOG, 1999).
   a. Sadovsky (1985b) developed the following protocol:
      (1) Normal
         (a) Assess FM for 30 minutes three times a day.
         (b) The perception of four or more FMs in a 30-minute period is normal; assess FM during the next counting period.
      (2) Requiring follow-up
         (a) If fewer than four FMs are noted, the client should continue counting for up to 6 hours.
         (b) Additional assessment is warranted in the presence of a nonreassuring count (AGOC, 1999). This assessment may be a nonstress test (NST), contraction stress test (CST), or biophysical profile (BPP).
   b. The Cardiff method
      (1) Count the first 10 movements each morning.
      (2) Freda, Mikhail, Mazloom, Polizzotti, Damus, and Merkatz (1993) found no difference in compliance between the two methods.
      (3) The same follow-up as previously mentioned should be instituted if fewer than 10 movements are noted.

Biophysical Assessment

Ultrasonography

A. Introduction
   1. Overview: with the advent of imaging via ultrasound, tissue can be assessed in either static or real time; a wide variety of information can be gathered pertinent to both maternal and fetal issues in both low-risk and high-risk pregnancies.
   2. Principles
      a. Definition: ultrasonography is a method of tissue imaging based on graphic analysis of the spectral characteristics of reflected high-frequency sound waves (Sonek & Nicolaides, 1998).
      b. Equipment
         (1) Transducer
             (a) Most scanning in obstetrics is done with 3.5- and 5-MHz transducers.
             (b) The transducer contains crystals that emit ultrasound wave energy; it also receives the reflected sound energy as echoes.
         (2) Signal display (B-scan)
             (a) Reflected sound waves are converted first into electrical signals then into a spot on the oscilloscope.
             (b) The intensity (brightness) of the spot varies directly with the strength of the echo, which can be amplified by the gain controls.
   3. Safety concerns: dosage levels
      a. The ratio between emitting and receiving time with diagnostic ultrasonography is only 1:1000.
         (1) Total exposure time during 24 hours is less than 84 seconds.
         (2) Therefore a fetus that is 8 cm from the source receives an average of 0.01 to 0.03 mW per square centimeter (mW/cm^2), which is only 0.01% of the maximal safe level of 100 mW/cm^2.
      b. More than 25 years of follow-up by the American College of Radiology have shown no adverse effects of diagnostic ultrasonography.
   4. Routes
      a. Both abdominal and vaginal ultrasound can be used.
      b. Advantages of vaginal ultrasound include the following:
         (1) Earlier visualization of the products of conception
         (2) Increased detail
         (3) Better evaluation of extra-uterine pregnancies or masses (Chervenak & Gabbe, 2002)

B. Assessment
   1. History: obstetric ultrasound can assess the following:
      a. Gestational dating
      b. Placental evaluation and localization
      c. Fetal presentation
      d. Fetal number
      e. Fetal viability
      f. Amniotic fluid volume
      g. Survey of fetal anatomy for gross anomalies
      h. Detection and evaluation of maternal pelvic masses
   2. Physical findings
      a. Gestational dating
         (1) Because clients in some clinic populations have questionable menstrual histories, a more accurate method for determining EDC than that based on LMP was needed.

(2) This is especially true in high-risk pregnancies in which the fetal maturity estimate weighs heavily in the risk-benefit decision in planning a delivery.

(3) In 1985, Queenan developed the scoring system given in Table 8-1 to identify a term fetus.

(4) Using measurements of various parts of fetal anatomy according to the trimester, Sabbagha (1978) and others developed equations and reference tables for serial size and age determinations (Table 8-2).

b. Placental evaluation

(1) Grading criteria: Grannum, Berkowitz, and Hobbins (1979) reported on a method of categorizing maturation into grades 0 to III.

(a) This method was based on the identification and distribution of calcium deposits within the placenta and the increasing delineations with maturity, as in the appearance of the basal and chorionic plate of placenta and the placental substance (Figure 8-1).

(b) Clinical implications (Grannum, Berkowitz, & Hobbins, 1979)

(i) Grade 0: immature placenta of less than 12 weeks' gestation

(ii) Grade I: placenta of more than 12 weeks' gestation, associated with only 67.7% fetal lung maturity

(iii) Grade II: placenta of more than 12 weeks' gestation, associated with 87.5% fetal lung maturity

(iv) Grade III

■ Placenta of more than 36 weeks' gestation or presence of hypertension or growth-restricted fetus; this grade was

---

■ TABLE 8-1
■ ■ **Fetal Maturity Scoring***

Traits of Parameter	Maturity
Biparietal diameter (BPD)	>9 cm
Placental grading	II-III
Amniotic fluid volume (AFV)	Normal to crowding

Modified from Queenan, J., & Warsof, S. (1985). In J. Queenan (Ed.), *Management of high-risk pregnancy* (2nd ed.). Oradell, NJ: Medical Economics.
*See the related findings discussions for explanation of each parameter.

■ TABLE 8-2
■ ■ **Gestational Age Determination by Ultrasound Measurements**

Parameter	Stage of Pregnancy (week)	Accuracy (days)
Gestational sac (GS)	6-8	±0.5-3
Crown-rump length formula: cm + 6.5 = weeks	8-14	±0.5-3
Biparietal diameter (BPD)	15-26	±10
Femur length (FL)		
Abdominal circumference (AC)		
BPD, FL, AC	>30	±14-21

Modified from Queenan, J., & Warsof, S. (1985). Ultrasonography. In J. Queenan (Ed.), *Management of high-risk pregnancy* (2nd ed., p. 217). Oradell, NJ: Medical Economics.

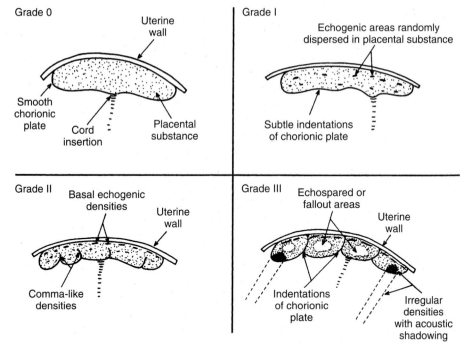

FIGURE 8-1 ■ Placental grading. (From Grannum, P., Berkowitz, R., & Hobbins, J. [1979]. The ultrasonic changes in the maturing placenta and the relation to pulmonic maturity. *American Journal of Obstetrics and Gynecology, 133*[8], 916.)

   associated in one study with 100% fetal lung maturity (Grannum, Berkowitz, & Hobbins, 1979) and in another with 93% lung maturity (Harman, Manning, Stearns, & Morrison, 1982).
- Placenta of more than 42 weeks' gestation; this grade has a 40% incidence of villous changes, which can reduce blood flow leading to fetal hypoxia (e.g., increased calcification, intervillous thrombosis, perivillous fibrin [Eden, 1990]).
(2) Localization
   (a) Placenta previa: in the presence of vaginal bleeding episodes, diagnostic ultrasonography is used to screen for low-lying placenta or placenta previa (implantation partially or completely over the cervical os).
   (b) Placental migration: with uterine growth and the development of the lower uterine segment as the pregnancy advances, the placenta may be carried away from the os.
      (i) Wexler and Gottesfeld (1977) found that, before the third trimester, 45% of pregnancies were characterized by a low-lying placenta; this finding contrasts with an incidence of placenta previa at birth of less than 1%.
      (ii) Clinical implication: because most cases of asymptomatic placenta previa found early are cured by placental migration, restriction of activity need not be practiced unless the placenta previa persists beyond 30 weeks or becomes clinically apparent before that time.

    c. Fetal presentation

        (1) Vertex: because malpresentations have a much higher incidence of morbidity associated with vaginal birth than do cephalic presentations, identifying the fetal presentation in labor accurately is crucial; visualization by ultrasonography of the fetal skull outline at the maternal pelvic brim is a reassuring finding.

        (2) Breech: because breech presentation in the last trimester may be manipulated into a vertex presentation by an external cephalic version procedure, antepartum assessment of presentation can also be of value in enabling a timely intervention to avoid a malpresentation at delivery.

    d. Multiple pregnancy

        (1) Risk of discordant growth: multiple pregnancies can be high risk, especially if monozygotic.

           (a) Two fetuses compete for nutrition from the same placenta.

           (b) The cords can become entangled in utero.

        (2) Mode of delivery planning

           (a) The third-trimester presentation of twin fetuses determines the mode of delivery; if vertex-vertex, many practitioners consider a vaginal birth to be safe.

           (b) If the first twin is vertex, some may do a version of the second transverse twin after the first has been born vaginally.

           (c) Cesarean birth is the preferred delivery method for all other presentations.

        (3) Clinical implication: antepartum surveillance of multiple pregnancies, starting at 28 weeks (Manning & Harman, 1990), is performed for the monitoring of serial growth patterns and adequate uteroplacental function.

    e. Fetal viability

        (1) Real-time ultrasonography can be used to confirm fetal death in utero by the presence of fetal scalp edema and the overlapping of the fetal cranial bones (Chervenak & Gabbe, 2002).

        (2) Fetal life can be confirmed by the visualization of the heart's beating and of fetal movements.

    f. Amniotic fluid volume

        (1) Most researchers agree that less than 500 ml of amniotic fluid at term is considered oligohydramnios, or decreased fluid, and more than 2000 ml is considered polyhydramnios (Brace, 1999); the exact ultrasonographic measurement that reflects a significant decrease has varied.

        (2) Amniotic fluid index (AFI)

           (a) The AFI is a method that was developed by Rutherford, Phelan, Smith, and Jacobs (1987) in which the depths (in centimeters) of amniotic fluid in all four quadrants surrounding the maternal umbilicus (in centimeters) are totaled.

           (b) The interpretation currently recommended is based on findings of an increased perinatal morbidity (low Apgar scores, meconium staining, fetal distress) in pregnancies with lower-than-normal measurements at term (Chervenak & Gabbe, 2002).

              (i) Normal: 5 to 19 cm

             (ii) Oligohydramnios: less than 5 cm

           (iii) Polyhydramnios: 20 cm or greater

(3) Severe oligohydramnios: Chamberlain, Manning, Morrison, Harman, and Lange (1984a, 1984b) reported severe oligohydramnios of 1 cm or less in less than 1% of more than 7500 pregnancies evaluated; this finding was associated with a 40-fold increase in perinatal mortality (187 of 1000) as compared with clients with normal fluid volumes; delivery is the preferred intervention as decreased amniotic fluid is associated with decreased placental perfusion and can result in meconium staining in the postterm pregnancy (ACOG, 1999).

(4) Hydramnios was observed in approximately 2.8% of pregnancies, and major fetal malformations were found in 18% of these cases; neural tube defects, obstruction of the fetal gastrointestinal tract, multiple gestations, and fetal hydrops are associated with hydramnios (Hobbins, Grannum, Berkowitz, Silverman, & Mahoney, 1979).

g. Congenital anomalies and follow-up directed (level-2) scans (refer to Chapter 2 on genetics and Chapter 17 on congenital abnormalities for additional discussion)

(1) Incidence

  (a) Based on 1995 Centers for Disease Control and Prevention (CDC) data (Chervenak & Gabbe, 2002), approximately 2% to 3% of live-born infants have a major anomaly.

  (b) At least 500 known developmental anomalies have been discovered.

  (c) Between 6% and 11% of all stillbirths and neonatal deaths is the result of aneuploid fetuses; morbidity as the result of chromosomal defects accounts for another 0.65% of newborns (ACOG, 2001a).

  (d) After 36 weeks, more than 85% of all major anomalies can be detected by ultrasound test (Manning, 1999b).

  (e) The recognition of an anomaly may influence the location and method of delivery so that neonatal outcome may be optimized (Chervenak & Gabbe, 2002).

  (f) Nuchal lucency has been added to the screening tests for Down syndrome, done between 11 and 14 weeks' gestation (Sonek & Nicolaides, 1998); congenital anomalies and heart disease, along with Down syndrome, have been associated with the increase in size of the normal clear area posterior to the fetal neck (ACOG, 2001a).

(2) Directed scans are performed as a thorough examination of a client suspected of carrying a physiologically or anatomically defective fetus, based on her history, clinical evaluation, or previous ultrasonography.

(3) Management of anomalies depends on consideration of variables such as:

  (a) Expected prognosis for the lesion

  (b) Demonstration of progressive pathophysiology

  (c) Availability of treatment modalities, if any

  (d) Fetal age at the time of diagnosis

h. Bleeding disorders—differentiation of placenta previa versus placenta abruptio (see Chapter 23 for complete discussion of hemorrhagic disorders)

Biophysical Profile and Modified Biophysical Profile
A. Introduction

The BPP was introduced in 1980 by Manning, Platt, and Sipos as a form of intrauterine Apgar score. The BPP provides an indication of fetal well being for the fetus who is at risk for altered oxygenation. Modification of the original procedure has recently been introduced.

B. Assessment

    1. History

        a. Physiology: perfusion to the uterus and across the placenta affects the delivery of fluids, nutrients, electrolytes, and oxygen; fetal hypoxemia and acidosis trigger a redistribution of cardiac output to the vital organs (brain, heart, adrenals, placenta) and away from those not essential to fetal life (lung, kidney, gut) (Manning, 1999a).

        b. The five criteria of the original BPP include (ACOG, 1999):

            (1) The four biophysical activities

                (a) Fetal movement

                (b) Fetal tone

                (c) Fetal breathing movements

                (d) Fetal heart rate activity (NST)

            (2) The semiquantitative measurement of amniotic fluid

            (3) The four biophysical parameters are indicative of acute CNS function.

                (a) In the presence of asphyxia, which causes CNS depression, these four variables become compromised, demonstrating decreased movement and tone, which in itself is a measure to conserve oxygen, thereby making it available for critical functioning.

                (b) The use of three criteria (fetal tone, movement, and breathing) has demonstrated accuracy similar to that when all four are used (Manning, 1999a).

                (c) An acute asphyxic episode demonstrates the resulting loss of fetal breathing, movement, tone, and heart rate reactivity while maintaining normal amniotic fluid volume.

                (d) Vintzileos, Fleming, Scorza Wolf, Balducci, Campbell, et al. (1991) further assessed cord gases and determined that fetal breathing movements and heart rate accelerations associated with movement seem to be the most sensitive of the variables affected, with fetal tone being the least sensitive.

            (4) Amniotic fluid volume has been identified as an indicator of chronic fetal compromise.

                (a) The resulting oligohydramnios may be a reflex induced by hypoxia, causing blood to be shunted away from the lung and kidney, thereby decreasing fetal urine output, which leads to a drop in amniotic fluid volume.

                (b) Oligohydramnios may also be related to a decrease in fluid perfusion across the placenta to the fetus.

        c. Modified biophysical profile—components include (ACOG, 1999):

            (1) NST—short-term indicator

            (2) AFI—long-term indicator of placental function

        d. Use of BPP: the following relationships have been made with the BPP:

            (1) Neonatal morbidity is increased as BPP score drops.

            (2) Low Apgar score is associated with low BPP score.

            (3) Cord pH shows an inverse relationship.

                (a) Normal BPP: pH of 7.28

      (b) Equivocal score: pH of 7.19

      (c) Abnormal score: pH of 6.99 (Vintzileos, Gaffney, Salinger, Campbell, & Nochemison, 1987)

   e. Variables influencing fetal breathing movements are as follows (Richardson & Gagnon, 1999):

     (1) Increasing fetal breathing movements (FBM)

      (a) Increased glucose concentration

      (b) Smoking

      (c) Chronic caffeine consumption (acute has no effect)

      (d) Tocolytics

     (2) Decreasing FBM

      (a) Ethanol alcohol (ETOH)

      (b) Chronic methadone use

2. Application, interpretation, reliability

   a. The BPP has been used in similar fashion to the Apgar score, with the evaluation of the five criteria having a total possible score of 10 (Table 8-3) (ACOG, 1999).

     (1) Normal: 8 to 10

     (2) Equivocal: 6

     (3) Abnormal: 4 or less

   b. In view of the fact that fetal tone, movement, and breathing demonstrate similar accuracy, as has the use of the three with fetal heart rate added, some practitioners base the results on four criteria only, without the fetal heart rate (NST); with this method, the maximum score becomes 8 (Manning, 1999a).

   c. McKenna, Tharma, Tnam, Mahsud, Baile, Harper, et al. (2003) suggest using ultrasound between 30 and 32 weeks' gestation in the low-risk population to identify a high-risk fetus and again between 36 and 37 weeks in the event that borderline intrauterine growth restriction (IUGR) has been identified.

   d. ACOG (1999) reports a negative predictive value at greater than 99.9% for both the BPP and the modified BPP; AAP/ACOG (2002) indicates that the

---

■ TABLE 8-3
■ ■ **Biophysical Profile**

Criteria	Points	
	None	Present
Reactive nonstress test	0	2
Fetal breathing movements (one or more episodes of 30 seconds or more in 30 minutes)	0	2
Fetal movements (three or more discrete body or limb movements in 30 minutes)	0	2
Fetal tone (one or more episodes of extension with return to flexion)	0	2
Quantitation of amniotic fluid volume (one or more pockets of 2 cm or more in two perpendicular planes)	0	2

Interpretation

Normal	8-10 (in the absence of oligohydramnios)
Equivocal	6
Abnormal	≤4

predictive value of the modified BPP to be as good as other biophysical fetal surveillance tests.

Doppler Ultrasound Blood Flow Assessment

A. Introduction

One of the major new advances in perinatal medicine is the ability to study blood flow noninvasively in the fetus and placenta, as well as heart motion. With the advanced technology of color coding, more in-depth assessment is possible. More commonly, in a fetus, the umbilical vessels are assessed. However, the vessels such as the aorta and cerebral blood flow can also be examined. The maternal uterine circulation can also be evaluated (Trudinger, 1999). The assessment of the growth-restricted fetus has been advanced with the use of Doppler blood flow assessment (AAP/ACOG, 2002; ACOG, 1999).

B. Assessment

    1. History: the Doppler principle

        a. When an ultrasound wave is directed at an acute angle to a moving target, as with blood flowing through a vessel, the frequency of the echoes is altered in response to the systolic and diastolic components of the cardiac cycle (Trudinger, 1999).

        b. This change, called the Doppler shift, indicates forward movement of blood within the vessel; Doppler shifts can be analyzed and displayed as velocity wave forms (Figure 8-2).

    2. Physical findings

        a. Visual representation of the blood flow can be calculated at the time of the procedure by dividing the systolic (S) peak by the end-diastolic (D) component (Trudinger, 1999).

        b. The normal S/D ratio declines from 2.8 to 2.2 between midpregnancy and term.

           (1) When uteroplacental perfusion is reduced, diastolic flow decreases, resulting in an elevated S/D ratio.

           (2) Elevations above 3 are abnormal.

           (3) The higher the S/D ratio, the lower the diastolic flow, leading to fetal growth restriction.

           (4) Reversed flow velocities lead to the most unfavorable fetal outcome (Karsdorp, van Vugt, van Geijn, Kostense, Arduini, Montenegro, et al., 1994), and birth weight below the 10th percentile in 84% of cases studied have been associated with a 5% to 10% incidence of fetal anomalies (Farrine, Kelly, Ryan, Morrow, & Ritchie, 1995).

Biochemical Assessment

Amniocentesis

A. Introduction

Amniocentesis can provide amniotic fluid to be studied for various high-risk fetal conditions. Initially, amniocentesis was used in assessing the color of the fluid. Advancement has been made to analyzing the cells, as well as the composition of the fluid, as the levels of components can deviate from the norm under certain circumstances.

B. Assessment

    1. History

        a. Definition: amniocentesis involves removal of amniotic fluid by a needle inserted transabdominally into the amniotic sac (Gilbert & Harmon, 2003) (Figure 8-3).

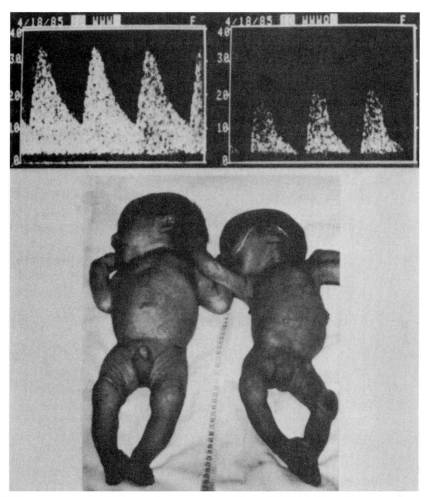

FIGURE 8-2 ■ Doppler ultrasound comparison of N1 twin to twin with intrauterine growth retardation (IUGR). (From Schulman, H. [1990]. Doppler ultrasound. In R. Eden & F. Boehm [Eds.], *Assessment and care of the fetus: Physiological, clinical and medicolegal principles* [p. 402]. Norwalk, CT: Appleton & Lange.)

b. Safety concerns: risks—amniocentesis is a relatively safe procedure with almost no severe maternal complications; the following are various risks and the reported incidence in experienced hands:

(1) Infection (amnionitis): 0.01% (Elias & Simpson, 1986)

(2) Pregnancy loss: 0.5% (Gardner & Sutherland, 1996)

(3) Needle injuries with ultrasound guidance: rare (ACOG, 2001a)

(4) Early amniocentesis (weeks 11 to 14) results in higher risks and other complications (leakage, loss) than procedures done after 14 weeks (Canadian Early and Mid-Trimester Amniocentesis Trial [CEMAT] Group, 1998), as well as an increased incidence of talipes equinovarus (Sunberg, Bang, Smidt-Jensen, Brocks, Lundsteen, Parner, et al., 1997) and therefore is not recommended by ACOG (2001a).

c. Accuracy: according to the National Institute of Child Health and Human Development (1976), the overall accuracy of prenatal diagnosis was 99.4%.

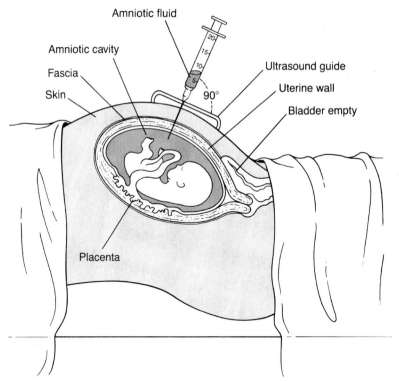

FIGURE 8-3 ■ Amniocentesis.

    d. Indications for amniocentesis include:
        (1) Detection of chromosomal abnormalities
        (2) Assessment of fetal lung maturity
        (3) Confirmation of amnionitis
        (4) Evaluation of Rh-sensitized pregnancies
        (5) Treatment of polyhydramnios (fluid reduction)
  2. Physical findings
    a. Detection of chromosomal abnormalities
        (1) Most common indication
        (2) Usually performed between 15 and 17 weeks to allow:
          (a) Uterus to be above the symphysis
          (b) Adequate amniotic fluid volume (150 to 300 ml)
          (c) Time for cell cultures and laboratory completion before it is too late for pregnancy termination at 20 weeks, if indicated
        (3) Early amniocentesis at 10 to 15 weeks
          (a) To minimize uterine irritability resulting from changes in fluid pressure after fluid withdrawal, total amount withdrawn is limited to 1 ml of fluid for each week of pregnancy (i.e., if the client is at 12 weeks, only 12 ml would be removed) (Rodriguez, 1991).
          (b) Earlier results make earlier termination possible, if so elected.
          (c) Advantages over chorionic villi sampling (CVS) (discussed later in the chapter) includes the ability to also measure fetal alpha-fetoprotein (AFP).

b. Tests to determine fetal lung maturity include the following (AAP/ACOG, 2002):

(1) Lecithin/sphingomyelin (L/S) ratio: the chance of lung maturity is 98% if the concentration of lecithin is twice that of sphingomyelin in lung surfactant secreted by the fetus into the amniotic fluid (L/S ratio over 2:1) in the nondiabetic client.

(2) PG: for diabetic clients, or in specimens contaminated with blood or vaginal fluids, the additional presence of PG, which appears after 35 weeks' gestation, is required for definitive maturity assessment.

(3) Lamellar body count (LBC)

(a) Lamellar bodies carry surfactant, are the same size as platelets, and can be counted via the same laboratory equipment that performs a platelet count (e.g., Coulter counter).

(b) The test requires 1 ml of amniotic fluid and takes less than 15 minutes (Greenspoon, Rosen, Roll, & Dubin, 1995).

(c) An LBC between 30,000/μl and 55,000/μl is highly predictive of pulmonary maturity (Druzin, Gabbe, & Reed, 2002).

(d) Ashwood, Palmer, Taylor, and Pingree (1993) found no cases of respiratory distress syndrome when the cutoff of 55,000/μl is used; lower acceptable values may be used as cutoff points based on varying the laboratory methods (Fakhoury, Daikoku, Benser, & Dubin, 1994).

(e) For tests yielding an immature result, further evaluation using the L/S ratio is recommended (Ashwood, Palmer, Taylor, & Pingree, 1993).

(f) The LBC test may become more prevalent based on the low amount of amniotic fluid required, the ready availability of the equipment used, and the speed in obtaining the test results.

(4) Foam stability index (FSI)

(a) Equal amounts of 95% ethanol, isotonic saline, and amniotic fluid are combined, and the test tube is shaken.

(b) The persistence of a complete ring of bubbles on the surface of the liquid after 15 minutes indicates a positive shake test result, signifying lung maturity (Jobe, 1999).

(5) Fluorescence polarization test (microviscosimetry, TDx test, surfactant/albumin ratio, FLM)

(a) The microviscosity of lipid aggregates in the amniotic fluid may be assayed by mixing the fluid with a specific fluorescent dye that incorporates into the hydrocarbon region of the lipids in the surfactant (Barkai, Reichman, Modan, Goldman, Serr, & Mashiach, 1988).

(b) The intensity of the fluorescence induced by polarized light is measured.

(c) Polarization value of 0.320 is associated with fetal lung maturity (Garite & Freeman, 1986).

(d) The technique is rapid and simple to perform, but the instrumentation is expensive.

(6) Optical density at 650 nm

(7) Saturated phosphatidylcholine

c. Confirmation of amnionitis: Gram stain of fluid for bacteria can confirm the presence of amnionitis in a pregnancy suspected of infection.

d. Evaluation of Rh-sensitized pregnancies

(1) Rationale

      (a) If an Rh-negative woman is exposed to Rh-positive blood, either through transfusion or a prior pregnancy, she produces immunoglobulin G (IgG) antibody (anti-Rh[D]).

      (b) She is then considered sensitized, and the amount of maternal Rh antibody produced (titer) can be measured; antibody titers of 16 or more as measured by albumin agglutination techniques indicate that the fetus is at risk (Morrison & Pryor, 1990).

      (c) If she becomes pregnant with an incompatible Rh-positive fetus, her Rh antibodies may cross the placenta and destroy fetal blood cells, causing hemolytic anemia in the fetus.

      (d) Concentrations of bilirubin and other breakdown products from destroyed (d) red blood cells (RBCs) can be detected in amniotic fluid by spectrophotometry (optical density [OD] reading at delta 450 mμ setting).

      (e) This measurement is then plotted on a Liley graph (by zones), which takes gestational age into consideration for the interpretation because a normal small amount of RBC breakdown decreases with fetal age (Liley, 1961).

   (2) Interpretation and management regimen

      (a) Zone I: the fetus is either unaffected or only mildly involved; no intervention is required, and another amniocentesis is needed in 2 to 3 weeks.

      (b) Zone II: there is moderate involvement and the need for closer observation by more frequent testing so the trend can be determined; the age of the fetus and trend in optical density determine the mode of therapy.

      (c) Zone III: there is severe fetal involvement necessitating either intrauterine transfusion or delivery if fetal maturity allows.

   (3) Test reliability

      (a) Although frequent, serial amniotic fluid OD 450 readings have been reported by Bowman (1999) to be 95% predictive of fetal anemia, a single reading may not be accurate.

      (b) Direct fetal blood sampling has been advocated as an alternative, especially in clients with histories of poor immunization or high zone II readings.

  e. Reduction of amniotic fluid volume: to decrease uterine overdistension, thereby decreasing the chance of preterm labor

Cordocentesis and Percutaneous Umbilical Blood Sampling (PUBS)

A. Introduction

Initially performed in the 1980s, this procedure permits direct access to fetal blood, which then can be analyzed. In the event of fetal anemia, a transfusion can be administered.

B. Assessment

  1. History

    a. Definition: cordocentesis involves obtaining fetal blood through ultrasound-guided puncture of the umbilical cord vessel (Harman, 1999).

    b. Indications

      (1) Detection of inherited blood disorders

      (2) Detection of fetal infection

      (3) Karyotyping of fetuses

      (4) RBC alloimmunization

      (5) Determination of acid-base balance of SGA fetuses (Harman, 1999)

(6) Nonimmune hydrops

(7) Twin-twin transfusion syndrome (TTTS)

(8) Neonatal thrombocytopenia

(9) Immune deficiencies

(10) Intrauterine fetal transfusion

c. Safety concerns:

(1) Complications include the following for cordocentesis (Harman, 1999):

(a) Fetal

(i) Bradycardia

(ii) Bleeding (incidence: up to 52%; minor in 50% to 60%)

(iii) Cord hematoma (less than 10%)

(iv) Failed procedure

(v) Infection

(b) Maternal

(i) Pain

(ii) Contractions

(iii) Anxiety

(iv) Preterm labor

(v) Maternal alloimmunization

(2) Risks for intrauterine transfusion (Bowman, 1999)

(a) Fetal

(i) Overtransfusion

(ii) Bleeding

(iii) Umbilical vein compression

(iv) Cerebral damage

(b) Maternal: same as for cordocentesis

(c) Fetomaternal: transplacental hemorrhage

d. Technique (Figure 8-4)

(1) Sampling

(a) With ultrasound-guided needle insertion, the cord is punctured close to its placental insertion, preferably the umbilical vein (Bowman, 1999).

(i) Between 1 and 4 ml of blood is removed for testing.

(ii) If the hemoglobin is normal, the needle is withdrawn.

(b) After needle withdrawal, the duration of bleeding from the umbilical cord usually is short and can be monitored ultrasonically; this depends on needle size and venous versus arterial puncture. About 50% to 60% will bleed for more than 15 seconds but less than 5 minutes (Harman, 1999).

(c) Daffos, Capella-Pavlovsky, and Forestier (1985) recommend continuous FHR monitoring for a few minutes and then a second ultrasound examination 1 hour later to ensure that no further bleeding or hematoma occurred.

(2) Intrauterine transfusion

(a) If the hemoglobin concentration is below the normal range, the tip of the needle is kept in the lumen of the umbilical cord vessel, and fresh, packed Rh-negative blood compatible with that of the mother is infused into fetal circulation through a 10-ml syringe.

(b) The FHR and flow of the infused blood are monitored continually by ultrasonography; at the end of the transfusion, a fetal blood sample is aspirated for determination of the hemoglobin concentration.

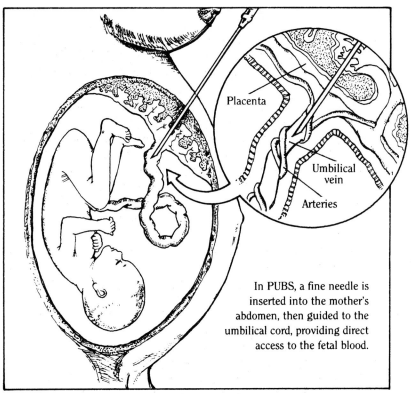

Placenta

Umbilical vein

Arteries

In PUBS, a fine needle is inserted into the mother's abdomen, then guided to the umbilical cord, providing direct access to the fetal blood.

FIGURE 8-4 ■ Percutaneous umbilical blood sampling (PUBS). (Drawing by Jonel Sofian for Pennsylvania Hospital, Philadelphia, PA.)

2. Physical findings
   a. Fetal infection
      (1) Viral particles may be identified directly by electron microscopy of fetal blood, ascites, or urine specimens.
      (2) Fetal blood and amniotic fluid may be cultured for further diagnosis (Weiner, 1988).
   b. Genetic disorders
      (1) An ultrasound-detected structural anomaly may be caused by fetal chromosome abnormalities.
      (2) Benefits of documenting an abnormal karyotype
         (a) Cesarean section for fetal distress may be avoided.
         (b) Recurrence risks are identified for counseling.
      (3) Advantages
         (a) A preliminary report not requiring specific confirmation is available within 48 hours.
         (b) Other causes of certain structural anomalies (e.g., congenital infections) may be sought.
         (c) The fetal metabolic condition can also be assessed (Weiner, 1988).
   c. RBC isoimmunization
      (1) Normal mean fetal hemoglobin values range from 11 g/dl at 16 weeks to 15.5 g/dl at more than 30 weeks (Harman, 1999).
         (a) Fetuses with hemoglobin deficits greater than 2 g/dl require transfusion.

(b) Severe isoimmunized fetuses may have deficits of greater than 7 g/dl (Nicolaides, Soothill, Clewell, Rodeck, Mibashan, & Campbell, 1988).

(2) Advantages

(a) Permits definition of fetal blood type and count precisely, including degree of fetal anemia.

(b) Avoids unnecessary further intervention if the fetus is antigen-negative.

(c) If fetus is antigen-positive, a direct Coombs test confirms the risk of hemolysis and need for further study (Ludomirski & Weiner, 1988).

Chorionic Villus Sampling

A. Introduction

CVS provides for analysis of fetal tissue for karyotyping during the first trimester before viability, at a time when termination of pregnancy is easier and poses fewer risks to the pregnant woman compared to waiting until the second trimester after karyotyping of cells obtained via amniocentesis (Scioscia, 1999)

B. Assessment

1. History

a. Rationale

(1) At the time that the CVS is performed (usually between 9 and 12 menstrual weeks), the placenta is a heterogeneous organ in which active and vigorous villus proliferation is noted in the central parts of the cotyledon (Golbus & Appelman, 1990).

(2) Proliferative villi at the embryonic pole that faces the decidua basalis constitute the chorion frondosum (Figure 8-5).

(3) Villi in the chorion frondosum are believed to reflect fetal chromosome, enzyme, and deoxyribonucleic acid (DNA) content, thereby permitting earlier diagnosis than can be obtained by amniocentesis (Brambati & Oldrini, 1985).

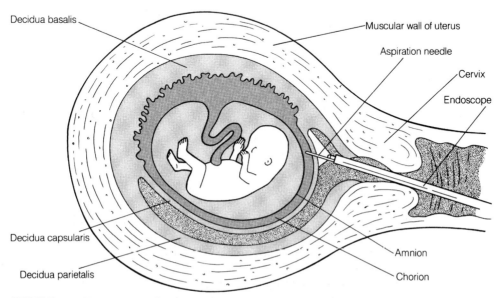

FIGURE 8-5 ■ Diagram of an 8-week pregnancy shows endoscopic needle aspiration of extraplacental villi. (From Rodeck, C.H., & Morsman, J.M. [1983]. First trimester biopsy. In M.A. Ferguson-Smith [Ed.], *Early prenatal diagnosis* [p. 338]. Edinburgh: Churchill Livingstone.)

    b. Indications

        (1) The most frequent indication for prenatal diagnosis via an invasive technique is advanced maternal age (Scioscia, 1999).

        (2) The other major indication for CVS involves biochemical or molecular assays or family history of genetic defect.

    c. Safety concerns: risks

        (1) Spotting or bleeding usually subsiding without consequences

        (2) Fetal loss (0.6% to 0.8% over amniocentesis)

        (3) Chorioamnionitis

        (4) Oligohydramnios

        (5) Rupture of membranes

        (6) Fetal-maternal hemorrhage

        (7) An increased risk of limb anomalies has been noted when CVS is performed under 10 weeks' gestation (Cunningham, MacDonald, Cant, Leveno, Gilstrap, Hauth, et al., 2001).

            (a) Performing CVS only after 10 weeks or more of gestation may be prudent (ACOG, 2001a).

            (b) In some areas, clinicians have been hesitant about performing CVS for this reason and instead have been advocating early amniocentesis (Henry & Miller, 1992).

    d. Techniques

        (1) Technique for transcervical sampling

            (a) The morning of the procedure, the client is asked to fill her bladder because displacement of an anteverted uterus may aid in positioning the uterus for catheter insertion.

            (b) A high-resolution linear-array or sector ultrasound is used to determine uterine position, cervical position, size of the gestational sac, and crown-rump length measurement, as well as to identify the area of placental formation and cord insertion.

            (c) The client is placed in the lithotomy position; the vulva, vaginal vault, and cervix are cleansed with povidone-iodine (Betadine); and a sterile speculum is inserted into the vagina.

            (d) The catheter with its encircled metal obturator is introduced transcervically under simultaneous ultrasonographic visualization.

            (e) The device is directed into the placenta, parallel to the long axis and away from either gestational sac or decidua.

            (f) The obturator is then removed, and the catheter connected to a 20- to 30-ml syringe containing 5 ml of tissue culture medium; by negative pressure, 10 to 25 ml of chorionic villi is aspirated (Elias, Simpson, Martin, Sabbagha, Bombard, Rosinsky, et al., 1986).

        (2) Transabdominal technique

            (a) Via concurrent ultrasonography, a spinal needle with stylet is passed into the placenta, with the device inserted lengthwise to the long axis of the placenta.

            (b) After removal of the stylet, the spinal needle is connected to a 20- to 30-ml syringe containing 5 ml of medium and heparin.

            (c) Using gentle suction, villi are aspirated (Scioscia, 1999).

(3) Precautions
   (a) To protect against infection, if more than one attempt is necessary, a new catheter should be used before each attempt at passage through the cervix in the transvaginal approach.
   (b) Rh-negative women should be given RhoGAM to avoid possible isoimmunization.
2. Physical findings
   a. Analysis of fetal cells
      (1) Chorionic villi cells divide so rapidly that metaphases can accumulate within hours and therefore take fewer days for growth than do amniotic fluid cells.
      (2) Therefore results are obtained in 3 hours to 7 days as compared with 2 to 4 weeks for amniocentesis.
   b. Results obtained in the first trimester enable:
      (1) Earlier counseling in the event of abnormal genetic findings
      (2) Earlier termination of pregnancy, if the family so chooses, in the case of abnormal results with fewer risks involved

Maternal Serum Alpha-Fetoprotein Screening

A. Introduction

During the 1980s, this test was introduced into the United States practice of perinatal medicine (Scioscia, 1999). The discovery that AFP is found in maternal serum led to the screening of this substance as the first line assessment for neural tube defects (NTDs). These anomalies occur in 1.4 to 2 per 1000 pregnancies (ACOG, 2003).

B. Assessment
1. History
   a. Background physiology
      (1) AFP is the major protein in the serum of the embryo and early fetus; initially produced by the yolk sac, it is primarily of hepatic origin by the end of the first trimester.
      (2) After 13 weeks, levels in fetal serum and amniotic fluid decrease rapidly, whereas those in maternal serum (msAFP) continue to rise until late in pregnancy (Cunningham, MacDonald, Cant, Leveno, Gilstrap, Hauth, et al., 2001).
   b. Rationale
      (1) Some of the most common reasons for an elevated AFP level in either amniotic fluid or maternal serum are in fetuses in whom the following circumstances occur:
         (a) A failure of neural tube closure during embryogenesis, as the result of multifactorial or polygenetic causes, that allows the protein to leak from capillaries into the amniotic fluid (anencephaly, spina bifida)
         (b) Increased amount leaked by the fetal kidney (hydronephrosis and other renal anomalies)
         (c) Abdominal wall (omphalocele and gastroschisis) and gastrointestinal defects (intestinal atresias)
         (d) Undetected fetal demise
         (e) Normal fetuses in conjunction with one or more of the following:
            (i) Amniotic fluid contaminated with fetal blood; most laboratories routinely perform a Kleihauer-Betke stain or hemoglobin phoresis on bloody amniotic fluid
            (ii) Underestimated gestational age
            (iii) Multiple gestation

(iv) Placenta that contains an increased number of thin-walled blood vessels that leak into the amniotic fluid

(v) Decreased maternal weight

(vi) Mother who has insulin-dependent diabetes

(2) Conditions associated with abnormally low levels include:

(a) Chromosomal trisomies

(b) Normal fetuses with:

(i) Overestimated gestational age

(ii) Increased maternal weight

(c) Gestational trophoblastic disease

c. In most states, the health care provider must offer msAFP screening at 15 to 18 weeks; the most sensitive time to test is 16 to 18 weeks; however, it can be done any time between 15 and 22 weeks' gestation (Cunningham, MacDonald, Cant, Leveno, Gilstrap, Hauth, et al., 2001).

2. Physical findings

a. Interpretation and diagnostic work-up

(1) Incidence of elevated AFP and follow-up

(a) About 5% of all women have abnormally high levels, defined as more than 2.5 multiples of the median (MOM) for the population being studied (MOM is defined by each laboratory).

(b) For initial high, abnormal results, some centers repeat the msAFP screen before follow-up testing is performed; according to Cunningham, MacDonald, Cant, Leveno, Gilstrap, Hauth, et al. (2001), 2% of the original 5% of cases are eliminated by repeated testing and the remaining 3% are referred for directed ultrasonography.

(c) For elevated or low levels of msAFP, follow-up ultrasound can be done to rule out or verify the following (Scioscia, 1999):

(i) Gestational age

(ii) Multiples

(iii) Genetic defects such as NTDs and Down syndrome

(iv) Intrauterine fetal death (IUFD)

(v) Other fetal anomalies (heart, gastrointestinal system, genitourinary system, CNS)

(d) In 1% of the total, multiple gestation, inaccurate gestational age, or missed abortion is identified, leaving only 2% of all women screened who undergo amniocentesis for acetylcholinesterase, which is present only if an open NTD occurs.

(2) Incidence of NTD and routine screening controversy

(a) Because the incidence of newborns with NTDs is 1.5 to 2 per 1000 in the general population in the United States (ACOG, 2001b), the cost-benefit ratio of routine screening for all prenatal clients as a public health screening policy is controversial.

(b) Some believe that only at-risk clients should be screened.

(i) Previous child with NTD

(ii) Close relatives (siblings, aunts, uncles) of a client with an NTD are at increased risk (Burton, Schulz, & Burd, 1992)

(3) Third-trimester complications have been reported with unexplained elevations of msAFP, which include (Scioscia, 1999):

(a) Low birth weight (LBW)

(b) Preeclampsia

(c) Placental abruption

(d) IUFD

    b. Anencephaly
       (1) Anencephaly is a malformation characterized by an absence of the skull and cerebral hemispheres that are either rudimentary or absent.
       (2) It is also the most common cause of gross hydramnios and may require therapeutic amniocentesis of as much as 2 to 3 L (2 to 3 qt) to reduce the risk of abruptio placentae after spontaneous rupture of the membranes with sudden loss of amniotic fluid and marked uterine decompression.
       (3) It is a lethal anomaly, with a 100% neonatal death rate.
    c. Spina bifida and meningomyelocele
       (1) Spina bifida consists of an opening in the lumbosacral vertebrae through which a meningeal sac may protrude, forming a meningocele.
       (2) If the sac contains the spinal cord, the anomaly is called a meningomyelocele.
       (3) Varying degrees of disability are displayed in 80% to 90% of these infants. The role for correcting these defects surgically during the fetal period is growing (ACOG, 2003).

Estriol Assays

A. Assessment
  1. Estriol levels were once evaluated as a measure of fetal well being because it takes:
    a. Adequate production of estrogen by the placenta
    b. An intact healthy fetus to metabolize estrogen into estriol (Buster & Carson, 2002)
  2. Estriol levels were evaluated on maternal 24-hour urine specimens and were costly.
  3. Fetal monitoring, sonography, or a combination of the two have now superseded the use of estriol levels because they are more cost effective and provide earlier indicators of fetal stress.
  4. Serum estriol has been combined with two other biochemical markers to evaluate the likelihood of Down syndrome; this test is known as the triple marker.

Triple Marker Test

A. Introduction
Use of the triple marker has further developed the screening for chromosomal anomalies.

B. Assessment
  1. History
    a. msAFP has been used in screening for neural tube defects since the mid-1980s; during this screening, it was identified that low msAFP levels were associated with Down syndrome (Cuckle, Wald, & Lindenbaum, 1984; Merkatz, Nitowsky, Macri, & Johnson, 1984).
    b. Other chromosomal anomalies, as well as trisomy 21, have been identified with levels of human chorionic gonadotropin (hCG) (Bogart, Pandiam, & Jones, 1987; Bogart, Jones, Felder, Best, Bradley, Butts, et al., 1991), as well as with unconjugated estriol (Canick, Knight, Palomaki, Haddow, Cuckle, & Wald, 1988).
    c. Biagiotti, Cariati, Brizzi, and D'Agata (1995) suggested that effective maternal serum screening be carried out in the first trimester so that prenatal diagnosis via CVS might allow for the identification of trisomy 21 and thus early pregnancy termination.
    d. Most screening is done in the early second trimester; however, it is more accurate when done between 16 and 18 weeks' gestation (ACOG, 2001a).

    e. Offering chromosomal screening for fetal aneuploidy to women over age 35 is common practice in the United States today (ACOG, 2001a).
   2. Physical findings
    a. Trisomy 18 was identified in a second-trimester population with the presence of the following values (Kellner, Weiss, Weiner, Neuer, Martin, Schulman, et al., 1995):
      (1) msAFP less than or equal to 0.75 MOM
      (2) Unconjugated estriol less than or equal to 0.60 MOM
      (3) hCG less than or equal to 0.55 MOM
    b. Down syndrome
      (1) Down syndrome is associated with the following values:
        (a) Low msAFP (approximately 0.75 MOM) (Haddow, 1990)
        (b) Elevated hCG (mean value 2.03 MOM) (Cuckle & Wald, 1992)
        (c) Low estriol levels (mean value 0.74 MOM) (Cuckle & Wald, 1992)
      (2) Adjustment of the values is recommended by O'Brien, Dvorin, Drugen, Johnson, Yarow, and Evans (1997) because they are ethnic-specific; Asians and blacks demonstrate higher AFP, hCG, and estriol levels than Hispanic and white populations do.
      (3) The triple marker test has identified 60% to 65% of fetuses with trisomy 21 with a false-positive rate of 5% to 10% (Haddow, Palomaki, Knight, Cunningham, Lustig, & Boyd, 1994).
      (4) A comparison of msAFP alone, hCG and msAFP (double marker), and the triple marker (msAFP with hCG and estriol) demonstrate a sensitivity of 91% and specificity of 94%; the triple marker is a better test than the double marker, as well as more cost-effective than an amniocentesis (Cheng, Luthy, Zebelman, Williams, Lieppman, & Hickok, 1993).
      (5) Analysis of free beta subunits has been added to the triple screen to increase the detection incidence to 67% to 76% (Wenstrom, Owen, Chu, Boots, 1999).
    c. Maternal serum screening is followed by amniocentesis and ultrasonography for more specific evaluation and to rule out the occurrence of false-positive serum results.

Fetal DNA in Maternal Circulation

Lo, Tein, Lau, Haines, Leung, Poon, et al. (1998) reports the analysis of fetal DNA retrieval from maternal serum. This has implications for earlier fetal assessment using a noninvasive technique. Bartha, Finney, and Soothill (2003) support this finding that the health care provider is able to provide earlier pregnancy management of an affected fetus. Lamvu and Kuller (1997) report identification of fetal RBCs, lymphocytes, granulocytes, and trophoblasts at various gestational ages. The role of the nurse has yet to be identified given that this testing is so new and not widely used as of this writing.

Electronic Assessment

A. Introduction
   1. Whereas first- and second-trimester antenatal assessment is directed primarily at the diagnosis of fetal congenital anomalies, the goal of third-trimester testing is to determine whether the intrauterine environment continues to be supportive to the fetus.
   2. The testing is often used to determine the timing of the delivery of clients at risk for uteroplacental insufficiency.

3. Both the regimen and interpretation of tests must always be done with consideration of the client's risk factors and the gestational age of the fetus (see Chapter 12 for additional material on fetal monitoring).

Nonstress Test

B. Assessment

  1. History

  a. Definition: the NST involves observation of accelerations of the fetal heart by the electronic fetal monitor, as they occur either spontaneously or in association with FMs, to determine adequacy of fetal oxygenation and autonomic function.

  b. Rationale

  (1) In the healthy fetus with an intact CNS, 92% of gross fetal body movements are associated with fetal heart accelerations (Richardson & Gagnon, 1999).

  (2) This response can be blunted by hypoxia or acidosis, drugs (analgesics, barbiturates, and beta-blockers), fetal sleep, and some congenital anomalies (Sonek, Reiss, & Gabbe, 1990).

  (3) Loss of reactivity can be caused by fetal sleep, CNS depression, and acidosis (ACOG, 1999).

  c. Advantages

  (1) The NST is easy to perform in an outpatient setting and can be performed in the home as well.

  (2) The test has no known contraindications.

  (3) The NST is relatively inexpensive, rapid, noninvasive, and therefore a good screening test.

  d. Disadvantages

  (1) The NST has a high false-positive rate for nonreactive findings, reportedly 80% (Parer, 1999), secondary to sleep cycles, medications, and fetal immaturity, yet its negative predictive value is 99.8% (ACOG, 1999).

  (2) The NST has slightly lower sensitivity to fetal compromise than the CST or biophysical profile.

  e. Technique

  (1) The client rests in a semi-Fowler or left-lateral position.

  (2) An external fetal heart ultrasound transducer and tocodynamometer are applied.

  (3) On sensing FM, the mother presses the marker, which records the time of movement on the same strip on which the FHR is recorded.

  (a) Some fetal hearts accelerate without perceived movement by the mother, and that acceleration is also a valid finding.

  (b) Because almost all accelerations are accompanied by FM, the movements need not be recorded for the test to be considered reactive (Huddleston, Williams, & Fabre, 1993).

  (4) Monitoring is continued for at least 40 minutes or until criteria for reactivity is met (see later discussion for criteria).

  (5) Acoustic stimulation test (ACOG, 1999) (also known as vibroacoustic stimulation [VAS])

  (a) Rather than require a 40-minute wait for a spontaneous fetal response, this technique uses sound stimulation to elicit accelerations.

  (b) Procedure

  (i) Establish the baseline measurement for at least 10 minutes without spontaneous accelerations.

(ii) If no spontaneous accelerations occur, apply an artificial larynx over the fetal head and stimulate for 1 to 2 seconds.

(iii) Restimulate if no acceleration occurs within 10 seconds (may be repeated up to three times), duration of stimulus up to 3 seconds.

(iv) Continue to monitor.

2. Physical findings

  a. Interpretation: ACOG (1999) and Devoe (1990) recommend the following threshold for grading reactivity:

    (1) Criteria for a reactive tracing (reassuring): two or more fetal heart rate accelerations of at least 15 beats per minute (each with a duration of at least 15 seconds) within a 20-minute period.

    (2) Nonreactive (nonreassuring): if the test does not meet the criteria in a minimum of 40 minutes, it is nonreactive and requires further evaluation.

    (3) Accelerations as the result of acoustic stimulation is also reassuring (AAP/ACOG, 2002).

  b. Suggested testing regimen

    (1) Weekly (ACOG, 1999) because reactive results are associated with fetal survival for 1 week or more in 99% of the cases (Parer, 1999)

    (2) Twice weekly in some of the higher risk conditions

      (a) Prolonged pregnancy (more than 41 weeks)

      (b) IUGR

      (c) Insulin-dependent diabetes

      (d) Hypertensive disorders

    (3) More frequently in the event of deterioration of maternal or fetal condition

    (4) This testing regimen is based partly on findings reported by Boehm, Salyer, Shah, and Waughn in 1986, which showed that by increasing the frequency of NSTs to twice weekly, the corrected stillbirth rate dropped from 6.1 to 1.9 per 1000 after a reactive test.

    (5) Some clinicians alternate an NST with a CST, or BPP, or both on a twice-weekly testing schedule.

Contraction Stress Test

A. Assessment

1. History

  a. Definition: a CST observes the response of the FHR to the stress of uterine contractions; a negative test result is desired (Olds, London, Ladewig, & Davidson, 2004).

  b. Rationale

    (1) The CST is based on the premise that fetal oxygenation that is only marginally adequate with the uterus at rest is transiently worsened by uterine contractions.

    (2) The resultant intermittent fetal hypoxemia, in turn, leads to the FHR pattern of late decelerations (ACOG, 1999).

  c. Technique

    (1) With the mother in a semi-Fowler or lateral position, the electronic fetal monitor's ultrasonic transducer and tocotransducer are applied to the maternal abdomen, and a baseline tracing is obtained for at least 15 minutes.

    (2) If three spontaneous, 40- to 60-second contractions of good quality occur in a 10-minute period, the results are evaluated and the test is concluded.

    (3) If inadequate contractions occur, nipple stimulation or intravenous (IV) oxytocin is used.
      (a) Nipple stimulation
        (i) The client brushes her palm across one nipple through her shirt for 2 to 3 minutes, stopping if a contraction begins.
        (ii) The nipple stimulation continues after a 5-minute rest period, with the same process repeated if no contractions occur.
        (iii) To avoid hyperstimulation (uterine contractions lasting more than 90 seconds or occurring more frequently than every 2 minutes), bilateral stimulation should not be instituted unless unilateral stimulation fails to induce contractions.
      (b) Oxytocin challenge test (OCT)
        (i) If the nipple stimulation test is either unsatisfactory or contraindicated, a titrated IV pitocin infusion can be initiated according to the institution's protocol.
        (ii) Oxytocin is administered until three contractions, each lasting 40 to 50 seconds, occur in a 10-minute period.
        (iii) Oxytocin is discontinued:
          ■ If no response occurs when levels reach 10 mu per minute
          ■ If repetitive late decelerations occur

2. Physical findings
  a. Interpretation of CST (ACOG, 1999; AAP/ACOG, 2002)
    (1) Positive results (nonreassuring)
      (a) Late decelerations after 50% or more of contractions
      (b) When the fetal PO_2 consistently falls below the critical level, late decelerations become persistent, and the CST result becomes positive
      (c) Associated with increased incidence of:
        (i) IUGR
        (ii) Low 5-minute Apgar scores
        (iii) Meconium-stained amniotic fluid
        (iv) Intrauterine fetal distress
        (v) Late decelerations in labor
        (vi) Intrauterine death (Druzin, Gabbe, & Reed, 2002)
    (2) Suspicious or equivocal results
      (a) Nonrepetitive late decelerations occurring with fewer than one half of contractions are inconclusive
      (b) When the oxygen level fluctuates between low and normal, late decelerations are intermittent, and the test result is equivocal
      (c) Significant variable decelerations
    (3) Hyperstimulation
      (a) Contractions closer than every 2 minutes apart or that last more than 90 seconds with a late deceleration indicate hyperstimulation.
      (b) A late deceleration that occurs after a contraction lasting more than 90 seconds may not indicate a diminished reserve because fetuses with normal reserves also decelerate with uteroplacental flow that has been interrupted for too long.
    (4) Negative results (reassuring)
      (a) Three contractions of good quality lasting more than 40 seconds without late decelerations is a normal result.

          (b) If the fetus never demonstrates a late deceleration when contractions are 3 minutes apart (three contractions in 10 minutes), last at least 40 to 60 seconds, and are of palpable strength, the test result is considered negative.

          (c) No significant variable decelerations

       (5) Unsatisfactory (less than three contractions in 10 minutes or a tracing unable to be interpreted) (ACOG, 1999)

    b. Consideration in interpretation

       (1) Even if a 10-minute window of three contractions occurs in which no decelerations occur, if a contraction is associated with a late deceleration elsewhere in the tracing, Freeman and Lagrew (1990) believe this should be considered a suspicious test result.

       (2) The perinatal mortality rate with this criterion for a negative result was 0 to 2.2 per 1000 compared with 10 per 1000 when the window interpretation was used. ACOG (1999) reports the negative predictive value at greater than 99.9%.

    c. Contraindications to performing a test include the following (ACOG, 1999):

       (1) Clients at high risk for preterm labor

       (2) Presence of premature rupture of membranes (PROM)

       (3) History of uterine surgery

       (4) Diagnosis of placenta previa

B. Nursing Diagnoses

  1. Risk for maternal-fetal injury related to test complications

  2. Deficient knowledge related to specific high-risk pregnancy condition and treatment options; fetal diagnostic tests and surveillance regimen

  3. Anxiety related to poor outcome from disease process; fear of pain and unknown outcome; lack of support in stressful circumstances; risk for fetal injury

  4. Risk for ineffective individual coping related to financial and time demands of serial testing regimen; denial of severity of health risk involved

  5. Risk for compromised family coping related to significant other excluded from testing sessions; fear of loss of fetus

  6. Impaired fetal gas exchange related to decreased placental perfusion; fetal anemia

  7. Risk for infection related to invasive procedures (i.e., amniocentesis and PUBS)

  8. Risk for deficient fluid volume related to amniocentesis and PUBS

  9. Decisional conflict related to adverse test outcome

  10. Situational low self-esteem related to abnormal test results

  11. Anticipatory grieving related to the loss of a normal pregnancy or fetus, or both

  12. Impaired comfort related to procedures

C. Interventions/Outcomes

  1. Risk for maternal-fetal injury related to test complications

    a. Interventions

       (1) Use sterile technique to prevent chorioamnionitis.

       (2) Position client properly (in lateral or wedged position) to avoid supine hypotension during fetal monitoring tests.

       (3) Have terbutaline, 0.25 mg, available for subcutaneous (or IV) injection for hyperstimulation response to CST.

    b. Outcomes

       (1) No complications were caused by diagnostic procedures.

2. Deficient knowledge related to specific high-risk pregnancy condition and treatment options; fetal diagnostic tests and surveillance regimen

    a. Interventions

       (1) Provide simple, clear explanations of the condition's pathophysiology and the maternal-fetal implications.

       (2) Clarify the treatment options.

       (3) Explain what the fetal test measures.

       (4) Describe the procedure for testing.

       (5) Describe the purpose and frequency of the tests, what the results mean, and the estimated length of the sessions.

    b. Outcomes

       (1) Client verbalizes awareness of the condition.

       (2) Client understands what treatments are available to improve her pregnancy outcome.

       (3) Client understands how, why, and when she is to be tested).

3. Anxiety related to poor outcome from disease process; fear of pain and unknown outcome; lack of support in stressful circumstances; risk for fetal injury

    a. Interventions

       (1) Allow the client to vent her frustrations with the discomfort, time-consuming demands, and limitations imposed by this high-risk pregnancy and fetal surveillance program.

       (2) Assist the client in setting realistic goals for progress in her pregnancy so that she experiences a sense of accomplishment.

          (a) Each day in utero is beneficial to the normal development of her fetus.

          (b) The fetus has improved chances for survival as long as the testing remains reassuring.

          (c) Compliance with treatment and testing regimens is beneficial to the fetus.

       (3) Encourage interaction (if appropriate) with other high-risk mothers in informal or structured groups.

       (4) Administer local anesthesia when starting an IV, as permitted by the institution's protocol.

       (5) Use comforting measures such as touch during difficult procedures.

       (6) Explain procedures step by step.

       (7) Encourage the client's significant others to be with her if she requests it during procedures.

       (8) Remain with the client if significant others are not available.

    b. Outcomes

       (1) Client verbalizes her fears and concerns, as well as her perception of care.

       (2) Client experiences minimal pain and fear during testing.

       (3) Client is comforted by the presence of her significant others.

       (4) Client agrees to continue treatment and testing regimens.

4. Risk for ineffective individual coping related to financial and time demands of serial testing regimen; denial of severity of health risk involved

5. Risk for compromised family coping related to significant other excluded from testing sessions; fear of loss of fetus

    a. Interventions

      (1) Review sources of conflict for the client, such as financial limitations and family commitments.

      (2) Arrange for social service counseling to help with problem solving.

      (3) Schedule testing appointments at the client's convenience when possible.

      (4) Follow up when the client does not keep an appointment.
        (a) Reinforce the value of testing.
        (b) Identify the cause of noncompliance.

      (5) Include significant others during testing and teaching sessions.

   b. Outcomes

      (1) Client attends all scheduled testing sessions and gains reassurance of fetal well being from the good results.

      (2) Significant others are coping well and being supportive.

6. Impaired fetal gas exchange related to decreased placental perfusion; fetal anemia

   a. Interventions

      (1) Instruct client in measures to increase uteroplacental perfusion, such as:
        (a) Lateral positioning
        (b) Adequate hydration
        (c) Decreasing environmental stressors

      (2) Instruct client in evaluating fetal movement.

      (3) Perform NST or CST as appropriate.

   b. Outcomes

      (1) Fetus will maintain greater than four movements per hour.

      (2) FHR will:
        (a) Have normal baseline between 110 and 160.
        (b) Demonstrate variability appropriate for gestational age.
        (c) Demonstrate reactivity.
        (d) Not have late or variable decelerations.

7. Risk for infection related to invasive procedures (i.e., amniocentesis, PUBS)

   a. Interventions

      (1) Employ good hand washing techniques.

      (2) Adhere to aseptic or sterile technique during invasive procedures.

   b. Outcomes

      (1) Client will remain afebrile.

      (2) Puncture site will be without redness, edema, ecchymosis, or drainage.

      (3) Baseline FHR will be between 110 and 160.

8. Risk for deficient fluid volume related to amniocentesis and PUBS

   a. Interventions

      (1) Assess puncture site for oozing.

      (2) Monitor FHR for signs and symptoms of decreasing blood volume (increased baseline heart rate).

      (3) Monitor maternal vital signs for signs and symptoms of hypovolemia.

   b. Outcomes

      (1) Puncture site will be intact without drainage.

      (2) FHR baseline will be between 110 and 160 with average variability and without variable decelerations.

      (3) No vaginal amniotic fluid is visible.

9. Decisional conflict related to adverse test outcome

   a. Interventions.

      (1) Provide information regarding choices available and potential outcomes.

(2) Listen and allow family to discuss options.

(3) Refer to genetic specialists, clergy, or social services as appropriate.

   b. Outcomes

(1) Client and family will make informed choice related to the progression of the pregnancy.

10. Situational low self-esteem related to abnormal test results

   a. Interventions

(1) Provide emotional support and stay with client.

(2) Allow client to vent feelings.

(3) Provide positive feedback for appropriate actions.

(4) Refer to community support groups.

   b. Outcomes

(1) Client will regain positive self-esteem and return to family or community with the ability to resume preexisting activities.

11. Anticipatory grieving related to the loss of a normal pregnancy or fetus

   a. Interventions

(1) Allow display of anger, disbelief, and blaming.

(2) Acknowledge the loss of normalcy.

(3) Be available to the client during notification.

(4) Refer to clergy or social services.

   b. Outcomes

(1) Client and family will accept and be able to resolve feelings so they can regain contribution to family or community, or be able to care for child after birth, or both.

12. Impaired comfort related to invasive procedure

   a. Interventions

(1) Provide privacy.

(2) Provide pillows for positioning.

(3) Allow choice of local anesthesia if appropriate.

(4) Use guided imagery or distraction if possible.

   b. Outcomes

(1) Client will report minimal discomfort during procedures.

(2) Client and fetus vital signs will remain within normal limits.

HEALTH EDUCATION

A. Several client education issues have already been addressed under the nursing diagnosis of knowledge deficit and during the description of the various tests; therefore these sections are provided for a complete review of this topic.

B. Because certain high-risk pregnancy conditions are preventable and relate to lifestyle choices that are hazardous to the fetus, counseling during some testing sessions can assist clients in making better choices.

   1. Obtain prenatal care within the first trimester.

   a. Prenatal care increases the accuracy of gestational age assessment.

   b. It allows more timely intervention in true cases of postterm pregnancies.

   c. It improves determination of inadequate fetal growth for a given fetal age.

   2. Avoid alcohol, illegal drugs, caffeine, and over-the-counter drugs during pregnancy, especially during the first trimester, to prevent teratogenic effects.

   3. Normal fetal growth can result if smoking is stopped during pregnancy.

CASE STUDIES AND STUDY QUESTIONS

Ms. J is a 37-year-old gravida 1, para 0 (G1, P0) whose last menstrual period was March 17. Her first prenatal visit was on July 3, at which time her fundal height was 22 cm. Fetal heart rate was audible by Doppler ultrasonography but not by DeLee stethoscope, and she has not yet felt fetal movement. Select from among the following items those that apply to Ms. J or the issue addressed.

1. High-risk factor(s)
   a. Fetal cardiac anomaly
   b. Advanced maternal age
   c. Size greater than dates
   d. IUGR
   e. Decreased fetal movement

2. Differential diagnosis for size greater than dates
   a. Oligohydramnios
   b. Polyhydramnios
   c. Twins
   d. Uterine fibroids
   e. Inaccurate date of LMP
   f. Pregnancy-induced hypertension

3. Diagnostic testing options
   a. CST
   b. Amniocentesis for genetics
   c. NST
   d. Ultrasonography for dating

4. Risk of miscarriage because of amniocentesis
   a. Less than 1%
   b. 10%
   c. 5%
   d. 8%

Ms. S is a 30-year-old G3 at 43 weeks' gestation (by poor dates) with late prenatal care. Her obstetrical ultrasonography at 42½ weeks showed a grade III placenta and biparietal diameter of 9.2 cm. She has complained of decreased FM since the previous night. Her next scheduled office visit is in 3 days. Select from among the following items those that apply to Ms. S or the issue addressed.

5. High-risk factor(s):
   a. Preterm labor
   b. Postdate pregnancy
   c. Abruptio placentae
   d. Decreased fetal movement
   e. Grand multipara

6. Possible diagnoses:
   a. Postterm pregnancy
   b. Term pregnancy
   c. Placenta previa
   d. Inaccurate maternal perception of fetal movement
   e. Uterine dystocia
   f. Fetal distress
   g. Preterm pregnancy

7. Diagnostic testing options:
   a. CVS
   b. PUBS
   c. Amniocentesis for L/S ratio
   d. NST
   e. CST
   f. AFI
   g. OD delta 450 reading
   h. Biophysical profile

8. Is it true or false that Ms. S is at no additional risk if she waits until her next scheduled office visit to be evaluated?

9. Is it true or false that all clients should be induced for postterm pregnancy at 42 weeks by dates, regardless of the accuracy of their EGA dating method, fetal surveillance results, or evidence of fetal maturity?

Ms. G is a 25-year-old G2, P1 at 32 weeks' EGA. She is Rh-negative and delivered an Rh-positive infant 2 years previously without receiving postpartum RhoGAM. Her current Rh titer is 1:30. Select from among the following items those that apply to Ms. G or the issue addressed.

10. High-risk factor(s)
    a. Preeclampsia
    b. Rh sensitization
    c. Maternal anemia
    d. IUGR

11. Diagnostic testing options for Rh-sensitized pregnancy
    a. Amniocentesis for OD delta 450 reading
    b. Early amniocentesis for genetics
    c. PUBS
    d. AFP screen
    e. NST

12. Is it true or false that if the results were zone III on the Liley graph, intrauterine transfusion would be an option for therapy in the absence of hydrops?

Ms. L is a 25-year-old G4, P3 at 34 weeks' gestation (by good dates) who has a history of drug abuse and smoking. Fetal serial ultrasound tests show poor interval growth, with a current biparietal diameter (BPD) of 7.8 cm and femur length of 6 cm, both consistent with 30 weeks' gestation. Select from among the following items those that apply to Ms. L or the issue addressed.

13. High-risk factor(s)
    a. Preeclampsia
    b. Diabetes
    c. IUGR
    d. Multiple pregnancy
    e. Substance abuse

14. Diagnostic testing for IUGR pregnancy and treatment planning
    a. Cervical culture

b. Biophysical profile
c. Amniocentesis for lung profile
d. Maternal urine toxicology screen
e. Maternal glucose testing
f. NST and AFI

15. Is it true or false that if Ms. L were to stop smoking now, her fetus would have an improved blood supply and would gain weight more rapidly?

Mrs. M, a 35-year-old G5, P3012, is 33 weeks' pregnant, has experienced a 7-lb weight gain in the last 4 weeks, and has 2+ protein in her urine. The physician has required her to quit work and maintain bedrest at home.

16. Because of the potential for uteroplacental insufficiency associated with pregnancy-induced hypertension, Mrs. M may have the following parameters evaluated in the home:
    a. AFI
    b. BPP
    c. CST
    d. NST
    e. Fetal movement

17. Two weeks later, she experiences spontaneous rupture of the membranes. She continues to leak amniotic fluid daily, and the AFI has just decreased by 50% at 36 weeks' gestation. To determine fetal maturity, which of the following tests might be performed?
    a. L/S ratio
    b. OD delta 450
    c. AFP
    d. LBC
    e. PG
    f. Triple marker

ANSWERS TO STUDY QUESTIONS

1. b, c	6. a, b, d, f	11. a, c, e	16. d, e
2. b, c, d, e	7. c, d, e, f, h	12. True	17. a, d, e
3. b, d	8. False	13. c, e	
4. a	9. False	14. b, c, d, f	
5. b, d	10. b	15. True	

REFERENCES

Adamsons, K., & Myers, R. (1977). Late decelerations and brain tolerance of the fetal monkey to intrapartum asphyxia. *American Journal of Obstetrics and Gynecology, 128*(8), 893-900.

American Academy of Pediatrics, American College of Obstetricians and Gynecologists. (2002). *Guidelines for perinatal care* (5th ed.). Washington, DC: AAP/ACOG.

American College of Obstetricians and Gynecologists. (1999). *Antepartum fetal surveillance. Practice Bulletin No. 9.* Washington, DC: ACOG.

American College of Obstetricians and Gynecologists. (2001a). *Prenatal diagnosis of fetal chromosomal abnormalities. Practice Bulletin No. 27.* Washington, DC: ACOG.

American College of Obstetricians and Gynecologists. (2001b). *Fetal surgery for open neural tube defects. Committee Opinion No. 252.* Washington, DC: ACOG.

American College of Obstetricians and Gynecologists. (2003). *Neural tube defects. Practice Bulletin No. 44.* Washington, DC: ACOG.

Ashwood, E.R., Palmer, S.E., Taylor, J.S., & Pingree, S.S. (1993). Lamellar body counts for rapid fetal lung maturity testing. *Obstetrics and Gynecology, 81*(4), 619-624.

Association of Women's Health, Obstetrics and Neonatal Nurses (AWHONN). (2002). *Fetal assessment: Clinical position statement.* Washington, DC: AWHONN

Association of Women's Health, Obstetrics and Neonatal Nurses (AWHONN). (1998). *Clinical competencies and education guide: Antepartum and intrapartum fetal heart rate monitoring.* Washington, DC: AWHONN.

Barkai, G. Reichman, B., Modan, M., Goldman, B., Serr, D., & mashiach, S. (1988). The influence of abnormal pregnancies on fluorescence polarization of amniotic fluid lipids. *Obstetrics and Gynecology, 67*(4), 566-568.

Bartha, J.L., Finney, K., & Soothill, P.N. (2003). Fetal sex determination from maternal blood at 6 weeks of gestation when at risk for 21-hydroxylase deficiency. *Obstetrics and Gynecology, 101*(5), 1135-1136.

Biagiotti, R., Cariati, E., Brizzi, L., & D'Agata, A. (1995). Maternal serum screening for Down's syndrome in the first trimester of pregnancy. *British Journal of Obstetrics and Gynaecology, 102*(8), 660-662.

Boehm, F., Salyer, S., Shah, D., & Waughn, W. (1986) Improved outcome of twice weekly nonstress testing. *Obstetrics and Gynecology, 67*(4), 566-568.

Bogart, M.H., Jones, O.W., Felder, R.A., Best, R.G., Bradley, L., Butts, W., et al. (1991). Prospective evaluation of maternal serum human chorionic gonadotropin levels in 3428 pregnancies. *American Journal of Obstetrics and Gynecology, 165*(3), 663-667.

Bogart, M.H., Pandian, M.R., & Jones, O.W. (1987). Abnormal maternal serum chorionic gonadropin levels in pregnancies with fetal chromosome abnormalities. *Prenatal Diagnosis, 7*(9), 623-630.

Bowman, J.M. (1999). Hemolytic disease. In R. Creasy & R. Resnick (Eds.), *Maternal-fetal medicine* (4th ed., pp. 736-767). Philadelphia: Saunders.

Brace, R. (1999). Dynamics and disorders of amniotic fluid. In R. Creasy & R. Resnick (Eds.), *Maternal-fetal medicine: Principles and practice* (4th ed., pp. 632-643). Philadelphia: Saunders.

Brambati, B., & Oldrini, A. (1985, May). CVS for first-trimester fetal diagnosis. *Contemporary OB/GYN, 25*, 94-97.

Burton, B., Schulz, C., & Burd, L. (1992). Limb anomalies associated with CVS. *Obstetrics & Gynecology, 79*(5, Pt 1), 726-730.

Buster, J.E., & Carson, S.A. (2002). Endocrinology and diagnosis of pregnancy.

In S.G. Gabbe, J.R. Niebyl, & J.L. Simpson (Eds.), *Obstetrics: Normal & problem pregnancies* (4th ed., pp. 3-36). New York: Churchill Livingstone.

Caldeyro-Barcia, R., Casacuberta, C., & Bustos, R. (1968). Correlation of intrapartum changes in fetal heart rate with fetal blood oxygen and acid-base state. In K. Adamsons (Ed.), *Diagnosis and treatment of fetal disorders* (pp. 25-37). New York: Springer-Verlag.

Canadian Early and Mid-Trimester Amniocentesis Trial (CEMAT) Group. (1998). Randomised trial to assess safety and fetal outcome of early and midtrimester amniocentesis. *Lancet, 351*(9098), 242-247.

Canick, J.A., Knight, G.J., Palomaki, G.E., Haddow, J.E., Cuckle, H.S., & Wald, N.J. (1988). Low second trimester maternal serum unconjugated oestriol in pregnancies with Down's syndrome. *British Journal of Obstetrics and Gynaecology, 95*(4), 330-333.

Chamberlain, P.F., Manning, F.A., Morrison, I., Harman, C.R., & Lange, I.R. (1984a). Ultrasound evaluation of amniotic fluid volume. Part I: The relationship of marginal and decreased amniotic fluid volumes to perinatal outcome. *American Journal of Obstetrics and Gynecology, 150*(3), 245-249.

Chamberlain, P., Manning F., Morrison I., Harman, C.R., & Lange, I.R. (1984b). Ultrasound evaluation of amniotic fluid volume. Part II: The relationship of increased amniotic fluid volume to perinatal outcome. *American Journal of Obstetrics and Gynecology, 150*(3), 250-254.

Cheng, E., Luthy, D., Zebelman, A., Williams, M., Lieppman, R., & Hickok, D. (1993). A prospective evaluation of a second-trimester screening test for fetal Down syndrome using maternal serum alpha-fetoprotein, human chorionic gonadropin, and unconjugated estriol. *Obstetrics and Gynecology, 81*(1), 72-77.

Chervenak, F., & Gabbe, S. (2002). Obstetric ultrasound: Assessment of fetal growth and anatomy. In S. Gabbe, J. Neibyl, & J. Simpson (Eds.), *Obstetrics: Normal and problem pregnancies* (4th ed., pp. 251-296). New York: Churchill Livingstone.

Cibils, L.A. (1981). *Electronic fetal-maternal monitoring: Antepartum and intrapartum.* Boston: PSG.

Cooper, R.L., Goldenberg, R.L., Creasy, R.K., DuBard, M.B., Davis, R.O., Entman, S.S.,

et al. (1993). A multicenter study of preterm birth weight and gestational age-specific mortality. *American Journal of Obstetrics and Gynecology. 168*(1, Pt 1), 78-84.

Cuckle, H.S., & Wald, N.S. (1992). hCG, estriol and other maternal blood markers of fetal aneuploidy. In S. Elias & J. L. Simpson (Eds.), *Maternal serum screening for fetal genetic disorders* (pp. 87-107). New York: Churchill Livingstone.

Cuckle, H.S., Wald, N.J., & Lindenbaum, R.H. (1984). Maternal serum alpha-fetoprotein measurement: A screening test for Down syndrome. *Lancet, 1*(8383), 926-929.

Cunningham, F.G., MacDonald, P.C., Cant, N.F., Leveno, K., Gilstrap, L. III, Hauth, J.C., et al. (2001). *Williams obstetrics* (21st ed.). Norwalk, CT: Appleton & Lange.

Daffos, F., Capella-Pavlovsky, M., & Forestier, F. (1985). Fetal blood sampling during pregnancy with the use of a needle guided by ultrasound: A study of 606 consecutive cases. *American Journal of Obstetrics and Gynecology, 153*(6), 655-660.

Devoe, L. (1990). The nonstress test. In R. Eden & F. Boehm (Eds.), *Assessment and care of the fetus: Physiological, clinical, and medicolegal principles* (pp. 365-383). Norwalk, CT: Appleton & Lange.

Druzin, M.L., Gabbe, S.G., & Reed, K.L. (2002). Antepartum fetal evaluation. In S.G. Gabbe, J.R. Niebyl, & J.L. Simpson (Eds.), *Obstetrics: Normal and problem pregnancies* (4th ed., pp. 313-352). New York: Churchill Livingstone.

Eden, R. (1990). Postdate pregnancy. In R. Eden & F. Boehm (Eds.), *Assessment and care of the fetus: Physiological, clinical and medicolegal principles* (pp. 767-778). Norwalk, CT: Appleton & Lange.

Elias, S., & Simpson, J.L. (1986). Amniocentesis. In A. Milunski (Ed.), *Genetic disorders and the fetus* (2nd ed., pp. 31-52). New York: Plenum.

Elias, S., Simpson, J.L., Martin, A.O., Sabbagha, R., Bombard, A., Rosinsky, B.J., et al. (1986). Chorionic villus sampling in continuing pregnancies. I: Low fetal loss rates in initial 109 cases. *American Journal of Obstetrics and Gynecology, 154*(6), 1349-1352.

Fakhoury, G., Daikoku, N.H., Benser, J., & Dubin, N.H. (1994). Lamellar body concentrations and the prediction of fetal pulmonary maturity. *American Journal of Obstetrics and Gynecology, 170*(1), 72-76.

Farrine, D., Kelly, E., Ryan, A., Morrow, R., & Ritchie, J. (1995). Absent and reversed umbilical artery and diastolic velocity in Doppler ultrasound. In J. Copel & K. Reed (Eds.), *Doppler ultrasound in obstetrics and gynecology* (pp. 187-188). New York: Raven.

Freda, M., Mikhail, M., Mazloom, E., Polizzotti, R., Damus, K., & Merkatz, I. (1993). Fetal movement counting: Which method? *Maternal Child Nursing, 18*(6), 314-321.

Freeman, R., & Lagrew, D. (1990). The contraction stress test. In R. Eden & F. Boehm (Eds.), *Assessment & care of the fetus: Physiological, clinical, and medicolegal principles* (pp. 351-363). Norwalk, CT: Appleton & Lange.

Gardner, R.J.M., & Sutherland, G.R. (1996). Prenatal diagnostic procedures. In *Chromosome abnormalities and genetic counseling* (2nd ed.). Oxford monographs on medical genetics, No 29. New York: Oxford University Press.

Garite, T. (1990). Theory of antepartum testing. Presentation at Advanced Fetal Monitoring Conference. Co-sponsored by Memorial Medical Center of Long Beach, University of California, Irvine, and Saddleback Memorial Hospital, Newport Beach, CA.

Garite, T., & Freeman, R. (1986). Fetal maturity cascade: A rapid and cost effective method for fetal lung maturity testing. *Obstetrics and Gynecology, 67*(4), 619-622.

Gilbert, E.S., & Harmon, J.S. (2003). *Manual of high risk pregnancy & delivery* (3rd ed.). St. Louis: Mosby.

Golbus, M., & Appelman, Z. (1990). Chorionic villus sampling. In R. Eden & F. Boehm (Eds.), *Assessment and care of the fetus: Physiological, clinical, and medicolegal principles* (pp. 259-265). Norwalk, CT: Appleton & Lange.

Grannum, P.A., Berkowitz, R.L., & Hobbins, J.C. (1979). The ultrasonic changes in the maturing placenta and their relation to fetal pulmonic maturity. *American Journal of Obstetrics and Gynecology, 133*(8), 915-922.

Greenspoon, J.S., Rosen, D.J., Roll, K., & Dubin, S.B. (1995). Evaluation of lamellar body number density as the initial assessment in a fetal lung maturity test cascade. *Journal of Reproductive Medicine, 40*(4), 260-266.

Haddow, J.E. (1990). Alpha-Fetoprotein. In M.R. Harrison, M.S. Golbus, & R.A. Filly (Eds.), *The unborn patient* (2nd ed., pp. 63-74). Philadelphia: Saunders.

Haddow, J.E., Palomaki, G.E., Knight, G.J., Cunningham, G.C., Lustig, L.S., & Boyd, P.A. (1994). Reducing the need for amniocentesis in women 35 years of age or older with serum markers for screening. *New England Journal of Medicine, 330*(1), 114-118.

Harman, C., Manning, F., Stearns, E., & Morrison, I. (1982). The correlation of ultrasonic placental grading and fetal pulmonary maturation in five hundred sixty-three pregnancies. *American Journal of Obstetrics and Gynecology, 143*(8), 941-943.

Harman, C.R. (1999). Percutaneous fetal blood sampling. In R. Creasy & R. Resnick (Eds.), *Maternal-fetal medicine* (4th ed., pp. 341-363). Philadelphia: Saunders.

Henry, G., & Miller, W. (1992). Early amniocentesis. *Journal of Reproductive Medicine, 37*(5), 396-402.

Hobbins, J.C., Grannum, P.A., Berkowitz, R.L., Silverman, R., & Mahoney, M.J. (1979). Ultrasound in the diagnosis of congenital anomalies. *American Journal of Obstetrics and Gynecology, 134*(3), 331-345.

Huddleston, J., Williams, G., & Fabre, E. (1993). Antepartum assessment of the fetus. In R. Knuppel & J. Drukker (Eds.), *High-risk pregnancy: A team approach* (2nd ed.). Philadelphia: Saunders.

Jobe, A.H. (1999). Fetal lung development, tests for maturation, induction of maturation, and treatment. In R. Creasy & R. Resnick (Eds.), *Maternal-fetal medicine* (4th ed., pp. 404-422). Philadelphia: Saunders.

Karsdorp, V.H., van Vugt, J.M., van Geijn, H.P., Kostense, P.J., Arduini, D., Montenegro, N., et al., (1994, December 17). Clinical significance of absent or reversed end diastolic velocity waveforms in umbilical artery. *Lancet, 344*(8938), 1664-1668.

Kellner, L.H., Weiss, R.R., Weiner, Z., Neuer, B.S., Martin, G.M., Schulman, H., et al. (1995). The advantages of using triple-marker screening for chromosomal abnormalities. *American Journal of Obstetrics and Gynecology, 172*(3), 831-836.

Krebs, H.B., Petres, R.E., Dunn, L.J., Jordaan, H.V., & Segreti, A. (1979). Intrapartum fetal heart rate monitoring. I: Classification and prognosis of fetal heart rate patterns. *American Journal of Obstetrics and Gynecology, 133*(7), 762-772.

Lamvu, G., & Kuller, J. (1997). Prenatal diagnosis using fetal cells from maternal circulation. *Obstetrics and Gynecology Survey, 52*(6), 433-437.

Liley, A. (1961). Liquor amnii analysis in the management of the pregnancy complicated by rhesus sensitization. *American Journal of Obstetrics and Gynecology, 82*(6), 1359-1370.

Little, G. (1990). Fetal growth and development. In R. Eden & F. Boehm (Eds.), *Assessment and care of the fetus: Physiological, clinical, and medicolegal principles* (pp. 3-15). Norwalk, CT: Appleton & Lange.

Lo, Y.M., Tein, M.S., Lau, T.K., Haines, C.S., Leung, T.N., Poon, P.M., et al. (1998). Quantitative analysis of fetal DNA in maternal plasma and serum: Implications for non-invasive prenatal diagnosis. *American Journal of Human Genetics, 62*(4), 768-775.

Ludomirski, A., & Weiner, S. (1988). Percutaneous fetal umbilical blood sampling. *Clinical Obstetrics and Gynecology, 31*(1), 19-26.

Manning, F. (1999a). Fetal assessment by evaluation of biophysical variables. In R. Creasy & R. Resnick (Eds.), *Maternal-fetal medicine* (4th ed., pp. 319-330). Philadelphia: Saunders.

Manning, F. (1999b). General principles and application of ultrasonography. In R. Creasy & R. Resnick (Eds.), *Maternal-fetal medicine* (4th ed., pp. 169-206). Philadelphia: Saunders.

Manning, F., & Harman, C. (1990). The fetal biophysical profile. In R. Eden & F. Boehm (Eds.), *Assessment and care of the fetus: Physiological, clinical, and medicolegal principles* (pp. 385-396). Norwalk, CT: Appleton & Lange.

Manning, F., Morrison, I., Lange, I., Harman, C., & Chamberlain, P. (1985). Fetal assessment based on fetal biophysical profile scoring: Experience in 12,620 referred high-risk pregnancies. *American Journal of Obstetrics and Gynecology, 151*(3), 343-350.

Manning, F., Platt, L., & Sipos, L. (1980). Antepartum fetal evaluation: Development of a fetal biophysical profile. *American Journal of Obstetrics and Gynecology, 136*(6), 787-795.

Martin, C., de Haan, J., van der Wildt, B., Jongsma, H., Dilleman, A., & Arts, T. (1979). Mechanisms of late decelerations in the fetal heart rate: A study with autonomic blocking agents in fetal lambs. *European Journal of Obstetrics, Gynecology and Reproductive Biology, 9*(6), 361-365.

McDuffie, R., & Haverkamp, A. (1991). Intrapartum fetal surveillance. In J. Frederickson & L. Wilkins-Haug (Eds.), *Ob-gyn secrets* (pp. 253-256). St. Louis: Mosby.

McKenna, D., Tharma, R.A., Tnam, M.B., Mahsud, S., Baile, C., Harper, A., et al. (2003). A randomized trial using ultrasound to identify the high risk fetus in a low risk population. *Obstetrics and Gynecology, 4*(101), 626-632.

Merkatz, I.R., Nitowsky, H.M., Macri, J.N., & Johnson, W.E. (1984). An association between low maternal serum alpha-fetoprotein and fetal chromosomal abnormalities. *American Journal of Obstetrics and Gynecology, 148*(7), 886-894.

Meschia, G. (1999). Placental respiratory gas exchange and fetal oxygenation. In R. Creasy & R. Resnick (Eds.), *Maternal-fetal medicine* (4th ed., pp. 260-269). Philadelphia: Saunders.

Morrison, J., & Pryor, J. (1990). Hemolytic disorders. In R. Eden & F. Boehm (Eds.), *Assessment and care of the fetus:\Physiological, clinical, and medicolegal principles* (pp. 737-748). Norwalk, CT: Appleton & Lange.

Murata, Y., Martin, C.B., Ikenoue, T., Hashimoto, T., Taira, S., Sagawa, T., et al. (1982). Fetal heart rate accelerations and late decelerations during the course of intrauterine death in chronically catheterized rhesus monkeys. *American Journal of Obstetrics and Gynecology, 144*(2), 218-223.

Myers, R., Beard, R., & Adamson, K. (1969). Brain swelling in the newborn rhesus monkey following prolonged partial asphyxia. *Neurology, 19*(10), 1012-1018.

National Institute of Child Health and Human Development, National Registry for Amniocentesis Study Group. (1976). Midtrimester amniocentesis for prenatal diagnosis: Safety and accuracy. *Journal of the American Medical Association, 236*(13), 1471-1476.

Nicolaides, K., Soothill, P., Clewell, W., Rodeck, C., Mibashan, R., & Campbell, S. (1988). Fetal haemoglobin measurement in the assessment of red cell isoimmunisation. *Lancet, 1*(8594), 1073-1075.

O'Brien, J.E., Dvorin, E., Drugen, A., Johnson, M.P., Yarow, Y., & Evans, M.I. (1997). Race-ethnicity-specific variation in multiple-marker biochemical screening: Alpha-fetoprotein, human chorionic gonadotropin and estriol. *Obstetrics and Gynecology, 89*(3), 355-358.

Olds, S., London, M., Ladewig, P., & Davidson, M.R. (2004). *Maternal-newborn nursing* (7th ed.). Upper Saddle River, NJ: Prentice Hall.

Parer, J. (1999). Fetal heart rate. In R. Creasy & R. Resnick (Eds.), *Maternal-fetal medicine: Principles and practice* (4th ed., pp. 270-299). Philadelphia: Saunders.

Porto, M. (1987). Comparing and contrasting methods of fetal surveillance. *Clinical Obstetrics and Gynecology, 30*(4), 956-967.

Queenan, J. (1985). *Management of high-risk pregnancy* (2nd ed.). Oradell, NJ: Medical Economics.

Richardson, B.S., & Gagnon, R. (1999). Fetal breathing and body movements. In R. Creasy & R. Resnick (Eds.), *Maternal-fetal medicine* (4th ed., pp. 231-246). Philadelphia: Saunders.

Robinson, H. (1980) Ultrasound measurements in the evaluation of the normal early pregnancy. In R. Sanders & A. James (Eds.), *The principles and practice of ultrasonography in obstetrics and gynecology* (pp. 121-130). New York: Appleton-Century-Crofts.

Rodriguez, H. (1991). *Early amniocentesis.* Paper presented at the PAC/LAC subregion VI monthly meeting, Pomona Valley Medical Center, Pomona, CA.

Rutherford, S., Phelan, J., Smith, C., & Jacobs, N. (1987). The four-quadrant assessment of amniotic fluid volume: An adjunct to antepartum fetal heart rate testing. *Obstetrics and Gynecology, 70*(3), 353-356.

Sabbagha, R. (1978). Standardization of sonar cephalometry and gestational age. *Obstetrics and Gynecology, 52*(4), 402-409.

Sadovsky, E. (1990). Fetal movements. In R. Eden & F. Boehm (Eds.), *Assessment and care of the fetus: Physiological, clinical, and medicolegal principles* (pp. 341-349). Norwalk, CT: Appleton & Lange.

Sadovsky, E. (1985a). Fetal movements. In J. Queenan (Ed.), *Management of high-risk pregnancy* (2nd ed., pp. 183-193). Oradell, NJ: Medical Economics.

Sadovsky, E. (1985b). Monitoring fetal movements: A useful screening test. *Contemporary OB/GYN, 25,* 123-127.

Schulman, H. (1990). Doppler ultrasound. In R. Eden & F. Boehm (Eds.), *Assessment and care of the fetus: Physiological, clinical and medicolegal principles* (pp. 397-407). Norwalk, CT: Appleton & Lange.

Scioscia, A.L. (1999). Prenatal genetic diagnosis. In R. Creasy & R. Resnick (Eds.), *Maternal-fetal medicine* (4th ed., pp. 40-62). Philadelphia: Saunders.

Silverman, F., Suidan, J., Wasserman, J., Antoine, C., Young, B.K. (1985). The Apgar score: Is it enough? *Obstetrics and Gynecology, 66*(3), 331-336.

Simpson, J. (2002). Genetic counseling and prenatal diagnosis. In S. Gabbe, J. Niebyl, & J. Simpson (Eds.), *Obstetrics: Normal and problem pregnancies* (4th ed., pp. 187-220). New York: Churchill Livingstone.

Sonek, J., Reiss, R., & Gabbe, S. (1990). Antenatal fetal assessment. In F. Zuspan & E. Quilligan (Eds.), *Manual of obstetrics and gynecology* (2nd ed., pp. 57-95). St. Louis: Mosby.

Sonek, J.D., & Nicolaides, K.H. (1998). The ultrasound examination. In N. Gleicher (Ed.), *Principles and practice of medical therapy in pregnancy* (3rd ed., pp. 48-70). Stamford, CT: Appleton & Lange.

Sunberg, K., Bang, J., Smidt-Jensen, S., Brocks, V., Lundsteen, C., Parner, J., et al. (1997). Randomised study of risk of fetal loss related to early amniocentesis versus chorionic villus sampling. *Lancet, 350*(9079), 697-703.

Trudinger, B. (1999). Doppler ultrasound assessment of blood flow. In R. Creasy & R. Resnick (Eds.), *Maternal-fetal medicine* (4th ed., pp. 216-229). Philadelphia: Saunders.

Vintzileos, A., Campbell, W., Ingardia, C., & Nochimson, D. (1983). The fetal biophysical profile and its predictive value. *Obstetrics and Gynecology, 62*(3), 271-278.

Vintzileos, A., Fleming, A., Scorza W., Wolf, E., Balducci, J., Campbell, W., et al. (1991). Relationship between fetal biophysical activities and umbilical cord blood gas values. *American Journal of Obstetrics and Gynecology, 165*(3), 707-713.

Vintzileos, A., Gaffney, S., Salinger, I., Campbell, W., & Nochemison, D. (1987). The relationship between fetal biophysical profile and cord pH in patients undergoing cesarean section before the onset of labor. *Obstetrics and Gynecology, 70*(2), 196-201.

Weiner, C. (1988). The role of cordocentesis in fetal diagnosis. *Clinical Obstetrics and Gynecology, 31*(2), 285-292.

Wenstrom, K.D., Owen, J., Chu, D., & Boots, L. (1999). Prospective evaluation of free beta-subunit of human chorionic gonadotropin and dimeric inhibin A for aneuploidy detection. *American Journal of Obstetrics and Gynecology, 181*(4), 887-892.

Wexler, P., & Gottesfeld, K.R. (1977). Second-trimester placenta previa: An apparently normal placentation. *Obstetrics and Gynecology, 50*(6), 706-709.

9 Environmental Hazards

ROXENA WOTRING

OBJECTIVES

1. Recognize potential environmental hazards and the possible risks to the fetus.

2. Identify persons who have had exposure to potential environmental hazards and refer for appropriate follow-up.

3. Recognize the need to take a complete occupational history on all prenatal clients.

4. Assist prenatal clients in handling their fears regarding environmental risks.

5. Use community resources for health education, or referral relevant to environmental hazards, or both.

6. Educate women of childbearing age regarding potential environmental hazards and how to protect against or minimize exposure.

INTRODUCTION

A. Scope of the problem: Hewitt and Tellier (1996) report that the estimate is that every year 20 million workers in the United States can be exposed to reproductive toxins; the National Institute of Occupational, Safety and Health (NIOSH) reports more than 5000 chemicals have possible reproductive toxicity; a simple health history tool with the mnemonic CH2 OP D2 can be used to identify persons who are at risk (Abelsohn, Gibson, Sanborn, & Weir, 2002) (Box 9-1).

    1. Exposure has reproductive implications for both parents.

    2. The embryo is most vulnerable during the first trimester.

    3. Negative outcomes include:

        a. Altered fertility

        b. Genetic defects

        c. Reproductive waste (spontaneous abortions, stillbirths, and neonatal deaths)

        d. Altered gestational lengths

        e. Growth restriction

        f. Congenital malformations

        g. Conditions that develop later in life (developmental disabilities, behavioral disorders, chronic diseases, and malignancies)

B. Consider the following when evaluating potential risks:

    1. Susceptibility varies with the developmental stage at the time of exposure.

    2. Susceptibility depends on the genetic makeup of the mother and embryo or fetus and the manner in which it responds to environmental factors.

    3. Outcome depends on the nature of the agent, amount and duration of the exposure, and mode of transmission.

    4. The benefits must be weighed against the potential risks.

■ BOX 9-1
■ **ENVIRONMENTAL HEALTH HISTORY TOOL**

> **CH2 OP D2 (Community, Home, Hobbies, Occupation, Personal Habits, Diet, and Drugs)**
> Community: Polluting industries? Toxic waste sites?
> Home: Water supply, heating source?
> Hobbies: Either parent exposed to any of the following?
> ■ Chemicals
> ■ Loud noise
> ■ Radiation
> ■ Heavy metals
> ■ Vibration
> ■ Prolonged standing
> ■ Extreme heat or cold
> Occupation: Either parent exposed to any of the items on the previous list?
> Personal habits: Either parent smoke? Is mother exposed to secondhand smoke? Does mother use hot tub or Jacuzzi?
> Diet: Fish, wild meat consumption by mother?
> Drugs: Does mother use prescription or over-the-counter medication?

5. Causal relationships between exposure and negative outcomes are difficult to confirm because exposure to more than one agent at a time may have occurred, and determining and quantifying exposures is difficult.

C. **Stages of susceptibility to exposure**
1. First stage is during the first 2 weeks before implantation; fetus is likely to experience little structural damage but lethality risk may be great.
2. Second stage is from 3 to 8 weeks' gestation during organogenesis.
   a. Fetus is very susceptible to structural damage.
   b. Major malformations usually occur from 14 to 56 days' gestation.
3. Third stage when organogenesis is complete; growth restriction and functional problems are the most common anomalies (Polifka & Friedman, 2002).

D. **Categories of environmental risks in this chapter include the following:**
1. Occupational hazards
2. Temperature extremes
3. Pharmaceuticals
4. Secondhand smoke

E. **Definition of terms used in this chapter**
1. Reproductive risk: probability that reproductive impairment and developmental impairment or death in the embryo, fetus, or child may result from exposure to a chemical, physical, or biologic agent; reproductive effects depend on the potential for the agent to cause harm, as well as the extent of exposure
2. Mutagen: chemical or physical agent that causes permanent alterations in deoxyribonucleic acid (DNA), changing the genetic material of the fetal cells
3. Teratogen: agents that act directly on developing fetuses, causing abnormal embryonic or fetal development
   a. Dosage
      (1) With low dose, no effect may occur.
      (2) With intermediate dose, malformation may result.
      (3) With high dose, death of embryo may occur.

    b. For teratogenesis to occur, the following must be present:
        (1) A particular dose of a toxic agent
        (2) A genetically susceptible host
        (3) An embryo in a susceptible stage of development
  4. Carcinogen: occurrence of cancer in children attributed to parental exposure

CLINICAL PRACTICE
Occupational Hazards

A. Introduction
  1. Labor force profile: according to the U.S. Census Bureau 2002, in the year 2000, over 60% of all women 18 to 64 years of age were in the civilian labor force and accounted for nearly 50% of the workforce.
  2. The workplace has been designed predominantly for men.
  3. Work exposures affect the reproductive health of both male and female workers.
  4. Inaccurate and incomplete exposure data during gestation make determining reproductive risk difficult.
  5. Occupational and nonoccupational exposures are difficult to separate.

B. Assessment
  1. History of occupational exposure
    a. Establish time of exposure (when in pregnancy).
    b. Establish duration of exposure.
    c. Establish mode of exposure (respiratory, gastrointestinal, skin).
    d. Evaluate precautions taken to control exposure (i.e., protective clothing, equipment used).
    e. Establish exposure levels in the workplace.
  2. Exposure agent
    a. Ethylene oxide: may produce mutagenic effects and spontaneous abortion.
        (1) Use
            (a) Production of ethylene glycol for antifreeze, polyester fibers and films, and detergents
            (b) In sterilizing equipment and supplies in health care facilities
            (c) As a fumigant in the manufacture of medical products and foodstuffs
            (d) In libraries and museums
        (2) Establish history of exposure: exposure during all stages of cell division is important.
    b. Colorants: implicated as teratogens with nearly double the risk of gastroschisis in the exposed fetus.
        (1) Use: permanent hair dyes, nail polish, and furniture paints or fabric dyes
        (2) Establish history and timing of exposure, either at work or with hobbies; especially risky during the first trimester.
    c. Ergonomics: design of the workplace is important to ensure safety of the pregnant woman, particularly in the second and third trimesters as body weight and girth increase.
        (1) Sitting at a desk, use of video display terminal, and other work-related activities may pose an ergonomic risk.
        (2) Establish history of exposure, either at work or with hobbies.
        (3) An ergonomic assessment may be helpful to determine risk.
        (4) Redesign of the workplace may effectively decrease the risk.

    d. Halogenated hydrocarbons: several have been implicated as:

      (1) Exposure

        (a) Paternal exposure may lead to early fetal death and birth defects.

        (b) Women may be more susceptible to the effects, reflecting their increased metabolic rate.

        (c) Paternal exposure before pregnancy in some cases may have a negative impact.

      (2) Use: laundry and dry cleaner industries; rubber industry

      (3) Establish history and timing of exposure of either mother or father to tetrachloroethylene, vinyl chloride, and chloroprene.

        (a) Mutagen: all stages of cell division.

        (b) Teratogen: exposure is most important during early differentiation.

        (c) Carcinogen: any time during pregnancy.

    e. Heavy metals: cadmium, lead, arsenic, and mercury may be teratogenic.

      (1) Effects

        (a) Cadmium may also affect male fertility.

        (b) Premature birth and early fetal death may result from lead exposure.

        (c) Perinatal lead exposure is associated with cognitive deficits (Myers & Davidson, 2000).

        (d) Lead and mercury may lead to spontaneous abortions.

        (e) Arsenic is implicated in spontaneous abortion, low birth weight, and fetal loss.

        (f) Mercury may result in spontaneous abortions, low birth weight, developmental disabilities, and cerebral palsy.

      (2) Use:

        (a) Cadmium: used in batteries, pigments, paints, soldering liquids, semiconductors, photocells, insecticides, and fungicides

        (b) Lead: used in gasoline, batteries, paints, ink, ceramics, pottery, ammunition, and textiles

        (c) Arsenic: used in the production of various alloys to improve characteristics such as corrosion resistance, to improve machinability, and to increase annealing temperatures

        (d) Mercury: used in mercury vapor lamps, paint, and thermometers

      (3) Establish a history and timing of exposure: exposure at any time may be dangerous, especially during first trimester.

    f. Herbicides: exposure to 2,4,5,-trichlorophenoxyacetic acid in the United States has been associated with an increased spontaneous miscarriage rate.

      (1) Use: used to control unwanted vegetation

      (2) Establish a history of exposure: exposure during the first trimester is important.

    g. Ionizing radiation: exposures to x-rays and gamma rays are usually well controlled and with proper protection do not pose a major threat; high-dose techniques—computed tomography (CT) and interventional radiology—require radiation protection

      (1) Use: used diagnostically and therapeutically in the health care industry

      (2) It has been recently recognized that female flight personnel and pregnant frequent flyers are exposed to cosmic radiation and may exceed recommended radiation exposure (Geeze, 1998).

      (3) Establish a history of exposure: a dose to a pregnant woman should not exceed 1.5 rad during pregnancy.

   (a) Timing of exposure
       (i) Mutagen: exposure is important at any stage of cell division.
       (ii) Teratogen: exposure is most important during early differentiation.
   (b) Establish workplace levels.
       (i) High doses may lead to:
           ■ Spontaneous abortion
           ■ Late fetal death
           ■ Neonatal death
           ■ Low birth weight
           ■ Microcephaly or mental retardation
           ■ Childhood mortality
       (ii) Low doses may lead to:
           ■ Altered sex ratio
           ■ Childhood malignancies: solid tumors and leukemia
           ■ Childhood mortality
 h. Noise: sound transmits to the fetus, but the effects on the fetus are inconclusive.
   (1) Exposure is linked to:
       (a) Growth restriction in the fetus
       (b) Low birth weight of infant
       (c) Prematurity
       (d) An increase in the child's risk of high-frequency hearing losses
   (2) Use: used in such areas as many manufacturing processes and heavy-equipment operation
   (3) Establish a history and timing of exposure.
       (a) Exposure above 85 decibels (dB) may be dangerous (Table 9-1).
       (b) Cumulative noise exposure must include exposure to recreational noise, such as to loud music.
       (c) Noise levels above 85 dB usually interfere with communication.
       (d) It is uncertain which time is most critical; may be dangerous at all stages.
 i. Nonionizing radiation: no reproductive data are available at this time to support concern for exposure to nonionizing radiation.

■ TABLE 9-1
■ ■ **Typical Noise Levels**

Level	Example
30 dB	Quiet library, soft whisper
40 dB	Quiet office, living room, bedroom away from traffic
50 dB	Light traffic at a distance, refrigerator
60 dB	Air conditioner at 6.1 m (20 ft) conversation, sewing machine
70 dB	Busy traffic, noisy restaurant (constant)
80 dB	Subway, heavy city traffic, alarm clock at 0.6 m (2 ft), factory noise; dangerous if more than an 8-hr exposure
90 dB	Truck traffic, noisy home appliances, shop tools, lawnmower; dangerous if more than 8-hr exposure
100 dB	Chainsaw, boiler shop, pneumatic drill; dangerous if more than a 2-hr exposure

j. Organic solvents
   (1) Effects
      (a) Benzene may act as a teratogen and carcinogen.
      (b) Propene and glycol may act as teratogens and have been found to double the risk of gastroschisis in the exposed fetus.
   (2) Use
      (a) Chemical laboratories
      (b) Auto work
      (c) Furniture stripping and painting
   (3) Establish a history of exposure.
      (a) Teratogen: exposure is most important during early differentiation.
      (b) Carcinogen: exposure is important during any stage.
k. Pesticides: can effect the neurobehavioral development of the fetus; exposure to chlorinated hydrocarbons, such as chlordane, may be mutagenic and carcinogenic
   (1) Use: used to control unwanted pests in crops; commonly used by farm workers
   (2) Establish a history of exposure: exposure at any stage may be important.
l. Polychlorinated biphenyls (PCBs) (found in some trout and salmon)
   (1) Exposure may be linked to:
      (a) Low birth weight
      (b) Low intelligence quotient (IQ) scores in the child
      (c) Possibly at least 2 years' lag in reading comprehension
      (d) Immunotoxic effect
   (2) Use
      (a) Dielectric in capacitors and transformers
      (b) Investment casting processes
      (c) Heat-exchange fluid and hydraulic fluid
   (3) Establish a history of exposure: timing of exposure may determine specific effect.
m. Physical energy demands: no *conclusive* evidence is available that links heavy work and pregnancy outcome.
   (1) Exertion may increase the risk of:
      (a) Early fetal death
      (b) Prematurity and low birth weight
   (2) Working long hours, lengthy periods of standing, and night work have been associated, in some studies, with increased risk for preterm delivery (Mozurkewich, Luke, Avni, & Wolf, 2000).
   (3) Reduced intrauterine growth has been associated with physically strenuous jobs requiring long hours of standing.
   (4) Heavy lifting has been linked with spontaneous abortion.
   (5) Exposure to vibration may be related to stillbirths.
   (6) Use: physical effort occurs at work or during prolonged standing
   (7) Establish a history and timing of exposure: tolerance of strenuous exertion, such as lifting, pulling, pushing, or climbing, varies greatly among women on the basis of physical fitness and strength, load handled, and the environment; exposure is important at any stage, especially late in pregnancy.

    n. Waste anesthetic gases: gases can cross the placental barrier.

      (1) Exposure may cause:

        (a) Early fetal death

        (b) Altered sex ratio

        (c) Late fetal death

        (d) Low birth weight

        (e) Birth defects

      (2) Exposure to *halogenated gases* may be carcinogenic, teratogenic, and mutagenic, and it may reduce fertility in men.

      (3) Use: common in health care workers, dentists, laboratory personnel, and veterinarians

      (4) Establish history and timing of exposure: may be important at any stage, including before pregnancy.

  3. Diagnostic procedures

    a. Establish client's level of exposure through review of records when possible; review biologic samples when appropriate (e.g., urine to determine levels of organic solvents and pesticides; blood to determine lead levels).

    b. Establish level of exposure through environmental monitoring of workplace (i.e., use of dosimeter for noise level).

C. Nursing Diagnoses

  1. Risk for fetal injury related to maternal exposure to environmental hazards

  2. Deficient knowledge and learning need related to prenatal exposure to environmental hazards

  3. Anxiety related to maternal exposure to environmental hazards

D. Interventions/Outcomes

  1. Risk for fetal injury related to maternal exposure to environmental hazards

    a. Interventions

      (1) Assess for exposure to potential hazards.

      (2) Evaluate risk, accounting for the specificity of the agent, the developmental stage, the dose and length of exposure, the health of the mother, and what type of protection was used to control exposure.

      (3) Use occupational health nurse and physician in the workplace to further assess and plan for exposure control.

      (4) Refer to health care provider for further evaluation.

      (5) Refer client to appropriate agencies for further information about the potential hazard or to report exposure.

      (6) Refer for genetic counseling as needed.

      (7) Reassure that not every exposure results in a negative outcome; many uncertainties exist.

    b. Outcomes

      (1) Client follows through on referrals made.

      (2) Client obtains information to more clearly understand exposure to potential hazards.

      (3) Client avoids exposure to potential hazards and controls exposure to minimize negative effects.

  2. Deficient knowledge and learning need related to prenatal exposure to environmental hazards

    a. Interventions

      (1) Provide client information about the possible effects of exposure to environmental hazards, putting the information in proper perspective.

(2) Refer client to material safety data sheets, available at the workplace, that describe possible hazards.

(3) Advise client to use appropriate safety precautions to control exposure when indicated.

(4) Advise client to inform the health care provider of possible or real exposure.

(5) Advise client to inform the occupational health office of pregnancy as soon as possible and discuss possible options to prevent or minimize exposures.

(6) Advise expectant father to also control exposure to potential reproductive hazards.

(7) Advise client to cooperate in biologic monitoring while at the workplace.

(8) Refer client to appropriate agencies for further information.

(9) Educate client about the importance of avoiding potential environmental hazards at all times, not just while pregnant.

(10) Advise client to plan pregnancies to avoid potentially harmful exposures before she becomes pregnant because the first trimester is important in determining outcome of exposure.

(11) Advise client to avoid prolonged standing and exertion.

(12) Encourage client to share information with others and serve as an advocate for healthy pregnancies.

b. Outcomes

(1) Client is able to describe potential harmful effects of exposures.

(2) Client uses protective equipment when advised to control exposure.

(3) Client follows through on referrals and advice.

(4) Client establishes healthy behaviors to maximize pregnancy outcome.

3. Anxiety related to maternal exposure to environmental hazards

a. Interventions

(1) Listen to client's fears.

(2) Reassure the client that not all exposures result in negative consequences to the fetus.

(3) Provide information honestly.

(4) Refer for counseling as needed.

(5) Assist in finding support system.

b. Outcomes

(1) Client is more calm and has realistic perspective.

(2) Client avoids further risks.

(3) Client is able to communicate concerns with appropriate health professionals and significant others.

Temperature Extremes

A. **Introduction**

1. Extreme heat and humidity may lead to impairment of alertness, mental function, and physical capacity.

2. Pregnant women may be more sensitive to heat and humidity.

3. Controversy exists about the possible risk to the fetus.

B. **Assessment**

1. History

a. Hyperthermia increases the body's core temperature, and prolonged, high temperature may affect the central nervous system (CNS) of the fetus (Araujo, 1997).

> (1) Hyperthermia is considered a suspected teratogen by some authorities; others have concluded that hyperthermia causes no reproductive hazard.
> (2) Exposure to hot tubs and Jacuzzis early in pregnancy may increase the risk of birth defects by two to three times; spina bifida and other neural tube defects are particularly associated with heat exposure.
> (3) Pregnant women should be advised to avoid hot tub or Jacuzzi temperature of 100° F or higher (Pergament, Schectman, & Rochanayon, 1997).
> (4) No evidence has been found that electric blankets pose a danger.
> (5) Use: hyperthermia may result from exposure to high temperatures in hot tubs, Jacuzzis, or from febrile illness.
> (6) Establish a history of exposure.
>> (a) Timing of exposure
>>> (i) As a suspected teratogen, the greatest harm is produced during early differentiation.
>>> (ii) Exposure during all stages of pregnancy may be dangerous.
>> (b) Establish temperature level of client and environment.

2. Physical findings

   a. Symptoms of heat exhaustion
   - (1) Syncope, dizziness, and weakness
   - (2) Nausea and vomiting
   - (3) Increased pulse rate
   - (4) Shortness of breath
   - (5) Skin moist and clammy

   b. Symptoms of heat stroke
   - (1) Hot, dry skin
   - (2) Confusion
   - (3) Convulsions
   - (4) Loss of consciousness

   c. Hypotension

3. Psychosocial findings

   a. Disorientation

   b. Diminished mental alertness and functioning

C. Nursing Diagnoses

1. Risk for fetal injury related to hyperthermia

2. Deficient knowledge and learning need related to effects of hyperthermia on fetus

D. Interventions/Outcomes

1. Risk for fetal injury related to hyperthermia

   a. Interventions
   - (1) Assess for exposure to extreme heat.
   - (2) Provide cooling measures immediately.
   - (3) Provide extra liquids.
   - (4) Refer to health care provider for further evaluation.

   b. Outcomes
   - (1) Client avoids exposure to extreme heat conditions.

2. Deficient knowledge and learning need related to effects of hyperthermia on fetus

   a. Interventions
   - (1) Provide information about the possible dangers of prolonged exposure to heat.
   - (2) Advise use of Jacuzzis or hot tubs at temperatures of less than 100° F.

(3) Discourage strenuous physical activities and exercise that might increase body temperature.
  b. Outcomes
    (1) Client is able to describe potential dangers of hyperthermia to pregnancy.
    (2) Client avoids exposure to extreme heat conditions.

Pharmaceuticals

A. **Introduction**
  1. Pharmaceuticals may be prescribed as part of a treatment regimen or may be taken as over-the-counter drugs to relieve symptoms.
  2. No safe dose has been determined in most cases.
  3. The most critical time for exposure to pharmaceuticals is during early differentiation.
  4. Drugs may have a variety of effects on the fetus; the dose of the agent, timing of exposure, agent synergism, rate of metabolism, and host susceptibility of both mother and fetus play a role in fetal outcome; polypharmacy use further complicates the problem.
  5. Dose and method of administration must also be considered in evaluating risk.
  6. Evaluation of each drug taken must be based on its potential effect as carcinogen, mutagen, or teratogen.
  7. Drugs that are either absorbed systemically or are known to be potentially harmful to the fetus are required by the U.S. Food and Drug Administration to be categorized according to one of five pregnancy categories as follows (the letter signifies the level of risk to the fetus):
    a. Category A: drugs that have failed to pose a demonstrated risk to the fetus in controlled studies in women
    b. Category B: drugs that have not posed a demonstrated fetal risk but for which no controlled studies in pregnant women have been conducted
    c. Category C: drugs that have revealed adverse effects on the fetus in animal studies, but no controlled studies in women have been conducted; category C also includes drugs for which no studies are available; most drugs are in this category because of the lack of available studies
    d. Category D: drugs for which positive evidence of human fetal risk exists, but the benefits might outweigh the risk if no safer effective drugs are available
    e. Category X: drugs deemed contraindicated in women who are or may become pregnant, and the risk of use clearly outweighs any possible benefit
  8. Because of space constraints, priority has been given to drugs found in categories D and X.
B. **Assessment**
  1. History
    a. Amphetamines
      (1) Action: CNS stimulant
      (2) Effects
        (a) Dextroamphetamine (Dexedrine): effects may include congenital heart defects (though no conclusive evidence is available to support this possibility).

(b) Methamphetamine: effects include:
  (i) Prematurity
  (ii) Placental abruption
  (iii) Fetal distress
  (iv) Postpartum hemorrhage
  (v) Developmental delays, tremulousness, increased startle reflex, and alterations in visual processing and quality of alertness in infants
  (vi) Frontal lobe dysfunction that manifests at school age
  (vii) Methamphetamine is also a teratogen.
(c) Benzphetamine hydrochloride (Didrex): effects in pregnant women have not been established.
(3) Timing of exposure: exposure is important at any stage, with greatest damage occurring during the stage of early differentiation.
b. Analgesics
(1) Action: nonnarcotic pain relievers
(2) Aspirin and phenylbutazone (Butagesic, Butazolidin) have been classified as category D drugs.
  (a) Safe use during pregnancy has not been demonstrated, particularly during the third trimester.
  (b) Both drugs should be avoided during pregnancy when possible.
(3) Effects of aspirin include:
  (a) A potential decrease in blood clotting time near delivery
  (b) Prolonged gestation
  (c) A quadrupled risk of gastroschisis when taken during the first trimester
(4) Ibuprofen, although classified as a category B drug, has been found to quadruple the risk of gastroschisis in the fetus, especially when the fetus is exposed during the first trimester; the drug should be avoided during pregnancy.
c. Antialcohol agents
(1) Action: deterrence of alcohol ingestion
(2) Disulfiram (Antabuse) is classified as a category X drug and is contraindicated during pregnancy; specific risks are not well documented.
d. Antibiotics
(1) Action: infection control
(2) Effects
  (a) Streptomycin: effects may include damage to the auditory nerve that leads to fetal deafness.
  (b) Ribavirin (tribavirin, Viramid): an antiviral; associated with fetal abnormalities
  (c) Quinine sulfate: an antimalarial drug; contraindicated as a category X drug
  (d) Tetracycline: when administered in the last half of pregnancy, effects may include tooth discoloration in infant.
  (e) The following antiinfective agents are included in category D: specific effects on the fetus have not been described.
    (i) Ethionamide (Trecator-SC)
    (ii) Kanamycin (Anamid, Kantrex, Klebcil)
    (iii) Povidone-iodine (Betadine)
    (iv) Tobramycin sulfate (Nebcin, Tobrex)

      (v) Netilmicin sulfate (Netromycin)

      (vi) Emetine hydrochloride

e. Anticoagulants

  (1) Action: decreases clotting time

  (2) Effects

    (a) Coumarin derivatives (warfarin, dicumarol) include decreased synthesis of the vitamin K–dependent clotting factors II, VII, IX, and X, as well as interference with protein binding of calcium; coumarin is also considered to be teratogenic.

    (b) Warfarin

      (i) Exposure during the first trimester produces the following effects:

- Increases the risk for warfarin embryopathy (nasal hypoplasia resulting from the lack of development of the nasal septum and stippling of the epiphyses).
- Effects may include the following:
  — Growth and developmental retardation
  — Scoliosis
  — Deafness
  — Congenital heart disease

      (ii) Exposure during the second and third trimesters is associated with the following:

- Eye anomalies
- Hydrocephaly and other CNS defects
- Spontaneous abortions
- Stillbirth
- Neonatal hemorrhage

f. Anticonvulsants

  (1) Action: treatment of tonic-clonic and psychomotor seizures; assigning teratogenic potential is difficult because epilepsy and anomalies may be interrelated.

  (2) Effects

    (a) Effects of exposure to anticonvulsants include:

      (i) Seizure-related hypoxia

      (ii) Acidosis in the developing embryo or fetus

    (b) Phenytoin (Dilantin), diazepam (Valium), and trimethadione have been implicated as teratogens.

    (c) Phenytoin: effects include:

      (i) Intrauterine and extrauterine growth restriction

      (ii) Mental impairment

      (iii) Congenital heart lesions

      (iv) Facial dysmorphisms (cleft lip or palate, low-set ears, depressed nasal bridge, and short nose)

      (v) Hernias

      (vi) Distal digital and nail hypoplasias and limb anomalies

      (vii) Also associated with increased risk for childhood neuroectodermal tumors and neonatal coagulopathy

    (d) Trimethadione may cause:

      (i) Developmental delay

      (ii) Mental impairment

      (iii) Craniofacial abnormalities

      (iv) Spontaneous abortion

(e) Diazepam has been associated with an increase in congenital malformations when taken during the first trimester.
(f) The following drugs are classified as category D drugs and should be used with caution:
  (i) Paramethadione (Paradione)
  (ii) Phenacemide (Phenurone)
  (iii) Phensuximide (Milontin)
  (iv) Primidone (Mysoline)
  (v) Valproic acid (Depakene)

(3) Timing of exposure
  (a) First trimester poses the greatest risk.
  (b) Use of anticonvulsants is contraindicated during any stage of pregnancy.

g. Antidepressants and psychotropics
  (1) Action: treatment of depression
  (2) Effects
    (a) Lithium has been linked to cardiac abnormalities.
    (b) Meprobamate (Equanil, Miltown) has been implicated in cardiac abnormalities.
    (c) Chlordiazepoxide hydrochloride (Librium) may cause:
      (i) Mental retardation
      (ii) Spastic diplegia
      (iii) Deafness
      (iv) Microcephaly
      (v) Duodenal atresia
    (d) Haloperidol (Haldol) has been implicated in limb deformity.
    (e) Other category D drugs include (specific risks have not been documented):
      (i) Nortriptyline hydrochloride (Aventyl)
      (ii) Alprazolam (Xanax)
      (iii) Lorazepam (Ativan, Alzapam)

h. Antiemetics
  (1) Action: control of nausea and vomiting
  (2) Thiethylperazine maleate (Torecan) is contraindicated during pregnancy as a category X drug; specific effects are not well documented.

i. Antihyperlipidemics and hypocholesterolemic agents
  (1) Action: lower levels of cholesterol and low-density lipoproteins
    (a) Fluvastatin sodium, lovastatin (formerly mevinolin), pravastatin sodium, and simvastatin are classified as category X drugs and should be avoided during pregnancy.

j. Antihypertensives
  (1) Action: treatment of hypertension
  (2) Effects
    (a) Reserpine may cause nasal congestion, lethargy, depressed Moro reflex, and bradycardia in infants.
    (b) Metolazone (Diulo, Zaroxolyn), benzthiazide (Hydrex, Aquatag, Marazide), or polythiazide (Renese) may result in neonatal jaundice, thrombocytopenia, and other adverse reactions.

k. Antimigraine agents
  (1) Action: prevention or abortion of migraine, cluster headache, and other vascular headaches

(2) Effects: exposure to ergotamine tartrate (Ergostat, Ergomar) is clearly contraindicated during pregnancy as a category X drug because of the potential uterotonic effects of the ergot alkaloids.

l. Antineoplastics
  (1) Action: alkylating agents commonly used in the treatment of cancers
  (2) Effects
    (a) Aminopterin is associated with a significant number of birth defects—hydrocephaly, cleft palate, meningomyelocele, and cranial abnormalities.
    (b) Methotrexate may cause fetal death, and congenital anomalies that have not been well described.
    (c) Most antineoplastics are classified as category X drugs and are clearly contraindicated during pregnancy; fetal death and unspecified congenital anomalies are the common risks of exposure.
  (3) Timing of exposure
    (a) Exposure is most critical during the first trimester.
    (b) Exposures during the second and third trimesters do not seem to be associated with congenital malformations.

m. Antithyroid drugs
  (1) Action: inhibit the excess production of thyroid hormone
  (2) Effects
    (a) Propylthiouracil (PTU) is capable of inducing mild fetal hypothyroidism, usually resolved within several days; enlargement of the thyroid gland in the fetus may also result.
    (b) Methimazole (Tapazole) and propylthiouracil can induce goiter and even cretinism in the developing fetus; therefore caution is recommended in determining a small but effective dose; it may be withdrawn 2 or 3 weeks before delivery.
    (c) Potassium iodide may cause the development of fetal goiter.
    (d) Radioactive iodine may result in congenital hypothyroidism in neonates; its use is contraindicated.
  (3) Timing of exposure
    (a) Exposure is most critical during the first or second trimester.
    (b) Minimal doses are recommended, especially in the third trimester.

n. Antiulcer agents
  (1) Action: inhibit gastric acid secretion and protect the gastric mucosa
  (2) Misoprostol is classified as a category X drug and should be avoided during pregnancy.

o. Antiviral agents
  (1) Action: block viral replication
  (2) Ribavirin is classified as a category X drug and is considered teratogenic and embryo lethal and is contraindicated during pregnancy; as an aerosol mist it is critical that a scavenging unit be used during administration.

p. Decongestants
  (1) Action: produce decongestion of respiratory tract mucosa
  (2) Pseudoephedrine and phenylpropanolamine, although identified as category C drugs, have been found to double the risk of having an infant with gastroschisis, particularly when exposed during the first trimester; it is recommended that they be avoided during pregnancy when possible.

q. Diethylstilbestrol (DES)
  (1) Action: a potent, synthetic nonsteroidal estrogen used widely between 1940 and 1971 for treating various pregnancy complications; all forms of estrogen contraindicated during pregnancy
  (2) Effects
    (a) Increased risk for female reproductive tract abnormalities
    (b) Increased risk for male reproductive tract defects, including epididymal cysts, hypotrophic testes, varicocele, and altered semen
    (c) Early fetal death and childhood malignancies
  (3) Timing of exposure: exposure is most critical during the first trimester, when it is most commonly associated with abnormalities.
r. Gallstone-solubilizing agents
  (1) Action: promote dissolution of uncalcified cholesterol gallstones
  (2) Chenodiol (chenodeoxycholic acid) is classified as a category X drug and is contraindicated during pregnancy.
s. Gonadotropic hormones
  (1) Action: in women, stimulate progesterone production and stimulate expulsion of the ovum from a mature follicle
  (2) Human chorionic gonadotropin (hCG), histrelin acetate, menotropins, nafarelin acetate, and urofollitropin for injection are classified as category X drugs and should be avoided during pregnancy.
t. Nicotine polacrilex (nicotine resin complex)
  (1) Action: smoking-deterrent gum
  (2) Nicorette, and Nicorette DS, and Nicorette Plus are classified as category X drugs and should be avoided during pregnancy.
u. Nicotine Transdermal System (Nicotine Patch) is classified as a category D agent and should be used in pregnancy only if the mother will not quit smoking and the potential benefit outweighs the potential risk of nicotine to the fetus.
v. Retinoids
  (1) Action: vitamin A analogues used for treating chronic cystic acne
    (a) Isotretinoin (Accutane) may cause:
      (i) Early or late fetal death
      (ii) Birth defects
        ■ Hydrocephalus
        ■ Craniofacial anomalies
        ■ Cardiovascular anomalies
        ■ Thymus abnormalities
    (b) Childhood mortality is high when exposed in utero.
      (i) Exposed infants are approximately 27 times more likely to die during the first year of life than are unexposed infants.
      (ii) Specific causes of death have not been well documented.
    (c) Retinoids are considered some of the most potent human teratogens; the risks of retinoic acid are similar to those posed by prenatal thalidomide exposure in the 1960s.
  (2) Timing of exposure is most critical during the first trimester of pregnancy, resulting in a risk of giving birth to an infant who has a CNS, cardiovascular, or craniofacial abnormality that is 25 times that of infants not exposed.
w. Sedatives and hypnotics
  (1) Action: control of agitation

(2) Effects
    (a) Exposure to barbiturates can cause fetal damage and is associated with a higher incidence of fetal abnormalities.
    (b) The highest concentration of barbiturates has been found in the placenta, fetal liver, and brain.
    (c) Withdrawal symptoms occur in infants born exposed.
(3) Examples of barbiturates: pentobarbital (Nembutal), phenobarbital, triazolam (Halcion), butabarbital (Barbased, Butatran), amobarbital (Amytal), estazolam, and quazepam
(4) Timing of exposure
    (a) Exposure is most critical during the first 6 weeks and is most significant in influencing fetal development.
    (b) Exposure during the third trimester is of concern for withdrawal symptoms in the infant at time of birth.

  x. Thalidomide
    (1) Action: widely used in the 1960s as a sedative in other countries but banned in the United States
    (2) Effects: exposure leads to birth defects.

2. Diagnostic procedures
  a. Take a urine sample from newborn to detect level of drug.
  b. Perform a fetal ultrasound evaluation as necessary.

C. Nursing Diagnoses
  1. Risk for fetal injury related to maternal ingestion of drugs
  2. Deficient knowledge and learning need related to effects of drugs on fetus
  3. Anxiety related to effects of drugs on fetus

D. Interventions/Outcomes
  1. Risk for fetal injury related to maternal ingestion of drugs
    a. Interventions
      (1) Advise of potential reproductive dangers of pharmaceuticals, whether prescribed or over the counter.
      (2) Advise client to consult health care provider before taking any drugs.
      (3) Refer pregnant women exposed to potentially hazardous pharmaceuticals before and early in the pregnancy to teratogen registries, March of Dimes, and other agencies who are interested in collecting data to generate or support hypotheses about the link between the use of pharmaceuticals and pregnancy outcome.
    b. Outcomes
      (1) Client obtains information about potentially hazardous pharmaceuticals.
      (2) Client informs health care provider of medications used.
      (3) Client discontinues all drugs not approved by health care provider.
      (4) Client follows through on all referrals.
  2. Deficient knowledge and learning need related to effects of drugs on fetus
    a. Interventions
      (1) Advise client of potential dangers during pregnancy of any drug use, including over-the-counter drugs or drugs prescribed by other health care providers.
      (2) Advise client to read all labels and adhere to their precautions.
      (3) Advise client to inform health care provider of plans for pregnancy to discuss implications of prescribed drugs.
    b. Outcomes
      (1) Client avoids drug use except those approved by a health care provider.

        (2) Client informs all health care providers of pregnancy.

        (3) Client reads drug labels.

        (4) Client uses drugs as directed.

        (5) Client disposes of drugs appropriately.

  3. Anxiety related to effects of drugs on fetus

    a. Interventions

        (1) Provide emotional support and factual information to provide a realistic perspective to pregnant women concerned about potentially hazardous exposures to pharmaceuticals.

        (2) Participate in or support research on the correlation between pharmaceutical use and pregnancy outcome.

    b. Outcomes

        (1) Client is calmer and has realistic perspective of dangers.

        (2) Client avoids further exposure.

        (3) Client communicates concerns with appropriate health professionals and significant others.

Secondhand Smoke (Environmental Tobacco Smoke and Passive Smoking)

A. Introduction

  1. Refers to exposure to approximately 15% of mainstream smoke (from smoker) and approximately 85% of sidestream smoke (from the cigarette).

  2. Smoke contains approximately 3800 chemicals.

  3. Evidence suggests that maternal exposure to secondhand smoke during pregnancy adversely affects the unborn child; measurable concentrations of cotinine (a metabolite of nicotine) have been found in the hair of infants born to mothers exposed to secondhand smoke (Joad, 2000).

  4. Exposure to secondhand smoke has been associated with elevated risks of prematurity, small-for-gestational age, and sudden infant death syndrome; studies on spontaneous abortion are suggestive of a role for secondhand smoke, but further work is needed.

  5. Approximately 25% of all pregnant women in the United States smoke during pregnancy (Slotkin, 1998).

B. Assessment

  1. History

    a. Effects: exposure to environmental tobacco smoke at work or at home increases the risk of:

        (1) Prematurity

        (2) Low birth weight and altered gestational length

        (3) Placental abruption

        (4) Sudden infant death syndrome

        (5) Possibly spontaneous abortion

    b. The length and frequency of exposure must be considered.

    c. Pregnant women should be advised not to smoke and to avoid exposure to secondhand smoke.

    d. Timing of exposure: exposure is important during any stage of pregnancy.

  2. Diagnostic procedures: none known

C. Nursing Diagnoses

  1. Risk for fetal injury related to exposure to secondhand smoke

  2. Deficient knowledge and learning need related to fetal exposure to secondhand smoke

D. Interventions/Outcomes
1. Risk for fetal injury related to exposure to secondhand smoke
   a. Interventions
      (1) Advise client to maintain a smoke-free environment during pregnancy.
      (2) Educate client about the adverse effects of smoking, active and passive, on the unborn child.
      (3) Inform of laws and legislation that provide smoke-free environments.
      (4) Encourage client to be assertive in not allowing smoking in environments she can control.
   b. Outcomes
      (1) Client protects fetus from exposure to secondhand smoke.
      (2) Client informs employer of potential dangers of exposure to secondhand smoke as indicated and demands a smoke-free environment.
2. Deficient knowledge and learning need related to fetal exposure to secondhand smoke
   a. Interventions
      (1) Advise client of potential dangers from both active and passive smoking.
      (2) Advise client to evaluate environments she is exposed to for potential hazards and avoid them as much as possible.
      (3) Advise client of increased risk of respiratory problems, ear infections, sudden infant death syndrome, and childhood cancers in infants and children resulting from exposure to secondhand smoke.
   b. Outcomes
      (1) Client avoids smoke-polluted environments.
      (2) Client selects nonsmoking areas in public places.
      (3) Client restricts smoking in personal environments at home and work.
      (4) Client is knowledgeable of the health risks associated with both active and passive smoking.

HEALTH EDUCATION

The following health educational needs have been identified. Refer to previous nursing interventions for additional detail. Community resources are listed in Box 9-2.

■ BOX 9-2
■ **COMMUNITY RESOURCES**

The following community resources may provide useful information on environmental hazards:
■ American Lung Association
■ Genetic Counseling Services
■ March of Dimes
■ National Institute of Occupational Safety and Health *(www.cdc.gov/niosh/homepage.html)*
■ National Service Center for Environmental Protection ([800] 490-9198)
■ Occupational Safety and Health Administration (federal/state)
■ Teratogen Registries
■ Pesticide Information ([800] 858-7378)

For each of the following categories, the client, or family, or both need to know the following:

A. Occupational hazards
1. Accurate, current information on potential reproductive risks in the workplace and possible negative outcomes
2. Importance of informing obstetrician of potential occupational exposures
3. Importance of informing occupational health office at work of pregnancy or plans for pregnancy
4. Safety precautions to take at work to minimize exposure
5. Importance of biologic monitoring for exposure levels in the workplace
6. Information regarding potential reproductive risks at work for spouse
7. Precautions to control exposures to environmental hazards at home (e.g., with chemicals and noise)

B. Pharmaceuticals
1. Dangers of taking any medication, over-the-counter or prescribed, unless discussed with health care provider
2. Importance of informing all health care providers of pregnancy before treatment is prescribed
3. Importance of taking drugs as directed
4. Dangers of drug interactions
5. Importance of planning pregnancies and avoiding use of potentially harmful drugs before becoming pregnant

C. Temperature extremes
1. Dangers of exposure to extreme hot or cold temperatures
2. Importance of avoiding hot tubs, spas, tanning booths, and saunas
3. Importance of avoiding strenuous physical activity, which may increase the body's core temperature

D. Secondhand smoke
1. Dangers of secondhand smoke to mother, fetus, and others exposed
2. Importance of selecting nonsmoking areas in public places
3. Importance of working in a smoke-free environment
4. Importance of being assertive in maintaining smoke-free environment
5. Importance of supporting legislation that limits smoking
6. Importance of attaining and maintaining nonsmoker status
7. Importance of informing friends and relatives of the dangers of smoking to fetus and children

---

CASE STUDIES AND STUDY QUESTIONS
OCCUPATIONAL HAZARDS

Mrs. M is a 25-year-old woman who has been employed by the research and development office of a major oil company for the last 2 years. Her work involves standing about 50% of the time. She has just learned that she is 6 weeks pregnant. Her husband is a chemist for the same company. Both individuals have graduate degrees and have planned this pregnancy. She plans to resume working after the child is born. She attends aerobic classes for exercise three times per week.

1. Which of the following would you include in an occupational history on Mrs. M?
   a. Chemicals with which she works
   b. Precautions taken to control exposure

    c. Chemicals with which Mr. M works

    d. Amount of time Mrs. M spends standing and sitting at work
      (1) a, b
      (2) a, b, c
      (3) a, b, d
      (4) All of the above

2. Which of the following would you include in health education for Mrs. M?

    a. Importance of reviewing material safety data sheets on each chemical to which she and her husband are exposed

    b. Importance of using recommended protective equipment

    c. Importance of informing health office of pregnancy

    d. Importance of taking 5- to 10-minute activity breaks every hour to avoid prolonged standing and sitting
      (1) a, b
      (2) a, b, d
      (3) a, c
      (4) All of the above

3. Which of the following would you advise regarding her recreational activities?

    a. Aerobic class activities should be evaluated to determine level of safety.

    b. Advise her to discontinue aerobic classes because they are too strenuous.

    c. Advise her to continue aerobic classes because they do not pose a potential health threat.

    d. Recommend that she discuss her pregnancy with her aerobics instructor.

PHARMACEUTICALS

Ms. J is a 33-year-old woman who is 8 weeks pregnant. This pregnancy is not wanted and she is extremely depressed. Her obstetrician referred her to a psychiatrist for evaluation. She has three other children and is currently unemployed. Her family physician prescribed lithium 2 years ago for "her nerves." She uses the drug when needed. Since she became pregnant, she has taken aspirin for headaches and antihistamines for allergy symptoms. She also uses antacids occasionally. Her husband is an executive for a savings and loan company.

4. Which of the following drugs that she may be using would concern you?

    a. Lithium

    b. Aspirin

    c. Antihistamines

    d. a and b

5. Which of the following would you recommend for her to ease her depression and manage stress?

    a. Become involved with a social support group.

    b. Follow through on referral for psychiatric evaluation and counseling.

    c. Learn and practice stress management techniques such as relaxation, meditation, and biofeedback.

    d. All of the above

TEMPERATURE EXTREMES

Mrs. D is a pregnant, 31-year-old mother of three children. She and her husband live in a large home in an affluent neighborhood. They have a swimming pool and hot tub. They enjoy relaxing in the hot tub nightly before retiring.

6. Which of the following would you advise her to do to control her exposure to high temperatures?
   a. Stop using the hot tub.
   b. Use the hot tub only if the temperature is 100° F or lower.
   c. Sit with only her legs or feet dangling in the hot water.
   d. Suggest that she take an evening walk with her husband instead of using the hot tub.
      (1) a
      (2) b
      (3) b, c, d
      (4) d

7. She inquires about the use of hot showers. Which of the following would you recommend?
   a. Hot showers should be avoided altogether.
   b. Hot showers are relatively safe if they last for only 5 minutes.
   c. Hot showers are safe.
   d. Refer her to her health care provider.

SECONDHAND SMOKE

Ms. R is a 22-year-old pregnant single mother who works for a metropolitan newspaper in the newsroom. She quit smoking when she first discovered she was pregnant with her second child. Smoking is permitted in the newsroom because most of the people in that department smoke: they claim that smoking relieves the tension of having deadlines to meet. Ms. R usually dates every Friday and Saturday evening. She especially enjoys dancing. She does not permit smoking in her home or car.

8. Which of the following responses to her work situation would you support?
   a. Quit her job and find one in a smoke-free workplace.
   b. Discuss with her employer the potential dangers of second-hand smoke to the fetus and request a separate office that would be smoke free.
   c. Use a fan to vent the smoke away from her.
   d. Request a transfer to a different department immediately.

9. What health teaching would you include relative to her social life?
   a. Suggest that she stop dating because of potential dangers to fetus.
   b. Advise her to avoid dancing because finding a dance floor free of smoke is impossible.
   c. Encourage her to discuss her concern regarding effects of passive smoking with her date and consider alternatives that would be safe.
   d. Do nothing because the dangers of secondhand smoke to the fetus have not been well documented.

ANSWERS TO STUDY QUESTIONS

1. 4	4. d	7. b
2. 4	5. d	8. b
3. a	6. 3	9. c

REFERENCES

Abelsohn, A., Gibson, B.L., Sanborn, M.D., & Weir, E. (2002). Identifying and managing adverse environmental health effects: 5. Persistent organic pollutants. *Canadian Medical Association Journal, 166*(12), 1549-1554.

Anderson, A., Vastrup, P., Wohlfahrt, J., Anderson, P., Olsen, J., & Melbye, M. (2002). Fever in pregnancy and risk of fetal death: A cohort study, *Lancet, 360*(9345), 1552-1556.

Anderson, H., & Wolff, M. (2000). Environmental contaminants in human milk. *Journal of Exposure Analysis and Environmental Epidemiology, 10*(6 Pt 2), 755-760.

Annesi-Maesano, I., Moreau, D., & Strachan, D. (2001). In utero and perinatal complications preceding asthma. *Allergy, 56*(6), 491-497.

Araujo, D. (1997). Expecting questions about exercise and pregnancy? *The Physician and Sportsmedicine, 27*(8), 51.

Arcadi, F.A., Costa, C., Imperatore, C., Marchese, A., Rapisarda, A., Salemi, M., et al. (1998). Oral toxicity of bis (2-Ethylhexyl) phthalate during pregnancy and suckling in the Long-Evans rate. *Food and Chemical Toxicology, 36*(11), 963-970.

Artal, R., & Sherman, C. (1999). Exercise during pregnancy: Safe and beneficial for most. *Physician and Sportsmedicine, 27*(8), 51.

Campbell, K.N., & Fisher, R. (1997). Occupational health nursing in the pharmaceutical industry, *Occupational Medicine: State of the Art Reviews, 12*(1), 160-179.

Cannon, R., Schmidt, J., Cambardella, B., & Browne, S. (2000). High risk pregnancy in the workplace: Influencing positive outcomes. *AAOHN Journal, 48*(9), 435-447.

Center for the Evaluation of Risk to Human Reproduction. (2002). *NTP-CERHR Expert Panel Report on the Reproductive and Developmental Toxicity of Ethylene Glycol*, National Toxicology Program. Washington, DC: U.S. Department of Health and Human Services.

Chetty, C.S., Reddy, G.R., Murthy, K.S., Johnson, J., Sajwan, K., & Desaiah, D. (2001). Perinatal lead exposure alters the expression of neuronal nitric oxide synthase in rat brain. *International Journal of Toxicology, 20*(3), 113-120.

Clement, J. (1997). Reproductive health hazards in the pharmaceutical industry. *Occupational Medicine: State of the Art Reviews, 12*(1), 131-143.

Committee on Drugs, American Academy of Pediatrics. (2000). Use of psychoactive medication during pregnancy and possible effects on the fetus and newborn. *Pediatrics, 105*(4 Pt 1), 880-887.

Fattibene, P., Mazzei, F., Nuccetilli, C., & Risica, S. (1999). Prenatal exposure to ionizing radiation: Sources, effects and regulatory aspects. *Acta Paediatrica, 88*(7), 693-702.

Felton, J.S. (2000). Occupational health in the USA in the 21st Century. *Occupational Medicine-Oxford, 50*(7), 523-531.

Fishbein, E., & Phillips, M. (1989). How safe is exercise during pregnancy? *Journal of Obstetrics and Neonatal Nursing, 19*(1), 45-49.

Geeze, D.S. (1998). Pregnancy and in-flight cosmic radiation. *Aerospace Medical Association, Aviation Space and Environmental Medicine, 69*(11), 1061-1064.

Gjere, N. (2000). Psychopharmacology in pregnancy, *Journal of Perinatal and Neonatal Nursing, 14*(4), 12-25.

Gray, L.E. (2000). Perinatal exposure to the phthalates DEHP, BBP, and DINP, but not DEP, DMP, or DOTP, alters sexual differentiation of the male rat. *Toxicology Sciences, 58*(2), 350-365.

Hewitt, J., & Tellier, L. (1996, Oct). A description of an occupational reproductive health nurse consultant practice and women's occupational exposures during pregnancy. *Public Health Nursing, 13*(5), 365-373.

Joad, J. (2000). Smoking and pediatric respiratory health. *Clinics in Chest Medicine, 21*(1), 37-46.

Johnson, B. (1999). A review of the effects of hazardous on reproductive health. *Agency for toxic substances and disease registry. Public Health Service, U.S. Department of Health and Human Services, 181*(1), S12-S16.

Koren, G., Pastuszak, A., & Ito, S. (1998). Drug therapy—drugs in pregnancy. *New England Journal of Medicine, 338*(16), 1128-1138.

Li, D.K., Janevic, R., Odouli, R., & Liu, L. (2001). Use of hot tub or Jacuzzi during pregnancy and the risk of spontaneous abortion (SAB). *Journal of Pediatric and Perinatal Epidemiology, 15,* A20.

Mozurkewich, E., Luke, B., Avni, M., & Wolf, F. (2000). Working conditions and adverse pregnancy outcome. *Health Sciences Research, Division of Maternal-Fetal Medicine and Department of Obstetrics and Gynecology A, 95*(4), 623-635.

Myers, D., & Davidson, P. (2000). Does methylmercury have a role in causing developmental disabilities in children? *Environmental Health Perspectives, 108*(3), 413-420.

Oncology News International. (1999). Fetus may be harmed by second-hand smoke, 8(7). Retrieved 2/23/2003 from *www.cancernetwork.com/journalsoncnews/n9907m.htm.*

Pastore, L., Hertz-Picciotto, I., & Beaumont, J. (1999). Risk of stillbirth from medications, illnesses and medical procedures, *Paediatric and Perinatal Epidemiology, 13*(4), 421-430.

Perera, F., Jedrychowski, W., Rauh, V., & Whyatt, R.M. (1999). Molecular epidemiologic research on the effects of environmental pollutants on the fetus. *Environmental Health Perspectives, 107* (Suppl 3), 451-460.

Pergament, E., Schechtman, A., & Rochanayon, A. (1997). Hyperthermia and pregnancy. *Risk Newsletter.* Retrieved February, 24, 2003 from *www.fetal-exposure.org/HYPERTH.html.*

Polifka, J., & Friedman, J.M. (2002). Medical genetics: Clinical teratology in the age of genomics. *Canadian Medical Association Journal, 167*(3), 265-273.

Rice, D., & Barone, S. (2000). Critical periods of vulnerability for the developing nervous system: Evidence from humans and animal models. *National Center for Environmental Assessment, U.S. Environmental Protection Agency, Washington, DC, 108*(3), 511-533.

Rubin, P. (1998). Drug treatment during pregnancy, *British Medical Journal, 317*(7171), 1503-1506.

Shiverick, K.T., & Salafia, C. (1999). Cigarette smoking and pregnancy 1: Ovarian, uterine and placental effects, *Placenta, 20*(4), 265-272.

Skakkebaek, N.E., & Niels, E. (1998). Trends in male reproductive health. Environmental aspects, *Advances in Experimental Medicine and Biology, 444,* 1-4.

Slotkin, T. (1998). Fetal nicotine or cocaine exposure: Which one is worse? *Pharmacology and Experimental Therapeutics, 285*(3), 931-945.

Stern, S., Cox, C., Cernichiari, E., Balys, M., & Weiss, B. (2001). Perinatal and lifetime exposure to methylmercury in the mouse: Blood and brain concentrations of mercury to 26 months of age. Department of Environmental Medicine School of Medicine and Dentistry, University of Rochester, NY, *Neurotoxicology, August 2294,* 467-477.

Thuvander, A., Sundberg, J., & Oskarsson, A. (1996). *Immunomodulating effects after perinatal exposure to methylmercury in mice.* Uppsala, Sweden: National Food Administration.

Tryphomas, H. (1998). The impact of PCBs and dioxins on children's health: Immunological considerations, *Canadian Journal of Public Health, 89*(1), S49-S57.

United States Census Bureau. (2002). *Civilian labor force and participant rates, with projections: 1980 to 2010.* Statistical abstract of the United States. Washington, DC: Census Bureau.

Warner, J., & Warner, J. (2000). Early life events in allergic sensitisation. *British Medical Bulletin, 56*(4), 883-893.

Watson, G.E. (1997). Influences of material lead ingestion on caries in rat pups, *Nature Medicine, 3*(9), 1024-1025.

Wyszynski, D.F., Duffy, D., & Beaty, T. (1997). Maternal cigarette smoking and oral clefts: A meta-analysis. *Journal of Cleft Palate Craniofacial, 34*(3), 206-210.

INTRAPARTUM PERIOD

10 Essential Forces and Factors in Labor

GAIL M. TURLEY

OBJECTIVES

1. List the forces affecting labor.
2. Identify the possible causes of the onset of labor.
3. Discuss the oxytocin release theory of labor onset.
4. Discuss the fetal prostaglandin theory of labor onset.
5. Describe the amount of uterine activity required to effect cervical changes.
6. Differentiate between muscle contraction and muscle retraction, and discuss the significance of both to the progress of labor.
7. List the techniques used for assessing uterine activity and uterine efficiency.
8. Differentiate between true labor and false labor, using information gathered by history and physical examination.
9. Identify the basic pelvic shapes.
10. Recognize adequate pelvic dimensions.
11. Describe methods for assessing pelvic capacity.
12. Compare and contrast the anticipated progress of labor for each of the four pelvic shapes.
13. Identify and discuss maternal conditions that may alter or influence pelvic capacity.
14. Analyze the relation between maternal posture and the pelvic passage.
15. Define fetal lie, attitude, presentation, presenting part, position, and station.
16. List the mechanisms of spontaneous vaginal delivery.
17. Discuss the significance of breech presentation or transverse lie to the progress of labor.
18. Recognize fetal variables that may interfere with the progress of labor.
19. Discuss the significance of fetal malpositioning to the course and outcome of labor.
20. Describe the characteristic emotions associated with labor.
21. Identify variables that determine a couple's expectations for the labor and birth experience.
22. Distinguish between adaptive coping and maladaptive coping during labor.
23. Identify the nursing diagnoses associated with the forces of labor.
24. Describe the nursing actions that maximize the forces of labor.
25. Predict when a woman is at risk for a difficult labor as the result of an alteration in one of the forces of labor.

INTRODUCTION

Traditionally, four essential forces or powers have been identified as the determinants of labor outcome. These "4 Ps," which are interrelated, are:

1. Power: the uterine muscle provides the power of labor, and the onset and establishment of a satisfactory contraction pattern is a readily recognized force of labor.
2. Passage: the bony boundaries of the pelvis define the labor passage, and its shape and configuration determine the ease with which the infant is expelled from the uterus.
3. Passenger: the infant, or passenger, is an active participant in the labor process as it moves and turns to accommodate to the maternal pelvis.
4. Psyche: finally, a woman's psyche, or emotional system, determines her total response to labor and influences both physiologic and psychologic functioning.

CLINICAL PRACTICE

Power of Labor

A. Assessment
   1. History
      a. Onset of contractions
         (1) Maternal factor theories
            (a) The uterus is stretched to threshold point, leading to synthesis and release of prostaglandin.
            (b) The pressure on the cervix and its nerve plexus reaches threshold point.
            (c) Oxytocin stimulation theory
               (i) Exogenous oxytocin is known to stimulate myometrial contractions, but no evidence clearly documents its role in the onset of labor.
               (ii) Progesterone inhibits myometrial response throughout pregnancy.
               (iii) Estrogen at term enhances myometrial sensitivity to oxytocin.
               (iv) A surge of oxytocin may be released by stretching of the cervix at term (Ferguson's reflex), but studies do not agree about this possibility.
            (d) Progesterone withdrawal theory
               (i) In animals, a decrease in progesterone is followed by evacuation of the uterus.
               (ii) In humans, no firm evidence documents that progesterone is decreased at term.
               (iii) Many researchers, however, support the view that an altered progesterone-estrogen ratio leads to increased myometrial contractility.
         (2) Fetal factor theories
            (a) Placental aging and deterioration trigger initiation of contractions.
            (b) Fetal cortisol theory
               (i) It is reasoned that normal fetal adrenal glands produce a steroid, cortisol, which stimulates the onset of labor.
               (ii) It is recognized that anencephaly causes adrenal dysfunction secondary to pituitary dysfunction.
               (iii) Empirically, anencephalic fetuses tend to have prolonged gestations.

    (c) Prostaglandin synthesis theory
        (i) Prostaglandins are known to stimulate uterine contractions at any gestational age.
        (ii) Prostaglandin is present in increased quantities in blood and amniotic fluid during labor.
        (iii) Prostaglandin production requires the precursor arachidonic acid.
        (iv) Esterified arachidonic acid is stored in fetal membranes.
        (v) It is postulated that free arachidonic acid is released at term and is then converted by agents in the uterine decidua to prostaglandin.
  b. Physiology of contractions
    (1) Myometrium
        (a) Uterine muscle is controlled by involuntary innervation.
        (b) Alpha-receptors stimulate uterine contractions.
        (c) Beta-receptors stimulate uterine relaxation.
        (d) Norepinephrine and epinephrine stimulate both alpha- and beta-receptors.
            (i) When progesterone is present, beta-receptors are stimulated.
            (ii) When estrogen is present, alpha-receptors are stimulated.
    (2) Contraction: the shortening of a muscle in response to a stimulus, with return to its original length (Figure 10-1)
        (a) Increment: building up; the longest phase of a contraction
        (b) Acme: peak
        (c) Decrement: letting up

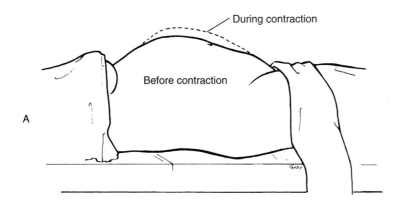

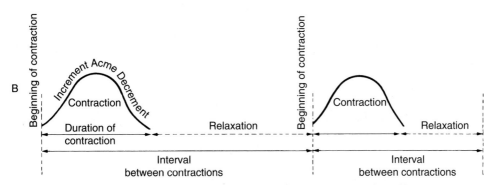

FIGURE 10-1 ■ Wavelike pattern of contractile activity. (From Lowdermilk, D.L., & Perry, S.E. [2004]. *Maternity & women's health* care [8th ed., p. 564]. St. Louis: Mosby.)

(3) Retraction: the shortening of a muscle in response to a stimulus, without return to its original length; muscle becomes fixed at a relatively shorter length, but no increase in baseline tension occurs after the contraction (also known as brachystasis)
  (a) With each uterine contraction, the upper segment of the uterus becomes shorter and thicker, and the lower segment of the uterus becomes longer, thinner, and more distended.
  (b) The division between the contractile upper segment of the uterus and the passive lower uterine segment is the physiologic retraction ring.
  (c) Longitudinal traction on the cervix by the upper portion of the uterus as it contracts and retracts leads to cervical effacement and dilatation.
  (d) The shortening and thickening of the upper uterine segment leads to fetal descent.
(4) Tonus: the degree of pressure exerted by the uterine musculature as measured by intrauterine pressure
  (a) Tonus is measured in millimeters of mercury (mmHg), which is also called torr.
  (b) Normal baseline tonus between contractions is 8 to 12 mmHg.
  (c) Pressure at peak of a contraction ranges from 35 to 75 mmHg.
(5) Intensity: the rise in intrauterine pressure above baseline brought about by a contraction
  (a) Intensity is measured as the difference between peak pressure and baseline pressure.
  (b) Normally, 30 to 50 mmHg intensity is necessary for effective labor.
(6) Pacemaker: the site of electrical activity responsible for triggering a uterine contraction
  (a) Pacemakers are generally located in the fundus of the uterus (fundal dominance).
    (i) Previous theories suggested that specialized cells existed that acted as pacemakers.
    (ii) Current research indicates that the cells responsible for initiating electrical stimuli are not different from surrounding myometrial cells.
    (iii) Because the fundus contains a greater number of myometrial cells, it is reasonable that the cells primarily responsible for triggering electrical activity would be located there.
  (b) The wave of the contraction begins in the fundus then proceeds downward to the rest of the uterus (descending gradient).
    (i) The duration of the contraction diminishes progressively as the wave moves away from the fundus; therefore during any contraction, the upper portion of the uterus is contracted for a longer time.
    (ii) The intensity of the contraction diminishes from top to bottom, so that the upper segment contracts more strongly than the lower segment.
    (iii) If the duration and intensity of the contraction were constant throughout, effacement and dilatation cannot occur.
  (c) Asymmetry results when the uterine halves function independently, leading to ineffective contractions with minimal dilatation.

(d) Ectopic pacemakers (i.e., pacemakers located outside of the uterine fundus) result in spasmodic myometrial contractions, which are disorganized and colicky, and rarely effective in producing dilatation (see Chapter 11 for a complete discussion of dysfunctional labor).

c. False labor

(1) Discomfort is perceived, but cervical changes do not occur.

(2) Discomfort is usually perceived more in lower abdomen than in back.

(3) Discomfort may be caused by uterine contractions, intestinal or bladder spasm, or abdominal wall muscle tension.

(4) Despite perceived discomfort, the uterus is often relaxed, although mild contractions may be palpated.

(5) Contractions are irregular and short in duration.

(6) The interval between contractions is long and irregular, and it does not decrease as discomfort continues.

(7) The intensity does not increase with time.

(8) Contractions are easily interrupted by medication and activity, such as walking.

(9) There is an absence of cervical bloody show.

(10) False labor is mentally and physically tiring for the client.

d. True labor

(1) By definition, true labor is the onset of contractions that leads to progressive cervical effacement and dilatation.

(2) Discomfort is perceived in both front and back.

(3) Hardening of the uterus is palpable.

(4) Contractions occur at regular intervals, usually begin 20 to 30 minutes apart, last 10 to 20 seconds, and are of mild intensity.

(5) Frequency, duration, and intensity increase as contractions continue.

(6) Medication does not easily disrupt true labor.

(7) Walking increases the intensity.

(8) Presenting part descends.

(9) Bulging of the membranes may occur.

(10) Bloody show is present.

2. Physical examination

a. Contraction strength

(1) Myometrial activity

(a) Myometrial activity is solely responsible for effacement and dilatation of the first stage of labor.

(b) Uterine contractions create increased intrauterine pressure, which exerts tension on cervix and pressure on the descending fetus.

(c) Myometrial effectiveness is improved by good uterine blood flow.

(i) Lateral positions avoid the vena caval syndrome.

(ii) Walking and activity increase circulating blood to the uterus.

(iii) Relaxation and sense of well being mitigates fight-or-flight response, avoiding diminished blood flow to the uterus.

(2) Expulsive activity

(a) During the second stage of labor, both involuntary and voluntary forces are present.

(b) Involuntary myometrial activity continues to create increased intrauterine pressure, which exerts pressure against the fetus.

   (c) Full dilatation causes involuntary reflex desire to bear down, which increases intraabdominal pressure, thereby increasing intrauterine pressure.
   (d) Voluntary efforts to bear down increase intraabdominal pressure, thereby increasing intrauterine pressure.
   (e) Positions that flex the legs on the abdomen increase intraabdominal pressure, thereby increasing intrauterine pressure.
   b. Contraction frequency
   (1) Contraction frequency is measured from the beginning of one contraction to the beginning of the next contraction.
   (2) Typical frequency of contractions during active labor is two to five contractions per 10 minutes.
   c. Contraction duration
   (1) Contraction duration is measured from the beginning of the increment to the end of the decrement.
   (2) Typical duration of contractions during active labor is 30 to 90 seconds.
3. Diagnostic studies and techniques
   a. Manual palpation of contractions
   (1) Judge indentability of the uterine wall and assign a rating of mild, moderate, or strong.
      (a) Mild: uterine wall easily indented
      (b) Moderate: uterine wall demonstrates resistance to pressure, though some indentation occurs
      (c) Strong: uterine wall cannot be indented
   b. External monitoring of contractions: tocotransducer
   (1) The tocotransducer reflects increased intraabdominal pressure.
   (2) Placement of the tocotransducer influences the accuracy of information.
   (3) Intraabdominal pressure does not directly correlate with intrauterine pressure; therefore it does not measure the actual intensity of contractions.
   (4) No known risks have been found of using the tocotransducer, but some women feel confined and uncomfortable.
   c. Internal monitoring of contractions: intrauterine pressure catheter
   (1) Allows direct measurement of intrauterine pressure.
   (2) Provides accurate measurement of actual intensity of uterine contraction.
   (3) Associated risks
      (a) Introduction of infection into uterine cavity
      (b) Uterine rupture caused by traumatic insertion
   d. Montevideo units:
   (1) Developed by Calderyo-Barcia to measure and quantify uterine work
   (2) Calculated by multiplying the frequency of contractions (as expressed by the number of contractions in 10 minutes) by their intensity
   (3) Expressed as mmHg per 10 minutes
   (4) Example
      (a) The client is contracting every 3 minutes; therefore three contractions occur in 10 minutes.
      (b) The intensity of the contraction at its peak is 35 mmHg.
      (c) 3 contractions ÷ 10 minutes × 35 mmHg ÷ contractions = 105 mmHg ÷ 10 minutes

B. **Nursing Diagnoses**
   1. Risk for infection related to the use of an intrauterine pressure catheter (IUPC)
   2. Risk for situational low self-esteem related to ineffective uterine contraction pattern

C. **Interventions/Outcomes**
   1. Risk for infection related to the use of an IUPC
      a. Interventions
         (1) Therapeutic
            (a) Use aseptic technique when assembling the pressure catheter.
            (b) Maintain asepsis during insertion of the pressure catheter.
            (c) Use aseptic technique during vaginal examinations.
            (d) Limit vaginal examinations to those necessary for clinical decision making.
         (2) Diagnostic
            (a) Every 2 to 4 hours, or as indicated by the stage of labor and the client's clinical status, obtain temperature.
            (b) As appropriate to the client's stage of labor and clinical status, assess fetal heart rate.
            (c) On an ongoing basis, assess characteristics of amniotic fluid.
            (d) On an ongoing basis, assess for uterine tenderness.
            (e) On an ongoing basis, monitor laboratory results.
      b. Outcomes: client does not develop chorioamnionitis, as evidenced by:
         (1) Temperature is within normal limits for parturition.
         (2) Fetal heart rate is within normal limits.
         (3) Amniotic fluid is not foul smelling.
         (4) Uterus is relaxed and nontender between contractions.
         (5) White blood cell count is within normal limits for parturition.
   2. Risk for situational low self-esteem related to ineffective uterine contraction pattern
      a. Interventions
         (1) Therapeutic
            (a) Facilitate effective uterine contractions.
         (2) Encourage the client to walk about as much as possible.
         (3) When the client is in bed, assist her to a lateral position with the head of the bed slightly elevated, using pillows and other supports.
            (a) Provide the client with encouragement and support.
               (i) Review the normal variations in labor patterns.
               (ii) Provide positive feedback regarding:
                  ∎ Improving contraction strength
                  ∎ Increasing frequency of contractions
                  ∎ Increasing duration of contractions
               (iii) Provide positive feedback for the client's attempts to use alternative positions.
            (b) Permit the client to exercise autonomy by allowing her to determine positions of comfort.
         (4) Diagnostic
            (a) On an ongoing basis, assess the client's level of satisfaction with her labor.
            (b) On an ongoing basis, assess the client's feelings of self-worth.

b. Outcomes
  (1) The client demonstrates positive self-esteem as evidenced by:
    (a) Verbalizing satisfaction and contentment with the progress of her labor
    (b) Verbalizing statements of self-worth

Labor Passage

A. Assessment

1. History
  a. Musculoskeletal deformities and diseases
    (1) A contracted pelvis may lead to disproportion between the pelvis and the fetus.
    (2) Uterine neoplasms (e.g., fibromyomas, ovarian cysts) may block the birth canal, impeding the passage.
    (3) Bicornuate uterus:
      (a) May lead to abortion, premature labor, or premature rupture of membranes.
      (b) Has been implicated in incompetent cervix.
      (c) May be causative factor of breech or transverse lie.
      (d) Vaginal delivery is possible but may be accompanied by uterine inertia or obstruction of descent.
    (4) Maternal dwarfism
      (a) This is defined as a height of less than 1473 cm (4 ft, 10 in) at maturity.
      (b) Pelvic dimensions may be favorable if dwarfism is proportionate.
    (5) Kyphoscoliosis
      (a) If the thoracic area is involved, little or no reduction of pelvic capacity occurs.
      (b) If the dorsolumbar or lumbosacral area is involved, marked pelvic deformity is common.
    (6) Bony disease of femurs or acetabula may result in abnormal pressures on the pelvis during development, leading to pelvic asymmetry and reduced pelvic capacity.
    (7) Nutritional deficiencies and diseases (e.g., rickets) may contribute to bone deformities that impede the passage.
  b. Pelvic trauma or injury may lead to asymmetry and reduced capacity.
  c. Cervical trauma or injury:
    (1) Includes accidental insults as well as those resulting from surgical procedures (e.g., dilatation and curettage [D&C], cone biopsy, uterine aspiration).
    (2) May result in loss of cervical integrity with resultant incompetence.
    (3) May result in cervical scarring and adhesions, with resultant failure to dilate.
    (4) Cervical abnormalities are frequently found among women exposed in utero to DES.
2. Physical examination
  a. Pelvic shapes (Figure 10-2)
    (1) Rigid classification is not possible.
      (a) Name assigned is based on classification of inlet.
      (b) Nonconforming characteristics are then described.
      (c) Shape and size of pelvis influence fetal position and attitude.

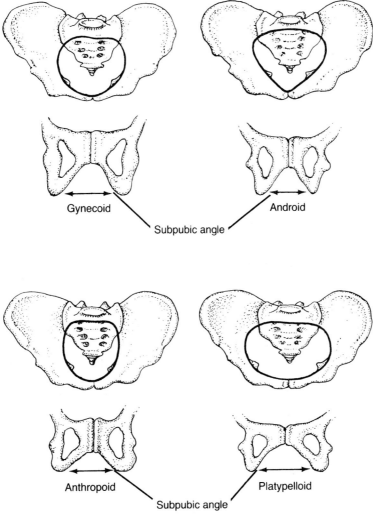

FIGURE 10-2 ■ Caldwell-Moloy classification of pelvis. (From Sloane, E. [2002]. *Biology of women* [4th ed.]. Albany, NY: Delmar.)

(2) Gynecoid: normal female
   (a) Uterine function is good.
   (b) Early and complete internal rotation occurs.
   (c) Labor prognosis is good.
   (d) This shape offers the optimal diameters in all three planes of the pelvis.
   (e) Approximate incidence is 50%.
(3) Android: male
   (a) Posterior segments are reduced in all the pelvic planes.
   (b) Deep transverse arrest is common.
   (c) Failure of rotation is common.
   (d) Labor prognosis is poor.
   (e) Approximate incidence is 20%, but it occurs more frequently among white women (30%) than nonwhite women (15%).

    (4) Anthropoid: apelike
        (a) Reduced transverse measurements are compensated by large anteroposterior diameters.
        (b) Prognosis is generally more favorable than android or platypelloid.
        (c) This shape may deliver occiput posterior.
        (d) Approximate incidence is 25%, but it occurs more frequently among nonwhite women (50%) than white women (25%).
    (5) Platypelloid: flat female
        (a) Arrest at inlet is common.
        (b) Labor prognosis is poor.
        (c) Approximate incidence is 5%.
b. Pelvic dimension
    (1) The measurements that define the obstetric capacity of the pelvis
    (2) Important measurements
        (a) Obstetric conjugate of the inlet (Figure 10-3):
            (i) Is the shortest diameter through which the infant must pass.
            (ii) Extends from the middle of the sacral promontory to the posterior superior margin of the symphysis pubis.
            (iii) Can be approximated by manually measuring the diagonal conjugate, extending from the subpubic angle to the middle of the sacral promontory, then subtracting 15 cm (0.6 in).
            (iv) Adequate measurement: 11 cm (4.4 in)
        (b) Transverse diameter between the ischial spines
            (i) The spines form the lateral boundaries of the pelvic cavity plane of least dimension (Figure 10-4).
            (ii) Adequate measurement: 10.5 cm (4.2 in)
        (c) Subpubic angle (see Figure 10-2):
            (i) Forms the apex of the anterior triangle of the pelvic outlet.
            (ii) Adequate measurement: 90 degrees or more
        (d) Bituberous diameter
            (i) Transverse diameter of the pelvic outlet.
            (ii) Adequate measurement: 11 cm (4.4 in)

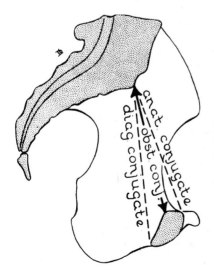

FIGURE 10-3 ■ Obstetric conjugate. (From Oxorn, H. [1986]. *Oxorn-Foote human labor and birth* [5th ed., p. 29]. New York: Appleton & Lange.)

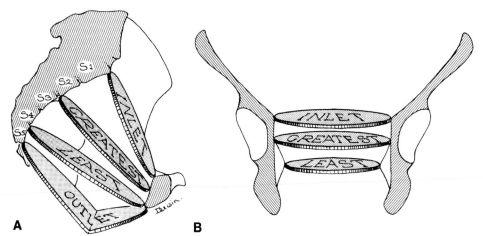

FIGURE 10-4 ■ Pelvic cavity planes. (From Oxorn, H. [1986]. *Oxorn-Foote human labor and birth* [5th ed., p. 27]. New York: Appleton & Lange.)

(e) Posterior sagittal diameters (Figure 10-5):
   (i) Extend from the intersection of the transverse and anteroposterior diameters to the posterior limit of the latter.
   (ii) Represent the back portion of the anteroposterior diameters:
      ■ Inlet: 4.5 cm (1.8 in)
      ■ Cavity: 4.5 to 5 cm (1.8 to 2 in)
      ■ Outlet: 9 cm (3.6 in)
(f) Curve and length of the sacrum
   (i) The sacrum forms the curved canal of the pelvic cavity.
   (ii) Posterior wall should be deep and concave.
   (iii) Sacrum should measure 10 to 15 cm (4 to 6 in).
(3) Maternal posture influences pelvic size and contours.
   (a) There is no correct position; each offers advantages and disadvantages.

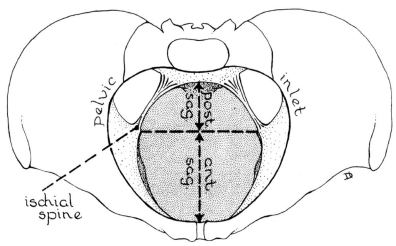

FIGURE 10-5 ■ Posterior sagittal diameters. (From Oxorn, H. [1986]. *Oxorn-Foote human labor and birth* [5th ed., p. 29]. New York: Appleton & Lange.)

(b) Walking and changing positions affects changes in pelvic joints, facilitating descent and rotation.

(c) Horizontal postures

    (i) Contribute to vena caval syndrome.

       ■ Decreased placental blood flow can lead to fetal compromise.

       ■ Decreased uterine blood flow can lead to uterine muscle hypoxia.

         — Decreased strength of uterine contractions

         — Increased pain perception

    (ii) Decrease the ability of the client to push voluntarily.

    (iii) Expulsive forces must work against gravity.

    (iv) Foster dependency and passivity of client; mirror is required for client to see birth.

    (v) Provide for ease of attendant.

    (vi) Associated with increased incidence of interventions.

       ■ Instrument-assisted delivery

       ■ Episiotomy

    (vii) Positions

       ■ Dorsal or supine

         — Legs may be extended or knees flexed.

         — Pelvic angle is 30 degrees, which directs the fetal head away from the pelvic inlet.

         — Probably best reserved for rare instances when delivery difficulties anticipated.

         — Lithotomy: client's legs are in stirrups.

         — Semi-Fowler's: head of bed is elevated.

       ■ Lateral

         — Relaxation of the pelvic muscles facilitates descent and rotation of the presenting part.

         — Avoids vena caval syndrome.

         — Left side lying may offer increased control of pushing efforts.

         — Requires a support person to hold the anterior leg.

         — May impede interaction with the attendant or infant, since the delivery occurs at the woman's back.

(d) Upright postures

    (i) Avoid venal caval syndrome.

    (ii) Abdominal muscles work in synchrony with uterine contractions, maximizing expulsive forces; associated with a shortened second stage.

    (iii) Abdominal wall relaxes, allowing the fundus to fall forward because of the force of gravity and straightening the longitudinal axis of the birth canal.

       ■ Fetus is well aligned with the angle of the pelvis.

       ■ Effect of gravity is maximized.

       ■ Fetal descent is enhanced.

    (iv) Pelvic angle is 90 to 120 degrees, directing the fetal head to enter the pelvis in the anterior position and enhancing application of the fetal head against the cervix.

    (v) Uterine contractions are more efficient.

       ■ Gravity increases pressure to cervix by 10 to 35 mmHg.

       ■ Contractions may be less frequent but of greater amplitude.

(vi) Fosters participation of client in the birth process.
- Increases client's perception of control.
- Facilitates interactions with care providers.
- May reduce anxiety.

(vii) Technically more difficult for some attendants.

(viii) Associated with fetal and newborn well being.
- Decreased incidence of abnormal fetal heart patterns.
- Decreased incidence of acidosis at birth.
- Decreased incidence of Apgar less than 7.

(ix) Epidural anesthesia is not an absolute contraindication to upright postures.
- Determined by agent used as well as dosing regimen.
- Requires sufficient leg strength to support maternal weight.

(x) Positions
- Squatting
  — Enlarges the pelvic outlet by approximately 28%.
  — Increases the efficiency and effectiveness of expulsive forces.
  — Often cited as *best* position for second stage of labor.
  — Efficacy of position requires less forceful pushing and may be less tiring.
  — Induces a slight separation of the lower symphysis pubis, resulting in an enlarged outlet.
  — Thighs are flexed and abducted, creating leverage on the innominate bones, thereby opening the bony outlet.
  — Without the pressure of a bed, the sacrum and coccyx are easily pushed back by the descending fetus, thereby enlarging the outlet.
  — Pressure of the thighs on the abdomen increase intraabdominal pressure.
  — Pressure is evenly distributed to the perineum, reducing the need for episiotomy.
  — Reduces visibility of perineum for the attendant.
  — Not a customary stance in Western societies.
  — Decreased muscle strength and joint flexibility can be fatiguing and uncomfortable.
  — Use of squatting bar provides opportunities for rest.
  — Playing tug-of-war with support person simulates squatting while minimizing stress on thighs.
- Sitting
  — Increases the pelvic diameters but not as much as squatting.
  — May increase edema of perineum and perineal blood loss.
  — Continuous pressure on lower buttocks leads to venous congestion and dependent edema.
  — More pronounced when using a molded birthing chair, which inhibits position changes and weight shifts.
  — Client can unintentionally slide into a semirecumbent posture if she relies too much on back support.
- Standing
  — Is tiring for the client.
  — Requires the assistance of two attendants or support persons.

(e) Kneeling postures
  (i) Assist rotation of a fetus to a posterior position.
  (ii) Coccyx is freely mobile, maximizing pelvic diameter.
  (iii) Are tiring for the client.
  (iv) May reduce participation in birth process and interaction with the infant because the woman may be using her arms and hands to support herself.

  c. Cervical changes
  (1) Effacement
    (a) Shortening of the cervix
    (b) Passive reduction in the length of the cervical canal from 2 cm (0.8 in) to a paper-thin orifice
    (c) Internal os disappears as cervical canal is drawn up into the lower uterine segment.
    (d) In nulliparas, effacement generally begins before the onset of labor.
    (e) In multiparas, effacement may not begin until labor ensues.
  (2) Dilatation (Figure 10-6)
    (a) Opening of the external os
    (b) Caused by two forces:
      (i) Pressure of the presenting part
      (ii) Contraction and retraction of the uterine muscle
3. Diagnostic studies and techniques
  a. Vaginal examination to assess cervical changes
  (1) Effacement
    (a) 0%: cervical canal is 2 cm (0.8 in) long.
    (b) 50%: cervical canal is 1 cm (0.4 in) long.
    (c) 100%: cervical canal is obliterated.

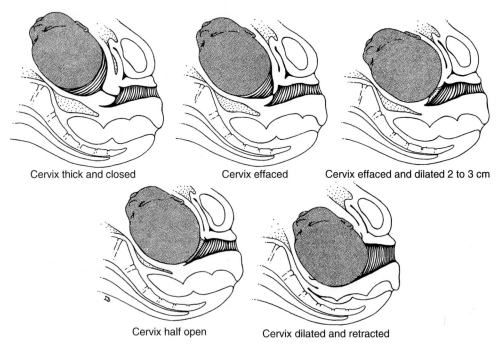

Cervix thick and closed   Cervix effaced   Cervix effaced and dilated 2 to 3 cm

Cervix half open   Cervix dilated and retracted

FIGURE 10-6 ■ Dilatation of the cervix. (From Oxorn, H. [1986]. *Oxorn-Foote human labor and birth* [5th ed., p. 119]. New York: Appleton & Lange.)

    (2) Dilatation

       (a) 0 cm: external os is closed.

       (b) 10 cm (4 in): external os is fully dilated and will permit passage of the fetus.

  b. Manual determination of pelvic capacity

    (1) Measurement of the diagonal conjugate permits calculation or estimation of the obstetric conjugate.

    (2) Engagement of the presenting part signals adequacy of the inlet but does not predict adequacy of the midpelvis or the pelvic outlet.

B. Nursing Diagnoses

  1. Risk for situational low self-esteem related to possible reduced pelvic capacity

C. Interventions/Outcomes

  1. Risk for situational low self-esteem related to possible reduced pelvic capacity

    a. Interventions

      (1) Therapeutic

        (a) Promote maximum pelvic capacity.

          (i) Help the client assume adaptive positions.

- Upright
- Squatting
- Sitting
- Modified knee-chest

          (ii) Encourage the client to change position frequently.

          (iii) Provide the client with encouragement and support.

          (iv) Provide positive feedback for the client's attempts to use alternate positions.

          (v) Remind the client that absolute pelvic measurements are less important than the relation between the pelvis and the infant.

      (2) Diagnostic

        (a) On an ongoing basis, assess the client's level of satisfaction with her labor.

        (b) On an ongoing basis, assess the client's feelings of self-worth.

    b. Outcomes

      (1) The client demonstrates positive self-esteem as evidenced by:

        (a) Verbalizing satisfaction and contentment with the progress of her labor

        (b) Verbalizing statements of self-worth

Passenger

A. Assessment

  1. History

    a. Previous pregnancies

      (1) Birth weight of previous children

      (2) Malpresentation or disproportion encountered during previous labors

    b. Current pregnancy: unusual perceptions by the client that suggest a large infant or atypical positioning

  2. Physical examination

    a. Fetal lie: relation of the long axis of the fetus to the long axis of the mother

(1) Longitudinal lie: the long axes of the fetus and of the mother are parallel.
(2) Transverse or oblique lie: the long axis of the fetus is perpendicular to the long axis of the mother.
b. Fetal attitude: the relation of fetal parts to one another
  (1) Flexion: the typical fetal attitude in utero
  (2) Extension: tends to present larger fetal diameters
c. Presentation: determined by the pole of the fetus that first enters the pelvic inlet
  (1) Cephalic: head first (95% of term deliveries)
  (2) Breech: pelvis first (3% of term deliveries)
  (3) Shoulder: shoulder first (2% of term deliveries)
d. Presenting part: the specific fetal structure lying nearest to the cervix
  (1) Determined by the attitude of the fetus.
  (2) Each presenting part has an identified denominator that is used to describe the fetal position in the pelvis.
  (3) Cephalic presentations (Figure 10-7)
    (a) Vertex (denominator is occiput)
      (i) Flexion
        ■ Normal fetal position, with infant's chin resting on its chest
        ■ Presents optimal fetal dimensions during labor
        ■ At term, the position of 95% of fetuses
      (ii) No flexion and no extension
        ■ Known as a *military attitude*
        ■ Presents slightly larger diameters than full flexion
        ■ Usually converts to flexion or full extension
        ■ Prognosis for labor and delivery generally favorable
    (b) Frontum or brow (denominator is frontum)
      (i) Partial extension
      (ii) Incidence less than 1%
      (iii) May be related to fetal anomaly
      (iv) May be associated with polyhydramnios or a small fetus
      (v) Presents relatively larger fetal diameters to pelvis
      (vi) Spontaneous delivery possible if pelvis is large, contractions are adequate, and infant is small
      (vii) Delivery expedited by conversion to vertex or face presentation
    (c) Face (denominator is mentum-chin)
      (i) Full extension
      (ii) Incidence less than 1%
      (iii) More frequent in multiparas
      (iv) May be secondary to fetal factors that cause hyperextension, such as enlarged thyroid or multiple nuchal cords
      (v) Fetal diameters essentially the same as with a vertex presentation
      (vi) Vaginal delivery possible only if mentum is anterior
  (4) Breech presentations (denominator is sacrum) (Figure 10-8)
    (a) Complete breech: flexion at hips, flexion at knees
    (b) Frank breech: flexion at hips, extension at knees

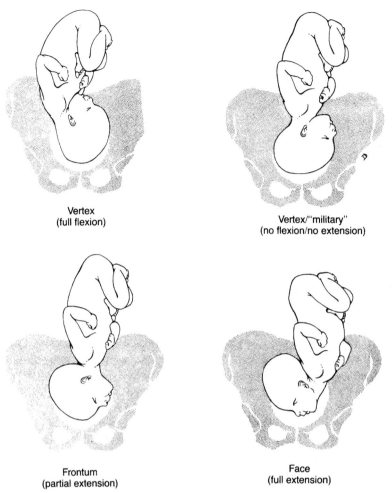

Vertex
(full flexion)

Vertex/"military"
(no flexion/no extension)

Frontum
(partial extension)

Face
(full extension)

FIGURE 10-7 ■ Cephalic presentations. (From Oxorn, H. [1986]. *Oxorn-Foote human labor and birth* [5th ed., p. 55]. New York: Appleton & Lange.)

(c) Footling breech: extension at one or both hips, extension at one or both knees
(d) Kneeling breech: extension at hips, flexion at knees
(e) Passage of meconium may occur secondary to pressure changes and does not necessarily indicate fetal stress or distress.
(f) Associated with prematurity, placenta previa, multiparity, pelvic abnormality, and some congenital anomalies, such as hydrocephaly
(g) Associated with increased fetal mortality and morbidity
   (i) Prematurity
   (ii) Malformations
   (iii) Asphyxia caused by prolonged compression of cord, prolapse of cord, or trauma to after-coming head, which does not have the opportunity to undergo molding
   (iv) Injury to brain and skull, resulting in minute hemorrhages or fractures

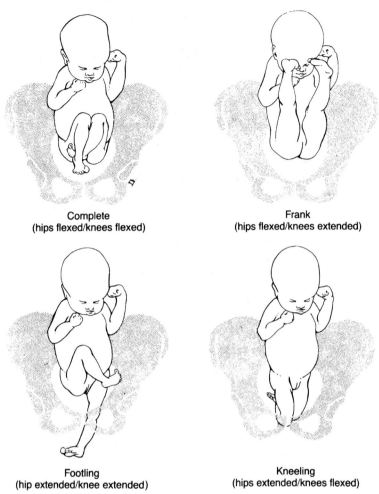

Complete
(hips flexed/knees flexed)

Frank
(hips flexed/knees extended)

Footling
(hip extended/knee extended)

Kneeling
(hips extended/knees flexed)

FIGURE 10-8 ■ Breech presentations. (From Oxorn, H. [1986]. *Oxorn-Foote human labor and birth* [5th ed., p. 57]. New York: Appleton & Lange.)

      (v) Trauma of manipulation during delivery, leading to cervical fractures, brachial plexus paralysis, liver rupture, and spinal cord traction

   (h) Associated with protracted and dysfunctional labor

      (i) Maternal positioning may facilitate conversion to cephalic presentation.

      (i) Not proven effective, though studies may have been confounded by noncompliance

      (ii) Elkins procedure: knee chest position for 15 minutes every 2 hours while awake for 5 days

      (iii) Modified Elkins procedure: knee chest position with a full bladder for 15 minutes three times a day for 7 days

(5) Transverse presentation (Figure 10-9)

   (a) Shoulder is the usual presenting part (denominator is scapula).

   (b) May be caused by anything that prevents descent of the head or the breech into the lower pelvis.

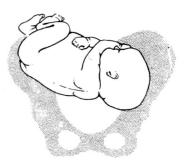

FIGURE 10-9 ■ Transverse presentation. (From Oxorn, H. [1986]. *Oxorn-Foote human labor and birth* [5th ed., p. 57]. New York: Appleton & Lange.)

- (i) Placenta previa
- (ii) Neoplasm
- (iii) Anomalies of the lower uterine segment
- (iv) Multiple gestation
- (v) Fetal anomalies
- (c) Associated with multigravidas, possibly secondary to increased relaxation of uterine and abdominal muscles
- (d) Vaginal delivery impossible without injury to mother and fetus
- (6) Compound presentation
    - (a) The infant assumes a unique posture, usually with the arm or the hand presenting alongside the presenting part.
    - (b) Presents increased fetal diameters.
    - (c) May interfere with the cardinal movements of labor.
- **e.** Fetal position: the relation of the denominator to the maternal pelvis
    - (1) In practice, eight points are demarcated.
    - (2) The denominator is assigned right or left, depending on which side of the maternal pelvis it is in.
    - (3) The denominator is assigned anterior, posterior, or transverse according to maternal front, back, or side (Figure 10-10).
    - (4) The occiput anterior position is most facilitative of vaginal delivery.
    - (5) The occiput transverse position typically requires rotation to anterior or posterior position for delivery.
    - (6) The occiput posterior position presents slightly larger diameters to pelvis.
        - (a) May slow progress of descent.
        - (b) Usually converts to anterior position during descent for delivery.
        - (c) An increased degree of internal rotation is required to align occiput beneath the maternal symphysis.
        - (d) Typically causes increased back pain during labor.
- **f.** Fetal station: the relation of the presenting part to an imaginary line drawn between the ischial spines
    - (1) Designations
        - (a) The ischial spines are 0 station.
        - (b) Above the spines is a negative value.
        - (c) Below the spines is a positive value.
    - (2) Engagement: when the widest diameter of the presenting part has passed the inlet
        - (a) Usually corresponds to a 0 station.
        - (b) Depth of the pelvis and amount of caput succedaneum that is present influence the actual station at engagement.

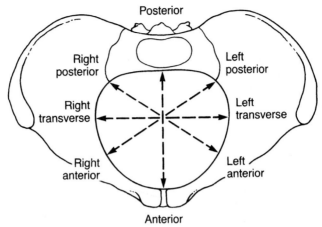

FIGURE 10-10 ■ Assignment of fetal position.

        (c) In primigravidas:
           (i) Often occurs before labor.
          (ii) When the fetus is unengaged at the outset of labor, disproportion is suggested.
        (d) Engagement may occur anytime in multigravidas.
     (3) Floating: when the presenting part is entirely out of the pelvis and freely movable in the inlet
     (4) Synclitism: when the biparietal diameter (BPD) of the fetal head is parallel to the planes of the maternal pelvis (Figure 10-11)
     (5) Asynclitism: when the biparietal diameter is not parallel to the maternal pelvis (i.e., the fetal head appears tilted); may lead to a disproportion or delayed descent (see Figure 10-11)
  g. Fetal size
     (1) Size alone is less significant than the relation between fetal size and pelvic dimensions.
     (2) Macrosomia
        (a) Defined as birth weight above 4000 g (8 lb, 14½ oz) (in some places, 4500 g [9 lb, 15 oz] is used [MacMillen, Brucker, & Zwelling, 1997]).
        (b) Incidence is between 0.5% and 1.8%.
        (c) Associated variables
           (i) Family history
          (ii) Multiparity
         (iii) Advanced maternal age
         (iv) Excessive maternal weight gain
          (v) Maternal diabetes
         (vi) Postterm gestation
        (vii) Male fetus
        (viii) Father of infant at least 10 years older than mother
        (d) Associated complications
           (i) Prolonged second stage of labor
          (ii) Maternal genital tract injury
         (iii) Postpartum hemorrhage related to atony

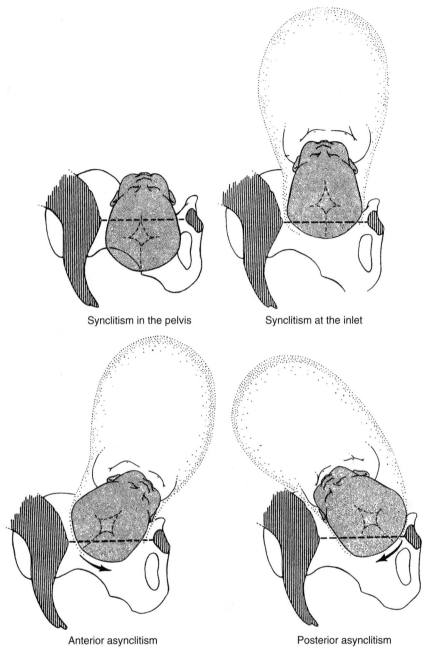

Synclitism in the pelvis

Synclitism at the inlet

Anterior asynclitism

Posterior asynclitism

FIGURE 10-11 ■ Synclitism and asynclitism. (From Oxorn, H. [1986]. *Oxorn-Foote human labor and birth* [5th ed., p. 71]. New York: Appleton & Lange.)

   (iv) Separation of pubic symphysis
   (v) Birth trauma
     ■ Skull fracture
     ■ Brachial plexus damage
     ■ Clavicle fracture
     ■ Asphyxia or depression (see Chapter 18 for risks associated with gestational age and birth weight)

      (3) Microsomia

         (a) Typically occurs in the preterm gestation but may be associated with intrauterine growth restriction.

         (b) Is associated with shortened second stage of labor.

         (c) May be possible to deliver the infant through an incompletely dilated cervix, predisposing to entrapment of the placenta or after-coming fetal parts and cervical lacerations or injury.

      (4) Fetal anomalies influencing fetal size

         (a) Hydrocephalus

         (b) Thyroid hypertrophy

         (c) Abdominal distension secondary to kidney disease

         (d) Omphalocele

         (e) Myelocele

   h. Fetal skull

      (1) The most important structure because it is the largest and least compressible

      (2) Landmarks

         (a) Cranial bones

            (i) At birth, they are thin, poorly ossified, and easily compressible.

            (ii) Occipital: located posteriorly

            (iii) Parietal (two): located laterally

            (iv) Temporal (two): located anteriorly

            (v) Frontal (two): located anteriorly

         (b) Sutures

            (i) The membranous tissue between the bones

            (ii) Sagittal: lies between the parietal bones, in an anteroposterior direction

            (iii) Lambdoidal: separates the occipital bone from the two parietal bones, and runs in a transverse direction

            (iv) Coronal: separates the parietal bones from the frontal bones and runs in a transverse direction

            (v) Frontal: lies between the frontal bones and is a continuation of the sagittal suture

         (c) Fontanelles

            (i) The intersections of the sutures

            (ii) Anterior (bregma)

               ■ Junction of the sagittal, frontal, and coronal sutures

               ■ Diamond shaped, 3×2 cm (1×1 in)

            (iii) Posterior (lambda)

               ■ Junction of the sagittal and lambdoidal sutures

               ■ Triangular shaped, 1×2 cm (0.5×1 in)

      (3) Molding

         (a) The ability of the fetal head to change shape to accommodate the maternal pelvis

         (b) Accomplished because of the lack of fusion of the cranial bones

         (c) May decrease dimensions by 0.5 to 1 cm (0.2 to 0.4 in)

      (4) Caput succedaneum

         (a) Soft-tissue edema caused by cervical pressure against the presenting head

         (b) If severe, may obscure the suture lines, making determination of fetal position difficult.

(c) May make determination of fetal station difficult.
  i. Cardinal movements
    (1) The manner in which the infant moves and rotates to accommodate to the maternal pelvis
    (2) Although often conceptualized as separate and sequential, the movements more typically are concurrent.
    (3) Engagement and descent
        (a) In nulliparas, engagement usually precedes the onset of labor, with additional descent occurring during labor.
        (b) In multiparas, engagement and descent may not occur before labor.
        (c) Absence of descent in a primigravida may signal disproportion or malpresentation.
        (d) The fetal head typically enters the pelvis with the sagittal suture aligned in the transverse diameter.
        (e) Responsible for *lightening*, the subjective sensation felt by the mother as the fetus settles into the lower uterine segment; more commonly perceived by primigravidas.
    (4) Flexion
        (a) Relative flexion is the natural posture of the fetus and is enhanced as the descending part encounters pelvic resistance.
        (b) Flexion achieves the smallest fetal diameters presenting to the maternal pelvic dimensions.
    (5) Internal rotation
        (a) Aligns the long axis of the fetal head with the long axis of the maternal pelvis.
        (b) The sagittal suture aligns in the anteroposterior diameter.
        (c) Occurs mainly during the second stage of labor.
    (6) Extension
        (a) Resistance of the pelvic floor causes the presenting part to pivot beneath the symphysis pubis.
        (b) Delivery is accomplished through extension of the head beneath the symphysis pubis.
    (7) Restitution
        (a) The sagittal suture returns to an oblique diameter.
        (b) The oblique position realigns the sagittal suture with the fetal trunk axis.
    (8) External rotation
        (a) Continuation of restitution, with the sagittal suture moving to a transverse diameter and the shoulders aligning in the anteroposterior diameter.
        (b) The sagittal suture maintains alignment with the fetal trunk as the trunk navigates through the pelvis.
    (9) Expulsion: after the delivery of the presenting part, the trunk typically follows easily.
3. Diagnostic studies and techniques
  a. Leopold's maneuvers (Figure 10-12)
    (1) Inspection and palpation of the maternal abdomen to determine the fetal position, station, and size
    (2) When performed by experienced clinicians, the maneuver is effective as a screening assessment for malpresentation.

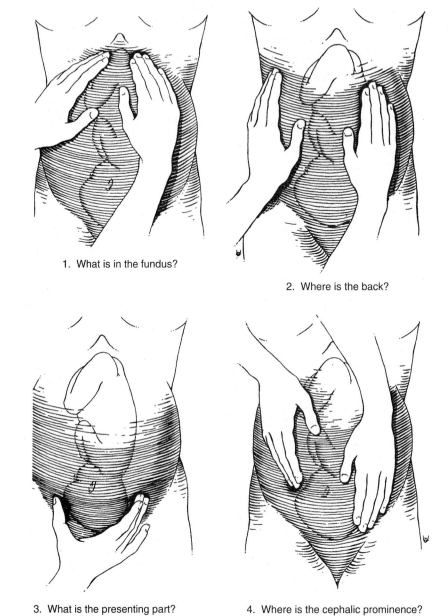

1. What is in the fundus?

2. Where is the back?

3. What is the presenting part?

4. Where is the cephalic prominence?

FIGURE 10-12 ■ Leopold's maneuvers. (From Oxorn, H. [1986]. *Oxorn-Foote human labor and birth* [5th ed., pp. 77-79]. New York: Appleton & Lange.)

   (3) First maneuver: what is in the fundus?
      (a) Stand at the client's side and palpate the fundus.
      (b) The head feels hard and smooth.
      (c) The breech feels more irregular.
   (4) Second maneuver: where is the back?
      (a) Face the client and place hands on the sides of her abdomen.
      (b) The back feels firm and smooth.
      (c) The small parts feel irregular.

(5) Third maneuver: what is the presenting part?
  (a) Move hands down the sides of the abdomen to grasp the lower uterine segment.
  (b) The breech feels soft and irregular.
  (c) The head feels globular and firm.
(6) Fourth maneuver: where is the cephalic prominence?
  (a) Face the client's feet and slide hands down the sides of the uterus to locate the side of greater resistance; this is the prominence.

b. Vaginal examination (Figure 10-13)
  (1) Determine presentation.
    (a) Cephalic
    (b) Breech
    (c) Shoulder
  (2) Determine station.
    (a) Presenting part at level of ischial spines: 0 station
    (b) Presenting part above level of ischial spines: −1, −2, −3 cm station
    (c) Presenting part below level of ischial spines: +1, +2, +3 cm station
  (3) Determine position.
    (a) Locate denominator by palpating sutures, facial features, or anatomic landmarks.
    (b) Define denominator in relation to the maternal pelvis (see Figure 10-10).

c. Ultrasonography
  (1) Size
    (a) BPD is measured with accuracy beginning at 13 weeks.
    (b) BPD is predictive of fetal age and fetal weight.

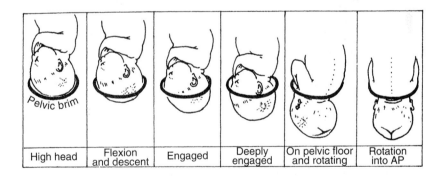

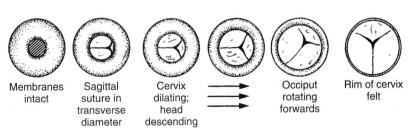

FIGURE 10-13 ■ Fetal head progressing through pelvis and changes in cervix. (From Fraser, D.M., & Cooper, M.A. [2003]. *Myles textbook for midwives* [14th ed., p. 448]. Edinburgh: Churchill Livingstone.)

    (2) Presentation: contents in lower pelvis are identified.

    (3) Morphology

        (a) Anencephaly is demonstrated by lack of cerebral formation.

        (b) Hydrocephaly is suggested if BPD is greater than 11 cm (4.4 in).

        (c) Microcephaly may be suspected but can be difficult to diagnose.

        (d) Anatomic structural defects may be recognizable.

B. Nursing Diagnoses

  1. Risk for injury (fetal trauma, uterine trauma, cervical trauma, fetal distress, or asphyxia) related to malpresentation

  2. Risk for situational low self-esteem related to impairment of cardinal movements

C. Interventions/Outcomes

  1. Risk for injury (fetal trauma, uterine trauma, cervical trauma, fetal distress, or asphyxia) related to malpresentation

    a. Interventions

      (1) Therapeutic

        (a) Report breech, transverse, and compound presentations promptly to the physician or nurse midwife.

        (b) Report arrest of the cardinal movements to the physician or nurse midwife.

        (c) Prepare the client for cesarean delivery as directed by the physician.

      (2) Diagnostic

        (a) As appropriate to the client's stage of labor and clinical status, perform a vaginal examination to assess presentation, station, and position.

        (b) As appropriate to the client's stage of labor and clinical status, assess fetal heart rate.

        (c) On an ongoing basis, assess for uterine tenderness.

    b. Outcomes: client and baby are not injured as evidenced by:

      (1) No uterine rupture

      (2) No cervical or vaginal lacerations

      (3) No newborn birth trauma

      (4) Newborn 5-minute Apgar score greater than 7

  2. Risk for situational low self-esteem related to impairment of cardinal movements

    a. Interventions

      (1) Therapeutic

        (a) Promote fetal descent and rotation.

          (i) Assist the client to assume adaptive positions.

            ■ Upright

            ■ Squatting

            ■ Sitting

            ■ Modified knee-chest

          (ii) Encourage the client to change position frequently.

          (iii) Provide the client with encouragement and support.

          (iv) Provide positive feedback regarding fetal descent and rotation.

          (v) Provide positive feedback for the client's attempts to use alternate positions.

      (2) Diagnostic
         (a) On an ongoing basis, assess the client's level of satisfaction with her labor.
         (b) On an ongoing basis, assess the client's feelings of self-worth.
   b. Outcomes: client demonstrates positive self-esteem as evidenced by:
      (1) Verbalizing satisfaction and contentment with the progress of her labor
      (2) Verbalizing statements of self-worth

Psyche

A. Assessment
   1. History
      a. Previous birth experiences
         (1) Complications of pregnancy, labor, and birth that occurred in previous pregnancies
         (2) Birth outcome of previous pregnancies
         (3) The degree to which the client's personal expectations for birth were achieved in previous pregnancies
      b. Current pregnancy experience
         (1) Planned versus unplanned pregnancy
            (a) A planned pregnancy imparts increased feelings of acceptance.
            (b) An unplanned pregnancy may be accompanied by anger and rejection.
         (2) Client age
            (a) Adolescent women must complete the developmental tasks of both adolescence and pregnancy.
            (b) Mature women are more accustomed to being in control of their lives and may be easily frustrated by the loss of control during pregnancy and birth.
         (3) Difficulty in conceiving
            (a) Relative infertility may result in increased anxiety about the well being of a *premium pregnancy*.
            (b) Technology to assist conception and maintenance of the pregnancy may reduce a client's sense of involvement and control.
         (4) Pregnancy discomforts may increase the client's anticipation of discomfort and difficulty during labor and birth.
         (5) High-risk pregnancy
            (a) The client may experience increased anxiety and fears about her own well being and the well being of the fetus.
            (b) The need for technology may interfere with the client's expectations for a natural birth.
         (6) Completion of the developmental tasks of pregnancy: failure to complete the developmental tasks of pregnancy may result in increased fears and anxiety about the birth experience.
      c. Cultural considerations (see Chapter 4 for a complete discussion of cultural considerations of childbearing)
         (1) Establish values and beliefs about sickness and health.
            (a) Pregnancy as physiologic process, a wellness experience
            (b) Pregnancy as a state of illness, a time of vulnerability

(2) Define the childbirth experience.
  (a) Shameful versus joyful experience
  (b) Intimate experience versus social event
  (c) Superstitions about pregnancy and birth
  (d) Prescribed behaviors and taboos influencing activities, food, and drink
(3) Define kinship structure and relationships.
  (a) Interaction between the couple
  (b) Parent-infant interactions
  (c) Role expectations of mother, father, and grandparents, for example
  (d) Involvement of support persons
  (e) Intergenerational behaviors
(4) Define pain.
  (a) Identifies the meaning and context of pain
  (b) Determines the acceptable response to pain (perceived pain is not always expressed as pain)
(5) Determine the significance of touch.
  (a) Soothing versus intruding
  (b) May be viewed as a symbol of intimacy

d. Expectations for birth experience
  (1) Childbirth can be viewed as either a meaningful or a stressful event.
  (2) Goals can be realistic and attainable or too idealistic and in conflict with reality, thus leading to disappointment.
  (3) Acceptable behavior for self and others is defined by cultural, as well as other, influences.
  (4) Labor may be viewed as a test.

e. Preparation for birth
  (1) Type of childbirth preparation
  (2) Familiarity with the institution and its policies and procedures
  (3) Type of relaxation techniques learned and practiced

f. Support system
  (1) The presence and support of a valued companion during birth is invaluable to most women.
    (a) The woman's spouse or partner is the most frequently chosen labor companion.
    (b) Woman's mother and other female relatives often provide additional support.
      (i) *Young* grandmothers may not be prepared to assume the grandparent role and thus may subconsciously withhold support.
      (ii) Grandparents may have misinformation and misperceptions, and may need knowledge of current practices.
  (2) The support of a trained labor attendant supplements and enhances familial support.
    (a) Types of attendants
      (i) Doula
        ■ From the Greek, meaning *in service of* or *woman's servant*.
        ■ Provides continuous physical and emotional support.
        ■ Does not assess maternal or fetal assessment well being.
        ■ Does not intervene to ensure safe outcome for mother or baby.
        ■ Relationship with client often begins before labor.

       (ii) Professional nurse
- Provides physical and emotional support, though not always on a continual basis.
- Assesses maternal and fetal well being.
- Intervenes to ensure safe outcome for mother and baby.

       (iii) Roles should be complementary, not adversarial.

    (b) Supportive activities

       (i) Emotional support
- Sustaining physical presence ("keeping company")
- Words of encouragement, reassurance, and praise

       (ii) Physical support
- Comfort measures and pain relief
- Hygiene
- Reassuring touch
- Application of heat or cold
- Calm environment (lighting, sounds, temperature)
- Therapeutic music
  - Anxiolytic music
  - Causes reduction or absence of anxiety
  - Typically characterized by no extremes of rhythm, melody, or dynamics
  - Selections chosen by client are best.

       (iii) Information and advice
- Provide information regarding progress of labor.
- Interpret medical language and jargon.

       (iv) Advocacy
- Support decisions.
- Ensure that others respect client's decisions.
- Manage visitors.

       (v) Support of partner
- Role model therapeutic interactions.
- Assist to meet own self-care needs (e.g., nutrition, hygiene).

    (c) Measurable effects on birth outcome

       (i) Reduced likelihood of needing pharmacologic pain relief

       (ii) Reduced likelihood of operative vaginal delivery, cesarean delivery, and oxytocin augmentation

       (iii) Increased likelihood that infant's 5-minute Apgar is greater than 7

       (iv) Increased likelihood of client satisfaction with birth experience

       (v) Increased likelihood of exclusive breastfeeding

       (vi) Increased likelihood of longer duration of breastfeeding

       (vii) Increased likelihood that client demonstrates positive mother-infant behaviors at birth

  (3) Religious values and spiritual faith also provide a supportive structure.

2. Psychosocial responses

  a. Emotions of labor

    (1) Latent phase

      (a) Is excited.

      (b) Is ready for anything.

      (c) Experiences anxiety and fear.

    (2) Active phase
        (a) Has decreased energy.
        (b) Experiences fatigue.
        (c) Turns attention to internal sensations.
        (d) Feels serious.
    (3) Transition
        (a) Is discouraged.
        (b) Is irritable or nasty.
        (c) Is panicky and overwhelmed by fears of death.
        (d) Is impatient.
        (e) Feels out of control.
    (4) Second stage
        (a) Is focused.
        (b) Has increased energy, though is still fatigued.
        (c) May subconsciously "hold back," resulting in decreased pushing efforts.
        (d) Is gratified that she can actively participate to bring about birth.
    (5) Immediate postpartum period:
        (a) Experiences joy and relief.
            (i) Is able to see and hold baby.
            (ii) Is eager to share the news with others.
        (b) Begins grief work:
            (i) Experiences loss of valued object (the pregnancy).
            (ii) Experiences loss of valued status (as a pregnant woman).
            (iii) May feel sense of failure at not achieving own expectations for labor and birth.
            (iv) Experiences loss of some aspect of self.
                ■ Altered body image
                ■ Changed self-esteem
                ■ Changed self-concept
                ■ Loss of former role
        (c) Fatigue: finally able to sleep after hours of work

b. Psychologic reactions to labor
    (1) Anxiety
        (a) Anxiety is defined as an uneasiness in response to a vague, nonspecific threat.
        (b) At mild to moderate levels, anxiety is an effective stimulant to action.
        (c) Excessive anxiety interferes with labor.
        (d) Somatic cues
            (i) Muscular pain and stiffness (especially in neck and back)
            (ii) Chest pain or tightness
            (iii) Nausea
            (iv) Flushing
            (v) Numbness in hands and face
        (e) Behavioral cues
            (i) Crying, tearfulness
            (ii) Tremulous voice
            (iii) Inability to focus or concentrate
            (iv) Jitteriness
        (f) Physiologic cues
            (i) Elevated blood pressure

        (ii) Elevated heart rate

        (iii) Dilated pupils

        (iv) Diarrhea

(2) Fear

    (a) Fear is defined as a painful, uneasy feeling in response to an identifiable threat.

    (b) Possible intrapartum threats

        (i) Labor is an unknown despite the best of preparations

        (ii) Maternal or fetal injury during labor and birth

        (iii) Pain

        (iv) Institutional procedures (e.g., IVs, shave preparation, enema, fetal monitor)

        (v) Impending irreversible lifestyle changes created by the birth of a baby

    (c) Fear causes peripheral vasoconstriction that may decrease uterine blood flow, decreasing uterine contractility.

    (d) Fear typically enhances pain perception, leading to increased fear.

(3) Loss of control and sense of helplessness

    (a) For many women, childbirth is their first hospitalization.

    (b) Personal belongings and clothing are removed.

    (c) Routine procedures are unfamiliar and intimidating.

    (d) Most clients recognize that, at some point in the labor process, they must depend on others for assistance.

(4) Feelings of aloneness or abandonment

    (a) Removal from familiar home environment

    (b) Restriction of support system

    (c) Changing patterns of communication

        (i) Increased reliance on nonverbal messages

           ■ Vision

           ■ Touch

           ■ Facial expression

           ■ Body movements

           ■ Vocal quality

        (ii) When verbal and nonverbal messages are out of synchrony, nonverbal communications are usually more accurate.

        (iii) As labor progresses, most women turn inward, which may lead to distorted message reception.

    (d) Isolation may decrease reality orientation, leading to increased anxiety and fear.

(5) Fatigue and weariness

    (a) Etiologic factors:

        (i) Sleep deprivation

        (ii) Sensory overload

        (iii) Generalized fatigue, which is common in late pregnancy

        (iv) Energy expended during labor

    (b) Fatigue generally leads to reduced energy and inability to focus and concentrate.

    (c) Fatigue may decrease myometrial activity.

c. Personality styles

(1) There is no one correct style, and a client may demonstrate aspects of each.

    (2) Controlling
       (a) The client seeks the opportunity to have influence in the decisions regarding her care.
       (b) The client explores the options and alternatives in a given situation.
       (c) The client relies on her knowledge base and relaxation skills.
       (d) The client's belief that she will succeed is affirmed.
       (e) Inability to participate in decision making leads to conflict.
    (3) Optimistic
       (a) The client freely releases the surge of energy that is generated by her emotions and feelings.
       (b) The client smiles, laughs, cries, and demonstrates increased activity levels.
       (c) The client accepts the expertise and assistance of those around her.
       (d) The client demonstrates basic trust in the outcome.
    (4) Fatalistic
       (a) The client focuses on her perceived loss of control.
       (b) The client avoids choosing options and participating in decision making.
       (c) The client becomes preoccupied with details.
       (d) The client has a heightened perception of danger, leading to increased fears.
       (e) The client displays hostility, aggression, and withdrawal.
       (f) The client demonstrates generalized distrust in the outcome and therefore views her own actions and those of others as meaningless.

  d. Behaviors
    (1) Effective coping
       (a) Rhythmic activity during contractions (rocking, swaying, self-stroking)
       (b) Attention-focusing activity during contractions
         (i) Tactile: touch, massage, stroking
         (ii) Auditory: music, murmuring, verbal encouragement
         (iii) Visual: partner's face, designated picture or object
         (iv) Kinesthetic: rocking, swaying, tapping
         (v) Mental: counting breaths, reciting verse, visualizing a favorite scene
         (vi) Vocalization: moaning, counting, chanting
       (c) Ritual
         (i) Repetition of the same rhythmic and attention focusing activities during each contraction
         (ii) May include use of introspective self-talk
    (2) Ineffective coping
       (a) Random or uncoordinated activity during contractions (wincing, writhing)
       (b) Unfocused or panicked activity during contractions
       (c) Absence of a consistent reaction to each contraction

B. Nursing Diagnoses
  1. Anxiety related to possible fetal conditions that are hindering labor, a strange environment, the disruption of normal routines and support systems, or the situational crisis of labor
  2. Ineffective coping related to the situational crisis of labor, inadequate support systems or absence of a support person, or conflict between

personal and cultural expectations and the health care system's
practices

3. Fear related to the unknown of labor, the threat of potential harm to self or fetus, or the anticipation of pain during labor

4. Deficient knowledge about the birthing process related to inadequate preparation or unanticipated circumstances

5. Disturbed sensory perception related to multiple environmental distracters

6. Social isolation related to changing patterns of communication, an unfamiliar environment, or inadequate support systems

C. **Interventions/Outcomes**

1. Anxiety related to possible fetal conditions that are hindering labor, a strange environment, the disruption of normal routines and support systems, or the situational crisis of labor

    a. Interventions

        (1) Therapeutic

            (a) Provide the client with factual information about the baby's condition.

                (i) Fetal heart rate

                (ii) Information regarding size and morphology gained from ultrasound examination

            (b) Reassure the client that cephalopelvic disproportion is not necessarily caused by fetal abnormalities.

            (c) Encourage the client to avoid engaging in unrealistic fantasies about the baby.

            (d) Explain all procedures and interventions to the client.

            (e) Provide a quiet, restful environment with minimal stimulation.

            (f) Remain with the client as much as possible.

            (g) Be direct and specific in communicating with the client, offering her a limited number of options.

            (h) Speak and behave calmly.

            (i) Do not communicate one's own problems and concerns to the client.

            (j) Encourage the client to remain focused on now and to avoid a past or future orientation.

        (2) Diagnostic

            (a) Every 4 hours or as appropriate for the stage of labor, obtain blood pressure, pulse, and respiration readings.

            (b) On an ongoing basis, evaluate the client's concerns about her fetus's well being.

            (c) On an ongoing basis, evaluate the client's ability to focus and concentrate.

            (d) On an ongoing basis, evaluate the client's ability to respond to messages.

            (e) On an ongoing basis, determine the synchrony between the client's verbal and nonverbal communications.

    b. Outcomes: client demonstrates minimal anxiety as evidenced by:

        (1) Having vital signs within normal limits

        (2) Verbalizing realistic expectations about the baby's condition

        (3) Using relaxation techniques

        (4) Verbalizing confidence in the health care providers

        (5) Understanding and responding correctly to messages

        (6) Demonstrating logical thought processes

2. Ineffective coping related to the situational crisis of labor, inadequate support systems or absence of a support person, or conflict between personal and cultural expectations and the health care system's practices

   a. Interventions

     (1) Therapeutic

       (a) Reinforce or teach relaxation techniques.

       (b) Encourage the use rhythmic and focused behaviors.

       (c) Keep the client informed about her condition and her progress.

       (d) Explain all procedures and interventions.

       (e) Assist the client in identifying her strengths, and praise her for her demonstration of adaptive coping skills.

       (f) Acknowledge the client's feelings of discouragement, then refocus her towards adaptive behaviors.

       (g) Provide physical comfort measures.

         (i) Cool cloth

         (ii) Mouthwash

         (iii) Back rub

         (iv) Sponge bath

         (v) Pillows

       (h) Control the environment to minimize sensory overload and intrusion.

       (i) Remain with the client as much as possible.

       (j) Identify things within the client's control and encourage her to be involved.

       (k) Be direct in communicating with the client, using a *take charge* style.

         (i) Maintain eye contact.

         (ii) Create a pacing rhythm.

         (iii) Develop a contraction ritual.

         (iv) Exude calm confidence.

       (l) Support the support person.

         (i) Provide nourishment.

         (ii) Provide episodic relief from responsibility.

         (iii) Provide praise and encouragement.

       (m) Discuss with the client her expectations and values and integrate them into the labor experience as much as possible.

         (i) Ask questions to determine the client's state of mind and point of view.

         (ii) During active labor, use directed questions ("Does this cool cloth help?") because open-ended questions become difficult for the client to answer ("How can I help?").

     (2) Diagnostic

       (a) On an ongoing basis, evaluate the client's use of relaxation techniques and coping behaviors.

       (b) On an ongoing basis, evaluate the client's patterns of communication.

       (c) On an ongoing basis, evaluate the client's ability to receive and use information that is provided.

       (d) On an ongoing basis, evaluate the client's degree of satisfaction with the experience.

    b. Outcomes: client demonstrates effective coping as evidenced by:
        (1) Verbalizing her perception that she is coping with the labor process
        (2) Participating in decision making about her own basic needs
        (3) Using relaxation techniques and adaptive coping behaviors in response to painful stimuli
        (4) Communicating effectively with her support person and health care personnel

3. Fear related to the unknown of labor, the threat of potential harm to self or fetus, or the anticipation of pain during labor
    a. Interventions
        (1) Therapeutic
            (a) Orient the client to the surroundings.
            (b) Familiarize the client with the usual routines and procedures, and keep her informed about what to expect.
            (c) Remain with the client as much as possible.
            (d) Inform the client of her status and progress, offering reassurance when everything is normal.
        (2) Diagnostic
            (a) Every 4 hours or as appropriate for the stage of labor and the client's labor progress, obtain blood pressure, pulse, and respirations.
            (b) On an ongoing basis, identify the client's concerns and expectations.
            (c) On an ongoing basis, determine the client's understanding of what is happening.
    b. Outcomes: client demonstrates minimal fear as evidenced by:
        (1) Having vital signs within normal limits
        (2) Verbalizing a realistic and accurate perception of the labor experience
        (3) Verbalizing a perception of being in a comforting environment
        (4) Verbalizing confidence in the health care provider's ability to safeguard her well being

4. Deficient knowledge about the birthing process related to inadequate preparation or unanticipated circumstances
    a. Interventions
        (1) Therapeutic
            (a) Explain the principles of labor and birth as related to the client's specific circumstances.
            (b) Explain all procedures.
            (c) Encourage the client to ask questions.
            (d) Answer questions honestly and promptly.
            (e) Identify changes in the client's status that might be misunderstood and offer anticipatory education.
        (2) Diagnostic
            (a) On an ongoing basis, determine the client's level of comprehension.
    b. Outcomes: client understands the birthing process as evidenced by:
        (1) Describing accurately what is happening and what is expected to happen
        (2) Asking questions that are reality oriented

5. Disturbed sensory perception related to multiple environmental distracters
    a. Interventions
        (1) Therapeutic

(a) Eliminate unnecessary lights and noises.
(b) Remove unnecessary equipment and supplies from the bedside.
(c) Avoid unnecessary conversation at the bedside.
(d) Speak calmly, quietly, and slowly to the client.
(e) Provide a single source of sensory input.
  (i) Music through earphones (in some clients, using earphones may contribute to isolation from their support system and health care providers).
  (ii) A focus point.
(2) Diagnostic
(a) On an ongoing basis, determine the client's reaction to the environment.
(b) On an ongoing basis, determine the client's patterns of communication.
(c) On an ongoing basis, determine the client's problem-solving abilities.
  b. Outcomes: client does not suffer sensory overload as evidenced by:
  (1) Describing self and situation accurately
  (2) Resting quietly between contractions, without restlessness, withdrawal, or agitation
  (3) Participating in decision making about her own basic need
6. Social isolation related to changing patterns of communication, an unfamiliar environment, or inadequate support systems
  a. Interventions
  (1) Therapeutic
  (a) Encourage the client to express her thoughts and feelings.
  (b) Respond to both verbal and nonverbal communications.
  (c) Validate the messages being received.
  (d) Decrease environmental distractions.
  (e) Speak in a simple, focused manner.
  (f) Communicate with the client in her own communication mode.
    (i) Return eye contact.
    (ii) Return touch.
    (iii) Answer questions.
  (2) Diagnostic
  (a) On an ongoing basis, determine the client's patterns of communication.
  (b) On an ongoing basis, determine the client's degree of satisfaction with the experience.
  b. Outcomes: client experiences adequate interaction with support persons and health care providers as evidenced by:
  (1) Verbalizing that her messages are being understood and her needs are being met

HEALTH EDUCATION

A. Optimizing labor power
1. Encourage normal activity and exercise patterns throughout pregnancy.
  a. Women with generally well-toned musculature tend to have more efficient uterine contractions.
  b. Good abdominal musculature assists during the second stage of labor.

  c. Women who exercise are generally more aware of their bodies and can more effectively control pushing efforts.

 2. Instruct the client in exercises specific to pregnancy and childbearing.

  a. Kegel exercise to tone perineal floor

  b. Pelvic tilt to tone abdominal muscles and relieve backache (Figure 10-14)

  c. Adductor stretching to tone thighs (tailor sitting)

 3. Instruct the client in intrapartum activities that strengthen uterine effort.

  a. Walk and remain active as long as possible.

  b. Lateral positions and an elevated head of the bed improve regularity and intensity of contractions.

  c. Avoid supine hypotension, which leads to decreased uterine blood flow and decreased muscle strength.

B. Maximizing labor passage

 1. Instruct the client in postures that increase pelvic capacity.

 2. Instruct support person in techniques to achieve alternative postures.

 3. Encourage the client to change positions frequently during labor.

  a. Provides dynamic pelvic capacity, which facilitates fetal passage.

  b. Avoids excessive stress and tension on a single muscle group.

C. Emotional preparation for birth

 1. Encourage attendance at childbirth preparation classes.

 2. Support self-study efforts, such as books and videos.

 3. Encourage rehearsal of coping behaviors and relaxation techniques.

 4. Encourage guidance and support of family members.

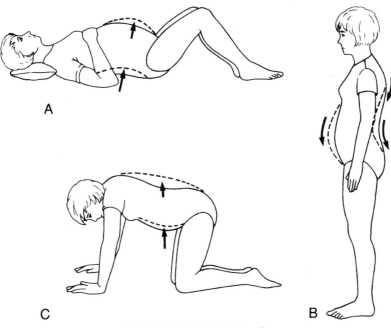

FIGURE 10-14 ■ Pelvic tilt.

CASE STUDIES AND STUDY QUESTIONS
PRIMIGRAVIDA IN EARLY LABOR

Mrs. W is a 37-year-old, gravida 1 (G1), who began experiencing irregular contractions late Tuesday afternoon. Throughout Tuesday evening, she and her husband diligently timed each contraction. They were very excited that labor had begun. They were equally excited that the baby's arrival had waited until the end of the academic year. She had recently been promoted to associate professor and took great pride in personally reviewing all of her students' papers before issuing final grades.

Near midnight, the contractions were 3 to 4 minutes apart, lasting 45 to 50 seconds. Her discomfort was increasing, although she remained able to focus on the relaxation breathing techniques she had learned. Her husband was becoming tired, but he remained excited and eager to time each new contraction. When her membranes ruptured at 12:30 AM, she phoned her physician, confident that her baby would be born soon.

Mr. and Mrs. W arrived in labor and delivery at 1:10 AM Wednesday. On arrival, she provided the nurse with a detailed summary of the previous 8 hours. She also shared with the nurse her goals for the birth experience, which included being permitted to breast-feed immediately after birth and going home as soon as possible. She was obviously uncomfortable with contractions, but she used her breathing techniques well.

The nurse escorted the couple to a labor-delivery-recovery (LDR) room, oriented them to the hospital environment, and assisted Mrs. W in changing into a hospital gown. Her initial assessment findings included:

- Maternal vital signs within normal limits
- Fetal heart rate of 136
- Contractions every 4 to 5 minutes, lasting 45 to 50 seconds, and of moderate intensity
- Cervix 100% effaced and 3 to 4 cm dilated
- Baby at 0 station, in the right occipitoanterior (ROA) position

When the nurse informed Mr. and Mrs. W of her findings, Mrs. W was obviously distressed and disappointed, "How can I be only 3 cm? I've been in labor for hours. I should be almost finished by now." As she spoke, she became increasingly agitated, and each new contraction heightened her frustration. She became restless and had difficulty implementing her breathing techniques.

1. What factor is most responsible for Mrs. W's reaction to the nurse's information?
   a. Maternal age
   b. The frequency and duration of her contractions
   c. Unrealistic expectations
   d. Her unfamiliarity with the hospital environment

2. How should the nurse respond to her?
   a. Remind her that first babies usually take 18 to 24 hours.
   b. Assist her in resuming the relaxation techniques she had been using on admission.
   c. Inform her that the physician will be contacted to obtain something to help her relax.
   d. Obtain additional information about her birth plan.

3. How can the nurse assist her to cope adaptively with her labor and birth?
   a. Provide her with information and encouragement.
   b. Leave her and her husband alone as much as possible.
   c. Share with Mrs. W her own birth experience.
   d. Teach her how to time her contractions.

4. What immediate intervention does Mr. W. require?
   a. Provision of scrub attire
   b. Information about the early discharge procedure
   c. Instruction about how to time contractions
   d. Information about how best to support his wife

PRIMIGRAVIDA, MULTIPLE GESTATION

Mr. and Mrs. C, a couple in their mid-twenties, were thrilled when they first learned that Mrs. C. was pregnant. They had been married for more than a year, and Mrs. C. had quit her job at the local bookstore shortly after their marriage in anticipation of raising a family. Both individuals came from large families, and they hoped to continue the tradition. Despite their desire for children and plans for a large family, they were shocked when the physician informed them that they were expecting twins.

As the shock faded, Mrs. C began to revel in the specialness of her pregnancy and enjoyed the extra attention that her friends and family paid her. She was unprepared, however, for the increased discomfort she experienced. Her physician reassured her that both fetuses were healthy and that everything was normal. Nonetheless, with each new sensation, she worried that something was wrong.

At 37 weeks' gestation, she began having contractions. She telephoned her physician immediately and went to the hospital.

On admission to labor and delivery, she was quiet and reserved. She told the nurse that her contractions had begun 2 hours earlier. Her husband drove a delivery truck, and the company was trying to contact him to meet her at the hospital. She had tried to telephone her mother but was unable to reach her at home. The nurse also learned that Mr. and Mrs. C had not attended childbirth-preparation classes. According to Mrs.

C, "My husband's schedule is very unpredictable, and I couldn't go alone. Besides, most of the time I didn't have the energy to do much of anything."

The nurse's assessment revealed:
- Blood pressure 144/86, pulse 88, respirations 20
- Fetal heart tones, 124 in right lower quadrant (RLQ) and 136 in right upper quadrant (RUQ)
- Contractions every 10 minutes, lasting 20 seconds, and of mild intensity
- Cervix 80% effaced and 4 cm dilated
- Fetus A presented vertex, at 0 station; fetus B also was vertex

5. What factors should the nurse consider as contributing to Mrs. C's anxiety level?
   a. Her lack of attendance at childbirth preparation classes
   b. Multiple gestation
   c. Maternal age
   d. Inadequate support system
      (1) a, c
      (2) a, b, d
      (3) a, c, d
      (4) All of the above

6. What should the nurse do first to minimize Mrs. C's anxiety?
   a. Notify the physician, and obtain an order for medication.
   b. Instruct her in childbirth-preparation information.
   c. Permit her to listen to the fetal hearts, and reassure her that the fetuses are doing well.
   d. Remain with her.

7. What is the significance of fetus A's station?
   a. Suggestive of pelvic adequacy
   b. Indicative of malpresentation
   c. Suggestive of a short labor
   d. Indicative of the need to prepare for cesarean delivery

8. What actions can the nurse take to increase the likelihood of a vaginal delivery?

a. Encourage Mrs. C to walk around during the early stage of labor.
b. When Mrs. C is in bed, keep the head of the bed slightly elevated.
c. Assist Mrs. C in assuming upright positions.
d. Assist Mrs. C with relaxation breathing techniques.
(1) a, c
(2) b, c, d
(3) b, d
(4) All of the above

9. At the outset of her labor, what information would best assist Mrs. C in coping adaptively?
a. An explanation of the procedures she should expect
b. A discussion of the anatomy and physiology of labor
c. A description of the institution's policies about support persons' attendance at cesarean birth
d. Instruction in relaxation techniques
(1) a, c
(2) a, b, d
(3) a, c, d
(4) All of the above

MULTIGRAVIDA, ACTIVE LABOR

Mrs. A is a 34-year-old, 41-week-gestation, gravida 3, para 2 (G3, P2) who arrived in labor and delivery on Friday at 10:20 AM. She states that when she awoke she noticed some pelvic heaviness, but that she ignored it as she got her 9-year-old and 6-year-old children off to school. Once the house was quiet, she became aware that she was contracting regularly, though she describes the contractions as mild and cramplike. Because her previous labors were quick (first pregnancy, 11 hours; second pregnancy, 4 hours), she went right to the hospital without notifying her physician or husband: "The last time, it was over almost before it had begun." Throughout the admission process, she remained calm. When the nurse was finished, she remarked, "Well, I guess I should call my husband if I expect him to get here in time."

Admission assessment includes:
■ Maternal vital signs within normal limits
■ Fetal heart tones 148 RLQ
■ Contractions every 5 to 6 minutes, 30 to 45 seconds, and of mild-to-moderate intensity
■ Cervix 70% effaced and 2 cm dilated
■ Fetal position in right occipitoposterior (ROP), at a –1 station

10. What additional findings would reassure the nurse that Mrs. A was in true labor?
a. The presence of a bloody show
b. Bulging membranes
c. A progressive increase in the length of time between contractions
d. A progressive increase in the duration of the contractions
(1) a, c
(2) a, c, d
(3) a, b, d
(4) All of the above

11. What is the significance of the baby's station and position?
a. Of little significance at this time
b. Suggestive of cephalopelvic disproportion
c. Suggestive of a prolonged labor
d. Indicative of the need to prepare for cesarean delivery

12. What additional assessments would be helpful to the nurse in planning care for the family?
a. The gestational age and birth weight of Mrs. A's previous deliveries
b. The time and amount of Mrs. A's last oral intake

c. Mrs. A's preparation for this birth experience
d. Mrs. A's expectations about pain management
    (1) a, c
    (2) a, b, d
    (3) a, c, d
    (4) All of the above

13. Which cardinal movement is most affected when a baby is occipitoposterior?
    a. Flexion
    b. Internal rotation
    c. Extension
    d. External rotation

14. Which factors may contribute to the baby's presenting occiput posterior?
    a. Maternal pelvic shape
    b. Maternal age
    c. Fetal size
    d. Postmaturity
    (1) a, c
    (2) b, c, d
    (3) b, d
    (4) All of the above

ADDITIONAL STUDY QUESTIONS

15. Which of the following are characteristic of the powers of the first stage of labor?
    a. Controlled by the involuntary nervous system
    b. Responsible for cervical efface-ment and dilatation
    c. Responsive to nursing inter-ventions
    d. Quantified by calculating fre-quency times intensity
    (1) a, c
    (2) a, b, d
    (3) a, c, d
    (4) All of the above

16. True or false: women should be encouraged to go through labor in an upright position because this is the most facilitative posture for childbirth.

17. Which of the following describe the delivery of a macrosomic baby?
    a. The infant is at increased risk of birth trauma.
    b. Prolonged labor is likely.
    c. The mother is at increased risk of birth trauma.
    d. Postpartum hemorrhage is likely.
    (1) a, c
    (2) a, b, d

    (3) a, c, d
    (4) All of the above

18. Which of the following are characteristic of the anxiety and fear experienced during labor?
    a. Results in an elevated blood pressure and pulse rate
    b. Results in an improved ability to concentrate
    c. Results in increased pain perception
    d. May prolong labor
    (1) a, c
    (2) a, b, d
    (3) a, c, d
    (4) All of the above

19. Which of the following nursing interventions are indicated to reduce sensory overload?
    a. Keep the room's lighting sub-dued.
    b. Speak quietly and calmly to the client and her support person.
    c. Provide music in the room.
    d. Avoid doing a procedure dur-ing a contraction.
    (1) a, c
    (2) a, b, d
    (3) a, c, d
    (4) All of the above

ANSWERS TO STUDY QUESTIONS

1. c	6. d	11. c	16. True
2. b	7. a	12. 3	17. 4
3. a	8. 4	13. b	18. 3
4. d	9. 2	14. 1	19. 2
5. 2	10. 3	15. 4	

REFERENCES

Anderson, C. (1976). Operational definition of "support." *Journal of Obstetric, Gynecologic, and Neonatal Nursing, 5*(1), 17-18.

Angelini, D. (1978). Body boundaries: Concerns of laboring women. *Maternal-Child Nursing Journal, 7*(1), 41-46.

Bates, B., & Turner, A.N. (1985). Imagery and symbolism in the birth practices of traditional cultures. *Birth, 12*(1), 29-35.

Biancuzzo, M. (1993). Six myths of maternal posture during labor. *MCN The American Journal of Maternal Child Nursing, 18*(5), 264-269.

Block, C., & Block, R. (1975). The effect of support of the husband and obstetrician on pain perception and control in childbirth. *Birth and the Family Journal, 2*(2), 43-47.

Browning, C.A. (2000). Using music during childbirth. *Birth, 27*(4), 272-276.

Callister, L.C. (1995). Cultural meanings of childbirth. *Journal of Obstetric, Gynecologic, and Neonatal Nursing, 24*(4), 327-331.

Chiota, B.J., Goolkasian, P., & Ladewig, P. (1976). Effects of separation from spouse on pregnancy, labor and delivery, and the postpartum period. *Journal of Obstetric, Gynecologic, and Neonatal Nursing, 5*(1), 21-23.

Clark, A. (1978). *Culture, childbearing, health professionals.* Philadelphia: F. A. Davis.

Clark, A., & Affonso, D. (Eds.). (1979). *Childbearing: A nursing perspective* (2nd ed.). Philadelphia: Davis.

Coleman, A., & Coleman, L. (1978). *Pregnancy: The psychological experience* (2nd ed.). New York: Bantam.

Cunningham, F., Gant, N., Leveno, K., Gilstrap, L., Hauth, J., & Wenstrom, K. (2001). *Williams obstetrics* (21st ed.). New York: McGraw-Hill.

Dunn, P., & Feinberg, R. (1996). Oncofetal fibronectin: new insight into the physiology of implantation and labor. *Journal of Obstetric, Gynecologic, and Neonatal Nursing, 25*(9), 753-757.

Fenwick, L., & Simkin, P. (1987). Maternal positioning to prevent or alleviate dystocia in labor. *Clinical Obstetrics and Gynecology, 30*(1), 83-89.

Friedman, E.A. (1978). *Labor: Clinical evaluation and management* (2nd ed.). New York: Appleton-Century-Crofts.

Gagnon, A., & Waghorn, K. (1999). One-to-one nurse labor support of nulliparous women stimulated with oxytocin. *Journal of Obstetric, Gynecologic, and Neonatal Nursing, 28*(4), 371-376.

Gagnon, A., Waghorn, K., & Covell, C. (1997). A randomized trial of one-to-one nurse support of women in labor. *Birth, 24*(2), 71-80.

Gale, J., Fothergill-Bourbonnais, F., & Chamberlain, M. (2001). Measuring nursing support during childbirth. *MCN The American Journal of Maternal Child Nursing, 26*(5), 264-271.

Gay, J. (1978). Theories regarding endocrine contributions to the onset of labor. *Journal of Obstetric, Gynecologic, and Neonatal Nursing, 7*(5), 42-47.

Gilder, K., Mayberry, L.J., Gennaro, S., & Clemmens, D. (2002). Maternal positioning in labor with epidural analgesia—Results from a multi-site survey. *AWHONN Lifelines, 6*(1), 40-45.

Gilliland, A.L. (2002). Beyond holding hands: The modern role of the professional doula. *Journal of Obstetric, Gynecologic, and Neonatal Nursing, 31*(6), 762-769.

Golay, J., Vedam, S., & Sorger, L. (1993). The squatting position for the second stage of labor: Effects on labor and on maternal and fetal well-being. *Birth, 20*(2), 73-78.

Harris, C.J. (1985). Rheumatoid arthritis and the pregnant woman. *American Journal of Nursing, 85*(4), 414-417.

Hodnett, E. (1996). Nursing support of the laboring woman. *Journal of Obstetric, Gynecologic, and Neonatal Nursing, 25*(3), 257-264.

Horn, M., & Manion, J. (1985). Creative grandparenting: Bonding the generations. *Journal of Obstetric, Gynecologic, and Neonatal Nursing, 14*(3), 233-236.

Jordan, B. (1978). The hut and the hospital: Information, power, and symbolism in the artifacts of birth. *Birth, 14*(1), 36-40.

Kennell, J., Klaus, M., McGrath, S., Robertson, S., & Hinckley, C. (1991). Continuous emotional support during labor in a U.S. hospital: A randomized controlled trial. *Journal of the American Medical Association, 265*(17), 2197-2201.

Lehrman, E. (1985). Birth in the left lateral position: An alternative to the traditional delivery position. *Journal of Nurse-Midwifery, 30*(4), 193-197.

Liu, Y.C. (1989). The effects of the upright position during childbirth. *Image, 21*(1), 14-18.

Lowdermilk, D.L., & Perry, S.E. (2004). *Maternity & women's health care* (8th ed.). St. Louis: Mosby.

Lydon-Rochelle, M., Albers, L., Gurwoda, J., Craig, E., & Qualls, C. (1993). Accuracy of Leopold maneuvers in screening for malpresentation: A prospective study. *Birth, 20*(3), 132-135.

Mackey, M.C., & Lock, S.E. (1989). Women's expectations of the labor and delivery nurse. *Journal of Obstetric, Gynecologic, and Neonatal Nursing, 18*(6), 505-512.

MacMillen, N., Brucker, M., & Zwelling, E. (1997). High-risk childbirth. In F. Nichols & E. Zwelling (Eds.), *Maternal-newborn nursing* (pp. 862-931). Philadelphia: Saunders.

Manogin, T.W., Bechtel, G.A., & Rami, J.S. (2000). Caring behaviors by nurses: Women's perceptions during childbirth. *Journal of Obstetric, Gynecologic, and Neonatal Nursing, 29*(2), 153-157.

Mayberry, L.J., Strange, L.B., Suplee, P.D., & Gennaro, S. (2003). Use of upright positioning with epidural analgesia—findings from an observational study. *MCN The American Journal of Maternal Child Nursing, 28*(3), 152-159.

Mayberry, L.J., Wood, S.H., Strange, L.B., Lee, L., Heisler, D.R., & Neilsen-Smith, K. (2000). Managing second-stage labor—exploring the variables during the second stage. *AWHONN Lifelines, 3*(6), 28-34.

McKay, S. (1984). Squatting: An alternative position for the second stage of labor. *MCN The American Journal of Maternal Child Nursing, 9*(3), 181-183.

McKay, S., & Barrows, T. (1991). Holding back: Maternal readiness to give birth. *MCN The American Journal of Maternal Child Nursing, 16*(5), 251-254.

McKay, S., & Mahan, C. (1980). Laboring patients need more freedom to move. *Contemporary Obstetrics and Gynecology, 18*(7), 90-116.

Meissner, J.E. (1980). Predicting a patient's anxiety level during labor: A two-part assessment tool. *Nursing '80, 10*(7), 50-51.

Meleis, A., & Sorrell, L. (1981). Arab-American women and their birth experience. *MCN The American Journal of Maternal Child Nursing, 6*(5), 171-176.

Melender, H. (2002). Experiences of fears associated with pregnancy and childbirth: A study of 329 pregnant women. *Birth, 29*(2), 101-111.

Miltner, R.S. (2000). Identifying labor support actions of intrapartum nurses. *Journal of Obstetric, Gynecologic, and Neonatal Nursing, 29*(5), 491-499.

Miltner, R.S. (2002). More than support: nursing interventions provided to women in labor. *Journal of Obstetric, Gynecologic, and Neonatal Nursing, 31*(6), 753-761.

Nichols, F., & Zwelling, E. (Eds.). (1997). *Maternal-newborn nursing.* Philadelphia: Saunders.

Noller, K.L., Resseguie, L.J., & Voss, V. (1996). The effect of changes in atmospheric pressure on the occurrence of the spontaneous onset of labor in term pregnancies. *American Journal of Obstetrics and Gynecology, 174*(4), 1192-1197.

Olds, S., London, M., & Ladewig, P. (1999). *Maternal-newborn nursing—a family and community-centered approach* (6th ed.). Princeton: Prentice-Hall.

Oxorn, H. (1986). *Human labor and birth* (5th ed.). New York: Appleton-Century-Crofts.

Paciornik, M. (1990). Commentary: Arguments against episiotomy and in favor of squatting for birth. *Birth, 17*(2), 104-105.

Perez, P.G., & Herrick, L.M. (1998). Doulas: Exploring their roles with parents, hospitals, and nurses. *AWHONN Lifelines, 2*(2), 54-55.

Peter, E. (2000). Commentary: Ethical conflicts or political problems in intrapartum nursing care? *Birth, 27*(1), 46-48.

Pillitteri, A. (1998). *Maternal-newborn nursing: Care of the growing family* (3rd ed.). Boston: Little, Brown.

Regalia, A.L., Curiel, P., Natale, N., Galluzzi, A., Spinelli, G., Chezzi, G., et al. (2000). Routine use of external cephalic version in three hospitals. *Birth, 27*(1), 19-24.

Roberts, J. (1980). Alternative positions for childbirth. Part I: First stage of labor. *Journal of Nurse-Midwifery, 25*(4), 11-18.

Roberts, J. (1980). Alternative positions for childbirth. Part II: Second stage of labor. *Journal of Nurse-Midwifery, 25*(5), 13-19.

Roberts, J., & Van Lier, D. (1984, Spring). Debate: Which position for the second stage? *Childbirth Educator, lll*, 33-38.

Roberts, J., & Woolley, D. (1996). A second look at the second stage of labor. *Journal of Obstetric, Gynecologic, and Neonatal Nursing, 25*(5), 415-423.

Roberts, J.E., Goldstein, S.A., Gruener, J.S., Maggio, M., & Mendez-Bauer, C. (1987). A descriptive analysis of involuntary bearing-down efforts during the expulsive phase of labor. *Journal of Obstetric, Gynecologic, and Neonatal Nursing, 16*(1), 48-55.

Romond, J., & Baker, I. (1985). Squatting in childbirth. *Journal of Obstetric, Gynecologic, and Neonatal Nursing, 14*(5), 406-411.

Sauls, D.J. (2002). Effects of labor support on mothers, babies, and birth outcomes. *Journal of Obstetrics, Gynecologic, and Neonatal Nursing, 31*(6), 733-741.

Shermer, R.H., & Raines, D.A. (1997). Positioning during the second stage of labor: Moving back to basics. *Journal of Obstetric, Gynecologic, and Neonatal Nursing, 26*(6), 727-734.

Shorten, A., Donsante, J., & Shorten, B. (2002). Birth position, accoucheur, and perineal outcomes: Informing women about choices for vaginal birth. *Birth, 29*(1), 18-27.

Simkin, P. (1995). Reducing pain and enhancing progress in labor: A guide to non-pharmacologic methods for maternity caregivers. *Birth, 22*(3), 161-171.

Simkin, P. (2002). Supportive care during labor: A guide for busy nurses. *Journal of Obstetrics, Gynecologic, and Neonatal Nursing, 31*(6), 721-732.

Sleutel, M.R. (2000). Intrapartum nursing care: A case study of supportive interventions and ethical conflicts. *Birth, 27*(1), 38-45.

Smith, C., Crowther, C., Wilkinson, C., Pridmore, B., & Robinson, J. (1999). Knee-chest postural management for breech at term: A randomized controlled trial. *Birth, 26*(2), 71-75.

Stern, E.W., Glazer, G.L., & Sanduleak, N. (1988). Influence of the full and new moon on onset of labor and spontaneous rupture of membranes. *Journal of Nurse-Midwifery, 33*(2), 57-61.

Trainor, C. (2002). Valuing labor support—A doula's perspective. *AWHONN Lifelines, 6*(5), 387-389.

Tumblin, A., & Simkin, P. (2001). Pregnant women's perceptions of their nurse's role during labor and delivery. *Birth, 28*(1), 52-56.

VandeVusse, L. (1999). The essential forces of labor revisited: 15 Ps reported in women's stories. *MCN The American Journal of Maternal Child Nursing, 24*(4), 176-184.

Winslow, W. (1987). First pregnancy after 35: What's the experience? *MCN The American Journal of Maternal Child Nursing, 12*(2), 92-96.

Zhang, J., Bernasko, J.W., Leybovich, E., Fahs, M., & Hatch, M.C. (1996). Continuous labor support from labor attendant for primiparous women: A meta-analysis. *Obstetrics and Gynecology, 88*(4, Pt 2), 739-744.

11 Normal Childbirth

KATHLEEN V. SMITH

OBJECTIVES

1. Determine the potential for alteration in health status during the intrapartum period.
2. Recognize the signs and symptoms of labor.
3. Identify phases of the first stage of labor.
4. Describe the normal physiologic changes occurring in all four stages of labor.
5. Discuss methods of pain relief used during labor.
6. Use nursing interventions that reflect knowledge of standards of care.
7. Accurately record documentation of nursing care.
8. Identify variables that may alter the course of labor and delivery.
9. Modify the nursing plan of care to changes in client status.
10. Recognize the variables that influence the normal progress of labor.
11. Practice the concept of family-centered care during the intrapartum period.

INTRODUCTION

A. **The intrapartum period of pregnancy or labor begins with the first stage's uterine contractions and the progressive dilatation of the cervix.**
B. **From complete dilatation of the cervix to the infant's delivery is the second stage of labor.**
C. **The third stage of labor is completed with the expulsion of the placenta and membranes.**
D. **The fourth stage of labor is the first hour postpartum.**

CLINICAL PRACTICE

Premonitory Signs

A. **Assessment**
   1. History
      a. Lightening
         (1) On the average, lightening occurs 10 days before onset of labor in a primigravida.
         (2) Increased pressure of presenting part leads to:
            (a) Urinary frequency
            (b) Backache and leg pain
            (c) Increased vaginal discharge
            (d) Dependent edema
         (3) Lightening results in easier respirations
      b. Increased vaginal discharge
      c. Braxton Hicks contractions

           (1) Called false labor.
           (2) Walking lessens discomfort.
           (3) Is usually irregular.
           (4) No progressive shortening of interval between contractions
      d. Show
           (1) Late sign: occurs after the beginning of cervical changes and increased pressure of presenting part.
           (2) Blood-tinged cervical mucus
      e. Spontaneous rupture of amniotic sac: leakage of clear or cloudy amniotic fluid
      f. Burst of energy: often 24 to 48 hours before labor onset
      g. Gastrointestinal (GI) symptoms
           (1) Diarrhea
           (2) Indigestion
           (3) Nausea and vomiting
      h. Sleep disturbances
           (1) Change in sleep pattern
           (2) Restlessness
  2. Physical findings
      a. Lightening
           (1) The uterus and presenting part descend into pelvis.
           (2) Occurrence is determined by abdominal and pelvic examination.
      b. Braxton Hicks contractions
           (1) Movement of the cervix from a posterior position to an anterior position
           (2) Prime, or soften, cervix.
      c. Cervical changes
           (1) Ripening and softening of cervix resulting from hormonal changes
           (2) Effacement: thinning of the cervix
           (3) Dilatation: opening of the cervix
      d. Spontaneous rupture of the amniotic sac
           (1) Barrier to infection is gone.
           (2) There is danger of cord prolapse.
      e. Burst of energy: increased epinephrine release caused by decreased progesterone release
      f. Weight loss: client may experience a 0.9- to 1.36-kg (2- to 3-lb) weight loss 24 to 48 hours before onset of labor.
      g. Increased vaginal discharge
  3. Psychosocial: burst of energy may result in nesting urge
  4. Diagnostic procedures
      a. Spontaneous rupture of amniotic sac
           (1) Visible pooling of fluid is observed.
           (2) pH is tested with Nitrazine.
           (3) Sterile speculum examination is performed to obtain specimen for microscopic ferning pattern.
      b. Vaginal examination for cervical status
B. Nursing Diagnoses
  1. Anxiety related to uncertainty about onset of labor and ability to cope
  2. Fear of pain related to impending labor
  3. Risk for infection related to spontaneous rupture of membranes (SROM)
C. Interventions/Outcomes
  1. Anxiety related to uncertainty about onset of labor and ability to cope

      a. Interventions
        (1) Listen attentively to concerns.
        (2) Allow verbalization of feelings.
        (3) Provide information and support.
        (4) Reinforce prenatal education.
        (5) Provide an awareness of changes as labor begins.
        (6) Give clear, concise explanations, and repeat as necessary.
        (7) Use anxiety-reduction techniques.
          (a) Relaxation techniques
          (b) Guided imagery
        (8) Provide for the presence of a support person.
      b. Outcomes
        (1) Client's anxiety is reduced.
          (a) Relaxation techniques are demonstrated.
          (b) Early signs of labor are verbalized.
        (2) Client attended prenatal classes.
  2. Fear of pain related to impending labor
    a. Interventions
      (1) Encourage prenatal preparation for active labor participation.
      (2) Review and demonstrate relaxation techniques.
      (3) Discuss pain-relief methods.
      (4) Explain all nursing activities.
      (5) Answer questions presented.
    b. Outcomes
      (1) Client verbalizes her fears.
      (2) Client attended childbirth education classes.
      (3) Client discusses the methods of pain relief available during labor.
  3. Risk for infection related to SROM
    a. Interventions
      (1) Instruct the client and her family to notify medical personnel immediately after SROM.
      (2) Instruct the client to refrain from sexual intercourse after SROM (if client is at home).
      (3) Monitor the client's temperature every 2 hours for elevation.
      (4) Observe for foul-smelling vaginal discharge or amniotic fluid.
      (5) Educate the client about the need for perineal cleanliness.
        (a) Hand washing after voiding or defecation
        (b) Cleansing of perineal area from front to back
    b. Outcomes
      (1) Prompt medical notification occurs after SROM.
      (2) Temperature remains within normal limits.
      (3) Client washes hands and cleans perineum correctly.

First Stage of Labor: Dilatation

A. Assessment
  1. Physiologic changes during first stage of labor
    a. Cardiovascular changes
      (1) Cardiac output increases.
      (2) Slight pulse changes: may increase to more than 100 beats per minute as a result of exhaustion or dehydration.

    (3) Blood pressure (BP) changes very little.
     (a) Increases are noted if monitored during a contraction.
     (b) Hypotension may occur: vena caval syndrome or supine hypotension resulting from pressure of pregnant uterus on inferior vena cava.
    (4) White blood cell (WBC) count increases up to 20,000/mm^3 with strenuous labor.
  b. GI changes
    (1) Motility and absorption are decreased.
    (2) Gastric emptying time is decreased.
    (3) Nausea and vomiting are common.
    (4) Dry lips and mouth occur, resulting from mouth breathing.
  c. Renal changes
    (1) The tendency to concentrate urine results in specific gravity above 1.025.
    (2) Pressure of full bladder is felt.
     (a) Increased discomfort
     (b) Impedes labor and fetal descent
    (3) Pressure of presenting part on urethra may require catheterization to empty the urinary bladder.
    (4) Proteinuria
     (a) Caused by increased metabolic activity
     (b) May be sign of pregnancy-induced hypertension (PIH)
  d. Respiratory changes
    (1) Exhalation of more CO_2
    (2) Hyperventilation
     (a) Tingling and numbness of hands and feet
     (b) Dizziness
 2. Phases of labor
  a. Latent phase
    (1) Admission history
     (a) Identification of client
      (i) Date and time of arrival
      (ii) Reason for admission
      (iii) Time physician notified and time seen
      (iv) Last food intake
     (b) Prenatal history (prenatal record)
      (i) Estimated date of confinement (EDC)
      (ii) Pregnancies, births, abortions, and living children
      (iii) Allergies
      (iv) Medications taken during pregnancy
       ■ Time and amount of last dose
       ■ Frequency of use during pregnancy
      (v) Chronic conditions and medical-surgical history
      (vi) Illness during pregnancy, recent exposures, present infections
      (vii) Results of laboratory work done during pregnancy (see Chapters 5 and 8 for discussion and interpretation of pregnancy laboratory tests)
       ■ Complete blood count (CBC) and hemoglobin and hematocrit (H&H)
       ■ Blood type and Rh factor
       ■ Urinalysis

- Venereal disease research laboratory (VDRL) and serologic testing
- Gonorrhea culture (GC)
- Chlamydia culture
- Rubella titer
- Papanicolaou's stain test

(viii) Special tests
- Glucose screen
- Sickle cell screen
- Ultrasonography
- Chorionic villi sampling (CVS), amniocentesis, percutaneous umbilical blood sampling (PUBS)
- Genetic studies
- Lecithin/sphingomyelin (L/S) ratio, phosphatidylglycerol (PG)
- Maternal serum alpha-fetoprotein (msAFP)
- Human immunodeficiency virus (HIV) titer
- Hepatitis B surface antigen (HbsAg) titer for hepatitis screening
- Rh antibody screen
- Nonstress test (NST), oxytocin challenge test (OCT), or contraction stress test (CST)
- Biophysical profile (BPR)

(ix) Childbirth preparation
- Birth plan
- Support system
- Previous experience
- Cultural influences
- Coping skills

(2) Physical findings
  (a) Vital signs: BP, temperature, pulse, respirations, fetal heart rate (FHR), and fetal activity
  (b) Contraction status
    (i) Onset of contractions
    (ii) Present contraction status
- Frequency of contractions; contractions may be irregular and may occur every 5 to 10 minutes.
- Duration: 30 to 45 seconds
- Contraction strength
  — Mild by palpation
  — 25 to 40 mmHg by intrauterine pressure catheter (IUPC)

  (c) Vaginal examination if no abnormal vaginal bleeding
    (i) Cervix location (posterior, moving to anterior)
    (ii) Dilatation: 0 to 3 cm
    (iii) Effacement: 0% to 40%
    (iv) Fetal presentation, position, and station
    (v) Status of membranes
  (d) Vaginal discharge
    (i) Amniotic fluid
- Time of rupture
- Color, amount, and odor
- Consistency

                 (ii) Bloody show
                        ■ Characteristics
                        ■ Amount
             (e) Abdominal examination
                 (i) Fundal height
                 (ii) Leopold's maneuvers to determine fetal position and lie
                 (iii) Scars, ridges, or masses
             (f) Chest examination: heart and lung sounds
             (g) Deep tendon reflexes
                 (i) Patellar or brachial
                 (ii) Clonus
        (3) Psychosocial
             (a) Emotional status
                 (i) Confident, low anxiety level
                 (ii) Excited, talkative
                 (iii) Anticipatory, apprehensive
             (b) Support systems
             (c) Fears and concerns
             (d) Nonverbal clues (restlessness, muscle tension, frowning)
        (4) Diagnostic procedures
             (a) Urine screen
                 (i) Specific gravity
                 (ii) Protein
                 (iii) Glucose
             (b) Routine blood screen
                 (i) CBC (especially H&H)
                 (ii) Serologic testing
                 (iii) Blood type and Rh factor
   b. Active phase
        (1) Physical findings
             (a) Contraction pattern evaluated (by electronic fetal monitoring
                  [EFM] or by palpation) every 30 minutes
                 (i) Frequency: every 2 to 5 minutes
                 (ii) Duration: 45 to 60 seconds
                 (iii) Intensity
                        ■ Moderate to strong by palpation
                        ■ 50 to 70 mmHg by IUPC
             (b) Vaginal examination
                 (i) Dilatation: 4 to 7 cm
                 (ii) Effacement: 40% to 80%
                 (iii) Station: −2 to 0
                 (iv) Presenting part and position
                 (v) Status of membranes
                        ■ Intact
                        ■ If ruptured
                          — Color
                          — Consistency
                          — Odor
                 (vi) Progression of labor: suggested dilatation rate
                        ■ 1.2 cm/hr for primipara
                        ■ 1.5 cm/hr for multipara
                 (vii) Cervix location: anterior

(c) Intake and output (I&O)
   (i) Hydration status
      ■ Last oral intake
      ■ Intravenous (IV) fluid intake monitored
   (ii) Edema
   (iii) Nausea and vomiting
(2) Psychosocial findings
   (a) Absorbed in serious work of labor
   (b) Intense and quieter
   (c) Increased dependency
   (d) Wavering self-confidence
c. Transition phase
   (1) History
      (a) Childbirth preparation is important.
      (b) Time for relaxation between contractions decreases.
   (2) Physical findings
      (a) Dilatation: 8 to 10 cm
      (b) Effacement: 80% to 100%
      (c) Station: −1 to +1
      (d) Contractions
         (i) Frequency: every 2 to 3 minutes
         (ii) Duration: 60 to 90 seconds
         (iii) Intensity
            ■ Strong by palpation
            ■ 70 to 90 mmHg by IUPC
      (e) Strong urge to push if station is low
      (f) Backache
      (g) Nausea and vomiting
      (h) Trembling limbs
      (i) Vaginal discharge: bloody show increases.
      (j) I&O
         (i) Monitor oral and IV intake.
         (ii) Frequent bladder emptying is important to allow descent of fetus.
   (3) Psychosocial findings
      (a) Supportive needs increase, but client is agitated and irritable.
      (b) Client is increasingly discouraged because of fatigue and may want to give up.
      (c) Client's coping ability decreases because she feels overwhelmed.
      (d) Client relaxation is almost impossible.
3. Analgesia or anesthesia for first stage of labor
   a. Goal: change perception through:
      (1) Relaxation to decrease tension
      (2) Medication to increase pain threshold
   b. Pain receptors are stimulated by uterine contractions that result in:
      (1) Myometrial anoxia
      (2) Cervical stretching or dilatation
      (3) Distension of lower uterine segment
      (4) Pressure on pelvic nerves
      (5) Traction on supporting and nearby structures
      (6) Distension of pelvic floor

    c. Pain perception is affected by:
      (1) Experience
      (2) Cultural expectations
      (3) Psychosexual development
      (4) Fatigue, anemia
      (5) Fear, anxiety, and emotional stress
      (6) Environment
      (7) Support system
      (8) Pain anticipation
    d. Medications
      (1) Barbiturates (phenobarbital [Nembutal], secobarbital [Seconal]):
        (a) Provide sedation or sleep.
        (b) Reduce tension and fear.
        (c) Are used for rest.
      (2) Tranquilizers (hydroxyzine [Vistaril], promethazine [Phenergan]):
        (a) Are antianxiety agents.
        (b) Provide muscle relaxation.
        (c) Have antiemetic properties.
        (d) May potentiate narcotics.
      (3) Narcotics (meperidine [Demerol], morphine, butorphanol [Stadol], nalbuphine [Nubain], fentanyl [Sublimaze], sufentanil):
        (a) Increase pain threshold: client's ability to tolerate or cope with discomfort increases.
        (b) May increase or decrease uterine activity.
        (c) May cause drowsiness.
        (d) Have narcotic antagonist available.
    e. Regional anesthesia
      (1) Paracervical block (Note: this anesthesia is rarely used anymore and is described here only for historic purposes.)
        (a) Local anesthesia is injected transvaginally lateral to cervix at dilatation of 4 to 6 cm.
        (b) Lower uterine segment, cervix, and upper vagina are affected.
        (c) Effect on fetus is transient bradycardia.
      (2) Epidural or caudal
        (a) Local anesthesia is injected into epidural or caudal space.
        (b) Nerves leaving the spinal cord are blocked.
        (c) Entire pelvis and lower extremities are affected so that the client perceives touch but not pain.
        (d) Fetal effect: uterine blood flow is decreased if maternal hypotension occurs, leading to potential fetal distress.
      (3) Intrathecal narcotic
        (a) Narcotic injected into subarachnoid space
        (b) Given at approximately 5 cm of dilatation
        (c) Provides pain relief; able to maintain mobility and sensation.
        (d) Side effects: pruritus, nausea and vomiting, and urinary retention
    f. Nonpharmacologic methods
      (1) Transcutaneous electrical nerve stimulation (TENS)
        (a) Electrodes are placed on either side of client's lower spine.
        (b) Client provides electrical stimulation during contractions.
        (c) TENS provides alternate sensation to decrease perception of pain from contractions.

      (2) Touch
        (a) Acupressure: increases endorphin release and reduces sensation.
        (b) Cutaneous stimulation: effleurage provides an alternative sensation.
        (c) Massage and counterpressure
        (d) Hot or cold application
        (e) Therapeutic touch
      (3) Relaxation techniques
        (a) Biofeedback
        (b) Visual imagery
        (c) Controlled breathing patterns
        (d) Shower or Jacuzzi
        (e) Movement, position changes, and ambulation

B. Nursing Diagnoses
1. Risk for ineffective maternal tissue perfusion related to position in labor
2. Impaired urinary elimination related to progression of labor
3. Anxiety related to labor and birth
4. Fatigue related to prolonged labor
5. Fear related to discomfort of labor
6. Ineffective individual coping related to progress of labor
7. Pain related to uterine contractions and cervical dilatation
8. Risk for deficient fluid volume related to decreased intake or abnormal loss
9. Risk for infection related to vaginal examinations following SROM

C. Interventions/Outcomes
1. Risk for ineffective maternal tissue perfusion related to position in labor
  a. Interventions
    (1) Discourage supine position to prevent supine hypotension or vena caval syndrome.
    (2) Assess BP between contractions for an accurate reading.
    (3) Encourage frequent position changes.
  b. Outcomes
    (1) Vital signs and FHR remain stable.
    (2) No supine hypotension occurs.
2. Impaired urinary elimination related to progression of labor
  a. Interventions
    (1) Maintain an accurate I&O record.
    (2) Encourage adequate intake of oral fluids.
    (3) Monitor IV fluid intake.
    (4) Encourage bladder elimination every 2 hours.
  b. Outcomes
    (1) I&O is balanced.
    (2) Bladder is emptied regularly.
    (3) Bladder is not palpable.
3. Anxiety related to labor and birth
  a. Interventions
    (1) Orient the client to her environment.
    (2) Call the client by her name.
    (3) Encourage verbalization of feelings.
    (4) Listen attentively.
    (5) Provide information about routine procedures.
    (6) Monitor vital signs and labor status, and keep the client and her family informed.

(7) Encourage participation of support system.
(8) Encourage relaxation techniques.
(9) Respect the client's privacy.
   b. Outcomes
      (1) Client identifies stressors.
      (2) Client remains in control and relaxed.
      (3) Support system is stable and present.
   4. Fatigue related to prolonged labor
      a. Interventions
         (1) Encourage rest in latent phase and promote relaxation.
         (2) Encourage rest between contractions in active phase and transition.
         (3) Minimize environmental stimuli.
         (4) Offer comfort measures.
         (5) Offer and explain analgesia or anesthesia, if indicated and desired.
      b. Outcomes
         (1) Client rests and relaxes.
         (2) Client accepts analgesia or anesthesia.
         (3) No adverse effects of medication occur in mother or fetus.
   5. Fear related to discomfort of labor
      a. Interventions
         (1) Offer anticipatory guidance.
         (2) Orient the client to her surroundings.
         (3) Give clear explanations of what is to come (the labor process and possible interventions).
         (4) Maintain support system.
         (5) Allow and encourage verbalization of source of fear.
      b. Outcomes
         (1) Confidence and control are exhibited.
         (2) Support system is strong.
   6. Ineffective individual coping related to progress of labor
      a. Interventions
         (1) Encourage expression of feelings.
         (2) Reinforce previously learned coping methods.
         (3) Maintain and assist support system.
         (4) Present new methods of coping with the situation.
         (5) Provide comfort measures.
      b. Outcomes
         (1) Client communicates feelings about situation.
         (2) Client's confidence is restored.
         (3) Client uses learned coping skills.
   7. Pain related to uterine contractions and cervical dilatation
      a. Interventions
         (1) Document uterine activity and labor progress.
         (2) Provide comfort measures.
            (a) Encourage breathing and relaxation techniques.
            (b) Encourage bladder emptying.
            (c) Encourage frequent position changes.
            (d) Provide back rubs.
         (3) Use nonpharmacologic measures of pain relief.
         (4) Administer analgesia as ordered.
         (5) Assist with anesthesia as needed.
            (a) Monitor vitals according to standard of care.
            (b) Monitor IV fluid intake per anesthesia protocol.

  b. Outcomes
  (1) Discomfort is decreased.
  (2) No adverse side effects are observed from analgesia or anesthesia in mother or infant.
 8. Risk for deficient fluid volume related to decreased intake or abnormal loss
  a. Interventions
  (1) Monitor hydration status.
  (2) Monitor vital signs for deviations from normal.
   (a) Monitor BP, pulse, and respirations every 30 to 60 minutes.
   (b) Signs may indicate bleeding (e.g., elevated pulse, decreased BP).
   (c) Monitor temperature every 4 hours (every 2 hours after rupture of membranes [ROM]) for elevation, which may indicate dehydration.
  (3) Monitor FHR for signs of distress caused by decreased uteroplacental perfusion (see Chapter 12 for further discussion of fetal assessment in labor).
   (a) May be done continuously with EFM.
   (b) Monitor every 15 minutes if no EFM.
  (4) Monitor I&O.
   (a) Encourage voiding every 2 hours.
   (b) Test urine for specific gravity (normal is 1.010 to 1.025).
   (c) Administer oral or IV fluids as indicated.
  (5) Observe for obvious vaginal bleeding.
  b. Outcomes
  (1) Vital signs and FHR remain stable.
  (2) Adequate hydration is maintained.
  (3) No obvious signs of bleeding are observed.
 9. Risk for infection related to vaginal examination after ROM
  a. Interventions
  (1) Maintain good perineal hygiene.
  (2) Document time of ROM and characteristics of amniotic fluid.
  (3) Monitor temperature every 2 hours after ROM.
  (4) Monitor laboratory data as indicated.
  (5) Perform vaginal examinations only when necessary.
  (6) Ensure aseptic technique during procedures.
  (7) Observe FHR for tachycardia, often an early indication of maternal infection.
  b. Outcomes
  (1) No evidence of infection is present.
   (a) Vital signs and FHR remain normal.
   (b) Laboratory data are within normal limits.
  (2) Time and date of ROM are documented.
  (3) Character of amniotic fluid is documented.
  (4) No foul-smelling fluid is observed.

Second Stage of Labor: Infant Expulsion

A. Assessment
 1. Physical findings
  a. Vaginal examination
  (1) Dilatation: 10 cm (complete cervical dilation)
  (2) Effacement: 100%
  (3) Station: 0 to +2

    b. Contractions
        (1) Frequency: every 2 to 3 minutes
        (2) Duration: 60 to 90 seconds
        (3) Intensity
            (a) Strong by palpation
            (b) 80 to 100 mmHg by IUPC
    c. Diaphoresis
    d. Methods to facilitate fetal descent
        (1) Laboring down
            (a) Second stage rest period for clients with epidural
            (b) Begin pushing when the urge to push is felt.
        (2) The urge-to-push method, in which the mother bears down as she feels the urge and in a manner that feels right to her
            (a) Most women make three to five brief (4- to 6-second) pushes with each contraction.
            (b) Most pushes are accompanied by the release of air.
        (3) Traditionally, women have been taught to push in the following manner:
            (a) Hold the breath.
            (b) Bear down on the rectum for a count of 10.
            (c) Inhale again, push again, and repeat the process three or four times for each contraction.
            (d) Assume a C-shaped position around the fetus, with the chin on the chest.
            (e) Pushing in this fashion leads to hemodynamic changes in the mother from the resultant Valsalva maneuver and may also produce abnormalities in the FHR.
        (4) The open-glottis method in which air is released during pushing so that no intrathoracic pressure builds up, which would be helpful for women with cardiac or hypertensive conditions for which a prolonged Valsalva effect is contraindicated
    e. Signs of descent of presenting part
        (1) Bulging of perineum occurs.
        (2) Anal changes occur.
            (a) Passing of flatus or stool
            (b) Rectal mucosa exposed
        (3) Opening of the vaginal introitus occurs.
        (4) The presenting part is visible (crowning).
        (5) Burning or stretching sensation is felt in the perineal area.
        (6) Urine is expressed during pushing.
    f. Anesthesia for delivery
        (1) Continuation of caudal or epidural anesthesia
        (2) Pudendal anesthesia:
            (a) Is a transvaginal block of the pudendal nerve near ischial spines.
            (b) Affects vaginal and perineal area.
            (c) Has little or no fetal effect.
        (3) Saddle block: low spinal anesthesia
            (a) Local anesthesia is introduced into the subarachnoid space.
            (b) Motor and sensory nerves are blocked.
            (c) Effect on fetus is decreased blood flow with maternal hypotension secondary to peripheral vasodilation.

      (4) Local infiltration
        (a) Perineal body is injected with local anesthesia.
        (b) Performed just before delivery at site of episiotomy.
        (c) Has no fetal effect.
  g. Episiotomy: incision in perineum to provide more space for presenting part
    (1) Indications
      (a) To prevent tearing
      (b) To prevent undue stretching of bladder and rectal supports
      (c) To reduce time and stress of second stage
      (d) To allow for ease in manipulation with a forceps or breech delivery
    (2) Types
      (a) Median or midline
        (i) Advantages
          ■ Heals quickly
          ■ Easily repaired
          ■ Less discomfort
          ■ Less dyspareunia
        (ii) Disadvantage: extension can involve rectal area.
      (b) Mediolateral: 45-degree angle to left or right
        (i) Advantages
          ■ Is used for large infant.
          ■ Has no rectal involvement.
        (ii) Disadvantages
          ■ Heals more slowly.
          ■ Is more painful.
          ■ Causes greater blood loss.
  h. Lacerations
    (1) First degree: involves perineal skin and vaginal mucous membrane.
    (2) Second degree: involves skin and mucous membrane plus fascia of perineal body.
    (3) Third degree: involves skin, mucous membrane, and muscle of perineal body; extends into rectal sphincter.
    (4) Fourth degree: extends into rectal mucosa to expose the lumen of the rectum.
2. Psychosocial
  a. Client is less irritable and agitated.
  b. Client is more cooperative.
  c. Try to maintain client's modesty, often not a priority with her.
  d. Client may doze off between contractions.
  e. Client is intent on work of pushing.
3. Diagnostic procedures
  a. Method for controlled vaginal vertex delivery
    (1) Maintain gentle pressure on presenting part.
    (2) Provide perineal support.
    (3) Support fetal head as it is delivered.
    (4) Check for nuchal cord.
    (5) Suction infant's mouth, then nose.
    (6) Deliver anterior shoulder under symphysis.
    (7) Deliver posterior shoulder over coccyx.

(8) Rest of infant delivers easily.

(9) Note time of delivery, the point at which the entire infant body is free of the mother.

  b. Assisted delivery

    (1) Indications for forceps or vacuum use

      (a) Maternal

        (i) Progress of second stage stops as the result of:

          ■ Inadequate contraction strength

          ■ Poor pushing efforts

          ■ Excessive infant size

          ■ Fetal position: posterior or asynclitic

        (ii) Maternal condition that warrants a shortened second stage (e.g., cardiac problems)

        (iii) Extreme fatigue of mother after prolonged labor, particularly second stage

      (b) Fetal

        (i) Preterm infant (potential for cranial damage with prolonged pushing)

        (ii) Distress that warrants a shortened second stage

    (2) Prerequisites

      (a) No cephalopelvic disproportion (CPD) is present.

      (b) Head is engaged.

      (c) Membranes are ruptured.

      (d) Cervix is completely dilated.

      (e) Bladder is empty.

    (3) Types of assisted deliveries

      (a) Low/outlet forceps: used when the head is visible at the perineum

      (b) Midforceps

        (i) Head is at the ischial spines.

        (ii) Often needed for rotation to anteroposterior position

      (c) Vacuum

        (i) Head is visible.

        (ii) Silastic suction cup is applied to presenting part and gentle traction is exerted while the mother pushes.

    (4) After any assisted delivery, the infant should be examined thoroughly for possible injuries.

      (a) Bruising

      (b) Cephalhematoma (area of edema of scalp at location of Silastic cup is usual with vacuum extractions)

      (c) Facial nerve damage

    (5) Use of forceps or vacuum may predispose the client to lacerations of the vagina or perineum.

B. Nursing Diagnoses

  1. Impaired urinary elimination related to pressure of presenting part

  2. Ineffective tissue perfusion related to expulsive efforts

  3. Impaired tissue integrity related to delivery process

  4. Ineffective individual coping related to second stage of labor

  5. Pain related to descent of fetus and perineal stretching

  6. Risk for infection related to prolonged second stage

C. Interventions/Outcomes

  1. Impaired urinary elimination related to pressure of presenting part

    a. Interventions

      (1) Encourage emptying of bladder.

      (2) Catheterize distended bladder if the client is unable to void.

      (3) Monitor the client's I&O.

  b. Outcomes

      (1) Bladder does not become distended.

      (2) I&O is adequate.

      (3) Complications are avoided or minimized.

2. Ineffective tissue perfusion related to expulsive efforts

  a. Interventions

      (1) Encourage side-lying or pillow-propped position because dorsal recumbent position occludes the inferior vena cava.

      (2) Closely monitor vital signs after analgesia or anesthesia.

      (3) Discourage prolonged Valsalva maneuvers while pushing.

      (4) Administer oxygen as indicated.

      (5) Maintain adequate fluid intake.

  b. Outcomes

      (1) Vital signs and FHR remain within normal limits.

      (2) Gentle pushing is used.

      (3) No signs of dizziness or syncope are noted.

3. Impaired skin integrity related to delivery process

  a. Interventions

      (1) Encourage upright rather than recumbent position for pushing.

      (2) Encourage gentle pushing efforts to allow for gradual stretching of tissue.

      (3) Avoid precipitous or uncontrolled delivery when possible.

      (4) Position the client to facilitate perineal floor relaxation and increased pelvic diameters (see Chapter 10 for a complete discussion of optimal positions for expulsion).

  b. Outcomes

      (1) No lacerations occur.

4. Ineffective individual coping related to second stage of labor

  a. Interventions

      (1) Support and direct coach related to second stage of labor.

      (2) Encourage rest periods between pushing contractions.

      (3) Provide comfort measures.

      (4) Provide mirror to observe progress of pushing.

      (5) Provide encouragement.

  b. Outcomes

      (1) Client uses effective coping skills.

      (2) Client is actively involved in her care.

      (3) Client uses effective breathing and expulsive methods.

5. Pain related to descent of fetus and perineal stretching

  a. Interventions

      (1) Assist with nonpharmacologic techniques.

        (a) Breathing patterns

        (b) TENS

      (2) Provide information and analgesia or anesthesia as necessary.

      (3) Monitor response to medications used.

      (4) Put side rails up after analgesia or anesthesia has been administered.

  b. Outcomes

      (1) Comfort is attained.

6. Risk for infection related to prolonged second stage

  a. Interventions

      (1) Use clean or aseptic technique as appropriate.

(a) Keep the perineal area clean.
(b) Using institution's designated solutions, cleanse perineal area before delivery.
(2) Monitor temperature and pulse for deviations.
  b. Outcomes
   (1) Clean, aseptic conditions are maintained.
   (2) No evidence of infection is observed.

Third Stage of Labor: Placental Expulsion

A. Assessment
  1. Physical findings
    a. Signs of separation of placenta
     (1) Gush of blood occurs.
     (2) Cord lengthens at vaginal opening.
     (3) Fundus rises in abdomen.
     (4) Uterine shape changes from flat to firm and globular as placenta drops into lower uterine segment.
    b. Types of placental delivery
     (1) Spontaneous
       (a) Schultz's mechanism: fetal side delivers first.
       (b) Duncan's mechanism: maternal side delivers first.
     (2) Manual extraction: delivery attendant assists with placental separation and removal.
    c. Placental abnormalities (Figure 11-1)
     (1) Battledore: cord is inserted at or near the placental margin, rather than in the center.
     (2) Circumvellate: the fetal surface of the placenta is exposed through a ring of chorion and amnion opening around the umbilical cord.
     (3) Succenturiate: one or more accessory lobes of fetal villi have developed.
       (a) Only the membranes support the vessels from the major to the minor lobe, increasing the risk of retention of the minor lobe during the third stage.
       (b) Blood loss may also occur if these vessels are nicked during intrauterine procedures.
     (4) Velamentous insertion of cord: fetal vessels separate in the membranes before reaching the placenta.
       (a) If bleeding is visible, it should be tested for fetal hemoglobin by means of Kleihauer-Betke or APT test to determine if fetal or maternal blood.
       (b) Fetus may become hypovolemic.
       (c) Fetus is most vulnerable during labor and delivery.
       (d) Condition is more common with:
          (i) Multiple gestation
          (ii) Placental anomalies (Olds, London, & Ladwig, 1996)
     (5) Vasa previa: associated with velamentous insertion of the cord
       (a) The umbilical vessels in the membranes cross the region of the internal os and present ahead of the fetus.
       (b) Potential danger to the fetus is considerable if rupture of the membranes is accompanied by rupture of a fetal vessel.
       (c) In severe cases, vasa previa can lead to exsanguination of the fetus (Wong & Perry, 1998).

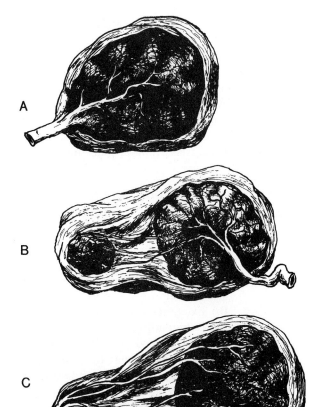

FIGURE 11-1 ■ Placental variations: **A,** battledore placenta; **B,** placenta succenturiate; and **C,** velamentous insertion of the umbilical cord. (From Lowdermilk, D.L., & Perry, S.E. [2004]. *Maternity & women's health care* [8th ed.]. St. Louis: Mosby.)

       (d) Vasa previa may be diagnosed by:
          (i) Vaginal examination
          (ii) Amnioscopy
          (iii) Palpation of a vessel pulsating synchronously with the FHR in the membranes in front of the fetus
       (e) Cesarean delivery may be indicated if the health care provider believes the risk of hemorrhage to be great.

B. Nursing Diagnoses
   1. Anxiety related to concern for the newborn
   2. Risk for deficient fluid volume related to blood loss

C. Interventions/Outcomes
   1. Anxiety related to concern for well being of newborn
     a. Interventions
       (1) Provide early infant contact as soon as possible: place the infant on the mother's abdomen after delivery if not contraindicated.
       (2) Encourage touching and holding of the infant.
       (3) Explain any procedures for stimulation or resuscitation of the infant to allay anxiety.
       (4) Reassure the mother about the infant's status and well being.
     b. Outcomes
       (1) Infant is placed on the mother's abdomen.
       (2) Mother holds the infant.
       (3) Mother reports assurance of the infant's well being.

2. Risk for deficient fluid volume related to blood loss
  a. Interventions
    (1) Ensure that placenta is delivered within 30 minutes.
    (2) Monitor vaginal bleeding with delivery of the placenta.
    (3) Monitor firmness of the uterus.
    (4) Administer oxytocin as indicated.
  b. Outcomes
    (1) Blood loss is less than 500 ml.
    (2) Uterus is firm after placental delivery.

Fourth Stage of Labor: Immediate Postpartum Period

A. **Assessment**
  1. Physical findings
    a. Vital signs
      (1) BP is taken every 15 minutes.
        (a) Transient changes are secondary to decreased blood volume after delivery.
        (b) Excitement may elevate BP.
        (c) Low reading is often a late sign of blood loss.
      (2) Pulse is checked every 15 minutes.
        (a) Bradycardia may occur to compensate for decreased vascular bed and decreased intraabdominal pressure.
        (b) Tachycardia may indicate an increase in blood loss or a temperature elevation.
      (3) Temperature: slight elevation is normal (100° F [37.8° C]) as the result of dehydration and the fatigue of labor.
    b. Fundal checks are made every 15 minutes.
      (1) Fundus is firm and well contracted.
      (2) Fundus is midway between umbilicus and symphysis after delivery of placenta.
      (3) Fundus rises slowly to the level of umbilicus during the first hour after placental delivery.
    c. Lochia estimation is performed every 15 minutes.
      (1) Nature of flow
        (a) Intermittent
        (b) Trickle
        (c) Clots
      (2) Amount of flow: greater than 500 ml indicates postpartum hemorrhage (see Chapter 30 for further discussion of postpartum hemorrhage).
        (a) Weigh peripads or Chux (1 g = 1 ml)
        (b) Saturated peripad in less than 1 hour (see Chapter 13 for more details regarding lochial flow and evaluation)
      (3) Character and odor of flow
    d. Perineal inspection
      (1) Episiotomy, lacerations, or both
        (a) Intact: edges approximated
        (b) No hematomas, redness, or edema
      (2) Clean
  2. Psychosocial
    a. Joy: sense of peace and excitement

      b. Excitement: wide awake, talkative, hungry, and thirsty
      c. Attachment process begins
        (1) Mother inspects the newborn.
        (2) Mother wants to cuddle the infant and begin breastfeeding.
        (3) Mother feels the need to "let the world know."

B. Nursing Diagnoses
  1. Risk for interrupted family processes related to acceptance of newborn
  2. Impaired urinary elimination related to process of labor and delivery
  3. Pain related to early uterine involution
  4. Risk for deficient fluid volume related to fluid shift in early postpartum period
  5. Risk for infection related to labor and delivery

C. Interventions/Outcomes
  1. Risk for interrupted family processes related to acceptance of newborn
    a. Interventions
      (1) Provide for early infant contact.
      (2) Assist with early breastfeeding.
      (3) Call attention to quiet, alert state of infant.
      (4) Provide information about infant's ability to see and hear.
      (5) Postpone eye prophylaxis.
    b. Outcomes
      (1) Parental exploration of infant takes place.
      (2) Infant is cuddled and breastfed if desired.
  2. Impaired urinary elimination related to process of labor and delivery
    a. Interventions
      (1) Encourage emptying of the bladder.
      (2) Monitor fundal height.
      (3) Catheterize distended bladder if the client is unable to void.
      (4) Monitor I&O.
    b. Outcomes
      (1) Bladder does not become distended.
      (2) No displacement of uterus is visible.
      (3) I&O is adequate.
      (4) Complications are avoided or minimized.
  3. Pain related to early uterine involution
    a. Interventions
      (1) Assist with nonpharmacologic methods of relief.
        (a) Apply an ice bag to soothe perineum.
        (b) Supply a warm blanket if client is chilled.
      (2) Provide medication as ordered.
    b. Outcomes
      (1) Comfort is attained.
      (2) Client verbalizes pain reduction.
  4. Risk for deficient fluid volume related to fluid shift in early postpartum period
    a. Interventions
      (1) Monitor vital signs.
      (2) Administer IV and oral fluids as indicated.
      (3) Monitor vaginal discharge for excessive bleeding.
      (4) Monitor fundal height and firmness.
    b. Outcomes
      (1) Vital signs are within normal limits.

(2) Hydration is maintained.
(3) Blood loss is less than 500 ml.
(4) Uterus remains firmly contracted.
5. Risk for infection related to labor and delivery
   a. Interventions
      (1) Use clean or aseptic technique, as appropriate.
         (a) Apply a sterile perineal pad after delivery.
         (b) Clean the perineal area from front to back.
      (2) Inspect the perineal area for breakdown.
      (3) Emphasize good hand-washing technique to client.
      (4) Monitor client's pulse and temperature for deviations.
   b. Outcomes
      (1) Clean and aseptic conditions are maintained.
      (2) Skin condition is documented.
      (3) No evidence of infection is visible.
      (4) Client washes her hands.

Variables Influencing Labor and Delivery

Induction or Augmentation

Initiation or augmentation of uterine contractions will accomplish delivery.
A. Assessment
   1. History
      a. Relative indications for induction or augmentation
         (1) Maternal
            (a) Diabetes
            (b) PIH
            (c) Slowed progress of labor
            (d) History of precipitate labor
            (e) Chorioamnionitis
         (2) Fetal
            (a) Prolonged ROM
            (b) Postmaturity
            (c) Rh sensitization
            (d) Fetal death
      b. Relative contraindications for induction or augmentation
         (1) Maternal
            (a) Previous classic uterine incision
            (b) Placenta previa
            (c) Grand multipara
            (d) Overdistended uterus
            (e) Active genital herpes
         (2) Fetal
            (a) CPD
            (b) Severe fetal distress
            (c) Fetal malposition
            (d) Fetal immaturity
   2. Physical findings: the Bishop score measures physiologic readiness of cervix (Table 11-1).
      a. Dilatation
      b. Effacement
      c. Station

■ TABLE 11-1
■ ■ **Bishop Score**

	0	1	2	3
Dilatation	Closed	1-2 cm	>3-4 cm	≥5 cm
Effacement	30%	40%-50%	60%-70%	≥80%
Station	−3	−2	−1/0	+1
Cervical consistency	Firm	Medium	Soft	
Cervical position	Posterior	Middle	Anterior	

Total possible score is 13. High score indicates a greater chance for successful outcome. With a score of 9, successful induction is likely; with 7, success is likely for a primigravida; and with 5, success is likely for a multipara. However, a high score at early gestation forewarns of possible premature labor.

From Nurses' Association of the American College of Obstetricians and Gynecologists (NAACOG) (1991). *Inpatient obstetrics certification review manual.* Washington, DC: NAACOG.

   d. Cervical consistency
   e. Cervical position
 3. Diagnostic findings
   a. Maternal readiness
     (1) Informed consent
     (2) Bishop score of 5 to 7 indicates probable induction success.
   b. Fetal readiness
     (1) Gestational age established by early ultrasound test or measurement of appropriate parameters
     (2) Acceptable L/S ratio (usually 2:1 or higher)
     (3) Presence of PG in amniotic fluid (see Chapter 8 for a complete discussion)
 4. Methods of induction or augmentation
   a. Amniotomy: mechanical
     (1) Allows for pressure of presenting part on cervix.
     (2) Side effects
       (a) Increased risk of infection
       (b) Increased risk of prolapsed cord
   b. Prostaglandin
     (1) Used as suppository or gel to ripen cervix to improve the Bishop score.
     (2) Side effects
       (a) Nausea and vomiting
       (b) Diarrhea
       (c) Fever
   c. Oxytocin: goal is to mimic natural labor.
     (1) Given intravenously (diluted in an isotonic electrolyte solution) in secondary line with an infusion pump
     (2) Side effects
       (a) Tetanic contractions
       (b) Maternal hypotension
       (c) Antidiuretic effect
       (d) Neonatal hyperbilirubinemia has been reported (Wong & Perry, 1998).

B. Nursing Diagnoses
1. Anxiety related to induction or augmentation
2. Pain related to uterine contractions
3. Risk for excess fluid volume related to use of oxytocin
4. Risk for injury related to induction

C. Interventions/Outcomes
1. Anxiety related to induction or augmentation
   a. Interventions
      (1) Present procedure with clear explanations.
      (2) Maintain frequent presence, with continuous EFM for fetus and maternal contractions.
      (3) Reassure the client of fetal status and progress of labor.
   b. Outcomes
      (1) Client verbalizes understanding of situation and plan of care.
      (2) Client is involved in alternative birth plan.
      (3) Client uses effective coping methods.
2. Pain resulting from uterine contractions
   a. Interventions
      (1) Anticipate that the client will feel the pain from contractions sooner than with naturally occurring labor.
      (2) Provide comfort measures.
      (3) Promote the use of breathing and relaxation techniques.
      (4) Support the birthing coach.
      (5) Provide and monitor analgesia or anesthesia, as appropriate.
      (6) Use nonpharmacologic means of pain control.
   b. Outcomes
      (1) Client reports increased comfort.
      (2) Support person is actively participating.
      (3) No adverse effects of medication occur in mother or infant.
3. Risk for excess fluid volume related to use of oxytocin
   a. Interventions
      (1) Monitor I&O strictly.
      (2) Maintain an accurate record of the amount of oxytocin administered.
      (3) Observe for signs of water intoxication.
         (a) Altered consciousness
         (b) Excessive fluid intake compared with output
         (c) Edema
   b. Outcomes
      (1) Adequate I&O is maintained.
      (2) Water intoxication is avoided.
4. Risk for injury related to induction
   a. Interventions
      (1) Observe institution's written policy or protocol for medication use; a suggested oxytocin protocol follows.
         (a) Dilute 10 U of oxytocin in 1000 ml of lactated Ringer's solution or other physiologic electrolyte solution so that each ml contains 10 mU of oxytocin.
         (b) Administer by means of infusion pump as secondary line, connected as close as possible to the primary IV site.
         (c) Initial dose is usually 0.5 to 1 mU/min.
         (d) Dose may be gradually increased in increments of 1 to 2 mU/min every 30 to 60 minutes.

  (e) Once the desired frequency of contractions is reached (usually every 3 minutes), the rate may be maintained (a client seldom requires more than 20 to 40 mU/min).
 (2) Nurse-client ratio should be 1:1 or 1:2.
 (3) During administration, accurate monitoring is required for:
  (a) Uterine contractions for frequency, duration, and intensity
  (b) Uterine resting tone
  (c) FHR response to contractions
  (d) Maternal vital signs
 (4) Discontinue oxytocin infusion:
  (a) With a tetanic contraction (one lasting longer than 90 seconds)
  (b) With uterine hyperstimulation (contractions occurring less than 2 minutes apart)
  (c) With elevated uterine resting tone
  (d) With nonreassuring FHR patterns (see Chapter 12 for complete discussion of FHR patterns)
 (5) Suggested protocol for prostaglandin (misoprostol [Cytotec] is a prostaglandin E analog frequently used for induction of labor or ripening of unripe cervix; see institutional policy for specific protocols).
  (a) In all clients, an IV should be started and continuous electronic fetal monitoring begun.
  (b) Supine or nearly side-lying bed rest for 1 to 2 hours after cervical ripening agent with vital signs.
  (c) Continuous FHR and contraction monitoring for 1 to 4 hours.
  (d) Oxytocin may be initiated no sooner than 4 hours before or after the last misoprostol dose (if this drug is being used).
  (e) If uterine hyperstimulation occurs, notify health care provider.
  (f) If FHR indicates fetal compromise, institute measures to remove the tablet and improve fetal oxygenation (Murray, 1996).
 b. Outcomes
  (1) Oxytocin is administered via infusion pump.
  (2) Prostaglandin gel or tablet is inserted appropriately.
  (3) Accurate documentation is made of medication dosage and method of administration.
  (4) No adverse effects of medication are visible in mother or fetus.

Dysfunctional Labor
A. Assessment
 1. History
  a. Abnormal progress of labor (some overlapping exists between classifications)
   (1) Nulliparous women are more subject to conditions that occur in early labor.
    (a) Hypertonic uterine dysfunction
    (b) Primary inertia
    (c) Prolonged latent phase
   (2) Multiparous women more often demonstrate problems that occur in the active phase.
    (a) Hypotonic uterine dysfunction
    (b) Secondary inertia
    (c) Protraction or arrest of the active phase

    b. Altered Friedman curve (Figure 11-2)
        (1) Friedman demonstrated a normal labor pattern by plotting, on a graph, cervical dilatation and degree of descent against lapsed time.
        (2) Categories of delayed progression according to his terminology:
            (a) Prolonged latent phase
            (b) Protraction disorders
            (c) Arrest disorders
2. Physical findings
    a. Hypertonia (primary inertia)
        (1) Uncoordinated uterine activity: no normal resting phase
        (2) More than one uterine pacemaker sending signals
        (3) Frequent contractions
        (4) Occurs in latent phase (protracted latent phase).
        (5) Painful because of uterine anoxia
        (6) Management with therapeutic rest (Lowdermilk & Perry, 2004)
    b. Hypotonia (secondary inertia)
        (1) Ineffective tightening and pressure
        (2) Contractions insufficient to dilate cervix
        (3) Poor contraction intensity
        (4) Occurs in active phase (protracted active phase).
        (5) Management with labor augmentation (Lowdermilk & Perry, 2004)
    c. Precipitate labor
        (1) Labor of less than 3 hours
        (2) Low maternal tissue resistance
        (3) Often rapid transit of fetus through birth canal
3. Diagnostic findings
    a. Pathologic retraction ring (Bandl's ring) (Figure 11-3)
        (1) A normal physiologic retraction ring develops at the junction of the active upper and passive lower segments of the uterus.
        (2) A pathologic ring is an exaggeration of this physiologic ring; it grips the fetus, preventing descent.
        (3) Labor is arrested at this point.
        (4) The uterus above the ring becomes thicker, and the lower segment thins out and ruptures unless the obstruction is relieved.
        (5) Tocolytic drugs to relax the uterus are often used.

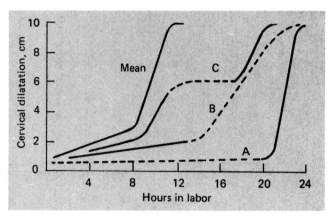

FIGURE 11-2 ■ Abnormal Friedman curve. (From Friedman, E. [1965]. In J.P. Greenhill [Ed.], *Obstetrics* [13th ed.]. Philadelphia: Saunders.)

FIGURE 11-3 ■ Bandl's ring. Left, normal second stage; right, abnormal second stage—dystocia. (Redrawn from Cunningham, G., MacDonald, P., & Gant, N. [1988]. *Williams obstetrics* [18th ed., p. 214]. Norwalk, CT: Appleton & Lange.)

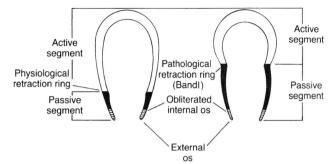

        (6) If drug therapy is not successful, delivery must be made by cesarean birth.
  b. Fetus in occiput posterior position
        (1) A larger diameter presents to the pelvis.
        (2) The degree of flexion is altered.
        (3) Cervical dilatation and fetal descent are slowed.
B. Nursing Diagnoses
  1. Anxiety related to abnormal progress of labor
  2. Deficient knowledge related to dysfunctional labor
  3. Pain related to abnormal labor pattern
  4. Risk for infection related to prolonged labor
C. Interventions/Outcomes
  1. Anxiety related to abnormal progress of labor
    a. Interventions
        (1) Monitor progress of labor.
            (a) Document contraction pattern.
            (b) Perform vaginal examinations to determine cervical dilatation and fetal descent.
            (c) Communicate deviations from normal to physician or midwife.
        (2) Explain unknown or unplanned situations in an easily understood manner.
        (3) Identify how this situation may alter birth plan.
        (4) Maintain a positive attitude about ability to cope.
        (5) Reassure the client as to the status of the fetus.
    b. Outcomes
        (1) Client verbalizes understanding of the situation and the options available.
        (2) Client has a positive attitude and realistic expectations about outcome.
  2. Deficient knowledge related to dysfunctional labor
    a. Interventions
        (1) Provide factual information about dysfunctional labor.
        (2) Explain expected treatment and outcome.
            (a) Oxytocin use for hypotonic labor
            (b) Sedation
            (c) Regional anesthesia for hypertonic labor
        (3) Encourage questions and expression of feelings.
    b. Outcomes
        (1) Client verbalizes understanding of dysfunctional labor.
        (2) Client is cooperative and involved in alternative to birth plan.
        (3) Informed consent has been given.

3. Pain related to abnormal labor pattern
   a. Interventions
      (1) Provide analgesia or anesthesia as appropriate.
      (2) Use counterpressure with low back pain or other nonpharmacologic techniques.
      (3) Document contractions and response and coping ability.
   b. Outcomes
      (1) Reduction of client's tension and anxiety provides comfort.
      (2) Client verbalizes decreased discomfort.
      (3) No adverse effects of medications occur in mother or fetus.
4. Risk for infection resulting from prolonged labor
   a. Interventions
      (1) Monitor and document vital signs and FHR.
      (2) Maintain good aseptic technique.
         (a) Minimize vaginal examinations.
         (b) Maintain perineal cleanliness.
      (3) Monitor characteristics and odor of amniotic fluid.
      (4) Administer antibiotics as indicated.
   b. Outcomes
      (1) Temperature, FHR, and WBC count are within normal limits.
      (2) No sign of infection occurs.

Cesarean Birth

Delivery is through incision in abdominal and uterine walls.

A. **Assessment**
1. History
   a. Previous uterine surgery
   b. Maternal condition (e.g., hemorrhage)
   c. Maternal illness
2. Physical findings
   a. Indications for cesarean birth
      (1) Fetal distress, disease, or anomaly
      (2) Fetal malposition or malpresentation
      (3) Fetal macrosomia
      (4) Active herpes genitalia
      (5) CPD
      (6) Placental abnormality
         (a) Placenta previa
         (b) Abruptio placentae
   b. Vaginal birth after cesarean (VBAC)
      (1) Decision making
         (a) Nonrepeating condition
         (b) Desire to avoid cesarean birth
         (c) Ability to perform emergency cesarean birth
         (d) Benefits mother by shortening recovery time
      (2) Risks
         (a) Small possibility of uterine rupture
         (b) Need for close monitoring during labor
3. Psychosocial
   a. Relief after long labor with failure to progress
   b. Fear if fetus or mother is stressed
   c. Helplessness if birth plan is altered
   d. Disappointment if vaginal delivery is not achieved

4. Diagnostic findings
  a. Preoperative CBC, urinalysis, blood typed and crossmatched
  b. Fetal lung maturity and gestational age if elective
  c. Ultrasonography for fetal position and placental placement
5. Anesthesia (see Chapter 26 for complete discussion of anesthesia and surgery during pregnancy)
  a. General
    (1) General anesthesia usually is used only in emergency situations or when regional anesthesia is contraindicated.
    (2) General anesthesia leads to central nervous system (CNS) depression of mother and fetus.
    (3) Mother must take nothing by mouth.
    (4) Nonparticulate antacids are given before surgery.
    (5) Because of the resulting hypoxia in the infant, it is recommended that induction time to birth be less than 8 minutes.
  b. Regional
    (1) Spinal
      (a) Local anesthesia is injected into the subarachnoid space.
      (b) Motor and sensory block ensues.
      (c) Spinal anesthesia has the potential for causing severe headaches during recovery period.
    (2) Epidural
      (a) Local anesthesia is injected into epidural space.
      (b) Sensory block of entire pelvis and legs ensues.
      (c) Epidural block has the potential for hypotensive episode if the mother is not well hydrated first.
      (d) If hypotension occurs, fetus may suffer distress.
B. Nursing Diagnoses
  1. Anxiety related to surgical delivery
  2. Deficient knowledge related to cesarean birth
  3. Pain related to surgical intervention
  4. Risk for deficient fluid volume related to surgical procedure and blood loss
  5. Risk for infection related to surgical procedure
  6. Situational low self-esteem related to change in birth plan
C. Interventions/Outcomes
  1. Anxiety related to surgical delivery
    a. Interventions
      (1) Assist client with appropriate coping techniques.
      (2) Encourage active participation in decision making.
      (3) Provide clear explanations of all proposed treatment options.
      (4) Facilitate involvement of support person.
      (5) Reassure client about infant if surgery is performed for fetal distress.
    b. Outcomes
      (1) Client uses effective coping methods.
      (2) Client verbalizes understanding of the situation and the options available.
  2. Deficient knowledge related to cesarean birth
    a. Interventions
      (1) Provide factual information about cesarean birth and informed consent.
      (2) Explain expected procedures.
        (a) Anesthesia preparation

         (i) IV fluid
         (ii) Client takes nothing by mouth
         (iii) Nonparticulate antacid administered if general anesthesia planned
     (b) Foley catheter
     (c) Skin preparation
   (3) Encourage questions and verbalization of situation.
  b. Outcomes
   (1) Client verbalizes understanding and acceptance of situation not a part of birth plan.
   (2) Client is cooperative and involved in preparation for cesarean birth.
3. Pain related to surgical intervention
  a. Interventions
   (1) Use nonpharmacologic methods for relief as appropriate.
   (2) Provide analgesia or anesthesia as appropriate.
   (3) Position for comfort.
  b. Outcomes
   (1) Reduction of tension and anxiety provides comfort.
   (2) Client reports decreased discomfort.
   (3) No adverse effects from medication occur.
4. Risk for deficient fluid volume related to surgical procedure and blood loss
  a. Interventions
   (1) Monitor I&O and hydration status.
   (2) Observe and document blood loss.
   (3) Monitor vital signs for impending shock.
  b. Outcomes
   (1) Hydration is maintained.
   (2) No excessive blood loss occurs.
   (3) Vital signs remain within normal limits.
5. Risk for infection as a result of cesarean birth
  a. Interventions
   (1) Monitor and document vital signs and FHR.
   (2) Monitor characteristics and odor of amniotic fluid.
   (3) Maintain good aseptic technique during:
     (a) Vaginal examinations
     (b) Catheterization
     (c) Preoperative skin preparation
     (d) Postoperative wound care and assessment for developing infection
   (4) Monitor blood loss.
   (5) Administer antibiotics as indicated.
  b. Outcomes
   (1) Temperature and WBC count are within normal limits.
   (2) Wound has no signs of infection.
   (3) Client has no infection at any site.
6. Situational low self-esteem related to change in birth plan
  a. Interventions
   (1) Discuss changes in birth plan.
   (2) Encourage verbalization of feelings about a cesarean birth rather than a vaginal delivery.
   (3) Involve the client in decision making.
   (4) Provide positive reassurances.

    b. Outcomes
        (1) Client verbalizes self-confidence.
        (2) Client verbalizes positive attitude and realistic expectations.

HEALTH EDUCATION

A. Intrapartum health education should provide the following:
  1. Information about the process of labor
  2. Clear explanations about the procedures (risk versus benefits) performed during the process of labor and delivery
  3. Information about the available pain-relief methods
  4. Methods of involvement and participation during the intrapartum period
  5. Preoperative teaching for cesarean birth
  6. Information about variables that may alter or influence a birth plan

---

CASE STUDY AND STUDY QUESTIONS

Mrs. V, a 24-year-old gravida 2, para 1 (G2, P1), is admitted to labor and delivery at 39 weeks' gestation. A vaginal examination indicates her cervix is 80% effaced and 3 cm dilated. The presenting vertex is at −1 station. The amniotic sac is not palpated, and Mrs. V says she thinks it has ruptured.

1. What should the nurse ask about the amniotic sac?
  a. The time the membranes ruptured
  b. The color and amount of fluid, if observed
  c. The presence of back pain
  d. The presence of bloody show

2. During this early phase of labor, how often should the FHR be evaluated?
  a. Every 5 minutes
  b. At least every 15 minutes
  c. At least every 30 minutes
  d. At least every hour

3. To promote comfort, she is encouraged to assume certain positions while in labor and to avoid others. Which of the following position should not be used during labor?
  a. Lateral position
  b. Squatting position
  c. Standing position
  d. Supine position

4. As her labor progresses to 5 cm, she becomes increasingly uncomfortable and requests an epidural anesthetic. After this is in place, to what should the nurse be particularly alert?
  a. Possible hypertensive rebound
  b. Possible hypotensive episode
  c. Increased thirst
  d. Signs of water intoxication

When she is comfortable from the epidural, it is observed that her contractions have spaced out to a frequency of every 5 to 6 minutes and are only mild to palpation. An oxytocin infusion is started to augment her labor.

5. What would be the most likely classification for the dysfunctional labor?
  a. Pathologic retraction ring
  b. Hypertonic labor
  c. Protracted active phase
  d. Prolonged latent phase

6. All of the following are possible side effects of oxytocin administration except:
  a. Fetal hyperglycemia
  b. Fetal hyperbilirubinemia
  c. Hyperstimulation of the uterus
  d. Water intoxication

7. When should the oxytocin infusion be discontinued?

a. When the client is comfortable with her contractions
b. When signs of fetal distress are observed on the fetal monitor
c. When the contractions are 3 minutes apart
d. When the client is ready to push

8. On assessment, Mrs. V is found to be completely dilated and effaced and at a +1 station. Which of the following findings suggest transition to the second stage of labor?
   a. Decreased urge to push
   b. Decreased bloody show
   c. FHR accelerations
   d. Bulging of the perineum

Because of the epidural anesthetic, she is not able to push as effectively. She pushes the infant to a +3 station but cannot bring it under the symphysis to effect delivery. It is decided to assist her by use of the vacuum extractor.

9. Which of the following are prerequisites for use of the vacuum?
   a. Membranes intact
   b. Presenting part engaged
   c. Cervix completely dilated
   d. Documentation of gestational age
   e. Empty bladder
      (1) a, b, c
      (2) b, d, e
      (3) b, c, e
      (4) c, e

10. For what should the infant be carefully examined after this procedure?
    a. Brachial plexus injury
    b. Respiratory distress
    c. Facial bruising
    d. Cephalhematoma

11. Which of the following structures are involved when an episiotomy is performed?

a. Vaginal mucosa
b. Levator ani muscle
c. Glans clitoris
d. Cardinal ligament
e. Fourchette

12. Which of the following signs would indicate that delivery is imminent?
    a. The mother has the desire to defecate.
    b. An increase in frequency, duration, and intensity of uterine contractions.
    c. The mother begins to bear down spontaneously with uterine contractions.
    d. Bulging of the perineum occurs.
    e. There is an increase in the amount of blood-stained mucus flowing from the vagina.
       (1) d
       (2) a, c, d
       (3) b, d, e
       (4) b
       (5) All of the above

13. The nurse caring for the mother and infant in the fourth stage of labor would do which of the following?
    a. Keep the mother warm and out of drafts.
    b. Massage the uterus every 15 minutes, or more often, if needed.
    c. Massage the uterus continuously.
    d. Check maternal vital signs every 15 minutes.
    e. Administer oxytocin as ordered.
       (1) a, b, d
       (2) b, d, e
       (3) c, d
       (4) b, d
       (5) a, d, e

14. Identify and match the most important risks of the various

methods of obstetrical anesthesia listed below:
a. General anesthesia
b. Regional conduction anesthesia
c. Paracervical block
  (1) Fetal bradycardia
  (2) Aspiration of stomach contents
  (3) Maternal hypotension

15. Match each term or phrase with the definition that best fits it:
a. Enlargement of the external os to 10 cm in diameter
b. Maximum shortening of the cervical canal

c. A condition caused by failure of the uterine muscle to stay contracted after delivery
d. Surgical incision of the perineum during the second stage of labor
e. Settling of the infant's head into the brim of the pelvis
  (1) Uterine atony
  (2) Complete dilatation
  (3) Lightening
  (4) Complete effacement
  (5) Episiotomy

ANSWERS TO STUDY QUESTIONS

1. a	5. c	9. 3	13. 2
2. c	6. a	10. d	14. (a) 2, (b) 3, (c) 1
3. d	7. b	11. a	15. (a) 2, (b) 4, (c) 1, (d) 5, (e) 3
4. b	8. d	12. 5	

REFERENCES

Callister, L.C., & Hobbins-Garbett, D. (2000). Cochrane pregnancy and childbirth database: Resource for evidence-based practice. *Journal of Obstetric, Gynecologic, and Neonatal Nursing, 29*(2), 123-128.

Clayworth, S. (2000). The nurse's role during oxytocin administration. *MCN The American Journal of Maternal Child Nursing, 25*(2), 80-85.

Davies, B.L., & Hodnett, E. (2002). Labor support: Nurses' self-efficacy and views about factors influencing implementation. *Journal of Obstetric, Gynecologic, and Neonatal Nursing, 31*(1), 48-56.

Faucher, M.A., & Brucker, M.C. (2000). Intrapartum pain: Pharmacologic management. *Journal of Obstetric, Gynecologic, and Neonatal Nursing, 29*(2), 169-180.

Gagnon, A.J., & Waghorn, K. (1999). One-to-one nurse labor support of nulliparous women stimulated with oxytocin. *Journal of Obstetric, Gynecologic, and Neonatal Nursing, 28*(4), 371-376.

Gale, J., Fothergill-Bourbonnais, F., & Chamberlain, M. (2001). Measuring nursing support during childbirth. *MCN The American Journal of Maternal Child Nursing, 26*(5), 264-271.

Gilder, K., Mayberry, L.J., Gennaro, S., & Clemmens, D. (2002). Maternal positioning in labor with epidural analgesia: Results from a multi-site survey. *AWHONN Lifelines, 6*(1), 40-45.

Kardong-Edgren, S. (2001). Using evidence-based practice to improve intrapartum care. *Journal of Obstetric, Gynecologic, and Neonatal Nursing, 30*(4), 371-375.

Lowdermilk, D.L., & Perry, S.E. (2004). *Maternity & women's health care* (8th ed.). St. Louis: Mosby.

Mayberry, L.J., Wood, S.H., Strange, L.B., Lee, L., Heisler, D.R., & Neilsen-Smith, K. (2000). Managing second-stage labor: Exploring the variables during the second stage. *AWHONN Lifelines, 3*(6), 28-34.

McCartney, P.R. (1998). Caring for women with epidurals using the "laboring down" technique. *MCN The American Journal of Maternal Child Nursing, 23*(5), 274.

McRae-Bergeron, C.E., Andrews, C.M., & Lupe, P.J. (1998). The effect of epidural analgesia on the second stage of labor. *Journal of the American Association of Nurse Anesthetists, 66*(2), 177-182.

Minato, J.F. (2000). Is it time to push? Examining rest in second-stage labor. *AWHONN Lifelines, 4*(6), 20-23.

Murray, M. (1996). *Advanced fetal monitoring: Maternal/fetal challenges for the caregiver.* Albuquerque, NM: Learning Resources International, Inc.

Olds, S., London, M., & Ladwig, M. (1996). *Maternity newborn nursing: A family-centered approach* (5th ed.). Redwood City, CA: Addison-Wesley.

Ruchala, P.L., Metheny, N., Essenpreis, H., & Borcherding, K. (2002). Current practice in oxytocin dilution and fluid administration for inducting of labor. *Journal of Obstetric, Gynecologic, and Neonatal Nursing, 31*(5), 545-550.

Searing, K.A. (2001). Induction vs. post-date pregnancies: Exploring the controversy of who's really at risk? *AWHONN Lifelines, 5*(2), 44-48.

Simpson, K.R., & Knox, G.E. (2001). Fundal pressure during the second stage of labor: Clinical perspectives and risk management issues. *MCN The American Journal of Maternal Child Nursing, 26*(2), 64-71.

Sleutel, M., & Golden, S.S. (1999). Fasting in labor: Relic or requirement. *Journal of Obstetric, Gynecologic, and Neonatal Nursing, 28*(5), 507-512.

Sprague, A., & Trèpanier, M.J. (1999). Charting in record time: Setting guidelines for documenting FHR enhances care for laboring women. *AWHONN Lifelines, 3*(4), 35-40.

Wilson, C. (2000). The nurse's role in misoprostol induction: A proposed protocol. *Journal of Obstetric, Gynecologic, and Neonatal Nursing, 29*(6), 574-583.

Wong, D., & Perry, S. (1998). *Maternal child nursing care.* St. Louis: Mosby.

12 Intrapartum Fetal Assessment

KEIKO L. TORGERSEN

OBJECTIVES

1. Identify techniques and methods of fetal assessment.
2. Identify baseline (BL) features, including rate, rhythm, and variability.
3. Identify, interpret, and discuss probable causes of periodic patterns of variable, late, early, and combined decelerations and accelerations.
4. Identify, interpret, and discuss probable cause of nonperiodic (episodic) patterns of variable and prolonged decelerations and accelerations.
5. Assess probable fetal status.
6. Discuss strategies to document fetal heart rate (FHR) events accurately and completely for the client record.
7. Reiterate the critical values of fetal blood gases and pH, and relate these to fetal outcome.
8. State appropriate physiologic interventions for deceleration patterns and altered variability in relation to fetal outcome.

INTRODUCTION

Intrapartum fetal assessment is essential to providing critical information regarding fetal well being and the fetal response to labor. FHR and uterine activity (UA) data can be collected by nonelectronic or electronic methods. Regardless of the method chosen to assess fetal status, the nurse is accountable for knowing and responding to both auditory and electronically obtained data (Moffatt & Feinstein, 2003). Nonelectronic assessment uses auscultation and palpation to assess the FHR and UA. Electronic assessment or electronic fetal monitoring (EFM) uses electronic techniques, such as tocodynamometer, ultrasound, fetal scalp electrode (FSE), or intrauterine pressure catheter (IUPC) to monitor FHR and UA. The technique provides a permanent record that can be observed and discussed instantaneously or retrospectively by professional care providers. Events that cannot be heard or measured by auscultation, such as variability, are available through EFM. Therefore EFM is another tool available to the care provider to easily provide information that would otherwise consume many hours of care and yield less complete data. The ability to monitor using short- or long-distance telemetry influences nursing care management and client comfort and may aid consultation and transport practices. The reader should also be aware of research in progress to refine or augment interpretation of fetal status and probable outcomes. One such method that is currently available for use is fetal pulse oximetry. Other methods that may be available for future use include oxicardiotocograph, computer analysis of fetal electrocardiogram, near-infrared spectroscopy for high-risk pregnancies, lactate measurement as a replacement for pH fetal blood sampling, and artificial intelligence to assess all fetal data and clinical events. Today, proper interpretation of FHR patterns may be the best method to reliably determine fetal status.

In 1995-1996 the U.S. National Institute of Child Health and Development (NICHD) pulled together EFM experts to discuss EFM terminology. In 1997 this group of experts published new EFM terminology (nomenclature) that was based on "clinical, laboratory, manufacturing, and published research" (Cypher, Adelsperger, & Torgersen, 2003, p. 113). Use of this standardized nomenclature may offer improved predictive value for EFM because it can significantly improve the ability to compare research studies. Although AWHONN is delighted to support this concept, readers must be aware that it takes time before research is ready to be translated into evidence-based practice. Because further research is needed before universal adoption of the NICHD nomenclature, AWHONN continues to use standardized terminology in their Fetal Heart Monitor Principles and Practices programs. However, the NICHD nomenclature system is very similar and is often used in conjunction with current terminology. The language used in this chapter, then, is consistent with the most recently understood interpretations of EFM tracings in general use and is inconsistent with the current Fetal Heart Monitoring Principles and Practices workshops, recently revised in 2003.

"Regardless of the practice setting or the terminology, the process of interpreting a FHR monitoring tracing includes (a) examining the tracing for trends of FHR and uterine activity parameters and (b) answering the question 'At the present time, what is the likely status of this fetus?'." (Cypher, Adelsperger, & Torgersen, 2003, p. 115) Nurses using EFM should know the capabilities, benefits, limitations, and troubleshooting of the assessment modalities employed.

A. **Nonelectronic methods of FHR assessment**
  1. Auscultation (Feinstein, Sprague, & Trepanier, 2000; Moffatt & Feinstein, 2003)
    a. Fetoscope:
      (1) Detects FHR BL.
      (2) Detects FHR rhythm.
      (3) Verifies presence of a dysrhythmia visualized on EFM tracing.
      (4) Detects increases and decreases from FHR baseline.
      (5) Clarifies halving or doubling on the EFM tracing.
      (6) Differentiates fetal and maternal heart rates, eliminating errors related to fetal demise and EFM equipment errors.
    b. Doptone:
      (1) Detects FHR BL.
      (2) Detects FHR rhythm.
      (3) Detects increases and decreases from FHR BL.
    c. Benefits (Feinstein, Sprague, & Trepanier, 2000)
      (1) Outcomes are comparable to those with EFM based on current randomized clinical trials (RCTs).
      (2) Lower cesarean birth rates have been associated more with auscultation than EFM in some RCTs.
      (3) Noninvasive
      (4) Widespread application
      (5) Clients have increased freedom of movement and ambulation.
      (6) Allows for FHR assessment during water immersion.
      (7) Equipment costs less than EFM.
      (8) Caregiver present by bedside to allow for 1:1 nurse-client ratio recommended based on RCTs comparing auscultation and EFM; hands-on time increased with client.

   d. Limitations (Feinstein, Sprague, & Trepanier, 2000)
      (1) May limit ability to hear FHR resulting from maternal obesity, increased amniotic fluid volume, and maternal or fetal movement.
      (2) Uterine tension disrupts assessment.
      (3) Certain FHR characteristics associated with EFM cannot be detected (e.g., variability, types of decelerations).
      (4) Some clients may believe that auscultation is more intrusive.
      (5) Is not automatically documented on paper.
      (6) Creates a potential need to increase or realign staff to meet 1:1 nurse-client ratio.
      (7) Requires education, practice, and skill in auditory assessment.
   e. Documentation
      (1) Numerical BL rate
      (2) Rhythm
      (3) Increases and decreases (abrupt or gradual) in BL rate
      (4) Timing related to contraction
      (5) Frequency (ACOG, 1995a; AWHONN, 2002; Society of Obstetricians & Gynaecologists of Canada [SOGC], 2002b)
         (a) AWHONN: auscultation and EFM
             (i) Low risk: every 30 minutes during active phase, every 15 minutes during second stage
            (ii) High risk: every 15 minutes during active phase, every 5 minutes during second stage
         (b) SOGC
             (i) Auscultation: every 15 to 30 minutes in active labor, every 5 minutes in active portion of the second stage
            (ii) EFM: every 15 minutes during the active phase of labor, at least every 5 minutes during the second stage of labor
 2. Palpation
   a. Detects relative uterine resting tone (Moffatt & Feinstein, 2003).
   b. Detects relative frequency, duration, and relative strength of uterine contractions (UCs) (Moffatt & Feinstein, 2003).
   c. Benefits
      (1) Noninvasive; allows for hands-on assessment or care of client.
      (2) Widely used; not limited by access to equipment.
      (3) Client has increased freedom of movement and ambulation.
      (4) Allows for *touch* therapy that may be reassuring to some clients.
   d. Limitations
      (1) Actual intrauterine pressures cannot be detected.
      (2) Certain conditions may limit ability to palpate contractions (e.g., maternal size, large amount of adipose tissue).
      (3) Subjective assessment that may result in different UA interpretations.
      (4) No permanent record is provided.
B. Electronic methods of FHR assessment
 1. Doppler ultrasound for FHR assessment
   a. Detects FHR BL rate, accelerations, decelerations, and long-term variability (LTV) of the FHR.
   b. Benefits
      (1) Is noninvasive.
      (2) Rupture of membranes is not required.
      (3) Creates a permanent record via hard copy, electronic disks, or microfilm process.

      (4) Can be observed from many locations when visual screens are used as a central display or as a bedside monitor to track all clients.

    c. Limitations (Moffatt & Feinstein, 2003)

      (1) Signal transmissions may be influenced by maternal obesity, occiput posterior fetal position, anterior placenta, and fetal movement (e.g., weak, absent, or false signal).

      (2) Maternal movement may be restricted.

      (3) Maternal and fetal movement may interfere with continuous record.

      (4) Artifact may artificially increase variability.

      (5) Monitor may half- or double-count, especially if FHR tachycardia or bradycardia is present.

      (6) May detect maternal aorta movement and trace as FHR, especially if fetus is small.

  2. FSE for FHR assessment

    a. Detects FHR BL rate, variability (LTV short-term variability [STV]), accelerations, and decelerations.

    b. Detects FHR dysrhythmias.

    c. Benefits

      (1) Provides continuous detection of FHR.

      (2) Accurately detects variability (LTV and STV).

      (3) Maternal position change does not alter assessment ability or tracing quality.

      (4) Provides a permanent record.

      (5) Can be observed from many locations when visual screens are used.

    d. Limitations

      (1) The procedure is invasive.

      (2) Rupture of membranes, cervical dilatation, and accessible or appropriate fetal presenting part is required.

      (3) Moist environment is required for detection of FHR.

      (4) Potential small risk of infection, fetal hemorrhage, or fetal injury is presented.

      (5) May not be accurate when fetal demise occurs; maternal heart rate will be detected and traced.

      (6) Fetal dysrhythmias may not be evident if logic or electrocardiogram (ECG) button is turned on or engaged.

      (7) Electronic interference and artifact may occur.

  3. Tocodynamometer (tocotransducer) for UA assessment

    a. Detects relative uterine resting tone.

    b. Detects relative frequency and duration of UCs.

    c. Benefits

      (1) Is noninvasive.

      (2) Is easily placed.

      (3) Ruptured membranes or cervical dilatation is not required.

      (4) Creates a tracing via hard copy, electronic disks, or microfilm process for future assessment and for permanent medical record.

    d. Limitations

      (1) Subjective assessment.

      (2) Cannot detect UC intensity and resting tone.

      (3) May be unable to accurately detect exact UC frequency and duration in some conditions (e.g., maternal obesity or preterm labor).

      (4) Location sensitive; placement may lead to false information.

(5) Sensitive to maternal or fetal motion that may be superimposed on the waveform.

(6) Transducer presence or position may be uncomfortable for mother.

(7) Maternal movement and ambulation during labor may be limited.

4. IUPC for UA assessment

   a. Detects actual uterine resting tone.

   b. Detects actual frequency, duration, and strength of UCs.

   c. Access for amniotic fluid testing (e.g., amniotic fluid sampling).

   d. Allows for amnioinfusion.

   e. Benefits

     (1) Objective; accurate assessment of UC frequency, duration, intensity, and resting tone

     (2) Correlation of timing of FHR changes with UA is more accurate.

     (3) Provides a tracing via hard copy, electronic disks, or microfilm process for future assessment and for permanent medical record.

     (4) Provides means for aspiration of amniotic fluid to assess for chorioamnionitis.

     (5) Provides means for amnioinfusion as intervention for oligohydramnios or thick meconium-stained amniotic fluid.

     (6) Solid-state IUPC is easily zeroed to atmospheric pressure.

     (7) Solid-state IUPC design avoids pressure artifacts that may be caused by a catheter containing air, becomes kinked, or lodged against the uterine wall (e.g., fluid-filled IUPC).

   f. Limitations

     (1) General

       (a) Rupture of membranes (ROM) or adequate cervical dilatation required.

       (b) Is an invasive procedure.

       (c) Maternal ambulation may be limited during labor.

       (d) Increased risk of uterine perforation (rupture), placental abruption or perforation, infection, or umbilical cord prolapse.

       (e) IUPC reading may be different between fluid- or air-filled and sensor-tipped catheters.

       (f) May be contraindicated with infections in which ROM is discouraged to prevent maternal-fetal transmission (e.g., group B-streptococcus, genital herpes, human immunodeficiency virus [HIV]).

       (g) May be contraindicated in presence of vaginal bleeding.

     (2) Fluid- or air-filled IUPC

       (a) Catheter tip may become wedged against uterine wall or fetal part; might prevent production of pressure data or produce distorted or truncated waveform.

       (b) Catheter tip may affect pressures, especially as related to external pressure transducer.

       (c) Catheter may become obstructed with meconium, vernix, or blood.

       (d) Pressure readings may be lower than solid-state (sensor-tipped) IUPC transducer.

       (e) Air may dissipate or pass through balloon at tip; may change pressure waveform or provide inaccurate pressure data (air-filled IUPC).

          (3) Solid-state IUPC

               (a) Pressure readings, including uterine resting tone, may be higher than fluid- or air-filled IUPCs.

               (b) Larger tip may require further dilatation for insertion when compared to fluid- or air-filled IUPCs.

C. Fetal factors influencing the FHR

  1. Parasympathetic nervous system

    a. Slows FHR and variability.

    b. Provides variability; greatest influence on STV.

    c. Is of vagal origin.

    d. Increases with increasing gestational age.

    e. Effect on FHR may be exaggerated during hypoxemia.

    f. Blocking (e.g., with atropine) produces increased FHR and loss of variability.

  2. Sympathetic nervous system

    a. Increases FHR and cardiac output.

    b. Some influence on variability (LTV) in conjunction with parasympathetic nervous system.

    c. Influences epinephrine and norepinephrine (epinephrine secreted in significantly smaller amounts than norepinephrine).

    d. Effect on FHR may be stimulated during hypoxemia.

    e. Blocking the sympathetic system, as with maternal medication, produces decrease in the BL FHR.

  3. Baroreceptors

    a. Located in carotid artery and aortic arch.

    b. Responds rapidly to fetal blood pressure (BP) changes; transfers information to sympathetic and parasympathetic systems.

    c. An increase in fetal BP produces decrease in the FHR, which decreases fetal cardiac output and BP.

    d. Decreases in fetal BP results in sympathetic stimulation to increase FHR.

  4. Chemoreceptors (Feinstein & Atterbury, 2003; Feinstein, Torgersen, & Atterbury, 2003)

    a. Located in aortic arch and carotid artery.

    b. Consists of peripheral receptors in the central nervous system (CNS).

    c. Responds to fetal oxygen or carbon dioxide changes and in pH levels of blood and cerebrospinal fluid; transfers information to sympathetic and parasympathetic nervous systems.

    d. Least-understood factor influencing FHR.

    e. Stimulation caused by mild increases in carbon dioxide or mild decreases in oxygen produces an increase in fetal BP and FHR; more severe changes can produce bradycardia.

  5. CNS

    a. Is responsible for variations in FHR and variability in response to fetal sleep state and body movements; in fetal sleep cycles of 20 to 40 minutes, variability and reactivity decrease.

    b. In alert states, FHR variability and reactivity increase.

    c. Is integrative center for central and peripheral neural influences that produces variability and net increase or decrease in BL FHR.

  6. Hormonal influences

    a. Catecholamines facilitate hemodynamic changes in response to hypoxemia and adaptational changes in neonate at birth (Lagercrantz & Slotkin, 1986; Parer, 1976, 1999).

   b. Epinephrine increases FHR and blood flow to skeletal muscle.
   c. Norepinephrine
      (1) Associated with initial increase in FHR (Lagercrantz & Slotkin, 1986; Parer, 1999).
      (2) Increases blood flow to vital organs and away from nonvital organs.
      (3) Hemodynamic changes elevate BP and may cause parasympathetic response resulting in decreased FHR (norepinephrine cannot overcome this parasympathetic response).
      (4) Secreted in greater amounts than found in resting adult.
   d. Vasopressin
      (1) Secreted by pituitary; increases during hypoxemia and hemorrhage.
      (2) Helps regulate BP.
      (3) Produces rise in BP by increasing peripheral vascular resistance and decreasing FHR.
      (4) Decreases blood flow to nonvital organs.
   e. Renin-angiotension system
      (1) Renin secreted by kidneys; increases in response to hemorrhage
      (2) Angiotension II
         (a) Secreted by kidneys; increases in response to hemorrhage and hypovolemia.
         (b) Exerts vasoconstriction on peripheral vascular bed resulting in maintenance of systemic arterial BP and umbilical-placental blood flow.
         (c) Increased level produces marked increase in BP with initial decrease in FHR followed by increase to higher than previous FHR; produces increased cardiac output and blood flow to heart.
         (d) Decreases renal blood flow.

CLINICAL PRACTICE
Baseline Characteristics
Baseline Fetal Heart Rate
A. Assessment
Normal rate ranges from 110 to 160 beats per minute (bpm); assessed when mother has no UC and fetus is not having periodic or nonperiodic (episodic) FHR changes; minimum of 10 minutes is needed to establish an FHR BL (Figure 12-1).
   1. Tachycardia
      a. History: possible causes
         (1) Maternal causes
            (a) Fever
            (b) Infection
            (c) Dehydration
            (d) Hyperthermia
            (e) Hyperthyroidism
            (f) Endogenous adrenaline or anxiety
            (g) Medication or drug response
               (i) Ketamine, atropine, and phenothiazines
               (ii) Hydroxyzine (Visteral and Atarax)
               (iii) Beta-sympathomimetic drugs
               (iv) Sympathomimetic bronchodilators used in asthma clients (albuterol)
               (v) Epinephrine

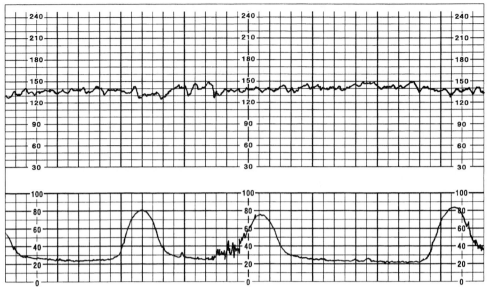

FIGURE 12-1 ■ Normal baseline FHR and average/within normal limits LTV (moderate variability).

(vi) Selected positive inotropes (e.g., dobutamine, positive chronotropic drugs)
(vii) Over-the-counter medications (e.g., decongestants, appetite suppressants, stimulants or caffeine)
(h) Illicit drugs
(i) Anemia
(j) Nicotine, if inhaled (if inhaled by smoking, may increase the FHR; if absorbed through nicotine patch, may decrease FHR [Cypher, Adelsperger, & Torgersen, 2003; Muller, Antunes, Behle, Teixeira, & Zielinsky, 2002; Oncken, Kranzler, O'Malley, Gendreau, & Campbell, 2002; Oncken, Hardardottir, Hatsukami, Lupo, Rodis, & Smeltzer, 1997]).
(2) Fetal causes (Cypher, Adelsperger, & Torgersen, 2003; King & Simpson, 2001)
(a) Infection
(b) Activity or stimulation
(c) Compensatory effort following acute hypoxemia
(d) Chronic hypoxemia
(e) Fetal hyperthyroidism
(f) Fetal tachyarrhythmias (e.g., supraventricular tachycardia [SVT])
(g) Prematurity
(h) Congenital abnormalities
(i) Cardiac abnormalities or heart failure
(j) Anemia
b. Physical findings (Figure 12-2)
(1) Persistent FHR above 160 bpm
(2) Duration of a minimum of 10 minutes with no maximum (days or weeks are possible); if persists greater than 200 to 220 bpm for extended period, can result in fetal hydrops or fetal demise (Cypher, Adelsperger, & Torgersen, 2003).

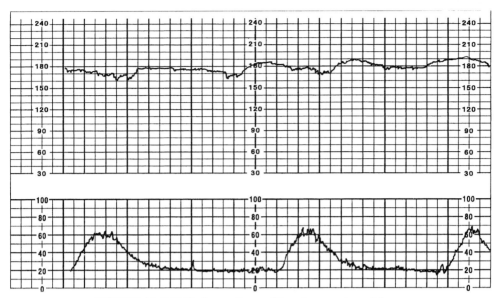

FIGURE 12-2 ■ Tachycardia resulting from maternal fever.

(3) Decreased variability common as rate increases, especially at rates above 180 bpm (Torgersen, 2003)

(4) Tachyarrhythmias and dysrhythmias more frequent

c. Related physiology

(1) Increased sympathetic tone

(2) Decreased parasympathetic tone

(3) Persistently high rate associated with fetal hydrops or fetal demise (e.g., SVT, atrial flutter, atrial fibrillation)

2. Bradycardia (Figure 12-3)

a. History: possible causes

(1) Maternal causes

(a) Mother lying in supine position

(b) Hypotension

(2) Anesthetic agents (e.g., epidural, spinal, pudendal, paracervical)

(3) Adrenergic-receptor blocking agents (e.g., propranolol)

(4) Connective tissue disease (e.g., systemic lupus erythematosus) (Hohn & Stanton, 2002; Tucker, 2000)

(5) Prolonged maternal hypoglycemia

(6) Conditions that cause acute maternal cardiopulmonary compromise (e.g., pulmonary embolus, anaphylactoid syndrome of pregnancy [formally amniotic fluid embolism], trauma, uterine rupture)

(7) Fetal causes

(a) Mature parasympathetic nervous system

(b) Acute hypoxemia

(c) Hypothermia

(d) Umbilical cord occlusion

(e) Congenital complete heart block (CCHB)

(f) Cardiac structural defect (resulting from maternal cytomegalovirus infection)

(g) Excessive parasympathetic nervous system tone (i.e., vagal stimulation) resulting from chronic head compression in a vertex

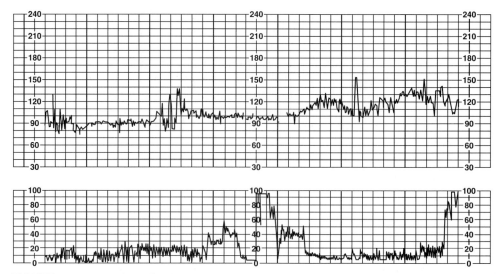

FIGURE 12-3 ■ Bradycardia. (From Feinstein, N.F., Torgersen, K.L., & Atterbury, J.L. [Eds.]. [2003]. *Fetal heart monitoring principles and practices* [3rd ed.]. Dubuque, IA: Kendall-Hunt Publications.)

presentation, occiput posterior, or transverse position; FHR usually does not decrease to less than 90 to 100 bpm in this situation (Cypher, Adelsperger, & Torgersen, 2003).
   (h) Late or profound hypoxemia
   b. Physical findings
      (1) FHR below 110 bpm
      (2) Bradycardia accompanied by adequate variability may be normal (fetal dependent).
      (3) Duration of at least 10 minutes
      (4) If physiologic bradycardia during labor, found to have bradycardia in the nursery; considered well oxygenated and normal (Garite, 2002)
      (5) Average (moderate) variability less likely if FHR persists at rate less than 90 bpm for more than 10 minutes; if variability and accelerations present, is considered benign or reassuring and not associated with acidemia (Freeman, Garite, & Nageotte, 1991; King & Parer, 2000).
      (6) Bradycardia accompanied by loss of variability and late decelerations may indicate current or impending fetal hypoxia (NICHD Research Planning Workshop, 1997).
   c. Related physiology
      (1) Excessive parasympathetic nervous system tone
      (2) Rate of approximately 60 to 70 bpm in second trimester and 50 to 60 bpm at term without variability may indicate CCHB (Eronen, Heikkila, & Teramo, 2001).
      (3) Bradycardia may be related to maternal hypotension secondary to supine hypotension, hypovolemia, vasodilatation following epidural anesthesia, or maternal catecholamine production.
      (4) The lower the FHR gets, the lower the fetal cardiac output (Cypher, Adelsperger, & Torgersen, 2003).

(5) Bradycardia less than 60 bpm or associated with decreased variability requires immediate attention and collaborative management (Cypher, Adelsperger, & Torgersen, 2003).
(6) Rate must be differentiated from maternal rate (use real time ultrasound or palpate maternal apical pulse and compare to FHR).
(7) Rate must be differentiated from prolonged deceleration (prolonged deceleration duration is more than 2 minutes but less than 10 minutes; if deceleration is more than 10 minutes, bradycardia occurs).

B. Nursing Diagnoses
1. Risk for impaired fetal gas exchange related to intrapartum physiologic changes that reduce oxygen levels
2. Maternal anxiety related to fetal status
3. Impaired maternal comfort related to immobility

C. Interventions/Outcomes
1. Risk for impaired fetal gas exchange related to intrapartum physiologic changes that reduce oxygen levels
  a. Interventions
    (1) Tachycardia
      (a) Monitor maternal vital signs, specifically temperature and pulse.
      (b) Increase or initiate hydration with intravenous fluids as needed.
      (c) Initiate interventions to decrease maternal temperature, if elevated (e.g., antipyretics).
      (d) Assess for possible tachyarrhythmias or dysrhythmias; administer appropriate medications to lower FHR (e.g., cardiac agents for SVT, tocolytic agents or discontinuation of uterine-stimulating agents to enhance placental blood flow).
      (e) Perform scalp stimulation for tachyarrhythmias or dysrhythmias.
        (i) Vagal stimulation may lower tachycardic FHR.
        (ii) FHR accelerations following scalp stimulation usually rule out an acidotic fetus.
      (f) Reduce anxiety, offer explanations, provide comfort measures, and assist with breathing and relaxation techniques (Adelsperger & Waymire, 2003).
      (g) Change or maintain maternal position that optimizes uteroplacental perfusion (e.g., side lying, walking).
      (h) Administer oxygen (8 to 10 L/min via snug face mask) as needed.
      (i) Assess for use of illicit and legal drugs and alcohol.
      (j) If auscultating, intervene as needed and consider application of EFM to further assess FHR, variability, and periodic and nonperiodic (episodic) changes.
    (2) Bradycardia
      (a) Assess maternal vital signs, specifically BP.
      (b) Validate FHR versus maternal HR.
      (c) Evaluate fetal movement.
      (d) Perform vaginal examination for possible cord prolapse; if prolapse evident, elevate fetal presenting part off of cord.
      (e) Note: scalp stimulation has been noted in the past as an intervention for bradycardia. In a nonreassuring FHR (bradycardia or prolonged decelerations without variability or accelerations), scalp stimulation is not recommended. Scalp stimulation in this instance will elicit a vagal response that overrides the sympathetic response and results in a further drop

in the FHR (Harvey, 1987; Murray, 2001; Reddy, Paine, Gegor, Johnson, & Johnson, 1991).
  (f) Accurately document FHR findings and interventions.
  b. Outcomes
    (1) No evidence of fetal tachycardia or bradycardia on the fetal monitor
    (2) Maternal vital signs (to include blood pressure) remain within or return to normal limits.
    (3) No cord felt on vaginal examination
    (4) Use of all drugs assessed and documented
    (5) FHR tracing is actually fetal.
  2. Maternal anxiety related to fetal status
    a. Interventions
      (1) Provide information and reassurance as needed regarding the possible changes in BL FHR.
      (2) Provide information and reassurance about current fetal status and care process.
      (3) Explain the reasons for the interventions; give directions clearly and calmly (e.g., repositioning desired).
      (4) Remain with the client, and encourage a significant other to remain when possible.
      (5) Guide maternal breathing techniques to prevent hyperventilation (hyperventilation causes hypocapnia [increased carbon dioxide in blood] that can lead to hypoventilation) (Adelsperger & Waymire, 2003).
      (6) Encourage and coach mother to use open glottis pushing during second stage labor (helps to decrease prolonged breath holding thus improving oxygen availability to mother and fetus).
    b. Outcomes
      (1) Mother reports a decrease in anxiety.
      (2) Support person remains at the bedside.
      (3) Body posture is less tense.
      (4) Fetus maintains stable FHR with adequate variability.
  3. Impaired maternal comfort related to immobility
    a. Interventions
      (1) Change her position frequently.
      (2) Use comfort measures (e.g., pillows, blankets, back rubs, ice).
      (3) Explain why certain positions may be necessary to maintain or improve favorable fetal heart characteristics.
      (4) Encourage mother to ambulate, or use alternative methods of labor management, or both (e.g., labor ball, squatting position, rocking chair, shower).
    b. Outcomes
      (1) Mother changes positions when requested and as desired for her own comfort.
      (2) Mother indicates an understanding of the necessity for certain position changes.
      (3) Mother ambulates or uses alternative methods of labor management.

Variability

A. Assessment
  1. Variability is defined as "the variations or fluctuations of the FHR during a steady state (in the absence of contractions, decelerations, and accelerations)" (Cypher, Adelsperger, & Torgersen, 2003, p. 120). The two branches of the

autonomic nervous system (parasympathetic and sympathetic nervous systems) have opposite effects on the FHR. The parasympathetic nervous system slows the FHR, and the sympathetic nervous system speeds the FHR. This continual *push-and-pull* effect produces the moment-to-moment change in the FHR that is called variability. Variability is interpreted as a single combined term (NICHD Research Planning Workshop, 1997); however, it is important to understand the different types of variability, specifically LTV and STV. These two types provide for us the visual tracing that is recorded on the EFM. This section, as others, is written to agree with the AWHONN Fetal Heart Monitoring Principles and Practices course content.

a. History (variability)

　(1) Described as normal irregularity of cardiac rhythm (Tucker, 2000).

　(2) Influenced by fetal oxygenation status, cardiac output regulation, fetal behavior during fetal sleep-wake states, humoral regulation, and drug effects (Freeman, Garite, & Nageotte, 1991; Martin, 1982; Parer, 1997; Petrie, 1991). Also influenced by alcohol and illicit drugs that can cause fetal neurological damage thus affecting variability: morphine (Kopecky, Ryan, Barrett, Seaward, Ryan, Koren, et al., 2000), methadone (Anyaegbunam, Tran, Jadali, Randolph, & Mikhail, 1997), anomalies, and previous insults damaging the fetal brain (Wadhwa, Sandman, & Garite, 2001).

　(3) Impulse transmission to the FHR is influenced by CNS oxygenation

　(4) Adequate oxygenation and a mature and functioning autonomic nervous system contribute to production of variability (LTV and STV) (Cypher, Adelsperger, & Torgersen, 2003).

　(5) Absent or decreased (minimal) variability may be associated with preterm fetus (under 28 to 32 weeks' gestation), alteration in the function of the nervous system, inadequate oxygenation, or any combination (Cypher, Adelsperger, & Torgersen, 2003).

　(6) NICHD nomenclature describes and communicates variability as one unit (versus LTV and STV); however, it is still important to understand the physiology of both LTV and STV.

　　(a) LTV characterized by oscillations and described as cycles per minute. Frequency of cycles are 3 to 6 per minute (Hammacher, 1969; Martin, 1982; King & Simpson, 2001; Parer, 1997). LTV is measured by amplitude (bpm) and the number of cycles per minute in BL rate not to include accelerations or decelerations. Consensus has yet to be achieved for standardization for categories of LTV; however, the LTV categories definitions correspond to the NICHD definitions for combined variability (Cypher, Adelsperger, & Torgersen, 2003). Information below also adapted from Cypher, Adelsperger, and Torgersen.

　　　(i) Amplitude < 3 bpm; description = undetectable, LTV category = decreased or minimal; NICHD category = absent variability (Figure 12-4)

　　　(ii) Amplitude 3 to 5 bpm; description = > undetectable but < 5 bpm; LTV category = decreased or minimal; NICHD category = minimal variability (Figure 12-5)

　　　(iii) Amplitude 6 to 25 bpm; description = 6 to 25 bpm; LTV category = average or within normal limits; NICHD category = moderate variability (see Figure 12-1)

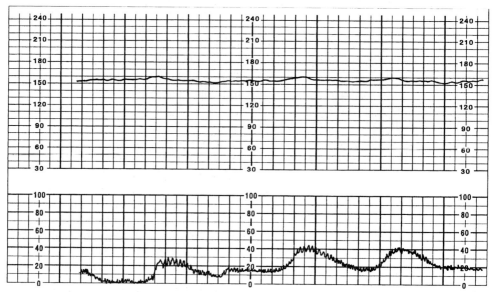

FIGURE 12-4 ■ Absent variability.

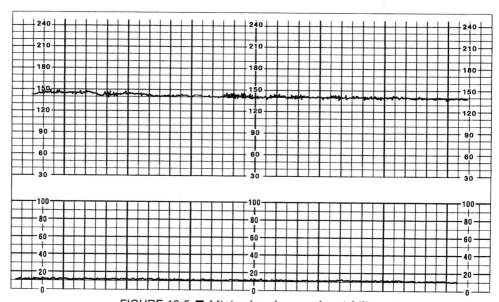

FIGURE 12-5 ■ Minimal or decreased variability.

     (iv) Amplitude > 25 bpm; description = > 25 bpm; LTV
         category = marked or saltatory; NICHD category = marked
         variability (Figure 12-6)
  (b) STV is defined as "the moment-to-moment changes (reflecting
     R-to-R intervals) in the FHR that, when printed on EFM, generally
     produce a small, irregular nature of the BL" (Cypher, Adelsperger,
     & Torgersen, 2003, p. 124).
     (i) Indicative of well-oxygenated, nonacidemic fetus
     (ii) Influenced by parasympathetic nervous system

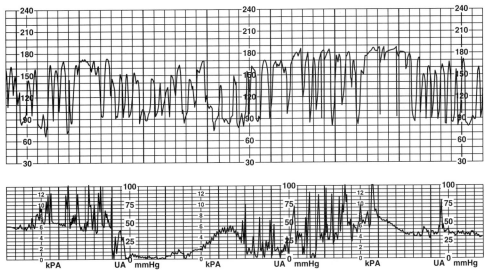

FIGURE 12-6 ■ Marked or saltatory variability.

(iii) If hypoxia is present, impulse transmission is decreased resulting in decreased variability, indicating the fetal compensatory mechanisms have failed in their job to maintain fetal cerebral oxygenation (Parer, 1999).

(iv) Fetal spiral electrode (FSE) provides an accurate assessment of STV (Garite, 2002); and because of the rapid and sometimes subtle changes, the more accurate method to assess STV is with internal (FSE), continuous monitoring (ACOG, 1995b; Cypher, Adelsperger, & Torgersen, 2003; May & Mahlmeister, 1994).

(v) Evaluated for the roughness or smoothness of the tracing.
- Tracing appears rough = present STV (Figure 12-7)
- Tracing appears smooth = absent STV (Figure 12-8)

(7) Because of interrelated physiologic components of LTV and STV, can be interpreted as a single entity. This concept is known as combined variability (Cypher, Adelsperger, & Torgersen, 2003; NICHD Research Planning Workshop, 1997).

(8) Undulating patterns
  (a) Defined as "repeating cycles or changes in the FHR that result in an upward increase in the rate followed by a decrease in the rate" (Cypher, Adelsperger, & Torgersen, 2003, p. 126).
  (b) BL rate is usually within 110 to 160 bpm, frequency of 3 to 5 cycles and amplitude undulations 5 to 15 bpm above and below the baseline.
  (c) Described as pseudosinusoidal or sinusoidal.
  (d) It can be difficult to differentiate pseudosinusoidal from sinusoidal; therefore, in those instances, the pattern is described as undulating.
  (e) Pseudosinusoidal characteristics (Figure 12-9)
    (i) Saw-toothed appearances; BL rate 110 to 160 bpm
    (ii) Less uniform oscillations
    (iii) Periods of normal (moderate) variability (LTV and STV)

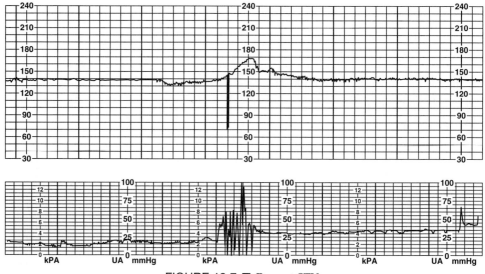

FIGURE 12-7 ■ Present STV.

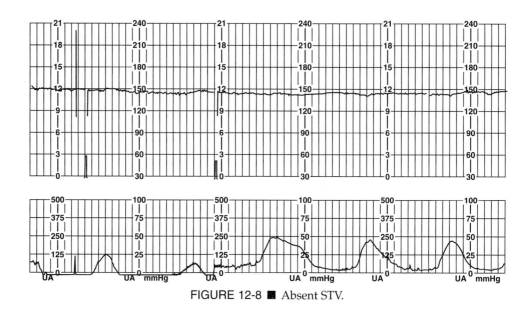

FIGURE 12-8 ■ Absent STV.

     (iv) Accelerations may be present.

     (v) Associated with:

         ▪ Narcotic or analgesic administration or ingestion

         ▪ Fetal thumb sucking

         ▪ Unknown causes

  (f) Sinusoidal characteristics (Figure 12-10)

     (i) Persistent oscillating pattern; BL rate 110 to 160 bpm

     (ii) Amplitude of undulations usually 5 to 15 bpm above and below BL rate

     (iii) Frequency of undulation usually 2 to 5 cycles per minute

     (iv) Absent STV

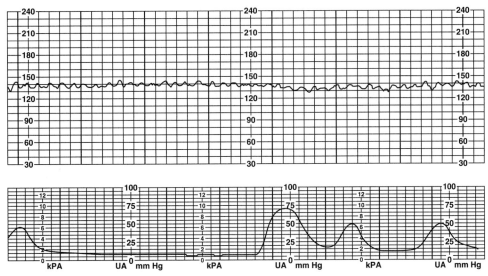

FIGURE 12-9 ■ Undulating pattern (pseudosinusoidal).

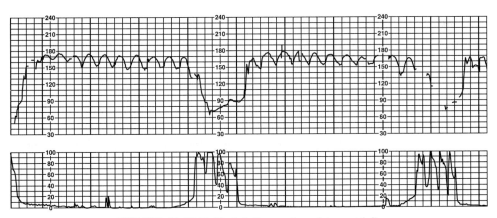

FIGURE 12-10 ■ Undulating pattern (sinusoidal).

   (v) No accelerations present even in response to fetal stimulation
       or fetal movement
  (vi) Associated with:
       ▪ Severe fetal anemia (Rh isoimmunization; abruptio
         placentae; fetal-maternal hemorrhage; severe fetal acidosis)
         (Garite, 2002; King & Simpson, 2001; Parer, 1997)
       ▪ Unknown causes
2. Arrhythmias and dysrhythmias
   a. History
      (1) Approximately 2% to 14% of all pregnancies exhibit fetal dysrhythmic
          patterns (Chan, Woo, Ghosh, Tang, & Lam, 1990; Copel, Buyon, &
          Kleinman, 1995; DeVore, Siassi, & Platt, 1984; Southall, Arrowsmith,
          Oakley, McEnergy, Anderson, & Shinebourne, 1979). Of these, 90% are
          benign, requiring little or no intervention; however, 10% are

potentially life threatening (Bianchi, Crobleholme, & D'Alton, 2000; Drose, 1998).

(2) Terms dysrhythmia and arrhythmia often used interchangeably; however, they represent two distinct patterns.

　(a) Arrhythmia = FHR without rhythm; describes sporadic, irregular beats; associated with variability of the R-to-R intervals; on ECG, shows normal P wave occurring in normal association with each QRS complex (Torgersen, 2003)

　(b) Dysrhythmia = fetal heart rhythm associated with disordered impulse formation, impulse conduction, or a combination of both (Cabaniss, 1993); on ECG, shows early P waves, or bizarre-looking QRS complexes, or both

(3) Dysrhythmias and arrhythmias derive their names from the anatomic site of variant impulse formation, conduction, or both (Torgersen, 2003).

b. Physical findings

(1) A pattern irregularity is audible by auscultation and usually by ultrasound and electrode methods; pattern irregularity can be observed with internal EFM using FSE.

(2) Causes:

　(a) Conduction system defects

　(b) Cardiomyopathy

　(c) Cardiac tumors

　(d) Cardiac structural disease

　(e) Maternal collagen disease

　(f) Infections such as cytomegalovirus or Coxsackie B viruses

　(g) Most return to normal sinus rhythm shortly after birth.

　(h) Diagnosis may be aided by Doppler velocimetry, fetal echocardiogram (EchoCG), fetal magnetocardiography, M-mode EchoCG, or pulsed Doppler EchoCG.

c. Fetal arrhythmias

(1) Sinus node variants

　(a) Sinus bradycardia (see Figure 12-3)

　　(i) FHR < 110 bpm lasting for > 10 minutes; from standpoint of arrhythmia, some describe as FHR < 100 bpm (Crosson & Brenner, 1999; Shaffer & Wiggins, 1998; Sharland, 2001; Strasburger, 2000)

　　(ii) Normal P-QRS complex

　　(iii) Most common cause is head compression; less frequent causes are hypothermia, hypoxia, and response to drugs such as beta-blocking agents.

　　(iv) Persistent rates of < 100 bpm is considered unusual and associated with intrauterine growth restriction (IUGR), increased vagal tone, maternal beta-blocker therapy, prolonged QT syndrome or severe hydrops (Allan, Crawford, Anderson, & Tynan, 1984; Ferrer, 1998; Meijboom, van Engelen, van de Beek, Weijtens, Lautenschutz, & Benatar, 1994; Shaffer & Wiggins, 1998; Sharland, 2001; Southall, Arrowsmith, Oakley, McEnergy, Anderson, & Shinebourne, 1979).

　(b) Sinus tachycardia (see Figure 12-2)

　　(i) FHR > 160 bpm lasting > 10 minutes; from standpoint of arrhythmia, some describe as FHR >180 bpm (Crosson &

Brenner, 1999; Shaffer & Wiggins, 1998; Sharland, 2001; Strasburger, 2000)
   (ii) Normal P-QRS complex
  (iii) Most common cause = continuous fetal activity, maternal fever, or certain medications such as betasympathomimetic drugs (terbutaline or ritodrine) or parasympatholytic medications (atropine, hydralazine [Apresoline], or hydroxyzine hydrochloride [Atarax]; other causes = compensatory response to hypoxia, secondary to baroreceptor or chemoreceptor stimulation (Shaffer & Wiggins, 1998), acidosis, myocarditis, maternal drug ingestion, and hormone or catecholamine transfer (Mucklow, 1986; Pickoff, 1998)
 (c) Marked sinus arrhythmia (Figure 12-11)
   (i) FHR pattern shows changes as much as 120 bpm within 5-second intervals.
  (ii) Unless repetitive, no significant change in fetal oxygenation is noted (Reiss, Gabbe, & Petrie, 2001).
  (iii) Most common cause = parasympathetic response to fetal hypoxemia (Cabaniss, 1993; Murray, 2001); often seen with increased UA; commonly associated with bradycardia and seen preceding prolonged or nonreassuring variable decelerations (King & Simpson, 2001; Tucker, 2000)
  d. Fetal dysrhythmias
   (1) Supraventricular—pattern originates above the ventricles
    (a) Premature atrial contractions (PAC) (Figure 12-12)—associated with redundancy or an aneurysm of the foraminal flap (Fyfe, Meyer, & Case, 1988; Stewart & Wladimiroff, 1988) and maternal use of caffeine, cigarettes, or alcohol (Nyberg & Emerson, 1990; Strasburger, 2000); premature P wave followed by narrow,

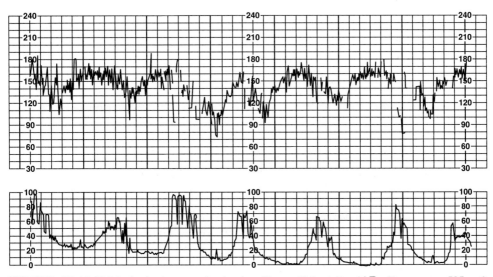

FIGURE 12-11 ■ Marked sinus arrhythmia. (From Feinstein, N.F., Torgersen, K.L., & Atterbury, J.L. [Eds.]. [2003]. *Fetal heart monitoring principles and practices* [3rd ed.]. Dubuque, IA: Kendall-Hunt Publications.)

normal-appearing QRS complex; EFM tracing shows vertical spikes above and below the BL FHR; upper line = premature beat (often above 180 bpm); lower line = partial (incomplete) compensatory pause and is short distance from FHR BL; middle line = FHR

(i) PAC with bigeminy (Figure 12-13)
- PAC occurs with every other beat (e.g., normal beat followed by one premature beat [PAC]).
- Most frequent type of intrapartum fetal dysrhythmia (Cabaniss, 1993; Strasburger, 2000)

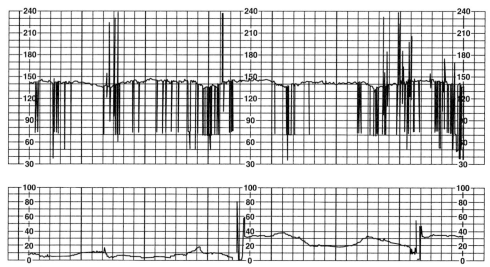

FIGURE 12-12 ■ Premature atrial contraction (PAC). (From Feinstein, N.F., Torgersen, K.L., & Atterbury, J.L. [Eds.]. [2003]. *Fetal heart monitoring principles and practices* [3rd ed.]. Dubuque, IA: Kendall-Hunt Publications.)

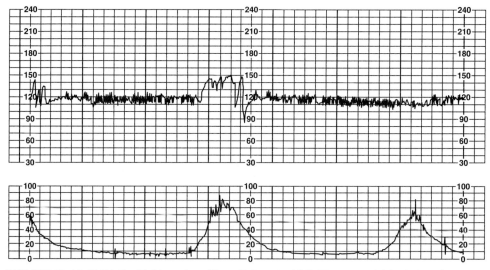

FIGURE 12-13 ■ PAC with bigeminy. (From Feinstein, N.F., Torgersen, K.L., & Atterbury, J.L. [Eds.]. [2003]. *Fetal heart monitoring principles and practices* [3rd ed.]. Dubuque, IA: Kendall-Hunt Publications.)

- EFM tracing shows two horizontal parallel lines; upper line = rate between normal and premature beats; lower line = partial (incomplete) compensatory pause; BL FHR obscured.
  (ii) PAC with trigeminy (Figure 12-14)
  - PAC occurs every third beat (e.g., two normal beats followed by one premature beat [PAC]).
  - EFM tracing shows vertical spikes with long upward strokes and short downward strokes (Cabaniss, 1993; Torgersen, 2003); upward stroke = premature beat; downward stroke = partial (incomplete) compensatory pause; FHR BL seen intermittently.
  (iii) PAC with bigeminy and trigeminy
  - Bigeminal pattern will dominate.
  - EFM tracing will show uninterrupted parallel vertical lines with FHR BL obscured (Cabaniss, 1993; Murray, 2001; Strasburger, 2000).
  (iv) Nonconducted PAC (Figure 12-15)
  - Premature beat too premature to conduct through atrioventricular (AV) junction.
  - EFM tracing shows upper line = FHR BL; lower line = pause produced by nonconducted premature beat; FHR BL is visible.
  - Because of slow ventricular rate produced, it may be difficult to differentiate nonconducted PAC from complete heart block (Sharland, 2001).
(b) SVT (Figure 12-16)
  (i) Sustained, rapid, regular dysrhythmia in excess of 180 to 210 bpm
  (ii) May occur suddenly or in waves or spasms (paroxysmal) or may be continuous.

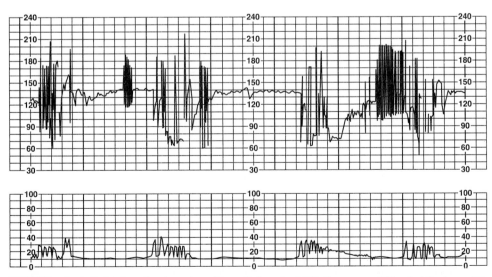

FIGURE 12-14 ■ PAC with trigeminy. (From Feinstein, N.F., Torgersen, K.L., & Atterbury, J.L. [Eds.]. [2003]. *Fetal heart monitoring principles and practices* [3rd ed.]. Dubuque, IA: Kendall-Hunt Publications.)

(iii) If rate < 210 bpm, may show variability within BL rate around 5 to 15 bpm (Shaffer & Wiggins, 1998); EFM may half count the FHR.

(iv) ECG = fixed R-to-R interval with P waves preceding each QRS complex

(v) May contribute to increased birth weight, heavier placenta and neonatal diuresis of a few day's duration (often related to hydrops fetalis) (Crosson & Brenner, 1999); also associated with beta-mimetic therapy (terbutaline or ritodrine) (Cabaniss, 1993).

(vi) Can come directly from atria without relying on ventricles to sustain tachycardic rate = primary atrial tachycardia; if

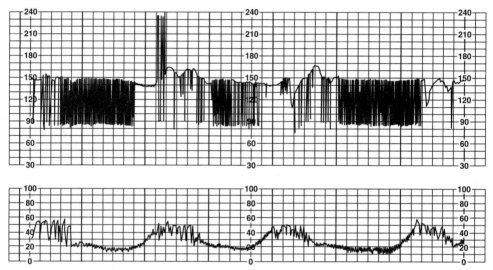

FIGURE 12-15 ■ Nonconducted PAC. (From Feinstein, N.F., Torgersen, K.L., & Atterbury, J.L. [Eds.]. [2003]. *Fetal heart monitoring principles and practices* [3rd ed.]. Dubuque, IA: Kendall-Hunt Publications.)

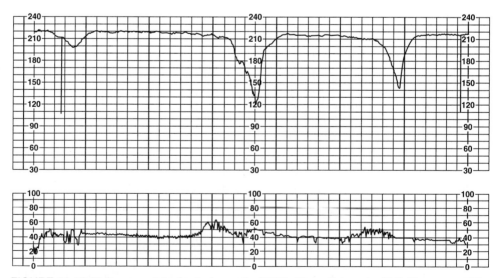

FIGURE 12-16 ■ Supraventricular tachycardia (SVT). (From Feinstein, N.F., Torgersen, K.L., & Atterbury, J.L. [Eds.]. [2003]. *Fetal heart monitoring principles and practices* [3rd ed.]. Dubuque, IA: Kendall-Hunt Publications.)

occurs, fetus usually manifests Wolff-Parkinson-White syndrome (Crosson & Brenner, 1999).

(c) Atrial flutter (Figure 12-17)

(i) Incidence low; associated with high fetal mortality because of difficulty in controlling the pattern and its association with congenital cardiac anomalies (Kleinman, Nehgme, & Copel, 1999; Shaffer & Wiggins, 1998; Strasburger, 2000).

(ii) Rates range from 400 to 500 bpm for fetus and 300 to 360 bpm for neonate.

(iii) ECG = regularly recurring saw-toothed atrial activity instead of normal P wave; EFM may half count the FHR.

(iv) Associated with reentrant SVT, atrial septal defect, hypoplastic left heart syndrome; Ebstein's malformation of the tricuspid valve, cardiomyopathy; although very rare, is associated with familial rickets and dislocated hip (Ferrer, 1998; Kleinman, Donnerstein, Jaffe, DeVore, Weinstein, Lynch, et al., 1983; Shenker, 1979).

(d) Atrial fibrillation

(i) More rare than atrial flutter (Kleinman, Nehgme, & Copel, 1999; Strasburger, 2000)

(ii) Associated with fetomaternal hemorrhage, neonatal Wolff-Parkinson-White syndrome, and cardiac structural abnormalities.

(iii) In antepartum period, variable degree of AV block will cause ventricular rate to vary from 60 to 200 bpm.

(iv) ECG = low-amplitude irregular atrial activity with complexes of various sizes (Cabaniss, 1993; Torgersen, 2003)

(2) Ventricular—ventricular in origin; result of premature electrical discharge below the AV junction; considered benign; tend to disappear in late labor or soon after birth; require no treatment in utero or postnatally; if present, mother should avoid cardiac stimulants (Strasburger, 2000).

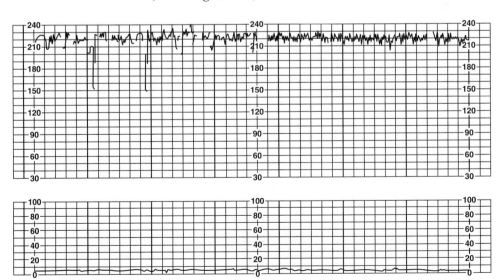

FIGURE 12 17 ■ Atrial flutter. (From Feinstein, N.F., Torgersen, K.L., & Atterbury, J.L. [Eds.]. [2003]. *Fetal heart monitoring principles and practices* [3rd ed.]. Dubuque, IA: Kendall-Hunt Publications.)

(a) Premature ventricular contractions (PVC) (Figure 12-18)—
extremely rare in the fetus (Murray, 2001; Strasburger, 2000);
associated with cardiomyopathy, long QT syndrome, complete AV
block with rates < 55 bpm, hydrops fetalis, myocarditis, digitalis
toxicity, cocaine use, hyperkalemia resulting from hyperemesis
(rare in pregnancy), structural cardiac anomalies or unknown
reasons (Allan, Crawford, Anderson, & Tynan, 1984; Cabaniss,
1993; Ferrer, 1998; Murray, 2001; Silverman, Kleinman, Rudolph,
Copel, Weinstein, Enderlein, et al., 1985; Southall Arrowsmith,
Oakley, McEnergy, Anderson, & Shinebourne, 1979); frequency
may be increased by maternal use of caffeine, nicotine or alcohol
(Cabaniss, 1993).

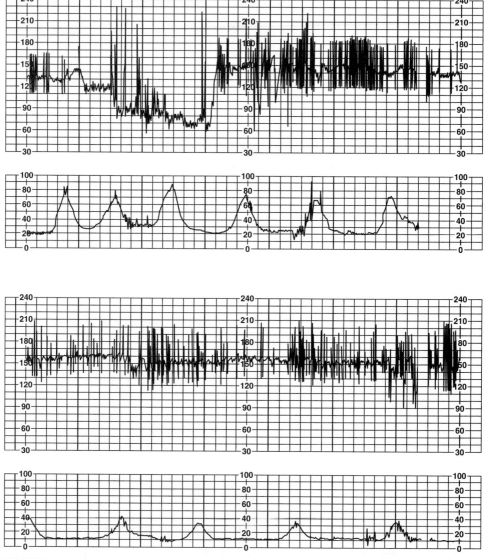

FIGURE 12-18 ■ Premature ventricular contraction (PVC). (From Feinstein, N.F., Torgersen, K.L., & Atterbury, J.L. [Eds.]. [2003]. *Fetal heart monitoring principles and practices* [3rd ed.]. Dubuque, IA: Kendall-Hunt Publications.)

(i) PVC with bigeminy (Figure 12-19)
- Will show no middle line.
- FHR or variability obscured

(ii) PVC with trigeminy (Figure 12-20)
- Top line = premature beat
- Bottom line = full compensatory pause
- Middle line = FHR; because of only every third beat being seen, middle line does not represent true beat-to-beat variability (Cabaniss, 1993).

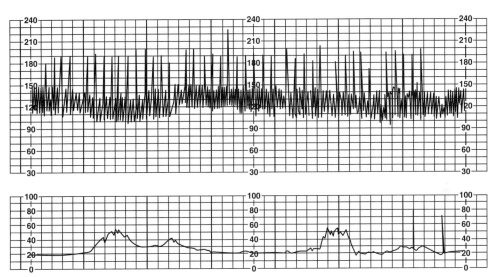

FIGURE 12-19 ■ PVC with bigeminy. (From Feinstein, N.F., Torgersen, K.L., & Atterbury, J.L. [Eds.]. [2003]. *Fetal heart monitoring principles and practices* [3rd ed.]. Dubuque, IA: Kendall-Hunt Publications.)

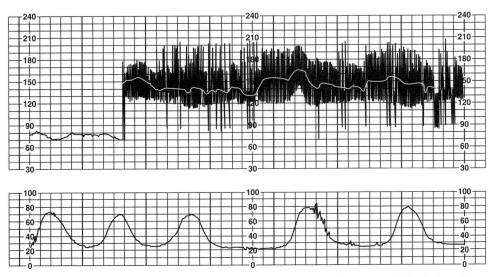

FIGURE 12-20 ■ PVC with trigeminy. (From Feinstein, N.F., Torgersen, K.L., & Atterbury, J.L. [Eds.]. [2003]. *Fetal heart monitoring principles and practices* [3rd ed.]. Dubuque, IA: Kendall-Hunt Publications.)

- Upward and downward strokes are of unequal distance from FHR BL, with upward stroke appearing longer than downward stroke (Torgersen, 2003).
    (iii) PVC with bigeminy and trigeminy (Figure 12-21)—BL FHR can appear as uninterrupted line; gives appearance of dotted line between PVCs.
  (b) Ventricular tachycardia
    (i) Rare fetal abnormality
    (ii) FHR varies between 170 and 500 bpm.
    (iii) May or may not require treatment (Kleinman, Nehgme, & Copel, 1999; Shaffer & Wiggins, 1998; Strasburger, 2000).
(3) Atrioventricular—result from AV conduction defect; first-degree AV block is difficult to recognize in the fetus and has no known pathophysiology (Cabaniss, 1993). Second-degree heart block, Mobitz type I (Wenckebach) is not seen in the fetus.
  (a) Second-degree heart block (Mobitz type II)—difficult to diagnose in the fetus because of atrial and ventricular rates appearing as the same rate
    (i) Associated with rapid atrial rate resulting from SVT, atrial flutter, or atrial fibrillation.
    (ii) Associated with maternal collagen vascular disease and cardiac structural defects (Crosson & Brenner, 1999; Kleinman, Nehgme, & Copel, 1999; Strasburger, 2000).
  (b) Third-degree (complete) heart block (Figure 12-22)
    (i) Caused by maternal anti-SSA (B) antibodies or congenital heart disease (Torgersen, 2003); associated with fetal cytomegalovirus infection and antiphospholipid antibody syndrome (Kleinman, Nehgme, & Copel, 1999; Strasburger, 2000).
    (ii) Two categories: (a) CCHB associated with complex congenital heart disease or (b) complete heart block secondary to

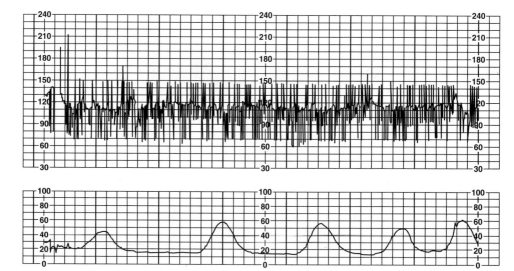

FIGURE 12-21 ■ PVC with bigeminy and trigeminy. (From Feinstein, N.F., Torgersen, K.L., & Atterbury, J.L. [Eds.]. [2003]. *Fetal heart monitoring principles and practices* [3rd ed.]. Dubuque, IA: Kendall-Hunt Publications.)

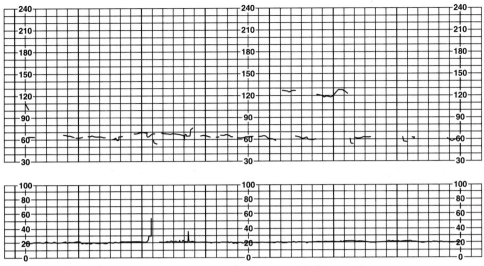

FIGURE 12-22 ■ Third-degree (complete) heart block. (From Feinstein, N.F., Torgersen, K.L., & Atterbury, J.L. [Eds.]. [2003]. *Fetal heart monitoring principles and practices* [3rd ed.]. Dubuque, IA: Kendall-Hunt Publications.)

autoimmune disease-producing autoantibodies that destroy fetal cardiac conductive tissue (Freidman, Zervoudakis, & Buyon, 1998; Horsfall, Venables, Taylor, & Maini, 1991; Litsey, Noonan, O'Connor, Cottrill, & Mitchell, 1985; Moodley, Vaughan, Chuntarpursat, Wood, Noddeboe, & Schwarting, 1986; Schmidt, Ulmer, Silverman, Kleinman, & Copel, 1991; Tanel & Rhodes, 2001; Taylor, Scott, Gerlis, Esscher, & Scott, 1986)

(iii) Fetuses do well in utero and usually require intervention only after delivery.

B. Nursing Diagnoses

1. Risk for impaired fetal uteroplacental gas exchange and hypoxia
2. Risk for ineffective fetal perfusion related to hypoxic myocardial dysfunction or anomaly
3. Risk for neurogenically mediated fetal loss of variability
4. Risk for postdelivery fetal interventions resulting from myocardial dysfunction
5. Maternal anxiety related to fetal status

C. Interventions/Outcomes

1. Risk for impaired fetal gas exchange related to intrapartal reduction of oxygen levels
   a. Interventions
      (1) For decreased LTV
         (a) Change maternal position to a lateral position.
         (b) Administer oxygen (8 to 10 L/min) via snug face mask.
         (c) Assess hydration and initiate or increase intravenous fluids.
         (d) Assess maternal hemoglobin and hematocrit; if levels indicate anemia, notify primary care provider for preparation and administration of blood as ordered.
         (e) If oxytocin is being administered, discontinue the infusion.

(f) If hyperstimulation is observed, and because of oxytocin or other uterotonics, discontinue oxytocin; if hyperstimulation unresolved or not a result of oxytocin or other uterotonics, administer tocolytics (e.g., terbutaline), as ordered or per protocol.

(g) Investigate maternal medication intake and possible use of therapeutic or illicit drugs, alcohol, or tobacco.

(h) Observe for alternating periods of average (moderate) variability and accelerations; determine if the fetus is in a sleep cycle; attempt to awaken fetus only when immediate evaluation is necessary.

(i) Encourage mother to alter her breathing, or pushing patterns, or both.

(j) Communicate findings to primary care provider; document findings.

(2) For marked or saltatory LTV

(a) Change maternal position to lateral position.

(b) Assess hydration and initiate or increase intravenous fluids.

(c) Discontinue oxytocin or other uterotonic drugs; administer tocolytics if no change in UA occurs.

(d) Administer oxygen (8 to 10 L/min) via snug face mask.

(e) Coach mother to alter her breathing or pushing techniques.

(f) Communicate findings to primary care provider; document findings.

(3) For Absent STV (variability)

(a) Change maternal position to lateral position.

(b) Assess hydration and initiate or increase intravenous fluids.

(c) Discontinue oxytocin or other uterotonic drugs; administer tocolytics if no change in UA occurs.

(d) Administer oxygen (8 to 10 L/min) via snug face mask

(e) Palpate uterus to assess relaxation between UCs.

(f) Assess tracing for accelerations; assess tracing for other nonreassuring signs (e.g., late, variable, or prolonged decelerations; rising BL FHR).

(g) Assess maternal vital signs.

(h) Perform scalp stimulation, vibroacoustic stimulation, or scalp sampling to assess fetal acid-base status.

(i) Attach fetal scalp oximeter (if available).

(j) Communicate findings to primary care provider; document findings.

(k) Plan for expedited delivery and possible resuscitation of the neonate.

(4) For undulating patterns: pseudosinusoidal patterns require observation. However, sinusoidal patterns may require the following interventions:

(a) Change maternal position to lateral position.

(b) Assess hydration and initiate or increase intravenous (IV) fluids.

(c) Administer oxygen (8 to 10 L/min) via snug face mask.

(d) Notify primary health care provider.

(e) Further interventions are dependent on cause of pattern.

(i) Kleihauer Betke test

(ii) Expeditious delivery

(iii) Intrauterine blood transfusion to fetus via cordocentesis (requires tertiary care facility and skilled staff)

(5) For arrhythmic patterns—interventions are the same as discussed in previous FHR BL section.
(6) For dysrhythmic patterns
  (a) SVT
    (i) Observation if pregnancy near term, if tachycardic episodes are short-lived, and if fetal cardiac failure is not evident (Torgersen, 2003)
    (ii) Early delivery (before term) dependent on gestational age and presence of fetal cardiac failure
    (iii) Prenatal drug therapy dependent on gestational age, presence of cardiac failure, duration of pattern, and parental desires
    (iv) Intrapartum period—scalp stimulation
    (v) Antepartum period—pharmacologically converted with digoxin monotherapy (drug of choice), adenosine, verapamil, procainamide, quinidine or propranolol via maternal route or percutaneous umbilical route
  (b) Atrial flutter and fibrillation
    (i) Intrapartum period—scalp stimulation
    (ii) Antepartum period—pharmacologically converted with digoxin or propranolol initially (Kleinman, Nehgme, & Copel, 1999; Schmolling, Renke, Richter, Pfeiffer, Schlebusch, & Holler, 2000; Shaffer & Wiggins, 1998; Strasburger, 2000; Vautier-Rit, Dufour, Vaksmann, Subtil, Vaast, Valat, et al., 2000; Vlagsma, Hallensleben, & Meijboom, 2001). If unsuccessful, flecainide, quinidine or procainamide, sotalol, amiodarone, or diltiazem can be used (Kleinman, Nehgme, & Copel, 1999; Schmolling, Renke, Richter, Pfeiffer, Schlebusch, & Holler, 2000; Shaffer & Wiggins, 1998; Strasburger, 2000; Tanel & Rhodes, 2001; Vautier-Rit, et al., 2000).
  (c) Ventricular tachycardia
    (i) Transplacental treatment with amiodarone or sotalol (Strasburger, 2000)
    (ii) If fetus in congestive heart failure, lidocaine can be administered via umbilical cord (Cuneo & Strasburger, 2000; Ferrer, 1998; Kleinman, Nehgme, & Copel, 1999). Intracordal lidocaine is often followed by maternal oral therapy of propranolol, mexiletine, quinidine, procainamide, amiodarone, or sotalol (Kleinman, et al., 1999).
  (d) AV block
    (i) Increase FHR with atropine, isoproterenol, or terbutaline.
    (ii) If left ventricular failure, digoxin can be used.
    (iii) Fetus without hydrops fetalis and ventricular rate > 55 bpm is managed similar to normal pregnancy; monitor for hydrops fetalis and cardiac function, specifically left ventricular function.
    (iv) Fetus with hydrops fetalis is difficult to manage; successful conversion may be found with maternal administration of isoproterenol, terbutaline, or digoxin (Crosson & Brenner, 1999; Pinsky, Gillette, Garson, & McNamara, 1982).
    (v) Postdelivery temporary transplacental pacing with fetal epicardial or endocardial leads (Weindling, Saul, Triedman,

Burke, Jonas, Gamble, et al., 1994). Following temporary pacing, permanent pacing is usually required in neonates with structural cardiac disease.

  b. Outcomes
    (1) Likely cause of decreased or absent variability is identified and treated as needed.
    (2) Likely cause of undulating pattern is identified and treated as needed.
    (3) Maternal position is changed and FHR and variability improves.
    (4) Oxygen is administered and FHR and variability improves.
    (5) Oxytocin is discontinued, or tocolytics are administered; uterine activity decreases and FHR and variability improves.
    (6) Fetus responds to stimulation with accelerations in FHR.
 2. Risk for ineffective fetal perfusion related to hypoxic myocardial dysfunction or anomaly
 3. Risk for neurogenically mediated fetal loss of variability
 4. Risk for postdelivery fetal interventions resulting from myocardial dysfunction
 5. Maternal anxiety related to fetal status
  a. Interventions
    (1) Reassure and provide information about fetal condition.
    (2) Explain the interventions in terms of improving fetal well being.
  b. Outcomes
    (1) Mother reports decreased anxiety.
    (2) Client verbalizes understanding of interventions.

PERIODIC PATTERNS

Periodic patterns are FHR patterns that have a direct relation to UCs.

Accelerations

A. **Assessment**
 1. History: probable causes
  a. Repetitive fetal stimulation or movement
  b. Direct sympathetic stimulation
  c. Mild umbilical cord compression stimulating fetal compensatory acceleration
 2. Physical findings (Figure 12-23)
  a. Pattern characteristics
    (1) FHR abruptly increases > 15 beats above the BL FHR for a minimum of 15 seconds but not longer than 2 minutes (King & Simpson, 2001; NICHD Research Planning Workshop, 1997; Parer, 1997).
    (2) NICHD defines abrupt increase as onset to peak being < 30 seconds (NICHD Research Planning Workshop, 1997).
    (3) Preterm fetuses < 32 weeks' gestation, acceleration defined as > 10 beats above the BL FHR for a minimum of 10 seconds (Garite, 2002; King & Simpson, 2001; NICHD Research Planning Workshop, 1997; Tucker, 2000).
    (4) Variability is usually present.
    (5) Accelerations are considered to be benign patterns, indicate fetal well being (well oxygenated), and require no interventions.
    (6) May be a forerunner of variable decelerations.

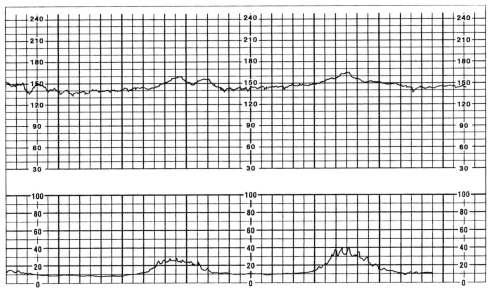

FIGURE 12-23 ■ Acceleration with UC (periodic).

(7) May be biphasic or triphasic.

(8) Shoulders = compensatory acceleration that may precede or follow deceleration; increase in rate generally < 20 bpm and lasting < 20 seconds (Cypher, Adelsperger, & Torgersen, 2003).

(9) Overshoot or rebound overshoot = blunt acceleration that follows deceleration; gradual, smooth acceleration that lasts > 60 to 90 seconds with increase in rate 10 to 20 bpm; has no variability, no abruptness, and returns to BL FHR gradually; if repetitive and STV absent, pattern is considered nonreassuring (Cypher, Adelsperger, & Torgersen, 2003).

b. Clinical findings

(1) When associated with fetal activity or stimuli that meet established criteria, accelerations are called reactivity.

(a) Observed in an active fetus or a fetus stimulated tactally, by fetal scalp stimulation, or by vibroacoustic stimulation.

(b) Fetal reactivity is expected by 28 to 30 weeks' gestation; once fetus demonstrates reactivity, should continue through gestation.

(2) When associated with variable decelerations, they are called shoulders or overshoots.

(3) Prolonged acceleration is defined as FHR that abruptly increases > 15 beats above the BL FHR for > 2 minutes and < 10 minutes (King & Simpson, 2001; NICHD Research Planning Workshop, 1997; Parer, 1997).

Variable Decelerations

A. Assessment

1. History: probable causes

a. Decreased umbilical cord perfusion

b. Umbilical cord compression

    c. Baroreceptor stimulation with vagal response; depth of deceleration depends on fetal baroreceptor stimulation; depth is reflex mediated and not related to degree of fetal hypoxia or fetal acid-base status (Cypher, Adelsperger, & Torgersen, 2003).

    d. Hypoxia and hypercarbic states

    e. Associated with clinical observation of nuchal cord, body cord entanglement, prolapsed cord, short cord, decreased amniotic fluid, second-stage descent of fetus, true knot of cord, and decreased Wharton's jelly.

    f. Acceleration that precedes or follows deceleration is a physiologic compensatory response to hypoxemia (oxygen deprivation).

2. Physical findings

    a. Pattern characteristics

      (1) Varies in depth, duration, nadir, and timing.

      (2) Variable onset

      (3) Variable shape: resembles W, U, V shapes or mimic other patterns (Figures 12-24 and 12-25).

      (4) Often drops abruptly and significantly below the BL of the FHR; NICHD defines as onset to nadir < 30 seconds (NICHD Research Planning Workshop, 1997).

      (5) Shoulders and overshoots may be present with variable decelerations (see definition as previously noted).

      (6) Often classified as reassuring or nonreassuring

        (a) Reassuring = duration < 60 seconds; rapid return to FHR BL; accompanied by normal baseline rate and variability

        (b) Nonreassuring = prolonged return to FHR BL; presence of overshoots; tachycardia; absence or loss of STV, or LTV, or both; persistent to < 60 bpm and > 60 seconds (ACOG, 1995b)

    b. Indicative of fetal well being

      (1) Variability present in baseline of FHR

      (2) Fetal recovery rapid

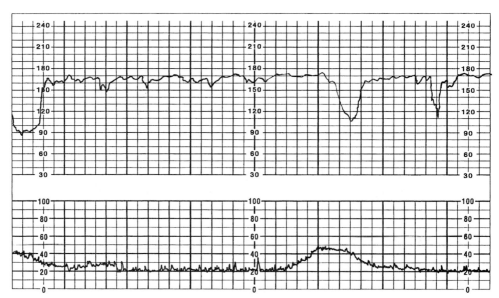

FIGURE 12-24 ■ Periodic variable decelerations tolerated well by fetus as evidenced by recovery and average LTV and present STV (moderate variability).

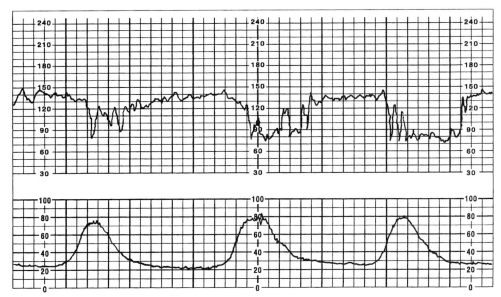

FIGURE 12-25 ■ Periodic variable deceleration, with slow recovery to baseline.

   c. Indicative of fetal compromise
      (1) Variability absent in BL FHR
         (a) STV is usually lost first at the nadir of deceleration because of the arrest phenomenon.
         (b) STV is lost next during the recovery of deceleration.
         (c) STV is lost last between decelerations (in BL rate).
      (2) Slow recovery or failure to recover to baseline
      (3) Compensatory overshoots of FHR
         (a) Without variability and persistent
         (b) Change of FHR BL with decreased variability (e.g., rising or falling FHR BL)
B. Nursing Diagnoses
   1. Risk for impaired fetal gas exchange related to inadequate umbilical cord perfusion, hypoxia, and hypercarbia
   2. Maternal anxiety related to fetal status
C. Interventions/Outcomes
   1. Risk for impaired fetal gas exchange related to inadequate umbilical cord perfusion, hypoxia, and hypercarbia
      a. Interventions
         (1) Change maternal position that maintains FHR in reassuring pattern (left or right lateral, upright, hands and knees or knee-chest).
            (a) Change pressure on umbilical cord.
            (b) May abolish, improve, or worsen FHR pattern.
            (c) Avoid supine hypotension and maximize uteroplacental and umbilical blood flow.
         (2) Administer oxygen if variable decelerations are persistent, BL FHR is increasing and variability is decreased, or if overshoots are present; oxygen administered via snug face mask at 8 to 10 L/min.
         (3) Perform vaginal examination to assess for prolapsed cord or imminent delivery; if prolapsed cord, elevate presenting part off cord.
         (4) Perform amnioinfusion according to hospital protocol.

(a) Increases cushion effect for the umbilical cord.

(b) Relieves or lessens variable decelerations when effective.

(c) Dilutes thick, particulate meconium, if it is present.

(d) Sample protocol (see own institutional guidelines)

    (i) Most protocols recommend initial bolus of 800 ml; follow up bolus by maintenance infusion to replace lost amniotic fluid (ACOG, 1995a; Adelsperger & Waymire, 2003).

    (ii) Some protocols recommend titration of fluid bolus at 15 to 20 ml per minute until deceleration resolves, followed by an additional 250 ml.

    (iii) Warming of solution not required for full term fetuses; appropriate for preterm or growth-restricted fetuses; keep temperature between 34° to 37° C (93° to 96° F) (Adelsperger & Waymire, 2003).

    (iv) Infusion may be discontinued when variables are abolished, the meconium is diluted, 800 ml are infused, or the amniotic fluid index (AFI) is used to determine infusion amounts.

    (v) Maintenance fluid is 120 to 180 ml per hour (Adelsperger & Waymire, 2003).

    (vi) Amnioinfusion should reach therapeutic result or increase the amniotic fluid index in approximately 30 minutes (ACOG, 1995a; Snell, 1993).

    (vii) It is important to monitor maternal vital signs, FHR and variability, resolution of decelerations, and uterine tone.

(5) Discontinue oxytocin or other uterotonics; obtain order for and administer tocolytics (terbutaline) if UA continues.

(6) Access for accelerations.

(7) Perform scalp stimulation or fetal scalp sampling or attach fetal pulse oximeter.

(8) Instruct mother to alter her breathing or pushing technique.

(9) Communicate findings to primary care provider; document events on the client's record.

(a) Note the duration and depth of the variable deceleration.

(b) Recovery time: if slow, note the recovery time in seconds.

(c) Note BL rate and variability; note variability within deceleration itself, including the nadir.

(d) Note persistency of pattern.

(e) Document in trends; use hospital-approved abbreviations (see examples in Box 12-1).

(10) Plan for expedited delivery if unresolved despite interventions.

(11) If auscultating and abrupt decreases in the FHR are heard, change maternal position and reauscultate; consider placing EFM to assess FHR variability and possible deceleration pattern.

  b. Outcomes

    (1) Improvement or resolution in variable deceleration pattern

    (2) Improvement of FHR BL variability and reactivity

    (3) Improvement of recovery time to BL

    (4) Improvement or resolution of oligohydramnios thus relieving variable deceleration pattern

2. Maternal anxiety related to fetal status

  a. Interventions

    (1) Maintain a calm manner.

■ BOX 12-1
■ **ABBREVIATIONS FOR CHARTING ELECTRONIC FETAL MONITORING**

EFM	Electronic fetal monitoring
FHM	Fetal heart monitoring
FM	Fetal movement
FMC	Fetal movement counting
FHR	Fetal heart rate or rhythm
US	Ultrasonography (external)
TOCO	Tocodynamometer (external)
SE	Spiral electrode (internal)
FSE	Fetal spiral electrode (internal)
IUPC	Intrauterine pressure catheter (internal)
UC	Uterine contraction
UA	Uterine activity
RT	Resting tone
Palp	Palpated/via palpation
Mod	Moderate
MVU	Montevideo Units
BL	Baseline (refers to FHR and sometimes to baseline tonus)
bpm	Beats per minute
LTV ↓	Long-term variability is decreased or minimal, 0 to 5 beats amplitude, and < 3 cycle changes per minute; also var ↓ (NICHD)
LTV +	Long-term variability is present, 6 to 25 beats amplitude, and 3 to 6 cycle changes per minute; also var + (NICHD)
LTV ↑	Long-term variability is increased > 25 beats amplitude per minute—also called marked or saltatory pattern; also var ↑ (NICHD)
STV +	Short-term variability is present; roughness of actual tracing line can be visualized; SE mode is most accurate to evaluate STV
STV Ø	Short-term variability is absent; actual tracing line is smooth
Var	Variability absent (NICHD)
Late decel	Late deceleration pattern
Early decel	Early deceleration pattern
Var decel	Variable deceleration pattern
Prolonged decel	Deceleration more than 2 minutes but less than 10 minutes
Late-Var decel	Late variable deceleration pattern

    (2) Provide clear explanations to the client and family of events and interventions.
    (3) Explain how dramatic variable deceleration patterns may be well tolerated by the fetus.
    (4) Reassure and prepare the client for the necessity to act rapidly if fetal status dictates.
  b. Outcomes
    (1) Client reports decreased anxiety and increased confidence in caregivers.
    (2) Client verbalizes understanding of interventions.

Late Decelerations

A. Assessment
  1. History
    a. Probable cause is fetal response to transient alterations in oxygen transport produced or attenuated by UC (Cypher, Adelsperger, &

Torgersen, 2003); all leading to decreased uteroplacental blood flow related to one of the following:

(1) Uteroplacental insufficiency or diminished placental function that alters maternal-fetal gas exchange; associated with decreased variability, fetal myocardial depression, and fetal acidosis
   (a) Hypertension as a result of gestational or chronic hypertension; medications (illicit drugs such as amphetamines or cocaine)
   (b) Placental changes such as postmaturity; premature aging (calcification or necrosis); old or new abruptio placentae sights; placenta previa; or placental malformation
   (c) Uterine hyperstimulation or hypertonus with or without oxytocin, misoprostol, or prostaglandin administration
   (d) Increased association with other high-risk pregnancy conditions such as chronic maternal diseases (diabetes and collagen disease); maternal smoking; poor maternal nutrition; multiple gestation (usually monochorionic); or maternal anemia
   (e) Cardiopulmonary disease that may decrease maternal arterial hemoglobin or oxygen saturation

(2) Impeded maternal blood flow to placenta or diminished maternal arterial oxygen saturation; associated with normal pH and variability for at least the first 30 minutes of blood flow impedance; also called reflex late decelerations resulting from:
   (a) Maternal hypotension from:
      (i) Supine hypotension
      (ii) Trauma or blood loss
      (iii) Regional anesthesia
      (iv) Drug use
   (b) Maternal hyperventilation or hypoventilation

2. Physical findings: pattern characteristics of late decelerations (Figures 12-26 to 12-28)
   a. Shape is uniform.

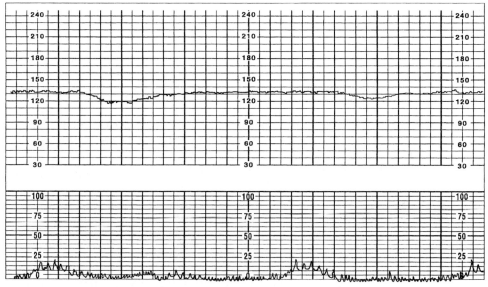

FIGURE 12-26 ■ Late decelerations with external ultrasound, ↓ LTV (minimal variability).

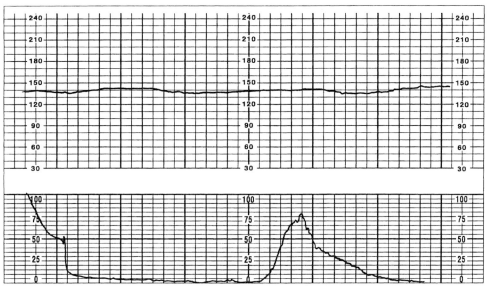

FIGURE 12-27 ■ Late decelerations with internal FSE, ↓ LTV, ØSTV (absent variability).

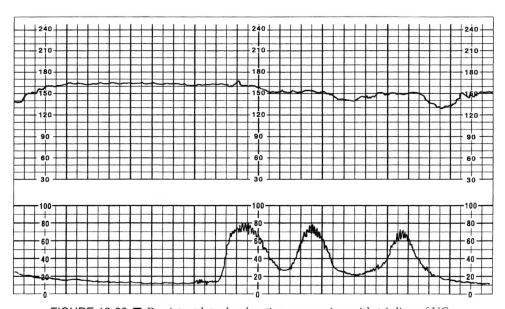

FIGURE 12-28 ■ Persistent late decelerations, occurring with tripling of UCs.

b. Pattern is smooth and can be repetitive (or persistent meaning occurring in > 50% of UC).

c. Onset is gradual; NICHD defines gradual onset as > 30 seconds from beginning to nadir; nadir (lowest point of deceleration) is offset (usually occurs after acme [peak] of UC).

   (1) Deceleration usually begins 20 to 30 seconds after the UC begins.

   (2) Nadir commonly decreases 5 to 30 bpm; rarely 30 to 40 bpm below BL (Cypher, Adelsperger, & Torgersen, 2003).

   (3) NICHD = to be classified as late deceleration, FHR required to decrease below the BL FHR for a minimum of 15 bpm and last for minimum of 15 seconds.

    d. BL often has absent or decreased variability (STV and LTV); BL may increase with repetitive late decelerations.

    e. The intensity of the client's UC is reflected in the depth of the deceleration.

B. Nursing Diagnoses

    1. Risk for impaired fetal gas exchange related to factors that diminish adequate blood supply to placenta combined with common intrapartal events that reduce fetal oxygen levels

    2. Maternal anxiety related to fetal status and impeding medical interventions

C. Interventions/Outcomes

    1. Risk for impaired fetal gas exchange related to factors that diminish adequate blood supply to placenta combined with common intrapartal events that reduce fetal oxygen levels

      a. Interventions

        (1) Position the client in lateral position to:

          (a) Maximize uteroplacental blood flow.

          (b) Avoid supine hypotension effect.

        (2) Discontinue oxytocin or other uterotonic medications.

        (3) Assess hydration; initiate or increase intravenous fluids.

          (a) Correct hypotension.

          (b) Increase volume to maximize uteroplacental blood flow.

        (4) Administer oxygen via snug face mask at 8 to 10 L/min to maximize fetal oxygenation.

        (5) Palpate uterine resting tone to ensure uterine relaxation; consider or request order for tocolytic medication.

        (6) Assist with scalp stimulation or fetal pulse oximetry (if available); scalp stimulation should be limited to use as assessment tool to assess fetal acid-base status; not considered an action to correct late decelerations.

        (7) Communicate the irreversibility or worsening pattern of late decelerations to the appropriate personnel and care providers to include anesthesia and neonatal resuscitation team.

          (a) The likelihood of hypoxia, acidosis, and asphyxia increases as duration of the late deceleration pattern increases.

          (b) Variability usually reflects fetal status.

          (c) Plan for expedited delivery and possible neonatal resuscitation.

        (8) Documentation (Boxes 12-2 and 12-3)

          (a) Document the depth, duration, and persistence of the deceleration pattern and their timing in relationship to UCs.

          (b) Document BL FHR and variability.

          (c) Document interventions and outcomes.

          (d) Document notification of the primary care provider.

          (e) Use hospital-approved nomenclature and abbreviations (see Box 12-1).

      b. Outcomes

        (1) Late deceleration pattern is improved or corrected by interventions as previously noted.

        (2) FHR and variability (STV and LTV) return to uncompromised state.

        (3) Fetus is delivered expeditiously, if warranted, and resuscitation team is present at delivery and resuscitation performed expeditiously as warranted by neonatal cardiorespiratory status.

■ BOX 12-2
■ **INFORMATION INCLUDED IN DOCUMENTATION**

BL FHR
Variability: LTV and STV (if possible)
Accels: periodic or nonperiodic (episodic)
Decels: periodic or nonperiodic (episodic)
Type or shape (describe if uncertain of what to call deceleration)
Depth (nadir)
Duration (of nadir)
Recovery time (duration): timed from end of nadir to when FHR returns to BL
UC pattern to include frequency, duration, intensity, and resting tone: if using IUPC, should also
  validate information via palpation, especially intensity and resting tone
Interventions
Maternal-fetal responses to intervention
Notification of primary care provider (include understanding from provider re: report)
Understanding of client

■ BOX 12-3
■ **DOCUMENTATION EXAMPLES OF EFM EVENTS**

1. BL FHR 130-140 bpm; reassuring Var decel to 80 bpm × 30 seconds; return to BL of 130-
   140 bpm after decel; LTV +, STV + (var moderate); UC q 3-4 minutes, lasting 50-60 seconds, intensity 50-60 mmHg/palp mod, and RT 10-15 mmHg/palp soft between UC. Pt
   turned to left side; var decels ↓ in depth/duration; Pt tolerating labor; breathing with contractions, father at bedside. Dr.____ notified of above information, he verbalized understanding.
2. BL FHR 120-124 bpm; repetitive late decels to 110 bpm × 40 seconds; return to BL of 130-
   132 bpm after decel; STV Ø, LTV ↓ (var ↓); UC q 1-2 minutes, lasting 30-45 seconds, intensity strong by palp, and RT palp firm between UCs. Pt on right side; no change in
   deceleration pattern, turned to left side; oxygen 8-10 L/min per snug face mask applied to
   pt; oxytocin infusion d/c'd; Dr. ____ paged to come to L&D now; explained to pt and family that fetus is not tolerating labor; pt and family verbalized understanding.
3. FHR BL 150-160 bpm; nonreassuring Var decel to 50 to 60 bpm × 60 to 70 seconds, with
   recovery from nadir to BL × 30 seconds; overshoots present to 180 bpm x 20-30 seconds;
   BL now 140-143 bpm after decel, BL STV intermittent between + and Ø, LTV ↓(var ↓); UC
   not seen on external monitor; none palp; none perceived by pt; pt turned to left side; oxygen 8-10 L/min per snug face mask applied to pt; IVF D_5LR increased; MD called and told
   of fetal and uterine status as noted above; MD stated he is coming right over and to prepare
   the client for emergent delivery.
If any one of the examples above continues as written, the subsequent note would state, *pattern continues*. Need to chart today as if you had to recall the entire labor and delivery process
two to twenty years in the future.

   2. Maternal anxiety related to fetal status and impeding medical interventions
      a. Interventions
         (1) Explain interventions to the client.
         (2) Reassure the client regarding observation of fetal status and care.
         (3) Anticipate events and explain possible treatment options.

  b. Outcomes
    (1) Client reports a decrease in anxiety and increased confidence in caregivers.
    (2) Client verbalizes understanding of situation and interventions.

Early Decelerations

A. **Assessment**
  1. History: probable causes
    a. Head compression that results in vagal response
    b. Vagal stimulation via pushing against cervix; compression of head during pushing; forceps or vacuum application
    c. Considered to be benign, requiring no intervention (Cypher, Adelsperger, & Torgersen, 2003).
    d. Factors associated with early decelerations include cephalopelvic disproportion (CPD), unengaged presenting part, or persistent occiput posterior presentation.
  2. Physical findings: pattern characteristics (Figure 12-29)
    a. Gradual decrease in FHR; nadir coincides with peak of UC.
    b. NICHD further describes the decrease in FHR as > 30 seconds from onset to nadir (NICHD Research Planning Workshop, 1997).
    c. Nadir is rarely more than 30 to 40 beats below BL (Garite, 2002; NICHD Research Planning Workshop, 1997).
    d. Are usually associated with variability.
    e. Occur more frequently with primigravidas; occurs more often in early active labor usually between 4 and 7 cm and may also be seen between 8 and 10 cm secondary to head compression.
    f. Can be confused with or not identified as late decelerations.

B. **Nursing Diagnoses**
  1. Maternal anxiety related to fetal status
  2. Risk for progressive fetal hypoxic changes in pattern

C. **Interventions/Outcomes**
  1. Maternal anxiety related to fetal status

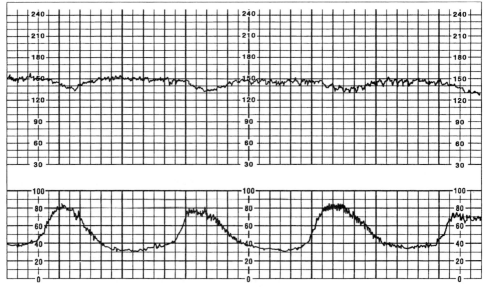

FIGURE 12-29 ■ Early deceleration.

a. Interventions
   (1) Assess progress of labor and perform vaginal examination for dilatation, fetal position, and station (assessing for dilatation and descent).
   (2) Reassure regarding fetal status.
   (3) Continue observation for fetal hypoxia patterns.
   (4) Documentation
       (a) Document characteristics of the early deceleration (e.g., onset, offset, depth, duration, persistency).
       (b) Document BL rate and variability.
       (c) Document the maternal position.
       (d) Document the fetal station and presenting part, if possible.
       (e) Use hospital-approved nomenclature and abbreviations (see Box 12-1).
b. Outcomes
   (1) Pattern resolves or does not deteriorate.
   (2) LTV is average (variability moderate).
   (3) Client reports low anxiety.
2. Risk for progressive fetal hypoxic changes in pattern
   a. Interventions
      (1) Assess for variability and fetal response to stimulation (scalp stimulation, abdominal, or vibroacoustic stimulation).
   b. Outcomes
      (1) Pattern should not deteriorate.
      (2) LTV is average (variability is moderate).

Combined Decelerations

A. Assessment
1. History: probable causes
   a. Fetal monitoring terminology suggests only one physiologic mechanism occurring at one time hence early, late, or variable decelerations.
   b. Pregnancy is a complex physiologic state; more than one physiologic mechanism may occur at the same time.
2. Physical findings (Figure 12-30)

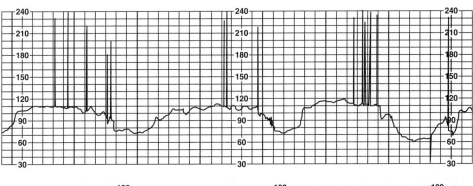
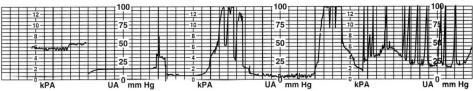

FIGURE 12-30 ■ Combined deceleratory pattern, late decelerations, and late variable decelerations.

   a. Contain characteristics of early, late, or variable decelerations.
   b. May occur separately in the same tracing or superimposed on each other.
   c. No agreement on terminology for recognition of these patterns; sometimes referred to as late variable decelerations, early variable decelerations, or combined deceleration patterns

B. Nursing Diagnoses
   1. Same as those for early, late, or variable decelerations; see previous sections

C. Interventions/Outcomes
   1. Same as those for early, late, or variable decelerations; see previous sections.
   2. Further assessment of FHR BL rate, presence of variability, and presence of accelerations
   3. Documentation, including description of the pattern similar to description of early, late, and variable decelerations

NONPERIODIC PATTERNS

Nonperiodic patterns are FHR patterns that do not have a direct relation to UCs.

Accelerations

A. Assessment
   1. History: probable causes
      a. Environmental stimuli (e.g., vibroacoustic stimulation)
      b. Fetal movement
      c. Actions or events that may stimulate sympathetic nervous system (e.g., scalp stimulation, occiput posterior presentation, application of FSE)
   2. Physical findings (Figure 12-31)
      a. Pattern characteristics
         (1) FHR abruptly increases > 15 beats above the BL FHR for a minimum of 15 seconds but not longer than 2 minutes (Cypher, Adelsperger, & Torgersen, 2003; King & Simpson, 2001; NICHD Research Planning Workshop, 1997; Parer, 1997).
         (2) NICHD defines abrupt increase as onset to peak being < 30 seconds (NICHD Research Planning Workshop, 1997); often more peaked or abrupt than periodic accelerations.
         (3) Preterm fetuses < 32 weeks' gestation—acceleration defined as > 10 beats above the BL FHR for a minimum of 10 seconds (Cypher, Adelsperger, & Torgersen, 2003; Garite, 2002; King & Simpson, 2001; NICHD Research Planning Workshop, 1997; Tucker, 2000).

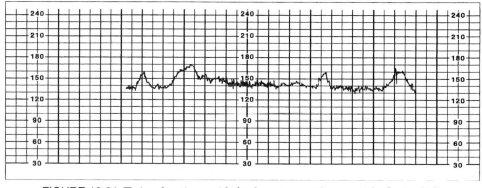

FIGURE 12-31 ■ Accelerations with fetal movement (nonperiodic [episodic]).

    (4) Variability is usually present.

    (5) Accelerations are considered to be benign patterns, indicate fetal well being (well oxygenated), and require no interventions.

    (6) Do not occur in consistent manner.

  3. Clinical findings

    a. When associated with fetal activity or stimuli that meet established criteria, accelerations are called reactivity.

      (1) Observed in an active fetus or a fetus stimulated tactally, by fetal scalp stimulation, or by vibroacoustic stimulation.

      (2) Fetal reactivity is expected by 28 to 30 weeks' gestation; once fetus demonstrates reactivity, it should continue through gestation.

    b. Prolonged acceleration is defined as FHR that abruptly increases > 15 beats above the BL FHR for > 2 minutes and < 10 minutes (Cypher, Adelsperger, & Torgersen, 2003; King & Simpson, 2001; NICHD Research Planning Workshop, 1997; Parer, 1997).

Variable Decelerations

A. Assessment

  1. History

    a. Decreased umbilical cord perfusion

    b. Umbilical cord compression

    c. Decreased amniotic fluid

    d. Baroreceptor stimulation with vagal response; depth of deceleration depends on fetal baroreceptor stimulation; depth is reflex mediated and not related to degree of fetal hypoxia or fetal acid-base status (Cypher, Adelsperger, & Torgersen, 2003).

    e. Hypoxia and hypercarbic states

    f. Acceleration that precedes or follows deceleration is a physiologic compensatory response to hypoxemia (oxygen deprivation).

  2. Physical findings (Figure 12-32): same as periodic variable decelerations in addition to the following:

    a. May occur before labor.

    b. Unlike periodic variable decelerations, if deceleration decreases > 15 bpm or has a duration of at least 15 seconds, further evaluation is warranted (ACOG, 1995b).

    c. Umbilical cord compression

    d. Decreased amniotic fluid

    e. Varies in depth, duration, nadir, and timing.

    f. Variable onset

    g. Variable shape: resembles W, U, V shapes or mimic other patterns.

    h. Often drops abruptly and significantly below the BL of the FHR; NICHD defines as onset to nadir < 30 seconds (NICHD Research Planning Workshop, 1997).

B. Nursing Diagnoses

  1. Risk for impaired fetal gas exchange related to inadequate umbilical cord perfusion, hypoxia, and hypercarbia

  2. Maternal anxiety related to fetal status

C. Interventions/Outcomes

  1. Risk for impaired fetal gas exchange related to inadequate umbilical cord perfusion, hypoxia, and hypercarbia

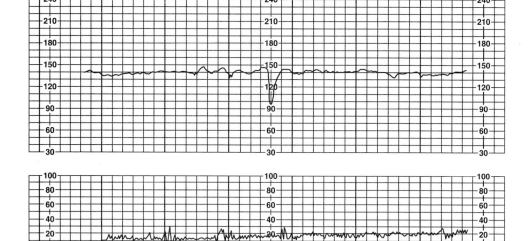

FIGURE 12-32 ■ Nonperiodic (episodic) variable deceleration. (From Feinstein, N.F., Torgersen, K.L., & Atterbury, J.L. [Eds.]. [2003]. *Fetal heart monitoring principles and practices* [3rd ed.]. Dubuque, IA: Kendall-Hunt Publications.)

    a. Interventions

        (1) Change maternal position that maintains FHR in reassuring pattern (left or right lateral, upright, hands and knees or knee-chest).

            (a) Change pressure on umbilical cord.

            (b) May abolish, improve, or worsen FHR pattern.

            (c) Avoid supine hypotension and maximize uteroplacental and umbilical blood flow.

        (2) Administer oxygen if variable decelerations are persistent, BL FHR is increasing, and variability is decreased. Oxygen administered via snug facemask at 8 to 10 L/min.

        (3) Perform vaginal exam to assess for prolapsed cord or imminent delivery; if prolapsed cord, elevate presenting part off cord.

        (4) Perform amnioinfusion according to hospital protocol (see previous variable deceleration section).

        (5) Assess for accelerations.

        (6) Perform scalp stimulation.

        (7) Communicate findings to primary care provider; document events on the client's record.

            (a) Note the duration and depth of the variable deceleration.

            (b) Recovery time: if slow, note the recovery time in seconds.

            (c) Note BL rate and variability; note variability within deceleration itself, including the nadir.

            (d) Note persistency of pattern.

            (e) Document in trends; use hospital-approved abbreviations (see Box 12-1).

        (8) If auscultating and abrupt decreases in the FHR are heard, change maternal position and reauscultate; consider placing EFM to assess FHR variability and possible deceleration pattern.

    b. Outcomes

        (1) Improvement or resolution in variable deceleration pattern

        (2) Improvement of FHR BL variability and reactivity

(3) Improvement of recovery time to BL

(4) Improvement or resolution of oligohydramnios thus relieving variable deceleration pattern

2. Maternal anxiety related to fetal status

    a. Interventions

        (1) Maintain a calm manner.

        (2) Provide clear explanations to the client and family of events and interventions.

        (3) Explain how dramatic variable deceleration patterns may be well tolerated by the fetus.

        (4) Reassure and prepare the client for the necessity to act rapidly if fetal status dictates.

    b. Outcomes

        (1) Client reports decreased anxiety and increased confidence in caregivers.

        (2) Client verbalizes understanding of interventions.

Prolonged Decelerations

A. Assessment

1. History: probable causes

    a. Any mechanism that has been previously identified for other decelerations (e.g., cord compression, head compression, uteroplacental insufficiency (Garite, 2002)

    b. Profound changes in fetal environment (e.g., abruptio placentae, uterine hypertonus or hyperstimulus, terminal fetal conditions, maternal death, cord accidents)

    c. Hypotension associated with drug responses or maternal positioning (e.g., sympathetic blockade with anesthesia, paracervical block)

    d. Vagal stimulation with vaginal examination; Valsalva maneuver

    e. Cord impingement, cord prolapse, or cord compression for substantial periods; oligohydramnios with decreased Wharton's jelly allowing for possible cord compression

    f. Uterine rupture

    g. Maternal seizures, status asthmaticus, or maternal cardiorespiratory collapse

    h. Rapid fetal descent

    i. Procedures (e.g., vaginal examination, fetal blood capillary sampling, application of internal fetal monitoring devices)

2. Physical findings (Figure 12-33)

    a. Decrease in FHR > 2 minutes but < 10 minutes

    b. A decrease lasting longer than 10 minutes is considered a BL change.

        (1) In the absence of hyperstimulation, numerical intrauterine pressure catheter values are not a diagnostic aid.

        (2) Hyperstimulation is usually defined as UCs that occur more frequently than every 2 minutes, uterine relaxation < 30 seconds between UCs, or UCs that are longer than 90 to 120 seconds; hypertonus is defined as elevated resting tone > 20 to 25 mmHg, depending on type of IUPC used (Cypher, Adelsperger, & Torgersen, 2003).

B. Nursing Diagnoses

1. Risk for impaired fetal gas exchange related to inadequate umbilical cord perfusion, hypoxia, hypercarbia, and factors that diminish adequate blood

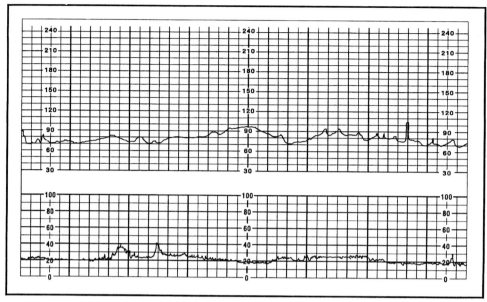

FIGURE 12-33 ■ Prolonged deceleration.

supply to placenta combined with common intrapartal events that reduce fetal oxygen levels
  2. Maternal anxiety related to fetal status and impeding medical interventions
C. **Interventions/Outcomes**
  1. Risk for impaired fetal gas exchange related to inadequate umbilical cord perfusion, hypoxia, hypercarbia, and factors that diminish adequate blood supply to placenta combined with common intrapartal events that reduce fetal oxygen levels
    a. Interventions
      (1) Change maternal position that maintains FHR in reassuring pattern (left or right lateral, upright, hands and knees or knee-chest).
        (a) Change pressure on umbilical cord.
        (b) May abolish, improve, or worsen FHR pattern.
        (c) Avoid supine hypotension and maximize uteroplacental and umbilical blood flow.
      (2) Discontinue oxytocin or other uterotonics; obtain order for and administer tocolytics (terbutaline) if UA continues.
      (3) Assess hydration; initiate or increase IV fluids.
      (4) Evaluate presenting part to rule out breech presentation.
      (5) Perform vaginal examination to assess for prolapsed cord or imminent delivery; if prolapsed cord, elevate presenting part off cord.
      (6) Perform amnioinfusion as needed or ordered (see previous section for protocol).
      (7) Administer oxygen if variable decelerations are persistent, BL FHR is increasing, and variability is decreased or if overshoots are present; oxygen administered via snug facemask at 8 to 10 L/min.
      (8) Communicate findings to primary care provider; document events on the client's record.

(a) Note the duration and depth of the prolonged deceleration.
(b) Recovery time: if slow, note the recovery time in seconds.
(c) Note BL rate and variability; note variability within deceleration itself, including the nadir.
(d) Note persistency of pattern.
(9) Plan for expedited delivery if unresolved despite interventions.
(10) If auscultating and abrupt decreases in the FHR are heard, change maternal position and reauscultate; consider placing EFM to assess FHR variability and possible deceleration pattern.
b. Outcomes
(1) Improvement or resolution of prolonged deceleration
(2) Improvement of FHR BL variability and reactivity
(3) Improvement of recovery time to BL
2. Maternal anxiety related to fetal status and impeding medical interventions
a. Interventions
(1) Maintain a calm manner.
(2) Provide clear explanations to the client and family of events and interventions.
(3) Explain how dramatic prolonged deceleration patterns may be well tolerated by the fetus.
(4) Reassure and prepare the client for the necessity to act rapidly if fetal status dictates.
b. Outcomes
(1) Client reports decreased anxiety and increased confidence in caregivers.
(2) Client verbalizes understanding of interventions.
D. **Documentation** (see Box 12-2)
1. Fetal vital sign assessment
a. FHR BL rate
b. Variability (LTV and STV)
c. Periodic changes (accelerations, decelerations, or both): use descriptive names.
d. Nonperiodic changes (accelerations, decelerations, or both): use descriptive names.
e. Persistency of patterns (repetitive): pattern occurs with > 50% of UCs.
2. UA (frequency, duration, intensity and resting tone)
3. Pertinent events and actions
4. Nursing interventions
5. Maternal-fetal responses to interventions
6. Notification of primary care provider
7. Confusing patterns
a. Depth of decelerations
b. Height of accelerations
c. Timing in relation to UC
d. Duration
e. BL variability; BL FHR following deceleration
8. Chain of command
a. Is a communication mechanism established by institutions to facilitate problem resolution (Simpson & Knox, 2003).
b. Should be present in all institutions to resolve conflicts or problems in a timely and effective manner.
c. Protects the best interests of the client, family, and staff.

UTERINE ACTIVITY

A. Introduction (see Chapter 10 for a complete discussion)
1. Ultimate definition of adequate labor is based on cervical effacement and dilatation and fetal descent (Norwitz, Robinson, & Repke, 2002).
2. Assess three *P*s of labor to ensure adequacy: power (UCs), passenger (fetus), and passage (pelvis).
3. Montevideo units (MVU): quantitative measurement of UCs over a 10-minute period
   a. Subtract resting tone of uterus from the peak pressure of UC (in mmHg) for each contraction in the 10-minute period.
   b. Calculated numbers are then added together.
   c. Ranges from 95 to 395 MVUs; average range for adequate labor is 180 to 250 MVUs.
4. Dysfunctional contractions physiologically described as subnormal (or hypotonic, hypertonic, or abnormal) (see Chapter 11 for a complete discussion)
5. Factors affecting labor (UA) that can be changed:
   a. Hydration
   b. Maternal psychologic status and anxiety
   c. Intensity and duration of UCs
   d. Maternal positioning and pushing efforts
   e. Drugs or medications taken by or given to mother
B. Assessment (Figures 12-34 and 12-35)
1. Frequency: beginning of one UC to beginning of next UC; described in minutes.
2. Duration: time from beginning of UC to the end of UC; measured in seconds or minutes.
3. Intensity: strength of UC; measured externally via palpation (mild, moderate, or strong) or internally with IUPC; IUPC annotated as mmHg or MVUs.
4. Resting tone: also referred to as BL resting tone; pressure in uterus between UCs; measured externally by palpation (soft or firm) or internally with IUPC in mmHg.

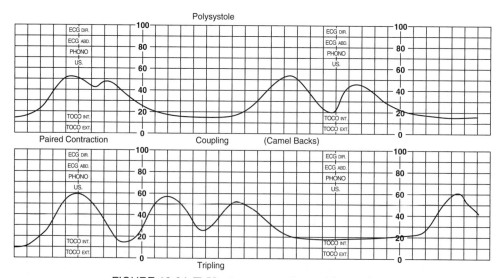

FIGURE 12-34 ■ Uterine contractions with coupling.

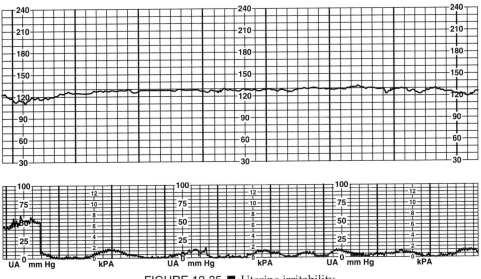

FIGURE 12-35 ■ Uterine irritability.

5. Cervical changes as appropriate
   a. Presence of factors affecting UCs
   b. Changes in UA in response to interventions
C. **Documentation**
   1. Frequency
   2. Duration
   3. Intensity
      a. Can use mmHg with IUPC or MVUs.
      b. Palpated as mild, moderate, or strong with external monitoring; also palpated with internal monitoring to validate internal IUPC reading.
   4. Resting tone
      a. Can use mmHg with IUPC.
      b. Palpated as soft or firm with external monitoring; also palpated with internal monitoring to validate internal IUPC reading.

FETAL SCALP SAMPLING

A. **Introduction**
   1. A sample of fetal scalp blood is obtained to measure the acid and base levels of the fetus.
      a. pH is measured.
      b. Evaluates fetal status when intrapartum compromise is suspected.
      c. Fetal capillary scalp blood pH is usually lower than umbilical venous blood and similar to umbilical arterial blood values.
   2. Samples must be obtained by correct procedure, and attempts are made to collect the sample during BL of the FHR rather than at the nadir of a deceleration.
   3. Scalp sampling is a supplement to EFM and is not meant to replace it.
   4. BL values for acidemia determination vary with institutions, and agreement is not universal.

5. The use of fetal blood sampling is decreasing, and its necessity has been dramatically reduced by using other noninvasive test, such as fetal scalp stimulation (Ecker & Parer, 1999).
6. FHR patterns and characteristics indicative of fetal scalp sampling
   a. Unexplained, decreased, minimal, or absent variability (LTV and STV) without periodic or nonperiodic changes
   b. Undulating or sinusoidal pattern of unknown origin
   c. Late decelerations with absent or decreasing variability (LTV and STV)
   d. Abnormal or unusual FHR patterns or characteristics
7. Contraindications for use
   a. Fetal coagulopathy, determined or suspected (e.g., hemophilia, thrombocytopenia)
   b. Active maternal genital infections (e.g., herpes, group B streptococcus)
   c. Suspected or documented HIV or hepatitis
   d. Chorioamnionitis

B. **Assessment**
1. When the fetal scalp pH is less than 7.15, 80% of the newborns have an Apgar score less than 6.
2. When the pH is greater than 7.25, 92% of newborns have an Apgar score greater than 7.
3. When the pH is 7.15 to 7.25, agreement on fetal status varies and other factors—such as variability, biophysical profile scores, any other technology available, fetal activity, and maternal status—are used to determine intervention and action.
4. Serial scalp sampling via several fetal scalp blood samples shows the trend and verifies the accuracy.
5. Maternal alkalosis and acidosis influence quality of blood available to the fetus; fetal pH values and comparison values of fetal and maternal pH may be helpful when the acid-base balance of the mother is in question.
6. Near-infrared spectroscopy and other technologies cited at the beginning of this chapter are less invasive, are more cost-effective, and (with further study and refinement) will likely replace fetal scalp blood sampling.

C. **Nursing Diagnoses**
1. Risk for impaired fetal gas exchange related to intrapartal reduction of oxygen levels
2. Maternal anxiety related to fetal status and procedure to obtain sampling

D. **Interventions/Outcomes**
1. Risk for impaired fetal gas exchange related to intrapartal reduction of oxygen levels
   a. Interventions
      (1) Provide optimal intrauterine environment with position, fluids, oxygen, and other treatments and medications, as needed.
      (2) Continue to interpret FHR tracing.
      (3) Prepare for and assist with sampling procedure according to protocol.
      (4) Assist with the accurate assessment of blood pH evaluation according to hospital protocol.
   b. Outcomes
      (1) Fetal pH and presence of acidosis is assessed by scalp sampling.
2. Maternal anxiety related to fetal status and procedure to obtain sampling
   a. Interventions
      (1) Explain the necessity for the procedure in terms of the assessment of fetal well being.

(2) Explain the procedure, from client perspective, step by step.
(3) Provide support by significant other or another nurse during the procedure.
(4) Anticipate future events and explain the possible treatment options based on results of scalp sampling.
  b. Outcomes
  (1) Client reports decreased anxiety and is able to follow instructions during the procedure.
  (2) Support person is at bedside.
  (3) Client discusses reasons for the procedure or asks questions.
  (4) Client understands possible interventions after results obtained.

FETAL PULSE OXIMETRY

A. Introduction
  1. In May 2000 the U.S. Food and Drug Administration (FDA) approved fetal pulse saturation ($FSpO_2$) as an additional method of assessing fetal oxygen status during labor.
  2. FDA approved fetal pulse oximetry is to be used as an adjunct to EFM, not as a stand-alone assessment tool.
  3. Currently, fetal pulse oximetry in clinical practice has not been adopted as a standard of care and has not been endorsed by the American College of Obstetricians and Gynecologists or the Society of Obstetricians and Gynaecologists of Canada (SOGC, 2002a).
  4. Normal oxygen saturation for the fetus is 30% to 65% saturation (Dildy, Thorp, Yeast, & Clark, 1996; Nijland, Jongsma, Nijhuis, van den Berg, & Oeseburg, 1995; Richardson, Carmichael, Homan, & Patrick, 1992; Seelbach-Göbel, Heupel, Kühnert, & Butterwegge, 1999).
  5. Oxygenation saturation rate between 30% and 65% indicates the fetus is adequately oxygenated with a fetal scalp blood pH of at least 7.2.
  6. Metabolic acidosis does not develop until the saturation level falls below 30% for at least 10 to 15 minutes (Cypher & Adelsperger, 2003); known as critical threshold (the point below which hypoxia would likely cause metabolic acidosis or above which there would be no risk for acidosis) (Garite & Porreco, 2001).
  7. Currently no standards or guidelines from ACOG on frequency of assessment or documentation of data during labor; use of device implies higher-risk fetal status; therefore fetal assessment should occur every 15 minutes during active phase of labor and every 5 minutes during the second stage of labor (Cypher & Adelsperger, 2003).
  8. Sensor usually descends with the fetus (Simpson, 1998).

B. Assessment
  1. Criteria for nonreassuring FHR patterns (Cypher & Adelsperger, 2003; Garite, Dildy, McNamara, Nageotte, Boehm, Dellinger, et al., 2000; Cypher & Adelsperger, 2003; Simpson & Porter, 2001)
  a. FHR BL between 100 to 110 bpm without accelerations
  b. FHR BL < 100 bpm with accelerations
  c. Increased variability > 25 bpm for > 30 minutes
  d. Mild or moderate variable deceleration for > 30 minutes
  e. Late decelerations (at least one in every 30-minute period)
  f. Decreased variability < 5 bpm for > 30 minutes that cannot be explained by clinical situation (e.g., narcotic administration)

      g. Persistent late decelerations (> 50% of UC) for > 15 minutes

      h. Tachycardia > 160 bpm with LTV < 5 bpm

      i. Sinusoidal pattern

      j. Variable decelerations with any of the following:

        (1) Relative drop of > 70 bpm or an absolute drop to < 70 bpm for > 60 seconds

        (2) Persistent slow return to FHR BL

        (3) Variability of < 5 bpm

        (4) Tachycardia of > 160 bpm

        (5) Recurrent prolonged decelerations (two decelerations of < 70 bpm for > 90 seconds in 15 minutes)

  2. Criteria for use (Cypher & Adelsperger, 2003)

      a. Singleton fetus

      b. > 36 weeks' gestation

      c. Vertex presentation

      d. Ruptured membranes

      e. Cervix > 2 cm dilated

      f. Fetal station of < −2 cm

      g. Nonreassuring FHR pattern as defined by FDA and US clinical trials

  3. Contraindications (Cypher & Adelsperger, 2003)

      a. Documented or suspected placenta previa

      b. Ominous FHR pattern requiring immediate intervention

      c. Need for immediate delivery (unrelated to FHR pattern), such as active uterine bleeding

      d. Certain infectious disease (e.g., HIV, active genital herpes, hepatitis B or hepatitis E seropositivity)

  4. Warnings (Cypher & Adelsperger, 2003)

      a. Do not use with an electrosurgical unit.

      b. Do not use in presence of flammable anesthetics.

      c. Sensor can be used during maternal defibrillation; data may be inaccurate.

      d. Do not use to monitor clients immersed in water (e.g., water births).

      e. Do not leave in place during vacuum extraction or forceps or cesarean delivery.

      f. Do not attempt to insert if cervix < 2 cm dilated or if membranes are not ruptured.

C. Nursing Diagnoses

  1. Risk for impaired fetal gas exchange related to intrapartal reduction of oxygen levels

  2. Maternal anxiety related to fetal status and procedure to obtain sampling

D. Interventions/Outcomes

  1. Risk for impaired fetal gas exchange related to intrapartal reduction of oxygen levels

      a. Interventions

        (1) Provide optimal intrauterine environment with position, fluids, oxygen, and other treatments and medications, as needed.

        (2) Continue to interpret FHR tracing; identify nonreassuring tracing according to exclusion and inclusion criteria (as previously noted).

        (3) Prepare for and assist with fetal pulse oximeter insertion according to protocol; providers should demonstrate expertise in determining fetal presentation and head position, and proficiency in placing FSEs and IUPCs.

(4) Use monitor display, audible fetal pulse tones, and feedback from $FSpO_2$ machine to ensure optimal placement achieved.

(5) Interpret data, document procedure and data collection in client's medical record, and communicate findings to primary care provider; documentation should include ranges of $FSpO_2$ values, intrauterine resuscitation techniques (if used), and notification of provider.

b. Outcomes

(1) Fetal oxygenation saturation is assessed; mode of delivery and expediency of delivery may change in light of saturation findings.

2. Maternal anxiety related to fetal status and procedure to obtain sampling

a. Interventions

(1) Explain the necessity for the procedure in terms of the assessment of fetal well being.

(2) Explain the procedure, from client perspective, step by step.

(3) Provide support by significant other or another nurse during the procedure.

(4) Anticipate future events and explain the possible treatment options based on results of fetal oxygen saturation.

b. Outcomes

(1) Client reports decreased anxiety and is able to follow instructions during the procedure.

(2) Support person is at bedside.

(3) Client can verbalize understanding for the procedure or ask questions.

(4) Client verbalizes understanding of possible interventions, to include possible expedited delivery, once results obtained.

UMBILICAL CORD BLOOD SAMPLING

A. Introduction

1. Considered the most reliable indication of fetal oxygenation and acid-base condition at birth (Thorp & Rushing, 1999).

2. Finding of normal umbilical blood gas measurement precludes the presence of asphyxia at or immediately before delivery (Gregg & Weiner, 1993); more objective than Apgar score.

3. Indications include:

a. Nonreassuring FHR characteristics or tracing

b. Thick meconium

c. Low Apgar scores

d. Preterm birth

e. Instrumented (forceps or vacuum extraction) or emergency cesarean delivery

f. Newborn depression (Thorp & Rushing, 1999)

B. Assessment

1. Identify normal, respiratory, and metabolic acidemia ranges (Table 12-1).

2. Interpret normal, respiratory and metabolic acidemia with single-digit values (Table 12-2).

3. Respiratory acidemia: excess carbon dioxide in fetal system

4. Metabolic acidemia: excess lactic acid in fetal system

5. Mixed acidemia: excess carbon dioxide and lactic acid in fetal system

6. Diagnosis of intrapartum asphyxial brain damage

a. FHR pattern with absent FHR variability at birth after asphyxial event; evidenced by severe variable and late decelerations or bradycardia

b. Umbilical artery pH < 7.0

■ TABLE 12-1
■ ■ Normal Ranges of Umbilical Cord Arterial Blood Gas Values

Arterial Measure[a]	Normal Mean Value Range[b]	Range (± 2 SD)
Ph	7.20-7.29	7.02-7.43
pCO_2 (mmHg)	49.2-56.3	21.5-78.3
Bicarbonate (mEq/L)	22.0-24.1	14.8-29.2
Base deficit (mEq/L)	2.7-8.3	−2.0-16.3
pO_2 (mmHg)	15.1-23.7	2.0-37.8

From Cypher, R., Adelsperger, D. (2003). Assessment of fetal oxygenation and acid-base status. In N.F. Feinstein & K.L. Torgersen (Eds.), *Fetal heart monitoring: Principles and practice* (3rd ed.). Dubuque, IA: Kendall/Hunt.
[a]Venous values reflect maternal acid-base status; they are generally higher than arterial values; arterial values reflect fetal acid-base status. Venous values may be normal (due to reflecting maternal acid-base status being normal) despite arterial values reflecting fetal acidemia.
[b]Represent range of normal mean values reported in a review of studies of umbilical arterial cord blood gases (Thorp & Rushing, 1999).

■ TABLE 12-2
■ ■ Single-Digit Acid-Base Values

	Single-Digit Value Guideline for Initial Assessment of Normal and Abnormal Umbilical Cord Blood Acid-Base Values*		
	Normal Values	Metabolic Acidemia	Respiratory Acidemia
pH	> 7.10	< 7.10	< 7.10
pO_2 (mmHg)	> 20	< 20	Variable
pCO_2 (mmHg)	< 60	< 60	> 60
Bicarbonate (mEq/L)	> 22	< 22	> 22
Base deficit (mEq/L)	> 10	> 10	< 10
Base excess (mEq/L)	< −10	< −10	> −10

From Feinstein, N.F., & Torgersen, K.L. (2003). *Fetal heart monitoring: Principles and practice* (3rd ed.). Dubuque, IA: Kendall/Hunt.
*Values are suggested as a guide for evaluating acid-base status.

    c. Umbilical artery base excess < 15 mEq/L
    d. Apgar score < 3 at 5 minutes
    e. Neurologic sequelae: hypotonia or seizure activity
    f. Multiorgan damage in newborn
C. Nursing Diagnoses
    1. Risk for impaired neonatal gas exchange related to intrapartal reduction of oxygen levels
    2. Maternal anxiety related to neonatal status, procedure to obtain sample, or possible neonatal resuscitation procedures
D. Interventions/Outcomes
    1. Risk for impaired neonatal gas exchange related to intrapartal reduction of oxygen levels
      a. Interventions
        (1) Provide optimal intrauterine environment with position, fluids, oxygen, and other treatments and medications, as needed.
        (2) Prepare for and gather umbilical cord blood samples according to protocol; arterial and venous samples should be obtained; if only one sample, it should be the arterial sample.

(3) Interpret data, document procedure and data collection in client's medical record, and communicate findings to primary care provider.

b. Outcomes
(1) Fetal acid-base status is assessed.

2. Maternal anxiety related to neonatal status, procedure to obtain sample, or possible neonatal resuscitation procedures

a. Interventions
(1) Explain the necessity for the procedure.
(2) Explain the procedure, from client perspective, step by step; often resulting from expediency to collect sample, procedure may need to be explained after sample is collected.
(3) Provide support by significant other.
(4) Anticipate future events and explain the possible treatment options based on results of umbilical cord blood sample.

b. Outcomes
(1) Client reports decreased anxiety and is able to follow instructions during the procedure.
(2) Support person is at bedside.
(3) Client can verbalize understanding for the procedure or ask questions.
(4) Client verbalizes understanding of possible interventions, to include possible expedited delivery, once results obtained.

HEALTH EDUCATION

A. **Use a holistic approach for maternal support and education throughout the pregnancy and prenatal period.**
   1. Assess the client's family and support system.
   2. Assess the educational level, educational needs, language level, and language needs of the client.
B. **Employ standards of care, as identified by AWHONN and agency or institution protocols and procedures.**
C. **Evaluate client's previous experiences with fetal assessment**
D. **Assess client instruction needs regarding fetal assessment technology and purpose.**
E. **Explain the technique used, its purpose, and the appropriate client compliance needed.**
F. **Answer questions and explain the data obtained, as appropriate, at the client's level of understanding.**
   1. Anxiety level and educational needs affect outcome.
   2. Catecholamine release and physiologic stress responses are associated with observable changes in FHR.

CASE STUDIES AND STUDY QUESTIONS

Mrs. S, a 30-year-old gravida 6, para 3 (G6, P3003) arrives at the labor and delivery room of a local hospital, which performs approximately 125 to 150 deliveries per month. She states she has undergone one previous cesarean section for fetal distress, has had no prenatal care, and believes that she is due in 2 weeks, which, according to her last menstrual period, appears to be accurate. Her FHR is 144 by Doppler ultrasound; she has intact membranes and is 3 cm dilated, 80% effaced, at −1 station, vertex presentation; BP, 120/80; pulse,

76; respirations, 18; temperature, 36.6° C (97.8° F). EFM was applied via the tocodynamometer and Doppler ultrasound.

1. According to the EFM tracing A (Figure 12-36), the BL FHR is the following:
   a. 130 to 150 bpm
   b. 140 to 150 bpm
   c. LTV ↑ (variability marked)
   d. BL cannot be determined

2. The periodic pattern of tracing A is:
   a. No periodic pattern is shown
   b. Normal BL tracing
   c. Variable decelerations
   d. Early decelerations

3. The UCs are:
   a. Every 1 to 1½ minutes × 50 seconds
   b. Every 2½ minutes × 50 to 60 seconds
   c. Hypotonic
   d. Hypertonic

4. During tracing B (Figure 12-37), Mrs. S suddenly says, "I have to push," and "something is wrong." The nurse performs a vaginal examination and finds that Mrs. S

is 3 cm dilated and notes that her fetal heart tracing (via tocodynamometer and Doppler ultrasound) shows:
   a. A need for more tracing to determine FHR BL; at end of tracing appears to be FHR BL rate of 140 to 150 bpm and LTV + (variability moderate)
   b. A BL FHR of 150 to 170 bpm, LTV ↓ (variability minimal)
   c. An agonal FHR pattern
   d. Second-stage labor with impending delivery

5. Her uterine contraction tracing in Figure 12-37 shows:
   a. UCs every 1½ minutes × 40 to 50 seconds
   b. UCs every 30 seconds × 30 to 40 seconds
   c. Increased uterine activity (irritability); requires further assessment via palpation
   d. Uterine hypotonus

6. In tracing C (Figure 12-38), 9 minutes later, an abrupt change in the FHR occurs; Mrs. S's nurse applies oxygen, changes the maternal position, gives a fluid

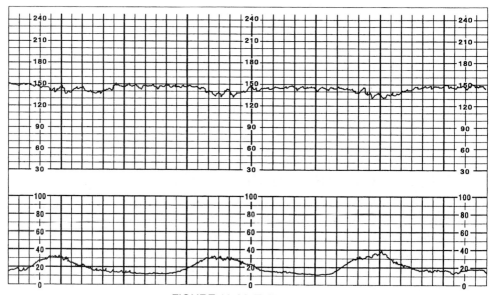

FIGURE 12-36 ■ Tracing A.

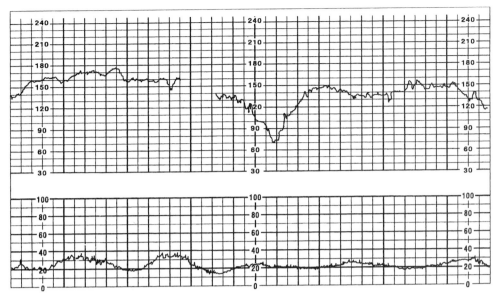

FIGURE 12-37 ■ Tracing B.

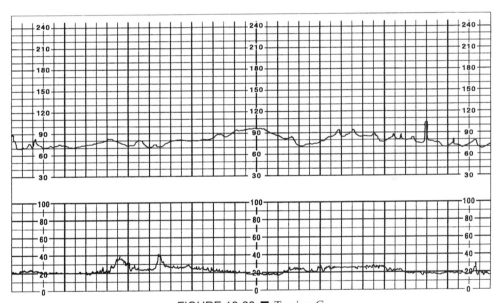

FIGURE 12-38 ■ Tracing C.

bolus, and applies a fetal spiral electrode. Uterine activity is still being monitored via tocodynamometer. In addition, preparations for a cesarean delivery have begun. The primary rationale underlying these interventions is:

a. Enhance maternal status in preparation for a surgical delivery

b. Suspicion of an abruptio placentae

c. Maximize oxygenation and uteroplacental blood flow

d. To show that, legally, everything possible was done

7. In tracing D (Figure 12-39), the surgery team is preparing for a cesarean delivery while the physician is en route to the

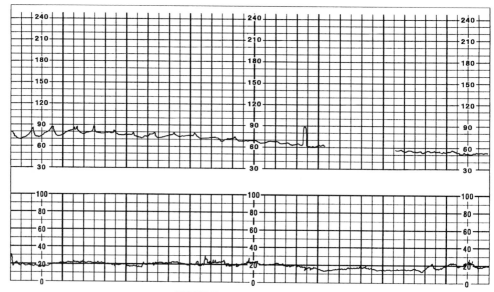

FIGURE 12-39 ■ Tracing D.

delivery room. The pattern is extremely nonreassuring. This situation means:

a. The fetus will die no matter what occurs.

b. The fetus is in immediate need of delivery and expedient interventions may produce a viable newborn that may need resuscitation at delivery.

c. The fetus will have permanent compromise if it lives.

d. The fetus will be asphyxiated at birth.

The physician arrived a few minutes after this tracing (see Figure 12-39) had been made and delivered a nonviable fetus that was floating in the abdomen. The entire lower uterine segment had separated from the body of the uterus and the placenta was wedged against this lower segment. The maternal toxicology report was positive for amphetamines and negative for cocaine.

8. Ms. K, a 27-year-old G1, P0 who is 5 days post dates, is admitted in spontaneous labor. Her vital signs at admission are FHR, 160 bpm; BP, 124/84; pulse, 112; respirations, 20;

and temperature, 38.2° C (100.8° F). Her vaginal examination at admission shows a 2- to 3-cm posterior cervix, 50% effacement, – 1 station, and a light meconium-stained amniotic fluid. At admission, an IV solution of lactated Ringer's was started and opened for a fluid bolus. EFM is being accomplished via tocodynamometer and Doppler ultrasound. Assess tracing E (Figure 12-40), which began 1 hour after admission.

a. LTV + (variability moderate), FHR 160 to 170 bpm

b. LTV ↓ (variability minimal), FHR 160 bpm × 2 accelerations to 170 bpm

c. LTV ↓ (variability minimal), FHR 170 bpm × 2 prolonged decelerations

d. LTV ↓ (variability minimal), no reactivity (accelerations), FHR 168 to 170 bpm progressing to 158 to 160 bpm

9. In tracing F (Figure 12-41), an arrow indicates scalp stimulation of the fetus. This fetal response implies:

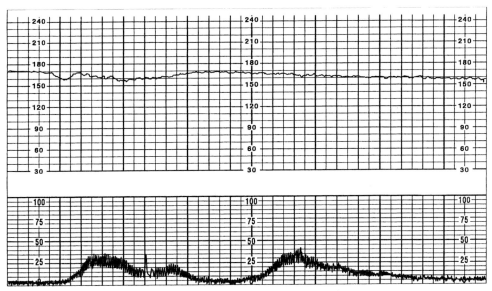

FIGURE 12-40 ■ Tracing E.

a. An anomalous fetus
b. A sleeping fetus
c. A nonacidotic fetus
d. An acidotic fetus

Mrs. H is a 35-year-old G2, P1001 who has type 2 (gestational) diabetes, is at 38 weeks' gestation, and is planning a vaginal birth after cesarean (VBAC). At admission, the FHR is 130 bpm; BP, 158/72; pulse, 80; respirations, 20; and temperature, 36.8° C (98.2° F). Her vaginal examination shows a thick cervix, ballottable vertex, and intact membranes. EFM is being accomplished via tocodynamometer and Doppler ultrasound.

10. Tracing G (Figure 12-42) began within minutes of her admission to the labor and delivery room. The tracing shows which of the following?

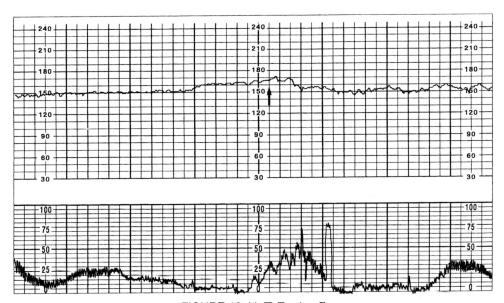

FIGURE 12-41 ■ Tracing F.

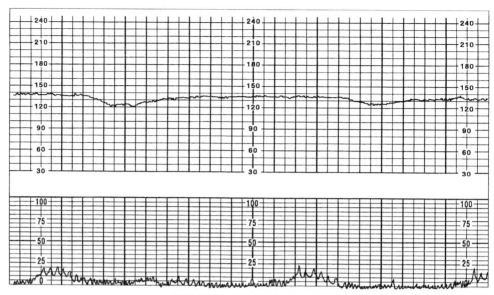

FIGURE 12-42 ■ Tracing G.

a. Late decelerations
b. Variable decelerations
c. Reassuring variability and BL features
d. Diabetic acidosis

11. Interventions for tracing G (see Figure 12-42) would be expected to:
a. Change maternal position and administer oxygen (8 to 10 L/min) via snug face mask to maximize oxygenation and uteroplacental blood flow.
b. Initiate adequate intravenous fluids and oxytocin augmentation to improve hydration status and adequate labor.
c. Administer oxygen (8 to 10 L/min) via snug face mask to maximize oxygenation.
d. Notify anesthesia and prepare for labor epidural anesthesia.

Anesthesia was immediately available, and an epidural was initiated for a cesarean delivery. Mrs. H was delivered of a male infant weighing 3997 g (8 lb, 13 oz). The Apgar score Mrs. H was 2 and 4 at 1 and 5 minutes, respectively, and umbilical blood gases revealed mixed respiratory and metabolic acidosis.

12. Tracing H (Figure 12-43) represents which of the following?
a. Machine malfunction
b. Fetal dysrhythmia
c. Fetal demise
d. Maternal heart rate

13. Tracing I (Figure 12-44) occurred approximately 1 hour following an amniocentesis while the fetus was undergoing routine observation. Interpretation of the tracing is:
a. Reactive nonstress test
b. Increased LTV (variability)
c. Machine artifact
d. Undulating pattern

Tracing J (Figure 12-45) is of a G1, P0 who is receiving oxytocin at 4 mU per minute. She is 5 to 6 cm dilated, 90% effaced, and at −1 station. EFM is being accomplished via fetal spiral electrode and tocodynamometer.

14. During the first 1½ minutes of the strip, which of the following interpretations can be made?
a. LTV + (variability moderate) and + fetal reactivity
b. LTV ↑ (variability marked); saltatory pattern

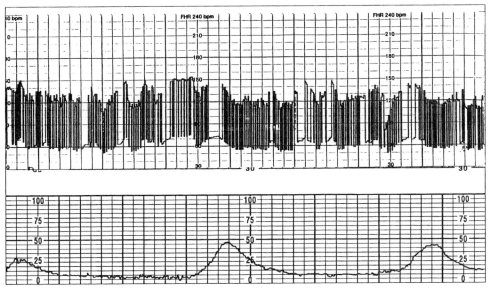

FIGURE 12-43 ▪ Tracing H.

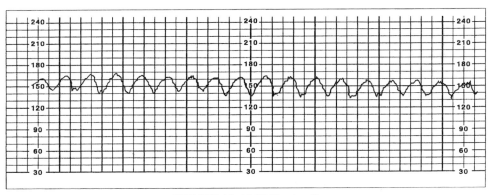

FIGURE 12-44 ▪ Tracing I.

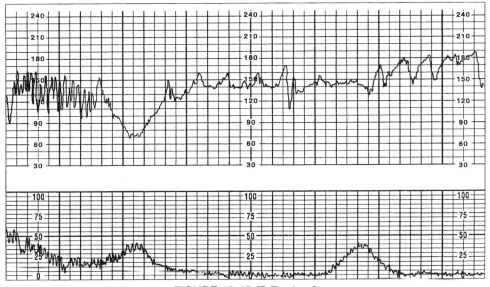

FIGURE 12-45 ▪ Tracing J.

c. Fetal atrial fibrillation
d. Fetal SVT (supraventricular tachycardia)

15. In tracing J (see Figure 12-45), during the last 1½ minutes of the strip, the FHR is likely demonstrating:
   a. A prolonged acceleration
   b. Overshoots
   c. Nonreassuring variable decelerations
   d. Compensatory sympathetic response to previous 1½ minutes of tracing

Ms. A is a G1, P0 in labor at 6 to 7 cm of dilatation, 90% effaced, and −1 station. EFM is accomplished via fetal spiral electrode and tocodynamometer.

16. Tracing K (Figure 12-46) shows her to have which of the following?
   a. LTV +, STV + (variability moderate), reactivity
   b. LTV ↓, overshoots
   c. Non–rapid-eye-movement fetal sleep-wake state
   d. Variable decelerations

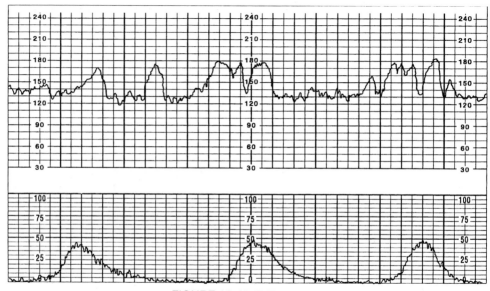

FIGURE 12-46 ■ Tracing K.

ANSWERS TO STUDY QUESTIONS

1. b	5. c	9. c	13. d
2. d	6. c	10. a	14. b
3. b	7. b	11. a	15. d
4. a	8. d	12. b	16. a

REFERENCES

Adelsperger, D., & Waymire, V. (2003). Physiological interventions for fetal heart rate patterns. In N. Feinstein, K.L. Torgersen, & J.L. Atterbury (Eds.), *Fetal heart monitoring principles and practices* (3rd ed., pp. 159-172). Dubuque, IA: Kendall-Hunt Publications.

Allan, L.D., Crawford, D.C., Anderson, R.H., & Tynan, M. (1984). Evaluation and treatment of fetal arrhythmias. *Clinical Cardiology, 7*(9), 467-473.

American College of Obstetricians and Gynecologists (ACOG). (1995a). *Fetal heart rate patterns: Monitoring, interpretation, and management* (Technical Bulletin No. 207). Washington, DC: ACOG.

American College of Obstetricians and Gynecologists (ACOG). (1995b). *Fetal heart rate patterns: Monitoring, interpretation, and management* (Technical Bulletin No. 207). Washington, DC: ACOG.

Anyaegbunam, A., Tran, T., Jadali, D., Randolph, G., & Mikhail, M.S. (1997). Assessment of fetal well-being in methadone-maintained pregnancies: Abnormal nonstress tests. *Gynecologic and Obstetric Investigations, 43*(1), 25-28.

Association of Women's Health, Obstetric, and Neonatal Nurses. (2002). *Fetal assessment (clinical position statement)*. Washington, DC: AWHONN.

Bianchi, D., Crobleholme, T., & D'Alton, M. (2000). *Fetology: Diagnosis and management of the fetal patient*. Philadelphia: McGraw-Hill.

Cabaniss, M. (1993). *Fetal monitoring interpretation*. Philadelphia: Lippincott.

Chan, F.Y., Woo, S.K., Ghosh, A., Tang, M., & Lam, C. (1990). Prenatal diagnosis of congenital fetal arrhythmias by simultaneous pulsed Doppler velocimetry of the fetal abdominal aorta and inferior vena cava. *Obstetrics & Gynecology, 76*(2), 200-205.

Copel, J.A., Buyon, J.P., & Kleinman, C.S. (1995). Successful in utero therapy of fetal heart block. *American Journal of Obstetrics and Gynecology, 173*(5), 1384-1390.

Crosson, J.E., & Brenner, J.I. (1999). Fetal arrhythmias. In D.K. James, P.J. Steer, C.P. Weiner, & B. Gonik (Eds.). *High-risk pregnancy: Management options* (2nd ed., pp. 371-378). London: Saunders.

Cuneo, B.F., & Strasburger, J.F. (2000). Management strategy for fetal tachycardia. *Obstetrics and Gynecology, 96*(4), 575-581.

Cypher, R., & Adeslperger, D. (2003). Assessment of fetal oxygenation and acid-base status. In N. Feinstein, K. L. Torgersen, & J. L. Atterbury (Eds.), *Fetal heart monitoring principles and practices* (3rd ed., pp. 177-196). Dubuque, IA: Kendall-Hunt Publications.

Cypher, R., Adelsperger, D., & Torgersen, K.L. (2003). Interpretation of the fetal heart rate. In N. Feinstein, K.L. Torgersen, & J.L. Atterbury (Eds.), *Fetal heart monitoring principles and practices* (3rd ed., pp. 113-154). Dubuque, IA: Kendall-Hunt Publications.

DeVore, G.R., Siassi, B., & Platt, L.D. (1984). Fetal echocardiography. IV. M-mode assessment of ventricular size and contractility during the second and third trimesters of pregnancy in the normal fetus. *American Journal of Obstetrics and Gynecology, 150*(8), 981-988.

Dildy, G.A., Thorp, J.A., Yeast, J.D., & Clark, S.L. (1996). The relationship between oxygen saturation and pH in umbilical blood: Implications for intrapartum fetal oxygenation monitoring. *American Journal of Obstetrics and Gynecology, 175*(3), 682-687.

Drose, J.A. (1998). *Fetal echocardiography*. Philadelphia: Saunders.

Ecker, J.L., & Parer, J. T. (1999). Obstetric evaluation of fetal acid-base balance. *Critical Reviews in Clinical Laboratory Sciences, 36*(5), 407-451.

Eronen, M., Heikkila, P., & Teramo, K. (2001). Congenital complete heart block in the fetus: Hemodynamic features, antenatal treatment, and outcome in six cases. *Pediatric Cardiology, 22*(5), 385-392.

Feinstein, N.F., & Atterbury, J.L. (2003). Intrinsic influences on the fetal heart rate. In N. Feinstein, K.L. Torgersen, & J.L. Atterbury (Eds.), *Fetal heart monitoring principles and practices* (3rd ed., pp. 39-56). Dubuque, IA: Kendall-Hunt Publications.

Feinstein, N.F., Sprague, A., & Trepanier, M.J. (2000). *Fetal heart rate auscultation*. Washington, DC: AWHONN.

Feinstein, N.F., Torgersen, K.L., & Atterbury, J.L. (2003). *Fetal heart monitoring principles and practices* (3rd ed.). Dubuque, IA: Kendall-Hunt Publications.

Ferrer, P.L. (1998). Fetal arrhythmias. In B.J. Deal, G.S. Wolff, & H. Gelband (Eds.), *Current concepts in diagnosis and management of arrhythmias in infants and children* (pp. 17-63). Armonk, NY: Futura.

Freeman, R.K., Garite, T.J., & Nageotte, M.P. (1991). *Fetal heart rate monitoring* (2nd ed.). Baltimore: Williams & Wilkins.

Freidman, D.M., Zervoudakis, I., & Buyon, J.P. (1998). Perinatal monitoring of fetal well-being in the presence of congenital heart block. *American Journal of Perinatology, 15*(12), 669-673.

Fyfe, D.A., Meyer, K.B., & Case, C.L. (1988). Sonographic assessment of fetal cardiac arrhythmias. *Journal of the American College of Cardiology, 12*, 1292-1297.

Garite, T.J. (2002). Intrapartum fetal evaluation. In S.G. Gabbe, J.R. Niebyl, & J.L. Simpson (Eds.), *Obstetrics: Normal and problem pregnancies* (4th ed., pp. 395-429). New York: Churchill Livingstone.

Garite, T.J., Dildy, G.A., McNamara, H., Nageotte, M.P., Boehm, F.H., Dellinger, E.H., et al. (2000). A multicenter controlled trial of fetal pulse oximetry in the intrapartum management of nonreassuring fetal heart rate patterns. *American Journal of Obstetrics and Gynecology, 138*(5), 1049-1058.

Garite, T.J., & Porreco, R.P. (2001). Evaluating fetal hypoxia with pulse oximetry. *Contemporary OB/GYN, 46*(7), 12-26.

Gregg, A.R., & Weiner, C.P. (1993). "Normal" umbilical arterial and venous acid-base and blood gas values. *Clinical Obstetrics and Gynecology, 36*(1), 24-32.

Hammacher, K. (1969). The clinical significance of cardiotocography. In P. Huntingford, K. Hüter, & E. Saling (Eds.), *Perinatal medicine: 1st European Congress, Berlin* (p. 81). Stuttgart, Germany: Thieme.

Harvey, C. J. (1987). Fetal scalp stimulation: Enhancing the interpretation of fetal monitor tracings. *Journal of Perinatal Nursing, 1*(1), 13-21.

Hohn, A., & Stanton, R. (2002). The cardiovascular system. In A. Fanaroff, & R. Martin (Eds.), *Neonatal-perinatal medicine: Diseases of the fetus and infant* (7th ed., pp. 883-940). St. Louis: Mosby.

Horsfall, A.C., Venables, P.J., Taylor, P.V., & Maini, R.N. (1991). Ro and La antigens and maternal anti-La idiotype on the surface of myocardial fibres in congenital heart block. *Journal of Autoimmunity, 4*(1), 165-176.

King, T.L., & Parer, J.T. (2000). The physiology of fetal heart rate patters and perinatal asphyxia. *Journal of Perinatal and Neonatal Nursing, 14*(3), 19-39.

King, T.L., & Simpson, K.R. (2001). Fetal assessment during labor. In K.R. Simpson & P. Creehan (Eds.), *Perinatal nursing* (2nd ed., pp. 378-416). Philadelphia: Lippincott.

Kleinman, C.S., Donnerstein, R.L., Jaffe, C.C., DeVore, G.R., Weinstein, E.M., Lynch, D.C., et al. (1983). Fetal echocardiography: A tool for evaluation of in utero cardiac arrhythmias and monitoring of in utero therapy: Analysis of 71 patients. *American Journal of Cardiology, 51*(2), 237-243.

Kleinman, C.S., Nehgme, R., & Copel, J.A. (1999). Fetal cardiac arrhythmias: Diagnosis and therapy. In R.K. Creasy & R. Resnick (Eds.), *Maternal-fetal medicine* (4th ed., pp. 301-318). Philadelphia: Saunders.

Kopecky, E.A., Ryan, M.L., Barrett, J.F., Seaward, P.G., Ryan, G., Koren, G., et al. (2000). Fetal response to maternally administered morphine. *American Journal of Obstetricians and Gynecologists, 183*(2), 424-430.

Lagercrantz, H., & Slotkin, T.A. (1986). The "stress" of being born. *Scientific American, 254*(4), 100-107.

Litsey, S. E., Noonan, J.A., O'Connor, W.N., Cottrill, C.M., & Mitchell, B. (1985). Maternal connective tissue disease and congenital heart block. *British Heart Journal, 60*, 512-515.

Martin, C.B. Jr. (1982). Physiology and clinical use of fetal heart rate variability. *Clinics in Perinatology, 9*(2), 339-352.

May, K., & Mahlmeister, L. (1994). *Comprehensive maternity nursing*. Philadelphia: Lippincott-Raven.

Meijboom, E.J., van Engelen, A.D., van de Beek, E.W., Weijtens, O., Lautenschutz, J.M., & Benatar, A.A. (1994). Fetal arrhythmias. *Current Opinions in Cardiology, 9*(1), 97-102.

Moffatt, F.W., & Feinstein, N. (2003). Techniques for fetal heart assessment. In N. Feinstein, K. Torgersen, & J. Atterbury (Eds.), *Fetal heart monitoring principles and practices* (3rd ed., pp. 77-106). Dubuque, IA: Kendall-Hunt Publications.

Moodley, T.R., Vaughan, J.E., Chuntarpursat, I., Wood, D., Noddeboe, Y., & Schwarting, F. (1986). Congenital heart block detected in utero. A case report. *South African Medical Journal, 70*(7), 433-434.

Mucklow, J.C. (1986). The fate of drugs in pregnancy. *Clinics of Obstetrics and Gynaecology, 13*(2), 161-175.

Muller, J.S., Antunes, M., Behle, I., Teixeira, L., & Zielinsky, P. (2002). Acute effects of maternal smoking on fetal-placental-maternal system hemodynamic. *Arquivos Brasileiros De Cardiologia, 78*(2), 148-155.

Murray, M.L. (2001). *Antepartal and intrapartal fetal monitoring* (2nd ed.). Albuquerque: Learning Resources International, Inc.

National Institute of Child Health and Development (NICHD) Research Planning Workshop. (1997). Electronic fetal heart rate monitoring: Research guidelines for interpretation. *Journal of Obstetric, Gynecologic and Neonatal Nursing, 26*(6), 635-640.

Nijland, R., Jongsma, H.W., Nijhuis, J.G., van den Berg, P.P., & Oeseburg, B. (1995). Arterial oxygen saturation in relation to metabolic acidosis in fetal lambs. *American Journal of Obstetrics and Gynecology, 172*(3), 810-819.

Norwitz, E.R., Robinson, J.N., & Repke, J.T. (2002). Labor and delivery. In S.G. Gabbe, J.R. Neibyl, & J.L. Simpson (Eds.), *Obstetrics: Normal and problem pregnancies* (4th ed., pp. 353-394). New York: Churchill Livingstone.

Nyberg, D.A., & Emerson, D.S. (1990). Cardiac malformations. In D.A. Nyberg, B.S. Mahony, & D.H. Pretorius (Eds.), *Diagnostic ultrasound of fetal anomalies: Test and atlas* (pp. 300-341). Chicago: Yearbook Medical.

Oncken, C.A., Hardardottir, H., Hatsukami, D.K., Lupo, V.R., Rodis, J.F., & Smeltzer, J.S. (1997). Effects of transdermal nicotine or smoking on nicotine concentrations and maternal-fetal hemodynamics. *Obstetrics and Gynecology, 90*(4, Pt 1), 569-574.

Oncken, C.A., Kranzler, H., O'Malley, P., Gendreau, P., & Campbell, W.A. (2002). The effect of cigarette smoking on fetal heart rate characteristics. *Obstetrics and Gynecology, 90*(5, Pt 1), 751-755.

Parer, J.T. (1976). Physiological regulation of the fetal heart rate. *Journal of Obstetric, Gynecologic, and Neonatal Nursing, 5*(Suppl 5), 26s-29s.

Parer, J.T. (1997). *Handbook of fetal heart monitoring* (2nd ed.). Philadelphia: Saunders.

Parer, J.T. (1999). Fetal heart rate. In R.K. Creasy & R. Resnick (Eds.), *Maternal-fetal medicine* (4th ed., pp. 270-300). Philadelphia: Saunders.

Petrie, R. (1991). Intrapartum fetal evaluation. In S. Gabbe, J. Neibyl, & J. Simpson (Eds.). *Obstetrics: Normal and problem pregnancies* (2nd ed., p. 457). New York: Churchill Livingstone.

Pickoff, A.S. (1998). Developmental electrophysiology in the fetus and neonate. In R.A. Polin & W.W. Fox (Eds.), *Fetal and neonatal physiology* (2nd ed., pp. 891-913). Philadelphia: Saunders.

Pinsky, W.W., Gillette, P.C., Garson, A. Jr., & McNamara, D.G. (1982). Diagnosis, management, and long-term results of patients with congenital complete atrioventricular block. *Pediatrics, 69*(6), 728-733.

Reddy, U.M., Paine, L.L., Gegor, C.L., Johnson, M.J., & Johnson, T.R.B. (1991). Fetal movement during labor. *American Journal of Obstetrics and Gynecology, 165*(4 Pt 1), 1073-1076.

Reiss, R.E., Gabbe, S.G., & Petrie, R.H. (2001). Intrapartum fetal evaluation. In S.G. Gabbe, J.R. Niebyl, & J.L. Simpson (Eds.), *Obstetrics: Normal and problem pregnancies* (4th ed., pp. 396-424). New York: Churchill-Livingstone.

Richardson, B.S., Carmichael, L., Homan, J., & Patrick, J. (1992). Electrocortical activity, electrocular activity, and breathing movements in fetal sleep with prolonged and graded hypoxemia. *American Journal of Obstetrics and Gynecology, 167*(2), 533-558.

Schmidt, K.G., Ulmer, H.E., Silverman, N.H., Kleinman, C.S., & Copel, J.A. (1991). Perinatal outcome of fetal complete atrioventricular block: A multicenter experience. *Journal of the American College of Cardiology, 17*(6), 1360-1366.

Schmolling, J., Renke, K., Richter, O., Pfeiffer, K., Schlebusch, H., & Holler, T. (2000). Digoxin, flecainide, and amiodarone transfer across the placenta and the effects of an elevated umbilical venous pressure on the transfer rate. *Therapeutic Drug Monitor, 22*(5), 582-588.

Seelbach-Göbel, B., Heupel, M., Kühnert, M., & Butterwegge, M. (1999). The prediction of fetal acidosis by means of intrapartum fetal pulse oximetry. *American Journal of Obstetrics and Gynecology, 180*(1 Pt 1), 73-81.

Shaffer, E.M., & Wiggins, J.W. (1998). Fetal dysrhythmias. In J.A. Drose (Ed.), *Fetal echocardiography* (pp. 279-290). Philadelphia: Saunders.

Sharland, G. (2001). Fetal cardiography. *Seminars in Neonatology, 6*(1), 3-15.

Shenker, L. (1979). Fetal cardiac arrhythmias. *Obstetrics and Gynecologic Survey, 34*(8), 561-572.

Silverman, N.H., Kleinman, C.S., Rudolph, A.M., Copel, J.A., Weinstein, E.M., Enderlein, M.A., et al. (1985). Fetal atrioventricular valve insufficiency associated with nonimmune hydrops: A two-dimensional echocardiographic and pulsed Doppler ultrasound study. *Circulation, 72*(4), 825-832.

Simpson, K.R. (1998). Intrapartum fetal oxygen saturation monitoring. *Lifelines, 3*(2), 20-24.

Simpson, K.R., & Knox, G.E. (2003). Communication of fetal heart monitoring information. In N. Feinstein, K.L. Torgersen, & J.L. Atterbury (Eds.), *Fetal heart monitoring principles and practices* (3rd ed., pp. 201-232). Dubuque, IA: Kendall-Hunt Publications.

Simpson, K.R., & Porter, M.L. (2001). Fetal oxygen saturation monitoring: Using this new technology for fetal assessment during labor. *Lifelines, 5*(2), 26-33.

Snell, B.J. (1993). The use of amnioinfusion in nurse-midwifery practice. *Journal of Nurse Midwifery, 38*(2 Suppl), 625-715.

Society of Obstetricians and Gynaecologists of Canada (SOGC). (2002a). *SOGC Policy Statement: Fetal health surveillance in labour* (SOGC Clinical Practice Guidelines No. 112). Ottawa, Ontario, Canada: SOGC.

Society of Obstetricians and Gynaecologists of Canada (SOGC). (2002b). Fetal health surveillance in labour (SOGC Clinical Practice Guidelines No. 112). *Journal of Obstetrics and Gynaecology in Canada, 112*(March), 1-13.

Southall D.P., Arrowsmith, W.A., Oakley, J.R., McEnergy, G., Anderson, R.H., & Shinebourne, E.A. (1979). Prolonged QT interval and cardiac arrhythmias in two neonates: Sudden infant death syndrome in one case. *Archives of Disease in Childhood, 54*(10), 776-779.

Southall, D.P., Richards, J., Hardwick, R.A., Shinebourne, E.A., Gibbens, G.L., Thelwall-Jones, H., et al. (1980). Prospective study of fetal heart rate and rhythm patterns. *Archives of Disease in Childhood, 55*(7), 506-511.

Stewart, P.A., & Wladimiroff, J.W. (1988). Fetal atrial arrhythmias associated with redundancy/aneurysm of the foramen ovale. *Journal of Clinical Ultrasound, 16*(9), 643-650.

Strasburger, J.F. (2000). Fetal arrhythmias. *Progress in Pediatric Cardiology, 11*(1), 1-17.

Tanel, R.E., & Rhodes, L.A. (2001). Fetal and neonatal arrhythmias. *Clinics in Perinatology, 28*(1), 187-207.

Taylor, P.V., Scott, J.S., Gerlis, L.M., Esscher, E., & Scott, O. (1986). Maternal antibodies against fetal cardiac antigens in congenital complete heart block. *New England Journal of Medicine, 315*(11), 667-672.

Thorp, J.A., & Rushing, R.S. (1999). Umbilical cord blood gas analysis. *Obstetrics and Gynecology Clinics of North America, 26*(4), 695-709.

Torgersen, K.L. (2003). Fetal arrhythmias and dysrhythmias. In N. Feinstein, K.L. Torgersen, & J.L. Atterbury (Eds.), *Fetal heart monitoring principles and practices* (3rd ed., pp. 289-324). Dubuque, IA: Kendall-Hunt Publications.

Tucker, S.M. (2000). *Pocket guide to fetal monitoring and assessment* (4th ed.). St. Louis: Mosby.

Vautier-Rit, S., Dufour, P., Vaksmann, G., Subtil, D., Vaast, P., Valat, A.S., et al., (2000). Fetal arrhythmias: Diagnosis, prognosis, treatment, apropos of 33 cases. *Gynecologic & Obstetric Fertility, 28,* 729-737.

Vlagsma, R., Hallensleben, E., & Meijboom, E.J. (2001). Supraventricular tachycardia and premature atrial contractions in the fetus. *Ned Tijdschr Genneskd, 145*(7), 295-299.

Wadhwa, P.D., Sandman, C.A., & Garite, T.J. (2001). The neurobiology of stress in human pregnancy: Implications for prematurity and development of the fetal central nervous system. *Progress in Brain Research, 133,* 131-142.

Weindling, S.N., Saul, J.P., Triedman, J.K., Burke, R.P., Jonas, R.A., Gamble, W.J., et al. (1994). Staged pacing therapy for congenital complete heart block in premature infants. *American College of Cardiology, 74,* 412-413.

POSTPARTUM PERIOD

13 Physical and Psychologic Changes

JANET SCOGGIN

OBJECTIVES

1. Identify normal physiologic changes in the reproductive system after childbirth.
2. Describe systemic physiologic changes after childbirth.
3. Describe common emotional changes in the family in response to childbirth.
4. Recognize normal attachment behaviors in parents and infants.
5. Differentiate between "baby blues" and postpartum depression.
6. Prevent postpartum complications using assessment data.
7. Design individualized client education based on assessed needs.
8. Develop a discharge teaching plan designed to facilitate competent self-care and assumption of the parenting role.

INTRODUCTION

A. **Postpartum period (puerperium)**
   This period encompasses the time from the delivery of the placenta and membranes to the return of the woman's reproductive system to its nonpregnant condition.
B. **Maternal system changes**
   1. Reproductive system
      a. Uterus
         (1) Involution (retrogressive return to normal condition after pregnancy)
            (a) Immediately after delivery
               (i) Weight is approximately 1000 g (2 lb, 4 oz).
               (ii) Fundal height is midway between symphysis and umbilicus in midline.
               (iii) Afterpains (contractions) are common, especially for multiparas and breastfeeding mothers.
            (b) At 1 hour postpartum
               (i) Fundal height is at the umbilicus in midline.
               (ii) Consistency is firm and contracted.
            (c) Within 12 hours—1 cm above the umbilicus
            (d) At day 2 and after
               (i) Fundal height decreases by 1 cm (0.4 in)/day and is no longer palpable in the abdomen by day 10.
               (ii) Afterpains decrease in frequency after the first few days and usually are associated with
                  ▪ Breastfeeding
                  ▪ Multiparity

- Multiple fetuses
- Conditions producing overdistension of the uterus
- (e) Postpartum hemorrhage is the leading cause of maternal morbidity and mortality (see Chapter 30 for a complete discussion).
- (2) Lochia
  - (a) Composition
    - (i) Endometrial tissue
    - (ii) Blood
    - (iii) Lymph
  - (b) Stages
    - (i) Rubra (red): 1 to 3 days
      - Scant: less than 2.5 cm (1 in) on menstrual pad in 1 hour
      - Light: less than 10 cm (4 in) on menstrual pad in 1 hour
      - Moderate: less than 15 cm (6 in) on menstrual pad in 1 hour
      - Heavy: saturated menstrual pad in 1 hour
      - Excessive: menstrual pad saturated in 15 minutes
    - (ii) Serosa (pink, brown-tinged): 3 to 10 days
    - (iii) Alba (yellowish-white): 10 to 14 days but can last 3 to 6 weeks and remain normal
  - (c) A danger sign is the reappearance of bright red blood after lochia rubra has stopped.
  - (d) Odor is normally that of menstrual flow; foul-smelling lochia might indicate infection.
  - (e) Amount might increase temporarily on standing because of pooling in uterus and vagina.
  - (f) Amount of lochia might be less after cesarean section, but stages remain unchanged.
  - (g) Average amount of lochial discharge is 240 to 270 ml (8 to 9 oz).
- (3) Return of the menstrual cycle
  - (a) Nonlactating women
    - (i) At 6 to 8 weeks (40% to 45%)
    - (ii) At 12 weeks (75%)
    - (iii) Within 6 months (100%)
  - (b) Lactating women: some resume menstruation as early as 12 weeks, but some might not resume menstruation for as long as 18 months.
- (4) Ovulation: depends on prolactin levels.
  - (a) For lactating women, 80% of the first few cycles are anovulatory.
  - (b) For nonlactating women, 50% of the first few cycles are anovulatory.
- **b.** Cervix
  - (1) Cervix is edematous immediately postdelivery.
  - (2) Cervix is easily distensible for several days postdelivery.
  - (3) Internal os returns to normal by 2 weeks.
  - (4) External os widens and appears as a slit.
- **c.** Vagina
  - (1) Rugae reappear in 3 weeks.
  - (2) Vagina returns to near prepregnant size at 6 to 8 weeks postdelivery, but will always remain slightly larger.
  - (3) Normal mucus production usually returns with ovulation.

  d. Perineum
  - (1) Episiotomy is normally without redness, discharge, or edema; most healing takes place within the first 2 weeks.
  - (2) Intact perineum might have ecchymosis, edema, or both.
  - (3) Lacerations might be present.
    - (a) First degree: through skin and structures that are superficial to muscle
    - (b) Second degree: extends through perineal muscles
    - (c) Third degree: continues through anal sphincter muscle
    - (d) Fourth degree: also involves anterior rectal wall

2. Breasts
  - **a.** Changes of pregnancy regress in 1 to 2 weeks' postpartum if mother is not breastfeeding.
  - **b.** Nipples become erect when stimulated.
  - **c.** Breasts increase in vascularity and swell in response to presence of prolactin at the second or third postpartum day (engorgement).
  - **d.** Nonbreastfeeding engorgement will subside in 2 to 3 days (see Chapter 14 for a complete discussion of lactation).

3. Endocrine system
  - **a.** Placental hormones
    - (1) Human chorionic gonadotropin (HCG) levels are nonexistent at the end of the first postpartum week.
    - (2) Human chorionic somatomammotropin (HCS) (human placental lactogen [HPL]) is undetectable by 24 hours postdelivery.
    - (3) Plasma progesterone levels are undetectable by 72 hours postdelivery; production is reestablished with the first menstrual cycle.
    - (4) Plasma estrogen levels decrease to 10% of the prenatal value within 3 hours after delivery and reach the lowest levels by day 7.
  - **b.** Pituitary hormones
    - (1) Serum prolactin levels rise significantly during the first 2 weeks and rapidly decline to prepregnant levels in the absence of breastfeeding.
    - (2) Follicle-stimulating hormone (FSH) and luteinizing hormone (LH) are absent during the first few weeks of the postpartum period.

4. Cardiovascular system
  - **a.** Heart
    - (1) Returns to normal position because of shift in diaphragm and abdominal contents.
    - (2) Cardiac output increases during first and second stages of labor and declines rapidly after delivery, returning to normal within 2 to 3 weeks.
    - (3) Cardiac load is increased because as uterine blood flow is redirected into the general circulation.
  - **b.** Blood volume
    - (1) There is an immediate decrease at delivery related to blood loss (normal blood loss at delivery is 200 to 500 ml for a vaginal delivery and 600 to 800 ml for a cesarean delivery; another 800 ml is lost during the first postpartal week).
    - (2) Return to normal prepregnant volume takes 3 to 4 weeks.
  - **c.** Hematologic changes
    - (1) Hematocrit
      - (a) Rises immediately after delivery and is related to a decrease in plasma volume and to dehydration.
      - (b) Returns to prepregnant value (37% to 47%) in 4 to 5 weeks.

        (2) Hemoglobin
- (a) Degree of blood loss is reflected in postpartum hemoglobin levels (500 ml blood loss equals 1 gm hemoglobin reduction; Blackburn, 2003).
- (b) Stabilizes in 2 to 3 days and returns to nonpregnant values 4 to 6 weeks' postpartum.

        (3) White blood cell count
- (a) Might increase to 20,000/mm³ or more during the first 10 days postpartum (average is 14,000 to 16,000/mm³).
- (b) Increase is primarily in neutrophils.
- (c) Might increase without the presence of infection; however, an increase of more than 30% over a 6-hour period is suggestive of infection (see Chapter 30 for further discussion).

    d. Vital signs

        (1) Blood pressure readings immediately postdelivery should be the same as those taken during labor.
- (a) Increased blood pressure might suggest pregnancy-induced hypertension.
- (b) Decreased blood pressure might suggest orthostatic hypotension or uterine hemorrhage.

        (2) Temperature might be slightly elevated because of dehydration: 36.2° to 38° C (98° to 100.4° F).

        (3) Pulse rate: bradycardia is normal in early postpartum period.
- (a) Normal range is 40 to 80 beats per minute (bpm).
- (b) Tachycardia is abnormal and might indicate uterine hemorrhage or infection.

5. Respiratory system

    a. Pulmonary function

        (1) Is affected primarily by change in thoracic cage.
- (a) Diaphragm descends.
- (b) Organs revert to normal positions.

        (2) Returns to prepregnant levels by 6 to 8 weeks' postpartum.

        (3) Respirations are usually in the range of 16 to 24/min.

    b. Acid-base balance returns to prepregnant levels by 3 weeks' postdelivery.

    c. Basal metabolic rate remains elevated for as long as 14 days' postpartum.

6. Gastrointestinal system

    a. Appetite returns to normal immediately postdelivery.

    b. Gastric motility might remain decreased, leading to constipation.

    c. Normal bowel elimination resumes at 2 to 3 days postdelivery.

    d. Average weight loss is 12 lb (5.5 kg) at time of delivery; another 5 lb (2.3 kg) is lost during the first postpartal week because of diuresis.

7. Urinary system

    a. Postdelivery edema of bladder, urethra, and urinary meatus is common because of delivery trauma.

        (1) Urinary retention might occur.

        (2) An elevated or laterally displaced uterus is a common sign of urinary retention after delivery.

    b. Kidney function

        (1) Mild proteinuria might persist related to catabolism in early postpartum period.

        (2) Diuresis begins within 12 hours postdelivery and continues throughout the first week of the postpartum period.

        (3) Normal function returns by 4 weeks after delivery.

8. Musculoskeletal system
   a. Abdominal musculature
      (1) Muscles relaxed because of stretching during pregnancy.
      (2) Separation of the rectus muscle (diastasis recti), usually 2 to 4 cm (1 to 2.5 in), can resolve by 6 weeks with gentle exercise.
   b. Joints stabilize again after 6 to 8 weeks' postpartum.
9. Integumentary system
   a. Hyperpigmentation gradually disappears after delivery.
   b. Diaphoresis is common, especially at night, for the first week.
      (1) Can become profuse at times.
      (2) Is a mechanism to reduce the fluids retained during pregnancy.
10. Immune system
    a. For women with Rh incompatibility, anti-RhD immunoglobulin is administered within 72 hours after delivery to prevent antibody formation if the mother is nonsensitized.
    b. Blood group incompatibility: ABO incompatibility should be detected early to prevent neonatal complications.
    c. If the rubella titer is 18 or less, the woman should receive a rubella virus vaccine and instructions to avoid pregnancy for the next 3 months.

C. **Psychologic changes**
   1. Role change is an important psychologic change for the mother.
      a. The mother must relinquish other roles and take on the role of mother.
      b. New mothers typically progress through a series of developmental stages: the rate of progression through these stages is unique to each mother.
         (1) Dependent and "taking in" phase of mother (Rubin, 1975)
            (a) Increase in dependent behavior of mother; wants care for herself.
            (b) Mother asks many questions and talks a great deal about delivery experience.
            (c) Phase typically lasts 1 to 2 days.
            (d) Might be the only phase observed by nurse during hospitalization because of a trend toward a shortened inpatient stay for obstetric clients without complications.
         (2) Dependent-independent or "taking-hold" phase of mother
            (a) Begins to focus on needs of infant.
            (b) Relinquishes pregnant role.
            (c) Takes on maternal role.
            (d) Is interested in learning to care for infant.
            (e) Experiences a period of high fatigue and increased demands by infant.
            (f) Might experience baby blues.
            (g) Is typically in this phase 4 to 5 weeks.
         (3) Interdependent or letting-go phase of mother
            (a) Lets go of perception of infant as extension of herself, and views infant as separate.
            (b) Refocuses on relationship with partner.
            (c) Might return to work and relinquish part of child care to other caretakers.
   2. Attachment
      a. Attachment is the enduring emotional bond between a parent (or parent figure) and an infant (Klaus & Kennell, 1982).
      b. Attachment is essential to the infant's growth and survival.

    c. The mother-infant bond is the basis on which all subsequent attachments are formed and plays a major role in the infant's developing sense of self (Bowlby, 1969).

    d. Besides the mother, infants also attach to the father, siblings, and other significant caregivers.

  3. Baby blues

    a. Baby blues or postpartum blues are described as a mild, transient mood disturbance that frequently begins on the third postpartum day and lasts 2 or 3 days.

    b. Approximately 60% to 80% of women experience baby blues during the postpartum period.

    c. The onset of postpartum blues coincides with the normal physiologic drop in estrogen and progesterone, which is a possible cause of this emotional change.

CLINICAL PRACTICE

Physical Changes

A. Assessment

  1. Frequency of postpartum checks according to protocol or as follows

    a. First hour: every 15 minutes; second hour: every 30 minutes

    b. First 24 hours: every 4 hours

    c. After 24 hours: every 8 hours

  2. Vital signs and blood pressure

  3. Breasts

    a. Soft, filling, or firm

    b. Engorged, reddened, or painful

    c. Nipples: erectility, possible cracks and redness

  4. Uterus

    a. Consistency and tone

    b. Position

    c. Height

    d. Size

  5. Cesarean section incision site, if appropriate

    a. Dressing and incision

    b. Drainage

    c. Edema, color changes, or both (redness or ecchymosis)

  6. Bladder and urinary output

    a. Voiding pattern and amounts voided

    b. Distension

    c. Pain

  7. Bowel

    a. Bowel movements

    b. Hemorrhoids

    c. Bowel sounds: auscultate all four quadrants, especially after cesarean section

  8. Lochia

    a. Type and amount

    b. Presence of odor

    c. Presence of clots

  9. Perineum

    a. Episiotomy, lacerations, and hemorrhoids

  b. Bruising, hematoma, edema, discharge, and loss of approximation
  c. Reddened areas indicative of infection
 10. Extremities for thrombophlebitis
  a. Homans' sign (calf pain from passive dorsiflexion of foot)
  b. Check for redness, tenderness, and warmth.
 11. Diagnostic studies commonly ordered: complete blood count (CBC), hemoglobin and hematocrit (Hgb/HCT) levels, and urinalysis (UA)

B. Nursing Diagnoses
 1. Impaired tissue integrity related to episiotomy or laceration
 2. Risk for urinary retention related to perineal edema
 3. Risk for constipation related to perineal discomfort and slowed peristalsis
 4. Pain related to episiotomy, hemorrhoids, or cesarean section incision

C. Interventions/Outcomes
 1. Impaired tissue integrity related to episiotomy or laceration
  a. Interventions
   (1) Monitor episiotomy for redness, edema, bruising, hematoma, intact sutures, and bleeding.
   (2) Apply ice packs for 2 hours to decrease edema (can be used later for analgesic effect for up to 24 hours).
   (3) Apply heat three or four times daily after 24 hours postdelivery.
    (a) Dry: heat lamp
    (b) Moist: sitz bath
   (4) Pain relief
    (a) Analgesia: oral
    (b) Analgesia: topical
  b. Outcomes: improved tissue integrity as indicated by:
   (1) Signs that episiotomy is healing
   (2) Signs of infection absent
   (3) Discomfort being kept at tolerable levels
 2. Risk for urinary retention related to perineal trauma
  a. Interventions
   (1) Check for bladder distension, encourage voiding, and catheterize if indicated.
   (2) Encourage early ambulation.
   (3) Ensure adequate fluid intake.
   (4) Offer warm sitz bath, if needed.
  b. Outcomes: urinary elimination reestablished as indicated by:
   (1) First void within 4 to 8 hours after delivery
   (2) Nondistended bladder
   (3) Voidings more than 200 ml in first two voids
    (a) Less than 100 ml/void suggests retention with overflow; catheterization for residual is suggested.
    (b) No complaints of still feeling urge to void immediately after voiding
   (4) No pain or discomfort with voiding
 3. Risk for constipation related to perineal discomfort and slowed peristalsis
  a. Interventions
   (1) Encourage adequate intake of fluids (maximum intake of 2000 ml/day).
   (2) Encourage diet high in fiber and roughage.
   (3) Encourage ambulation.
   (4) Administer stool softener, laxative, enema, or suppository if needed.

(5) Encourage warm sitz baths.

(6) Apply topical anesthetics.

(7) Teach methods to avoid constipation and importance of bowel movement within 2 to 3 days (especially important with early discharge practices).

(8) Acknowledge client's fear associated with first postdelivery bowel movement.

(9) Monitor bowel sounds following cesarean section.

b. Outcomes: bowel elimination reestablished as indicated by:

(1) Bowel movement (soft, formed stool) by second or third postpartum day

(2) Return of bowel sounds in cesarean section client

(3) Reports of minimal discomfort

4. Pain related to episiotomy, hemorrhoids, or cesarean section incision

    a. Interventions

(1) Inspect condition of perineum.

(2) Administer cold or hot perineal treatment.

(3) Administer analgesic medication, as ordered.

(4) Monitor cesarean section delivery clients for incisional pain.

(5) Explain cause of pain and how long pain will last.

(6) Explore various methods of nonpharmaceutical pain relief (e.g., relaxation techniques).

    b. Outcomes: minimal pain is experienced when client:

(1) Reports only tolerable discomfort.

(2) Does not demonstrate signs of discomfort.

(3) Communicates need for pain relief.

Psychologic Changes

A. Assessment

    1. Maternal role

        a. History: factors influencing transition to the maternal role

(1) Condition of mother

    (a) Prolonged labor

    (b) Use of drugs during labor

    (c) Type of delivery (e.g., cesarean section birth)

    (d) Other complications at time of delivery

(2) Condition of infant

    (a) Gestational age

    (b) Admission to neonatal intensive care unit (NICU) for other reasons

    (c) Physical anomalies

(3) Socioeconomic factors

    (a) Economic resources

    (b) Degree of maternal social support

(4) Familial factors

    (a) Demands of infant's other siblings

    (b) Quality of maternal relationship with partner

(5) Maternal age or parity

    (a) Previous experience with maternal role

        (i) Very young mothers might not be informed about infant care.

          (ii) Older mothers might face conflicts related to meeting demands of all family members.

      (6) Role conflict related to career demands: active career women might have difficulty in adjusting to role changes and conflicting demands of infant, family, and job (see Chapter 7 for a complete discussion of age-related concerns).

2. Baby blues
   a. History: onset typically occurs on the third postpartum day.
   b. Observable symptoms
      (1) Irritability
      (2) Restlessness
      (3) Crying spells
      (4) Sleeplessness
      (5) Anger toward family members, including infant
      (6) Anxiety
      (7) Moodiness
   c. Psychosocial responses occurring in postpartum depression and psychosis include:
      (1) Exaggerated and prolonged irritability
      (2) Labile behavior
      (3) Withdrawal
      (4) Inability to cope
      (5) Inappropriate responses to infant and family
      (6) Psychotic (out of touch with reality) behavior (see Chapter 30 for further discussion)
3. Attachment
   a. History: factors influencing attachment
      (1) Maternal factors
         (a) Past experience with one's own mother
         (b) Cultural and ethnic background
         (c) Socioeconomic status
         (d) Wanted versus unwanted status of infant
         (e) Quality of relationship with infant's father
         (f) Degree of paternal support
         (g) Age and maturity level
         (h) Circumstances surrounding delivery
            (i) High-risk versus low-risk delivery
            (ii) Type of delivery
            (iii) Prolonged separation from infant after delivery
         (i) Physical health
         (j) Intelligence
         (k) Degree to which infant matches expectations
      (2) Infant factors
         (a) Gender
         (b) Appearance
         (c) Presence or absence of abnormalities
         (d) Temperament
         (e) Degree of alertness
      (3) Paternal factors
         (a) Age
         (b) Maturity
         (c) Past experiences with infants

           (d) Degree to which infant matches expectations

           (e) Quality of the relationship with infant's mother

           (f) Degree to which father has been included in prenatal and birth experiences

  b. Observable attachment behaviors

    (1) Definition: social signals designed to increase proximity of parent and child

    (2) Observable behaviors in mother toward infant

        (a) Touching

        (b) Holding

        (c) Gazing

        (d) Cuddling

        (e) Kissing

    (3) Behaviors observable in infant

        (a) Signaling behaviors (nondiscriminatory before 8 weeks)

          (i) Crying

          (ii) Smiling

          (iii) Babbling

          (iv) Grasping

          (v) Following with eyes and gazing

        (b) Approach behaviors (require locomotion and are not observed before 6 months of age)

          (i) Clinging

          (ii) Moving toward mother

          (iii) Following mother

  c. Maternal malattachment behaviors

    (1) Prenatally

        (a) Excessive mood swings

        (b) Emotional withdrawal

        (c) Excessive preoccupation with appearance

        (d) Numerous physical complaints

        (e) Failure during last trimester to prepare for infant's birth

    (2) Postnatally

        (a) Negative comments about infant's appearance

        (b) Disappointment about infant's gender

        (c) Failure to look at infant

        (d) Failure to touch or stroke infant

        (e) Failure to respond to infant's signaling behaviors

        (f) Failure to name infant

        (g) Limited handling of infant

        (h) Failure to meet infant's physical needs

B. Nursing Diagnoses

  1. Risk for impaired parenting related to failure to take on role of mother

  2. Risk for ineffective coping related to mood alteration

  3. Risk for psychologic injury related to failure to achieve parent-infant attachment

C. Interventions/Outcomes

  1. Risk for impaired parenting related to failure to take on role of mother

    a. Interventions

      (1) Meet mother's "taking in" needs; allow mother to express feelings about being a mother.

      (2) Allow mother to participate in infant's care and have infant in room with mother, if conditions permit.

(3) Provide nursing care for infant if mother is too exhausted to participate.

(4) Provide teaching related to physical caretaking skills.

    (a) Teach mother techniques of infant feeding.

    (b) Demonstrate and supervise mother's physical care activities (e.g., diapering and bathing).

    (c) Discuss normal infant rhythm and ways in which infants communicate needs.

(5) Provide community-health follow-up for mother identified to be at risk for failure to assume maternal role; for example, mothers who:

    (a) Are adolescents.

    (b) Have inadequate social support.

    (c) Fail to demonstrate interest in caring for infant.

(6) Follow up with a phone call 2 days postdischarge for clarification of any of mother's questions.

b. Outcomes

(1) No evidence of impaired parenting at time of discharge

2. Risk for ineffective coping related to mood alteration

a. Interventions

(1) Observe and document alteration in maternal mood.

(2) Provide supportive environment.

(3) Provide adequate opportunities for mother to rest and sleep.

(4) Provide mother with relief from infant care.

(5) Educate client's partner or significant other about expected behavior.

(6) Reassure mother that negative emotions are normal.

(7) Provide appropriate psychiatric referrals if symptoms have progressed to postpartum depression or psychosis.

b. Outcomes

(1) Client copes with mood alterations immediately after delivery

3. Risk for psychologic injury related to failure to achieve parent-infant attachment

a. Interventions

(1) Provide time for parent-infant interaction as soon after birth as mother's and infant's conditions permit.

(2) Provide environment that encourages questions and expression of feelings.

(3) Encourage early and frequent skin-to-skin and eye-to-eye contact between mother and infant (touching, unwrapping, examining infant).

(4) Provide sufficient time for nurse to give information to parents about their infant's condition and to assist them in caretaking.

(5) Encourage parents to participate in infant's care.

(6) Develop a team approach for support and encouragement of positive parent-infant interactions.

(7) Provide daily information about infant's condition if infant is admitted to the NICU or transferred to another institution.

b. Outcomes

(1) Positive parent-infant attachment indicated by observed positive reciprocal relationship between parents and infant

(2) Community health follow-up ensured after hospitalization if problems related to parent-infant attachment are observed

HEALTH EDUCATION

A. Introduction

1. As economic constraints for families and decreased reimbursement for hospitals from third-party payers continue, the national trend toward shortened in-hospital stays for uncomplicated obstetric care, discharge planning, and patient teaching become even more vital components of the nurse's role.
2. These economic factors also increase the need for the hospital-based nurse to provide postdischarge follow-up.
3. Communication with community agencies for referral and follow-up of identified problems is essential for the health and welfare of the new family unit.

The teaching plan should include the following components:

B. Physiologic changes

1. Involution of uterus and stages of lochia
2. Diaphoresis
3. Weight loss
   a. Usual loss of 10 to 12 lb (4.5 to 5.5 kg) occurs after delivery
   b. Additional 5- to 8-lb (2.3- to 3.6-kg) loss occurs from diuresis and involution
4. Breast changes occur, whether nursing or not nursing
5. Discomforts and measures to provide comfort
   a. Incisional healing (use ice packs, sitz bath, local or topical anesthetic or analgesic)
   b. After pains (administer analgesic)
   c. Breast engorgement (provide supportive brassiere or binder, ice packs, or analgesic)
   d. Hemorrhoids (use ice packs, sitz baths, heat lamp, or topical anesthetic; avoid constipation)

C. Psychologic changes

1. Discuss role changes experienced by all family members
2. Discuss plans for maternal reentry into the work force (if applicable) and provision of criteria for evaluation of daycare centers
3. Discuss danger signs of postpartum depression

D. Self-care measures

1. Personal hygiene, including perineal care
2. Postpartum exercises, including Kegel exercises
3. Schedule activities to avoid fatigue
4. Diet instructions
5. Special instructions
   a. Breast and nipple care; nursing or nonnursing instructions
   b. Incisional care; post–cesarean section care

E. Danger signs

1. Temperature higher than 100.4° F (38° C)
2. Excessive vaginal bleeding (2 or more pads saturated in 1 hour)
3. Resumption of bright-red bleeding after lochia has already turned brown, especially if accompanied by clots
4. Vaginal discharge that has a foul odor
5. Increased swelling, redness, or tenderness of breasts, legs, or incision
6. Burning sensation upon urination, or inability to urinate
7. Severe headaches, blurred vision
8. Severe mood swings or thoughts of harming self or infant

F. **Care of the newborn**
  1. Description of characteristics of a normal newborn
  2. Description of infant-feeding techniques
  3. Demonstration and supervision of physical care of the infant
     a. Bathing
     b. Changing
     c. Holding
     d. Feeding
  4. Discuss normal rhythms and cues of infant related to:
     a. Hunger
     b. Sleep
     c. Socialization
     d. Discomfort
  5. Discuss signs and symptoms of illness.
  6. Discuss balance of maternal and infant needs, as well as those of other household members.
  7. Discuss normal growth and development and appropriate approaches to encourage development.
G. **Importance of scheduling a postpartum checkup with health care provider for self and infant**
H. **Resumption of sexual intercourse:** may be safely resumed when there is no active bleeding and episiotomy has healed (approximately 3 weeks).
I. **Family planning and birth control**
  1. Explore her feelings about family planning.
  2. Provide information about various methods.
  3. Discuss methods to use with intercourse before postpartum check (e.g., condoms and foam) (see Chapter 15 for a complete discussion of contraception)

CASE STUDIES AND STUDY QUESTIONS

Ms. B, 15, delivered her first infant 1 hour ago. It was a normal vaginal delivery. She plans to bottle-feed her infant.

1. What progression can she expect in the stages of the lochia?
   a. Rubra, alba, serosa
   b. Alba, rubra, serosa
   c. Serosa, alba, rubra
   d. Rubra, serosa, alba

2. On examination, where would the uterus normally be located?
   a. At the level of the symphysis pubis
   b. Midway between the umbilicus and symphysis
   c. At the level of the umbilicus
   d. At the level of the xiphoid process

3. She might experience diaphoresis for the first few days of the postpartum period. Diaphoresis occurs because of which of the following?
   a. An infection in the reproductive tract
   b. The restoration of prepregnant body fluid levels
   c. The establishment of lactation
   d. The toxic side effects of certain pain medications

4. Because she is not breastfeeding, what breast changes can she expect during the postpartum period?
   a. The breasts will immediately return to the prepregnant state.
   b. Engorgement might occur for 24 to 36 hours.

c. Engorgement occurs only with breastfeeding.
d. The breasts will return to the prepregnant state in 1 to 2 weeks.

5. On her second postpartum day, the nursing assessment indicated the following findings. Which finding is considered abnormal?
   a. Uterus firmly contracted at the level of the umbilicus and shifted to the right
   b. Lochia rubra and a moderate flow without clots
   c. Diaphoretic state
   d. Breast discharge that is clear and yellowish

Ms. S, 31, delivered her third child by planned cesarean section 3 hours ago. She will breastfeed this infant as she has her other children.

6. Her afterpains are caused by which of the following?
   a. Analgesic drugs
   b. Surgical incision into the uterus
   c. Contractions of the uterus
   d. Multiparity

7. Which answer best describes the routine postpartum assessment for Ms. S?
   a. Should be the same as that for any multipara.
   b. Should be unnecessary because she already knows what to expect.
   c. Should be expanded to include a postoperative check.
   d. Should be limited to a postoperative check.

Ms. J, a 16-year-old primigravida, gave birth to a 3005-g (6-lb, 10-oz) infant girl 15 hours ago. She delivered her daughter vaginally with no complications after a 12-hour labor. She is unmarried and has been living with her father since her parents' divorce. She did not receive prenatal care until the last trimester of her pregnancy because she was attempting to conceal her pregnancy from her father. She attended no preparation for childbirth classes. Until delivery, she was ambivalent about keeping her infant. However, she has now decided she wants to keep the child. She has had no previous experience in caring for children and is expressing concern about her ability to care for her child.

8. Which of the following factors predispose Ms. J to problems in the area of maternal-infant attachment?
   a. Her marital status
   b. Her lack of prenatal care
   c. Her ambivalence about keeping her infant
   d. Her age
   e. All of the above

9. A plan of care designed to assist her in taking on the maternal role would include which one of the following?
   a. Allowing her periods of rest when she feels unable to care for her infant.
   b. Insisting that she breastfeed her infant on demand.
   c. Allowing her to merely observe the nurse as she provides physical care for her infant.
   d. Questioning her about whether she is sure she wants to keep her infant.

10. During the mother's first contact with her infant, the nurse observes a number of behaviors. Select all of the behaviors that are commonly observed during the introductory phase of attachment.
    a. Describing the infant as looking just like her mother.
    b. Touching the infant with her finger tips.
    c. Examining the infant's fingers and toes.
    d. Looking directly at the infant's eyes.

11. Which of the following is significantly correlated with malattachment?
    a. Cesarean delivery
    b. Multiparity
    c. Child abuse
    d. Age of mother

Ms. C is a 34-year-old multipara being cared for in your labor delivery postpartum recovery (LDRP) unit. She delivered a 3969-g (8-lb, 12-oz) boy 10 hours ago. She and her infant are in stable condition after an uncomplicated delivery. Ms. C has requested rooming-in, and you have been assigned the care of this mother and infant. Mr. C has also been present while you are caring for Ms. C.

12. In thinking about your priorities for caring for Ms. C and her infant, in which of the following stages of the parenting role would you expect her to be?
    a. Taking in
    b. Taking hold
    c. Interdependent
    d. Independent-dependent

13. Select the typical behaviors included during this phase.
    a. Focusing on relationship with partner.
    b. Expressing a desire to be cared for physically.
    c. Focusing on needs of infant.
    d. Focusing on one's own physical needs.

14. Ms. C is very happy about her successful delivery of a healthy infant. On the second day you care

for her, she begins to ask you many questions about infant care. Select the important content areas to be included in your discharge teaching plan.
    a. Physical care of infant
    b. Infant-feeding techniques
    c. Ways in which infants communicate needs
    d. Need for proper rest and nutrition for the mother
    e. All of the above

15. After Ms. C's discharge from the hospital, you receive a call from her. She is upset and worried. She was so happy when she left the hospital and cannot understand why she is feeling anxious and sad, crying frequently, and having difficulty in sleeping. Which of the following problems is most likely the explanation of Ms. C's behavior?
    a. Postpartum depression
    b. Marital problems
    c. Baby blues
    d. Exhaustion

16. Which of the following would you include in your advice to Ms. C?
    a. Advise that she seek marital counseling.
    b. Advise that she seek personal counseling.
    c. Advise her that her emotional response is common in the early postpartum period and should be self-limiting.
    d. Advise that she arrange for additional help with infant care until she is less exhausted.

ANSWERS TO STUDY QUESTIONS

1. d	5. a	9. a	13. b, d
2. c	6. c	10. b, c, d	14. e
3. b	7. c	11. c	15. c
4. b, d	8. e	12. a	16. c

REFERENCES

Ainsworth, M.D.S., Bleher, M.C., Waters, E., & Wall, S. (1978). *Patterns of attachment.* Hillsdale, NJ: Erlbaum.

American Academy of Pediatrics and American College of Obstetricians and Gynecologists. (1997). *Guidelines for perinatal care* (4th ed.). Elk Grove Village, IL: American Academy of Pediatrics.

Beck, C.T., & Gable, R.K. (2000). Postpartum depression screening scale: Development and psychometric testing. *Nursing Research, 49*(5), 272-282.

Blackburn, S.T. (2003). *Maternal, fetal, and neonatal physiology: A clinical perspective* (2nd ed.). Philadelphia: Saunders.

Bowlby, J. (1959). The nature of the child's tie to his mother. *International Journal of Psychoanalysis, 39,* 350.

Bowlby, J. (1969). *Attachment and loss: Vol. I. Attachment.* New York: Basic.

Brazelton, T.B. (1974). The origins of reciprocity: The early mother-infant interaction. In M. Lewis & L.A. Rosenblum (Eds.), *The effect of the infant on its caregiver.* New York: Wiley.

Cunningham, F.G., et al. (2002) *Williams obstetrics* (21st ed.). Norwalk, CT: Appleton & Lange.

Kennell, J.H, & Klaus, M.H. (1998). Bonding: Recent observations that alter perinatal care. *Pediatric Review, 19*(1), 4-12.

Klaus, M., & Kennell, J. (1982). *Parent-infant bonding* (2nd ed.). St. Louis: Mosby.

Luegenbiehl, D. (1997). Improving visual estimation of blood volume on peripads. *MCN American Journal of Maternal Child Nursing, 22*(6), 294-298.

Rubin, R. (1975). Maternal tasks in pregnancy. *Maternal-Child Nursing Journal, 4*(3), 143-153.

Ruchala, P. (2000). Teaching new mothers: Priorities of nurses and postpartum women. *Journal of Obstetric, Gynecologic, and Neonatal Nursing, 29*(3), 265-273.

Scoggin, J., & Morgan, G. (1997). *Practice guidelines in obstetrics and gynecology.* Philadelphia: Lippincott.

Varney, H. (1997). *Varney's midwifery* (3rd ed.). Boston: Jones and Bartlett.

14 Breastfeeding

SUSAN SAFFER ORR

OBJECTIVES

1. Identify the two hormones necessary for synthesis of milk and the milk ejection reflex.
2. List two strategies to correct flat or inverted nipples.
3. State two subjective findings that can contribute to a poor initial feeding.
4. Demonstrate criteria for correct positioning of the infant at the breast.
5. List three objective findings that contribute to poor "latching on."
6. List four strategies to decrease breast and nipple pain related to engorgement, plugged ducts, mastitis, or all three.
7. Identify effective swallowing of infant at the breast.
8. Describe two interventions to assist a lactating mother in each of the following special circumstances: infant of a cesarean birth; reluctant or sleepy infant; irritable or fussy infant; infant with physiologic jaundice; preterm or hospitalized infant; multiple-birth infants; or special-needs infant.
9. List three suggestions to increase an inadequate milk supply.
10. State expected nutritional needs of the lactating woman.
11. Identify which infants might benefit from supplemental lactation aids.
12. Participate as a team member in planning care for infants and mothers with special needs in collaboration with a lactation specialist or consultant, physical therapist, occupational therapist, and other health care professionals.
13. Develop a source of referrals for families with special needs.
14. Access advanced education and training specialization in lactation services according to individual interest.

INTRODUCTION

An understanding of anatomy and physiology of breastfeeding is essential for the nurse who is assisting families during the immediate newborn period. The knowledge the nurse imparts provides the foundation for long-term success with lactation. The encouragement and practical skills shared assist the mother and infant in establishing a positive basis for their breastfeeding experience. Successful breastfeeding can help prevent hospital readmission of an infant for dehydration and can promote infant health. Encouraging frequent and efficient feedings (at least every 2 to 3 hours) of unlimited length, with the infant correctly positioned and latched on, promotes an adequate supply of breast milk and prevents many common breastfeeding problems.

CLINICAL PRACTICE

A. **Physiology** (Figure 14-1)
   1. Hormonal influences during pregnancy begin in the first trimester related to the following:
      a. Ductal sprouting (estrogen)

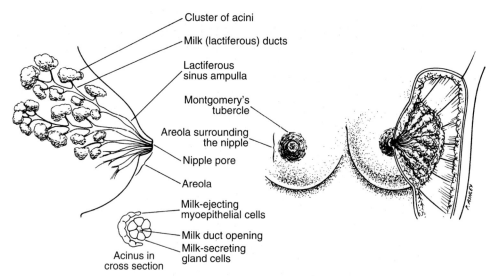

FIGURE 14-1 ■ Anatomy of the breast. (From Burroughs, A. [1992]. *Maternity nursing: An introductory text* (p. 15). Philadelphia: W.B. Saunders.)

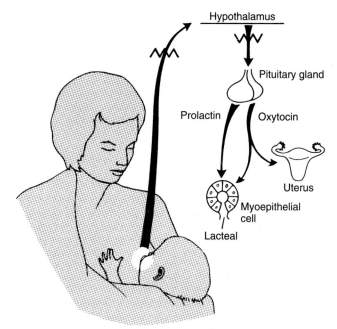

FIGURE 14-2 ■ Hormonal stimulation of milk production and milk ejection. (From Lawrence, R.A. [1989]. Breast-feeding: A guide for the medical profession [3rd ed.; p. 112]. St. Louis: Mosby.)

    b. Ductal branching (estrogen)
    c. Lobular formation (progesterone)
  2. Initiation of milk production (Figure 14-2)
    a. Prolactin level increases (at term, 200 to 400 ng/ml).
    b. Estrogen and progesterone levels decrease after delivery.
    c. Suckling provides continued stimulus for prolactin and oxytocin release.

    d. Prolactin is released from the anterior pituitary and initiates milk production; removal of the milk from the breast facilitates continued production of milk. Prolactin levels diminish over time in the lactating woman, but they do not return to baseline until 14 days of non–breastfeeding have occurred.

    e. Oxytocin is released from the posterior pituitary and initiates milk ejection ("let-down reflex"); let-down reflex is triggered by the infant's suckling at the nipple, the mother's emotional response to the infant, or both; alveoli contract and eject milk into the ducts and then into sinuses and out through the nipple. There are several let-downs during a feeding; most mothers notice only the first one (this is usually not perceptible in the very early weeks of breastfeeding); the first let-down occurs during the first 1 to 3 minutes of a feeding; let-down can also be diminished by stress and anxiety. Frequency and intensity of letdowns can be variable between feedings and between mothers.

  3. Stages of human milk

    a. Colostrum: is present at first postpartum days 1 to 5; thick and yellow; the volume varies from 2 to 20 ml per feeding (increased volume in parous women); higher in protein and lower in fat and sugar than mature breast milk.

    b. Transitional milk: is present 2 to 5 days to 2 weeks of postpartum period; not as yellow as colostrum; protein levels drop as fat, lactose, and calories increase.

    c. Mature milk: is present after transitional milk; whiter and thinner than transitional milk.

    d. Foremilk (a component of mature milk): immediate milk received in feeding; satisfies infant's initial thirst (no normal need to supplement breastfed infant with water).

    e. Hindmilk (a component of mature milk): later milk received in feeding; higher in fat content (four times higher than fore milk); satisfies hunger and promotes infant weight gain.

B. Assessment

  1. History

    a. Previous maternal breastfeeding experience

    b. Desire of mother to breastfeed and anticipated duration of breastfeeding

    c. Exposure of mother to breastfeeding education

    d. Cultural influences on mother

    e. Maternal support system

    f. Previous and current maternal infections and sexually transmitted diseases

    g. Any preexisting maternal health condition (such as breast surgery, thyroid dysfunction, HIV)

    h. Previous and current maternal use and abuse of tobacco, alcohol, and drugs (illicit, prescription, or over-the-counter)

    i. Difficult labor/delivery, cesarean section, or all

    j. Fetal distress

    k. Preterm infant or multiple births

    l. Hospitalized or special needs infant, or both

    m. Infant with poor sucking reflex

    n. Infant with poor latching on

    o. Maternal complaints of pain

      (1) Nipple

      (2) Breast

      (3) Related to incision, episiotomy, or position

2. Physical findings
   a. Inspect nipples for the following changes (when edge of areola is compressed at opposite sides):
      (1) Protracted: protrude slightly at rest; when stimulated, become erect and are easy for infant to grasp.
      (2) Flat: are difficult for infant to grasp and unchanged or retract with compression of areola.
      (3) Inverted: are rare; retract at rest as well as when areola is compressed.
      (4) Traumatized: are cracked, blistered, fissured, or bleeding; are painful when infant nurses.
   b. Inspect breast for the following
      (1) Previous surgery
         (a) Augmentation: client has the ability to breastfeed as long as milk ducts have not been severed (need to consult with surgeon about specific procedure performed; mother with poor milk production might benefit from supplemental lactation device).
         (b) Reduction: variable lactation success and depends on extent of tissue removed; if nipple has been relocated, ducts usually have been severed (check with surgeon); client might need supplemental lactation device.
         (c) Previous surgery for removal of cysts or lumps: incisions that could disrupt milk ducts
         (d) Mastectomy: infant can feed from remaining breast.
      (2) Size and condition of breast
         (a) Asymmetry of breasts is not uncommon; severe difference in size might indicate reduced milk glands in smaller breast.
         (b) Size of breast not related to ability to produce milk; large-breasted mother might need to hold breast back so infant can grasp nipple.
         (c) Fibrocystic breasts: might go into remission during lactation; might improve with decrease in caffeine intake; hand expression of milk might be uncomfortable in fibrocystic breasts, but mechanical pumping is effective.
         (d) Engorgement: breasts are tender, swollen, firm, and warm to the touch; mother might have fever; typically occurs 2 to 4 days postpartum, frequent breastfeeding and ice packs might alleviate condition.
         (e) Plugged duct: blocked milk duct; might have palpable lump and localized tenderness, swelling, and redness in area; warm compresses or shower before frequent breastfeeding might help alleviate condition.
         (f) Breast infection or mastitis: might be associated with unresolved plugged duct, cracked nipple, or both; mother might have more severe symptoms similar to those of influenza (fever, chills, joint pain, headache, nausea, and vomiting); usually only one breast with localized redness is involved; heat to the breast before frequent feedings, pumping following feedings, and rest for the mother may alleviate condition; antibiotic therapy might be required.
   c. Observe maternal positioning of infant; four positions are possible.
      (1) Cradle-hold position
      (2) Cross-cradle hold position
      (3) Football-hold position
      (4) Side-lying position

    d. Observe suckling infant

       (1) Check placement of lips, gums, and tongue.

       (2) Listen for infant's swallowing pattern.

       (3) Observe shape of nipple immediately after infant is removed from the breast.

C. Nursing Diagnoses

  1. Inadequate knowledge and skill related to maternal inexperience in positioning infant

  2. Risk for impaired maternal comfort related to incorrect latching on secondary to flat or inverted nipples, nipple confusion, or both

  3. Risk for maternal anxiety related to initial feeding secondary to inexperience

  4. Impaired maternal comfort related to breast or nipple pain because of nipple trauma, engorgement, plugged ducts, mastitis, or all of these conditions

  5. Anxiety about breastfeeding ability related to unexpected birth experience secondary to infant of cesarean section; irritable or fussy infant; sleepy or reluctant infant; infant with physiologic jaundice; preterm or hospitalized infant; multiple-birth infants; or special-needs infant

  6. Risk for maternal situational low self-esteem and self-concept related to inability to provide an adequate milk supply for infant

  7. Risk for maternal imbalanced nutrition: less than body requirements related to increased nutritional demands during lactation and/or depression

  8. Risk for maternal anxiety related to altered role change and sexual identity as a lactating mother

D. Interventions/Outcomes

  1. Inadequate knowledge or skill related to maternal inexperience in positioning infant

    a. Interventions for positioning (Mother needs to be in a relaxed position; as she supports her infant, the infant must grasp behind the nipple and keep the nipple drawn to the back of the mouth; the combination of proper positioning of infant, correct hand position on breast, and correct latching on prevents or decreases incidence of sore nipples; when choosing a position for breastfeeding, first ensure that mother is comfortable and well supported with pillows before attempting to position infant.)

       (1) Cradle-hold position (Figures 14-3 and 14-4)

          (a) Infant's head is held in the crook of mother's elbow.

          (b) Infant and mother should be tummy to tummy.

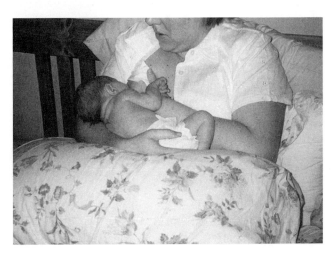

FIGURE 14-3 ■ Cradle hold position. (Courtesy Susan Saffer Orr, Long Beach, CA.)

(c) Grasp infant's thigh with hand, and tuck infant's lower arm next to mother's stomach.

(d) Support breast with opposite hand, fingers behind areola, index finger under breast, lift up under breast until nipple tips down slightly toward infant; continue to support breast during the early weeks of feeding (Figure 14-5).

(e) Bring infant to breast with pressure at the infant's upper back; do not push breast into infant; infant's chin should be positioned deeply under breast (pillows positioned under infant might be helpful).

(2) Cross-cradle hold offers the mother more control over the infant's head position (Figures 14-6 and 14-7).

(a) Place infant across mother's stomach similar to the cradle hold described above; hold the infant with the opposite hand placing mother's hand at the infant's upper back, supporting the back of his or her neck. The infant's body is held close to mother by

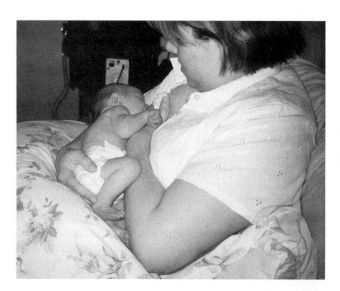

FIGURE 14-4 ■ Cradle hold position. (Courtesy Susan Saffer Orr, Long Beach, CA.)

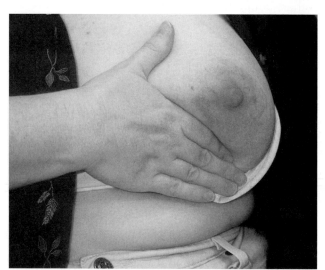

FIGURE 14-5 ■ Hand placement for cradle hold. (Courtesy Susan Saffer Orr, Long Beach, CA.)

tucking her forearm around the infant's bottom and pulling the infant close.

    (b) The hand that is supporting the breast is positioned in a "V" shape with the thumb and index finger coming up from the bottom of the breast; the nipple should gently tip toward the infant's mouth (Figure 14-8).

    (c) Once the infant has a wide, open mouth, he/she can be brought on to the breast with the mouth well behind the nipple.

(3) Football-hold position offers a good control of infant's head and is helpful after cesarean birth (Figure 14-9).

    (a) Place infant on pillow at mother's side.

    (b) Have mother support infant's upper back with arm and support infant's neck in hand.

    (c) Have infant's head level with the breast.

    (d) Have mother use opposite hand to support breast, fingers off areola with index finger under breast, palm should remain facing the mother's rib cage, nipple should gently tip down toward infant's mouth (Figure 14-10).

(4) Side-lying position (Figure 14-11)

    (a) Place infant on side, facing mother's abdomen.

    (b) Have mother support breast with opposite hand.

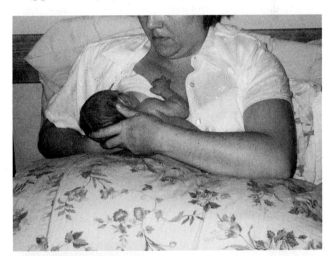

FIGURE 14-6 ■ Cross-cradle position. (Courtesy Susan Saffer Orr, Long Beach, CA.)

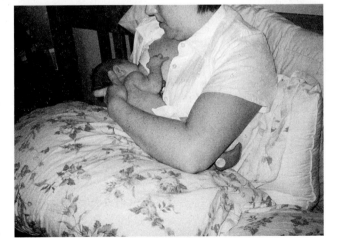

FIGURE 14-7 ■ Cross-cradle position. (Courtesy Susan Saffer Orr, Long Beach, CA.)

(c) Infant should be pulled into breast with pressure at the infant's upper back.

(d) Infant's chin should be positioned deep into breast.

b. Outcomes

(1) Mother reports absence of shoulder, neck, or back pain.

(2) Mother reports absence of nipple pain.

(3) Nipple protrudes evenly and shows no evidence of trauma.

(4) Mother appears relaxed and verbalizes confidence with positioning infant.

(5) Infant remains attached to breast.

2. Risk for impaired maternal comfort related to incorrect latching on secondary to flat or inverted nipples, nipple confusion, or both

a. Interventions for latching on (Correct placement of the infant's mouth behind the nipple ensures good stimulation for milk supply, promotes good milk transfer to the infant, and decreases or prevents sore nipples.)

(1) Have mother tickle infant's bottom lip with nipple.

(2) Allow mouth to open wide and center breast in mouth.

(3) Have mother pull infant in close (push infant in with pressure on infant's upper back or neck), place jaw behind nipple on areola with lips flanged; chin is positioned deep into breast.

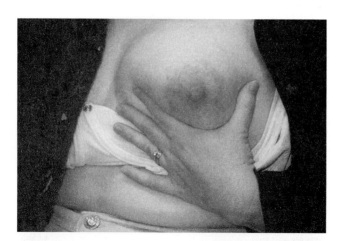

FIGURE 14-8 ■ Hand placement for cross-cradle hold. (Courtesy Susan Saffer Orr, Long Beach, CA.)

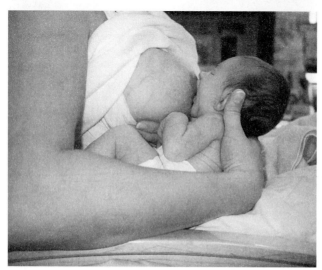

FIGURE 14-9 ■ Football hold. (Courtesy Susan Saffer Orr, Long Beach, CA.)

(4) Mother can remove infant from breast by breaking the suction: insert a finger gently into the corner of infant's mouth, between infant's gums.

b. Outcomes

(1) Infant's mouth is opened wide; lips are not tucked or curled.

(2) Lips are placed behind nipple on areola.

(3) Tongue is placed under breast.

(4) Infant is not sucking on own tongue.

(5) Few or no complaints of sore nipples occur.

(6) Infant does not slip off breast.

c. Interventions for flat or inverted nipples

(1) Have client wear breast shells/breast cups during third trimester: gentle pressure stretches and encourages nipple to protrude; can also be worn during postpartum period.

(2) Have client place her thumbs on either side of the areola and gently stretch the areola (Hoffman's exercise); thumbs should be rotated around edge of areola to stretch all areas; Hoffman's exercise can be performed several times per day.

(3) Have mother apply ice to nipple a few minutes before feeding to increase nipple erection.

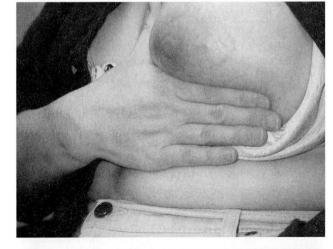

FIGURE 14-10 ■ Hand placement for football hold. (Courtesy Susan Saffer Orr, Long Beach, CA.)

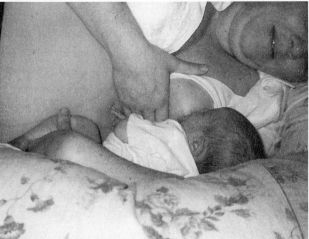

FIGURE 14-11 ■ Side-lying position in bed. (Courtesy Susan Saffer Orr, Long Beach, CA.)

---

(4) Have mother use breast pump for a few minutes before latch on to increase nipple protrusion.

(5) Silicon nipple shields can be used to assist in feeding only if the mother has a good milk supply and she is followed closely by a lactation specialist to ensure that the infant is getting adequate nutrition. A mother who is using a nipple shield will need to pump in addition to breastfeeding to compensate for the reduced stimulation to the breast that occurs when using a nipple shield until her milk supply is very well established.

d. Outcomes
(1) Improved ability of infant to grasp nipple
(2) Few or no complaints of sore nipples
(3) Signs of effective breastfeeding observed

e. Interventions for nipple confusion (Associated with infant having been fed supplements from rubber nipples; the placement and action of feeding from rubber nipples require the tongue to be up and back; an infant does not need to use the tongue to hold the artificial nipple in the mouth; when suckling at the breast, the tongue thrusts forward over the lower gum to grasp the nipple and pulls the nipple into the mouth, the lips flange around the areola, and the gums compress the milk sinuses; the tongue then creates a wavelike backward motion to extract milk.)
(1) Have mother avoid the use of rubber nipples during the first 4 weeks.
(2) Have mother use a supplemental lactation device if additional fluids are medically necessary.
(3) Encourage frequent feedings (every 2 to 3 hours) for practice.
(4) Have mother begin regular pumping to maintain or increase her milk supply if the infant is not breastfeeding adequately.

f. Outcomes
(1) Infant accepts breast without pulling away and swallows are heard during the breastfeeding period.
(2) Milk supply is adequate.
(3) Infant weight gain is appropriate.
(4) There is little or no nipple pain.

3. Risk for maternal anxiety related to initial feeding secondary to inexperience
a. Interventions for initial feeding
(1) Evaluate maternal discomfort and institute relief measures (medicate if indicated) for source of pain (incision, episiotomy, or uterus).
(2) Initiate feeding as soon as possible with alert mother and infant (ideal to initiate breastfeeding in delivery or recovery area).
(3) Position mother for comfort and provide back, neck, and arm support according to choice of position.
(4) Initiate correct latching on and positioning.
(5) Reassure mother if infant appears disinterested; some newborns are not immediately ready to nurse. Encourage her to snuggle, hold, and enjoy her infant instead; 1 hour of skin-to-skin contact in darkened, quiet room has been shown to enhance breastfeeding interest in the infant.
(6) Encourage frequent trials at the breast to enhance practice and confidence.
(7) Support and encourage mother to verbalize any feelings of disappointment, rejection, or unmet expectations related to initial feeding.

b. Outcomes

  (1) There is an increase in length of time the infant nurses at breast with both breasts being offered; breastfeeding sessions might last 30 to 60 minutes.

  (2) There are frequent feedings; most infants nurse between 8 and 12 times a day during the first month.

  (3) Client states that she has little or no nipple pain.

  (4) Infant weight gain is appropriate.

  (5) Client verbalizes confidence; increased breastfeeding skill is observed.

4. Impaired maternal comfort related to nipple or breast pain because of nipple trauma, engorgement, plugged ducts, mastitis, or all of these conditions

  a. Interventions for sore nipples (Nipple tenderness is usually associated with breastfeeding incorrectly; contributing factors are: waiting too long between feedings, poor positioning, poor latching on, or sucking dysfunction; limiting length of feeding times does not prevent sore nipples; infant thrush might be a cause of nipple soreness if the infant is older than 1 week.)

   (1) Inspect nipple tissue for redness, fissures, or blisters.

   (2) Have mother apply ice to nipple immediately before feeding to allow easier grasping of nipple and to produce a numbing effect.

   (3) Application of moist heat to the breast for 10 minutes before feeding encourages milk flow.

   (4) Have mother express a few drops of milk before feeding so that infant does not need to nurse as vigorously.

   (5) Have mother pump for 2 to 3 minutes before latching on to increase nipple protrusion.

   (6) Have mother change positions with each feeding so that area of tissue breakdown does not undergo repeated mechanical trauma. The football-hold position is especially helpful in encouraging infant to open mouth wide.

   (7) Check correct positioning of infant.

   (8) Check latching on and placement of tongue, lips, and gums (tongue under nipple, gums well behind nipple, chin deep into the breast, and lips flared out on the breast).

   (9) Correct and prevent engorgement.

   (10) Offer client a mild analgesic 30 minutes before feeding (if indicated).

   (11) Have mother use only cotton breast pads; plastic-lined breast pads retain moisture and paper pads might stick to irritated nipple.

   (12) Discontinue use of soap; rinse breast with water.

   (13) Have the client discontinue feeding before she falls asleep.

   (14) Do not use lanolin if client is allergic to wool.

   (15) Short (10-minute) and more frequent feedings (every 1½ to 2 hours) might be helpful; emphasize importance of active suckling to discourage infant from pacifying at the breast with a sore nipple.

   (16) Detach infant by breaking suction with finger.

   (17) After feeding, apply a few drops of breast milk to nipple and let dry. Breast milk is very healing unless thrush is noted on the infant's tongue and cheeks. Thrush (yeast infection) appears as a white coating on the tongue or the mucous membranes of the cheeks.

   (18) Instruct client to keep nursing bra flaps down to allow air to reach nipple between feedings (wearing breast shells with multiple holes for good air flow will also keep fabric away from the nipple when bra flaps are closed).

  b. Outcomes

    (1) Nipple pain is decreased.

    (2) Nipple area decreases in redness, cracking, bleeding, blisters, or fissures.

  c. Interventions for engorgement (As breast starts to change from production of colostrum to mature milk—the breasts might swell. A normal fullness is expected in the first days of breastfeeding, but engorgement is generally an exaggerated response related to one of the following: rigid feeding schedules, delayed first feeding, use of supplements, limited time at each feeding, ineffective infant suckle; the breasts are painful, swollen, and firm and the nipple is difficult for the infant to grasp because of areolar fullness.)

    (1) Encourage early feedings.

    (2) Encourage frequent feedings: every 2 to 3 hours; continue feeding until the infant cannot be persuaded to eat any longer.

    (3) Instruct mother to listen to the infant swallows (a soft exhalation sound) and promote active swallowing during a feeding; infant should be skin to skin with mother to enhance alertness, mother might need to take the infant off the breast, reawake, and relatch several times.

    (4) Discourage or discontinue use of supplements unless medically indicated.

    (5) Administer a mild analgesic 30 minutes before feeding, if indicated.

    (6) Instruct mother to apply warm compress to breast or offer a shower before feeding.

    (7) Instruct mother in gentle massage of her breast to encourage let-down and soften areolar tissue.

    (8) Encourage and instruct in use of breast pump to soften areolar tissue (caution: excessive pumping can aggravate the problem).

    (9) Apply ice packs to breast for 10 to 15 minutes after feedings.

    (10) Instruct client to wear breast shells between feedings to prevent areolar swelling.

  d. Outcomes

    (1) There is decreased pain, swelling, and tenderness within 12 to 24 hours.

    (2) Areolar tissue softens, and nipple is easier for infant to grasp.

    (3) Swallows can be heard while infant nurses.

  e. Interventions for plugged ducts (A decrease in the flow of milk results in a localized obstruction; area might be palpable and reddened.)

    (1) Administer a mild analgesic as indicated.

    (2) Apply a warm compress to breast, have mother soak in a warm bath or shower before feeding.

    (3) Offer and show technique for gentle breast massage before feeding.

    (4) Have infant feed at involved breast first.

    (5) Position infant's nose or chin in line with palpable lump.

    (6) Ensure frequent feedings (every 2 to 3 hours) and encourage infant to suckle actively as long as possible.

    (7) Avoid supplementary bottles or pacifier use until plug is resolved.

    (8) Suggest pumping, which might be necessary if infant is ill or reluctant to nurse.

    (9) Caution mother to check that her bra is not too tight or to determine if underwires are contributing to the problem.

    (10) Encourage mother to increase fluid intake.

  f. Outcomes
   (1) Decrease in pain, tenderness, and swelling
   (2) Resolution of palpable lump
 g. Interventions for mastitis (Reddened and painful area of the breast is accompanied by any or all of the following: fever, symptoms similar to those of influenza, joint pain, headache, and nausea.)
   (1) Encourage bed rest for 24 to 48 hours.
   (2) Administer antibiotics as indicated/ordered (usually if not resolved within 24 hours).
   (3) Increase fluid intake and ensure adequate nutrition.
   (4) Administer an analgesic as indicated.
   (5) Evaluate hygiene and encourage good handwashing.
   (6) Reassure mother that she can continue breastfeeding.
   (7) Apply warm compress to breast or have mother take warm bath or shower before feeding.
   (8) Encourage frequent feedings (every 2 to 3 hours); encourage prolonged active suckling and swallowing in the infant.
   (9) Vary infant's position at the breast.
   (10) Express milk with pump or hand if infant does not empty breast.
 h. Outcomes
   (1) Pain, swelling, and tenderness decrease.
   (2) Fever decreases.
   (3) Inflammation and infection process resolve.
5. Anxiety about breastfeeding ability related to unexpected birth experience secondary to infant of a cesarean section, irritable or fussy infant, sleepy or reluctant infant, infant with physiologic jaundice, preterm or hospitalized infant, multiple-birth infants, or special-needs infant.
 a. Interventions for infant of a cesarean section
   (1) Reassure women who have undergone cesarean sections that they can and do breastfeed as successfully as women who have delivered vaginally.
   (2) Medicate 15 to 30 minutes before feedings to minimize transmission of medication in milk to infant.
   (3) Encourage mobility and self-care for mother.
   (4) Position infant in football hold to avoid incision discomforts, or help mother into side-lying position.
   (5) Encourage night feedings to increase milk supply and decrease engorgement.
   (6) Encourage good nutrition, as essential for healing needs.
   (7) Encourage frequent rest periods for mother.
   (8) Encourage mother to obtain help for home responsibilities.
   (9) Allow expressions of any feelings of disappointment.
 b. Outcomes
   (1) Client demonstrates ability to latch and feed her infant independently.
   (2) Client demonstrates increasing competence with self-care and asks for assistance as needed.
   (3) Client demonstrates knowledge of nutritional needs by diet choices.
   (4) Client verbalizes confidence with breastfeeding ability.
   (5) Client has a plan for assistance if needed at discharge.
 c. Interventions for sleepy or reluctant infant (Infant is difficult to awaken, loses interest quickly, and does not feed vigorously.)
   (1) Wake infant after 2 to 3 hours during day time and after 4 to 5 hours at night.

(2) Encourage at least eight feedings per 24 hours.

(3) Use arousing techniques: unwrap blankets, undress infant, change diapers, burp frequently; lay sleepy infant down on firm surface, naked, to stretch and arouse for next breast.

(4) Place drops of sterile water on infant's lips to alert infant.

(5) Avoid use of rubber nipple and pacifiers.

(6) Encourage rooming-in so that when infant is awake, mother is available.

(7) Having 30 to 60 minutes of skin-to-skin contact between mother and infant in a dark, quiet room prior to feeding might enhance interest.

(8) Have mother reduce stimulation to infant, and limit visitors between feedings (overstimulated infants frequently shut down and will not arouse to feed well).

d. Outcomes

(1) Interest and time spent at breast increase.

(2) Infant swallows heard while breastfeeding becomes more frequent.

(3) Infant weight gain follows expected curve.

(4) Maternal confidence in meeting infant needs increases.

e. Interventions for a fussy or irritable infant (Infant might have strong sucking need, might become frantic when beginning feeding, or might want to breastfeed more often than every 2 hours.)

(1) Assess infant's feeding technique to ensure that infant is actively swallowing and nutritional needs are met.

(2) Use slow, gentle movements.

(3) Provide a quiet environment (e.g., quiet music, dim lights, rocking chair, cradle).

(4) Reduce visitors and activity in household.

(5) Use infant massage and skin-to-skin contact.

(6) Use soft, cloth infant carriers.

(7) Follow infant's preference for swaddling.

(8) Burp infant frequently (might swallow air when fussing).

(9) Allow infant's nonnutritive sucking needs to be met with sucking of own fingers or pacifier if infant has good weight gain and good latch-on skills.

(10) Have mother keep diet history (irritable behavior might be associated with an offending food, although this is not as common as once thought), excessive intake of acidic foods bother some infants.

(11) Eliminate caffeine and nicotine.

(12) Avoid using supplements with rubber nipples; this will reinforce impatience and increase the risk of nipple confusion.

(13) If infant gulps or chokes at breast, have mother pump for 2 to 3 minutes before latch-on to reduce overactive initial let-down (hyperlactation syndrome can be treated in the long term by having the infant nurse on one breast per feeding; reducing the amount of foremilk received on both breasts can reduce fussiness due to fast let-down with increased air swallowing).

(14) Educate mother on normal infant behavior and normal fussiness.

f. Outcomes

(1) Irritability and fussiness decrease.

(2) Infant is able to wait at least 2 hours between most feedings.

(3) Awareness of mother to infant cues increases.

g. Interventions for physiologic jaundice (A healthy newborn might show signs of physiologic jaundice [increased bilirubin values, yellowing of the skin, and sclera are objective findings] on the second or third day of life; treatment with sunlight or phototherapy assists in decreasing bilirubin levels; encouraging water supplements does not facilitate a decrease in bilirubin levels; bilirubin can be reabsorbed in the intestines; frequent breastfeeding promotes increased bowel movements and decreased reabsorption.)

    (1) Encourage frequent feedings (every 2 to 3 hours), with a minimum 8 to 10 feedings per day.

    (2) Have mother use techniques to arouse infant if he or she is sleepy or uninterested (undress infant, switch positions frequently).

    (3) Discourage use of rubber nipples for supplements (might cause increased nipple confusion, might decrease interest in breastfeeding, and might decrease the number of infant stools); discontinue use of a pacifier, which might reduce infant's willingness to eat. If supplementation is required, consider use of supplemental lactation device. Encourage pumping to maintain or increase milk supply.

    (4) Encourage/consider use of phototherapy in mother's hospital room and/or home phototherapy.

    (5) Encourage mother to verbalize concerns.

h. Outcomes

    (1) There is a decrease in bilirubin levels.

    (2) There is an increase in infant's interest in feedings.

i. Interventions for preterm or hospitalized infant (Can be an overwhelming experience for most parents; the concern about immediate needs, financial costs, and long-term outcomes is of most importance; the immunologic advantages, nutritional components, and digestibility of breast milk are of great value to a preterm or hospitalized infant; preterm infants who receive breast milk tend to have shorter hospital stays.)

    (1) Encourage and praise client's decision to breastfeed.

    (2) Provide an electric breast pump while infant is hospitalized (with attachment kit to pump both breasts simultaneously), and instruct in use and cleaning.

    (3) Begin pumping as soon as possible.

    (4) Have mother use relaxation techniques, use warm compresses, massage breasts, and visualize (or gaze at a picture of) her infant before beginning to pump.

    (5) Provide mother with time to touch infant before pumping: as infant's condition improves and stabilizes, just holding the infant helps with let-down.

    (6) Pump at least 8 to 10 times daily (with a minimum of 10 minutes for each breast); pump at least once during the night (use of a pump that can be used on both breasts at once is especially helpful when long-term pumping is necessary).

    (7) Provide mother with written instructions for pumping, milk collection, and storage at discharge.

    (8) Encourage mother to bring pumped milk to the hospital to be used for infant feedings when infant is ready to eat.

    (9) Provide referral for electric pump rental or purchase upon discharge.

    (10) Give mother instructions to rest, drink fluids, and maintain adequate nutrition.

    (11) Refer mother to lactation specialist or consultant when necessary for help with immature suck reflex or nipple confusion when infant is put to breast.

    (12) Use supplemental lactation device to increase caloric volume without using rubber nipple (Figure 14-12).

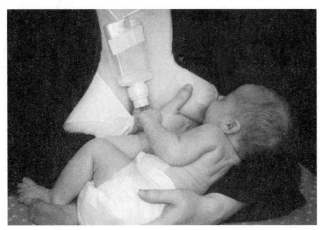

FIGURE 14-12 ■ Supplemental Nursing System by Medela, Inc., McHenry, IL. (Courtesy Susan Saffer Orr, Long Beach, CA.)

  j. Outcomes
    (1) Volume of collected breast milk is increasing.
    (2) Client expresses increasing confidence and skill when infant is put to breast.
    (3) There is a successful transition of infant to complete breastfeeding.
  k. Interventions for multiple births (The client might have to cope with the challenges of a cesarean section, preterm infants, and providing for long-term follow-up of more than one newborn; breastfeeding can reduce feeding and medical costs and assist in bonding with and meeting the individual needs of each infant.)
    (1) Reassure mother that milk supply is determined by milk demand and that the supply adjusts to infants' demands.
    (2) Instruct client in using "round robin" technique to feed sleepy babies in first weeks (i.e., put one infant to the breast until swallows slow down or stop; then have helper burp and arouse that infant while the mother nurses the other infant; mother continues to switch infants until both are completely fed, changed, and burped, thus making feeding time more efficient).
    (3) Assist client with positioning of two infants (both in cradle position, legs crossing; both in football position; or one in football position and one in cradle position); breastfeeding infants simultaneously might not be possible in early weeks, but as infants improve latch-on skills, this will become easier.
    (4) Assist client in anticipatory planning for rest and nutritional needs.
    (5) Provide client with a referral to a local chapter of Mothers of Twins or Mothers of Multiples.
    (6) Encourage client to feed infants concurrently to help her get needed rest.
    (7) Provide mother with referral to lactation specialist if breastfeeding problems persist.
  l. Outcomes
    (1) Client reports satisfaction with breastfeeding.
    (2) Infant's weight follows growth curve.
  m. Interventions for a special needs infant (When a family's dream of having a so-called perfect infant does not materialize, a period of grieving is appropriate and expected; breastfeeding enhances the bond between mother and child; providing breast milk might increase a mother's ability

to nurture and comfort her infant as well as provide ideal nutrition for the infant.)
- (1) Encourage and listen to client's feelings of disappointment, disbelief, and anger.
- (2) Provide flexibility in hospital routine for family support.
- (3) Provide information for support groups specific to disability (e.g., cleft palate, Down syndrome, spina bifida).
- (4) Initiate a collaborative plan, and include a lactation specialist or consultant, occupational therapist, physical therapist, and any other pertinent health care providers to provide consistent, optimal care for specific maternal and infant needs.
- (5) Provide breast pump information as needed for infants with reduced feeding capability (see the discussion of preterm infants).
- **n.** Outcomes
  - (1) Client has realistic approach to infant's ability to breastfeed and to maternal time and effort needed to explore alternatives (e.g., long-term pumping and/or supplemental nursing device).
  - (2) Client expresses increasing acceptance and understanding of infant's disability.
  - (3) Mother expresses increasing confidence and ability with breastfeeding skills.
  - (4) Infant demonstrates acceptable growth for condition.
- **6.** Risk for maternal situational low self-esteem and self-concept related to inability to provide an adequate milk supply for infant.
  - **a.** Interventions related to milk supply. (The amount of breast milk produced is related to the demand put on the breast by a suckling infant or to a lesser degree by a breast pump; supply is impacted by multiple factors such as inadequate transfer of milk out of the breast by ineffective suckling by the infant, infrequent or shortened feedings, maternal fatigue and/or depression, low thyroid function in the mother, retained placenta, previous surgical history of the breast, or inadequate glandular development of the breast.)
    - (1) Ensure sufficient stimulation with frequent feedings (every 2 to 3 hours, with a minimum of 10 to 15 minutes of effective suckling/swallowing at each breast).
    - (2) Encourage rooming-in.
    - (3) Evaluate for any missed or supplemented feedings.
    - (4) Wake infant if asleep longer than 3 hours.
    - (5) Avoid use of pacifier.
    - (6) Use lactation supplemental device if it is medically indicated that infant requires additional calories.
    - (7) Evaluate for poor latching on.
    - (8) Listen for infant swallowing, and keep infant aroused at breast.
    - (9) Follow feeding with 10 minutes of pumping with a double electric pump to further increase stimulation to the breast.
    - (10) Ensure adequate maternal fluid intake of 1920 ml (2 qt) daily.
    - (11) Evaluate maternal activity level, and encourage rest.
    - (12) Consider underlying maternal health condition if poor milk supply continues.
    - (13) Refer to lactation specialist.

b. Outcomes
   (1) Mother hears consistent infant swallows during breastfeeding.
   (2) Infant younger than 1 month has minimum of one stool per day.
   (3) There are six to eight wet diapers a day.
   (4) Infant has regular patterns of wakefulness, sleep, and feeding.
   (5) Infant's weight loss is not more than 5% to 10% during the first week.
   (6) Infant's weight follows a normal growth curve.
7. Risk for maternal imbalanced nutrition: less than body requirements related to increased nutritional demands during lactation and/or depression
   a. Interventions related to the following—*Nutrition:* a wide selection of foods can be offered, according to a mother's individual tastes and preferences; any food, in moderation, can be part of a diet during lactation (unless intolerance is noted by the infant—dairy products, soy, and peanuts have been found to bother some infants); the average diet during lactation consists of 2200 calories daily; it takes between 500 and 700 calories to produce milk; fat stores from pregnancy help provide some of these additional calories; 1920 ml (2 qt) of liquids and the following servings from all food groups are to be encouraged: protein, three or four; dairy, four to six; fruit, four; grains, four; vegetables, four; *Alcohol:* alcohol passes readily into milk; even moderate amounts of alcohol might slow brain growth in the infant and inhibit let-down; occasional intake of one serving of alcohol probably does not constitute considerable danger; *Drugs and medications:* several factors affect excretion of maternal medications in breast milk (solubility, route of administration, accumulation of substance, oral bioavailability of medication, duration of use, weight of infant, and amount and number of times infant breastfeeds); for specific prescription and over-the-counter medications, see Hale (2002); *Tobacco:* smoking of 20 cigarettes/day or more might cause nausea and vomiting in the infant and cause decrease in milk supply; breast milk of smoking mothers has lower level of vitamin C, and any infant exposure to second-hand smoke is detrimental; parents should not allow smoking when infant is present; *Caffeine:* might be taken in moderate amounts; infants who are frequently colicky, wakeful, or hyperactive might be consuming excessive amounts of caffeine in their breast milk, and maternal consumption of caffeine should be decreased or stopped.
   (1) Review dietary choices.
   (2) Provide consultation with a dietitian as needed.
   (3) Offer sample menus.
   (4) Plan menus according to cultural or religious preferences.
   (5) Inform mother of Women, Infants, and Children (WIC) program, a supplemental food and nutritional counseling program for pregnant, postpartum, and lactating mothers with children (pending income and risk qualifications).
   (6) Eliminate foods suspected of aggravating colic, and evaluate effect by keeping a food intake and infant behavior diary.
   (7) Encourage decrease in or elimination of maternal use of tobacco; eliminate infant's exposure to second-hand smoke.
   (8) Discourage moderate to excessive alcohol intake.
   (9) Provide physician with alternative medications that are compatible with breastfeeding.

b. Outcomes
(1) Mother makes good dietary choices from menu, and maintains an adequate level of fluids.
(2) There is an increase in maternal energy levels.
(3) There is adequate healing of episiotomy or other incisions.
(4) Client has adequate milk supply.
(5) There is a decrease in or elimination of tobacco use.
(6) Alcohol intake is limited to one to two servings maximum per week.
(7) Mother may continue breastfeeding while taking needed medication.
8. Risk for maternal anxiety related to altered role change and sexual identity as a lactating mother.
a. Interventions related to sexuality (New parents need time to adjust to each other sexually after the birth of their child; time schedules, fatigue, responsibilities, and role changes are all factors that might affect sexual desires and needs.)
(1) Allow client to express her concerns and feelings.
(2) Use of a water-soluble lubricant might be helpful for decreased vaginal lubrication related to lowered estrogen levels during lactation.
(3) Reassure client that many women notice a let-down reflex during orgasm.
(4) Reassure client that some women find their breasts are very sensitive while lactating; reassure her that an erotic response to breastfeeding can occur and has no particular significance.
(5) Reassure her that some women feel overwhelmed by partner's touch after caring for an infant all day.
(6) Encourage parents to find time for themselves as a couple.
(7) Reaffirm that menstruation might be delayed during lactation, but pregnancy can still occur.
(8) Provide client with information on methods of contraception.
b. Outcomes
(1) Parents express realistic expectations for coping with individual sexual needs.
(2) Parents have a plan for contraception, if an immediate pregnancy is not desired.

HEALTH EDUCATION

A. The health care provider can offer educational assistance about the following topics through written materials, audio-visual materials, and individual or group instruction.
1. Preparation for breastfeeding
a. Normal physiology
b. Correction of flat or inverted nipples
c. Production of milk
d. Let-down (milk ejection reflex)
e. Stages of human milk
2. Initial feeding
a. Correct positioning
b. Correct latching on
3. Correction and prevention of common breastfeeding problems
a. Sore nipples
b. Engorgement

    c. Plugged ducts
    d. Mastitis
    e. Building and maintaining a milk supply
4. Typical newborn behavior related to feeding in early weeks
5. Resource and referral information available for special situations
    a. Cesarean birth
    b. Irritable or fussy infant
    c. Sleepy or reluctant infant
    d. Infant with physiologic jaundice
    e. Preterm or hospitalized infant
    f. Infants of a multiple birth
    g. Special-needs infant
6. Nutritional guidelines for lactation
7. Sexuality and contraception during lactation

B. Outcomes: the mother can:
1. Demonstrate correct latching on and positioning for breastfeeding before discharge.
2. State measures to correct common breastfeeding problems (with the help of written material).
3. Provide information about resources available that are appropriate for special circumstances.
4. Make good nutritional choices.
5. Begin discussions with partner for planning contraceptive needs.

CASE STUDY AND STUDY QUESTIONS

Mrs. M is a 27-year-old gravida 2, para 1 (G2, P1) woman. She had an uncomplicated spontaneous vaginal delivery at 39 weeks' gestation, and her daughter weighed 3629 g (8 lb) with Apgar scores of 8 and 9. She had previously attempted to breastfeed her first daughter, but quit after 2 weeks because of cracked nipples and poor milk supply. She states, "I really want to breastfeed this infant at least 6 months."

1. What additional information is needed to help plan for her care?
    a. Previous breastfeeding experience
    b. Previous use of drugs, tobacco, and alcohol
    c. Maternal support systems
    d. Previous breast surgery
       1. a, b
       2. b, d
       3. c, d
       4. a, d
       5. All of the above

2. On physical examination you observe that Mrs. M's nipples are inverted. What would be helpful to make the nipples easier for the infant to grasp?
    a. Application of ice before feeding.
    b. Use of breast shells or milk cups.
    c. Toughening nipples with wash cloth.
    d. Use of pump before feeding.
       1. a, b, d
       2. a, b, c
       3. b, c, d

3. How soon after delivery should she be encouraged to attempt to breastfeed her daughter?
    a. Immediately after delivery
    b. Between 3 and 6 hours after delivery

c. Between 6 and 12 hours after delivery

d. At 12 hours after delivery

4. She expresses concern about how to prevent sore nipples. Which of the following is helpful?
   a. Limiting feedings to 5 minutes at each breast.
   b. Checking for correct latching on.
   c. Checking for positioning of infant.
   d. Using a supplemental bottle.
   e. Air-drying nipples after feeding.
      1. All of the above
      2. a, b, c, e
      3. b, c
      4. b, d, e
      5. b, c, e

5. What two hormones most affect milk synthesis and the milk ejection/let-down reflex?
   a. Progesterone
   b. Estrogen
   c. Oxytocin
   d. Follicle-stimulating hormone (FSH)
   e. Prolactin
      1. a, b
      2. b, e

3. c, d
4. d, e
5. c, e

6. List three strategies to prevent and decrease engorgement.

7. List five comfort measures to resolve engorgement.

8. List three strategies to increase milk supply.

9. What two breastfeeding aids might be helpful to a mother with a preterm or hospitalized infant?

10. Which of the following are true about a cesarean-section birth mother and breastfeeding?
    a. Usually cannot breastfeed until the fourth postpartum day.
    b. Needs help positioning infant during first few days.
    c. Might find football-hold position comfortable.
    d. Should pump milk while taking pain medication.
       1. All of the above
       2. All but a
       3. b, c
       4. a, c
       5. a, c, d

ANSWERS TO STUDY QUESTIONS

1. 5
2. 1
3. a
4. 5
5. 5
6. Frequent feedings (every 2 to 3 hours); sufficient length feeding; effective suckling of infant; avoidance of supplements
7. Analgesia; warm compresses before feeding; hand expression/pumping to soften areolar tissue; frequent feedings (every 2 to 3 hours); sufficient length with effective suckling of infant; avoidance of supplements; application of ice after feeding
8. Frequent feedings (every 2 to 3 hours); sufficient length with effective suckling of infant; additional use of a breast pump following feedings for stimulation to the breast; adequate maternal nutrition and fluid intake; adequate maternal rest
9. Electric breast pump; supplemental lactation device.
10. 3

RESOURCES

Advanced Breastfeeding Education for Health Care Professionals

Academy of Breast-Feeding Medicine, PO Box 15945-284, Lenexa, KS 66285

Health Education Associates, 211 S. Easton Road, Glenside, PA 19038

International Board of Lactation Consultant Examiners (IBLCE), PO Box 2348, Falls Church, VA 22042, (703) 560-7332

International Lactation Consultant Association, 1500 Sunday Drive, Suite 102, Raleigh, NC 27607, (919) 861-5577

Lactation Study Center, University of Rochester Medical Center, (716) 275-0088

La Leche League International, 1400 N. Meacham Road, Schaumburg, IL 60173, (800) LALECHE

Lactation Institute and Breastfeeding Clinic, 16430 Ventura Boulevard, Suite 303, Encino, CA 91436, (818) 995-1913

UCLA Extension, Department of Health Sciences, Room 614, 10995 Le Conte Avenue, Los Angeles, CA 90024

Wellstart International, PO Box 80877, San Diego, CA 92138-0877, (619) 295-5192

Printed and Audio-Visual Breastfeeding Materials

Birth and Life Bookstore, Inc., PO Box 70625, Seattle, WA 98107, (206) 789-4444

Childbirth Graphics, PO Box 21207, Waco, TX 76702-1207, (800) 299-3366, ext. 287

La Leche League International, 1400 N. Meacham Road, Schaumburg, IL 60173

Breast Pumps and Related Supplies

Hollister Inc., 2000 Hollister Dr, Libertyville, IL 60048, (800) 323-4060

Medela Inc., PO Box 660, McHenry, IL 60051, (800) 435-8316

Whittlestone, PO Box 2237, Antioch, CA 94531, (877) 608-6455

Supplemental Lactation Systems

Lact-Aid, PO Box 1066, Athens, TN 37371-1066

Supplemental Nursing System, Medela, Inc., PO Box 660, McHenry, IL 60051

REFERENCES

Abbott Laboratories. (1997). *Health care professional's annotated edition of guide for the breast-feeding mother.* Columbus: Ross Products Division.

Hale, T. (2002). *Medications and mother's milk* (10th ed.). Amarillo, TX: Pharmasoft Publishing.

Huggins, K. (1999). *The nursing mother's companion.* Boston: Harvard Common Press.

Lawrence, R.A., & Lawrence R.M. (1999). *Breast-feeding: A guide for the medical profession* (5th ed.). St. Louis: Mosby.

Osterman, K., & Rahm, V. (2000). Lactation mastitis: Bacterial cultivation of breast milk symptoms, treatment, and outcome. *Journal of Human Lactation, 16*(4), 297-302.

Martin, C. (2000) *The nursing mother's problem solver.* New York: Simon & Schuster.

Meier, P., Borucki, L., Brown, L., Engstrom, J., Hurst, N., Krause, A., et al. (2000) Nipple shields for preterm infants: Effect on milk transfer and duration of breast-feeding. *Journal of Human Lactation, 16*(2), 106-114.

Palmer, M. (2002). Recognizing and resolving infant suck difficulties. *Journal of Human Lactation, 18*(2), 166-167.

Riordan, J., & Averbach, K. (1993). *Breast-feeding and human lactation.* Boston: Jones and Bartlett.

15 Family Planning

DENISE G. LINK

OBJECTIVES

1. Describe the mechanism of action of various methods of birth control.
2. Compare the effectiveness ratings of the various methods of birth control.
3. Obtain a contraceptive history from a woman.
4. Describe the risks and benefits of each method of birth control.
5. Rank the various contraceptives in order of their appropriateness for an individual woman.
6. Explain how postpartum status affects choice of contraception.
7. Identify ethnocultural considerations that can affect the choice of contraception for a woman in postpartum status.
8. Identify social and psychologic considerations that help determine the appropriate choice of a contraceptive method after childbirth.

INTRODUCTION

Helping women make decisions about family planning is an important role for the nurse who provides care for women during the postpartum period. Short hospital stays for women after childbirth means that they might have limited contact with health care providers during the initial days following childbirth. If decisions are not made early in the postpartum period, women might use contraceptive methods that are inappropriate and, therefore, ineffective for the postpartum period. Nursing practice must include assessment of contraceptive knowledge, attitudes toward contraception, attitudes toward future pregnancies, and the need for family planning methods before the woman's hospital discharge.

CLINICAL PRACTICE

A. Assessment
  1. Contraceptive history
    a. Previous contraceptive use
      (1) Identify dissatisfaction with any of the methods.
      (2) Identify satisfaction with any of the methods.
      (3) Identify the method of choice.
      (4) Identify accuracy of knowledge base about methods used and methods rejected.
  2. Obstetric and gynecologic history
    a. Previous physical complications associated with contraceptive use
    b. Problems with current pregnancy or delivery that affect the choice of contraception
      (1) Hypertension
      (2) Thrombophlebitis
      (3) Diabetes
      (4) Infection

      c. Problems with current delivery that affect the timing of resumption of sexual intercourse
- (1) Operative delivery
- (2) Episiotomy/lacerations
- (3) Infection
- (4) Cultural beliefs and practices
- (5) Hemorrhage

  3. Breastfeeding plans
- **a.** Planned length
- **b.** Perceived importance
- **c.** Previous use of contraception while breastfeeding

  4. Psychosocial responses regarding family planning
- **a.** Attitude toward timing of resumption of sexual activities
- **b.** Religious or cultural views about contraception
  - (1) Identify religious or cultural barriers to contraception or to the use of particular contraceptive methods.
  - (2) Identify differences in beliefs or values between the woman and her partner.
  - (3) Identify conflicts between a desire to avoid conception and religious or cultural values that affect choice.
- **c.** Attitudes toward future pregnancies and their appropriate timing
- **d.** Motivation to avoid future pregnancy

  5. Contraceptive knowledge
- **a.** Postpartum fertility
- **b.** The use and effectiveness of various methods
- **c.** Methods of choice
- **d.** Partner's methods of choice
- **e.** Recommended physiologic minimum spacing between pregnancies for best outcome
- **f.** Costs of various methods
- **g.** Short-term versus long-term contraception
- **h.** Confidence in methods

B. Nursing Diagnoses
  1. Deficient knowledge related to postpartum fertility
  2. Deficient knowledge related to proper use of contraceptive method of choice
  3. Risk for unintended pregnancy related to selection of inappropriate contraceptive method
  4. Interrupted family processes related to value differences between the woman and her partner about contraceptive choices

C. Interventions/Outcomes
  1. Deficient knowledge related to postpartum fertility
- **a.** Interventions
  - (1) Explain variations in timing of the return of ovulation and menses during the postpartum period.
  - (2) Explain lack of reliable effectiveness of lactation in preventing conception during the postpartum period.
  - (3) Explain the possibility that pregnancy can occur because ovulation occurs before the resumption of menses.
- **b.** Outcomes
  - (1) Client states that 4 to 6 weeks after delivery is the usual time for the return of menses in the nonlactating woman.

   (2) Client explains that breastfeeding on demand (at least six to seven times daily) without supplementing the infant's diet with formula or other food delays the resumption of ovulation and menses for some, but not all, women.
   (3) Client acknowledges that pregnancy can occur with the first postdelivery ovulation although no menses have occurred.
   (4) Client states an understanding of the risk of pregnancy during the postpartum period and the need to use contraception if pregnancy is not desired.
2. Deficient knowledge related to proper use of contraceptive method of choice
   a. Interventions (Table 15-1)
      (1) Assess client's knowledge of selected method.
      (2) Identify appropriateness and effectiveness of selected method for the postpartum period.
      (3) Describe or review proper use of the method.
      (4) Identify advantages and disadvantages of selected method.
      (5) Determine client's access to selected method.
      (6) Review complications of selected method and the signs and symptoms of various complications.
      (7) Explain steps the client should take if complications occur.
      (8) Explain importance of consistent use.
      (9) After teaching, evaluate the client's comfort with use and confidence in selected method.
   b. Outcomes
      (1) Client explains how her method of choice is to be used.
      (2) Client identifies advantages and disadvantages of her method.
      (3) Client states how she plans to obtain her method of choice.
      (4) Client identifies signs and symptoms of complications related to her method of choice.
      (5) Client states her planned action if problems occur with her method of choice.
      (6) Client states her understanding of the importance of consistent use of her method of choice to prevent pregnancy.
      (7) Client states that she feels capable of comfortable use of the selected method.
3. Risk for unintended pregnancy related to selection of inappropriate contraceptive method
   a. Interventions
      (1) Identify client's level of commitment to avoiding pregnancy.
      (2) Identify client's attitude toward contraception and her selected method.
      (3) Identify partner's acceptance of the selected method.
   b. Outcomes
      (1) Client identifies how highly she values avoiding pregnancy.
      (2) Client describes how she feels about contraception.
      (3) Client describes use of her selected method of contraception.
      (4) Client describes her partner's willingness to accept use of her selected method.
4. Interrupted family processes related to value differences between the woman and her partner about contraceptive choices

Text continued on p. 416

TABLE 15-1
Methods of Contraception

Method	Accidental Pregnancy Rate (Typical Use in First Year)	Postpartum Use	Risks/Disadvantages	Benefits
Abstinence	0%	Is the method of choice for the first 4 to 6 weeks, especially for operative deliveries, complications, and lacerations	Might be unacceptable to client or partner; might cause relationship problems if there is disagreement	Promotes healing and involution
Vasectomy or male sterilization	0.15%	Has no contraindications	Is permanent; requires minor surgery	No further monitoring required after verification that all sperm in system have been ejaculated
Bilateral tubal ligation or female sterilization	0.5%	Can be performed during cesarean section; can be performed soon after vaginal delivery	Is permanent; might cause surgical complications	Requires no further monitoring
Oral contraceptives (two types: combined pill [estrogen plus progestin] and mini-pill [progestin only])	5% for each type	Might interfere with lactation by decreasing milk supply; if lactating, use mini-pill or wait until lactation is well established	Minor side effects are breast tenderness, nausea, and irregular bleeding (especially with mini-pill); women who weigh more than 155 lbs might have a slightly higher pregnancy rate on lower dose pills; major risks are rare in women ages 35 and younger who do not smoke, but they may include deep vein thrombosis, liver tumor, cerebrovascular accident (CVA), myocardial infarction (MI), and gallbladder disease; requires regular monitoring by a health care provider	Acceptable for healthy women ages 36 to 50 years who do not smoke; menses are lighter and shorter, and there are fewer cramps; might protect against ovarian and uterine disease

Method	Rate	Considerations	Side Effects/Risks	Advantages
Transdermal contraceptive skin patch	0.88%	Might interfere with lactation by decreasing milk supply; if lactating, wait until lactation is well established	Increased breakthrough bleeding and more breast discomfort in first two cycles than with pills; application site reactions; risk profile similar to combined pills; slightly less effective in women who weigh more than 198 lbs; ethinyl estradiol and norelgestromin	No daily pill required; improved compliance; good skin adhesion in humidity/exercise
Vaginal ring	0.65%	Might interfere with lactation by decreasing milk supply; if lactating, wait until lactation is well established	Risk profile similar to combined pills; ethinyl estradiol and etonogestrel	Less breakthrough bleeding than with pills; good lipid profile; no fitting required; can be removed for intercourse and replaced within 3 hours
Spermicide with condom (used together)	5%	Has no contraindications	Irritation and allergic reactions are rare; must be inserted/put on just before intercourse, is messy and might decrease sensation	As effective as the pill when used together; foam is a lubricant; available over the counter; provides protection against sexually transmitted diseases
Diaphragm with spermicide	20%	Decreased levels of estrogen make the vagina thinner and drier than normal and insertion more difficult; must be refitted after a pregnancy; proper fit is not possible until involution is complete	Causes irritation, allergic reactions, and bladder irritation; must be inserted before intercourse and left in place for 6 hours; some positions might dislodge it	Not appropriate during the early postpartum period
Copper intrauterine device (IUD)	0.7%	Can be inserted up to 48 hours after delivery; expulsion rates are higher in the early postpartum period	Might increase menstrual flow and cramps	Once in place, requires little monitoring by the woman; in a suitable candidate, can be inserted during first menses after childbirth; approved for up to 10 years of use

Continued

■ TABLE 15-1
■ **Methods of Contraception—cont'd**

Method	Accidental Pregnancy Rate (Typical Use in First Year)	Postpartum Use	Risks/Disadvantages	Benefits
Levonorgestrel intrauterine system (LNG-IUS)	0.2%	Can be inserted 6 weeks after delivery; expulsion rates are higher in the early postpartum period; contraindicated in women with acute liver disease or tumor; active thrombophlebitis or thromboembolic disorders	Irregular periods for 3 to 6 months after insertion; 20% of women using LNG-IUS will be amenorrheic after 12 months of use	Less cramping and bleeding; once in place, requires little monitoring by the woman; for a suitable candidate, can be inserted during first menses after childbirth; approved for up to 5 years of use
Spermicide alone	26%	Might cause irritation because of decreased levels of estrogen	Might cause allergic reactions; messy; inserted just before intercourse	Available over the counter
Condoms alone	14%	No contraindications in nonallergic individuals or partners	Irritation and allergic reactions are rare; might break or leak; might decrease sensation	Available over the counter; affords some protection against sexually transmitted diseases
Female condom	21%	No contraindications	Available over the counter	Can be inserted up to 8 hours before intercourse
Natural family planning, fertility awareness, and periodic abstinence	24%	Requires signs and symptoms of hormone fluctuation during normal cycling; this cycling does not occur during the postpartum period, especially during lactation	No risks; requires practice and education from a trained professional; requires self-monitoring and record-keeping as well as varying periods of abstinence	Requires no devices or chemicals; might be acceptable for couples who do not wish to use other methods because of religious or other reasons
Withdrawal	19%	Has no contraindications	Requires interruption of sexual response cycle; fluid with sperm is often released before ejaculation	Requires no devices or chemicals

Method	Failure rate	Considerations	Characteristics
Norplant	0.05%	Requires insertion and removal of implants by a trained health care provider; a change in bleeding pattern is common; risks similar to mini-pill; expensive	Contains progestin only; circulating hormone level less than that with mini-pill; lasts 5 years; little monitoring required after insertion
Depo-Provera	0.3%	Not recommended until lactation is well established unless the client is likely to be lost to follow-up; Requires injection every 3 months; change in bleeding pattern common; risks similar to mini-pill; weight gain averages 5 lb/year	Contains progestin only; amenorrhea common; requires no monitoring between injections
Combination estrogen/progesterone injection	0.2%	Not recommended until lactation is well established; Requires injection every month; estradiol cypionate plus medroxyprogesterone acetate; side effects similar to combined oral contraceptives; requires regular monitoring by a health care provider	No daily pill to remember; acceptable for healthy women ages 36 to 50 who do not smoke; menses are lighter and involve shorter, less frequent cramps; might protect against ovarian and uterine disease
Emergency contraception: High-dose combined estrogen/progesterone pills	3.2%	Must be taken within 72 hours of unprotected intercourse; Nausea and vomiting; ethinyl estradiol plus DL-norgestrel or equivalent in two doses 12 hours apart; antiemetic to be taken 1 hour before each dose	Effective for prevention of unintended pregnancy following unprotected intercourse
High-dose progesterone-only IUD	1.1% 1%	Must be taken within 72 hours of unprotected intercourse; Must be inserted within 5 to 7 days of unprotected intercourse; Rare side effects; levonorgestrel in two doses 12 hours apart; Same as for IUD or IUS	Effective for prevention of unintended pregnancy following unprotected intercourse

Data from Hatcher, R., Trussell, J., Stewart, F., Kowal, D., Guest, F., Cates, W., et al. (2003). *Contraceptive technology* (18th ed.). New York: Irvington Publishers.

a. Interventions
  (1) Discuss with client her partner's anticipated reaction to her contraceptive plans.
  (2) Encourage discussion of contraceptive goals between the client and her partner.
  (3) Encourage active participation of the partner in contraceptive planning.
  (4) Recognize that conflict regarding contraception between the client and her partner can lead to increased risk of noncompliance; it can also increase the stress of adjustment during the postpartum period.

b. Outcomes
  (1) Client and her partner discuss contraceptive goals with each other.
  (2) Client's partner discusses his reaction to her contraceptive plans.
  (3) Client's partner actively participates in decisions regarding contraceptive use.
  (4) Client and her partner identify any areas of conflict and their potentially negative effects on contraceptive use and family adjustment.

HEALTH EDUCATION

The health education component of family planning is shown in Table 15-1.

CASE STUDIES AND STUDY QUESTIONS

Ms. T, 36, delivered her first child 12 hours ago. She will be discharged after an overnight stay. Her delivery was uncomplicated, and she has no serious medical problems except that her social history reveals a habit of smoking two packs of cigarettes per day. She tells you that her partner is anxious to resume sexual relations, and she plans to begin taking birth control pills immediately.

1. What additional information would you need to help her determine whether or not her plans to use the pill are appropriate?
   a. Her breastfeeding plans
   b. Family history of breast or uterine cancer
   c. The type of pill she used before
   d. Presence of lacerations or episiotomy

2. She tells you that she plans to breastfeed her infant for at least 1 year and that the breastfeeding experience is very important to her.

What would be her best option in using birth control pills?
   a. Begin taking the same pill she used before pregnancy.
   b. Change to a different brand of birth control pill.
   c. Use an alternative method until lactation is well established.
   d. Use abstinence until lactation is well established.

3. Additional teaching will be planned for her based on your knowledge that
   a. Her risk of developing serious side effects from birth control pills is greater because she is older than 35, and she smokes.
   b. It is unknown whether she is motivated to avoid an immediate pregnancy.
   c. Her delivery experience makes a minimum 6-week period of abstinence essential to avoid postdelivery complications.

d. She is unwilling to consider other methods of contraception.

4. Which of the following groups of contraceptive methods have the highest typical use effectiveness rates?
   a. Intrauterine device (IUD), fertility awareness, or contraceptive ring
   b. Abstinence, DepoProvera, or foam and condoms used together
   c. Levonorgestrel IUD, diaphragm, or birth control pills
   d. Condoms, abstinence, or sterilization

5. Which of the following risks is not associated with oral contraceptive use?
   a. Clotting disorders
   b. Benign liver tumor
   c. Breast cancer
   d. Gallbladder disease

6. Which one of the following is associated with the copper IUD?
   a. Amenorrhea
   b. Ectopic pregnancy
   c. Increased flow and duration of menses
   d. Clotting disorders

7. Which of the following methods of contraception has the highest rate of unintended pregnancies during the first year of typical use?
   a. Fertility awareness
   b. Withdrawal
   c. Condoms only
   d. Sterilization

8. Which one of the following contraceptive methods is available only with a prescription?
   a. Condoms
   b. Spermicide

c. Contraceptive patch
d. Natural family planning

Mrs. N, 28, has just delivered her third child without difficulty. She plans a long breastfeeding experience. She states that after a 3- to 4-week period of sexual abstinence, she plans to use a diaphragm that she has had for several years.

9. Which of the following is correct?
   a. Contraception is not necessary as long as she breastfeeds because she cannot become pregnant while breastfeeding.
   b. It is appropriate to use the current diaphragm unless it is torn or has obvious holes.
   c. A diaphragm is difficult to use during involution, especially while nursing, because of problems with fit and irritation.
   d. A tubal ligation is a better choice because she already has three children.

Mrs. J, 24, has given birth to her second daughter in 12 months. Jane is crying and tells you that her husband "cannot wait to try again for a boy" and "is glad he does not have to wait any longer for sex." She says she does not feel "like a real woman anymore" because she feels "too tired and sore even to think about making love," and she does not want another baby right away.

10. Which of the following should you not encourage Mrs. J to do?
    a. Talk honestly with her partner about her feelings.
    b. Discuss her concerns about family planning with her partner.
    c. Continue to practice abstinence until she feels ready to resume sexual activities.
    d. Sign a consent for bilateral tubal ligation.

ANSWERS TO STUDY QUESTIONS

1. a	4. b	7. a	10. d
2. c	5. c	8. c	
3. a	6. c	9. c	

REFERENCES

Burkman, R. (August 2002). Rationale for new contraceptive methods. *The Female Patient,* (Suppl), 4-13.

Carlson, K., & Eisenstat, S. (2002). *Primary care for women* (2nd ed.). Philadelphia: Elsevier Science.

Hatcher, R., Trussell, J., Stewart, F., Kowal, D., Guest, F., Cates, W., & Policar, M. (2003). *Contraceptive technology* (18th ed.). New York: Irvington Publishers.

Lowdermilk, D.L., & Perry, S. (2004). *Maternity & women's health care* (8th ed.). St. Louis: Mosby.

SECTION SIX

THE NEWBORN

16 Adaptation to Extrauterine Life and Immediate Nursing Care

NATALIE DIANE CHEFFER

OBJECTIVES

1. Describe the cardiovascular, pulmonary, thermal, and gastrointestinal adaptation of the newborn.
2. Identify indications for instituting neonatal resuscitation.
3. Identify parameters used in the Apgar scoring of a newborn.
4. Describe the importance of maintaining a neutral thermal environment for the newborn, and discuss interventions to achieve a neutral thermal environment.
5. Define nutritional needs of the normal newborn, and assess readiness and ability of the newborn to feed orally.
6. Identify possible nursing diagnoses for the neonate, and develop a management plan.
7. Devise a health education plan for a particular situation.

INTRODUCTION

Transition from fetus to neonate requires profound physiologic adaptation. Most neonates make this transition without difficulty during the first 6 to 10 hours of life (Verklan, 2002). Key elements in the birth transition are: (1) shift from maternally dependent oxygenation to continuous respiration; (2) change from fetal circulation to mature circulation with increase in pulmonary blood flow and loss of left-to-right shunting; (3) commencement of independent glucose homeostasis; (4) independent thermoregulation; and (5) oral feedings (Gluckman, Sizonenko, & Basset, 1999; Verklan, 2002). Physiologic adaptation is considered complete when vital signs, feeding, and gastrointestinal and renal function are normal (Kelly, 1999). Close observation of the infant's adaptation to extrauterine life is imperative to identify problems in transition and initiate interventions.

A. Transition from fetus to neonate
  1. Respiratory adaptation
    a. Mechanical stimuli: compression of the fetal chest during vaginal delivery creates negative pressure by which air is drawn into the lung fields as the thorax recoils to its original size when the fetus exits the mother's body. Air fills the alveoli by replacing the lung fluids that have been expelled by chest compression during the vaginal delivery. The remaining lung fluids are removed through reabsorption by the

lymphatics. Infant crying creates intrathoracic positive pressure, keeping the alveoli open.

b. Chemical stimuli: with cessation of placental blood flow, the neonate's lungs must initiate and maintain gas exchange. The stress on the fetus during delivery leads to mild hypoxia, elevated carbon dioxide, and acidosis. Aortic and carotid bodies contain chemoreceptors that stimulate the medulla to trigger respiration. Surfactant, a phospholipid coating the alveolar epithelium, reduces the surface tension of the lung mucosa and allows exhalation without lung collapse.

c. Thermal stimuli: sudden chilling of the moist infant after delivery stimulates skin sensory receptors to transmit impulses to the respiratory center.

d. Sensory stimuli: normal handling after delivery (e.g., vigorous drying of the newborn) provides strong tactile stimulation to initiate breathing. Exposure to lights, sounds, touch, smell, and pain after the delivery continue to stimulate the infant to continue breathing after birth (Askin, 2002).

2. Cardiovascular adaptation: the neonate's circulatory system undergoes several physiologic changes after birth. The termination of fetal circulation and the transition to newborn circulation involve the closure of the three fetal shunts—the ductus venosus, the foramen ovale, and the ductus arteriosus.

a. The physiologic changes associated with lung inflation after delivery cause an increase of pressure in the left heart and increase systemic resistance.

b. With neonatal respiration, oxygenated blood enters the pulmonary musculature. This dilates the pulmonary artery and decreases the pulmonary vascular resistance.

c. The ductus arteriosus closes within 12 hours in the full-term infant due to decreasing pressure in the pulmonary vasculature and the increased pressure in the aorta (Moore, Brooke, & Heymann, 2001). This stops the flow of blood through the ductus arteriosus.

d. Vascular dilation along with the equalization and eventual overriding left atrial pressure forces functional closure of the foramen ovale. The foramen ovale, which acts like a flap valve, closes with the decreased pulmonary vascular resistance and increased left heart pressure due to termination of placental blood flow.

3. Thermoregulation

a. Thermoregulation: a critical component in the physiologic adaptation to extrauterine life. Thermoregulation is the means by which the neonate's body temperature is maintained by balancing heat generation and heat loss in a changing environment.

b. Normal temperature range: preferred temperatures for term infants are between 36° C and 36.5° C (axillary) for the first few hours of life. Temperature regulation is poor in the newborn for several reasons:
   (1) The ratio of large body surface to body mass
   (2) Limited ability to generate heat from muscular movement (Altimier et al., 1999)
   (3) Limited subcutaneous fat

c. Mechanisms of heat loss
   (1) Convection: heat is lost to air or fluid around the infant that is cooler than infant's temperature (e.g., air drafts on infant from open door in delivery room).

(2) Radiation: heat is lost to solid objects near infant that are cooler than infant's temperature (e.g., windows to the outside not covered by draperies).

(3) Conduction: heat is lost to cold surfaces or to objects with which the infant has contact (e.g., x-ray plate or unheated mattress or scale).

(4) Evaporation: heat is lost when water evaporates from the infant's skin surface or respiratory tract (e.g., infant not dried immediately after birth).

d. Newborns attempt to regulate body temperature through flexed fetal positioning, which decreases body surface area; peripheral vasoconstriction; increased metabolic rate; and nonshivering heat production by brown fat metabolism (Altimier et al., 1999; Hackman, 2001).

e. Neutral thermal environment: a neutral thermal environment is the temperature range in which normal body temperature can be maintained with minimal metabolic demands and oxygen consumption.

(1) Achieving a neutral thermal environment

(a) Incubator: usually single-walled plastic boxes that warm the infant by convection

(b) Radiant warmers: an open bed with radiant heat panels placed above the infant; convective and evaporative heat losses are increased

(c) Kangaroo care: direct skin-to-skin contact by placing the infant against the mother's skin to provide thermal support

(d) Open crib: once an infant's temperature is normalized, infant is placed in an open crib with hats and blankets, providing thermal support.

4. Gastrointestinal transition

a. Gastrointestinal system: the newborn's digestive tract becomes functional and able to process foodstuff via digestion, absorption, and metabolism.

b. Infants born beyond 32 to 34 weeks' gestation have adequate suck-and-swallow coordination for oral feedings unless neurologic damage has occurred or the infant is too ill to safely handle feedings.

c. Energy requirements: the goal of feeding is to provide energy for metabolic requirements and growth.

(1) Breastfed term infants: need 85 to 100 kcal/kg body weight per day

(2) Formula-fed term infants: need 100 to 110 kcal/kg body weight per day

d. Feeding newborn infants

(1) Breastfeeding: the preferred feeding for all infants and should begin as soon as possible after birth, usually within the first hour and continue for at least 12 months (American Academy of Pediatrics [AAP], 1997). (See Chapter 14 for a complete discussion of breastfeeding.)

(a) Provides 20 kcal/oz (30 ml).

(b) Advantages of breast milk

(i) Lower incidence of illness, including diarrhea, lower respiratory tract infections, otitis media, bacteremia, bacterial meningitis, urinary tract infections (AAP, 1997), and gastroesophageal reflux (Slusser & Powers, 1997)

(ii) Possible protective effect against sudden infant death syndrome, insulin-dependent diabetes mellitus, Crohn's disease, and possible improvement of cognitive development (AAP, 1997)

    (iii) Economic benefit for the family related to reduced health care costs and the cost of purchasing formula

    (iv) Psychologic benefits related to improved infant and maternal bonding and attachment

  (c) Disadvantages

    (i) Breast-related problems such as sore or cracked nipples, engorged breasts, or poor let down (Binns & Scott, 2002a)

    (ii) Difficulty with actual breastfeeding techniques of positioning and attachment.

    (iii) Might be inconvenient or limit activities outside the home for the mother.

(2) Bottle-feeding: commercially prepared formulas are based on cow's milk and have been modified to closely resemble human milk.

  (a) Provides 20 kcal/oz (30 ml).

  (b) Advantages of formula

    (i) Ability to share feedings with partner, family, and friends.

    (ii) Lack of physical problems (i.e., sore nipples, nipple confusion, etc.)

  (c) Disadvantages of formula

    (i) Is more costly, especially if purchased in ready-to-serve concentrations.

    (ii) Must be prepared if not purchased in ready-to-serve concentration.

    (iii) Is more difficult to digest and forms harder curds because of higher casein content.

(3) Pacifiers

  (a) Advantage: can be used to provide nonnutritive sucking and for comforting a crying infant.

  (b) Disadvantages: might decrease long-term breastfeeding (Howard et al., 1999) and is probably associated with oral candidiasis, increase incidence of respiratory and gastrointestinal illness, dental caries and dental malocclusions (Post & Goessler, 2001).

  (c) If pacifiers are going to be used, they should be given after 6 weeks of age (Binns & Scott, 2002b), and parents should limit their use to transitional periods or times of stress (Post & Goessler, 2001).

e. General considerations for feeding the newborn

(1) Breastfeeding:

  (a) Alert, healthy infants may have their first feeding in the delivery room.

  (b) Feed every 2 to 3 hours or on demand when infant is awake, alert, and shows signs of hunger. Each session should last 10 to 15 minutes on each breast. Burp infant between and after each breast.

  (c) Do not supplement the breastfed infant with feedings of water, glucose water, or formula, which might actually discourage breastfeeding.

(2) Bottle-feeding:

  (a) The first feeding should be initiated in the nursery. Infant should be offered several sips of sterile water before formula to assess for aspiration.

         (b) Bottle-fed infants should be fed 15 to 30 ml of formula every 3 to 4 hours on first day of life increasing to 75 to 90 ml by day 4 or 5.

         (c) Always hold infant during feedings; this provides vital human contact. Bottle-propping can lead to aspiration and middle-ear infections

         (d) Discard all unused formula left in bottle after feeding.

   f. Cultural considerations related to feeding practices

     (1) The prevalence of the initiation of breastfeeding and breastfeeding until 6 months of age in the United States have reached their highest levels recorded to date (Ryan, Wenjun, & Acosta, 2002). Despite these statistics, cultural, and economic barriers to breastfeeding should be identified and addressed. Barriers to the initiation and continuation of breastfeeding might include:

         (a) Giving formula promotion materials to mothers at discharge from the hospital (Ryan et al., 2002).

         (b) Breastfeeding is not the feeding method of choice among African-American women (Ludington-Hoe, McDonald, & Satyshur, 2002). African-American adolescents tend to lack role models and maternal encouragement for breastfeeding. (Wiemann, DuBois, & Berenson, 1998).

         (c) African-American and Latina adolescents identified perceived fear or pain, embarrassment with public exposure, and unease with the act of breastfeeding as significant barriers (Hannon, Willis, Bishop-Townsend, Martinez, & Scrimshaw, 2002).

         (d) Full-time maternal employment is associated with early weaning, whereas mothers working part-time were more likely to initiate and continue breastfeeding (Ryan et al., 2002).

         (e) Low-income mothers identified lack of support from health care providers, social disapproval of breastfeeding in public, ridicule by friends, and difficulties associated with employment as barriers to breastfeeding (Guttman & Zimmerman, 2000).

CLINICAL PRACTICE

A. Assessment

  1. Delivery-room assessment

    a. Identify the infant at risk.

     (1) Review maternal history.

     (2) Review prenatal course.

     (3) Review fetal well-being during labor and delivery.

         (a) Indications for ventilation

            (i) Apnea

            (ii) Heart rate (HR) absent or less than 100 beats per minute (bpm)

            (iii) Central cyanosis

         (b) Indications for chest compressions

            (i) HR absent or remains less than 60 bpm despite adequate assisted ventilation for 30 seconds.

            (ii) Two-thumb method is preferable because it allows better compression of the heart between the spine and the sternum (Price, 2001).

(c) Indications for medication: epinephrine at a dose of 0.01 to 0.03 mg/kg is administered if the heart rate remains slower than 60 bpm after a minimum of 30 seconds of adequate ventilation and chest compressions.
(d) Indications for intubation
  (i) Meconium-stained amniotic fluid
  (ii) Ineffectiveness of bag and mask ventilation (BMV)
  (iii) Need for prolonged ventilation (e.g., for an extremely small infant)
(4) Apgar scoring
  (a) This scoring system, initially developed by Virginia Apgar in 1952, provides practitioners with a standardized approach for evaluating the physical condition of newborns shortly after delivery. Studies have found that Apgar scoring is just as useful today as it was 50 years ago. In preterm and term infants, survival increases as Apgar scores increase (Casey, McIntire, & Leveno, 2001).
  (b) Scoring is done at 1, 5, and sometimes 10 minutes of life; the newborn is given a score from 0 to 2 for each category, based on the elements described in Table 16-1.

2. Admission to the nursery
   a. History
   b. Complete head-to-toe assessment
   c. Eye prophylaxis: regardless of route of delivery, topical antimicrobial therapy for prevention of gonococcal ophthalmia should be administered within an hour of delivery (Committee on Infectious Diseases and AAP, 1997).
   d. Umbilical cord care: topical antibiotic therapy is applied to the umbilical cord and surrounding skin after the bath to prevent bacterial colonization. The cord clamp can be removed after 24 hours (Kelly, 1999).
   e. Vitamin K: newborn infants have low levels of active vitamin K–dependent clotting factors. Hemorrhagic disease of the newborn can be prevented by administration of vitamin K, given intramuscularly within 1 hour of birth (AAP Committee on Fetus and Newborn and American College of Obstetricians and Gynecologists [ACOG] Committee on Obstetric Practice, 1997).

TABLE 16-1
Components of Apgar Scoring

Sign	Score 0	1	2
Heart rate	Absent	Below 100 bpm	Over 100 bpm
Respiratory effort	Absent	Weak, irregular	Good crying
Muscle tone	Flaccid	Some flexion of extremities	Well flexed
Reflex irritability (catheter in nose or slap sole of foot)	No response	Grimace	Cry
Skin color	Blue/pale	Body pink, extremities blue	Completely pink

   f. Blood glucose screening: using Dextrostix or Chemstrip, test any infant with symptoms attributable to hypoglycemia such as jitteriness, irritability, lethargy, hypotonia, poor feeding, diaphoresis, vomiting, apnea, temperature instabilities (Askin, 2002; Kelly, 1999). Inability to maintain normal blood glucose levels might necessitate more frequent feedings.
   g. Temperature regulation
      (1) Care must be taken during bathing to minimize heat loss.
      (2) Dress infant in shirt, diaper, and hat or cap.
      (3) Wrap in double blanket until infant can maintain temperature without second blanket (usually about 24 hours).
      (4) Assess infant's temperature every hour until stable.

B. **Nursing Diagnoses**
   1. Risk for hypothermia related to infant's poor ability to regulate temperature and moist body surface immediately after delivery
   2. Risk for ineffective airway clearance related to inability to adequately clear secretions from airways
   3. Risk for ineffective breathing pattern related to shallow or periodic breathing and apnea
   4. Risk for impaired gas exchange related to poor respiratory effort and retained lung fluid
   5. Risk for ineffective tissue perfusion; decreased, related to decreased cardiac output
   6. Risk for infection related to infant's poor physiologic response to pathogens
   7. Risk for imbalanced nutrition: less than body requirements related to infant's poor suck-and-swallow coordination
   8. Deficient knowledge in parents related to inexperience with newborn care and lack of parenting skills

C. **Interventions/Outcomes**
Delivery room and nursery interventions have been combined in this section. See Figure 16-1 for sequential steps for resuscitative interventions in the delivery room and Table 16-2 for medications used during resuscitation.
   1. Risk for hypothermia related to infant's inability to regulate temperature and moist body surface immediately after delivery
      a. Interventions
         (1) Close door to delivery rooms and nursery and place radiant warmer away from traffic patterns and air drafts.
         (2) Upon delivery, place infant under preheated radiant warmer.
         (3) Dry infant thoroughly and quickly; remove wet linens and wrap in preheated blankets.
         (4) Check infant's temperature every 15 to 20 minutes until stable, then every 4 to 8 hours.
         (5) In the nursery, pre-warm incubators and radiant warmers.
         (6) Some suggest postponing the admission bath until the infant's temperature is within normal range (Hackman, 2001); however, studies have found that early bathing did not demonstrate any negative effect on early adaptation of healthy newborns (Nako, Harigaya, Tomomasa, Morikawa, Amada, Kijima, et al., 2000).
         (7) During the bath, wash one area at a time; dry it, keeping the infant covered at all times. Place hat on infant's head to decrease heat loss (Hackman, 2001).

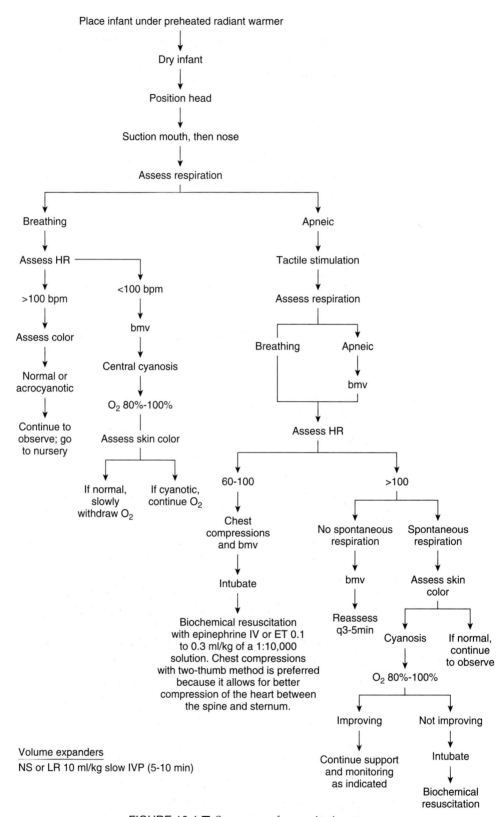

FIGURE 16-1 ■ Summary of resuscitation steps.

    (8) To warm infant, set incubator temperature at 1.5° C (2.6° F) higher than infant's temperature until infant's temperature begins to stabilize.

    (9) Use warming devices, such as heat lamps, sparingly and for only 15-minute intervals to prevent over warming the infant.

  b. Outcomes

    (1) Skin temperature is 36.4° C to 37° C (97.6° F to 98.6° F).

    (2) Temperature stabilizes within 4 hours.

2. Risk for ineffective airway clearance related to inability to adequately clear secretions from airways

  a. Interventions

    (1) Upon delivery, position infant's head in "sniff" position or slight extension.

    (2) Suction mouth, then the nose.

    (3) After feedings, position infant on side with head elevated and face and head in view of caregiver.

  b. Outcomes

    (1) Respiratory effort is good, and infant has lusty cry.

    (2) Fluid in airways has been removed to allow for normal breathing.

    (3) Infant is able to clear airway of regurgitated stomach contents.

3. Risk for ineffective breathing pattern related to shallow or periodic breathing and apnea

  a. Interventions

    (1) Upon delivery, position head in "sniff" position or slight extension.

    (2) Suction mouth, then nose.

    (3) Assess respiratory effort and HR.

    (4) Provide tactile stimulation (slap foot, flick heel with finger, or rub back).

    (5) Provide BMV with 100% oxygen for apnea, HR absent or less than 100 bpm, or central cyanosis.

  b. Outcomes

    (1) Respiratory effort is within normal limits after 30 seconds and free from retraction, grunting, and nasal flaring.

    (2) HR is greater than 100 bpm.

    (3) Skin color is normal with or without acrocyanosis.

4. Risk for impaired gas exchange related to poor respiratory effort and retained lung fluid

  a. Interventions

    (1) Upon delivery, position head in "sniff" position or slight extension.

    (2) Suction mouth, then nose.

    (3) Assess respiratory effort and HR.

    (4) Provide tactile stimulation (slap foot, flick heel with finger, or rub back).

    (5) Provide BMV with 100% oxygen for apnea, HR absent or less than 100 bpm, or central cyanosis.

  b. Outcomes

    (1) HR improves to more than 100 bpm.

    (2) Skin color becomes normal with or without acrocyanosis.

5. Risk for ineffective tissue perfusion; decreased, related to decreased cardiac output

  a. Interventions

    (1) Assess respiratory rate and HR.

    (2) Begin BMV with 100% oxygen if HR absent or less than 100 bpm, or central cyanosis.

TABLE 16-2
Medications for Neonatal Resuscitation

Medication	Concentration to Administer	Preparation	Dosage/Route	Total Dose/Infant			Rate/Precautions
Epinephrine	1:10,000	1 ml	0.1-0.3 ml/kg IV or ET	**Weight** 1 kg 2 kg 3 kg 4 kg	**Total ml** 0.1-0.3 ml 0.2-0.6 ml 0.3-0.9 ml 0.4-1.2 ml		Give rapidly May dilute with normal saline to 1-2 ml if giving ET
Volume expanders	O-Negative CBC Whole blood Normal saline Ringer's lactate	40 ml	10 ml/kg IV	**Weight** 1 kg 2 kg 3 kg 4 kg	**Total ml** 10 ml 20 ml 30 ml 40 ml		Give over 5-10 minutes
Sodium bicarbonate	0.5 mEq/ml (4.2% solution)	Two 10-ml prefilled syringes	2 mEq/kg IV	**Weight** 1 kg 2 kg 3 kg 4 kg	**Total Dose** 2 mEq 4 mEq 6 mEq 8 mEq	**Total ml** 4 ml 8 ml 12 ml 16 ml	Give slowly, over a rate of no more than 1 mEq/kg/min Give only if infant is being effectively ventilated

Drug	Concentration		Dose	Weight	Total Dose	Total ml	Comments
Naloxone hydrochloride	0.4 mg/ml	1 ml	0.1 mg/kg (0.25 ml/kg) IV, ET IM, SQ	1 kg	0.1 mg	0.25 ml	Give rapidly
				2 kg	0.2 mg	0.50 ml	IV, ET preferred
				3 kg	0.3 mg	0.75 ml	IM, SQ acceptable
				4 kg	0.4 mg	1.00 ml	
	1.0 mg/ml	1 ml	0.1 mg/kg (0.1 mg/kg) IV, ET IM, SQ	1 kg	0.1 mg	0.1 ml	
				2 kg	0.2 mg	0.2 ml	
				3 kg	0.3 mg	0.3 ml	
				4 kg	0.4 mg	0.4 ml	

Drug		Dose	Weight	Total µg/min	Comments
Dopamine	$\dfrac{\text{mg of dopamine}}{\text{per 100 ml of solution}} = \dfrac{6 \times \text{Weight (kg)} \times \text{Desired dose (µg/kg/min)}}{\text{Desired fluid (ml/h)}}$	Begin at 5 µg/kg/min (may increase to 20 µg/kg/min if necessary) IV	1 kg	5-20 µg/min	Give as a continuous infusion using an infusion pump
			2 kg	10-40 µg/min	
			3 kg	15-60 µg/min	Monitor heart rate and blood pressure closely
			4 kg	20-80 µg/min	Seek consultation

Data from the American Academy of Pediatrics. *IM,* Intramuscular; *ET,* endotracheal; *IV,* intravenous; *SQ,* subcutaneous.

(3) Begin chest compressions if HR absent or remains less than 60 bpm despite adequate assisted ventilation for 30 seconds. Two-thumb method is preferable because it allows better compression of the heart between the spine and the sternum (Price, 2001).

(4) Administer epinephrine at a dose of 0.01 to 0.03 mg/kg if the heart rate remains lower than 60 bpm after a minimum of 30 seconds of adequate ventilation and chest compressions.

b. Outcomes

(1) Improvement in cardiac output will be evidenced by the following:

(a) HR improving and more than 100 bpm

(b) Skin color improving to within normal limits

6. Risk for infection related to infant's poor physiologic response to pathogens

a. Interventions

(1) Consider performing initial temperature assessment via axillary mode after infant has been bathed to reduce risk of exposure to HIV via rectal mucosa.

(2) Be certain that traces of maternal blood have been removed from infant's skin surface before injections or invasive procedures.

(3) Clean injection sites with alcohol and friction before injections.

(4) Clean and observe any scalp monitoring sites for abscesses, redness, or drainage.

(5) Use alcohol for umbilical-stump care.

(6) Instill topical antibiotic for eye prophylaxis per protocol (silver nitrate, erythromycin, and tetracycline are most common).

(7) Check circumcision site with every diaper change, and remove petroleum jelly–covered gauze after 4 hours.

b. Outcomes

(1) Infant has minimal exposure to pathogens.

(2) Temperature of infant remains within normal limits.

(3) Signs of infection are absent at any areas where skin integrity has been disturbed.

(4) Eyes remain free of any purulent drainage.

(5) Circumcision site remains free of swelling, excess redness, or excess drainage.

7. Risk for imbalanced nutrition: less than body requirements related to infant's poor suck-and-swallow coordination

a. Interventions

(1) Assess ability to feed by giving first feeding using sterile water or assist/observe with first breastfeeding.

(2) Select iron-fortified formula if infant is to be formula-fed.

(3) Begin feedings at breast or with bottle.

b. Outcomes

(1) Infant is able to initiate and sustain suck-and-swallow coordination.

(2) Color and respiratory effort remain normal during feeding.

(3) Infant consumes 15 to 30 ml (½ to 1 oz) formula or nurses at each breast for 10 minutes/feeding.

8. Deficient knowledge in parents related to inexperience with newborn care and lack of parenting skills

a. Interventions

(1) Assess for prior parenting and infant-care experience.

(2) Instruct in and assess ability to establish breastfeeding or bottle-feeding pattern.

(3) Instruct in newborn nutrition and bathing.

     (4) Instruct in use of bulb syringe and thermometer.
     (5) Instruct in infant safety techniques.
     (6) Provide information on community resources.
     (7) Review follow-up plan for pediatric and well-baby care.
  b. Outcomes
     (1) Parent-infant dyad is able to establish oral feedings to desired amount and frequency of intake.
     (2) Parent verbalizes important factors to remember about nutrition.
     (3) Parent demonstrates and verbalizes safety measures pertinent to the newborn's care.
     (4) Parent demonstrates use of bulb syringe and thermometer, as well as bathing techniques.
     (5) Parent verbalizes knowledge of resources as appropriate to needs.

HEALTH EDUCATION

Health education centers on the preparation of parents for care of their newborn infant. Educational topics include general newborn care, nutrition, safety, and community resources to aid the family.

A. Delivery room care

When resuscitative efforts occur in the delivery room, parents become concerned about the activity occurring around the infant.

  1. It is important to discuss the normal course of events of birth and care of the newborn infant with parents before delivery so that they are not alarmed by normal delivery-room events.
  2. If there is a need for more in-depth resuscitation, provide parents with information as soon as possible.

B. General newborn care

  1. How to bathe while conserving heat and providing for safety
  2. How to take a temperature
  3. How to use bulb syringe
  4. How to diaper
  5. How to care for circumcision site: ordinary cleaning of the diaper area and inspection for bleeding, swelling, or decreased urine output; petroleum jelly gauze applied during the procedure removed after 4 hours
  6. How to clean genitalia
    a. Girls: separating the labia and cleaning from front to back
    b. Boys: wiping under scrotum and penis
  7. How to care for umbilical cord: keeping clean and dry; cleaning around cord with alcohol three times a day and as necessary; folding diaper underneath cord
  8. How to detect signs of illness and when to contact the physician

C. Newborn safety

  1. Place on his or her back to sleep.
  2. Never leave unattended on changing table or bed.
  3. Learn first aid for choking.
  4. Always use a car seat in the back seat; must be rear-facing until the infant is 1 year of age and 20 lbs.
  5. Avoid bottle propping.
  6. Wash hands before handling newborn; avoid exposure to others and to illness.
  7. Never leave infant alone in bathtub.
  8. Never shake an infant; shaking can cause severe brain damage.

D. Newborn nutrition
1. Preparation and storage of formulas; collection and storage of breast milk
2. Cleaning of bottles and nipples
3. Reasons to avoid honey and corn syrup
4. Feeding schedules versus on-demand feedings
5. Expected amounts of intake
6. Color, consistency, and frequency of stools
7. Initial weight loss and subsequent gain

E. Community resources
1. Local chapters of La Leche League or other lactation support groups
2. Home health supply companies (e.g., for breast pumps)
3. Referrals to local county and state agencies for such concerns as medical insurance, nutritional support (Women, Infants, and Children [WIC]), parenting classes, and early child development and education

F. Pediatric health maintenance and follow-up
1. First health care provider visit should be within 2 days if infant is breastfed (AAP, 1997) or 2 weeks if infant is formula-fed.
2. Schedule and teach importance of immunizations (generally first hepatitis B vaccine given in nursery).

CASE STUDIES AND STUDY QUESTIONS

A 39-weeks-gestation, 3270 g (7 lb, 2 oz) infant was born to a 17-year-old Latina, gravida 1, para 1 (G1, P1) mother. Labor and birth events were unremarkable and Apgar scores were 9 and 9 at 1 and 5 minutes, respectively. The infant exhibited nasal flaring and mild retractions, and color was acrocyanotic in the delivery room. The infant was admitted to the nursery for further observation. Admitting vital signs were temperature 35.7° C (96.2° F); heart rate 148 bpm; and respirations 68/min. After stabilization, the infant was taken to her mother, who had indicated that she wished to breastfeed. You help her with positioning the infant and "latching-on." When you return 5 minutes later, the mother states that she has no milk and requests a bottle of formula.

1. What is the most frequent mechanism of heat loss in the newborn infant?
   - a. Convection
   - b. Conduction
   - c. Radiation
   - d. Evaporation

2. The mother believes she does not have enough milk, and she wants to provide a supplement. Which of the following is the best response to her?
   - a. The nutritional requirements of the infant are minimal at this time and she has enough milk in the form of colostrum.
   - b. The infant should suck at the breast to stimulate milk production.
   - c. Colostrum is beneficial to the infant's health.
   - d. All of the above.

3. Which of the following is not true about breast milk?
   - a. Breast milk contains 30 kcal/oz.
   - b. Breast milk is economical.
   - c. Breast milk provides protection against diarrhea.
   - d. Breast milk provides protection against otitis media.

An infant born by emergency cesarean section was limp, had a weak cry, had gasping respirations, had an HR of 80 bpm, and was cyanotic at 1 minute of life.

4. What was the initial 1-minute Apgar score?
   a. 2
   b. 3
   c. 4
   d. 5

5. When should resuscitation be started in the delivery room?
   a. After the 1-minute Apgar score is obtained
   b. Immediately, if respirations are absent or ineffective
   c. Immediately, if HR is below 80 bpm

   d. After 90 seconds of attempted tactile stimulation

6. In what sequence (1 to 5) should the activities occur for initial resuscitation of an infant?
   ____ Position infant's head
   ____ Suction mouth
   ____ Dry infant
   ____ Place infant under preheated radiant warmer
   ____ Suction nose

ANSWERS TO STUDY QUESTIONS

1. d   4. b
2. d   5. b
3. a   6. 4, 3, 1, 2, 5

REFERENCES

Altimier, L., Warner, B., Amlung, S., & Kenner, C. (1999). Neonatal thermoregulation: Bed surface transfers. *Neonatal Network, 8*(4), 35-38.

American Academy of Pediatrics. (1997). Breastfeeding and the use of human milk. *Pediatrics, 100*(6), 1035-1039.

American Academy of Pediatrics Committee on Fetus and Newborn and American College of Obstetricians and Gynecologists Committee on Obstetric Practice. (1997). Postpartum and follow-up care. In J.C Hauth, & G.B. Merenstein (Eds.), *Guidelines for perinatal care* (4th ed., p. 155). Elk Grove Village, IL: American Academy of Pediatrics and American College of Obstetricians and Gynecologists.

American Academy of Pediatrics Committee on Infectious Diseases, American Academy of Pediatrics. (1997). Prevention of neonatal ophthalmia. In G. Peter, C.B. Hall, N.A. Halsey, S.M. Marcy, & L.K. Pickering (Eds.). *Report on the committee on infectious diseases* (24th ed., p. 601). Elk Grove Village, IL: American Academy of Pediatrics.

Askin, D. (2002). Complications in the transition from fetal to neonatal life. *Journal of Obstetric, Gynecologic, and Neonatal Nursing, 31*(3), 318-327.

Binns, C.W., & Scott, J.A. (2002a). Breastfeeding: Reasons for starting, reasons for stopping and problems along the way. *Breastfeeding Review, 10*(2), 13-19.

Binns, C.W., & Scott, J.A. (2002b). Using pacifiers: What are breastfeeding mothers doing? *Breastfeeding Review, 10*(2), 21-25.

Casey, B., McIntire, D., & Leveno, K. (2001). The continuing value of the Apgar score for the assessment of newborn infants. *New England Journal of Medicine, 344*(7), 467-471.

Gluckman, P.D., Sizonenko, S.V., & Bassett, N.S. (1999). The transition from fetus to neonate: An endocrine perspective. *Acta Paediatrica Supplementum, 428,* 7-11.

Guttman, N., & Zimmerman, D.R. (2000). Low-income mothers' views on breastfeeding. *Social Science Medicine, 50*(10), 1457-1473.

Hackman, P. (2001). Recognizing and the understanding the cold: Stressed term infant. *Neonatal Network, 20*(8), 35-41.

Hannon, P.R., Willis, S.K., Bishop-Townsend, V., Martinez, I.M., & Scrimshaw, S.C. (2000). African-American and Latina adolescent mothers' infant feeding decisions and breastfeeding practices: A qualitative study. *Journal of Adolescent Health, 26,* 299-407.

Howard, C.R., Howard, F.M., Lanphear, B., deBlieck, E.A., Eberly, S., & Lawrence, R.A. (1999). The effects of early pacifier use on breastfeeding duration. *Pediatrics, 103*(3), E33.

Ludington-Hoe, S., McDonald, P., & Satyshur, R. (2002). Breastfeeding in African-American women. *Journal of National Black Nurses Association, 3*(1), 56-64.

Kelly, J.M. (1999). General care. In G. Avery, M.A. Fletcher, & M.G. MacDonald (Eds.), *Neonatalogy: Pathophysiology and management of the newborn* (5th ed., pp. 333-343). Philadelphia: Lippincott, Williams & Wilkins.

Moore, P., Brook, M., & Heymann, M. (2001). Patent ductus arteriosus. In H.D. Allen, H.P. Gutgessel, E.B. Clark, & D.J. Driscoll (Eds.), *Heart disease in infants, children, and adolescents* (6th ed., pp. 652-669). Philadelphia: Lippincott, Williams & Wilkins.

Nako, Y., Harigaya, A., Tomomasa, T., Morikawa, A., Amada, M., Kijima, C., et al. (2000). Effects of bathing immediately after birth on early neonatal adaptation and morbidity: A prospective randomized comparative study. *Pediatrics International, 4*(5), 517-522.

Post, J., & Goessler, M. (2001). Is pacifier use a risk factor for otitis media? *Lancet 357*(9259), 823-824.

Price, D. (2001). New neonatal resuscitation program guidelines. *Canadian Family Physician, 47*(June), 1263-1264.

Ryan, A., Wenjun, Z., & Acosta, A. (2002). Breastfeeding continues to increase into the new millennium. *Pediatrics, 110*(6), 1103-1109.

Sansoucie, D., & Cavaliere, T. (1997). Transition from fetal to extrauterine circulation. *Neonatal Network, 16*(2), 5-12.

Slusser, W., & Powers, N. (1997). Breastfeeding update 1: Immunology, nutrition, and advocacy. *Pediatrics in Review, 18*(4), 111-119.

Verklan, M.T. (2002). Physiologic variability during transition to extrauterine life. *Critical Care Nursing Quarterly, 24*(4), 41-56.

Wiemann, C.M., Dubois, J.C., & Berenson, A.B. (1998). Racial/ethnic differences in the decision to breastfeed among adoloescent mothers. *Pediatrics, 101*(6). Available online at *www.pediatrics.org/cgi/contents/full6/e11/1-8.*

17 Newborn Biologic/ Behavioral Characteristics and Psychosocial Adaptations

NATALIE DIANE CHEFFER AND DEBRA ANN RANNALLI

OBJECTIVES

1. Identify normal physical characteristics of the newborn.

2. Interpret physical and neurologic findings for gestational age classification.

3. Define sensory capabilities of the newborn.

4. Distinguish sleep and wake cycles of the newborn.

5. Identify physical characteristics specific for common congenital abnormalities in the newborn.

6. Identify the incidence, risk factors, pathophysiology, and associated complications for the following congenital abnormalities: congenital heart disease, gastrointestinal and abdominal wall defects, and neurologic and musculoskeletal defects.

7. Describe specific initial nursing interventions that are appropriate for each type of congenital abnormality.

8. Relate health educational topics commonly needed for families of newborn infants.

9. Devise a health education plan for a particular situation.

INTRODUCTION

Within the first 24 hours after delivery, a thorough and systematic assessment of the newborn is necessary to identify the state of health of the neonate and detect congenital anomalies, which might suggest problems with extrauterine adaptation. It is important to determine whether physical assessment findings are normal variations or indicators of more serious congenital malformations or syndromes. Assessment of the neonate would be incomplete if the clinician failed to identify behavioral characteristics, such as infant states, sleep cycles, crying, and the sensory capacities of the normal newborn. Physical examination of the term infant should be performed with one or both parents in attendance. This fosters discussion with parents about expected physical and behavioral characteristics of their newborn.

CLINICAL PRACTICE
A. Assessment of expected findings in full-term neonates
  1. Growth parameters:
      a. Weight : 2500 to 4000 g (5 lb, 8 oz to 8 lb, 13 oz)
      b. Length from head to heel: 48 to 53 cm (19 to 21 in)
      c. Chest circumference: 30.5 to 33 cm (12 to 13 in)
      d. Head circumference: 33 to 35.5 cm (13 to 14 in)
  2. Vital signs:
      a. Temperatures should stabilize between 36.4° C to 37° C.
      b. Respiratory patterns are irregular, with respiratory rates between 30 to 60 inspirations per minute.
      c. Heart rates are regular, with rates between 110 to 160 beats per minute (bpm) depending on the infant's state.
      d. Blood pressure measurements are usually not assessed as part of the newborn examination.
  3. Physical examination:
      a. General survey: periods of alertness, symmetric features and movements, easily consolable
      b. Skin: smooth, pink-to-reddish with possible flaking in areas of major creasing. Vernix caseosa, a cheesy, white substance, can be found on the entire body but is more intense between folds. Lanugo, a fine hair, might be seen, especially on the back.
          (1) Benign skin conditions:
              (a) Acrocyanosis: cyanosis of hands and feet
              (b) Cutis marmorata: transient mottling, especially when exposed to cool temperatures
              (c) Erythema toxicum: pink, papular rash with vesicles on chest, abdomen, back, buttocks, and extermities
              (d) Capillary hemangioma: "stork bite" and "angel kiss" are flat, deep pink areas over eyelids, forehead, or nape of neck in infants with fair skin.
              (e) Mongolian spots: bluish-black hyperpigmented areas usually located on the back and buttocks in infants with dark skin
      c. Head:
          (1) Molding of the head might occur as the result of the delivery and usually resolves within a few weeks. Bruising is common.
              (a) Caput succedaneum: presents at birth with pitting edema of the scalp crossing suture lines as a result of accumulation of blood or serum above the periosteum (Fuloria & Kreiter, 2002a).
              (b) Cephalohematoma: occurs several hours after birth from bleeding between the periosteum and skull, causing swelling that does not cross suture lines; might take several weeks to resolve.
      d. Eyes
          (1) Eyelids are usually edematous immediately after birth.
          (2) Color of iris: slate gray, dark blue, or brown
          (3) Pupils reactive to light; red reflex present; focuses on objects and follows to midline.
          (4) Mucoid discharge is normal with absence of tears.
          (5) Scleral hemorrhages are possible.
      e. Ears
          (1) Position: top of pinna is horizontal to outer canthus of eye.

(2) Pinna: is flexible and well formed with cartilage present.
(3) Loud noise elicits startle reflex.
f. Nose
(1) Obligate nose breather.
(2) Nares are patent with no evidence of choanal atresia.
g. Mouth
(1) Intact palate with midline uvula
(2) Normal frenulum of tongue and lip
(3) Minimal or absent salivation
(4) Suck, root, and gag reflexes present
h. Neck
(1) Full range of motion without torticollis (a unilateral contracture of the sternocleidomastoid muscle) (Alexander & Kuo, 1997)
(2) Tonic neck reflex present
(3) Intact clavicles with no tenderness, swelling, or crepitation
(4) Absence of webbing
i. Chest/lungs
(1) Symmetric, barrel-shaped, with equal anteroposterior and lateral diameters.
(2) Slight subcostal and intercostal retractions are common.
(3) Breast enlargement and engorgement in either sex with physiologic galactorrhea. Resolves within several weeks.
(4) Bilateral bronchial breath sounds. Fine crackles and transient hoarseness are normal (Colyar, 2003).
j. Cardiac
(1) Apex or point of maximal impulse (PMI) at left third or fourth intercostal space.
(2) Murmurs that are present after the first 12 hours of life should be evaluated to rule out underlying structural abnormalities (Fletcher, 1999).
k. Abdomen
(1) Mildly protuberant
(2) Liver normally palpable 1 to 3 cm below costal margin in the mid-clavicular line.
(3) Kidneys: 1 to 2 cm above and to both sides of umbilicus and felt with deep palpation.
(4) Bowel sounds present, but might be hypoactive on first day of life.
(5) Three vessels in cord.
l. Genitals
(1) Female: labia and clitoris edematous; hymenal tag often present; labia majora larger than labia minora; urethral meatus located below clitoris; vaginal discharge whitish or blood-tinged
(2) Male: scrotum large, edematous and pendulous; testes palpable; urethral opening at tip of glans penis; foreskin tightly adhered (phimosis)
m. Extremities
(1) Symmetric
(2) Full range-of-motion
(3) All 10 fingers and toes present without webbing
(4) Brachial and femoral pulses present and equal
(5) Pink nail beds or acrocyanosis
(6) Creases on anterior two thirds of sole

(7) Scarf sign present
(8) Normal hip abduction without clicks
n. Back
(1) Spine intact without openings, masses, curves, dimples, or hairy tufts
(2) Patent anal opening
(3) Even gluteal folds
(4) Trunk incurvation reflex present
o. Neurologic
(1) Posture: general flexed position similar to that maintained in utero
(2) Tone: extremities have brisk recoil to flexion; infant able to hold head erect momentarily while sitting.
(3) Tremors or jitteriness: momentary quivering or tremors might occur as a result of immature nervous system.
(4) Newborn reflexes: Box 17-1
4. Behavioral states: These characteristics, combined with the infant's appearance, evoke responses in the parents that help facilitate the attachment process. Identifying infant's behavioral state is helpful in determining the infant's ability to perceive stimuli and interact with others. Behavioral states are as follows (Brazelton, 1999):
a. Quiet sleep: quiet sleep without movement except for sudden, jerky movements; hard to awaken from this state
b. Active sleep: eyes closed with some eye movement seen under lids, active body movements; sucking might be present
c. Drowsy: eyes open or closed, lids usually heavy; active body movements with occasional fussing
d. Alert inactivity: alert with eyes open; attentive to close objects; little body movement
e. Fussing: Alert inactivity with mild, agitated vocalizations
f. Crying: eyes tightly closed at times with crying, thrashing, and movements of head and extremities
5. Crying
a. Crying in the newborn period is usually not specific to the type of discomfort. The newborn tends to cry in response to hunger, pain, or disturbing stimuli.

■ BOX 17-1
■ **NEWBORN REFLEXES**

Name of Reflex	Expected Response
Sucking	Strong sucking movements of mouth can be elicited and might occur during sleep.
Swallow	Follows sucking, usually at pauses, and can be seen at the neck.
Rooting	When cheek is touched or stroked, infant turns head toward stroked side and opens mouth to receive nipple.
Moro (startle)	General body response to sudden stimulus that is a combination of full extension and abduction of limbs.
Babinski	Upward stroking of sole and across ball of foot causes great toes to hyperextend and foot to dorsiflex.
Palmar and plantar grasps	Touching palms of hands and feet causes flexion of fingers or toes.

      b. During the neonatal period, crying is an important behavior for organizing the day and reducing disturbance in the central nervous system (CNS) (Brazelton, 1999).

6. Sleep
      a. After the delivery, newborns have a period of alertness lasting for a variable amount of time, after which the infant will typically sleep for 2 to 3 hours at a time.
      b. Newborns will usually sleep between 16 to 18 hours in a 24-hour period.

7. Sensory capabilities
      a. Hearing: well-developed at birth; responds to noise.
      b. Vision: focuses on close-up objects (e.g., the mother's face when at breast); tracks with eyes to midline or beyond.
      c. Taste: distinguishes between sweet and sour at 3 days of age.
      d. Smell: distinguishes between mother's breasts and breast milk and those of another by fifth day of age and frequently sooner.
      e. Touch: sensitive to pain, usually responds to tactile stimuli.

9. Gestational age assessment (see Chapter 18 for a discussion of gestational age significance/risks).
      a. Reliable assessment of gestational age is based on neurologic development and physical characteristics found by direct examination of the infant.
      b. Classification of infant allows clinician to anticipate clinical problems and apply early diagnostic testing.
      c. Classifications: infant's weight and weeks of gestation are classified as follows:
        (1) Appropriate to gestational age (AGA): characterizes approximately 80% of the neonatal population.
        (2) Small for gestational age (SGA): fewer than 2500 g (5 lb, 8 oz) for term neonate due to less growth in utero than expected; associated risks include hypoglycemia, asphyxia, respiratory distress syndrome, meconium aspiration, intrauterine infection, and hyperbilirubinemia.
        (3) Large for gestational age (LGA): more than 4000 g (8 lb, 13 oz) for term neonate due to accelerated growth for length of gestation; associated risks include birth trauma, hypoglycemia, hypocalcemia, hyperbilirubinemia, meconium aspiration, intrauterine infection, and polycythemia.
      d. Assessing for gestational age (see Chapter 8 for a complete discussion of antepartum fetal assessment)
        (1) Guides are frequently used in the nursery to determine neuromuscular and physical maturity. Table 17-1, Box 17-2, and Figure 17-1 are commonly used.
        (2) A guide is frequently used to assess neurologic characteristics and maturity (Figure 17-2).

COMMON CONGENITAL ABNORMALITIES
Neural-Tube Defects
Hydrocephalus
A. Introduction
    1. Congenital hydrocephalus is an enlargement of the cerebral ventricles or subarachnoid spaces.

Text continued on p. 446

TABLE 17-1

Scoring System of External Physical Characteristics*

External Sign	0	1	2	3	4
			Score†		
Edema	Obvious edema of hands and feet; pitting over tibia	No obvious edema of hands and feet; pitting over tibia	No edema		
Skin texture	Very thin, gelatinous	Thin and smooth	Smooth; medium thickness; rash or superficial peeling	Slight thickening; superficial cracking and peeling, especially of hands and feet	Thick and parchmentlike; superficial or deep cracking
Skin color	Dark red	Uniformly pink	Pale pink; variable over body	Pale; only pink over ears, lips, palms, or soles	
Skin opacity (trunk)	Numerous veins and venules clearly seen, especially over abdomen	Veins and tributaries seen	A few large vessels clearly seen over abdomen	A few large vessels seen indistinctly over abdomen	No blood vessels seen
Lanugo (over back)	No lanugo	Abundant; long and thick over whole back	Hair thinning, especially over lower back	Small amount of lanugo and bald areas	At least half of back devoid of lanugo
Plantar creases	No skin creases	Faint red marks over anterior half of sole	Definite red marks over >anterior half; indentations over >anterior third	Indentations over >anterior third	Definite deep indentations over >anterior third

Nipple formation	Nipple barely visible; no areola	Nipple well defined; areola smooth and flat, diameter <0.75 cm	Areola stippled, edge not raised, diameter <0.75 cm	Areola stippled, edge raised, diameter >0.75 cm
Breast size	No breast tissue palpable	Breast tissue on one or both sides, <0.5 cm	Breast tissue on both sides, one or both 0.5 to 1.0 cm	Breast tissue on both sides, one or both >1 cm
Ear form	Pinna flat and shapeless; little or no incurving of edge	Incurving of part of edge of pinna	Partial incurving of whole of upper pinna	Well-defined incurving of whole of upper pinna
Ear firmness	Pinna soft, easily folded, no recoil	Pinna soft, easily folded, slow recoil	Cartilage to edge of pinna but soft in places, ready recoil	Pinna firm, cartilage to edge, instant recoil
Genitals: male	Neither testis in scrotum	At least one testis high in scrotum	At least one testis right down	
Genitals: female (with hips half abducted)	Labia majora widely separated, labia minora protruding	Labia majora almost cover labia minora	Labia majora completely cover labia minora	

Adapted by Dubowitz, L., Dubowitz, V., & Goldberg, C. (1970). Clinical assessment of gestational age in the newborn infant. *Journal of Pediatrics, 77,* 1-10.

*To be used in conjunction with Figure 17-2.

†If score differs on two sides, take the mean.

■ TECHNIQUES OF NEUROLOGIC ASSESSMENT*

Posture

With the infant supine and quiet, score as follows
Arms and legs extended = 0
Slight or moderate flexion of hips and knees = 1
Moderate to strong flexion of hips and knees = 2
Legs flexed and abducted, arms slightly flexed = 3
Full flexion of arms and legs = 4

Square Window

Flex the hand at the wrist. Exert pressure sufficient to get as much flexion as possible. The angle between the hypothenar eminence and the anterior aspect of the forearm is measured and scored. Do not rotate the wrist.

Ankle Dorsiflexion

Flex the foot at the ankle with sufficient pressure to get maximum change. The angle between the dorsum of the foot and the anterior aspect of the leg is measured and scored.

Arm Recoil

With the infant supine, fully flex the forearm for 5 seconds, then fully extend by pulling the hands and release. Score the reaction as follows:
Remain extended or random movements = 0
Incomplete or partial flexion = 1
Brisk return to full flexion = 2

Leg Recoil

With the infant supine, the hips and knees are fully flexed for 5 seconds, then extended by traction on the feet and released. Score the reaction as follows:
No response or slight flexion = 0
Partial flexion = 1
Full flexion (less than 90° at knees and hips) = 2

Popliteal Angle

With the infant supine and the pelvis flat on the examining surface, the leg is flexed on the thigh and the thigh fully flexed with the use of one hand. With the other hand the leg is then extended and the angle attained scored.

Heel-to-Ear Maneuver

With the infant supine, hold the infant's foot with one hand and move it as near to the head as possible without forcing it. Keep the pelvis flat on the examining surface. Score.

Scarf Sign

With the infant supine, take the infant's hand and draw it across the neck and as far across the opposite shoulder as possible. Assistance to the elbow is permissible by lifting it across the body. Score according to the location of the elbow:
Elbow reaches the opposite anterior axillary line = 0
Elbow between opposite anterior axillary line and midline of thorax = 1
Elbow at midline of thorax = 2
Elbow does not reach midline of thorax = 3

Head Lag

With the infant supine, grasp each forearm just proximal to the wrist and pull gently to bring the infant to a sitting position. Score according to the relationship of the head to the trunk during the maneuver:
No evidence of head support = 0
Some evidence of head support = 1
Maintains head in the same anteroposterior plane as the body = 2
Tends to hold the head forward = 3

Ventral Suspension

With the infant prone and the chest resting on the examiner's palm, lift the infant off the examining surface and score.

*To be used in conjunction with Figure 17-2.
If score differs on two sides, take the mean.
Adapted by Dubowitz, L., Dubowitz, V., & Goldberg, C. (1970). Clinical assessment of gestational age in the newborn infant. *Journal of Pediatrics, 77,* 1-10.

Neuromuscular Maturity

	0	1	2	3	4	5
Posture						
Square Window (wrist)	90°	60°	45°	30°	0°	
Arm Recoil	180°		100°-180°	90°-100°	<90°	
Popliteal Angle	180°	160°	130°	110°	90°	<90°
Scarf Sign						
Heel to Ear						

Apgars _____ 1 min _____ 5 min

Age at Exam _____ hrs

Race _____ Sex _____

B.D. _____

LMP _____

EDC _____

Gest. age by Dates _____ wks

Gest. age by Exam _____ wks

B.W. _____ gm. _____ %ile

Length _____ cm. _____ %ile

Head Circum. _____ cm. _____ %ile

Clin. Dist. None _____ Mild _____

　　　　　Mod. _____ Severe _____

PHYSICAL MATURITY

Skin	gelatinous red, trans- parent	smooth pink, vis- ible veins	superficial peeling &/or rash few veins	cracking pale area rare veins	parchment deep cracking no vessels	leathery cracked wrinkled
Lanugo	none	abundant	thinning	bald areas	mostly bald	
Plantar Creases	no crease	faint red marks	anterior transverse crease only	creases ant. 2/3	creases cover entire sole	
Breast	barely percept.	flat areola no bud	stippled areola 1–2 mm bud	raised areola 3–4 mm bud	full areola 5–10 mm bud	
Ear	pinna flat, stays folded	sl. curved pinna; soft with slow recoil	well-curv. pinna; soft but ready recoil	formed & firm with instant recoil	thick cartilage ear stiff	
Genitals ♂	scrotum empty no rugae		testes descend- ing, few rugae	testes down good rugae	testes pendulous deep rugae	
Genitals ♀	prominent clitoris & labia minora		majora & minora equally prominent	majora large minora small	clitoris & minora completely covered	

MATURITY RATING

Score	Wks
5	26
10	28
15	30
20	32
25	34
30	36
35	38
40	40
45	42
50	44

FIGURE 17-1 ■ Neuromuscular maturity and physical maturity. (Adapted by Dubowitz, L., Dubowitz, V., & Goldberg, C. [1970]. Clinical assessment of gestational age in the newborn infant. *Journal of Pediatrics*, 77[1], 1-10.)

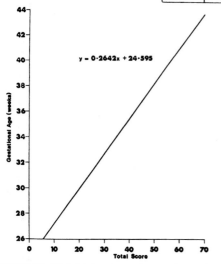

NEUROLOGICAL SIGN	SCORE					
	0	1	2	3	4	5
POSTURE						
SQUARE WINDOW	90°	60°	45°	30°	0°	
ANKLE DORSIFLEXION	90°	75°	45°	20°	0°	
ARM RECOIL	180°	90–180°	<90°			
LEG RECOIL	180°	90–180°	<90°			
POPLITEAL ANGLE	180	160°	130°	110°	90°	<90°
HEEL TO EAR						
SCARF SIGN						
HEAD LAG						
VENTRAL SUSPENSION						

$$y = 0.2642x + 24.595$$

FIGURE 17-2 ■ Scoring of neurologic findings in the infant and graph for ascertaining gestational age from the total score of physical and neurologic development. (Modified from Klaus, M.H., & Fanaroff, A.A. [1986]. *Care of the high-risk neonate* [3rd ed. p. 81]. Philadelphia: Saunders.)

    2. Incidence of congenital hydrocephalus is 1 in every 2000 newborns (Sujansky, Stewart, & Manchester, 1997).

B. Assessment
    1. History
        a. Fetal ultrasound testing shows an enlarged head.

      b. Cephalopelvic disproportion (CPD)

      c. Cesarean delivery

  2. Physical findings

      a. Head circumference greater than the 90th percentile for gestation equates to a 95% likelihood of ventricular dilatation.

      b. Enlarged or full fontanelles

      c. Wide or split suture lines

      d. Excessive rate of head growth

      e. Vomiting might occur.

C. Diagnostic procedures

  1. Sequential ultrasound testing to evaluate ventricular size and rate of dilatation

  2. Magnetic resonance imaging (MRI) and computed tomography (CT) for evaluation of cerebral parenchyma

D. Nursing Diagnoses (for immediate care)

  1. Risk for impaired skin integrity related to increased size and weight of the head

E. Interventions/Outcomes

  1. Interventions

      a. Clean and dry skin creases after feeding or vomiting.

      b. Use sheepskin under head or place infant on a waterbed or an egg-crate mattress.

      c. Reposition neonate's head frequently.

      d. Monitor any reddened areas, and position infant away from any questionable areas.

  2. Outcomes

      a. Neonate's skin will remain intact and show no signs of beginning breakdown.

Spina Bifida

A. Introduction

  1. Spina bifida is a general term used to describe defects in closure of the neural tube associated with malformations of the spinal cord and vertebrae.

  2. Spina bifida is the most common congenital malformation of the CNS.

  3. Spina bifida cystica includes three main types of defects:

      a. Meningocele

         (1) Presence of a sac containing meninges and cerebrospinal fluid (CSF); however, the spinal cord and nerve roots are normal in their structure and positioned within spinal canal.

         (2) Typically infants will not show neurologic deficits.

      b. Myelomeningocele (MN) (Figure 17-3)

         (1) Most common form of spina bifida cystica; occurrence rate is 1 to 1.5 per 1000 live births (Boyd & Gudeman, 1997).

         (2) Presence of a sac containing meninges, CSF, spinal cord and/or nerve roots

         (3) Typically infants will show neurologic deficit below level of lesion.

         (4) Associated with Arnold Chiari syndrome, which is the leading cause of death in patients with MN (Shurtleff, 2000) and hydrocephaly.

      c. Myeloschisis: most severe; no cystic covering; the spinal cord is open and exposed.

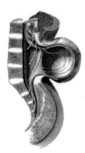

FIGURE 17-3 ■ Myelomeningocele. (From Ross Laboratories: *Clinical education aid*. Columbus, OH: Ross Laboratories.)

B. **Assessment**
   1. History
      a. Elevated maternal serum alpha-fetoprotein levels
      b. Ultrasound visualization of the defect
      c. Familial history of spina bifida
      d. Hydrocephalic fetus
   2. Physical findings
      a. Presence of a spinal lesion
      b. Enlarged head circumference: hydrocephalus
      c. Lack of spontaneous movement of the lower extremities
      d. Hip clicks secondary to congenital hip dislocation
      e. Clubfoot and scoliosis
      f. Flaccid or spastic muscles in the lower extremities
      g. Urine and stool leakage
C. **Nursing Diagnoses** (for immediate care in the delivery room)
   1. Risk for infection related to presence of sac or open lesion
D. **Interventions/Outcomes**
   1. Interventions
      a. Place neonate only in prone or side-lying position.
      b. Place neonate into sterile bowel bag, secure top at level of axilla; or cover defect with warm, normal saline–moistened sterile gauze, and place plastic wrap over dressing.
      c. Keep meconium or urine away from lesion.
      d. Administer antibiotics per orders.
   2. Outcomes
      a. Membranous sac stays intact.
      b. Aseptic environment is maintained around and over the lesion.
      c. Neonate does not show any signs of infection.

Gastrointestinal Congenital Anomalies

Cleft Lip and Cleft Palate
A. **Introduction**
   1. Cleft lip with or without cleft palate is the most common craniofacial anomaly affecting approximately 1 of every 700 live births (Thomas, 2000).
   2. Cleft palate alone occurs in 1 of every 1000 newborns (Thomas, 2000) and occurs more frequently in females.
   3. Cleft lip might be unilateral or bilateral (Figures 17-4, 17-5, and 17-6).
   4. Cleft palate might involve just the soft palate (Figure 17-7), or both the soft and the hard palates (Figures 17-8 and 17-9).

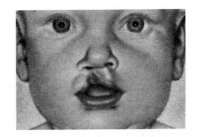

FIGURE 17-4 ■ Unilateral cleft lip, incomplete. (From Ross Laboratories: *Clinical education aid*. Columbus, OH: Ross Laboratories.)

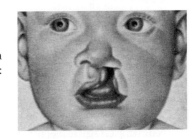

FIGURE 17-5 ■ Unilateral cleft lip, complete. (From Ross Laboratories: *Clinical education aid*. Columbus, OH: Ross Laboratories.)

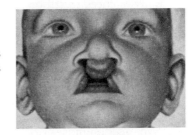

FIGURE 17-6 ■ Bilateral cleft lip, complete. (From Ross Laboratories: *Clinical education aid*. Columbus, OH: Ross Laboratories.)

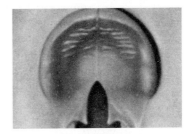

FIGURE 17-7 ■ Soft palate cleft. (From Ross Laboratories: *Clinical education aid*. Columbus, OH: Ross Laboratories.)

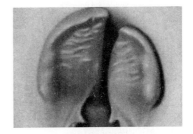

FIGURE 17-8 ■ Unilateral cleft palate, complete. (From Ross Laboratories: *Clinical education aid*. Columbus, OH: Ross Laboratories.)

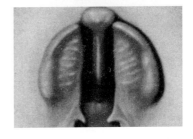

FIGURE 17-9 ■ Bilateral cleft palate, complete. (From Ross Laboratories: *Clinical education aid*. Columbus, OH: Ross Laboratories.)

5. Facial clefting is associated with an increased incidence of other abnormalities, such as congenital heart disease.

B. Assessment

1. History
   a. Maternal use of phenytoin, alcohol, retinoic acid, cigarette smoking
   b. Family history of cleft lip and/or palate in siblings
   c. Other physical anomalies (Sandberg, Magee, & Denk, 2002). More than 150 recognized syndromes include cleft lip and palate as a characteristic.

2. Physical findings
   a. Unilateral or bilateral visible defect
   b. Flattening or depression of midfacial contour in cleft lip
   c. Fissure connecting oral and nasal cavities in cleft palate
   d. Difficulty in sucking
   e. Expulsion of formula or breast milk through the nares
   f. Dehydration
   g. Poor weight gain or weight loss

C. Nursing Diagnoses (for immediate care)

1. Imbalanced nutrition: less than body requirements related to inability to adequately suck and swallow
2. Risk for impaired parenting related to inadequate bonding secondary to failure to accept impaired infant

D. Interventions/Outcomes

1. Interventions
   a. Feed with a special nipple and bottle set.
   b. Burp frequently.
   c. Feed in upright position with head and chest tilted slightly back to aid swallowing and discourage aspiration.
   d. Limit feedings to 30 to 45 minutes to avoid poor weight gain due to fatigue.
   e. Feed high-calorie-per-ounce formula to increase caloric intake.
   f. Have mother attempt breastfeeding if only cleft lip is present (Nichols & Zwelling, 1997).
   g. Support parental coping and assist parents with grief over loss of idealized baby.
   h. Encourage parents to verbalize feelings about the defect and the feeding frustrations.
   i. Provide role modeling while interacting with the neonate so that parents can internalize positive interaction.
   j. Refer parents to community agencies and support groups.

2. Outcomes
   a. Neonate is gaining weight appropriate to age.
   b. Neonate is not vomiting feedings.
   c. Neonate is not excessively fatigued after feeding.
   d. Parents are able to freely verbalize their feelings and frustrations about their infant.
   e. Parents are involved in the neonate's care in the hospital and frequently seek information about the infant's progress.
   f. Parents exhibit bonding behaviors with their infant.

Abdominal Wall Defects

A. Introduction

1. Omphalocele
   a. Defect of the umbilical ring that allows evisceration of abdominal contents into an external peritoneal sac (Lockridge, Caldwell, & Jason, 2002)

   b. Incidence is 1 in 5000 live births (Engum & Grosfeld, 2001).
  2. Gastroschisis
   a. Defect of the umbilical ring that allows evisceration of bowel through a defect in the abdominal wall with no membrane covering (Weber, Au-Fliegner, Downard, & Fishman, 2002).
   b. The incidence is 1 in 6000 to 10,000 live births (Engum & Grosfeld, 2001).
B. Assessment
  1. History
   a. Polyhydramnios
   b. Visualization on fetal ultrasonography
   c. Elevated maternal serum alpha-fetoprotein
   d. Preterm labor in the case of gastroschisis
  2. Physical findings
   a. Visible defect over the abdominal area
    (1) Omphalocele is covered with a sac consisting of peritoneum and amniotic membrane.
    (2) Gastroschisis defect exposes viscera because of lack of any covering.
    (3) Gastroschisis occurs almost exclusively to the right of the umbilicus.
   b. About 50% of newborns born with omphalocele will have cardiac, gastrointestinal, genitourinary, musculoskeletal, and CNS anomalies (Engum & Grosfeld, 2001).
C. Nursing Diagnoses (for immediate care in the delivery room)
  1. Risk for hypothermia related to exposed abdominal contents
  2. Risk for deficient fluid volume related to lack of skin integrity and exposed abdominal contents
D. Interventions/Outcomes
  1. Interventions
   a. Place neonate feet first into sterile bowel bag, secure top at level of axilla.
   b. Monitor temperature closely.
   c. Place in isolette, and maintain neutral thermal environment (NTE).
   d. Administer IV fluids and albumin per protocol.
   e. Maintain NPO status.
   f. Maintain integrity of sterile bowel bag or moist sterile dressing.
   g. Monitor glucose levels and electrolytes.
   h. Insert nasogastric tube to decompress bowel.
  2. Outcomes
   a. Omphalocele sac remains intact.
   b. Herniated viscera remains normal in color and remains moist.
    (1) Hydration is maintained.
    (2) No further advancement of bowel herniation through defect.
   c. Neonate's temperature remains within normal limits.

Congenital Diaphragmatic Hernia

A. Congenital diaphragmatic hernia (CDH) is a malformation that consists of herniation of abdominal contents into the thorax cavity via a defect in the diaphragm. The exact etiology of CDH is not fully understood. CDH might be caused by maldevelopment of one or more components of the diaphragm occurring during the embryonic stage of development.
B. Incidence of CHD is approximately 1 in every 2500 live births with a mortality rate of 35% in live born infants (Lally, 2002). Abdominal contents in the thorax

cause a mediastinal shift, which can result in impairment of cardiovascular function:
1. Interference with venous return to the heart
2. Reduction in cardiac output
3. Metabolic acidosis

C. **Preoperative stabilization and management will require extracorporeal membrane oxygenation (ECMO) for a period of at least 12 hours** (Juretschke, 2001).

CLINICAL PRACTICE

A. **Assessment**
  1. History
     a. Term or postterm
     b. Polyhydramnios common
  2. Physical findings
     a. Large or barrel chest
     b. Scaphoid abdomen (Fuloria & Kreiter, 2002b)
     c. Respiratory distress (ranges from mild to life-threatening)
        (1) Difficulty in initiating respiration
        (2) Gasping respirations
        (3) Retractions and nasal flaring
        (4) Cyanosis
        (5) Decreased or absent breath sounds on the side of the hernia
     d. Displacement of the cardiac impulse to one side of the chest
     e. Bowel sounds heard in the chest
     f. Asymmetrical chest expansion
  3. Diagnostic procedures
     a. Chest radiograph film: diaphragmatic margin is absent on the defective side with presence of loops of intestine in the chest cavity, which might be gas filled, giving a multicystic appearance; mediastinal shift to the side opposite of defect.
     b. Arterial blood gas assay: hypoxemia, respiratory acidosis, and metabolic acidosis.

B. **Nursing Diagnoses** (for immediate care)
  1. Impaired gas exchange related to decreased ventilation secondary to pulmonary compromise
  2. Ineffective tissue perfusion related to cardiopulmonary dysfunction secondary to pulmonary hypertension

C. **Interventions/Outcomes**
  1. Impaired gas exchange related to decreased ventilation secondary to pulmonary compromise
     a. Interventions
        (1) Delivery room resuscitation
           (a) Neonate should be immediately intubated; bag-and-mask ventilation must be avoided because air can be forced into the intestine, which will further compromise lung space in the chest.
           (b) Mechanical ventilation pressures should be kept at a minimal level to avoid pneumothorax.
           (c) Administer 100% oxygen to increase the PaO_2 and decrease persistent pulmonary hypertension.
        (2) Gastric decompression should be immediately initiated by inserting a large-bore nasogastric tube and advancing it as far as possible.

(3) Positioning
    (a) Elevate head of bed to minimize abdominal organ pressure on diaphragm.
    (b) Turn the neonate onto the affected side to allow unaffected lung to expand.
b. Outcomes
    (1) Neonate's respiratory effort receives optimal support until emergency surgical intervention occurs.
2. Ineffective tissue perfusion related to cardiopulmonary dysfunction secondary to pulmonary hypertension
  a. Interventions
    (1) Hyperoxygenate to minimize hypoxemia.
    (2) Ventilate with small tidal volumes at a rapid respiratory rate to provide oxygenation and decrease risk of pneumothorax.
    (3) Administer IV vasopressors as ordered.
    (4) Sedate as needed to minimize oxygen needs.
  b. Outcomes
    (1) Neonate remains hyperoxygenated as evidenced by blood gases.
    (2) Blood pressure remains within the ordered parameters.
    (3) Adequate sedation is maintained.

CONGENITAL CARDIAC LESIONS

A. The incidence of congenital cardiovascular malformations is approximately 5 to 8 per 1000 live born infants. Genetic disorders that might cause heart defects are categorized into three major groups (Clark, 2001).
1. Chromosomal disorders, including Di George syndrome, trisomy 21 (Down syndrome), and Turner syndrome
2. Single-gene disorders, which might be either autosomal dominant or autosomal-recessive
3. Polygenic disorders resulting from multiple genetic or environmental influences
B. Cardiac defects or lesions are categorized as:
1. Acyanotic: oxygenated blood is shunted to the body, but the infant remains "pink."
2. Cyanotic: unoxygenated blood is shunted to the body causing the infant to be "blue."

PATENT DUCTUS ARTERIOSUS

A. Introduction
1. An anatomic and functionally open shunt exists between the pulmonary artery and the aorta (Figure 17-10).
2. Patent ductus arteriosus (PDA) occurs in 5% to 10% of all cases of congenital heart disease in full-term neonates (Moore, Brook, & Heyman, 2001).
3. PDA occurs in 45% of infants weighing less than 1750 g, and 80% in infants weighing less than 1200 g (Moore et al., 2001).
4. PDA becomes functionally closed within the first 12 hours of life in the full-term infant. The closure is complete by 2 to 3 weeks of life (Moore et al., 2001).
B. Assessment
1. Physical findings
  a. A harsh systolic murmur, which becomes continuous, is heard at the left upper sternal border and posteriorly.

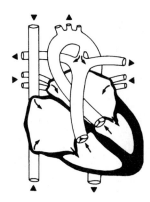

FIGURE 17-10 ■ Patent ductus arteriosus. (From Ross Laboratories: *Clinical education aid*. Columbus, OH: Ross Laboratories.)

    b. An active precordium is common.
    c. Bounding peripheral pulses
    d. Pulse pressure is widened with a low diastolic pressure.
    e. Signs associated with a large PDA
        (1) Tachypnea with retractions
        (2) Fine crackles from pulmonary edema
        (3) Diaphoresis with feeding
        (4) Left ventricular hypertrophy causing apnea
        (5) Hepatomegaly
  2. Diagnostic procedures
    a. Chest radiograph film: findings depend on shunt size; in moderate or large shunts, heart enlargement might be present.
    b. Electrocardiogram: might be normal or might show left ventricular hypertrophy with a deep Q wave and tall R waves.
    c. Echocardiogram: Doppler studies can reveal ductal flow; enlargement of left atrium and left ventricle is indicative of congestive heart failure
C. Interventions
  1. In preterm infants, administration of indomethacin (IV preferred) for three doses (Moore et al., 2001)
  2. Closure in the full-term infant might include coil closure done in the cardiac catheterization lab or surgical ligation via a lateral thoracotomy.

Atrial Septal Defects

A. Introduction
  1. An atrial septal defect (ASD) is an opening in the septum between the atria that occurs as a result of improper septal formation in early fetal cardiac development (Figure 17-11). An incompetent or malformed foramen ovale is the most common defect.
  2. Atrial septal defect occurs in approximately 0.19 in 1000 live births. Incidence in Down syndrome is 20% (Wolfe, Boucek, Schaffer, & Wiggins, 1997).
  3. Permits shunting of blood between the two atria.
  4. An incompetent or malformed foramen ovale is the most common ASD.
  5. A complete ASD involves a large septal defect that connects the atria and ventricles, also known as an atrioventricular septal defect.
  6. There are two types of partial ASDs:
    a. Ostium secundum
        (1) Most common form located in the area of the foramen ovale or central position on the atrial septum.

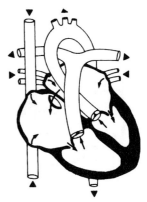

FIGURE 17-11 ■ Atrial septal defects. (From Ross Laboratories: *Clinical education aid*. Columbus, OH: Ross Laboratories.)

    b. Ostium primum
        (1) Positioned low in the atrial septum and is due to incomplete fusion of the embryonic endocardial cushions that form the lower portion of the atrial septum.
B. Assessment
    1. Physical findings—dependent on severity of defect
        a. Low-pitched diastolic murmur best heard at the left lower sternal border.
        b. Widely split S2
    2. Diagnostic procedures
        a. Chest radiograph film: cardiomegaly and increased vascular markings due to increased blood flow to the lungs as a result of shunting of blood from the left side of the heart to the right side.
        b. Electrocardiogram: usually sinus rhythm with ostium primum and secundum, but can show prolonged P-R interval with right atrial hypertrophy and P-wave changes.
C. Interventions
    1. Spontaneous closure is possible if lesion is small.
    2. Surgical repair might be necessary and require a primary closure by suturing the hole, but this still requires cardiopulmonary bypass. If this is not done, the child might eventually exhibit signs of congestive heart failure.
    3. Larger ASD will require placement of a patch while the infant is on cardiopulmonary bypass.

Ventricular Septal Defect

A. Introduction
    1. A ventricular septal defect (VSD) is an opening in the septum between the right and left ventricles that results from imperfect ventricular formation during early fetal development (Figure 17-12).
    2. VSD is the most commonly occurring form of congenital heart disease, with an incidence of 20% to 25% among neonates with cardiac defects.
    3. VSD frequently occurs in association with other congenital heart diseases.
    4. Perimembranous VSD is the most common, occurring 80% of the time (McDaniel & Gutgesell, 2001). It is located high in the septum below the aortic valve.
    5. A muscular VSD, which occurs 5% to 20% of the time, has multiple holes in the ventricular septum that resemble a "swiss cheese" septum (McDaniel & Gutgesell, 2001).

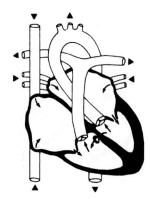

FIGURE 17-12 ■ Ventricular septal defects. (From Ross Laboratories: *Clinical education aid*. Columbus, OH: Ross Laboratories.)

6. Outlet VSD occurs in approximately 5% to 7% of cases. This septal defect is beneath the pulmonary valve (McDaniel & Gutgesell, 2001).
7. Inlet VSD occurs 5% to 8% and is inferior to the perimembranous VSD (McDaniel & Gutgesell, 2001).

B. Assessment
1. Physical findings
   a. Neonates with a small VSD usually show no signs other than a holosystolic murmur in area of left lower sternal border. The infant might have normal growth and development patterns.
   b. An infant with a large VSD will also have a holosystolic murmur that is frequently accompanied by a thrill. These infants will become symptomatic within several weeks of birth. Symptoms include:
      (1) Tachypnea
      (2) Excessive sweating
      (3) Fatigue with feedings
      (4) Symptoms of congestive heart failure are due to increases in blood flow to the lungs via the left-to-right shunting of blood in the ventricles.
2. Diagnostic procedures
   a. Chest radiograph film: might be normal with small VSD. If larger, will show cardiomegaly and increased vascular markings due to increased blood flow to the lungs as a result of the shunting from the left side of the heart to the right side.
   b. Electrocardiogram: left ventricular hypertrophy; right ventricular hypertrophy if pulmonary hypertension is present
   c. Echocardiogram: direct visualization of left to right shunting

C. Interventions
1. Infant might require management of CHF with furosemide and digoxin.
2. Infant might also require high-calorie formula or breast milk for failure to thrive until surgery can be performed, which includes a patch placed over the VSD (McDaniel & Gutgesell, 2001).

Coarctation of the Aorta

A. Introduction
1. Coarctation of the aorta is a narrowing of the upper thoracic aorta that produces an obstruction to the flow of blood through the aorta (Figure 17-13).

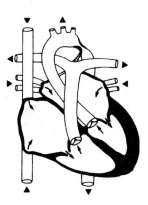

FIGURE 17-13 ■ Coarctation of the aorta. (From Ross Laboratories: *Clinical education aid*. Columbus, OH: Ross Laboratories.)

2. Simple coarctation presents with no other intracardiac lesions and can present with or without a PDA. Complex coarctation will present with other intracardiac lesions.
3. A coarctation of the aorta accounts for 6% to 8% of all cases of congenital heart disease (Beekman, 2001). About 35% percent of infants with Turner syndrome present with coarctation of the aorta (Beekman, 2001).
4. The coarctation can be juxtaductal, which is opposite to the location of the ductus arteriosus; preductal, which is proximal to the ductus arteriosus; or postductal, which is distal to the ductus arteriosus.

B. **Assessment**
1. Physical findings depend on location of the coarctation.
   a. Diminished or absent femoral pulses
   b. Blood pressure more than 20 mmHg; higher in upper extremities than in lower extremities (Wolfe et al., 1997)
   c. Blowing systolic murmur at the left upper sternal boarder and axilla area
   d. Respiratory distress
   e. Pallor
   f. Poor weight gain during the first 2 to 6 weeks of life
2. Diagnostic procedures
   a. Chest radiograph film: might show cardiomegaly with pulmonary venous congestion (Beekman, 2001).
   b. Electrocardiogram: might be normal. However, in symptomatic neonates, the electrocardiogram might show evidence of left ventricular hypertrophy.
   c. Echocardiogram: two-dimensional and color flow studies usually show site and extent of defect.

C. **Interventions**
1. Cyanotic infants require immediate treatment, including use of diuretics and inotropic therapy. Prostaglandin E1 can be used to keep a PDA open.
2. Depending on size and location, the infant might be taken to the cardiac catheterization lab for balloon angioplasty. Surgery will consist of resection and end-to-end anastomosis, patch aortoplasty, or opening the subclavian vein to form a flap aortoplasty (Beekman, 2001).

Tetralogy of Fallot

A. **Introduction**
1. Tetralogy of Fallot (TOF) is the most common type of cyanotic heart lesion, accounting for 10% to 15% of all cases of congenital heart disease (Wolfe et al., 1997), characterized by a combination of four defects (Figure 17-14).
   a. Ventricular septal defect

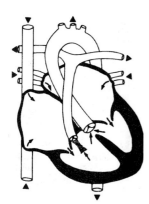

FIGURE 17-14 ■ Tetralogy of Fallot. (From Ross Laboratories: *Clinical education aid.* Columbus, OH: Ross Laboratories.)

    b. An overriding aorta
    c. Right ventricular outflow obstruction
    d. Hypertrophy of the right ventricle
B. Assessment
    1. Physical findings
        a. Respiratory distress, mainly tachypnea
        b. Cyanosis: degree is directly related to the extent of right ventricular outflow obstruction.
            (1) If there is severe right ventricular outflow tract obstruction and the ductus is patent, the neonate might have minimal cyanosis.
            (2) Spontaneous closure of the ductus arteriosus will result in a severe decrease in pulmonary blood flow and significant cyanosis.
            (3) Crying or feeding increases cyanosis and respiratory distress due to increased shunting of unoxygenated blood from the right side of the heart to the left as a result of pulmonary artery obstruction.
        c. Harsh systolic murmur located at the left upper and lower sternal borders (Siwik, Patel, & Zahka, 2001).
        d. Signs of congestive heart failure if the VSD is large.
        e. As the ductus arteriosus closes, the infant might exhibit hypoxemia if there is significant pulmonary stenosis.
    2. Diagnostic procedures
        a. Chest radiograph film: might be normal or decreased pulmonary vascular markings. Heart might have a boot-shaped appearance secondary to upturning of the apex related to right ventricular hypertrophy.
        b. Electrocardiogram: right atrial hypertrophy
        c. Echocardiogram: right ventricular wall thickening and visualization of the overriding aorta and the VSD
C. Interventions
    1. Current trend is complete repair of the TOF, which includes repair of pulmonary stenosis and closure of the VSD (Siwik et al., 2001).
    2. Palliative surgical interventions such as a Blalock-Taussig shunt and a central shunt can be used to control cyanosis. These shunts temporarily increase blood flow to the pulmonary artery from the aorta.

Transposition of the Great Arteries

A. Introduction
    1. Transposition of the great arteries (TGA) accounts for 5% to 7% of congenital heart disease (Wernovsky, 2001).

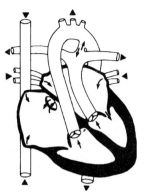

FIGURE 17-15 ■ Complete transposition of great vessels. (From Ross Laboratories: *Clinical education aid*. Columbus, OH: Ross Laboratories.)

2. The aorta originates from the right ventricle and the pulmonary artery originates from the left ventricle (Figure 17-15).
3. Survival is dependent on early diagnosis and aggressive treatment. An abnormal communication between the two separate circulations must be present or created if the infant is to survive. If the patent foramen ovale is closing, it should be reopened in the cardiac catheterization lab with a procedure called a balloon atrial septostomy. A PDA will also maintain blood flow between the two independent circulations.

B. **Assessment**
   1. If untreated, the infant will become critically ill, including hypoxemia and heart failure, which may result in death.
   2. As the communication between the independent circulations closes, the infant will become prominently cyanotic.
   3. Other symptoms might include progressive cyanosis that worsens with crying and feeding. Tachycardia, tachypnea, and a pansystolic murmur are present (Wernovsky, 2001).
   4. Diagnostic procedures
      a. Chest radiograph may initially be normal in the neonate, but will eventually show an oval cardiac silhouette, mild cardiomegaly, and increased pulmonary vascular markings (Wernovsky, 2001).
      b. Electrocardiogram might show ventricular hypertrophy.
      c. Echocardiogram is diagnostic and might show a small aorta and small left ventricle.

C. **Interventions**
   1. No supplemental oxygen to prevent closure of the PDA
   2. Correction of acidosis, inotropic therapy, and prostaglandin E1 via continuous intravenous infusion
   3. Immediate transport to an appropriate facility with cardiac expertise. Surgical, physiologic correction of the vessels called an arterial switch will need to be performed.

Hypoplastic Left Heart Syndrome or Single Ventricle

A. **Introduction**
   1. Hypoplastic left heart syndrome includes various defects that are either valvular or vascular obstructive lesions on the left side of the heart that impede left-sided filling or emptying. As a result of the obstruction during intrauterine growth, a very small quantity of blood fills the left ventricle, causing hypoplasia of the left ventricle (Wolfe et al., 1997).

2. Mitral atresia or aortic atresia rapidly causes congestive heart failure, and death can occur within a couple of days when ductus arteriosus typically closes.
3. Infants with communicating atrial and VSDs might live longer, but will require immediate surgical intervention.
4. Hypoplastic left heart syndrome accounts for 7% to 9% of all congenital heart defects (Freedom, Black, & Benson, 2001).
5. These neonates are dependent on the PDA, and, as it closes, the neonate's condition deteriorates rapidly, leading to death.

B. **Assessment**
1. Birth weight can be normal.
2. Neonate is commonly asymptomatic at birth but can become symptomatic within 1 to 2 days of life.
3. Respiratory distress includes tachypnea and dyspnea.
4. Diminished pulses, pallor, cyanosis, and mottling leading to vascular collapse and acidosis as the PDA begins to close.
5. Most neonates will have a soft, systolic, ejection murmur (Freedom et al., 2001).
6. Diagnostic procedures
   a. Chest radiograph film: radiograph may be normal. Vascular markings will be variable. Aortic arch to the right is common (Freedom et al., 2001).
   b. Electrocardiogram: sinus tachycardia and right ventricular hypertrophy

C. **Interventions**
1. This lesion was once thought to be a lethal abnormality and inoperable, but now, long-term, staged, palliative surgery is effective (Freedom et al., 2001). Other options also include cardiac transplantation.
2. The neonate requires immediate transfer to an appropriate pediatric facility with cardiac expertise.
3. Medical support might include inotropic therapy, prostaglandin E1 intravenous infusion to maintain a PDA, and hypoventilation (reduced oxygen concentration).
4. Maintenance of a delicate acid-base balance in the blood is essential for these fragile neonates.

HEALTH EDUCATION

New parents have many questions about the health and well-being of their infant. Health education should include a discussion of expected physical and behavioral characteristics as well as interventions that will foster infant attachment and development. It is important to discuss with parents situations that might require evaluation by a health care provider. Parents of infants with congenital anomalies will also need information regarding the infant's abnormality, treatment modalities, and surgical interventions. With all families, it is important to include information regarding community resources, which might pertain to a particular family situation. Specific teaching points to include are as follows:

A. **Infant growth and development**
1. Weight gain (1 oz/day)
2. Physical appearance: norms and slight departures that might apply to the individual infant
3. Newborn behavioral characteristics and sensory capabilities
4. Sleep and wake cycles to expect and opportunities for interaction

5. Calming and consoling activities including:
   a. Rocking infant
   b. Bringing infant's extremities into midline or swaddling the infant to provide security
   c. Speaking to the infant in soft, calm, and rhythmic tones
B. **Changes in behavior that might occur when an infant is ill** (Colyar, 2003)
   1. Fever (temperature higher than 100.4° F)
   2. Increased fussiness
   3. Decreased oral intake
   4. Persistent vomiting or diarrhea
   5. Any change in behavior or appearance that is concerning for the parents.
C. **Discussion of feeding practices** (see Chapter 16 for a complete discussion)
D. **Discussion of safety practices** (see Chapter 16 for a complete discussion)
E. **Community resources**
   1. Parent-child interactive programs
   2. Babysitting services or day-care organizations
   3. Red Cross or other agencies providing cardiopulmonary resuscitation (CPR) and first-aid education
   4. Local schools, hospitals, colleges, or recreation departments offering parenting and child development courses and support groups
   5. Referrals to support groups, appropriate literature and computer resources, and counseling (Bodurtha, 1999)

CASE STUDIES AND STUDY QUESTIONS

Baby L was born to a 21-year-old gravida 1, para 1 (G1, P1) Vietnamese mother. He was born vaginally after a difficult delivery due to shoulder dystocia. At admission, his weight was 4400 g (9 lb, 11½ oz). Physical and neurologic examination placed him at 40 weeks of gestation. His physical examination revealed an unequal Moro reflex with decreased movement of the left arm and crepitus at the left neck area. Bluish marking was also noted across the lower back.

1. What is the correct gestational classification for Baby L?
   a. LGA with risk for hypoglycemia
   b. AGA with risk for hypothermia
   c. SGA with risk for hypoglycemia
   d. LGA with risk for hyperglycemia

2. The historical and physical findings for Baby L might suggest:

   a. Torticollis
   b. Cystic hygroma
   c. Fractured clavicle
   d. Erb's palsy

3. What does the bluish marking across the lower back indicate?
   a. Purpura
   b. Birth trauma
   c. Blue nevi
   d. Mongolian spot

You enter Mrs. L's room to find both the mother and the infant crying. The infant is refusing to breastfeed, as he did earlier in the day. The infant cries each time he attempts to breastfeed. The mother is concerned she is not producing enough milk.

4. All of the following are true except:
   a. Mothers and babies often work these things out on their own.
   b. Feeding difficulties can affect attachment.
   c. The mother's misconception of the infant's not liking her milk

might affect her self-esteem as a parent.

d. Mrs. L might not know how to breastfeed, and might have little support at home to continue breastfeeding.

5. In this situation, which of the following actions should be taken?
   a. Give the mother a bottle of formula.
   b. Attempt to place the infant on the breast while the infant's mouth is fully open during crying.
   c. Attempt to calm the infant by talking softy, bringing his hand to midline and rocking him to bring him to a quiet state.
   d. Tell the mother not to worry; he will eat when he gets hungry enough.

Baby R is a 6-hour-old female born to a 28-year-old mother with a history of pregnancy-induced hypertension. Baby R was born 5 weeks premature and has a birthweight of 1450 g (3 lb, 3 oz). On admission to the newborn nursery, the infant's respiratory rate was 74, and she was noted to have mild intercostal and substernal retractions with adequate air entry on auscultation. Auscultation of her heart revealed a harsh murmur that was best heard in the area of the left upper sternal border.

6. Baby R's history and presentation are most indicative of:
   a. Coarctation of the aorta
   b. Atrial septal defect
   c. Patent ductus arteriosus
   d. Congenital diaphragmatic hernia

7. Based on your answer to question 6, further evaluation might reveal which of the following findings?

a. An active precordium
b. A widened pulse pressure
c. Bounding peripheral pulses
d. All of the above
e. None of the above

8. All of the following statements regarding gastroschisis are true, except:
   a. There is an increased incidence of preterm birth associated with gastroschisis.
   b. If the gastroschisis includes a defect in the abdominal wall, it is classified as an omphalocele.
   c. There is no skin covering the eviscerated organs.
   d. Intestinal atresias are frequently associated with gastroschisis.

9. A term infant develops severe respiratory distress immediately after birth. On physical examination, the chest is hyperexpanded, and the point of maximal impulse (PMI) is shifted to the right. Which of the following is the most likely cause for this infant's respiratory distress?
   a. Diaphragmatic hernia
   b. Congenital pneumonia
   c. Right pneumothorax
   d. Transposition of the great vessels

10. Signs in the neonate that might indicate a diaphragmatic hernia include:
    a. Respiratory distress
    b. Decreased breath sounds on the affected side
    c. Presence of a scaphoid abdomen
    d. Bile-stained emesis
    e. All except d

ANSWERS TO STUDY QUESTIONS

1. a	4. a	7. d	10. e
2. d	5. c	8. d.	
3. d	6. c	9. a	

REFERENCES

Alexander, M., & Kuo, K. (1997). Musculo-skeletal assessment of the newborn. *Orthopaedic Nursing, 16*(1), 21-31.

Beekman, R.H. (2001). Coarctation of the aorta. In H.D. Allen, H.P. Gutgessel, E.B. Clark, & D.J. Driscoll (Eds.), *Heart disease in infants, children, and adolescents* (6th ed., pp. 988-1010). Philadelphia: Lippincott Williams & Wilkins.

Bodurtha, J. (1999). Assessment of the newborn with dysmorphic features. *Neonatal Network, 18*(2), 27-29.

Boyd, S.B., & Gudeman, S. (1997). Spina bifida. In D.K. Nakayama, C.L. Bose, N.C. Chescheir, & R.D. Valley (Eds.), *Critical care of the surgical newborn* (pp. 527-541). Armonk, NY: Futura.

Brazelton, T. (1999). Behavioral competence. In G. Avery, M. Fletcher, & M. Mac-Donald (Eds.), *Neonatalogy: Pathophysiology and management of the newborn* (pp. 321-332). Philadelphia: Lippincott Williams & Wilkins.

Clark, E. (2001). Etiology of congenital cardiovascular malformations: Epidemiology and genetics. In H.D. Allen, H.P. Gutgessel, E.B. Clark, & D.J. Driscoll (Eds.), *Heart disease in infants, children, and adolescents* (6th ed.; pp. 64-77). Philadelphia: Lippincott Williams & Wilkins.

Colyar, M. (2003). *Well-child assessment for primary care providers.* Philadelphia: F.A. Davis.

Dubowitz, L., Dubowitz, V., & Goldberg, C. (1970). Clinical assessment of gestational age in the newborn infant. *Journal of Pediatrics, 77*(1), 1-10.

Engum, S.A., & Grosfeld, J.L. (2001). Pediatric surgery. In C.M. Townsend, R.D. Beauchamp, B.M. Evers, & K.L. Mattox (Eds.), *Sabiston textbook of surgery: The biological basis of modern surgical practice* (16th ed., pp. 1463-1517). Philadelphia: Saunders.

Fletcher, M.A. (1999). Physical assessment and classification. In G. Avery, M. Fletcher, & M. MacDonald (Eds.), *Neonatalogy: Pathophysiology and management of the newborn* (5th ed., pp. 301-320). Philadelphia: Lippincott Williams & Wilkins.

Freedom, R.M., Black, M.D., & Benson, L.N. (2001). Hypoplastic left heart syndrome. In H.D. Allen, H.P. Gutgessel, E.B. Clark, & D.J. Driscoll (Eds.), *Heart disease in infants, children, and adolescents* (6th ed., pp. 1011-1026). Philadelphia: Lippincott Williams & Wilkins.

Fuloria, M., & Kreiter, S. (2002a). The newborn examination: Part I. Emergencies and common abnormalities involving the skin, head, neck, chest, and respiratory and cardiovascular systems. *American Family Physician, 65*(1), 61-68.

Fuloria, M., & Kreiter, S. (2002b). The newborn examination: Part II. Emergencies and common abnormalities involving the abdomen, pelvis, extremities, genitalia, spine. *American Family Physician, 65*(2), 265-270.

Juretschke, L. (2001). Congenital diaphragmatic hernia: Update and review. *Journal of Obstetric, Gynecologic, and Neonatal Nursing, 30*(3), 259-268.

Klaus, M.H., & Fanaroff, A.A. (1993). *Care of the high-risk neonate* (4th ed.). Philadelphia: Saunders.

Lally, K. (2002). Congenital diaphragmatic hernia. *Current Opinion in Pediatrics, 14*(4), 486-490.

Lockridge, T., Caldwell, A.D., & Jason, P. (2002). Neonatal surgical emergencies: Stabilization and management. *Journal of Obstetric, Gynecologic, and Neonatal Nursing, 31*(3), 328-339.

McDaniel, N., & Gutgesell, H. (2001). Ventricular septal defects. In H.D. Allen, H.P. Gutgessel, E.B. Clark, & D.J. Driscoll (Eds.), *Heart disease in infants, children, and adolescents* (6th ed., pp. 636-651). Philadelphia: Lippincott Williams & Wilkins.

Moore, P., Brook, M., & Heyman, M. (2001). Patent ductus arteriosus. In H.D. Allen, H.P. Gutgessel, E.B. Clark, & D.J. Driscoll (Eds.), *Heart disease in infants, children, and adolescents* (6th ed.; pp. 652-669). Philadelphia: Lippincott Williams & Wilkins.

Nichols, F,. & Zwelling, E. (1997). *Maternal-newborn nursing*. Philadelphia: Saunders.

Sandberg, D., Magee, W., & Denk, M. (2002). Neonatal cleft lip and cleft palate repair. *AORN Journal, 75*(3), 490-499.

Shurtleff, D.B. (2000). 44 years of experience with management of myelomeningocele: Presidential address, society for research into hydrocephalus and spina bifida. *European Journal of Pediatric Surgery, 10*(suppl 1), 5-8.

Siwik, E.S., Patel, C.R., & Zahka, K.G. (2001). Tetrology of Fallot. In H.D. Allen, H.P. Gutgessel, E.B. Clark, & D.J. Driscoll (Eds.), *Heart disease in infants, children, and adolescents* (6th ed.; pp. 880-902). Philadelphia: Lippincott Williams & Wilkins.

Sujansky, E., Stewart, J., & Manchester, D. (1997). Genetics and dysmorphology. In W. Hay, J. Groothuis, A. Hayward, & M. Levin (Eds.), *Current pediatrics diagnosis and treatment* (13th ed., pp. 885-921). Stamford, CN: Appleton & Lange.

Thomas, P. (2000). Multidisciplinary care of the child born with cleft lip and palate. *ORL–Head and Neck Nursing, 18*(4), 6-16.

Weber, T.R., Au-Fliegner, M., Downard, C., & Fishman, S. (2002). Abdominal wall defects. *Current Opinion in Pediatrics, 14,* 491-497.

Wernovsky, G. (2001). Transposition of the Great Arteries. In H.D. Allen, H.P. Gutgessel, E.B. Clark, & D.J. Driscoll (Eds.), *Heart disease in infants, children and adolescents* (6th ed.; pp. 1027-1084). Philadelphia: Lippincott Williams & Wilkins.

Wolfe, R., Boucek, M., Schaffer, M., & Wiggins, J. (1997). Cardiovascular diseases. In W. Hay, J. Groothuis, A. Hayward, & M. Levin (Eds.), *Current pediatric diagnosis and treatment* (13th ed., pp. 474-536). Stamford, CT: Appleton & Lange.

18 Risks Associated with Gestational Age and Birth Weight

MARGARET A. PUTMAN

OBJECTIVES

1. Describe physical characteristics of preterm, postterm, small-for-gestational-age (SGA), and large-for-gestational-age (LGA) infants.
2. Recognize potential problems related to preterm, postterm, SGA, and LGA infants.
3. Identify maternal risk factors that may contribute to prematurity, postmaturity, and SGA and LGA infants.
4. Select appropriate nursing diagnoses for preterm, postterm, SGA, and LGA infants.
5. Describe appropriate nursing interventions for preterm, postterm, SGA, and LGA infants.

SMALL-FOR-GESTATIONAL-AGE INFANTS

Introduction

A. **An infant is defined as SGA when the weight is below the 10th percentile** (Avery & Richardson, 1998).
B. **The SGA infant may also be known as having intrauterine growth restriction (IUGR).**
C. **Not all IUGR infants are SGA;** IUGR from placental insufficiency usually reduces birth weight more than length and to a greater degree than head circumference; the greater the severity of IUGR, the greater is the deviation of weight, length, and (less so) head circumference as compared with population norms (Fanaroff & Martin, 2002).
D. **The SGA infant can be preterm, term, or postterm.**
E. **Conditions (alone or in combination) associated with SGA babies are as follows** (Kliegman & Das, 2002):
1. Maternal conditions, such as:
   a. Chronic hypertension (associated with a fourfold to eightfold increase in the incidence of abruptio placenta)
   b. Anemia
   c. Cardiorespiratory disease
   d. Connective tissue disorder
   e. Drug exposure (diethylstilbestrol, antineoplastics, narcotics, and illicit drugs)
   f. Lupus anticoagulant
   g. Renal disease and acidosis
   h. Smoking (frequently associated with abruptio placentae, placenta previa, prematurity, and respiratory distress) and alcohol consumption

       i. Young adolescent (10 to 14 years of age) or advanced maternal age (over 35 years)

       j. Asthma

  2. Fetal conditions, such as:

       a. Chromosomal abnormalities

       b. Heart disease and hemolytic disease

       c. Intrauterine infection: toxoplasmosis, rubella, cytomegalovirus, and herpes simplex (TORCH)

       d. Malformations

       e. Multiple gestation

       f. Inborn errors of metabolism

  3. Uterine conditions, such as:

       a. Arteriosclerosis of decidual spiral arteries

       b. Preeclampsia or eclampsia

       c. Decreased uteroplacental blood flow

       d. Diabetes mellitus

       e. Fibromyoma

       f. Morphologic abnormalities

  4. Placental conditions, such as:

       a. Abruptio placentae

       b. Placenta previa

       c. Chorioamnionitis

       d. Deciduitis, placentitis, and vasculitis

       e. Placental cysts

       f. Chorioangioma

       g. Edema and thrombosis

       h. Infarction (fibrin deposition)

       i. Prolonged pregnancy duration

  5. Environmental conditions, such as:

       a. High altitude

       b. Therapeutic x-ray exposure

F. Conditions altering fetal growth produce insults that affect all organ systems and are known to produce two patterns of growth that depend on the timing of the insult to the developing embryo or fetus (Kliegman & Das, 2002).

  1. Conditions affecting early gestation (generally less than 28 weeks) occur at a time when rapid cell proliferation (hyperplasia) occurs.

       a. An insult at this stage results in organs with cells of normal size but fewer numbers of cells than if the insult had not occurred.

       b. Infants are symmetrically grown (weight, length, and head circumference plot similarly on a growth curve) and all organ systems are small.

       c. Generally, these infants have the poorest long-term prognosis and are commonly associated with chromosomal abnormalities; postnatal nutrition is unable to correct for growth deficits; symmetrically grown SGA babies may never catch up in size when compared with unaffected children.

  2. Later in gestation (greater than 28 weeks), growth occurs as a combination of rapid cell proliferation (hyperplasia) but also as a result of increases in cell size (hypertrophy).

       a. An insult at this stage typically results in intrauterine malnutrition; organ systems have normal numbers of cells that are smaller.

b. The brain and heart are larger in proportion to body size as a whole, whereas the liver, spleen, adrenals, thymus, and placenta are small.

c. This type of infant is asymmetrically grown in that head size and length are spared, but overall weight and organ sizes are diminished.

d. Generally, the asymmetrically IUGR infant has a better prognosis than one who is symmetrically IUGR; in-utero malnutrition, however, is associated with increased risk of intrauterine death.

e. Optimal postnatal nutrition will generally restore normal growth potential because the number of body cells is normal.

G. **The SGA infant may present with problems from the moment of birth** (Townsend, 1999).

1. Fewer reserves are available to help the fetus tolerate the rigors of labor and delivery, leading to the development of fetal asphyxia or meconium passage in utero and the need for resuscitation at the time of delivery.

a. Uteroplacental circulation is often impaired in maternal and uterine conditions commonly associated with IUGR.

b. A small placenta may have diminished capability for gas exchange, nutrient delivery, and removal of waste products from the fetal circulation.

c. Cardiac glycogen stores may already be reduced, leading to the development of fetal bradycardia.

d. Uterine contractions may add an additional hypoxic stress on the chronically hypoxic fetus with a marginally functioning placenta.

2. The combination of intrapartum and neonatal asphyxia places the infant at increased risk for a continuum of central nervous system insults; the sequelae of perinatal asphyxia include the potential of multiple organ system dysfunction.

3. Decreased glycogen stores increase the potential for early development of hypoglycemia and temperature instability in the transition period (see discussion of preterm infants).

4. Polycythemia frequently occurs as a result of chronic subacute hypoxia and dehydration.

H. **Congenital anomalies occur more frequently associated with intrauterine insult early in gestation during organogenesis;** mortality rates for term SGA infants are five times that of term, appropriately grown infants resulting from the occurrence of major congenital anomalies (Fanaroff & Martin, 2002).

I. **The SGA infant is more frequently exposed to intrauterine infections such as rubella, cytomegalovirus (CMV), and toxoplasmosis;** risk for impaired fetal gas exchange related to inadequate umbilical cord perfusion, hypoxia, and hypercarbia; risk for impaired fetal gas exchange related to inadequate umbilical cord perfusion, hypoxia, and hypercarbia (Fanaroff & Martin, 2002).

J. **Immune function in the SGA infant may be depressed as in older children with postnatal onset of malnutrition** (Kliegman & Das, 2002).

K. **The prognosis for SGA infants must consider adverse perinatal consequences in addition to being SGA;** when perinatal problems are minimal or avoided because of early optimal obstetrical intervention, the SGA neonate may still demonstrate developmental handicaps, especially in the presence of relative head growth restriction; the reported incidence of neurologic handicaps and learning disabilities among preterm SGA infants is as high as 35% (Allen, 1998).

L. Socioeconomic status is the major determinant of developmental outcome at 2 years of age and older; SGA infants born to families of higher socioeconomic status demonstrate fewer developmental differences on follow-up, whereas those born to poorer families have significant developmental handicaps (Fanaroff & Martin, 2002).

Clinical Practice

A. Assessment
  1. History (Taeusch & Sniderman, 1998)
     a. Antenatal findings
        (1) Maternal weight gain
        (2) Age and socioeconomic status
        (3) Maternal illnesses or conditions
           (a) Renal
           (b) Cardiac
           (c) Hypertension
           (d) Phenylketonuria (PKU)
        (4) Substance use or abuse
           (a) Alcohol
           (b) Illicit drugs
           (c) Tobacco
        (5) Pregnancy conditions
           (a) Oligohydramnios
           (b) Multiple gestation
        (6) Elevated TORCH titers or other signs of infection
     b. Intrapartum findings
        (1) Length of gestation
        (2) Color, consistency, and amount of amniotic fluid
        (3) Fetal heart rate patterns suggestive of distress
  2. Physical findings (Taeusch & Sniderman, 1998)
     a. Soft-tissue wasting and dysmaturity
        (1) Decreased amount of breast tissue
        (2) Diminished subcutaneous fat tissue
        (3) Loose, dry, and cracked skin, with decreased turgor
        (4) Diminished muscle mass especially noticeable in the buttocks and extremities
        (5) Scaphoid abdomen resulting from shrinkage of the abdominal contents
     b. Smaller-than-average weight, length, and head circumference
        (1) The symmetrical IUGR infant is smaller in all growth parameters (weight, length, and head circumference).
        (2) The asymmetrical IUGR infant has smaller-than-average weight and average head circumference and length.
           (a) Large head-to-body ratio
           (b) Poor head control
  3. Presenting behavioral findings seen at or soon after delivery depend on the occurrence of asphyxia (postasphyxial encephalopathy) (Fashaw & Hernandez, 1999).
     a. Mild degree (duration under 24 hours) exhibited by hyperalertness and sympathetic overactivity

      b. Moderate degree exhibited by lethargy, stupor, hypotonia, suppressed primitive reflexes, and seizures

      c. Severe degree manifested by coma, flaccid tone, suppressed brainstem function, seizures, and increased intracranial pressure

    4. Placental examination (Sobl & Moore, 1998)

      a. Abnormal cord insertion

      b. Placental hemangiomas

      c. Circumvallate placenta

      d. Multiple infarcts

      e. Placenta previa

      f. Chronic abruptio placentae

    5. Diagnostic procedures (Townsend, 1999)

      a. Weight, length, and head circumference

      b. Gestational age assessment and plotting of growth parameters on curve

      c. Serial bedside glucose assessment

      d. Assessment for infection (see Chapter 22 for a complete discussion of sepsis)

        (1) Complete blood count (CBC) with differential and platelets (also assess for polycythemia)

        (2) Viral studies

          (a) TORCH titer

          (b) Urine for CMV titer and culture

          (c) Nasopharyngeal culture for rubella

        (3) Possible lumbar puncture

        (4) Possible total and direct bilirubin levels

        (5) Coagulation studies if indicated by thrombocytopenia or petechia

      e. Chromosome analysis if congenital anomalies are present

      f. Drug screen on meconium or urine if indicated by maternal history

      g. Cranial computed tomography (CT) to rule out hydrocephaly, microcephaly, and calcification

B. Nursing Diagnoses

    1. Risk for injury related to birth asphyxia

    2. Risk for hypothermia related to decreased glycogen stores and subcutaneous tissue

    3. Risk for imbalanced nutrition: less than body requirements related to increased metabolic expenditures, delayed feedings, or inadequate intake

    4. Risk for ineffective tissue perfusion related to polycythemia or hypothermia

    5. Risk for infection related to possible exposure to intrauterine infection and from compromised immune function

C. Interventions/Outcomes (Kabler & Delmore, 1997)

    1. Risk for injury related to birth asphyxia

      a. Interventions

        (1) Anticipate the need for and provide neonatal resuscitation according to Neonatal Resuscitation Program (NRP) guidelines as indicated by condition at the time of delivery.

        (2) Monitor and record trends in transition vital signs, blood pressure, and clinical parameters; anticipate clinical manifestations such as tachypnea, respiratory distress, acidosis, cardiovascular instability, cyanosis, and hypoxemia.

        (3) Provide stabilization care in a neutral thermal environment (NTE), and allow the infant to stabilize and self-correct mild acidosis, clear lung fluid, stabilize blood glucose, and stabilize blood pressure.

(4) Provide oxygen as indicated based on pulse oximeter saturation monitoring, blood gas values, and close observation.
   b. Outcomes
      (1) Infant's 5-minute Apgar score is 7 to 10.
      (2) Vital signs, blood pressure, blood glucose, and clinical parameters are stable and within normal limits.
      (3) Oxygen saturation is maintained within normal limits.

2. Risk for hypothermia related to decreased glycogen stores and subcutaneous tissue
   a. Interventions
      (1) Monitor incubator or warmer bed temperature and heater output; be concerned if heater output is constant.
      (2) Monitor infant's body temperature: axillary should be in the range of 36.4° to 37° C (97.6° to 98.6° F).
      (3) Examine the environment for potential sources of heat loss to prevent cold stress; for example, prewarm equipment, and avoid exposure to drafts.
      (4) Monitor blood glucose levels if temperature instability occurs (to determine if hypoglycemia is causing temperature instability); anticipate blood glucose instability and hypothermia if the infant is fasting or as the infant transitions to bolus feedings; administer intravenous glucose.
      (5) Monitor for signs and symptoms of respiratory distress and cyanosis.
   b. Outcomes
      (1) Normal body temperature is maintained.
      (2) Neutral thermal environment is maintained.
      (3) Infant shows no signs of cold stress; for example:
         (a) Increased oxygen consumption
         (b) Hypoglycemia
         (c) Respiratory distress

3. Risk for imbalanced nutrition: less than body requirements related to increased metabolic expenditures, delayed feedings, or inadequate intake
   a. Interventions
      (1) Monitor blood glucose level (normal > 40 mg%) using bedside testing system (e.g., One Touch, Accuchek, Chemstrip, and so on) with each check of vital signs until stable and within normal limits.
      (2) Anticipate blood glucose instability and hypothermia if the infant is fasting or as the infant transitions to bolus feedings.
      (3) Initiate early and frequent oral feedings (every 2 to 3 hours) if not contraindicated by respiratory status; provide a high-calorie formula (> 20 calories/oz [30 ml]) as ordered to provide additional nutrients.
      (4) Initiate and maintain peripheral intravenous (IV) access if indicated, and administer IV dextrose infusion as ordered.
      (5) Weigh infant daily.
      (6) Decrease metabolic requirements, when possible.
         (a) Feed by gavage.
         (b) Provide NTE.
         (c) Decrease iatrogenic stimuli and provide developmental care.
            (i) Swaddle.
            (ii) Offer pacifier.
            (iii) Cluster nursing and other care.
         (d) Ensure frequent and adequate rest for the infant.

b. Outcomes
- (1) Blood glucose levels will be maintained at greater than 40 mg%.
- (2) Oral feedings will be tolerated well.
- (3) IV dextrose infusion, if indicated, will maintain blood sugar within normal limits.
- (4) Infant's initial weight loss will stabilize within 3 to 5 days of life, and weight will increase thereafter at an average of at least 15 to 30 g (½ to 1 oz) per day.

4. Risk for ineffective tissue perfusion related to polycythemia or hypothermia
  a. Interventions
- (1) Obtain serum hemoglobin (normal 15 to 21.5 g/dl) and hematocrit (normal 45% to 65%) levels.
- (2) Observe for signs and symptoms of polycythemia.
  - (a) Ruddy appearance
  - (b) Cyanosis; may be more pronounced with activity or crying.
  - (c) Tachypnea
  - (d) Persistent hypoglycemia
  - (e) Apnea
  - (f) Bradycardia
  - (g) Jaundice
- (3) Consider IV dextrose infusion to provide hydration and glucose to prevent hypoglycemia and hyperviscosity syndrome.
- (4) Consider partial exchange transfusion when an infant is symptomatic to relieve capillary congestion and hyperviscosity.

  b. Outcomes
- (1) Serum hematocrit is less than 65%.
- (2) Signs and symptoms of hypoglycemia and polycythemia are absent.
- (3) Neonate's intake is sufficient to achieve a urine output greater than 1.5 ml/kg/hr.

5. Risk for infection related to possible exposure to intrauterine infection and from compromised immune function
  a. Interventions
- (1) Use Standard and Isolation Precautions when congenital infections are suspected.
- (2) Always use aseptic techniques as appropriate and good hand washing techniques.
- (3) Administer antibiotics as ordered after the initial workup is completed; check serum antibiotic levels as ordered.
- (4) Analyze laboratory values to determine trends.
  - (a) CBC with differential
  - (b) Platelet count
  - (c) Cultures
  - (d) Antibody titres
- (5) Assess infant's activity level and signs and symptoms suggestive of seizures.
- (6) Monitor infant's temperature for elevation or signs of hypothermia (above 37.2° C [99.6° F] or below 36.1° C [97° F] axillary).

  b. Outcomes
- (1) Neonate's blood culture is negative.
- (2) Temperature remains within normal limits.
- (3) Serum antibiotic levels are therapeutic.
- (4) Activity level and tone remain normal or return to normal.
- (5) Infection control principles and practices are followed to prevent nosocomial infection.

PRETERM INFANTS

Introduction

A. A preterm infant is one who is born before the end of 37 completed-weeks' gestation (Walker & Hull, 1998).

B. Preterm infants, particularly those born before 34 weeks' gestation, represent a prototype of high-risk infants because of immaturity of all organ systems, numerous physiologic handicaps, and significant morbidity and mortality (Thureen, Deacon, O'Neill, & Hernandez, 1999).

C. Risk factors (Ramsey & Goldenberg, 2002)
   1. Premature birth is frequently associated with maternal social deprivation and socioeconomic risk factors that promote catecholamine release, leading to decreased uterine blood flow and uterine irritability.
      a. Poverty, work away from home, teen pregnancy, and single motherhood have been identified as high-risk factors for preterm delivery.
      b. Race (especially black) continues to be a major risk factor for prematurity.
      c. Smoking and the use of illicit drugs, such as cocaine and crystal methamphetamines, have direct effects on placental and uterine blood flow and are commonly associated with uterine contractions, maternal hypertension, and placental abruption.
   2. Many women who deliver prematurely after spontaneous premature labor have an intraamniotic infection; bacterial vaginosis is a major risk factor for premature delivery, and early diagnosis and treatment of such infections has been shown to reduce the incidence of premature delivery.
   3. As the number of fetuses per pregnancy increases, the mean gestational age at delivery decreases; the mechanism of prematurity probably relates to the increase in intrauterine volume but also the increased rate of volume change with multiple gestation.
   4. Bicornate uterus and septate uterus are associated with increased incidence of prematurity.
   5. Prenatal maternal complications increase the risk for preterm birth.
      a. Maternal cardiorespiratory disease, hypoxia, hemorrhage, shock, hypotension, and hypertension
      b. Severe maternal anemia
      c. Maternal diabetes may result in preterm delivery because of fetal and maternal indications.
      d. Abnormal placental conditions affect oxygen transfer from mother to fetus and result in asphyxial insult to the developing fetal lung.

D. Clinical problems of the premature neonate are directly associated with the degree of organ maturity at birth; prematurity is not a disease but rather a lack of organ maturity (Kabler & Delmore, 1997).
   1. Without full development, organ systems are not usually capable of functioning at a level needed to maintain extrauterine homeostasis.
   2. The more immature or lower the gestational age, the greater the risk of complications and system failure.

E. Among organ systems, the respiratory system is one of the last to mature; therefore the preterm infant is at risk for numerous respiratory problems (Rodriguez, Martin, & Fanaroff, 2002) (see Chapter 19 for a complete discussion of respiratory distress).
   1. Prematurity is the most common factor in the occurrence of respiratory distress syndrome (RDS).

      a. Its incidence is inversely proportional to gestational age and occurs most frequently in infants of less than 1200 g (2 lb, 10½ oz) birth weight and 30 weeks' gestation.

      b. Surfactant deficiency is the principal factor leading to the development of RDS.

  2. Prenatal maternal complications increase the risk for preterm birth and increase the risk of respiratory distress in the preterm infant by negatively affecting the fetal pulmonary circulation.

  3. The ability to stabilize the chest wall is directly related to increasing gestational age; therefore the preterm infant is at risk for chest wall deformation and atelectasis, which can result in hypoxemia, hypercarbia, and apnea.

  4. Immaturity of the respiratory system and its control centers places the preterm infant at risk for apnea of prematurity, a paradoxic response to low oxygen, high carbon dioxide, or both in which the preterm infant fails to breathe more quickly but rather stops breathing.

  5. Other causes of respiratory problems in the preterm infant include (Miller, Fanaroff, & Martin, 2002):

      a. Transient tachypnea of the neonate (TTN), in which delayed clearance of fetal lung fluid occurs manifested by rapid breathing, retractions, grunting, and cyanosis

      b. Persistent pulmonary hypertension of the neonate (PPHN), in which hypoxemia and acidemia caused by failure to completely change from the fetal to the neonatal circulatory pattern occurs (see Chapter 19 for a complete discussion of respiratory distress)

      c. Bronchopulmonary dysplasia (BPD), in which oxygen therapy and intermittent mandatory ventilation combine to bring about chronic lung disease

F. The cardiovascular system undergoes transition at birth from the fetal to the neonatal circulatory pattern; preterm delivery can adversely affect this transition (McCollum, 1998).

  1. Transition is a response, in part, to the increased level of oxygen in the circulation once air breathing has begun; if oxygen levels remain low, the fetal pattern of circulation may persist, causing blood flow to bypass the lungs.

      a. Preterm infants have a high incidence of patent ductus arteriosus.

      b. The foramen ovale may remain open if pulmonary vascular resistance is high.

  2. The heart is relatively protected from hypoxia in utero; injury, if present, is generally reflected after delivery as cardiomegaly, with signs of cardiovascular insufficiency.

  3. Preterm infants may have impaired regulation of blood pressure in the face of apnea, bradycardia, mechanical ventilation, and other types of neonatal intensive care unit (NICU) care (Blackburn, 2003).

      a. Fluctuations in cerebral blood flow are common.

      b. These fluctuations predispose the fragile blood vessels in the brain to rupture, causing intracranial hemorrhage.

      c. Fluctuations can cause loss of brain blood flow, resulting in ischemia.

      d. These fluctuations also predispose the preterm infant to develop retinopathy of prematurity.

G. The immune system is both immature and inexperienced, making the preterm infant susceptible to infections (Blackburn, 2003).

1. Immunologic ability depends in part on immunoglobulins (Ig), such as IgG, IgM, and IgA.
2. Preterm infants often have a deficiency of IgG because of delivery before transplacental transfer (occurs at approximately 34 weeks' gestation).
3. IgA (the primary Ig in colostrum) is not available to the preterm infant if he or she does not receive breast milk or colostrum.
4. On occasion, preterm delivery comes about as a result of maternal infection with pathogenic bacteria; the preterm infant is especially prone to developing group B beta-hemolytic *Streptococcus* infection.
5. The risk for infection in the preterm infant is also increased because of disruption of skin integrity and instrumentation in the course of NICU care.

H. **The immature liver may be highly inefficient in conjugating bilirubin, leading to hyperbilirubinemia;** drug metabolism in the liver may be markedly altered, increasing the risk of drug intolerance (Blackburn, 2003).

I. **The preterm infant has great difficulty maintaining body temperature** (Blake & Murray, 2002).
   1. The preterm infant is at great risk for excessive heat loss resulting from the following:
      a. Decreased or inadequate subcutaneous fat
      b. Large head-to-body ratio
      c. Lack of muscle tone and flexion
      d. Increased transepidermal evaporative losses
   2. Brown fat is not available or is inadequate to generate heat because sufficient stores are not available for use until after approximately 30 weeks' gestation.
   3. Cold stress quickly depletes what brown fat and glycogen stores are present, resulting in the following:
      a. Increased metabolic needs
      b. Increased oxygen consumption
      c. Consequences that include metabolic acidosis, hypoxemia, and hypoglycemia
   4. Poor nutrient intake is commonly associated with temperature instability.

J. **The preterm renal system is immature, resulting in the following** (Blackburn, 2003):
   1. Decreased ability to concentrate urine
   2. Lack of selectiveness in filtration
   3. Decreased glomerular filtration rate (GFR)
      a. Decreased drug clearance
      b. Increased likelihood of fluid retention
      c. Increased likelihood to develop fluid and electrolyte disturbances

K. **Periventricular intraventricular hemorrhage (PIVH) and ischemic changes are of particular significance in the preterm infant weighing less than 1500 g** (see discussion under Cardiovascular System); more severe cases of PIVH tend to have poorer long-term neurodevelopmental outcomes (Moe & Page, 1998).

L. **Necrotizing enterocolitis (NEC) is of particular significance in preterm infants with birth weights less than 1500 g (3 lb, 5 oz) with time of onset inversely related to gestational age and birth weight;** signs and symptoms often begin with feeding intolerance and proceed to the classic signs and symptoms (similar to sepsis) and abdominal x-ray changes (Holland, Price, & Bensard, 1998).

M. **Hypocalcemia occurs in 30% to 90% of preterm infants.**

N. **Hypoglycemia is common among premature infants** (McGowan, Hagedorn, & Hay, 1998).

1. Functionally, hypoglycemia is defined as a serum glucose concentration of approximately 40 mg% or less.
2. Perinatal conditions commonly associated with hypoglycemia are common among preterm and SGA infants.
   a. Diabetic mother
   b. Prematurity or SGA status
   c. Perinatal stress or hypoxia
   d. Cold stress
   e. Congenital heart disease or congestive heart failure
   f. Maternal drug therapy (beta-sympathomimetics, propranolol)
3. Signs and symptoms, if present, are nonspecific and appear at various serum glucose concentrations in different infants; they are often confused with infection and respiratory distress.
   a. Abnormal cry
   b. Lethargy
   c. Apnea
   d. Hypothermia
   e. Hypotonia
   f. Jitters
   g. Tremors
   h. Tachypnea
   i. Seizures
   j. Cardiac arrest
4. Anticipating and preventing hypoglycemia are more important than treating the condition.
   a. Bedside blood glucose levels (e.g., Accuchek, One Touch, Chemstrip) should be routinely measured at specific intervals (every 1 to 4 hours) in premature infants and others who have risk factors for hypoglycemia through the first several days of life.
   b. Serum levels should be checked when the bedside value is less than 40 mg% in symptomatic infants.
   c. Continuous IV glucose infusion at maintenance rates (70 to 80 ml/kg/day), started early in symptomatic premature infants who are not yet hypoglycemic, will preclude the need for bolus glucose infusions that often result in flip-flopping serum glucose concentrations.
   d. Bolus IV glucose ($D_{10}W$ at 2 ml/kg over several minutes) followed by a continuous infusion at maintenance rates often restores the serum glucose level within several minutes without producing unwanted flip-flop of the serum glucose level.

Clinical Practice

A. Assessment

1. Maternal historical risk factors (Behrman & Shiono, 2002)
   a. Premature labor treated with bedrest and tocolytics
   b. Multiple gestation
   c. Infections
      (1) *Neisseria gonorrhoeae*
      (2) *Chlamydia*
      (3) *Trichomonas*
      (4) Group B beta-hemolytic *Streptococcus*
      (5) Pyelonephritis

    (6) CMV

    (7) Hepatitis A and B

  d. Antepartum bleeding

  e. Pregnancy-induced hypertension (PIH)

  f. Premature rupture of membranes

  g. Cervical insufficiency or incompetence

  h. Psychosocial stress or high-risk maternal behaviors

  i. No prenatal care

  j. Poor nutrition

  k. Use of illicit drugs

  l. Domestic abuse

  m. Motor vehicle accident

2. Physical findings (Katy & Nishioka, 1998) (see Chapter 17 for a complete discussion of gestational age assessment)

  a. Neurologic: hypotonic resting posture (predominance of extensor muscle tone and underdevelopment of flexor muscle tone)

  b. Head

    (1) Larger in proportion to the body compared with the term infant

    (2) Skull bones soft and spongy, especially along suture lines

    (3) Fontanelles wide and soft with overriding sutures

    (4) Ears lacking development of cartilage

    (5) Scalp hair matted and wooly in appearance

  c. Skin

    (1) Skin is thin and edematous at early gestations, but thickness and opacity increases with advancing gestational age.

    (2) Transparent in early gestations so that the underlying capillary bed shows through, giving the infant a ruddy look; veins are readily visible.

    (3) Lanugos fine and barely visible at early gestations, is thickest and abundant between 28 and 30 weeks, and slowly begins to disappear beginning in the lower back as gestation advances.

    (4) Skin is susceptible to breakdown because of decreased cohesion between the dermis and epidermis.

  d. Breasts and nipples

    (1) Are barely visible at early gestations.

    (2) Areola becomes raised at about 34 weeks and increases in size as the breast bud enlarges.

    (3) A small bud is palpable at about 36 weeks' gestation and slowly increases in size with advancing gestational age.

  e. Sole creases develop first in the anterior third of the sole and slowly advance downward with advancing gestational age.

  f. Genitalia

    (1) The preterm male has a small scrotum with few rugae and testes that are high in the inguinal canal; presence of rugae increases, and testes descend into the scrotum with advancing gestational age.

    (2) The preterm female has a prominent clitoris and labia minora; the labia majora enlarge with advancing gestational age.

  g. Thermal instability (at risk for heat loss) resulting from the following (Kabler & Delmore, 1997):

    (1) Larger surface-to-weight ratio

    (2) Immature muscle tone and decreased muscular activity

(3) Diminished stores of white fat and brown fat
(4) Poor nutrient intake
    (a) Infant has a scrawny appearance.
    (b) Lack of insulating properties of white fat allows for more rapid transfer of heat from the infant's core to the environment.
    (c) Reduced amounts of brown fat (deposited between 30 and 36 weeks' gestation) mean that chemical thermogenesis in the preterm infant (the usual, nonshivering method of heat production in newborns) is unreliable.

h. An immature respiratory control center is exhibited in periods of apnea, periodic breathing, or both.
(1) Apnea is an absence of respiration lasting more than 20 seconds accompanied by a fall in heart rate (usually to 80 beats per minute [bpm] or less) and with resultant cyanosis, hypotonia, and metabolic acidosis.
(2) Periodic breathing is exhibited as breathing pauses, sometimes lasting more than 20 seconds, but without bradycardia, cyanosis, hypotonia, or acidosis.

i. RDS, or hyaline membrane disease (HMD), may be present, is inversely related to gestational age, and is compounded when asphyxia is present.
(1) Surfactant reduces surface tension in the alveoli, preventing their collapse at end-expiration.
(2) Manifestations of RDS (see Chapter 19 for more information)
    (a) Retractions: supraclavicular, intercostal, and substernal
    (b) Tachypnea greater than 60 breaths per minute
    (c) Central cyanosis
    (d) Nasal flaring
    (e) Expiratory grunting
    (f) Diminished air exchange

j. Hypoglycemia may be present because of a lack of glycogen stores necessary to meet the infant's metabolic demands (see earlier discussion of hypoglycemia), exhibited by:
(1) Lethargy
(2) Tachycardia
(3) Increased respiratory effort
(4) Jitteriness

k. Presence of a patent ductus arteriosus, which may be intermittent, as evidenced by:
(1) Systolic cardiac murmur in area of upper left sternal border
(2) Desaturation on pulse oximetry with or without color change
(3) Increase in peripheral pulses
(4) Increase in respiratory rate

l. Signs and symptoms of infection may be present (see Chapter 22 for further discussion).
(1) Increase or decrease in white blood cell (WBC) count with a shift to the left
(2) Decrease in activity level; lethargy
(3) Acute change in oxygen requirements or an increase needed in ventilatory settings; episodes of apnea
(4) Feeding intolerance
(5) Temperature instability (usually subnormal)

      (6) Color changes
        (a) Cyanosis
        (b) Ashen color
        (c) Mottled complexion
  3. Diagnostic procedures (Taeusch & Sniderman, 1998)
    a. Heart and respiratory rates
    b. Axillary, skin, and rectal temperatures
    c. Oxygen saturation levels by pulse oximetry and arterial blood gas assays
      (1) Oxygen saturation should be 90% to 92% in most cases.
      (2) Normal PaO_2 should be in the 50s to 60s.
    d. Blood
      (1) Glucose
      (2) CBC with differential
      (3) Electrolytes including calcium
      (4) Blood urea nitrogen (BUN) and serum creatinine
      (5) Bilirubin concentrations
      (6) Cultures
    e. Urine
      (1) Output (normal 1 to 3 ml/kg/hr)
      (2) Specific gravity (normal 1.002 to 1.010)
    f. Chest radiographs
    g. Head and abdominal circumference
    h. Daily weights
    i. Feeding residuals

B. Nursing Diagnoses
  1. Ineffective thermoregulation related to large surface-to-body ratio and lack of fat stores
  2. Risk for imbalanced nutrition: less than body requirements related to diminished sucking reflex resulting from gestational immaturity
  3. Impaired skin integrity related to skin immaturity
  4. Risk for impaired urinary elimination and retention related to renal immaturity
  5. Risk for ineffective tissue perfusion related to impaired gas exchange
  6. Risk for alterated respiratory function related to respiratory immaturity
  7. Risk for infection related to immature immune system and lack of normal flora

C. Interventions/Outcomes
  1. Ineffective thermoregulation related to large surface-to-body ratio and lack of fat stores
    a. Interventions
      (1) Monitor temperature.
        (a) Place neonate on servo-control mode under radiant warmer or in isolette with thermistor located over the right upper quadrant of the abdomen) to achieve a neutral thermal environment.
        (b) Monitor heater output (be aware that continuous high heater output on servo-control mode in the face of normal skin surface temperatures is an alert to potential physiologic alterations in the neonate).
        (c) Measure axillary, skin, and core temperatures as necessary (axillary temperatures are preferable and are as accurate as a core temperature if taken correctly).

(2) Evaluate the environment for potential sources of heat loss or gain through conduction, convection, radiation, and evaporation.
  (a) Do not bathe the neonate without first evaluating the consequences of cold stress on the neonate's clinical condition.
  (b) Prewarm linens and equipment that will come in contact with the neonate.
  (c) Keep neonate's head covered with a cap.
  (d) Remain vigilant to the presence of radiant heat losses to cold walls or windows and convection heat losses in the path of air conditioning vents.

b. Outcomes
  (1) Neonate's axillary temperature is maintained within normal limits (36.4° to 37.1° C [97.6° to 98.8° F]).
  (2) Optimal equipment to maintain thermal neutrality for infant is provided.
  (3) No signs of cold stress are observed.

2. Risk for imbalanced nutrition: less than body requirements related to diminished sucking processes resulting from gestational immaturity
  a. Interventions
  (1) Monitor neonate's nutritional parameters.
    (a) Intake (IV and oral) and output (urine, stool, or other) on an hourly basis
    (b) Body weight on a daily basis
    (c) Head circumference and length on a weekly basis; document weight, length, and head circumference on a weekly basis on standard growth chart to assess for trends.
  (2) Offer oral feedings, as tolerated and as ordered.
    (a) Via premature nipple if suck, swallow, and breathing coordination is present, neonate is in an awakened state, and stamina is good
    (b) Via breastfeeding as tolerated
    (c) Via intermittent bolus gavage (via intermittent insertion or indwelling tube)
    (d) Via continuous gavage (via indwelling tube)
  (3) Offer opportunities for nonnutritive sucking on a premature-size pacifier and social interaction as tolerated during feedings.
  (4) Monitor for tolerance of feedings noting characteristics, amount, and frequency of alterations.
    (a) Vomiting or regurgitation
    (b) Abdominal distention
    (c) Gastric residual (aspirated before next feeding)
      (i) Color (bloody, bile-stained, or other)
      (ii) Partially digested or not
      (iii) Mucusy or not
    (d) Stools
      (i) Water loss
      (ii) Bloody
      (iii) Explosive
      (iv) Other
    (e) Apnea or bradycardia related to reflux
    (f) Signs and symptoms of hypoglycemia
      (i) Jitters and tremors

(ii) Lethargy and hypotonia

(iii) Abnormal cry and tachypnea

(iv) Bedside glucose screening test result less than 40 mg%

(5) Provide total parenteral nutrition (TPN), when enteral feedings are contraindicated, administered via peripheral vein IV (maximum dextrose concentration is 12.5%) or via central catheter (central line or percutaneous central line).

(a) Protein is supplied in the form of amino acids.

(b) Dextrose is the primary carbohydrate source.

(c) Minerals, vitamins, and trace minerals are factored into the solution.

(d) Fat is supplied as a lipid emulsion.

b. Outcomes

(1) The neonate gains 15 to 30 g (0.5 to 1 oz) of weight daily.

(2) Head circumference growth averages 0.5 to 1 cm (0.2 to 0.4 in) per week.

(3) The neonate is able to self-console by nonnutritive sucking on a pacifier and to show increased tolerance for social interaction.

(4) The infant does not exhibit signs and symptoms of feeding intolerance or hypoglycemia.

3. Impaired skin integrity related to skin immaturity

a. Interventions

(1) Turn and reposition neonate every 3 to 4 hours and check skin integrity if tolerated.

(2) Keep skin clean, dry, and free from abrasions.

(a) Never use oil-based lotions or creams, alcohol, or benzoin on the very low birth weight (VLBW) neonate or on dry skin of any neonate.

(b) Wipe off Betadine with sterile water and cotton balls after procedures when it is used.

(c) Use hydrogel products to affix thermistor probes or leads; do not use tape on VLBW neonates.

(d) Remove hydrogel products and tape with sterile water and soak them off; if adhesive remover must be used, wash it off with sterile water immediately after.

(e) Use baby soap, sterile water, and cotton balls for diaper care.

(f) Consider using commercial skin barrier products whenever repeated taping to the skin is required and over areas of skin breakdown.

(g) Use positioning aids (e.g., bolster, nest, rolled blanket) to position neonate for comfort and to relieve pressure over bony prominences.

(h) Avoid friction or tearing of skin surfaces.

(3) Evaluate environment for sources of excessive insensible water loss (IWL), and implement measures as needed to decrease IWL.

(a) Use heat shield or plastic wrap blanket under radiant warmer.

(b) Move to double-walled isolette as soon as possible after stabilization under radiant warmer.

(c) Provide warmed, humidified oxygen as needed.

(d) Ensure increased fluid intake under phototherapy as ordered.

b. Outcomes

(1) The neonate maintains good skin integrity as evidenced by lack of abrasions, skin breakdown, or local irritation or infection.

(2) The neonate does not have increased IWL.

4. Risk for impaired urinary elimination and retention related to renal immaturity
   a. Interventions
      (1) Monitor urine output (check for ml/kg/hr) by weighing each diaper.
      (2) Check dipstick (check for protein and blood) and specific gravity (check for concentration) on each voiding.
      (3) Monitor daily weight loss or gain.
      (4) Monitor for signs and symptoms of overhydration or fluid overload.
         (a) Peripheral edema; taut and shiny skin
         (b) Bounding pulses
         (c) Increased blood pressure
      (5) Monitor for signs and symptoms of dehydration.
         (a) Poor skin turgor
         (b) Dry mucous membranes
         (c) Sunken fontanelles
      (6) Estimate IWL when clinical conditions or therapies are present that increase IWL.
         (a) Radiant warmer
         (b) Phototherapy
         (c) Respiratory distress
         (d) Skin breakdown
         (e) Ambient temperature above thermoneutrality
         (f) Fever
         (g) Increased activity
      (7) Monitor enteral and parenteral nutrition/fluid intake as ordered.
   b. Outcomes
      (1) Urine output is greater than 1 to 2 ml/kg/hr.
      (2) Specific gravity ranges from 1.002 to 1.010.
      (3) Protein and blood are absent in the urine.
      (4) IWL is minimized or replaced with fluid intake.
      (5) Signs of dehydration or fluid overload are absent.

5. Risk for ineffective tissue perfusion related to impaired gas exchange
   a. Interventions
      (1) Auscultate heart for character, rate, and presence or absence of murmur or extra sounds.
      (2) Palpate radial, brachial, femoral, pedal, and palmar pulses for evidence of bounding.
      (3) Assess oxygen saturations from pre- and postductal sites (from right hand versus either foot).
      (4) Assess for color changes indicative of right-to-left shunting (may be subtle changes or dramatic from duskiness, circumoral cyanosis to mottling, and generalized cyanosis).
      (5) Monitor for widening pulse pressures.
      (6) Assess capillary refill time.
   b. Outcomes
      (1) Heart sounds are normal; appropriate interventions are provided for variations from normal.
      (2) Neonate does not experience desaturation.
      (3) Blood pressure remains within normal limits for gestational age.
      (4) Capillary refill time is less than 3 seconds.

6. Risk for altered respiratory function related to respiratory immaturity

    a. Interventions

       (1) Ensure ready availability of bag and mask setup and bulb and wall suction in the event that the infant requires intermittent mandatory ventilation or suction to clear the airway.

       (2) Assess the neonate's respiratory effort with regard to rate, character, effort, and signs of respiratory distress (see Chapter 19).

       (3) Maintain position of the neonate so that the upper airway is not obstructed.

       (4) Monitor continuously to determine trends.

         (a) Cardiorespiratory monitor with 15-second apnea delay

         (b) Oxygen saturation

       (5) Provide supplemental oxygen as needed to maintain optimal oxygen saturation; assist ventilations as needed for apnea.

       (6) Assist with obtaining and review diagnostic tests to determine likely causes of respiratory distress (including any or all of the following: hypoglycemia, pneumonia, and RDS).

         (a) Chest x-ray

         (b) Blood gas

         (c) CBC with differential

         (d) Blood glucose

    b. Outcomes

       (1) Neonate has respiratory rate within normal limits.

       (2) Neonate has no evidence of obstructive apnea, apnea, or respiratory failure.

       (3) Optimal oxygen saturation is maintained.

       (4) Blood glucose is within normal limits.

  7. Risk for infection related to immature immune system and lack of normal flora (see Chapter 22 for a complete discussion of sepsis in the newborn)

LARGE-FOR-GESTATIONAL-AGE INFANTS

Introduction

A. The LGA infant is one whose weight is above the 90th percentile for gestational age (Townsend, 1999).

B. LGA babies may be preterm, term, or postterm.

C. Birth weight over 4000 (8 lb, 14½ oz) often reflects a genetic predisposition, except for the infant of a diabetic mother (IDM).

  1. Large parents tend to have large babies.

  2. Some Native Americans are more likely to have LGA infants.

D. Large size of the fetus may predispose the mother to an operative delivery.

E. If an LGA infant is born vaginally, the incidence of operative vaginal delivery (forceps or vacuum-assisted delivery) is higher than in the non-LGA infant; birth trauma is higher when compared with non-LGA babies and may include:

  1. Fracture of the clavicle or humerus

  2. Brachial plexus injuries

  3. Facial palsy

  4. Depressed skull fracture

  5. Cephalohematoma

F. The LGA fetus may show evidence of nonreassuring fetal heart rate patterns during a prolonged and difficult second stage of labor; neonatal respiratory depression may occur at the time of the delivery.

1. Shoulder or body dystocia may occur.
   2. Particulate meconium-stained amniotic fluid may occur with risk of aspiration.
G. **LGA infants are at risk for hypoglycemia related to early depletion of glycogen stores** (see Chapter 24 for a complete discussion regarding the IDM).

Clinical Practice

A. **Assessment**
   1. History
      a. Maternal
         (1) Previous delivery of an LGA neonate
         (2) Large weight gain during pregnancy
         (3) Diabetes (classes A through C) during the pregnancy
         (4) Prolonged or difficult labor and birth, particularly a long second stage
         (5) Ultrasonography that confirms fetal macrosomia
         (6) Ethnic background
      b. Infant
         (1) Birth weight above the 90th percentile for gestational age
         (2) Type of delivery
            (a) Cesarean birth
            (b) Vaginal delivery with possible shoulder or body dystocia
            (c) Vacuum extraction or forceps assisted delivery
         (3) Apgar scores at 1 and 5 minutes suggestive of neonatal respiratory depression
         (4) Particulate meconium-stained amniotic fluid
   2. Physical findings (Townsend, 1999)
      a. Weight greater than 90th percentile for gestational age
      b. Presence of caput succedaneum on the head
         (1) Localized soft tissue swelling over the presenting scalp area
         (2) Is present at birth and does not increase in size.
         (3) Typically disappears within 12 to 48 hours.
      c. Presence of a cephalohematoma on the head
         (1) Increased incidence with vacuum extraction
         (2) Soft, fluctuant swelling in which the margins are limited to a cranial bone; does not cross suture lines.
         (3) Increases in size for 2 to 3 days after birth.
         (4) Disappears 6 to 8 weeks after birth.
         (5) Associated with complications
            (a) Jaundice, hyperbilirubinemia, or both
            (b) May be accompanied by a skull fracture with resultant subdural or subarachnoid hemorrhage.
            (c) May be accompanied by intracranial hemorrhage.
      d. Evidence of facial nerve damage, such as commonly occurs with intrapartum pressure on facial nerves as occurs with abnormal fetal position or forceps trauma
         (1) The eye on the affected side will not completely close as it normally does while the infant is crying.
         (2) The forehead does not wrinkle.
         (3) The side of the face is smooth.
         (4) The corner of the mouth droops.
         (5) Occasionally associated with intracranial damage, as evidenced by apnea, cyanosis, irritability, or birth depression.

    e. Evidence of brachial plexus injury as a result of overextension and torsion of the neck at the time of delivery resulting in overstretching, hemorrhage or tearing, or complete avulsion of the cervical nerve roots from the spinal cord

        (1) Erb's palsy (the most common type) as a result of upper cervical nerve root damage (C-5 and C-6)

            (a) Muscles of the upper arm are paralyzed.

            (b) The affected arm hangs limp, adducted, and internally rotated at the shoulder; movements that cannot be accomplished are:

                (i) Abduction and external rotation at the shoulder

                (ii) Flexion at the elbow and supination

            (c) Affected arm is pronated at the elbow and wrist is flexed, with strong palmar grasp present.

            (d) Deep tendon reflexes are absent.

            (e) Moro response is unilateral.

            (f) Occasionally associated with unilateral diaphragmatic paralysis, as evidenced by:

                (i) Asymmetry of chest expansion

                (ii) Tachypnea

                (iii) Cyanosis

                (iv) Dyspnea

        (2) Klumpke's palsy (rare) as a result of lower cervical root damage (C-8 to T-1 nerve roots)

            (a) The condition is limited to the wrist and hand.

            (b) The grasp reflex is abolished, the hand is held limply flexed, and voluntary movements of the wrist cannot be made.

            (c) Often associated with this are the manifestations of paralysis of the cervical sympathetic nerve (Horner's syndrome) on the same side.

                (i) Miosis of the pupil

                (ii) Slight lid droop

                (iii) Variations in local temperature, color, and sweating may be expected to appear later.

        (3) Complete brachial palsy (rare) as a result of injury to all roots from C-5 to T-1, producing entire paralysis of the arm and complete loss of sensation

    f. Evidence of clavicular or humeral fracture, either complete or incomplete

        (1) Decreased movement of affected side or arm; may be seen when startle reflex is elicited.

        (2) Infant may cry in pain when affected area is manipulated; crepitus may be elicited.

        (3) Visible angulation or hematoma over the fracture site

        (4) Hypermobility of the bone

        (5) X-ray study confirms the diagnosis.

    g. Evidence of hypoglycemia (see earlier discussion under Preterm Infants)

    h. Evidence of hypocalcemia, often resulting from birth asphyxia

        (1) Affects 50% of IDMs.

        (2) Symptoms include jitteriness, twitching, and convulsions (see earlier discussion under Preterm Infants).

    i. Signs of respiratory distress

        (1) Effort, character, and rate of respirations (increased, labored, greater than 60 breaths per minute [bpm])

        (2) Retractions: supraclavicular, intercostal, and substernal

        (3) Nasal flaring

        (4) Grunting

     j. Quality of breath sounds assessed by auscultation

     k. Possible barrel chest

  3. Diagnostic procedures

     a. Serum glucose

     b. X-ray study to assess for skeletal birth injuries

     c. X-ray study to assess for cause of respiratory distress

     d. Ultrasound scan or CT for possible head injuries if cephalohematoma or depressed skull fracture is noted

     e. Arterial blood gas assays if respirations are severely compromised

B. Nursing Diagnoses

  1. Risk for imbalanced nutrition: less than body requirements related to hypoglycemia

  2. Risk for altered respiratory function related to aspiration of meconium

  3. Risk for birth injury related to large size

C. Interventions/Outcomes

  1. Risk for imbalanced nutrition: less than body requirements related to hypoglycemia

     a. Interventions

        (1) Monitor for signs and symptoms of hypoglycemia; expect that the IDM will be entirely asymptomatic when hypoglycemic.

        (2) Monitor bedside blood glucose level (via products such as Accuchek, One Touch, and Chemstrip) every ½ to 1 hour initially until the blood glucose stabilizes.

        (3) If bedside glucose test result is less than 40 mg%, offer oral feeding immediately if not contraindicated.

          (a) Offer formula and $D_{10}W$ (to raise and sustain the blood glucose level) every 2 to 3 hours.

          (b) Gavage feed an infant who refuses to suck, has tachypnea (respiratory rate greater than 60), or has poor coordination of suck, swallow, and breathing.

          (c) Administer parenteral $D_{10}W$ if blood glucose is zero.

        (4) Monitor nutritional parameters.

          (a) Hourly intake and output

          (b) Daily weight

     b. Outcomes

        (1) Bedside blood glucose test results maintained above 40 mg%

        (2) Adequate urine output (greater than 1 ml/kg/hr)

        (3) Initial weight loss in the week following delivery minimized; adequate weight gain pattern (15 to 30 g/day [0.5 to 1 oz]) established as soon as possible

  2. Risk for altered respiratory function related to aspiration of meconium (see also Chapter 19)

     a. Interventions

        (1) Prepare for delivery using NRP guidelines.

        (2) Assist with intubation and suction of the trachea according to NRP guidelines.

        (3) Provide resuscitation according to NRP guidelines.

        (4) Provide appropriate follow-up respiratory support and monitoring as needed.

          (a) Endotracheal intubation

(b) Intermittent mandatory ventilation (IMV)
(c) Supplemental oxygen and oxygen saturation monitoring
(d) Chest physiotherapy
(5) Provide parenteral fluids and calories if oral feedings are contraindicated because of tachypnea or respiratory distress.
(6) Maintain infant in a neutral thermal environment to prevent increased oxygen consumption secondary to cold or heat stress.
   b. Outcomes
(1) Neonate shows no signs of aspiration and airway remains patent.
(2) Clear breath sounds are auscultated.
(3) Color remains pink without central cyanosis or desaturation.
(4) Respirations are regular in rate and rhythm.
3. Risk for birth injury related to large size
   a. Interventions
(1) On initial and repeat physical examination, note the following:
   (a) Size and position of caput or cephalohematoma
   (b) Evidence of skeletal bone fracture
   (c) Evidence of facial palsy or brachial plexus injury
(2) Observe for jaundice secondary to bruising or trauma.
   (a) Follow serum bilirubin levels (see Chapter 19 for further discussion of hyperbilirubinemia).
   (b) Begin phototherapy as ordered.
(3) Provide treatment for any incidence of palsy.
   (a) Begin physical therapy and splinting early to prevent formation of contractures.
   (b) Provide gentle range-of-motion exercises to the affected extremity periodically.
   (c) Teach parents how to handle the infant without causing additional injury, provide range-of-motion exercises, and put on and take off splints.
(4) Provide treatment for fractured clavicle.
   (a) Obtain x-ray film for confirmation.
   (b) Immobilize affected arm and shoulder.
   (c) Support back and arm when lifting the infant.
   (d) Teach parents to expect a small bump over the fracture site to appear as healing occurs.
   b. Outcomes
(1) Effects of trauma are minimized.
(2) Discomfort related to fracture is minimized or improved.
(3) Bilirubin levels remain within normal range or return to normal if phototherapy is instituted.

POSTTERM INFANTS
Introduction

A. A postterm pregnancy is one that extends beyond 41 completed weeks' gestation (Avery & Richardson, 1998).
B. Postterm neonates may be LGA, average for gestational age (AGA), SGA, or dysmature, depending on placental function.

1. If the placenta continues to function well, the fetus will continue to grow for the extra time in utero, which results in an LGA neonate with typical problems of LGA neonates (as previously stated).
2. If placental function decreases, the fetus may not receive adequate nutrition; wasting of subcutaneous fat, muscle, or both occurs (Charlton, 1998).
   a. As the placenta loses its ability to nourish the fetus (placental insufficiency), the fetus uses stored nutrients for nutrition and wasting occurs; the body is lean, with thin extremities and little subcutaneous fat.
   b. This condition occurs in three forms:
      (1) Chronic placental insufficiency
         (a) No meconium staining occurs.
         (b) Infant appears malnourished with skin changes.
         (c) Infant has an apprehensive look, reflecting hypoxia.
      (2) Acute placental insufficiency
         (a) Infant has a malnourished and apprehensive appearance.
         (b) Green meconium staining of the skin, umbilical cord, and placental membrane occurs.
      (3) Subacute placental insufficiency
         (a) Skin and nails are stained golden yellow (resulting from breakdown of green meconium to hydrolyzed meconium, which is golden or yellow).
         (b) Umbilical cord, placenta, and placental membranes may be greenish brown.
C. **Because of the incidence of placental degeneration, postterm neonates are susceptible to perinatal asphyxia and meconium passage** (American Heart Association, American Academy of Pediatrics, 2000).
   1. Prenatal asphyxia often results in meconium passage in utero with or without fetal gasping.
   2. Aspiration of particulate meconium is highly likely to occur at the time of delivery with the first breath.
   3. The maternal care providers and neonatal resuscitation team plan together to provide management of the meconium (see Chapter 19 for a complete discussion).
      a. With delivery of the fetal head, the mouth and nose are suctioned with DeLee catheter before delivery of the body.
      b. With delivery of the body, the infant may be intubated and suctioned with adherence to NRP guidelines for resuscitation.
      c. NRP guidelines are used to guide additional resuscitation care as. needed.
   4. Intrauterine hypoxia may trigger increased red blood cell (RBC) production, leading to polycythemia, which results in the following:
      a. Sluggish perfusion in organ systems
      b. Hyperbilirubinemia resulting from breakdown of excessive numbers of RBCs
D. **Postterm neonates are susceptible to hypoglycemia because of the rapid depletion of glycogen stores.**
E. **Postterm neonates experience skin and integument changes** (Katy & Nishioka, 1998).
   1. The skin is parchment-like and scaly.
   2. Loss of perfusion to the skin during prenatal asphyxia causes the top three layers of skin to die and slough, causing a macerated appearance.

3. Loss of subcutaneous fat predisposes the neonate to increased IWL (extrarenal fluid loss) and increased risk for hypothermia.
4. Hair is abundant; nails are abnormally long; Wharton's jelly is decreased, and the umbilical cord is thin.

F. **Amniotic fluid volume is decreased, leading to potential fetal distress while in labor** (Blackburn, 2003).
   1. Asphyxial renal changes cause fetal urine production to decrease; a low amniotic fluid index (AFI) may be present. (AFI < 5 suggests severe oligohydramnios.)
   2. In utero umbilical cord compression is more likely to occur if the amount of amniotic fluid to cushion the cord is reduced and the cord is thin, exhibited as decelerations, bradycardia, or both.
   3. Prenatal passage of meconium in the circumstance of reduced amniotic fluid volume means that the meconium is thicker and the risk of aspiration is increased.

Clinical Practice

A. **Assessment**
   1. History (Thureen, Hall, Townsend, O'Neill, & Hobbins, 1999)
      a. Estimated day of confinement (EDC)
      b. Gestational age assessment based on prenatal ultrasonography, if available
      c. Color, consistency, and amount of amniotic fluid
      d. Placental grading, if available (see Chapter 3 for further discussion regarding placental functioning)
         (1) Grades are based on deposits of calcium in the placenta that may interfere with adequate transfer of nutrients and oxygen to the fetus.
         (2) Grades II and III are mature.
      e. Fetal heart rate patterns in labor
         (1) Variable decelerations, which are often the result of decreased amniotic fluid volume
         (2) Late decelerations and decreased or absent variability, which are indicative of nonreassuring fetal heart rate patterns
         (3) Bradycardia
      f. Apgar scores
      g. Cord blood gases
   2. Physical findings (Katy & Nishioka, 1998) (see also Chapter 17 for complete gestational age assessment)
      a. Skin is leathery, wrinkled, cracked, and peeling and frequently stained with meconium.
      b. Vernix is absent except in protected areas (scant amounts in neck and groin creases only).
      c. Fingernails are long and frequently meconium stained.
      d. Lanugo is absent.
      e. Creases cover the entire soles of the feet.
      f. Breast buds are large (greater than 1 cm in diameter) and the areolae are full and raised.
      g. Ear cartilage is thick and firm; ears stand away from the head.
      h. Has a wide-eyed and alert appearance, with more time spent in alert states.

      i. Postterm SGA neonates frequently appear hungry, with frantic rooting and fist sucking.

      j. Postterm LGA infants may be lethargic and have poor sucking ability.

      k. Signs and symptoms of respiratory distress may be present.

      l. Signs of birth trauma may be present in large infants.

  3. Diagnostic procedures

      a. Gestational age assessment plotted by growth parameters on growth curve

      b. Bedside blood glucose test monitoring

      c. Chest x-ray film to evaluate possible aspiration

      d. If respiratory distress is present, monitor oxygenation.

        (1) Oxygen saturation monitoring

        (2) Arterial blood gas assay

B. Nursing Diagnoses

  1. Risk for alterated respiratory function related to meconium aspiration

  2. Risk for imbalanced nutrition: less than body requirements related to hypoglycemia

  3. Risk for impaired skin integrity related to absence of protective vernix and prolonged exposure to amniotic fluid

  4. Risk for ineffective thermoregulation related to loss of subcutaneous fat

C. Interventions/Outcomes

  1. Risk for altered respiratory function related to meconium aspiration

      a. Interventions

        (1) Use NRP guidelines to prepare for and intervene for particulate meconium-stained fluid.

        (2) Use NRP guidelines to provide immediate resuscitation and supportive care.

        (3) Perform chest physiotherapy and postural drainage with suctioning as needed to remove excessive meconium and secretions from the oropharynx.

        (4) Maintain a patent airway; position neonate to minimize respiratory effort.

        (5) Maintain in neutral thermal environment; check temperature every 4 hours.

        (6) Auscultate breath sounds for quality and distribution.

        (7) Offer supplemental oxygen via free flow, mask, hood, or endotracheal tube as needed; monitor oxygenation via saturation monitoring or arterial blood gas assay.

        (8) Provide enteral nutrition via gavage if nipple feeding is contraindicated; provide parenteral fluids and calories as indicated.

        (9) Provide nonnutritive sucking.

      b. Outcomes

        (1) Aspiration syndrome is prevented or minimized, as evidenced by the following:

          (a) Clear and equal breath sounds

          (b) Good air entry bilaterally

          (c) No respiratory distress

        (2) Adequate nutrition is maintained.

        (3) Optimal oxygenation is maintained.

  2. Risk for imbalanced nutrition: less than body requirements related to hypoglycemia (see same nursing diagnosis in discussion of LGA infants)

3. Risk for impaired skin integrity related to absence of protective vernix and prolonged exposure to amniotic fluid (see the same nursing diagnosis in the discussion of preterm infants)
4. Risk for ineffective thermoregulation related to loss of subcutaneous fat (see the nursing diagnosis risk for hypothermia in the discussion of SGA infants)

HEALTH EDUCATION

General Parental and Family Adaptation to an Ill Newborn (Siegal, Gardner, & Merenstein, 1998)

A. Orient parents or family members to the nursery environment, including nursing, medical, and ancillary staff who will come in contact with their newborn; visiting and operational policies and procedures that will affect them; and telephone numbers to call to access care providers.
B. Help parents or family members recognize that grief is an appropriate response to the loss of the fantasized newborn.
   1. Discuss stages of grief.
   2. Teach that reactions to loss have individual and cultural differences.
   3. Be alert for inappropriate denial, which signals a dangerous lack of progress through the stages of grief.
C. Encourage parents or family members to express feelings and to deal openly with feelings of anger, fear, sadness, guilt, blame, frustration, and loss of self-esteem.
D. Encourage parents or family members not to become trapped in feelings of guilt, blame, or low self-esteem.
E. Remind parents or family members to support each other in their unique reactions to the situation.
F. Help parents or family members obtain accurate information about the infant's treatment, care, prognosis, and outcomes.
G. Help mobilize support among the extended family, friends, and religious community.
   1. Provide information about local and national support groups.
   2. Refer the family to clergy and other social services as needed.
H. Promote attachment between parents or family members and infant.
I. Demonstrate safe methods of interaction and direct care that parents or family may provide.
J. Support and encourage the mother's attempts to express breast milk, if she desires.
K. Help parents or family members interpret infant responses and recognize cues of satisfaction, over stimulation, and distress.
L. Teach parents to bathe, clothe, position, feed, and monitor the newborn according to individual needs, and support and encourage parents as they learn new skills.
M. Teach the parents or family members infant cardiopulmonary resuscitation.
N. Perform discharge planning and teaching from the time of admission.
   1. Offer parents a rooming-in option as available in anticipation of discharge.
   2. Assist parents or family members to plan for care to be provided in the home.
O. Follow up with telephone calls and home visits after discharge.

Small-for-Gestational-Age Infants

A. Inform parents of possible causes of IUGR.
B. Assist parents with guilt if chronic illness is a factor or if mother used substances known to compromise fetal growth.
C. Make parents aware of the discharge parameters for their newborn.
D. Instruct parents or family members on managing infant at home.
   1. Preparation of higher caloric formula or frequent breastfeeding
   2. Performance of gavage feeding
   3. Use of developmental therapist to screen for developmental milestones and help optimize development

Large-for-Gestational-Age Infants

A. Remind parents of the infant's immaturity and fragility despite her or his large size.
B. If the delivery was traumatic for the mother, she may need extra recuperation time before assuming total care of the infant.
C. Assist the parents to lift, position, and care for their large infant, especially for breastfeeding.
D. Instruct parents or family members regarding birth trauma, expected resolution, handling or treatment, and follow-up.
E. Provide information about possible causes of macrosomia.
F. Provide feeding guidelines to prevent potential overfeeding or underfeeding.

Preterm Infants

A. Provide individualized instruction regarding the infant's respiratory diagnosis, handling and treatment considerations, and monitoring and treatment that will be continued in the home.
B. Teach parents to prepare high-calorie formulas or supplementation to breastfeeding to ensure adequate weight gain and growth, and instruct them if the infant is to be fed around the clock on a fixed schedule.
C. Teach parents to prepare and administer discharge medications.
D. Inform parents about the extent, outcome, and prognosis after PIVH or ischemic changes, as they may need referral for persistent neurodevelopmental delays.

Postterm Infants

A. Inform parents of the consequences or sequelae of resuscitation as it applies to their newborn.
B. Refer to neurodevelopmental follow-up as indicated.
C. Provide parents or family members with information about any trauma sustained at birth.
D. Explain that postterm infants may need to feed more frequently (i.e., every 2 to 3 hours).

CASE STUDIES AND STUDY QUESTIONS

A 2300-g (5-lb, 1½-oz) infant girl is born to a 25-year-old gravida 1, now para 1 (G1, P1) woman by spontaneous vaginal delivery. The infant's length is 44 cm (17.5 in), and her head circumference is 30.5 cm (12 in). No abnormalities are noted on physical examination. Maternal history and a gestational age assessment reveal the neonate to be at approximately 38 weeks' gestation and that she is SGA.

1. What might you expect to find in the mother's history?
   a. Positive culture for gonorrhea
   b. Weight gain of 15.9 kg (35 lb)
   c. A history of smoking one pack of cigarettes per day
   d. Documented class A diabetes

2. What implications do the infant's measurements have?
   a. The insult occurred late in gestation, during the hypertrophy phase.
   b. The insult occurred early in gestation, during the hyperplasia phase.
   c. The insult occurred during labor and delivery.
   d. The infant can catch up in weight with adequate nutrition.

3. To which of the following should the nurse be alert when caring for this infant?
   a. Projectile vomiting
   b. Possible skull fracture
   c. Positive drug screen
   d. Hypothermia

A 4100-g (9-lb, 1½-oz) boy is born after a difficult forceps delivery. The prenatal history reveals an uncomplicated pregnancy of 40 weeks' gestation. The infant's length is 53.3 cm (21 in), and his head circumference is 37 cm (14.6 in). Gestational age assessment reveals the infant to be LGA.

4. On physical examination, what might you expect to find with this infant?
   a. Club feet
   b. Brachial plexus injury
   c. Thin and transparent skin
   d. Diminished Babinski reflex

5. In actuality, the nurse finds the infant has a fractured clavicle, which is confirmed by x-ray. What may have led the nurse to this conclusion?
   a. Asymmetrical startle reflex
   b. Drooping left eye lid
   c. Extreme jitteriness
   d. History of forceps delivery

6. For what should the nurse be alert when caring for this infant?
   a. Hypothermia
   b. Congenital anomalies
   c. Respiratory distress
   d. Hypoglycemia

An 18-year-old G1, P1 woman is delivered of a 2000-g (4-lb, 6½-oz) boy by cesarean section. The infant is assessed to be appropriate for his gestational age of 34 weeks. No abnormalities are noted on physical examination.

7. This infant is at risk for which of the following conditions?
   a. Hyperglycemia
   b. Premature closure of the ductus arteriosus
   c. Respiratory distress syndrome
   d. Imperforate anus

8. What might the nurse expect to find in the mother's history?
   a. Premature labor treated with tocolytics
   b. Gestational diabetes
   c. Previous infant with Down syndrome
   d. Exposure to rubella in the first trimester

9. What might be detected in this infant during the first few days of life?
   a. Congenital syphilis
   b. Renal agenesis
   c. Cephalohematoma
   d. Hyperbilirubinemia

A 32-year-old gravida 3, now para 3 (G3, P3) is delivered of a 3250-g (7-lb, 3-oz) girl through meconium-stained fluid at 42 weeks' gestation. The infant's initial presentation is that she is limp, is cyanotic, has minimal respirations, and has a heart rate below 100 bpm. Her oropharynx was suctioned while the head was on the perineum, and she was intubated and suctioned by the neonatal team. Although she was suctioned through the endotracheal tube, no meconium was seen below the cords. With oxygen and stimulation, her Apgar scores at 1 and 5 minutes were 8 and 9, respectively.

10. What is the most serious consequence that might result from this delivery?

    a. Patent ductus arteriosus
    b. Meconium aspiration
    c. Hyaline membrane disease
    d. Depressed skull fracture

11. What would the nurse expect to see on examination of this infant?
    a. Abundant lanugo
    b. Absence of sole creases
    c. Leathery, cracked, and wrinkled skin
    d. Large caput succedaneum

12. What should the nurse do to protect this infant's skin from further trauma?
    a. Use powders and oils frequently.
    b. Restrain the infant so she will not scrape her knees and elbows.
    c. Wear gloves when handling the infant.
    d. Avoid the use of tape except when absolutely necessary.

ADDITIONAL STUDY QUESTIONS

13. Why is hyperbilirubinemia of special concern in preterm infants?
    a. Immature liver function
    b. Poor vascular system
    c. Decreased respiratory function
    d. Immature endocrine function

14. Which of the following physiologic factors contributes to greater risk for alterations in skin integrity in preterm infants?
    a. Immature immunologic system
    b. Malfunctioning of regulatory organs, such as the kidneys and respiratory tract
    c. Increased frequency of regurgitation
    d. Decreased cohesion between the dermis and epidermis

15. Gavage feedings are frequently needed to meet the nutritional needs of preterm infants because:
    a. Lactose enzyme activity is not adequate.
    b. Suck, swallow, and breathing reflexes are uncoordinated.
    c. Renal solute load must be considered.
    d. Hyperbilirubinemia is likely.

16. A 42-week postterm neonate was born with greenish discoloration of the nails and skin and greenish secretions in the nasal passages. Why might the infant be transferred to a level 3 nursery?
    a. To determine the reason for the postmaturity
    b. To observe more closely for skin color changes

c. To manage severe respiratory problems that develop

d. To manage the pulmonary hypotension that is likely to develop

17. Factors that contribute to impaired fetal growth include:
    a. Maternal obesity
    b. Class A and C maternal diabetes
    c. Grade III placenta
    d. Multiple births

18. The LGA infant may experience which of the following problems?

a. Patent ductus arteriosus
b. Facial nerve damage
c. Hypercalcemia
d. Poor suck, swallow, and breathing coordination

19. Which characteristic best describes an SGA infant?
    a. Lack of movement in the upper extremities
    b. Long fingernails that extend over the ends of the fingers
    c. Prone to meconium aspiration syndrome
    d. Wasted and thin at birth with loose and scaling skin

ANSWERS TO STUDY QUESTIONS

1. c	6. d	11. c	16. c
2. b	7. c	12. d	17. d
3. d	8. a	13. a	18. b
4. b	9. d	14. d	19. d
5. a	10. b	15. b	

REFERENCES

Allen, M.C. (1998). Outcome and follow-up of high-risk infants. In H. Taeusch & R. Ballard (Eds.), *Avery's diseases of the newborn* (pp. 413-428). Philadelphia: Saunders.

American Heart Association, American Academy of Pediatrics. (2000). Initial steps in resuscitation. In J. Kattwinkel (Ed.), *Textbook of neonatal resuscitation* (4th ed., pp. 2-1 to 2-25). Elk Grove Village, IL: AHA/AAP.

Avery, M.E., & Richardson, D. (1998). History and epidemiology. In H. Taeusch & R. Ballard (Eds.), *Avery's diseases of the newborn* (pp. 413-428). Philadelphia: Saunders.

Behrman, R.E., & Shiono, P.H. (2002). Neonatal risk factors. In A.A. Fanaroff & R.J. Martin (Eds.), *Neonatal-perinatal medicine: Diseases of the fetus and infant* (7th ed., pp. 17-26). St. Louis: Mosby.

Blackburn, S. (2003). *Maternal, fetal, and neonatal physiology: A clinical perspective* (2nd ed.). Philadelphia: Saunders.

Blake, W.W., & Murray, J.A. (2002). Heat balance. In G.B. Merenstein & S.L. Gardner (Eds.), *Handbook of neonatal intensive care* (5th ed., pp. 100-115). St. Louis: Mosby.

Charlton, V. (1998). Fetal growth: Nutritional issues (perinatal and long-term consequences). In H. Taeusch & R. Ballard (Eds.), *Avery's diseases of the newborn* (pp. 45-55). Philadelphia: Saunders.

Fanaroff, A.A., & Martin, R.J. (2002). *Neonatal-perinatal medicine: Diseases of the fetus and infant* (7th ed.). St. Louis: Mosby.

Fashaw, L., & Hernandez, J.A. (1999). Abnormal transition. In P. Thureen, J. Deacon, P. O'Neill, & J. Hernandez (Eds.), *Assessment and care of the well newborn* (pp. 101-113). Philadelphia: Saunders.

Goddard-Finegold, J., Mizrahi, E.M., and Lee, R.T. (1998). The newborn nervous system. In H. Taeusch & R. Ballard (Eds.), *Avery's diseases of the newborn* (pp. 839-891). Philadelphia: Saunders.

Holland, R.M., Price, F.N., & Bensard, D.D. (1998). Neonatal surgery. In G. Merenstein & S. Gardner (Eds.), *Handbook of neonatal intensive care* (4th ed., pp. 625-646). St. Louis: Mosby.

Kabler, J.L., & Delmore, P.M. (1997). Alterations in health status of newborns. In F. Nichols & E. Zwelling, (Eds.), *Maternal-newborn nursing: Theory and practice* (pp. 1331-1407). Philadelphia: Saunders.

Katy, K., & Nishioka, E. (1998). Neonatal assessment. In C. Kenner, J. Lott, & A. Flandermeyer (Eds.), *Comprehensive neonatal nursing: A physiologic perspective* (2nd ed., pp. 223-251). Philadelphia: Saunders.

Kenner, C., Lott, J., & Flandermeyer, A. (1998). *Comprehensive neonatal nursing: A physiologic perspective* (2nd ed.). Philadelphia: Saunders.

Kliegman, R.M., & Das, U.G. (2002). Intrauterine growth restriction. In A.A. Fanaroff & R.J. Martin (Eds.), *Neonatal-perinatal medicine: Diseases of the fetus and infant* (7th ed., pp. 228-262). St. Louis: Mosby.

McCollum, L.L. (1998). Resuscitation and stabilization of the newborn. In C. Kenner, J. Lott, & A. Flandermeyer (Eds.), *Comprehensive neonatal nursing: A physiologic perspective* (2nd ed., pp. 190-206). Philadelphia: Saunders.

McGowan, J.E., Hagedorn, M.Z.E., & Hay, W.W. (1998). Glucose homeostasis. In G. Merenstein & S. Gardner (Eds.), *Handbook of neonatal intensive care* (4th ed., pp. 259-274). St. Louis: Mosby.

Merenstein, G., & Gardner, S. (1998). *Handbook of neonatal intensive care* (4th ed.). St. Louis: Mosby.

Miller, M.J., Fanaroff, A.A., & Martin R.J. (2002). The respiratory system: Part 5: Respiratory disorders in preterm and term infants. In A.A. Fanaroff & R.J. Martin (Eds.), *Neonatal-perinatal medicine: Diseases of the fetus and infant* (7th ed., pp. 1025-1049). St. Louis: Mosby.

Moe, P., & Page, P. (1998). Neurologic disorders. In G. Merenstein & S. Gardner (Eds.), *Handbook of neonatal intensive care* (4th ed., pp. 571-603). St. Louis: Mosby.

Nichols, F., & Zwelling, E. (1997). *Maternal-newborn nursing: Theory and practice.* Philadelphia: Saunders.

Polin, R., & Spitzer, A. (2001). *Fetal and neonatal secrets.* Philadelphia: Hanley & Belfus.

Pomerance, J., & Richardson, C. (1993). *Neonatology for the clinician.* Norwalk: Appleton and Lange.

Ramsey, P.S., & Goldenberg, R.L. (2002). Obstetrical management of prematurity. In A. Fanaroff & R. Martin (Eds.), *Neonatal-perinatal medicine: Diseases of the fetus and infant* (7th ed., pp. 287-319). St. Louis: Mosby.

Reeder, S., Martin, L., & Koniak-Griffin, D. (1997). *Maternity nursing: Family, newborn, and women's health care* (18th ed.). Philadelphia: Lippincott.

Rodriguez, R.J., Martin, R.J., & Fanaroff, A.A. (2002). The respiratory system: Part 3: Respiratory distress syndrome and its management. In A.A. Fanaroff & R.J. Martin (Eds.), *Neonatal-perinatal medicine: Diseases of the fetus and infant* (7th ed., pp. 1001-1011). St. Louis: Mosby.

Rowland, L., & Iyer, P. (1995). *Patient outcomes in maternal-infant nursing.* Springhouse, PA: Springhouse.

Siegal, R., Gardner, S.L., & Merenstein, G.B. (1998). Families in crisis: Theoretical and practical approaches. In G.B. Merenstein & S.L. Gardner (Eds.), *Handbook of neonatal intensive care* (4th ed., pp. 647-672). St. Louis: Mosby.

Sobl, B., & Moore, T.R. (1998). Abnormalities of fetal growth. In H. Taeusch & R. Ballard (Eds.), *Avery's diseases of the newborn* (pp. 90-101). Philadelphia: Saunders.

Taeusch, H., & Ballard, R. (1998). *Avery's diseases of the newborn.* Philadelphia: Saunders.

Taeusch, H.W., & Sniderman, S. (1998). Initial evaluation and physical examination of the newborn. In H. Taeusch & R. Ballard (Eds.), *Avery's diseases of the newborn* (pp. 334-353). Philadelphia: Saunders.

Thureen, P., Deacon, J., O'Neill, P., & Hernandez, J. (1999). *Assessment and care of the well newborn.* Philadelphia: Saunders.

Thureen, P.J., Hall, D.M., Townsend, S.F., O'Neill, P., & Hobbins, J. (1999). Fetal assessment, labor, and delivery. In P. Thureen, J. Deacon, P. O'Neill, & J. Hernandez (Eds.), *Assessment and care of the well newborn* (pp. 24-38). Philadelphia: Saunders.

Townsend, S.F. (1999). The large-for-gestational-age and small-for-gestational- age infant. In P. Thureen, J. Deacon, P. O'Neill, & J. Hernandez (Eds.), *Assessment and care of the well newborn* (pp. 272-283). Philadelphia: Saunders.

Walker, M., & Hull, A. (1998). Preterm labor and birth. In H. Taeusch & R. Ballard (Eds.), *Avery's diseases of the newborn* (pp. 144-153). Philadelphia: Saunders.

19 Identification of the Sick Newborn

JACQUELINE M. MCGRATH

OBJECTIVES

1. Describe the signs of illness in the newborn, and distinguish well from ill.

2. Identify infants at risk for developing respiratory distress.

3. Explain the pathophysiology of respiratory distress syndrome (RDS).

4. Identify risk factors and the maternal and fetal history that are predictive of RDS.

5. Recognize signs and symptoms of RDS.

6. Describe specific nursing interventions that are appropriate for the infant with RDS.

7. Explain the pathophysiology of transient tachypnea of the newborn (TTN).

8. Identify risk factors and the maternal and fetal history that are predictive of TTN.

9. Recognize signs and symptoms of TTN.

10. Describe specific nursing interventions that are appropriate for the infant with TTN.

11. Explain the pathophysiology of meconium aspiration syndrome (MAS).

12. Identify risk factors and the maternal and fetal history that are predictive of MAS.

13. Recognize signs and symptoms of MAS.

14. Describe specific nursing interventions that are appropriate for MAS.

15. Explain the pathophysiology of persistent pulmonary hypertension of the newborn (PPHN).

16. Identify risk factors and the maternal and fetal history that are predictive of PPHN.

17. Recognize signs and symptoms of PPHN.

18. Describe specific nursing interventions that are appropriate for PPHN.

19. Identify neonatal complications that interfere with normal bilirubin conjugation in the neonate.

20. Describe the maternal and neonatal factors that contribute to jaundice in the neonate, and distinguish the differences between the various causal factors and related outcomes of jaundice in the neonate.

21. Describe the physiologic process of the production, conjugation, and elimination of bilirubin in the neonate, as well as the differences between conjugated and unconjugated bilirubin.

22. Identify the physical signs of hyperbilirubinemia in the neonate.

23. Analyze total, direct, and indirect values of bilirubin levels to determine their potential significance on the neonate's physical condition.

24. Discuss complications related to an interruption in the bilirubin conjugation process and identify strategies that would either eliminate or alter the interruption in the process.

25. Specify nursing interventions that are effective in providing nursing care to neonates with hyperbilirubinemia.

INTRODUCTION

Most newborns will transition to extrauterine life without a problem. However, even when transition is uneventful, the first 48 hours of life is a time when vigilant observation and anticipatory caregiving are essential. Most infants with serious illness present at birth or within the first 48 hours of life. The challenge for the caregiver is to be able to discriminate the subtle signs of disease from the dynamically changing characteristics of normal transition and adaptation to the extrauterine environment. Without excellent nursing care and good family education, early discharge might enable missing some of these infants and making them susceptible to poorer outcomes. Some of the most common disease processes that can appear in the newborn period include hypothermia, hypoglycemia, RDS, TTN, MAS, PPHN, sepsis, congenital heart disease, hyperbilirubinemia, and drug exposure of the infant. Hypothermia is discussed in Chapter 16, and hypoglycemia is discussed in Chapter 24. Newborn sepsis is discussed in Chapter 22, and the drug-exposed infant is covered in Chapter 27. Care of the infant with congenital heart disease is discussed in Chapter 17. Thus this chapter will discuss in detail RDS, TTN, MAS, PPHN, and hyperbilirubinemia. For ease of discussion, respiratory conditions will first be addressed followed by hyperbilirubinemia. However, it is important to note that these processes can occur concurrently, and in reality, often times, infants diagnosed with any one of the previously noted newborn disease processes are more susceptible to the others.

RESPIRATORY DISTRESS

Causes of Respiratory Distress

The causes of respiratory distress in the newborn may have its beginnings in the failure of one or more major body systems. Conditions that result in the structural and functional failure of a major body system result in mild to profound respiratory distress in the newborn, regardless of size and gestational age. The following is a discussion of the five most common body systems involved in the causes of respiratory distress.

A. **Cardiac diseases**
   1. Congenital heart disease (CHD)
   2. Congestive heart failure (CHF)
   3. Patent ductus arteriosus (PDA)
   4. Arrhythmias, such as supraventricular tachycardia (SVT)
   5. Heart failure, such as that related to arteriovenous malformation
B. **Hematologic disorders**
   1. Anemia
   2. Hemorrhage
   3. Polycythemia
C. **Metabolic disorders**
   1. Acidosis
   2. Hypoglycemia
   3. Hyperglycemia
   4. Hypocalcemia
   5. Hypothermia
   6. Hyperthermia
   7. Hypermagnesemia
   8. Congenital hyperthyroidism

D. Central nervous system disorders
  1. Hemorrhage
     a. Intracranial
     b. Intraventricular and periventricular hemorrhage (IVH and PVH)
     c. Subdural hemorrhage (SDH)
     d. Subarachnoid hemorrhage (SAH)
  2. Infection
  3. Neonatal depression related to maternal drugs given during labor
     a. Magnesium sulfate
     b. Analgesics
  4. Neonatal substance-withdrawal syndrome
  5. Malformations
  6. Asphyxia
  7. Neuromuscular involvement
     a. Spinal cord trauma
     b. Muscular dystrophies
E. Respiratory disorders
  1. Most common conditions
     a. RDS
     b. TTN
     c. Aspiration syndromes
        (1) MAS
        (2) Blood aspiration
        (3) Amniotic fluid aspiration
     d. PPHN
     e. Pneumonia
  2. Less common conditions
     a. Pulmonary hemorrhage
     b. Pulmonary air leak syndrome (PALS)
        (1) Spontaneous pneumothorax occurs in 1% to 2% of live births; only symptomatic in 1 in 1500 live births (Whitsett, Pryhuber, Rice, Warner, & Wert, 1999); symptoms may include tachypnea, minimal retractions, grunting, nasal flaring, and cyanosis; diminished air entry on affected side, shifting of cardiac impulse, muffled heart tones may also be noted.
        (2) Pneumomediastinum and pneumopericardium
        (3) Pulmonary interstitial emphysema (PIE)
  3. Rare conditions
     a. Upper airway obstruction
        (1) Choanal atresia
        (2) Pierre Robin syndrome
     b. Space-occupying lesions
        (1) Congenital diaphragmatic hernia (CDH)
        (2) Esophageal atresia, with or without tracheoesophageal fistula (TEF)

Clinical Practice

Although a knowledge and understanding of these conditions is helpful in diagnosing and treating respiratory distress, this section focuses specifically on several respiratory conditions, including RDS, TTN, MAS, and PPHN.

RESPIRATORY DISTRESS SYNDROME

A. Introduction: RDS is the major cause of respiratory distress in the newborn, and prematurity is the single most important risk factor (Whitsett et al., 1999)

1. RDS, sometimes referred to as hyaline membrane disease (HMD), accounts for 20% to 30% of all neonatal deaths and approximately 50% to 70% of all premature deaths (Hicks, 1995; Rizzo, Nisini, & Marzetti, 2002); RDS occurs in 60% of babies born at less than 28 weeks' gestation, 50% of those born at 28 to 34 weeks, and less than 5% of those born after approximately 34 weeks.

2. Pathophysiology: surfactant deficiency

   a. Surfactant is a complex mixture of phospholipids and proteins that binds to the alveolar surface of the lungs and forms a coat over the inner surface of the alveoli and decreases the surface tension, preventing collapse at the end of expiration (Hansen, & Corbet, 1998; Parmigiani, Panza, & Bevilacqua, 1997).

   b. Alveolar development occurs between 24 and 28 weeks' gestation, which results in the following (Hansen, & Corbet, 1998):
   (1) Increases in pulmonary vascularization
   (2) Development of ability for gas exchange
   (3) Development and proliferation of type II respiratory cells responsible for surfactant production and synthesis

   c. Surfactant deficiency results in the following (Hicks, 1995):
   (1) Increased surface tension, leading to alveolar collapse
   (2) Diffuse atelectasis
   (3) Loss of functional residual capacity
   (3) Decreased lung compliance
   (4) Right-to-left intrapulmonary shunting through the ductus arterious with increased pulmonary vascular resistance (PVR)

3. Complications of RDS include the following:

   a. PDA incidence increases with decreasing gestational age (see Chapter 17 for a complete discussion of PDA).

   b. Air leak syndromes (e.g., pneumothorax, pneumomediastinum, pneumopericardium) occur in 5% to 30% of infants with RDS (Whitsett et al., 1999).

   c. IVH occurs in approximately 15% to 20% of infants weighing less than 1500 g (3 lb, 5 oz) (Volpe, 2001).

   d. Bronchopulmonary dysplasia (BPD) occurs in approximately 23% of infants with RDS (Gracey, Talbot, Lankford, & Dodge, 2002).

   e. Retinopathy of prematurity (ROP) occurring in infants with RDS is increasing and is currently estimated to be between 20% and 25%; most of these cases regress, with the incidence of severe disease estimated to be between 5% and 10% (Quinn, 1998); prevention of premature birth is the best preventive of ROP; after a preterm birth, oxygen should be used only in amounts sufficient to avoid hypoxia.

   f. Necrotizing enterocolitis (NEC)

   g. PIE

   h. Oxygen toxicity

B. Assessment

1. History (risk factors) (Hicks, 1995; Whitsett et al., 1999)

   a. At less than 28 weeks' gestation, 60% of neonates demonstrate clinical signs of RDS.

    b. At 28 to 32 weeks' gestation, 50% of neonates demonstrate clinical signs of RDS.

    c. At 37 weeks' gestation and older, 3% to 5% of neonates demonstrate clinical signs of RDS.

    d. At birth, 10% to 15% of infants who weigh less than 2500 g (5 lb, 8 oz) demonstrate RDS; the highest incidence occurs among the group with the lowest birth weight (Whitsett et al., 1999).

    e. RDS is increased:

        (1) In males versus females (1.5 times higher incidence)

        (2) Among whites versus nonwhites

        (3) In infants of diabetic mothers (IDM); insulin is antagonistic to surfactant production

        (4) In the presence of asphyxia, regardless of gestational age

        (5) When birth is by cesarean section, especially in the absence of labor, related to the lack of a thoracic squeeze

        (6) In the second-born of twins, which may be related to the second-born's longer stay in the birth canal, with the second twin receiving an excess of amniotic fluid with the birth of the first twin

        (7) When prenatal maternal hypotension is present, with or without maternal hemorrhage

        (8) In the presence of rhesus (Rh) factor incompatibility, which retards surfactant production

    f. RDS is decreased with:

        (1) Prolonged or premature rupture of membranes (PROM)

        (2) Intrauterine growth restriction (IUGR)

        (3) Pregnancy-induced hypertension (PIH)

        (4) Maternal heroin addiction

        (5) Prenatal corticosteroids (Gibson, 2002)

2. Physical findings: symptoms of RDS frequently occur within 4 to 24 hours after delivery; symptoms are usually apparent in the delivery room; typically, the clinical course of RDS worsens during the first 48 hours after birth, and respiratory function generally begins to improve within 72 hours after birth.

    a. Intercostal, subclavicular, and substernal retractions occur because of the compliant chest wall of the preterm infant, in addition to relatively noncompliant lungs ("see-saw" respirations).

    b. Expiratory grunting, heard as a result of partial vocal cord closure, increases transpulmonary pressures in an attempt to improve lung volume capacity.

    c. Nasal flaring is often present as the infant attempts to decrease nasal airway resistance.

    d. Tachypnea with a respiratory rate of greater than 60 breaths per minute is common.

    e. Decreased breath sounds or unequal breath sounds are usually heard.

    f. Poor air entry is heard on auscultation.

    g. Fine rales may be heard bilaterally or unilaterally.

    h. Generalized cyanosis may be seen because of impaired ventilation and intrapulmonary and intracardiac shunting.

        (1) Peripheral cyanosis alone is common in newborns and is usually not significant.

        (2) The degree of cyanosis depends on the following (Berry, 2002):
           (a) Hemoglobin concentration
           (b) Status of the peripheral circulation
           (c) Color of the infant and the available light to visualize the cyanosis

  i. Tachycardia with a heart rate of 150 to 180 beats per minute (bpm) may occur.

  j. Hypothermia may occur despite a neutral thermal environment (NTE).

  k. Hypoglycemia with a glucose level of less than 20 mg/dl in the preterm infant may be noted.

  l. Hypotension is a frequent indication of severe RDS.

  m. Hypotonia results in a limp and flaccid infant.

  n. Apnea occurs frequently in the severely compromised infant.

3. Diagnostic procedures

  a. Apgar scores may not reflect the severity of RDS.

  b. Maturity assessment

    (1) Lecithin/sphingomyelin (L/S) ratio of greater than 2 indicates mature lungs in the absence of a diabetic pregnancy.

    (2) The presence of phosphatidylglycerol (PG) confirms maturity and is especially important to ascertain lung maturity in the presence of maternal conditions such as diabetes.
      (a) Is present at 37 weeks' gestation and levels rise to term.
      (b) If greater than 1%, indicates mature lungs.

    (3) Shake test or foam stability index (FSI) may be performed on amniotic fluid at the maternal bedside to quickly determine the presence of surfactant.

  c. Chest x-ray film initially may appear better than the clinical course would suggest; the classic chest x-ray film findings include the following:
    (1) Reticulogranular (ground-glass) pattern
    (2) Air bronchograms that demonstrate diffuse alveolar collapse surrounding open bronchi
    (3) Decreased lung volumes
    (4) Possible cardiomegaly

  d. Arterial blood gas (ABG) assays show hypoxemia and hypercapnia.

C. Nursing Diagnoses

1. Risk for respiratory complications resulting from prematurity

  a. Impaired ventilation and oxygenation in response to inadequate respiratory effort

  b. Impaired gas exchange related to decreased alveolar ventilation, increased pulmonary perfusion, or both

  c. Ineffective tissue perfusion related to cardiorespiratory immaturity

  d. Activity intolerance related to insufficient cardiorespiratory function and prematurity

2. Risk for complications of respiratory distress resulting from RDS

  a. Impaired respiratory function related to immobility of secretions

  b. Imbalance nutrition: less than body requirements related to increased energy requirements

  c. Imbalanced fluid volume related to a risk for fluid overload

D. Interventions/Outcomes

1. Risk for respiratory complications resulting from prematurity

a. Impaired ventilation and oxygenation in response to inadequate respiratory effort

b. Impaired gas exchange related to decreased alveolar ventilation, increased pulmonary perfusion, or both (Berry, 2002)

c. Ineffective tissue perfusion related to cardiorespiratory immaturity

d. Activity intolerance related to insufficient cardiorespiratory function and prematurity

e. Interventions

    (1) Provide appropriate supportive measures for the neonate to offer optimal respiratory support.

        (a) Intubate with the appropriate size of endotracheal tube (ETT); choice of tube size is determined by the neonate's weight, as follows (Klaus & Fanaroff, 2001):

           (i) Less than 1001 g: 2.5 mm

           (ii) 1001 to 2000 g: 3 mm

           (iii) 2001 to 3000 g: 3.5 mm

           (iv) More than 3001 g: 4 mm

        (b) Transfer infant to the neonatal intensive care unit (NICU) if mechanical ventilation is required.

        (c) Administer continuous positive airway pressure (CPAP) to infants, as needed, who do not require mechanical ventilation.

           (i) May be administered via ETT or nasal prongs.

           (ii) CPAP may resolve some of the atelectasis, decrease intrapulmonary shunting, and improve ventilation to alveoli already open.

        (d) Place infant in appropriate concentration of oxygen via oxygen hood or nasal cannula as determined by an ABG assay if mechanical ventilation or CPAP is not needed.

           (i) Oxygen should always be warmed and humidified to prevent infant heat loss and drying of mucous membranes.

           (ii) Oxygen concentrations should be monitored continuously and documented per facility protocol.

    (2) Provide continuous monitoring of infant's condition.

        (a) All infants should be connected to continuous cardiorespiratory monitors to detect abnormalities in heart rate and rhythm, as well as apnea and bradycardia.

        (b) Blood pressure should be monitored in all infants with RDS; normal blood pressure varies with size and gestational age (Klaus & Fanaroff, 2001).

           (i) 1000 to 2000 g (2 lb, 2 oz to 4 lb, 6½ oz): mean arterial blood pressure (MABP) = 30 mmHg

           (ii) 2000 to 3000 g (4 lb, 6½ oz to 6 lb, 10 oz): MABP = 35 mmHg

           (iii) 3000 to 4000 g (6 lb, 10 oz to 8 lb, 14 oz): MABP = 43 mmHg

           (iv) Systolic blood pressure in infants less than 2500 g (5 lb, 8 oz) = 50 mmHg

           (v) Systolic blood pressure in infants more than 2500 g (5 lb, 8 oz) = 60 mmHg

        (c) An ABG assay should be performed as needed.

        (d) Ongoing infant respiratory status should be assessed every 1 to 4 hours as needed.

           (i) Auscultation of breath sounds

       (ii) Quality of air entry

       (iii) Respiratory effort and spontaneous respiratory rate

    (e) Serial chest x-ray films should be obtained as appropriate to assess disease progression.

(3) Administer exogenous surfactant per physician or facility protocol as needed to support lung function until the infant's own supply is produced (Parmigiani, Panza, & Bevilacqua, 1997).

    (a) Administration in the delivery room (early) has been shown to be more beneficial than late administration (Plavka et al., 2002).

    (b) Administration protocol should be drug specific; not all surfactants are the same; dose, timing, and delivery systems may vary, as well as cost.

(4) Prevent or treat hypotension.

    (a) Systemic hypotension results in pulmonary and systemic vasoconstriction and will prevent adequate tissue perfusion and gas exchange.

    (b) Administer fluids to prevent or treat hypovolemia.

    (c) Administer pressor agents, such as dopamine, dobutamine, and epinephrine, as needed to maintain blood pressure within normal limits (WNL).

(5) Prevent or treat hypothermia.

    (a) Hypothermia causes cold stress in the neonate, which results in vasoconstriction and subsequent lowering of PaO_2.

    (b) Maintain an NTE: defined as the condition under which the amount of heat produced is equal to the least amount of heat lost to the environment, with the least metabolic stress.

    (c) Maintain a warm and humidified oxygen level.

    (d) Do not place infants on cold surfaces or in drafts.

    (e) Keep infant dry to prevent evaporative heat loss.

(6) Prevent or treat metabolic acidosis.

    (a) Metabolic acidosis causes constriction of pulmonary vessels and decreased lung perfusion.

    (b) Administer intravenous (IV) fluids, as indicated.

    (c) Prevent excessive water loss.

    (d) Administer buffer agents, as indicated (e.g., sodium bicarbonate [$NaHCO_2$], tromethamine [THAM]).

(7) Prevent or treat hypoglycemia.

    (a) Glucose is required with oxygen for normal function of the central nervous system (CNS).

    (b) Monitor glucose levels.

    (c) Administer dextrose via IV fluids.

(8) Prevent or treat anemia.

    (a) Anemia prevents adequate tissue perfusion and oxygenation.

    (b) Anemia is defined as a central venous hemoglobin level of less than 13 g/dl (hematocrit, 39%) or a capillary venous hemoglobin level of less than 14.5 g/dl (hematocrit, 45%).

    (c) Losses in excess of 10% blood volume (total volume calculated using 85 ml/kg) should be replaced (Klaus & Fanaroff, 2001).

    (d) Blood transfusions should be given to maintain a central venous hematocrit of at least 40% (hemoglobin value, 13.3 g/dl).

(9) Provide for minimal stimulation with appropriate sedation, if needed, to conserve energy stores.
  (a) Activity intolerance secondary to prematurity compromises effective ventilation, oxygenation, and caloric use.
  (b) Caretaking activities should be clustered to provide adequate periods of rest, but care should be taken to provide breaks between procedures when the infant demonstrates signs of stress.
  (c) Minimal handling should be observed by all personnel; unnecessary touching should be avoided to provide maximum opportunity for the parents for bonding (see Health Education).
  (d) Infant should be handled gently, with slow, purposeful movements rather than abrupt, jerky movements.
  (e) Sedation may be ordered for infants whose spontaneous activity level puts the infant at risk for respiratory distress.
  (f) Prone positioning has been shown to optimize respiratory status and decrease stress in the preterm infant (Sahni, Schulze, Kashyap, Ohira-Kist, Myers, & Fifer, 1999).
f. Outcomes
  (1) The neonate will be appropriately and adequately resuscitated in the delivery room with minimal asphyxia, hypothermia, shock, and acidosis.
  (2) The infant will receive the appropriate ventilatory support.
    (a) The appropriate size of ETT will be used, based on weight.
    (b) Mechanical ventilation, CPAP, or oxygen will be administered as needed.
  (3) The infant's vital signs will be WNL.
    (a) Heart rate of between 120 and 180 bpm.
    (b) Respiratory rate of between 40 and 60 breaths per minute.
    (c) Blood pressure WNL for size and gestational age.
  (4) The neonate will demonstrate minimal respiratory distress.
    (a) Bilateral breath sounds
    (b) Good air entry
    (c) Consistent respiratory effort with spontaneous respirations
    (d) Minimal retractions
    (e) Absence of grunting and nasal flaring
    (f) Absence of central or generalized cyanosis
  (5) The neonate will demonstrate adequate pulmonary and tissue perfusion.
    (a) Well oxygenated, with normal PaO_2
    (b) Absence of metabolic acidosis
    (c) Normal systemic blood pressure
    (d) Absence of hypothermia
    (e) Absence of hypoglycemia
    (f) Normal hematocrit and hemoglobin levels
  (6) The infant will receive minimal tactile stimulation.
    (a) Caretaking activities will be grouped together.
    (b) The infant will not be medically touched except to provide necessary care, and parental touch will be encouraged.
    (c) Parents will demonstrate knowledge of their infant's activity tolerance by minimizing stress during bonding activities.
    (d) The infant will be handled gently and carefully.

(e) Sedation will be given to infants who demonstrate excess activity resulting in failure to adequately ventilate or oxygenate and whose caloric expenditure is in excess of caloric intake.

2. Risk for complications of respiratory distress resulting from RDS
   a. Impaired respiratory function related to immobility of secretions
   b. Imbalanced nutrition: less than body requirements related to increased energy requirements
   c. Imbalanced fluid volume related to a risk for fluid overload
   d. Interventions
      (1) Provide airway patency by the removal of secretions using accepted guidelines per facility protocol (Youngmee & Yonghoon, 2003).
          (a) Use a catheter of appropriate size (a 5- or 6-mm catheter is recommended, if possible) to pass infant's airway.
          (b) Determine depth of suctioning by size of infant or length of ETT tube; never deep suction the infant, which may cause damage to the trachea tissues.
          (c) Set the vacuum gauge at 50 to 80 cm of water pressure.
          (d) Suction only as needed; assess need to suction by the following:
              (i) Breath sounds
              (ii) Tolerance to procedure
              (iii) Type and amount of secretions
              (iv) Clinical status
          (e) Have two people perform the procedure as necessary.
          (f) Preoxygenate and hyperinflate before suctioning.
              (i) Begin 1 minute before suctioning.
              (ii) Continue during and after procedure until the infant reaches presuctioning heart rate and oxygen saturation baseline.
          (g) Carefully pass the suctioning catheter, which will prevent damage to the mucosa; never deep suction, but rather, suction to ½ cm below the length of the ETT (Youngmee & Yonghoon, 2003).
          (h) Avoid repeated passes of the catheter if possible.
          (i) Irrigate (normal saline) only if secretions are thick and difficult to suction out.
      (2) To minimize the risk of suctioning, continuously monitor the infant's tolerance of the suctioning procedure by observing for the signs and symptoms of:
          (a) Hypoxia resulting in decreased oxygen saturation
          (b) Bradycardia, dysrhythmias, or both
          (c) Mucosal ulceration and hemorrhage secondary to the trauma of repeated suctioning (Youngmee & Yonghoon, 2003)
      (3) Provide sufficient calories to obtain optimal recovery, as well as growth and development (90 to 130 kcal/kg/day).
          (a) Infants less than 33 weeks' gestation should not be fed by nipple; alternatives include:
              (i) Gavage feedings
              (ii) Continuous nasogastric feedings
              (iii) Transpyloric feedings
          (b) Tachypneic infants may be fed carefully by gavage, with or without supplementary IV therapy.

        (c) Hypoxemia precludes enteral feedings, which necessitates IV
           therapy.

        (d) Preferred treatment in the face of intolerance to enteral feedings is
           nutrition via IV.

    (4) Provide for adequate hydration and observe for signs of fluid
       overload.

        (a) Edema

        (b) Excessive weight gain

        (c) Bulging anterior fontanelle

        (d) Worsening PDA, with or without audible murmur

    (5) Provide for adequate monitoring of fluid and electrolyte balance to
       prevent overhydration.

        (a) Take daily weight until stable, then weight three times a week or
           less as the infant becomes more stable.

           (i) Most important parameter to monitor

           (ii) Weight gain of more than 15 to 30 g/day (0.5 to 1 oz/day) is
              excessive.

        (b) Monitor serum glucose level

           (i) Bedside monitoring (Chemstrip, Dextrostix) every 4 hours
              and as needed to maintain serum glucose of 50 to 100 mg/dl

           (ii) Infants with RDS may experience erratic serum glucose levels
              and may need IV supplementation.

        (c) Monitor serum electrolyte values.

           (i) Sodium = 130 to 145 mg/dl

           (ii) Potassium = 4 to 6 mg/dl

           (iii) Chloride = 95 to 106 mg/dl

           (iv) Calcium = 8 to 10 mg/dl (preterm may be adequate at 7 to
              10 mg/dl)

        (d) Strict input and output: urine output (ml/kg/hr) should be
           calculated every 12 to 24 hours.

e. Outcomes

    (1) The infant will demonstrate improved respiratory function, as
       indicated by the following:

        (a) Minimal signs of respiratory distress

        (b) ABG assay WNL

        (c) Vital signs WNL

    (2) The infant will experience minimal negative side effects from the
       suctioning procedure.

        (a) The infant will remain well oxygenated.

        (b) The infant's heart rate will remain 100 bpm or higher with no
           observable dysrhythmia.

        (c) The infant will not exhibit negative outcomes associated with
           repeated suctioning attempts such as mucosal ulceration,
           hemorrhage, or both.

    (3) The infant will demonstrate intake of sufficient calories, as indicated
       by:

        (a) Weight gain of 15 to 30 g/day (0.5 to 1 oz/day)

        (b) Spontaneous activity level that does not compromise weight
           gain

    (4) The infant will be maintained on enteral feedings, as tolerated; if
       unable to tolerate enteral feedings, appropriate IV nutrition will be
       established and maintained.

    (5) Fluid and electrolyte levels will be monitored regularly as needed.
      (a) Weight
      (b) Bedside monitoring of serum glucose level
      (c) Serum electrolyte values
      (d) Physical examination to determine hydration status
    (6) The infant will demonstrate signs and symptoms of adequate hydration (absence of underhydration or overhydration).
      (a) Urine output between 1 and 2 ml/kg/hr
      (b) Electrolyte values WNL
      (c) Weight loss in the first few days of life, followed by a weight gain of 15 to 30 g/day (0.5 to 1.0 oz/day)
      (d) Absence of excessive generalized edema

TRANSIENT TACHYPNEA OF THE NEWBORN

A. Introduction: TTN is sometimes referred to as wet lung syndrome, retained lung fluid (RLF), and RDS type II.
  1. Pathophysiology: excess fluid in the lungs, failure to clear normal fetal lung fluid, or both
    a. Fluid accumulates in the peribronchial lymphatics and bronchovascular spaces.
    b. Excess fluid may be related to the following:
      (1) Aspiration
        (a) Amniotic fluid
        (b) Secretions
        (c) Tracheal fluid
      (2) Factors that promote the formation of interstitial lung fluid
        (a) Decreased plasma colloid osmotic pressure (hypoalbuminemia)
        (b) Increased interstitial colloid osmotic pressure (transudation of plasma proteins)
        (c) Increased capillary hydrostatic pressure
    c. Fetal lung fluid is normally cleared via the following:
      (1) Expulsion during delivery
      (2) Absorption after delivery
        (a) Pulmonary circulation
        (b) Lymphatic drainage
    d. Failure to clear fetal lung fluid is usually caused by the lack of a "thoracic squeeze" to expel the fluid during delivery, which may occur in:
      (1) Cesarean section
      (2) Breech birth
      (3) Second-born of twins
      (4) Small-for-gestational-age (SGA) infant
      (5) Rapid labor and delivery
  2. There is no known residual pulmonary dysfunction.
    a. Spontaneous pneumothorax may occur.
    b. Severe complications are rare.
B. Assessment
  1. History (risk factors)
    a. TTN infants tend to be term or near term (36 weeks' and longer gestation) with mature lungs, as indicated by L/S ratio.
    b. TTN is increased:
      (1) In large infants with a birth weight of more than 4000 g (8 lb, 14 oz)

(2) In infants born by cesarean section
(3) In breech births
(4) In the second-born of twins
(5) When labor and delivery are rapid and preclude the opportunity for an effective thoracic squeeze (especially in the small infant)
(6) With a maternal history of heavy sedation
(7) In infants with polycythemia, delayed cord clamping, or both; hyperviscosity of blood leads to sluggish circulation in the pulmonary vessels.
(8) In infants suffering from hypothermia at or shortly after birth
   (a) Hypothermia causes pulmonary vasoconstriction.
   (b) Vasoconstriction causes the infant to experience hypoxemia and increased oxygen consumption, which produces respiratory distress.

2. Physical findings: symptoms of TTN are usually present within the first hours of life (most often within 30 minutes); typically, the clinical course of TTN occurs during the first 12 to 72 hours of life and the disease is self-limiting.
  a. Transient tachypnea with a respiratory rate of 60 to 140 breaths per minute (rarely lasts longer than 48 to 96 hours)
  b. Grunting
  c. Mild intercostal retractions
  d. Possible mild cyanosis
  e. Breath sounds that may be slightly decreased because of reduced air entry
  f. Absence of rales
  g. Nasal flaring
  h. Chest that may appear hyperexpanded or barrel shaped
3. Diagnostic procedures: TTN is a diagnosis of exclusion.
  a. A diagnosis of TTN can be ascertained only after resolution of symptoms within the first 4 days.
  b. Chest x-ray film reveals the following:
   (1) Increased lung fluid, with fluid in the interlobar tissues
   (2) Prominent vascular marking (so-called hairy heart)
   (3) Flat diaphragm, with increased lung volume
   (4) Mild pleural effusions may be demonstrated
   (5) Occasional presence of mild cardiomegaly
   (6) Occasionally, the initial chest x-ray film (within the first 3 hours of life) appears similar to RDS.
  c. ABG assay
   (1) Mild hypoxemia
   (2) $PaCO_2$: normal to mildly elevated (less than 50 mmHg)
   (3) pH: usually normal

C. **Nursing Diagnoses**
1. Impaired oxygenation related to inadequate respiratory effort secondary to retained lung fluid
2. Imbalanced nutrition: less than body requirements related to respiratory distress

D. **Interventions/Outcomes**
1. Impaired oxygenation related to inadequate respiratory effort secondary to retained lung fluid (Berry, 2002)
  a. Interventions

(1) Assisted ventilation is seldom required.
(2) Provide appropriate oxygen therapy to maintain ABG values WNL.
  (a) Normal ABG assays for the term infant:
    (i) pH = 7.35 to 7.45
    (ii) $PaCO_2$ = 35 to 45 mmHg
    (iii) PaO_2 = 50 to 70 mmHg
  (b) TTN infants rarely require more than 70% fraction of inspired oxygen (FIO_2) (usually 35% to 40%).
  (c) Providing CPAP for the first few hours with severe pulmonary involvement may be useful.

b. Outcomes
(1) The infant will receive the appropriate concentration of oxygen.
(2) The infant's ABG values will be WNL.
(3) The infant will demonstrate minimal respiratory distress.
  (a) Respiratory rate between 40 and 60 breaths per minute
  (b) Minimal retractions
  (c) Bilateral breath sounds with good air entry
  (d) Absence of grunting and nasal flaring
  (e) Absence of generalized cyanosis

2. Imbalanced nutrition: less than body requirements related to respiratory distress
  a. Interventions
  (1) Care for TTN is largely supportive.
  (2) Enteral feedings may be established as the disease resolves.
    (a) Respiratory rate between 40 and 60 breaths per minute
    (b) Resolution of grunting and retractions
    (c) Adequate respiratory functioning with supplemental oxygen
  b. Outcomes
  (1) Enteral feedings will be initiated for the infant, with an intake of sufficient calories to promote optimal growth and development.

MECONIUM ASPIRATION SYNDROME

A. Introduction
1. Meconium aspiration is the most common of the aspiration syndromes.
2. Pathophysiology: two overlapping phenomena occur with MAS (Figure 19-1).
  a. Pneumonitis and pneumonia, with or without air leak
  (1) Bile salts and pancreatic enzymes and other particles in the meconium cause a chemical pneumonitis.
  (2) Meconium occludes the distal airways and acts as a ball-valve mechanism that allows air in but obstructs airflow out during expiration; this leads to air trapping and air leak (pneumothorax).
  b. Three general mechanisms in the fetus result in passage of meconium.
  (1) Direct hypoxic bowel stimulation
    (a) Passage of meconium into the amniotic fluid may be the result of some intrauterine insult that causes fetal distress.
    (b) Hypoxia and acidosis may result in relaxation of the anal sphincter and passage of meconium.
  (2) Spontaneous gastrointestinal (GI) motility: spontaneous normal physiologic defecation may occur in the term or postterm infant.
  (3) Vagal stimulation with or without specific cause (often the result of cord compression)

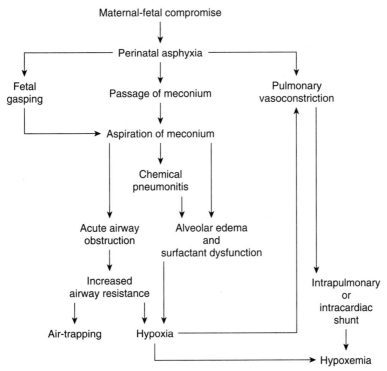

FIGURE 19-1 ■ Pathogenesis of meconium aspiration syndrome. (From Whitsett, J.A., Pryhuber, G.S., Rice, W.R., Warner, B.B., & Wert, S.E. [1999]. Acute respiratory disorders. In G.B. Avery, M.A. Fletcher, & M.G. MacDonald [Eds.], *Neonatology: Pathophysiology and management of the newborn* [5th ed., pp. 485-508]. Philadelphia: Lippincott.)

    c. After the passage of meconium into the amniotic fluid, the fetus may swallow or aspirate the meconium into the mouth, pharynx, and trachea.
       (1) With hypoxia, the fetus demonstrates normal or irregular respiratory movements.
       (2) Intrauterine aspiration can occur in infants with overwhelming distress.
       (3) The greatest risk for aspiration is at delivery, if meconium-stained fluid is present in the mouth and pharynx when the infant draws the first breath (Adhikari, Gouws, Velaphi, & Gwamanda, 1998).
    d. In addition to the mechanical damage done by the meconium itself, asphyxia is by far the most damaging aspect of MAS (MAS infants without asphyxia do better clinically) (Whitsett et al., 1999).
       (1) Meconium aspiration may be the primary presenting event but prolonged fetal asphyxia may have occurred before the meconium aspiration.
       (2) Asphyxia may lead to the following conditions:
         (a) Edema of the airways
         (b) Necrosis of the airways
         (c) Vascular collapse of the alveoli
         (d) Pulmonary hemorrhage
  3. Incidence of MAS
    a. Approximately 12% of all births include the presence of meconium-stained amniotic fluid (Whitsett et al., 1999).

  b. Meconium may be aspirated from the trachea in approximately 35% of these infants or approximately 4% of all live births.

  c. With better obstetric and pediatric management at birth, the incidence of MAS is decreasing.

  d. Infants who are depressed at birth or make poor attempts to take the first breath should be intubated in the delivery room and suctioning of the trachea should occur to remove meconium below the vocal cords; infants who do attempt to breathe and clear their own airway should be allowed to do so without intervention; approximately one third of infants with meconium below the vocal cords become ill and require intensive care (Whitsell et al., 1999; Wiswell et al., 2000).

 4. Prevention

  a. Antenatal diagnosis and treatment of fetal asphyxia is critical to the prevention of MAS (Adhikari et al., 1998).

  b. Intrapartum amnioinfusion, particularly when oligohydramnios is an issue, should be considered for prevention (Pierce, Gaudier, & Sanchez-Ramos, 2000; Whitsett et al., 1999).

   (1) Decreases rate of cesarean section.

   (2) Decreases morbidities related to MAS.

   (3) Decreases cord compression.

   (4) Dilutes meconium and may decrease its toxicity.

 5. Complications of MAS include:

  a. Air leak syndrome such as pneumothorax, pneumomediastinum, or both occurs in 20% to 30% of MAS infants (Whitsett et al., 1999).

  b. PIE

  c. Pulmonary hemorrhage

  d. PPHN

  e. Pneumonia

  f. Severe asphyxia

  g. Infection

  h. Thrombocytopenia

B. Assessment

 1. History

  a. MAS infants tend to be primarily term, postterm, or SGA; the condition rarely occurs before 38 weeks' gestation.

  b. Perinatal factors associated with or predisposing to MAS include (Liu & Harrington, 2002):

   (1) Prolonged labor

   (2) Fetal bradycardia and distress

   (3) Breech presentation

   (4) Presence of meconium-stained amniotic fluid

   (5) Delivery by cesarean section

   (6) Low Apgar scores (less than 6)

   (7) Lack of suction in the delivery room such as use of a DeLee suctioning on the perineum

   (8) IUGR

   (9) Decreased fetal movements

   (10) Maternal PIH, which leads to placental dysfunction

   (11) Prolapsed umbilical cord or placental abruption

 2. Physical findings

  a. Severity of MAS correlates with:

   (1) Consistency of meconium

(a) Early in the labor, heavy "pea soup" consistency

(b) Late in the labor, passage of large particles

(2) Amount of meconium

(a) More than 2 ml in pharynx

(b) More than 2 ml in trachea

b. Meconium staining of skin, umbilical cord, and nails

c. Hyperexpansion of the chest (barrel-shaped)

d. The following signs of respiratory distress occur in up to 50% of MAS infants:

(1) Grunting

(2) Retractions

(3) Nasal flaring

(4) Tachypnea

(5) Generalized cyanosis

(6) Irregular or gasping respirations or both

(7) Coarse, bronchial breath sounds, with audible rales heard on auscultation

e. Clinical signs of CHF

3. Diagnostic procedures

a. ABG assays show hypoxemia with respiratory or metabolic acidosis or both.

b. Chest x-ray film

(1) Lungs are hyperinflated (9 to 11 ribs expanded).

(2) Nonuniform, coarse, and patchy infiltrates radiate from one hilum into the peripheral lung fields.

(3) Infiltrates associated with focal areas of irregular aeration may be present; some appear atelectatic or consolidated, and others appear emphysematous (air trapping).

(4) Pleural effusions may be seen in MAS infants.

C. **Nursing Diagnoses**

1. Impaired ventilation and oxygenation in response to inadequate respiratory effort secondary to MAS

2. Risk for impaired respiratory function related to immobility of secretions

D. **Interventions/Outcomes**

1. Impaired ventilation and oxygenation in response to inadequate respiratory effort secondary to MAS

a. Interventions

(1) Perform amnioinfusion before delivery.

(2) Provide appropriate delivery room care to prevent aspiration of any meconium found in the mouth and pharynx.

(a) On the perineum, before delivery of the thorax:

(i) Suction mouth and hypopharynx.

(ii) Suction oropharynx and nares.

(b) Once delivered, if the infant is depressed (i.e., anticipated 1-minute Apgar of less than 7), the vocal cords should be visualized with a laryngoscope, and the trachea should be suctioned; this selective approach has decreased the need for intubation by 40% without an increase in incidence of MAS (Whitsett et al., 1999; Wiswell et al., 2000).

(3) Provide appropriate supportive measures for the neonate to offer optimal respiratory support.

(a) Provide ventilatory support and transport to a tertiary nursery, if needed.

(b) Provide for high oxygenation (PaO$_2$ of 75 to 90 mmHg) to prevent vasoconstriction.

(c) High-frequency oscillation ventilation, nitric oxide treatment, or extracorporeal membrane oxygenation (ECMO) may be required (Whitsett et al., 1999).

(d) Provide pharmacologic assistance, as needed, to achieve desired ventilation and oxygenation of the infant.
  (i) Surfactant inactivation can be overcome by instillation of exogenous surfactants; may require three or more doses (Bae, Takahashi, Chida, & Sasaki, 1998; Greenough, 2000).
  (ii) Sedation to prevent hyperactivity that can compromise oxygenation
  (ii) Vasodilators to increase pulmonary blood flow to allow for improved oxygenation

(4) Provide continuous monitoring of infant's condition.
  (a) Cardiorespiratory monitoring
  (b) Transcutaneous and oximetry monitoring
  (c) ABG assay
  (d) Ongoing respiratory status assessments
  (e) Serial chest films

(5) Prevent and treat conditions that may occur secondary to inadequate ventilation and oxygenation.
  (a) Systemic hypotension may be treated with the following:
    (i) Additional fluids
    (ii) Vasopressors
  (b) Persistent metabolic acidosis may be treated with the following:
    (i) Additional fluids
    (ii) Buffer agents as needed, to maintain a pH between 7.45 and 7.50
  (c) Anemia: transfuse with blood products, as indicated.
  (d) Infection
    (i) Meconium is an excellent growth medium for bacteria.
    (ii) Administration of prophylactic antibiotics may be indicated.

b. Outcomes

(1) The infant will receive adequate delivery room care to prevent MAS.
  (a) Suctioned on the perineum before delivery of the thorax
  (b) Intubation and tracheal suctioning after birth only if the infant is depressed

(2) The infant will be appropriately ventilated.
  (a) Mechanical ventilation, as needed
  (b) CPAP

(3) The infant will be adequately oxygenated, as evidenced by:
  (a) PaO$_2$ of 75 to 90 mmHg
  (b) The infant does not progress to or demonstrate signs of the severe consequences of MAS (persistent pulmonary hypertension, pneumonia, or air leaks).

(4) The infant will receive pharmacologic support, as needed, to achieve adequate ventilation and oxygenation.

(5) The infant will be continuously monitored.

(6) The infant will not demonstrate conditions secondary to inadequate ventilation and oxygenation.

(a) Hypotension

(b) Metabolic acidosis

(c) Anemia

(d) Infection

2. Risk for impaired respiratory function related to immobility of secretions

  a. Interventions

    (1) Intervene in the delivery room if the infant is depressed.

  b. Outcomes

    (1) The infant will be adequately suctioned in the delivery room as evidenced by minimal aspiration.

    (2) The infant will demonstrate improved respiratory function, as evidenced by:

      (a) Resolution of respiratory distress

      (b) Improving ABG assay values

      (c) Vital signs WNL

PERSISTENT PULMONARY HYPERTENSION OF THE NEWBORN

A. Introduction: PPHN is described as hypoxemia with "persistent physiologic characteristics of fetal circulation in the absence of recognizable cardiac, pulmonary, hematologic or central nervous system disease" (Whitsett et al., 1999, p. 497).

  1. Pathophysiology: failure to make the transition from high PVR and low pulmonary blood flow normally found in utero, to low pulmonary vascular resistance and high pulmonary blood flow normally found after transition to extrauterine life

  a. Usually, both the foramen ovale and ductus arterious remain open, with high blood flow shunting through these ducts that is sometimes bidirectional.

  b. Results in profound hypoxemia; mechanisms that maintain the fetal state are relatively unknown but may be related to alterations in nitric oxide, arachidonic acid metabolism, and systemic acidosis (Whitsett et al., 1999).

  c. Theories suggest that indomethacin and aspirin, which are cyclooxygenase blockers, may contribute because exposure of the fetus to these drugs may prevent the decrease in PVR that occurs after initiation of ventilation.

  d. Research suggests that increased levels of immunoreactive endothelin-1, as well as insufficient production of endogenous endothelium-derived relaxin factor, may contribute to continued vasoconstriction (Whitsett et al., 1999).

B. Assessment

  1. History (risk factors)

  a. MAS

  b. Birth asphyxia, post dates

  c. RDS

  d. Pneumonia

  e. Metabolic acidosis

  f. Infection (group B Streptococcus)

  g. Acute hypoxia with delayed resuscitation, hypoglycemia, or hypothermia

2. Physical findings: symptoms
   a. Cyanosis over entire body or differential cyanosis may be seen.
   b. Respiratory distress with tachypnea
   c. Normal or decreased blood pressure (BP) or asymmetric BP with right arm being greater than left lower extremity
   d. Tricuspid insufficiency murmur may be present (harsh).
3. Diagnostic procedures
   a. Hypoxia test: preductal and postductal PaO_2 with preductal and postductal oximetry
   b. Glucose status
   c. ABG assay: pH status; respiratory or metabolic or mixed acidosis usually present
   d. Chest x-ray film reveals variable heart size depending on cause of PPHN and whether heart defects are present; lung findings are also dependent on primary lung disease.
   e. Echocardiography may reveal:
      (1) Echo-increase in PA pressure, shunting right to left or bidirectional at foramen ovale; may be shunting right to left at ductus or bidirectional at ductus.
      (2) Tricuspid insufficiency
      (3) Right ventricular hypertrophy may be present.

C. **Nursing Diagnoses**
   1. Impaired oxygenation related to inadequate respiratory effort secondary to retained lung fluid
   2. Imbalanced nutrition: less than body requirements related to respiratory distress

D. **Interventions/Outcomes**
   1. Impaired oxygenation related to inadequate respiratory effort secondary to retained lung fluid
      a. Interventions
         (1) Prevention is best, with early and effective resuscitation and correction of acidosis and hypoxia.
         (2) Assisted ventilation with hyperoxia may be used as needed to increase passive oxygen diffusion across alveolar membrane and promote vasodilatation.
            (a) High frequency ventilation
            (b) ECMO
            (c) Inhaled nitric oxide
         (3) Provide appropriate oxygen therapy to maintain ABG values WNL, promote alkalosis, or both; alkalosis may play a role in relaxing the smooth muscle and thus reversing pulmonary vasoconstriction.
            (a) pH above 7.55
            (b) $PaCO_2$ between 25 and 35 mmHg
            (c) PaO_2 above 100 mmHg
         (4) Risks associated with hyperventilation to achieve alkalosis
            (a) Cerebrovascular vasoconstriction with reduction in cerebral blood flow
            (b) Increased barotrauma because of high inflating pressures
            (c) Increased risk of air leaks
            (d) Potential for overinflation with subsequent increase in PVR
            (e) Sensorineural hearing loss

    (5) Decrease environmental stimulation because these infants are often quite sensitive to handling and stress from the environment.
        (a) Decrease activity.
        (b) Decrease noise and light.
        (c) Cluster caregiving.
        (d) Use sedation as needed.
        (e) Manage and treat before painful procedures.
  b. Outcomes
    (1) The infant will receive the appropriate concentration of oxygen for PVR to decrease and pulmonary vascular blood flow to increase.
    (2) The infant's ABG values will be WNL.
    (3) The infant will demonstrate minimal respiratory distress.
        (a) Respiratory rate between 40 and 60 breaths per minute
        (b) Bilateral breath sounds with good air entry
        (c) Absence of generalized cyanosis
2. Imbalanced nutrition: less than body requirements related to respiratory distress
  a. Interventions
    (1) Nutritional care for PPHN is largely supportive.
    (2) The infant will demonstrate intake of sufficient calories, as indicated by:
        (a) Weight gain of 15 to 30 g/day (0.5 to 1 oz/day)
        (b) Spontaneous activity level that does not compromise weight gain
    (3) The infant will be maintained on enteral feedings, as tolerated; if unable to tolerate enteral feedings, appropriate IV nutrition will be established and maintained.
    (4) Fluid and electrolyte levels will be monitored regularly as needed.
        (a) Weight
        (b) Bedside monitoring of serum glucose level
        (c) Serum electrolyte values
        (d) Physical examination to determine hydration status
    (5) The infant will demonstrate signs and symptoms of adequate hydration (absence of underhydration or overhydration).
        (a) Urine output between 1 and 2 ml/kg/hr
        (b) Electrolyte values WNL
        (c) Weight loss in the first few days of life, followed by a weight gain of 15 to 30 g/day (0.5 to 1 oz/day)
        (d) Absence of excessive generalized edema
  b. Outcomes
    (1) Enteral feedings will be initiated for the infant, with an intake of sufficient calories to promote optimal growth and development.

HYPERBILIRUBINEMIA
Causes of Hyperbilirubinemia

Physiologic jaundice is a condition that is common in the term newborn infant during the second or third day of life (second to ninth day in preterm neonates) and is not considered to be pathologic unless bilirubin levels exceed the normal physiologic limitations of a healthy neonate; pathologic hyperbilirubinemia, which can be defined only by serum concentrations of unconjugated bilirubin, has diverse causes that are frequently, but not always, interlinked; jaundice is a manifestation of bilirubin accumulation in extravascular tissues.

A. Incidence of physiologic jaundice during the first week of life
   1. Almost all neonates have elevated serum bilirubin levels above 2 mg/dl (the normal level in adults is 1.3 mg/dl or less) (Hammond, 2000).
   2. Elevated serum bilirubin levels above 5 mg/dl occur in 60% of neonates (Dixit & Gartner, 2000).
   3. Hyperbilirubinemia, as it occurs in physiologic jaundice, may confer some biologic advantage to the neonate.
      a. Beneficial effects of bilirubin molecules might be noted at a cellular level (Yao & Stevenson, 1995).
      b. Bilirubin has a potent antioxidant effect.
      c. Neonates have deficient levels of most antioxidant substances.
   4. Breastfeeding jaundice appears in the first days of life and is called such because it appears to be related to early ineffective breastfeeding practices that lead to (Reiser, 2001):
      a. Decreased volumes
      b. Decreased caloric intakes
      c. Dehydration
      d. Delayed passage of meconium
   5. Breast milk jaundice occurs after 3 to 5 days of life, with a steady increase in serum bilirubin that usually peaks at approximately 2 weeks (5 to 10 mg/dl) and then decreases slowly; this type of jaundice appears to be related to the composition of the breast milk that results in enhanced enterohepatic circulation, although this is speculative (Halamek & Stevenson, 1998).

B. Bilirubin production and conjugation
   1. Bilirubin has two forms:
      a. Unconjugated or indirect
         (1) Fat soluble
         (2) Toxic to tissues
      b. Conjugated or direct
         (1) Water soluble
         (2) Nontoxic to tissues
   2. The majority of bilirubin comes from the destruction of hemoglobin.
      a. Catabolism of 1 g of hemoglobin results in the production of 34 mg of bilirubin.
      b. Destruction of circulating erythrocytes accounts for approximately 75% of the daily bilirubin production in the normal term neonate.
         (1) The neonate has a large red blood cell (RBC) mass per kilogram of body weight; the neonate's RBCs have a life span that is only two thirds that of an adult's RBCs.
         (2) The shortened life span of the neonate's RBCs accounts for the increased breakdown and subsequent increased production of bilirubin.
      c. The remaining 25% of the daily bilirubin production in the newborn originates from the following sources:
         (1) Destruction of heme proteins
         (2) Free heme from the liver
         (3) Destruction of the RBC precursor in bone marrow

3. Process of bilirubin conjugation (Figure 19-2)
   a. Within the circulatory system, unconjugated bilirubin tightly bound to albumin is transported to the liver, where the conjugation process takes place.
   b. Bilirubin is then released from the albumin binding site and undergoes the following:
      (1) Transfer across the hepatocyte membrane
      (2) Cytoplasmic protein binding
          (a) Within the liver, bilirubin is bound to ligandin and other hepatic proteins.
          (b) This binding helps prevent a backup of bilirubin into the general circulation.
      (3) Transport (while bound to protein)
          (a) Smooth endoplasmic reticulum is the site of conjugation process.
          (b) Process of conjugation transforms the poorly soluble, unconjugated bilirubin into a water-soluble form that can be excreted by the neonate; this process requires oxygen and glucose.
      (4) Excretion (after conjugation) into the bile, into the intestine, and finally mainly into the neonate's stool as stercobilin
          (a) Some bilirubin is excreted through the kidneys as urobilinogen.
          (b) In the intestine, the enzyme glucuronidase may break the ester linkage of the bilirubin, causing it to become unconjugated.

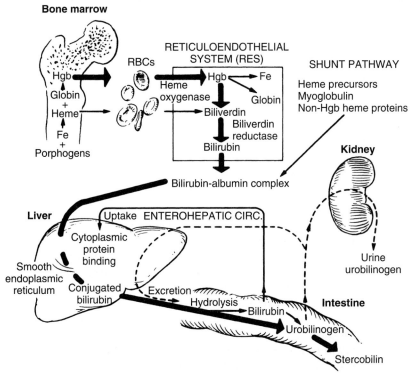

FIGURE 19-2 ■ Process of bilirubin conjugation. (From Gartner, L.M. [1972]. Disorders of bilirubin metabolism. In N.S. Assali (Ed.), *Pathophysiology of gestation* [Vol. 2, p. 457]. New York: Academic Press.)

(i) Can occur in the sterile (uncolonized) intestine.

(ii) Can be catalyzed if normal bacterial colonization has occurred.

(c) The newly unconjugated bilirubin may be reabsorbed into the neonate's circulation, necessitating a repetition of the entire conjugation process.

4. Neonatal hyperbilirubinemia can occur from the following:
   a. An increased load of circulating bilirubin resulting from the following:
      (1) Polycythemia
      (2) Isoimmune hemolytic disease
      (3) Structural and enzyme defects of RBCs
      (4) Drug toxicity (chemical hemolysis)
      (5) Extravascular hemolysis
         (a) Enclosed hemorrhage, as in cephalhematoma
         (b) Ecchymosis
   b. Impaired hepatic function (e.g., defective uptake, conjugation, or excretion)
      (1) Deficient glucuronyl transferase activity
      (2) Biliary obstruction or biliary atresia
      (3) Infection
      (4) Metabolic problems, such as:
         (a) Galactosemia
         (b) Breast milk jaundice
         (c) Hypothyroidism
   c. Perinatal complications, such as:
      (1) Asphyxia
      (2) Hypothermia
      (3) Hypoglycemia
   d. Decreased albumin binding sites, because of:
      (1) Preterm birth
      (2) Competition with drugs having an affinity for the binding sites
      (3) Acidosis
   e. Delayed meconium passage
      (1) Meconium contains 0.5 to 1 mg of bilirubin per gram.
      (2) Delayed meconium passage increases the amount of bilirubin that returns to the unconjugated state and is reabsorbed across the intestinal mucosa.

5. Rate of bilirubin level increase:
   a. Must exceed 4 to 6 mg/dl before it is visible as jaundice.
   b. In physiologic jaundice:
      (1) Bilirubin level increase first appears after 24 hours of age in term neonates and after 48 hours of age in preterm neonates.
         (a) Reaches peak at day 3 or 4 and returns to a normal level by the end of day 7 in term neonates.
         (b) Reaches peak at day 5 or 6 and returns to a normal level by the end of day 9 or 10 in preterm neonates.
         (c) Pattern for breastfed infants is slightly different; peak level often occurs on day 4 and the decline may be slower.
      (2) Indirect bilirubin value does not usually exceed 12 mg/dl.
      (3) Direct bilirubin does not usually exceed 1 to 1.5 mg/dl.
      (4) Daily increases of bilirubin do not usually exceed 5 mg/dl.

    c. In pathologic jaundice, elevated bilirubin levels:
      (1) Appear within the first 24 hours of life.
      (2) Persist beyond the age for return to a normal level in term and preterm neonates.
      (3) No specific serum level can be used for diagnosis.
    d. Kernicterus is a preventable neurologic syndrome with life long sequelae; it is caused by severe and inadequately treated hyperbilirubinemia during the neonatal period.
      (1) Bilirubin encephalopathy is the most serious complication of hyperbilirubinemia.
      (2) Yellow staining of brain tissue occurs and creates morphologic changes in brain cells, which results in irreversible damage.
      (3) Approximately one half of affected neonates do not survive.
      (4) Condition is generally thought to occur at bilirubin levels in excess of 20 mg/dl in full-term neonates.
      (5) Early signs include:
        (a) Extreme jaundice
        (b) Alterations in level of consciousness (lethargy)
        (c) Tone (hypotonia, then later, hypertonia)
        (d) Abnormal movement (opisthotonos)
        (e) Poor feeding
        (f) High-pitched crying
      (6) The long-term sequelae include:
        (a) Cerebral palsy
        (b) Sensorineural hearing loss
        (c) Gaze paresis
        (d) Dental dysplasia
        (e) Mental retardation

C. Phototherapy

  1. Treatment is widely used to manage and control rising bilirubin levels.
    a. Unclothed neonate, with eye shields, is placed in an infant incubator within 18 to 20 inches (45 to 50 cm) of the bank of lights and turned every 2 hours.
    b. Treatment can also be performed with a fiberoptic blanket attached to an illuminator and wrapped around the neonate's torso and extremities.
      (1) Allows use of an open crib.
      (2) Eye shields are not needed.
      (3) Neonate can be held.
      (4) Can be used for home phototherapy (Hammond & Perry, 2000).
  2. Mechanism of phototherapy action
    a. Treatment is thought to reduce serum bilirubin levels by facilitating biliary excretion of unconjugated bilirubin.
    b. Treatment causes the formation of photoisomers, which are more water soluble and therefore more easily excreted in stool and urine.
      (1) Unconjugated bilirubin is rapidly converted to photobilirubin and lumirubin.
      (2) Photobilirubin and lumirubin are rapidly taken up by the liver and transported into the bile.
      (3) Process occurs independent of hepatic conjugation of bilirubin.
    c. White, daylight, cool blue, and special blue are among the various types of phototherapy lights available.

(1) Lights with high-energy output, ranging between 420 and 450 nm in the blue spectrum, are the most effective.

(2) Optimal energy output light levels should be monitored to ensure that levels are maintained to achieve maximum efficiency.

d. Home monitoring and treatment

(1) Bilirubin levels can be determined in the hospital as well as during a home visit by using transcutaneous bilirubinometry (TcB).

(a) Procedure uses a noninvasive, portable instrument.

(b) Predicts serum bilirubin levels in the neonate by using reflective measurements on the skin to determine the amount of yellow color in the skin.

(c) Measurement can correlate well with serum bilirubin levels; however, error can be high because of a variety of neonatal factors (Dai, Parry, & Krahn, 1997).

(i) Gestational age of neonate

(ii) Birthweight

(iii) Skin pigmentation because of different ethnic origin

(iv) Phototherapy treatment (Linder et al., 1994)

(d) TcB should be used only as a screening tool to determine when a laboratory measurement of serum bilirubin is needed (Dai et al., 1997).

(2) In some circumstances, home phototherapy can be provided and thus avoid separation of neonate from parents.

D. **Treatment controversies surrounding physiologic jaundice exist.**

1. The trend has been to decrease interventions and to observe and manage neonates as outpatients.

2. Research has shown that healthy, full-term neonates in the absence of significant hemolysis or other underlying medical conditions with serum bilirubin levels of approximately 18 mg/dl do not have any detrimental effects with an expectant observation treatment approach (Haimi-Cohen, Merlob, Davidovitz, & Eisenstein, 1997; Torres-Torres, Tayaba, Weintraub, & Holzman, 1994).

3. The development of new drugs to modulate bilirubin production is the subject of ongoing research (Yao & Stevenson, 1995).

4. The American Academy of Pediatrics (AAP) Practice Guidelines for Management of Hyperbilirubinemia in the Healthy Term Newborn provides guidelines for identifying at risk infants and intervention and treatment strategies; in April 2001, the Joint Commission on Accreditation of Healthcare Organizations (JCAHO) issued a Sentinel Event Alert regarding the increased incidence of kernicterus; proposed risk reduction strategies include:

a. Predischarge bilirubin measurement, with standing orders allowing nurses to order total serum bilirubin (TSB) levels or TcB levels for newborns (Reiser, 2001)

b. Use of a percentile-based nomogram to predict the risk of hyperbilirubinemia and implement strategies for follow-up, which may be helpful in provision of care (Bhutani, Johnson, & Sivieri, 1999) (Figure 19-3)

c. Follow-up for all newborns within 48 hours after discharge by a physician or trained health care provider who is experienced in the care of newborns to provide follow-up physical assessment and ongoing lactation support to ensure adequacy of intake for breastfed infants (Bhutani, Gourley, Adler, Kreamer, Dalen, & Johnson, 2000)

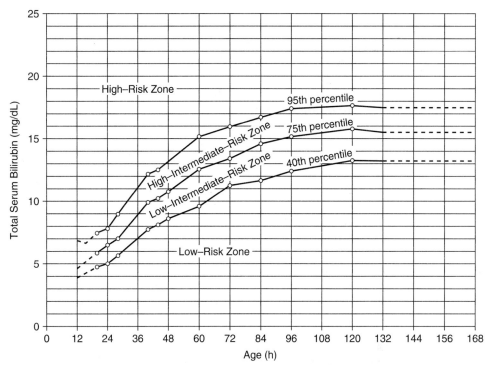

FIGURE 19-3 ■ Bilirubin risk designation based on age and current bilirubin level. (From Bhutani, V.K., Johnson, L.H., & Sivieri, E. [1999]. Ability of pre-discharge hour-specific serum bilirubin for subsequent significant hyperbilirubinemia in healthy term and near term infants. *Pediatrics, 103*[1], 6-14.)

d. Providing parents with adequate educational materials at discharge regarding jaundice, feeding adequacy and symptoms to watch for (see Health Education) (Dixit & Gartner, 2000; Jones, 1990; Reiser, 2001)

Clinical Practice

A. Assessment

1. History
   a. Maternal
      (1) Mother's blood type can have an impact on neonate's bilirubin levels by causing intravascular hemolysis via an antigen-antibody reaction.
          (a) Rh disease
          (b) ABO incompatibility
          (c) Positive Coombs' test result
      (2) Insulin-dependent diabetic mother
          (a) Neonate has an increased RBC mass at birth.
          (b) Breakdown of a high number of aged RBCs results in excessive amounts of bilirubin in the neonate.
      (3) Maternal and paternal ethnicity
          (a) Asian and Native American neonates have a higher incidence of hyperbilirubinemia.

(b) Mean serum levels of unconjugated bilirubin in Asian and Native-American neonates are higher than the mean levels for neonates of other ethnic origins (Hammond, 2000).
    (i) Mean serum levels of unconjugated bilirubin for the former are 10 to 14 mg/dl.
    (ii) This mean is approximately double that of neonates of other ethnic origins.
(c) Black and white neonates tend to have lower mean levels of bilirubin.
(4) Maternal drugs used during the last 3 months of pregnancy
    (a) The following drugs interfere with the binding of bilirubin to albumin in neonates:
        (i) Sulfonamides
        (ii) Salicylates
        (iii) Ibuprofen
    (b) Pitocin (synthetic oxytocin) is associated with a higher incidence of neonatal jaundice.
(5) A previous infant with diagnosed breast milk jaundice: a 70% possibility of recurrence occurs in subsequent siblings of an infant diagnosed with breast milk jaundice (Reiser, 2001).
    (a) Breast milk jaundice occurs in 0.5% to 2% of breastfed term infants (Lawrence & Lawrence, 1999).
    (b) Affected breast milk contains substances that inhibit the activity of glucuronyl transferase in the neonatal liver.
    (c) Bilirubin levels continue to rise on the fourth and fifth days, when physiologic jaundice should be subsiding.
        (i) Rise to peak concentrations of between 10 and 27 mg/dl between 10 and 15 days of age.
        (ii) Gradually decrease from peak levels to normal levels between 3 and 12 weeks of age (Reiser, 2001).

b. Labor and delivery history
(1) Use of the following drugs:
    (a) Pitocin (synthetic oxytocin)
    (b) Diazepam
    (c) Bupivacaine (in epidural anesthesia)
(2) Delayed umbilical cord clamping
    (a) Allows an excessive amount of blood to be transfused from the placenta to the neonate.
    (b) Increase in quantity of RBCs results in the following:
        (i) Sequestration of greater numbers of aged RBCs
        (ii) Excessive amounts of bilirubin from breakdown of aged RBCs (Korones & Bada-Ellzey, 1993)
(3) Operative delivery: ecchymosis and extravascular hemolysis may be increased by using forceps or vacuum extractor.

c. Perinatal complications
(1) Cephalhematoma
(2) Cerebral hemorrhage
(3) Pulmonary hemorrhage
(4) Any occult bleeding
(5) Maternal-fetal transfusion
(6) Hypoxia
    (a) Causes increase in free fatty acids.

          (b) Free fatty acids compete with bilirubin for albumin binding sites.

     (7) Infection and sepsis (bacterial, viral, or protozoal)

          (a) Hemolysis

          (b) Hemolytic anemia

     (8) Low Apgar scores at 1 minute and at 5 minutes may indicate a potential complication.

  d. Postnatal complications

     (1) Caloric deprivation, causing weight loss, results from:

          (a) Infrequent feedings

          (b) Poor suck-and-swallow reflex

          (c) Decrease in gastric motility and enzymatic activity

     (2) Glucose-6-phosphate dehydrogenase (G-6-PD) deficiency:

          (a) Is an enzymatic deficiency.

          (b) Disrupts erythrocyte metabolism and causes hemolysis.

          (c) Occurs primarily among blacks, Filipinos, Sephardic Jews, Sardinians, Greeks, and Arabs (Korones & Bada-Ellzey, 1993).

          (d) Manifests as jaundice on the second or third day of life and persists into the second or third week of life.

2. Physical findings

  a. Visible jaundice progresses in a cephalocaudal direction and can be seen first in facial skin, sclera, and gums, and later in the torso and lower extremities.

  b. Bilirubin levels

     (1) Elevated umbilical cord blood bilirubin level

     (2) Pattern of jaundice onset, length, and duration

  c. SGA condition that is associated with infection

  d. Small head circumference (microcephaly) that is associated with infection

  e. Cephalhematoma, ecchymosis, and abrasions are indicative of a traumatic delivery process.

  f. Pallor that is suggestive of hemolytic anemia

  g. Poor feeding or difficulty with breastfeeding

  h. Lethargy; difficult to awaken for feedings

  i. Petechiae that is suggestive of the following:

     (1) Congenital infection

     (2) Overwhelming sepsis

     (3) Severe hemolytic disease

  j. Plethora that is associated with polycythemia

  k. Vomiting that is suggestive of the following:

     (1) Sepsis

     (2) Pyloric stenosis

  l. Hepatosplenomegaly that is suggestive of the following:

     (1) Chronic intrauterine infection

     (2) Hemolytic anemia

  m. Congenital anomalies: increased incidence of jaundice is associated with infants with trisomies.

3. Diagnostic procedures

  a. Maternal blood group and indirect Coombs' test to rule out possibility of ABO or Rh incompatibility

  b. Serologic assays to rule out congenital syphilis

  c. Hemoglobin to rule out the following:

     (1) Anemia

     (2) Polycythemia: hemoglobin concentration higher than 22 g/dl

   d. Complete blood count (CBC) with differential
   (1) Elevated reticulocyte count suggests hemolytic disease.
   (2) RBC morphology
      (a) Spherocytes suggest ABO incompatibility.
      (b) RBC fragmentation suggests disseminated intravascular coagulopathy (DIC).
   (3) WBC count
      (a) Less than $5000/mm^3$ suggests infection.
      (b) Increase in bands to more than $2000/mm^3$ suggests infection.
   (4) Platelets: thrombocytopenia suggests infection.
   (5) Sedimentation rate values in excess of $5 mm^3$ during first 48 hours is suggestive of infection or ABO incompatibility.
   (6) Elevated direct bilirubin (conjugated) level suggests infection or severe Rh incompatibility.

B. Nursing Diagnoses
   1. Risk for deficient neonatal fluid volume related to phototherapy light exposure
   2. Ineffective neonatal thermoregulation related to phototherapy light exposure
   3. Risk for impaired neonatal skin integrity related to diarrhea, urinary excretions of bilirubin, and exposure to phototherapy lights
   4. Risk for injury of the neonatal cornea related to phototherapy light exposure and continuous wearing of protective eye shields
   5. Risk for impaired parenting related to parent-infant separation secondary to phototherapy treatments

C. Interventions/Outcomes
   1. Risk for deficient neonatal fluid volume related to phototherapy light exposure
   a. Interventions
      (1) Increase fluid intake to offset the following:
         (a) Increase in metabolic rate caused by phototherapy
         (b) Significant increase in water loss through the skin
         (c) Increase in water content of frequent stools
         (d) Water loss caused by hyperthermia
      (2) Offer neonate frequent feedings.
         (a) Feed as often as tolerated (approximately every 2 hours).
         (b) Increase calories to offset rapid intestinal transit time (frequent stooling) and decreased intestinal absorption of milk.
   b. Outcomes
      (1) Fluid intake is increased.
      (2) Neonate remains well hydrated while under phototherapy lights.
   2. Ineffective thermoregulation related to phototherapy light exposure
   a. Interventions
      (1) Maintain thermal homeostasis while infant is under phototherapy lights by using a servo control mechanism such as the following:
         (a) Isolette
         (b) Radiant warmer
      (2) Offer neonate fluids frequently and maintain dry bedding.
         (a) Hypothermia stimulates the release of free fatty acids, which compete for albumin binding sites.
         (b) Hyperthermia increases the neonate's metabolic rate.

    b. Outcomes
- (1) Neonate maintains a normal temperature while under the phototherapy lights.
- (2) Neonate's bedding is clean and dry.
- (3) Neonate is covered and kept warm when not under phototherapy lights (i.e., for feedings and other procedures).

3. Risk for impaired neonatal skin integrity related to diarrhea, urinary excretions of bilirubin, and exposure to phototherapy lights

    a. Interventions
- (1) Diapering of the neonate may be accomplished by using a paper face mask with the metal strip removed.
  - (a) Allows maximal skin exposure for phototherapy lights.
    - (i) Provides protection for genitals and bedding.
    - (ii) Shields a minimum of jaundiced skin.
  - (b) It is typical for stools to be loose, greenish, frequent, and expelled with force.
- (2) It is important to protect neonate's skin from excoriation by thoroughly removing urine and feces with each diaper change.
- (3) It is important to change diapers frequently.
- (4) It is important to keep neonate's skin clean and dry by frequently checking bedding for dampness or stool soiling.

    b. Outcomes
- (1) Neonate's skin remains clean and dry while under phototherapy lights.
- (2) No signs of redness or excoriation are present on the neonate's skin.

4. Risk for injury of the neonatal cornea related to phototherapy light exposure and continuous wearing of protective eye shields

    a. Interventions
- (1) Protect neonate's eyes from phototherapy lights by applying eye shields to prevent eye damage.
- (2) Secure placement of the eye shields tightly enough to prevent slippage and accidental eye exposure but not so tightly that constraint and excessive pressure are placed on the neonate's eyes.
- (3) Remove eye shields when neonate is not under phototherapy lights.
  - (a) For feedings
  - (b) For procedures not performed under phototherapy lights
- (4) Make sure the neonate's eyes are closed when applying the eye shields.
- (5) Change eye shields frequently and watch for any signs of conjunctivitis, such as:
  - (a) Purulent discharge
  - (b) Edema

    b. Outcomes
- (1) Neonate wears protective eye shields at all times while under phototherapy lights.
- (2) No signs of excessive eye shield pressure are present on neonate's skin around the eyes.
- (3) No signs of conjunctivitis are present in neonate.

5. Risk for impaired parenting related to parent-infant separation secondary to phototherapy treatments

    a. Interventions

(1) Encourage parents to participate in the caretaking responsibilities of their neonate.

(2) Encourage parents to hold their neonate for short periods.

(3) Encourage parents to provide gentle stroking and touching of the neonate while he or she is under phototherapy lights.

b. Outcomes

(1) Parents actively participate in caretaking activities with their neonate.

(2) Parents provide soothing tactile stimulation to their neonate while he or she is under phototherapy lights.

HEALTH EDUCATION

A. **The technologic advances made in newborn care during the last 30 years have markedly decreased morbidity and mortality in this group of high-risk infants.**

1. Technologic advances have brought a heightened sensitivity to the psychologic and emotional impact felt by the family of a sick neonate.

2. This awareness has introduced the need for a family-centered approach to newborn care.

3. In addition to the physiologic care of the sick neonate, health care workers need to address the psychologic needs of family members during this experience.

4. Parental attachment to the infant with respiratory distress, hyperbilirubinemia, or both is especially difficult.

   a. The infant may be premature.

   b. Normal interaction may be severely curtailed.

   c. An infant who is sick enough to be in a special care or intensive care unit on a ventilator, or receiving oxygen support, or phototherapy may not give cues adequate to arouse parental attachment.

5. Provide information in nontechnical terms to parents about serum bilirubin levels while the neonate is being monitored, and encourage their questions and concerns about their neonate's condition.

B. **The birth of a newborn who is sick represents a unique crisis for the family and perinatal health care team** (Siegel, Gardner, & Merenstein, 2002).

1. The family must simultaneously adjust to the immediate situation and begin the normal developmental process of parenthood.

2. Situational factors have an important bearing on the family's ability to cope with this present crisis and can affect the overall outcome.

   a. The behavior and attitude of the hospital staff

   b. The sensitivity used in the transfer process either to another facility or the NICU

   c. The flexibility in unit visitation and extended family involvement

   d. The instruction received by the family related to their infant's unique characteristics and behavior

   e. The staff's sensitivity to the family's responses and adaptation to crisis

   f. The use of emotionally supportive intervention programs in the nursery

   g. The development of appropriate discharge planning to provide adequate follow-up for the family

C. **Discharge planning for the infant with respiratory distress or hyperbilirubinemia may include the following:**
   1. Family education
      a. Use of equipment needed in the care of the infant (e.g., oxygen, suctioning devices, phototherapy)
      b. Praise for parents' caretaking abilities of infant while in the hospital; parents are not visitors
      c. When and how to perform chest physiotherapy
      d. Dosage, route of administration, side effects, and planned duration of use of all medications
      e. Nutritional information to maintain adequate calorie and fluid balance
         (1) Type of formula (if used instead of breast milk)
         (2) How and when to feed the infant
         (3) Possible alternative feeding methods
         (4) If and when to provide oxygen during the feedings
      f. Support for mother's or father's attempts to feed the neonate and encourage frequent feedings to provide neonate with adequate hydration and increased calories
      g. The use of home monitoring, if needed
      h. Infant cardiopulmonary resuscitation (CPR)
      i. Recognition of signs and symptoms of illness in the newborn
      j. Normal newborn care
   2. Acquisition and maintenance of specialized equipment that may be needed to care for the infant at home, including:
      a. Oxygen and oxygen equipment
      b. Suction machine and supplies
      c. Home monitoring equipment
      d. Phototherapy
   3. All information and education given to the family should be in written form, if possible; in addition, whenever possible, return demonstrations by the family reinforce learning.
   4. Parents should be instructed about signs, symptoms, and treatment of hyperbilirubinemia that may occur at home as a result of early discharge program (Bhutani et al., 2000 Dixit & Gartner, 2000; Jones, 1990).
      a. Monitoring neonate's behaviors that may be indicative of increasing bilirubin levels
      b. Blanching neonate's skin to determine degree of jaundice
      c. Placing the neonate's bassinet or cradle near a window during the daytime to take advantage of natural sunlight
      d. Monitoring feeding and level of consciousness
      e. Maintaining sufficient hydration level in neonate
      f. Advising when to bring the neonate to the health care provider for further evaluation of bilirubin levels
D. **Long-term follow-up of the infant with respiratory distress or hyperbilirubinemia is essential.**
   1. Parents must have telephone numbers of the medical facility and personnel to call 24 hours a day in case of problems or equipment failure.
   2. Before hospital discharge, parents need to have information regarding follow-up appointments and referrals for long-term care.

CASE STUDIES AND STUDY QUESTIONS

Ms. J, a gravida 2, para 1 (G2, P1), delivered an infant boy vaginally at 35 weeks' gestation. The infant weighed 2500 g (5 lb, 8 oz); the fetal heart rate appeared fine during labor, although an L/S ratio done was reported at 1.8/1. Ms. J has gestational diabetes.

1. Surfactant production for an infant with RDS will be inhibited owing to which of the following?
   a. Prematurity
   b. Water intoxication
   c. Alkalosis
   d. Drugs given to the mother

2. The best indicator of an infant's need for oxygen is which of the following?
   a. Respiratory rate
   b. Skin color
   c. Arterial PaO_2
   d. Pulse rate

3. Which of the following is characteristic of neonates with RDS?
   a. Have a deficiency of pulmonary surfactant
   b. Are postmature
   c. Have sternal excursions
   d. Demonstrate tachypnea and expiratory grunting
   e. a and d

4. Which of the following statement(s) is(are) true about RDS?
   a. It is characterized by atelectasis.
   b. Acidosis perpetuates the decreased production of surfactant.
   c. It may be induced by hypothermia in a preterm infant.
   d. With adequate supportive care, it is self-resolving in approximately 72 hours.
   e. All are correct except d.

5. In RDS, blood may not be oxygenated because of which of the following?
   a. A patent ductus arteriosus
   b. Failure of the foramen ovale to close
   c. Atelectasis of the alveoli
   d. Alkalosis
   e. a, b, and c

6. Which of the following prenatal factors predispose the neonate to development of respiratory distress?
   a. Maternal diabetes
   b. Breech presentation
   c. Fetal scalp pH of 7.20
   d. 43 weeks' gestation
   e. All of the above

7. True or false: acidosis and hypothermia may lead to decreased pulmonary blood flow, which perpetuates decreased production of surfactant and may cause RDS.

8. A condition that usually occurs in term infants and cesarean section deliveries, is manifested by tachypnea, and is caused by retained lung fluid is called which of the following?
   a. Pneumonia
   b. TTN
   c. Pulmonary hemorrhage
   d. Meconium aspiration

9. When suctioning the neonate born through meconium-stained amniotic fluid, which of the following is suctioned first?
   a. Both nares
   b. Stomach
   c. Trachea
   d. Oropharynx and nasopharynx (before the infant's body is delivered)

10. An infant with PPHN and a PDA is at risk for developing:
    a. Pulmonary hemorrhage
    b. Hepatomegaly
    c. Pleural effusions
    d. Hyperbilirubinemia

11. You are preparing to care for four infants just recently born. Which of the following infants is at greatest risk for TTN?
    a. Spontaneous vaginal delivery; 40 weeks' gestation
    b. Cesarean section delivery; 41 weeks' gestation
    c. Induced vaginal delivery; 43 weeks' gestation
    d. Vaginal delivery with maternal anesthesia; 38 weeks' gestation

Baby M was delivered after a 16-hour induced labor. Maternal membranes were artificially ruptured, fluid was clear, and a pitocin infusion was initiated. The mother was afebrile throughout the labor. The second stage of labor was 2 hours, 45 minutes. Review of the mother's prenatal and labor history yielded the following information:
Blood type is A+.
Venereal disease research laboratory (VDRL) is nonreactive.
Alpha-fetoprotein (AFP) is normal.
Average BP is 116-124/76-82.
Total weight gain was 12.25 kg (27 lb).
Medications are prenatal vitamins, iron, and aspirin for stress headaches.
Gestational age is 40 6/7 weeks.
Nonstress test is reactive.
Baby M had the umbilical cord wrapped twice around her neck and required stimulation to initiate breathing and administration of oxygen by face mask. Apgar scores were 7 at 1 minute and 8 at 5 minutes.

12. From this information, which of the following factors place Baby M at increased risk for hyperbilirubinemia?
    a. Ruptured membranes for 16 hours
    b. Postmaturity

    c. Mother's blood type is A
    d. Labor induced with pitocin

13. All of the following factors indicate that Baby M is at greater risk for hyperbilirubinemia except:
    a. The 1-minute Apgar score
    b. Gestational age of 40 6/7 weeks
    c. Mother taking aspirin for her headaches
    d. Respirations having to be stimulated and oxygen administered

On her second day of life, Baby M required phototherapy treatment. Her mother was being discharged from the hospital and came to the nursery to breastfeed her infant before leaving. Baby M's mother was crying and did not want to go home without her infant. Baby M's father was trying to comfort his wife.

14. While Baby M is under the phototherapy lights, it is important to do which of the following?
    a. Keep the infant under the lights continuously at all times so that there will be maximal effectiveness in the shortest period.
    b. Limit any unnecessary touch stimulation because Baby M's metabolism is already high and touch might further increase it.
    c. Discontinue Baby M's breastfeeding because the fluid content of breast milk is deficient for a neonate undergoing phototherapy.
    d. Prevent hypothermia, hyperthermia, or both in Baby M.

15. Baby M's mother is crying, expresses fear about her infant's health, and does not want to leave. Which intervention would be the least effective?
    a. Encourage the mother to come in to feed her infant as often as possible.

b. Emphasize the temporary nature of hyperbilirubinemia, and explain the monitoring of Baby M's bilirubin levels.

c. Remind the mother that newborns require demanding care, which is very fatiguing to a new mother, and that she should take this added opportunity to rest and recover.

ANSWERS TO STUDY QUESTIONS

1. a	5. d	9. d	13. b
2. c	6. d	10. a	14. d
3. e	7. True	11. b	15. c
4. e	8. b	12. d	

REFERENCES

Adhikari, M., Gouws, E., Velaphi, S.C., & Gwamanda, P. (1998). Meconium aspiration syndrome: Importance of the monitoring of labor. *Journal of Perinatology, 18*(1), 55-60.

Bae, C.W., Takahashi, A., Chida, S., & Sasaki, M. (1998). Morphology and function of pulmonary surfactant inhibited by meconium, *Pediatric Research, 44*(2), 187-199.

Berry, B.E. (2002). Assessing tissue oxygenation. *Critical Care Nurse, 22*(3), 22-42.

Bhutani, V.K., Gourley, G.R., Adler, S., Kreamer, B., Dalen, C., & Johnson, L.H. (2000). Noninvasive measurement of total serum bilirubin in a multiracial predischarge newborn population to assess the risk of severe hyperbilirubinemia. *Pediatrics, 106*(2), E17.

Bhutani, V.K., Johnson, L.H., & Sivieri, E. (1999). Ability of pre-discharge hour-specific serum bilirubin for subsequent significant hyperbilirubinemia in healthy term and near term infants. *Pediatrics, 103*(1), 6-14.

Dai, J., Parry, D., & Krahn, J. (1997). Transcutaneous bilirubinometry: Its role in the assessment of neonatal jaundice. *Clinical Biochemistry, 30*(1), 1-9.

Dixit, R., & Gartner, L. (2000). The jaundiced newborn: Minimizing the risks. *Patient Care, 34,* 45-69.

Gibson, A.T. (2002). Perinatal corticosteroids and the developing lung. *Paediatric Respiratory Reviews, 3*(1), 70-76.

Gracey, K., Talbot, D., Lankford, R., & Dodge, P. (2002). The changing face of bronchopulmonary dysplasia: Part 1. *Advances in Neonatal Care, 2*(6), 327-338.

Greenough, A. (2000). Expanded use of surfactant therapy. *European Journal of Pediatrics, 159*(9), 635-640.

Haimi-Cohen, Y., Merlob, P., Davidovitz, M., & Eisenstein, B. (1997). Renal function in full-term neonates with hyperbilirubinemia. *Journal of Perinatology, 17*(3), 225-227.

Halamek, L.P., & Stevenson, D.K. (1998). Kernicteric findings at autopsy in two sick near-term infants. *Pediatrics, 101*(1, Pt 1), 158-159.

Hammond, B. (2000). Physiology and physical adaptation of the newborn. In D. Lowdermilk, S. Perry, and I. Bobak (Eds.), *Maternity & women's health care* (7th ed., pp. 671-715). St. Louis: Mosby.

Hammond B., & Perry, S. (2000). Assessment of the newborn. In D. Lowdermilk, S. Perry, and I. Bobak (Eds.), *Maternity & women's health care* (7th ed., pp. 716-756). St. Louis: Mosby.

Hansen, T., & Corbet, A. (1998). Lung development and function. In H.W. Taeusch & R.A. Ballard (Eds.), *Avery's diseases of the newborn* (7th ed., pp. 541-551). Philadelphia: Saunders.

Hicks, M. (1995). A systematic approach to neonatal pathophysiology: Understanding respiratory distress syndrome. *Neonatal Network, 12*(8), 9-15.

Jones, M. (1990). A physiologic approach to identifying neonates at risk for kernicterus. *Journal of Obstetric, Gynecologic, and Neonatal Nursing, 19*(4), 313-318.

Klaus, M.H., & Fanaroff, A.A. (2001). *Care of the high-risk neonate* (5th ed.). Philadelphia: Saunders.

Korones, S.B., & Bada-Ellzey, H.S. (1993). *Neonatal decision making.* St. Louis: Mosby.

Lawrence, R.A, & Lawrence, R.M. (1999). *Breastfeeding: A guide for the medical profession* (5th ed.). St. Louis: Mosby.

Linder, N., Regev, A., Gazit, G., Carplus, M., Mandelberg, A., Tamir, I., et al. (1994). Noninvasive determination of neonatal hyperbilirubinemia: Standardization for variation in skin color. *American Journal of Perinatology, 11*(3), 223-225.

Liu, W.F., & Harrington, T. (2002). Delivery room risk factors for meconium aspiration syndrome. *American Journal of Perinatology, 19*(7), 367-378.

Parmigiani, S., Panza, C., & Bevilacqua, G. (1997). Evolution of respiratory mechanics in preterm infants after surfactant administration in the neonatal period. *Supplemento di Acta Bio-Medica de, 68,* 65-73.

Pierce, J., Gaudier, F.L., & Sanchez-Ramos, L. (2000). Intrapartum infusion for meconium-stained fluid: Meta-analysis of prospective clinical trials. *Obstetrics and Gynecology 95*(6, Pt 2), 1051-1056.

Plavka, R., Kopecky, P., Sebron, V., Leiska, A., Svihovec, P., Ruffer, J., et al. (2002). Early versus delayed surfactant administration in extremely premature neonates with respiratory distress syndrome ventilated by high-frequency oscillatory ventilation. *Intensive Care Medicine, 28*(10), 1483-1490.

Quinn, G.E. (1998). Retinopathy of prematurity. In H.W. Taeusch & R.A. Ballard (Eds.), *Avery's diseases of the newborn* (7th ed., pp. 1329-1342). Philadelphia: Saunders.

Reiser, D.J. (2001). *Hyperbilirubinemia: Identification and management in healthy term and near term newborns.* Chicago: Association of Women's Health, Obstetrical and Neonatal Nurses.

Rizzo, C., Nisini, R., & Marzetti, G. (2002). Respiratory distress syndrome in near-term infants. *Journal of Maternal, Fetal, and Neonatal Medicine, 11*(5), 350-351.

Sahni, R., Schulze, K.F., Kashyap, S., Ohira-Kist, K., Myers, M.M., & Fifer, W.P. (1999). Body position, sleep states, and cardiorespiratory activity in developing low birth weight infants. *Early Human Development, 54*(3), 197-206.

Siegel, R., Gardner, S.L., & Merenstein, G.B. (2002). Families in crisis: Theoretical and practical considerations. In G.B. Merenstein & S.L. Gardner (Eds.), *Handbook of neonatal intensive care* (5th ed., pp. 725-753). St. Louis: Mosby.

Torres-Torres, M., Tayaba, R., Weintraub, A., & Holzman, I. (1994). New perspectives on neonatal hyperbilirubinemia. *Mt Sinai Journal of Medicine, 61*(5), 424-428.

Volpe, J.J. (2001). *Neurology of the Newborn* (4th ed.). Philadelphia: Saunders.

Whitsett, J.A., Pryhuber, G.S., Rice, W.R., Warner, B.B., & Wert, S.E. (1999). Acute respiratory disorders. In G.B. Avery, M.A. Fletcher, & M.G. MacDonald (Eds.), *Neonatology: Pathophysiology and management of the newborn* (5th ed., pp. 485-508). Philadelphia: Lippincott.

Wiswell, T.E., Gannon, C.M., Jacob, J., Goldsmith, L., Szyld, E., Weiss, K., et al. (2000). Delivery room management of the apparently vigourous meconium-stained neonate: Results of the multi-center international collaborative trial. *Pediatrics, 105*(1, Pt 1), 1-7.

Yao, T., & Stevenson, D. (1995). Advances in the diagnosis and treatment of neonatal hyperbilirubinemia. *Clinical Perinatology, 22*(3), 741-758.

Youngmee, A., & Yonghoon, J. (2003). The effects of the shallow and the deep endotracheal suctioning on oxygen saturation and heart rate in high-risk infants. *International Journal of Nursing Studies, 40*(2), 97-104.

COMPLICATIONS OF CHILDBEARING

Intimate Partner Violence

SUSAN MATTSON

OBJECTIVES

1. Discuss the prevalence of violence against women in the United States.
2. Describe the cycle of violence, and differentiate between the various phases.
3. List behaviors of the abuser in each of the phases of the violence cycle.
4. Identify the types of physical injuries that battered women sustain, and discuss how pregnancy alters the body parts targeted by the abuser.
5. Discuss the psychologic injuries that battered women sustain.
6. Identify how cultural differences and socioeconomic status influence the prevalence of intimate partner violence (IPV) in the United States.
7. Describe common characteristics of men who are abusers and of women who are victims of abuse.
8. Recognize key elements to be included in the assessment of all women and additional data to be collected from a woman at high risk for abuse.
9. List physical, psychologic, and nonverbal findings in a woman that are consistent with abuse in her relationship.
10. Describe and discuss primary, secondary, and tertiary intervention strategies used to provide care to abused women.
11. Design a plan of care that maximizes the abused woman's ability to protect herself and her children and to make informed decisions on which she can act.
12. Identify resources and referrals that are available for victims of IPV.

INTRODUCTION

A. Intimate partner violence (IPV), family violence, battering, and spousal abuse are all terms used to describe a pattern of assaultive and coercive behaviors that include some or all of the following:
   1. Physical attack
   2. Sexual assault
   3. Psychologic attack
   4. Economic coercion (Rynerson, 1997)
B. The true incidence of IPV perpetrated against women in the United States is unknown because a large amount of it remains undetected and unreported.
   1. The mandatory reporting mechanism that detects the extent of child abuse does not exist in every state for the abuse of women (King et al., 1993).
   2. IPV is, however, considered a felony in all states.
   3. Battered women account for up to 35% of all women seeking care, for any reason, in an emergency room.
   4. Battered women account for 19% to 30% of all injured women seen in emergency departments (American College of Obstetricians and Gynecologists [ACOG], 1995).

5. Each year, 14% to 25% of women using primary care clinics report being physically assaulted by their partners (Rodriguez, 1994).
6. IPV has been recognized as a health problem of major proportions in the United States and Canada.
    a. In the United States, estimates are that 1.9 million women are assaulted annually by an intimate partner (Tjadin & Thoennes, 2000; Rynerson, 2000).
    b. In Canada, 3 of every 10 women have suffered assault in a current or previous marital relationship (Statistics Canada, 1993).
    c. Each year, more than 500,000 women injured as a result of IPV require medical treatment (Tjaden & Thoennes, 2000).
C. **Estimates of IPV during pregnancy vary widely.**
    1. Abuse of women is possibly the most common form of IPV occurring during the perinatal period (King et al., 1993).
    2. Parker, McFarlane, Soeken, Torres, and Campbell (1993) estimate that 40% to 60% of abused women are injured while pregnant; these numbers may be increasing (Rynerson, 2000); as many as 324,000 women each year experience IPV during a pregnancy (Gazmararian et al., 2000).
    3. Violence may induce preterm birth and may result in injury and even death for the fetus (Curry, 1998).
D. **The abuse often begins or escalates during pregnancy.**
    1. Many chronically abused women report an increase in violence directed at them during pregnancy.
    2. The specific types of injury inflicted on women tend to change during pregnancy; they are more likely to have multiple sites of injury and to be struck on the abdomen, leading to blunt trauma to the fetus.
E. **Cycle of violence**
    1. Pioneer research about abuse of women was conducted by Lenore Walker in 1979 (Walker, 1982).
        a. Her research gave detailed accounts of women's abuse and how the abuse progressed in a relationship.
        b. She discovered a cyclic pattern of progression of abuse in female-male relationships that is now identified as the cycle of violence (Figure 20-1).
    2. Battering behavior exhibits a three-phase cyclic pattern.
        a. Phase I is characterized as a period of increasing tension in the batterer, marked by the following behaviors:
            (1) Increased anger directed toward the woman
            (2) Increased blame attributed to the woman
            (3) Escalated arguments with the woman
        b. Phase II is the acute battering incident in which the batterer demonstrates an uncontrollable discharge of the built-up tension.
            (1) This phase can last from a few minutes to hours, sometimes even to several days.
            (2) Physical battering behaviors are as follows:
                (a) Slapping
                (b) Pinching
                (c) Kicking
                (d) Punching
                (e) Choking
                (f) Stomping
                (g) Pushing
                (h) Biting

Cycle of Violence

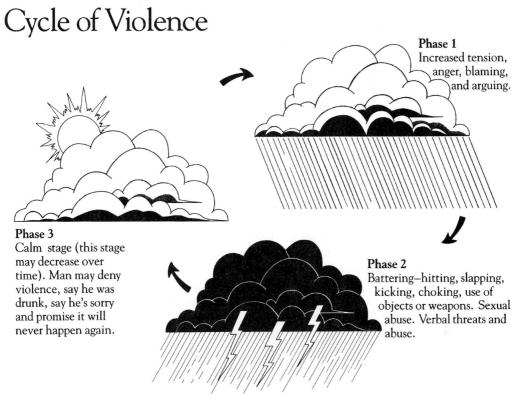

Phase 1
Increased tension, anger, blaming, and arguing.

Phase 3
Calm stage (this stage may decrease over time). Man may deny violence, say he was drunk, say he's sorry and promise it will never happen again.

Phase 2
Battering–hitting, slapping, kicking, choking, use of objects or weapons. Sexual abuse. Verbal threats and abuse.

FIGURE 20-1 ■ March of Dimes brochure on preventing battering during pregnancy. (Developed under a March of Dimes Birth Defects Foundation grant at Texas Woman's University, Houston.)

    (i) Throwing the woman across a room or up against a wall
    (j) Bone fracturing
    (k) Mutilating with objects such as knives, broken glass, razor blades, and tools
    (l) Burning with objects such as an iron, scalding liquids, cigarettes, or caustic substances
    (m) Shooting with a gun
    (n) Sexually abusing or mutilating
  (3) Psychologic battering behaviors are as follows:
    (a) Threats
    (b) Intimidation
    (c) Name calling
    (d) Destroying things of value to the woman
    (e) Destroying her personal belongings
    (f) Throwing her things out the door or window
    (g) Humiliation
    (h) Derogatory remarks
    (i) Verbal "put downs"
    (j) Remarks intended to decrease her self-esteem
    (k) Remarks to make her doubt her worth, her abilities, and her decision making
    (l) Taking away "privileges" normally afforded to adults and conditionally granting permission to temporarily get them back

    (m) Isolating her from family, friends, and adult contacts

    (n) Treating her as a child

   (4) The batterer frequently justifies his battering behaviors by stating that the purpose is to teach the woman a lesson.

   (5) Most injuries are to the woman's face, arms, and buttocks.

  c. Phase III is the calm stage; also called the honeymoon stage.

   (1) The batterer is usually remorseful and profusely apologetic.

   (2) He may shower her with gifts.

   (3) He solemnly promises that the abuse will never happen again.

   (4) He may deny or minimize the violence that occurred in phase II.

   (5) He promises the woman that everything will be different from this time on.

   (6) He may profess his intense love for her.

  d. The behaviors exhibited in phase III of the cycle of violence offer the woman hope and powerful, positive reinforcement for staying in the relationship.

   (1) This restores the woman's hope that he will change.

   (2) She has a tendency to deny the inevitable recurrence of the abuse.

F. Types of injuries

 1. Physical injuries to a battered woman may include the following:

  a. Bruises and abrasions

  b. Hematomas, particularly periorbital

  c. Bites

  d. Broken teeth

  e. Lacerations, particularly around the mouth, lips, eyes, and other parts of the face

  f. Perforation of the tympanic membrane

  g. Scalp lacerations, hematomas, tufts of hair missing

  h. Fractured ribs

  i. Fractured limbs

  j. Fractured nose

  k. Concussion

  l. Stab wounds

  m. Gun shot wounds

  n. Death

 2. Battered women report an increased prevalence of gastrointestinal disorders, sleep disorders, and chronic pain disorders (Rodriguez, 1994).

 3. Psychologic injuries to a battered woman may include the following:

  a. Anxiety and increased fear

  b. Insomnia

  c. Lethargy

  d. Feelings of helplessness and hopelessness

  e. Severe mood swings

  f. Panic attacks

  g. Night terrors

  h. Depression

  i. Posttraumatic stress syndrome

  j. Self-abuse

   (1) Alcoholism; initiated after the start of IPV

   (2) Drug abuse; initiated after the start of IPV

   (3) Eating disorders

  k. Diminished self-esteem

  l. Suicide attempts

G. Cultural and socioeconomic differences
  1. Violence against women cuts across all socioeconomic and ethnic lines (Rodriguez, 1994).
  2. Poverty and oppression are significant factors in the prevalence of violent behavior; the following factors have been associated with a higher incidence of IPV:
     a. Low income with subsequent stress
     b. Limited resources of all kinds
     c. Unemployment
     d. Low-prestige jobs
  3. The meaning of violence in various cultures is difficult to determine because cultures vary in their perceptions and definitions of abuse (Hanrahan, Campbell, & Ulrich, 1993; Mattson & Rodriguez, 1999).
  4. Minority women, in general, are less likely to use shelters and more likely to use the health care system combined with support from family and friends (Noel & Yam, 1992).
  5. Cultural influences on awareness of abuse
     a. Black American
        (1) No convincing evidence has been found that greater violence against women exists among this group; however, women are more likely to report violence when it does occur.
        (2) Men are more likely to be psychologically, socially, and economically oppressed.
        (3) IPV may occur as a result of anger from social stresses and limited resources (Rynerson, 1997).
        (4) The risk of abuse is thought to be highest when the woman has more education than the man, or when he is unemployed, has difficulty keeping a job, or both: a familiar scene with many black families (Barnes, 1999).
     b. Hispanic
        (1) Families tend to be hierarchical, with authority given to men.
        (2) Generally, sex roles are clearly defined.
        (3) Mexican-American women perceive fewer types of behavior as being abusive (Torrés, 1991).
        (4) Women typically seek health care from their families first and are not likely to seek assistance from professionals.
        (5) Through religious and cultural images, Hispanic women often believe abuse is the "lot in life to suffer"; they are defined by their family roles, and their primary obligation is to preserve the family at all costs (Flores-Ortiz, 1993; Mattson & Rodriguez, 1999).
        (6) The culture is viewed as an oppressed group, and access to health care can be very limited (Rynerson, 1997; Suarez & Ramirez, 1999).
     c. Native American
        (1) Reported prevalence rates for battering of women are high (Rynerson, 1997); however, cruelty to women and children continues to be viewed as a social disgrace (Green, 1996).
        (2) Social oppression, poverty, limited resources, isolation, and disenfranchisement are thought to be significant factors in the prevalence of violence within Native-American families (Rynerson, 1997).
        (3) Many communities in Canada have recently developed programs specifically designed to address family violence and facilitate healing at individual, family, and community levels (Green, 1996).

(4) Abuse within the culture is traditionally handled within the family; thus the abused woman may be reluctant to seek outside help because it would shame her with both families; variables to be considered in a discussion of options include the woman's social support system, her cultural value system, and her financial status (Lauderdale, 2003).

H. Characteristics of abusers

1. The progression of aggression continuum (O'Leary, 1993)
   a. Verbal aggression, such as yelling and name calling
   b. Followed by lesser forms of physical aggression, such as pushing and slapping
   c. Followed by true violent behavior, such as punching and beating
   d. In extreme situations, continuum ends with murder.

2. Intergenerational transmission of violence
   a. Both abuser and woman generally learn about IPV in their family of origin.
      (1) Approximately 30% of abused children become abusers as adults; exposure to violence in the home is predictive of a child's violent behavior.
      (2) Most abusers report childhood memories of harsh physical punishment as a means of discipline (Rynerson, 1997).
   b. Women typically have a history of having been beaten as a child (ACOG, 1995).
   c. An acceptable awareness is—as a child in a violent family—that people who love each other can be violent.
   d. Children who witness parental violence are especially susceptible to psychologic and social consequences with lifelong impact, including:
      (1) Posttraumatic stress disorders
      (2) Depressive disorders
      (3) Attention-deficit hyperactive disorder
      (4) Irritability, aggression, and quickness to anger
      (5) Boys are more likely to act out; girls are more likely to internalize (Ruiz & Mattson, 2003).
   e. Some research suggests that exposure of very young children to violence alters central nervous system development, predisposing the child to more impulsive, reactive, and violent behavior (Ruiz & Mattson, 2003).

3. Family structure can shape the attitude toward IPV.
   a. Gender inequality with ascribed gender roles
      (1) A woman's place is in the home.
      (2) A woman is dependent on a man as provider and protector.
   b. Power and violence serve to maintain a patriarchal view that gives authority to men.

4. Possible causes of aggression in an abuser (O'Leary, 1993)
   a. Verbal aggression
      (1) Need to control (Figure 20-2)
      (2) Misuse of power
      (3) Jealousy
      (4) Relationship discord
   b. Physical aggression
      (1) Violence an acceptable means to use to remain in complete control of the relationship
      (2) Modeling of violent behavior seen or experienced as a child
      (3) Alcohol abuse, drug abuse, or both

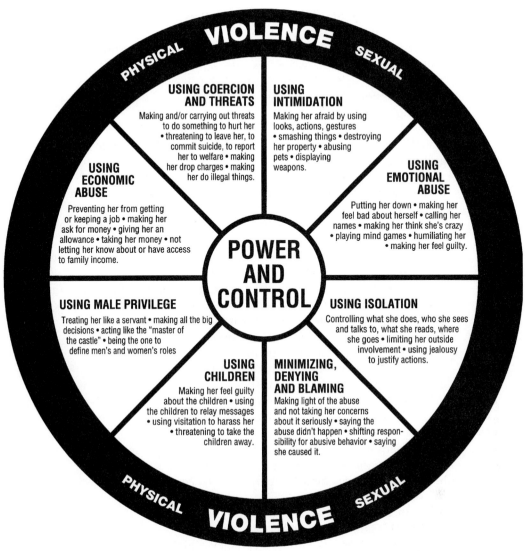

FIGURE 20-2 ■ "Power and Control" wheel. (From Domestic Abuse Intervention Project, 206 West Fourth St., Duluth, Minnesota 55806.)

    c. Severe physical aggression
        (1) Severe personality disorder
        (2) Emotional lability
        (3) Poor self-esteem with a fragile sense of self
        (4) Aggressive personality
    d. Fear of abandonment a common trait among abusers
I. Characteristics of women in battering relationships
    1. A battered woman frequently accepts blame and responsibility for the violence.
    2. She believes she is not a "good enough" wife or partner in the relationship.
    3. She believes she needs to try harder to please her abuser.
    4. She exhibits a blend of loyalty, fear, terror, and learned helplessness.

5. Most battered women have a very low self-esteem and fear societal rejection if they reveal the abuse.
6. Battered women seem to demonstrate a high level of traditional feminine traits, which are as follows:
   a. Nurturing
   b. Compassion
   c. Sympathy
   d. Yielding
7. Abused women who are more likely to seek help are divided into three groups (Rynerson, 1997):
   a. Women who are beaten frequently and severely
   b. Women who have not experienced or witnessed family violence in their family of origin
   c. Women who can see an alternative to life in their abusive relationships
J. **IPV during pregnancy**
   1. Pregnancy is often the trigger for the beginning or escalation of violence in a relationship.
      a. Stresses of pregnancy may strain a troubled relationship beyond normal coping abilities.
      b. The abuser may harbor jealousy of the fetus.
         (1) Resents intrusion into the relationship.
         (2) Resents the woman's attention to the fetus.
      c. Physical violence may be an attempt to end the pregnancy.
      d. A pregnant woman who is battered is unlikely to have strong social support on which she can rely (Christian, 1995).
   2. The body parts targeted for abuse tend to change when pregnancy is present.
      a. Pregnant women are likely to have more multiple injury sites than nonpregnant women (King et al., 1993).
      b. Physical abuse is directed to the breasts, genitalia, and especially to the abdomen.
      c. An increase in sexual assault is common.
      d. Risk of injury to the fetus is very high.
   3. When battering occurs during pregnancy, a high risk exists of the following sequelae:
      a. Continued battering after the birth
      b. Child abuse
   4. Pregnancy presents a unique opportunity for health care providers to recognize abuse and to appropriately intervene.

CLINICAL PRACTICE

A. **Assessment**
   1. The first task is for providers to examine their own feelings and beliefs about abuse, which may be difficult.
      a. Physical abuse has long been minimized by the public.
      b. The media portray violence in music, magazines, videos, and films.
      c. Many people believe that IPV is a private affair and should be worked out by the couple.
      d. Many people believe that abuse is justified in certain circumstances.
      e. To effectively ask women about abuse, the care provider must believe that IPV is a serious health problem.

2. History of abuse can be obtained from a chart or from the woman.
   a. Approach the topic of assessment by telling the woman that all women are screened for abuse.
   b. If she hesitates when asked to answer *yes* or *no,* offer her the choice of *sometimes.*
   c. Do not pressure her to respond to the abuse questions; she will choose when and where to share her history.
   d. Look for the following indicators:
      (1) Previous assault; a man who abuses a woman before pregnancy is likely to continue the abuse during pregnancy.
      (2) Injuries inflicted by weapons; look for scars from blunt traumas, as well as weapon wounds.
      (3) Injuries consistent with assault that are inadequately explained, which may include bruises to the upper arm, neck, and face; breast and genital mutilation; mouth and dental trauma; teeth marks; burns; clumps of hair missing; bruises on the pregnant abdomen; and history of broken bones, especially arms and nose
      (4) Multiple medical visits for injuries or anxiety symptoms; look for repeated visits for somatic complaints, including headaches, insomnia, back, chest or pelvic pain, or choking sensation.
      (5) History of depression, substance use, and suicide attempts by the woman or her male partner
         (a) Many violent episodes involve the use of alcohol or drugs by the abuser.
         (b) Abused women may use alcohol and drugs to cope with the abuse.
         (c) Both abuser and abused have a higher incidence of suicide attempts.
      (6) Eating disorders
      (7) Tranquilizer or sedative use
      (8) Complications of previous pregnancies, which include:
         (a) Spontaneous abortions
         (b) First- or second-trimester bleeding
         (c) Poor weight gain
         (d) Preterm labor or birth
         (e) Low birth weight
         (f) Abruptio placentae
      (9) Late or inadequate prenatal care; abused women are twice as likely as nonabused women to delay entry into prenatal care.
      (10) Sexually transmitted diseases, pelvic inflammatory disease, or both
      (11) Change in appointment pattern
         (a) Appointments that are missed
         (b) Increase in appointments for vague, but often somatic, complaints (McFarlane & Parker, 1995)
      (12) Reports of pet abuse
         (a) Abuse of women's pets, children's pets, or both may occur as a method of "keeping them in line."
         (b) Some women will not seek help because they worry about leaving pets behind.
3. Physical findings and observations that may indicate abuse:
   a. Early signs of abuse take many forms and may be considered warning signs.

(1) Partner is overly possessive and jealous.
(2) Partner is threatened by the woman's success or by her pregnancy.
(3) Partner is cruel and violent in other relationships.
(4) Partner may enjoy teasing or scaring the woman.
(5) Partner may be impatient or rough with the woman.
  b. Look for the following indicators:
(1) Injuries consistent with assault that are inadequately explained (see earlier discussion for assault-like injuries)
(2) Painful vaginal examination; women with a history of child or sexual abuse may experience difficulty, including pain and tenseness.
(3) Anxious behaviors
  (a) Crying
  (b) Sighing
  (c) Minimizing statements
  (d) Searching and engaging eye contact (fear)
  (e) No eye contact (not applicable in certain cultures)
  (f) Inappropriate laughing, giggling, or both
(4) Comments about emotional abuse
(5) Comments about a "friend" who is abused
(6) Woman's behavior in presence of her male partner
  (a) The woman may obviously be afraid of him.
  (b) She defers to him.
  (c) She checks out her responses with him.
(7) Partner's behavior in presence of the woman
  (a) He may hover and be very unwilling to leave her unattended.
  (b) He may speak for her.
  (c) He may make derogatory comments about her appearance and behavior.
  (d) He is anxious and wants to minimize the woman's time with the care provider (McFarlane & Parker, 1995).
B. Nursing Diagnoses
1. Risk for maternal and fetal injury related to physical abuse
2. Deficient knowledge related to lack of information regarding options for services and legal protection
3. Ineffective individual coping related to physical abuse (Bayer & Fein, 1997)
C. Interventions/Outcomes
The overall goal is that the mother and fetus do not suffer injury; thus the interventions are directed at acknowledging the abuse (assessment screening), ensuring the woman's and the fetus's safety (information concerning protection), and empowering the woman to make changes (increase her coping skills); assessing for abuse carries the responsibility for intervention after a positive response; at a minimum, all agencies should have referral sources available, as well as information on available legal options; in working with abused women, the nurse must be aware of state reporting procedures and be available to assist the woman in filing a report if she so requests.
1. Primary prevention includes assessing all women for potential or actual abuse.
  a. This intervention should occur at the first contact with the health care delivery system (i.e., prenatal care, labor and delivery suite, emergency room).
  b. Assessment for abuse at each visit is important.

   (1) Because of guilt, shame, embarrassment, and fear, some abused
       women deny the abuse during the initial assessment, but later the
       woman may feel comfortable in sharing the information.
   (2) Some abuse may not occur until the second or third trimester.
  c. A suitable atmosphere of quiet, privacy, and trust should be created for
     this questioning, away from the partner, whose presence might endanger
     the woman.
   (1) Assure her that her disclosure is confidential.
   (2) All states do not have mandatory reporting laws; if in a state that
       does not, inform her that the legal authorities will not be notified
       unless she wishes it.
  d. Ask specific, nonjudgmental, open-ended questions that encourage the
     woman to disclose abuse and yet do not label her as an "abused woman."
   (1) The questions should reflect the full spectrum of abuse.
   (2) Questions should be concrete and direct (King et al., 1993).
  e. An abuse assessment screen has been developed by the Nursing Research
     Consortium on Violence and Abuse (McFarlane & Parker, 1995) and
     addresses the following three questions:
   (1) Within the last year, have you been hit, slapped, kicked, or otherwise
       physically hurt by someone? If *yes*, by whom?
   (2) Since you've been pregnant, have you been hit, slapped, kicked, or
       otherwise physically hurt by someone? If *yes*, by whom?
   (3) Within the last year, have you been forced by anyone to have sexual
       activities? If *yes*, by whom?
  f. Prefacing the assessment by comments can convey the message that the
     nurse cares about a woman who is abused and is prepared to help her;
     examples of comments are as follows:
   (1) "Many women experience abuse."
   (2) "You are not alone."
   (3) "Sometimes abuse happens for the first time during pregnancy."
  g. An essential intervention for all abused women is assessing for their
     safety, including the safety of the woman, her infant and other children,
     and family members.
   (1) Asking directly about whether she feels safe is crucial; abused women
       can judge their own safety.
   (2) The Danger Assessment tool can be used to help the woman
       determine the danger she and others may be in (King et al., 1993)
       (Figure 20-3).
   (3) If a woman's safety is in question, this concern should be shared with
       her.
     (a) Desired assistance should be provided.
     (b) An important point to keep in mind is that a woman is in most
         danger of homicide when she leaves her partner or makes it clear
         that the relationship is ending (Parker, 1993).
   (4) Women should also be assessed for thoughts of suicide.
2. After the woman has told her story of abuse, it is important to validate her
   experience and empower her to discuss her options and decisions.
  a. Her decision may or may not be to leave the abuser; only she knows
     when it is feasible or safe.
  b. Secondary intervention should be aimed at assisting the woman in
     choosing what is best for her from many options.
  c. A crucial intervention is helping abused women mobilize social support.

Danger Assessment

Several risk factors have been associated with homicides (murder) of both batterers and battered women in research that has been conducted after the killings have taken place. We cannot predict what will happen in your case, but we would like you to be aware of the danger of homicide in situations of severe battering and for you to see how many of the risk factors apply to your situation. (The "he" in the question refers to your husband, partner, ex-husband, ex-partner, or whoever is currently physically hurting you.)

Please check YES or NO for each question below.

YES	NO	
_____	_____	1. Has the physical violence increased in frequency over the past year?
_____	_____	2. Has the physical violence increased in severity over the past year and/or has a weapon or threat with a weapon been used?
_____	_____	3. Does he ever try to choke you?
_____	_____	4. Is there a gun in the house?
_____	_____	5. Has he ever forced you into sex when you did not wish to do so?
_____	_____	6. Does he use drugs? By drugs I mean "uppers" or amphetamines, speed, angel dust, cocaine, "crack," street drugs, heroin, or mixtures.
_____	_____	7. Does he threaten to kill you and/or do you believe he is capable of killing you?
_____	_____	8. Is he drunk every day or almost every day? (In terms of quantity of alcohol.)
_____	_____	9. Does he control most of all your daily activities? For instance, does he tell you whom you can be friends with, how much money you can take with you shopping, or when you can take the car?
		(If he tries, but you do not let him, check here _____.)
_____	_____	10. Have you ever been beaten by him while you were pregnant?
		(If never pregnant by him, check here _____.)
_____	_____	11. Is he violently and constantly jealous of you?
		(For instance, does he say, "If I can't have you, no one can.")
_____	_____	12. Have you ever threatened or tried to commit suicide?
_____	_____	13. Has he ever threatened or tried to commit suicide?
_____	_____	14. Is he violent outside of the home?

_____ **TOTAL YES ANSWERS**

THANK YOU. PLEASE TALK TO YOUR NURSE, ADVOCATE, OR
COUNSELOR ABOUT WHAT THE DANGER ASSESSMENT
MEANS IN TERMS OF YOUR SITUATION.

FIGURE 20-3 ■ March of Dimes "Danger Assessment" questionnaire. (From Campbell, J. [1986]. Nursing assessment for risk of homicide with battered women. *Advances in Nursing Science, 8*[4], 36-51.)

(1) Identify other friends or relatives that might have been in a similar situation or who may be willing to help.
(2) Referrals can be made to local shelters, battered women's organizations, and legal advocacy resources (see Resources for Professionals).

    d. Another intervention is to provide adequate documentation of the abuse in the medical records.

      (1) The record should show that the woman revealed that she was abused by her partner and sought help.

      (2) The record should include the relationship of the abuser to the woman and detail the specifics of the emotional, sexual, or physical abuse.

      (3) Injuries should be explicitly described, with photographs if appropriate; a body map can be used to sketch the location of old and new injuries.

3. Tertiary intervention means assisting the abused woman in making long-term plans for her life.

    a. Constant support and intervention, coupled with advocacy by shelter staff or formerly battered women, are most effective in mobilizing a woman's resources.

    b. When a woman is ready to leave the relationship, she needs affirmation of her choice and encouragement in her independence; she should have the following available:

      (1) Telephone numbers for a shelter and the police

      (2) Plan for quick escape

      (3) Packed bag with keys, money, and important papers (see Health Education for a safety plan)

    c. Women experiencing repeated abuse may feel emotionally unstable and depressed and harbor feelings of low self-esteem.

      (1) Nurses can advocate for individual or group counseling to help women address these reactions.

      (2) Nurses can help women strengthen their emotional health while learning new coping strategies.

    d. It is important to ensure continued health care for the woman and her infant, as well as her other children.

HEALTH EDUCATION

A. The top priority of health education is to emphasize safety for the abused woman, her fetus, and her other children whether she decides to leave or to stay in the relationship; she should have the following items immediately ready for use at any time:

1. Domestic Violence Hot Line: (800) 572-SAFE

2. Safety plan

    a. Hide money.

    b. Hide extra set of house and car keys.

    c. Establish code with family and friends.

    d. Ask neighbor to call police if violence begins.

    e. Remove weapons.

    f. Have the following documents available:

      (1) Social security numbers (his, hers, children's)

      (2) Rent and utility receipts

      (3) Birth certificates (hers and children's)

      (4) Driver's license

      (5) Bank account numbers

      (6) Insurance policies and numbers

      (7) Marriage license

    g. Have prescription drugs and refill numbers for her and children.
    h. Have valuable jewelry and keepsakes.
    i. Have important telephone numbers.
    j. Hide bag with extra clothing.
B. Women need to be educated that abuse of any kind is a violation of their basic human rights.
    1. They need to know how to access protective services.
    2. They also need to know how to access affordable legal services.
C. Educate the woman about the cycle of violence and how to recognize signs of escalating danger.
D. Provide referrals for support services to empower the battered woman.
E. Encourage the woman to consider the following:
    1. Self-defense courses
    2. Assertiveness courses
    3. Self-help groups
    4. Educational or skills development courses

RESOURCES FOR PROFESSIONALS

Health Resource Center on Domestic Violence: Technical assistance to individuals or organizations setting up IPV training programs or developing IPV protocols; provides assistance in how to respond to IPV in a safe and effective manner; (800) 313-1310

National Directory of Shelters: National listing of shelters, safe homes, and community programs; (303) 839-1852
Prepared program for educating health professionals about intimate partner violence; AWHONN; (800) 673-8499; *www.awhonn.org*

CASE STUDY AND STUDY QUESTIONS

Ms. S is 20 years of age, unmarried, and 6 months pregnant. She lives with her boyfriend, Mr. K, who is also 20 years of age and is the father of her unborn infant. Mr. K works at a local restaurant where he washes dishes. Ms. S does not work, and their income is very limited. She has come to the clinic for her first prenatal visit. Mr. K is with her and says he wants to stay with her throughout the visit.

1. Ms. S is late in seeking prenatal care. This is one of the indicators of potential abuse for which of the following reasons?
  a. She may not value her unborn child.
  b. She may not have realized that she should seek early prenatal care.
  c. She may have been trying to conceal signs of abuse before this visit.
  d. She did not want her family to know she was pregnant.

2. Mr. K has some potential indicators of an abuser, which include all of the following except:
  a. His young age
  b. His low-paying job
  c. His constant presence during her clinic visit
  d. He is not her husband

Mr. K leaves the room briefly to go to the bathroom. When asked about her relationship with Mr. K, Ms. S says that it is good most of the time. She says he has a bad temper and sometimes gets very mad at her. She says it is usually over some dumb thing she has done or said, so she deserves it. She said she thinks she just needs to try harder not to do and say those things anymore.

3. Her response is typical of abused women because they frequently:
    a. Cannot admit to others that abuse is taking place
    b. Take the blame for invoking the abuse
    c. Are trying harder to be a better partner or wife to the abuser
    d. All of the above

4. Ms. S 's pregnancy is high risk because of late prenatal care. If physically abused, what added risk occurs?
    a. Fetus might have a genetic disorder.
    b. Gestational diabetes
    c. Polyhydramnios
    d. Fetus might be physically injured.

Ms. S returned to the clinic 2 weeks later for a scheduled ultrasound examination. Mr. K was unable to be with her. He insisted that she reschedule her appointment, but she did not. She was anxious to find out the sex of the infant. Exposure of her abdomen revealed several bruises, all in various states of healing. She tried to explain the presence of the bruises as merely the result of her clumsiness. With further questioning, she broke down in tears and admitted that Mr. K slapped her, pulled her by her hair, kicked her, and hit her in the stomach. He was extremely mad that she did not reschedule the appointment. She said that she had sure learned her lesson and would never do that again. She also said he is all over it now and has been wonderfully sweet to her. He promised to never do that again.

5. Mr. K 's actions are examples of all of the phases of:
    a. The circle of abuse
    b. The cycle of violence
    c. The abuser-abuse-victim syndrome
    d. The abuse, cover-up, make-up theory

6. The abuser typically tries to minimize the acute abuse episode. This was evident when Ms. S said:
    a. He is all over it now.
    b. He has been wonderfully sweet to her.
    c. She sure learned her lesson.
    d. He promised never to do that again.

7. The abdominal trauma she endured is:
    a. Not dangerous to the fetus because labor did not start and no vaginal bleeding occurred
    b. A typical target for the physical abuse of a pregnant woman
    c. Usually harmless because of the amniotic sac and fluid
    d. Less painful for a woman who is pregnant because of the extra cushioning for her vital organs

ANSWERS TO STUDY QUESTIONS

1. c	3. d	5. b	7. b
2. a	4. d	6. c	

REFERENCES

American College of Obstetricians and Gynecologists. (1995). *Technical bulletin on domestic violence* (No. 209). Washington, DC: ACOG.

Barnes, S. (1999) Theories of spouse abuse: Relevance to African Americans. *Issues in Mental Health Nursing, 20*(4), 357-371.

Bauer, H., Rodriguez, M., Quiroga, S., & Flores-Ortiz, Y. (2000). Barriers to health care for abused Latina and Asian immigrant women. *Journal of Health Care for the Poor & Underserved, 11*(1), 33-44.

Bayer, M., & Fein, E. (1997). High-risk pregnancy. In F. Nichols & E. Zwelling (Eds.), *Maternal-newborn nursing* (pp. 622-700). Philadelphia: Saunders.

Christian, A. (1995). Home care of the battered pregnant woman: One battered woman's pregnancy. *Journal of Obstetric, Gynecologic, and Neonatal Nursing, 24*(9), 836-842.

Curry, M. (1998). The interrelationships between abuse, substance use, and psychosocial stress during pregnancy. *Journal of Obstetric, Gynecologic, and Neonatal Nursing, 27*(6), 692-699.

Flores-Ortiz, Y. (1993). La mujer y la violencia: A culturally based model for the understanding and treatment of domestic violence in Chicana/Latina communities. In Mujeres Activas en Letras y Cambio Social (Ed.), *Chicana critical issues* (pp. 169-182). Berkeley, CA: Chicana/Latina Research Center.

Gazmararian, J., Lazorick, S., Spitz, A., Ballard, T., Saltzman, L., & Marks, J. (1996). Prevalence of violence against pregnant women. *Journal of the American Medical Association, 275*(24), 1915-1920.

Gazmararian, J., Petersen, R., Spitz, A., Goodwin, M., Saltzman, L., & Marks, J. (2000). Violence and reproductive health: Current knowledge and future research directions. *Maternal & Child Health Journal, 4*(2), 79-84.

Green, K. (1996). *Family violence in aboriginal communities: An aboriginal perspective.* Ottawa: National Clearing House on Family Violence.

Hanrahan, P., Campbell, J., & Ulrich, Y. (1993). Theories of violence. In J. Campbell & J. Humphreys (Eds.),

Nursing care of survivors of family violence (pp. 5-42). St. Louis: Mosby.

King, M., Torres, S., Campbell, D., Ryan, J., Sheridan, D., Ulrich, Y., et al. (1993). Violence and abuse of women: A perinatal health care issue. *AWHONN Clinical Issues in Perinatal and Women's Health Nursing, 4*(2), 163-173.

Lauderdale, J. (2003). Transcultural perspectives in childbearing. In M. Andrews & J. Boyle (Eds.), *Transcultural concepts in nursing care* (4th ed., pp. 95-131). Philadelphia: Lippincott Williams & Wilkins.

Lazzaro, M., & McFarlane, J. (1991). Establishing a screening program for abused women. *Journal of Nursing Administration, 21*(10), 24-29.

Limandri, B.J., & Tilden, V.P. (1993). Domestic violence: Ethical issues in the health care system. *AWHONN's Clinical Issues in Perinatal and Women's Health Nursing, 4*(3), 493-502.

Martin, S., English, K., Clark, K., Cilenit, D., & Kupper, L. (1996). Violence and substance use among North Carolina pregnant women. *American Journal of Public Health, 86*(7), 991-998.

Mattson, S., & Rodriguez, E. (1999). Battering in pregnant Latinas. *Issues in Mental Health Nursing, 20*(4), 405-422.

McFarlane, J., & Parker, B. (1994). Preventing abuse during pregnancy: An assessment and intervention protocol. *American Journal of Maternal Child Nursing, 19*(6), 321-324.

McFarlane, J., & Parker, B. (1995). *Abuse during pregnancy: A protocol for prevention and intervention. March of Dimes Nursing Monograph.* White Plains, NY: March of Dimes.

McFarlane, J., Parker, B., Soeken, K., & Bullock, L. (1992). Assessing for abuse during pregnancy. *Journal of the American Medical Association, 267*(23), 3176-3178.

National Council for Research on Women. (1995). Intervening: Immigrant women and domestic violence. *Issues Quarterly, 1,* 12-13.

Noel, N., & Yam, M. (1992). Domestic violence: The pregnant battered woman. *Nursing Clinics of North America, 4*(27), 871-884.

O'Leary, K. (1993). Through a psychological lens: Personality traits, personality disorders, and levels of violence. In R. Gelles & D. Loseke (Eds.), *Current controversies on family violence* (pp. 142-180). Newbury Park, CA: Sage.

Parker, B. (1993). Abuse of adolescents: What can we learn from pregnant teenagers? *AWHONN's Clinical Issues in Perinatal and Women's Health Nursing, 4*(3), 363-370.

Parker, B., McFarlane, J., & Soeken, K. (1994). Abuse during pregnancy: Effects on maternal complications and birth weight in adult and teenage women. *Obstetrics and Gynecology, 84*(3), 323-328.

Parker, B., McFarlane, J., Soeken, K., Torres, S., & Campbell, J. (1993). Physical and emotional abuse in pregnancy: A comparison of adult and teen women. *Nursing Research, 42*(3), 173-178.

Pinn, V., & Chunko, M. (1997). The diverse faces of violence: Minority women and domestic abuse. *Academic Medicine, 72* (1 suppl), S65-S71.

Rodriguez, M. (1994). Domestic violence. *Western Journal of Medicine, 161*(1), 60-61.

Ruiz, E., & Mattson, S. (2003). Observation, self-efficacy and anger: Latino children and domestic violence. In *Communicating nursing research conference proceedings: Responding to societal imperatives through discovery & innovation* (Vol. 3, p. 291). Portland, OR: Western Institute of Nursing.

Rynerson, B. (1997). Violence against women. In D. Lowdermilk, S. Perry, & I. Bobak (Eds.), *Maternity & women's health care* (6th ed., pp. 1220-1242). St. Louis: Mosby.

Rynerson, B. (2000). Violence against women. In D. Lowdermilk, S. Perry, & I. Bobak (Eds.), *Maternity & women's health care* (7th ed., pp. 225-246). St. Louis: Mosby.

Statistics Canada. (1993). The violence against women survey. Accessed January 18, 2002, at *http://stcwww.statcan.ca./english/sdds/3896.htm.*

Suarez, L., & Ramirez, A. (1999). Hispanic/Latino health and disease. In R. Huff & M. Kline (Eds.), *Promoting health in multicultural populations* (pp. 115-136). Thousand Oaks, CA: Sage Science Press.

Taggart, L., & Mattson, S. (1996). Delay in prenatal care as a result of battering in pregnancy: Cross-cultural implications. *Health Care for Women International, 17*(1), 25-34.

Titus, K. (1996). When physicians ask, women tell about domestic abuse and violence. *Journal of the American Medical Association, 275*(24), 1863-1874.

Tjaden, P., & Thoennes, N. (2000). *Extent, nature, and consequences of intimate partner violence.* Washington, DC: U.S. Department of Justice.

Torrés, S. (1991). A comparison of wife abuse between two cultures: Perceptions, attitudes, nature, and extent. *Issues in Mental Health Nursing, 12*(1), 113-131.

Walker, L. (1982). *The battered woman.* New York: Harper & Row.

21 Hypertensive Disorders in Pregnancy

JUDITH H. POOLE

OBJECTIVES

1. Define the hypertensive states in pregnancy.
2. Discuss theories about the causes and pathophysiology of preeclampsia and eclampsia, as well as hemolysis, elevated liver enzymes, and low platelets (HELLP) syndrome.
3. Identify factors that place women at greater risk for preeclampsia.
4. Correlate history and physical findings with signs and symptoms of preeclampsia, eclampsia, and HELLP syndrome.
5. Associate hypertensive pathophysiology with potential maternal and fetal complications.
6. Formulate nursing interventions to alleviate or prevent potential problems identified in the nursing assessment.
7. Summarize the treatment of preeclampsia, eclampsia, and HELLP syndrome.
8. Analyze the drug regimen to be used and its maternal and fetal effects.

INTRODUCTION

A. **Hypertensive disorders of pregnancy can result in life-threatening complications for the mother and fetus.**
   1. Hypertensive disorders of pregnancy are the most common medical conditions reported during pregnancy (Martin, Hamilton, Ventura, Menacker, Park, & Sutton, 2002).
   2. Hypertension complicates 12% to 20% of all pregnancies not terminating in first trimester miscarriages, with a higher incidence among populations at greatest risk for preeclampsia (American College of Obstetricians and Gynecologists, 2002; Egerman & Sibai, 1999b; Walker, 1998).
   3. Rate of pregnancy-associated hypertension has risen steadily, approximately 30% to 40%, since 1990 for all ages, races, and ethnic groups (Martin et al., 2002).
      a. Current rate of 37.7 per 1000 live births is a slight decline since 2000 (38.8 per 1000); rate had steadily risen since 1990 (from 27.2) until decline noted in 2001.
      b. Rates for chronic hypertension have increased moderately to 7.6 per 1000 live births.
      c. Rate for eclampsia has declined to 3.1 per 1000 live births.
      d. Age distribution remains U-shaped with highest rates of occurrence in women < 20 years of age or > 40 years of age.

      e. Highest rates seen among Native American (47.7), black (40.6), and white (38.0) women; lowest rates seen among Asian or Pacific Islander women (21.4).

    4. Hypertension during pregnancy is one of the leading causes of maternal morbidity and mortality in the United States and worldwide (Chang et al., 2003; Minino, Kochanek, Murphy, & Smith, 2002).

      a. Reported death rate in 2000 was 9.8 per 100,000 live births.

      b. Hypertension was the leading cause-specific cause of maternal death; rate is 1.8 deaths per 100,000 live births.

      c. Black women have the highest rate of maternal death secondary to hypertension during pregnancy.

    5. Therapy is aimed at controlling hypertension and seizures, preventing long-term morbidity, and preventing maternal, fetal, or neonatal death.

    6. Preeclampsia places the woman at increased risk of potentially lethal complications, including, but not limited to, eclampsia, abruptio placentae, disseminated intravascular coagulation (DIC), acute renal failure, hepatic failure, pulmonary edema, acute adult respiratory distress syndrome (ARDS), and cerebral hemorrhage or stroke.

    7. Preeclampsia depends on the presence of trophoblastic tissue thus the only cure is delivery.

B. Terminology describing the hypertensive disorders of pregnancy can be imprecise and confusing.

    1. The classification system most commonly used in clinical practice today is based on reports from the American College of Obstetricians and Gynecologists (ACOG, 2002) and the National High Blood Pressure Education Program, Working Group on High Blood Pressure in Pregnancy (2000).

      a. Classification differentiates between hypertensive disorders that predate pregnancy and preeclampsia (a potentially more ominous disease).

      b. The cardinal pathophysiologic feature of chronic hypertension is elevation of blood pressure above identified normal values as defined by the National Heart, Lung, and Blood Institute (Joint National Committee [JNC], 2003).

      c. With preeclampsia, hypertension is a sign of the underlying syndrome and is a potential cause of maternal morbidity.

    2. Hypertension may predate the pregnancy (chronic hypertension) or present for the first time during the pregnancy (gestational hypertension).

    3. Gestational hypertension

      a. Replaces the term *pregnancy-induced hypertension* (PIH), which was an umbrella term that encompassed many classifications of hypertension during pregnancy; serves as a presumptive diagnosis during the pregnancy.

      b. Blood pressure elevation is detected for first time after midpregnancy, at approximately 20 weeks.

      c. In a previously normotensive woman, gestational blood pressure elevation defined as:

        (1) Systolic blood pressure (SBP) of 140 mmHg or greater, or

        (2) Diastolic blood pressure (DBP) of 90 mmHg or greater, or

        (3) Mean arterial pressure (MAP) of 105 mmHg or greater

        (4) New onset of hypertension based on two elevated measurements within 7 days

   d. Gestational hypertension and chronic hypertension may occur independently or simultaneously; final diagnosis is made postpartum.
   e. Gestational hypertension is further classified according to maternal organ dysfunction (preeclampsia, eclampsia).
   f. A definitive diagnosis of transient hypertension is made postpartum in a woman who did not develop preeclampsia and who demonstrated resolution of gestational hypertension by 12 weeks' postpartum; if hypertension persists, a definitive diagnosis of chronic hypertension is made.
4. Preeclampsia
   a. Pregnancy-specific syndrome that develops after the twentieth week of gestation
   b. Represents a multi-organ, vasospastic process of reduced organ perfusion (hypoperfusion) and activation of the coagulation cascade (National High Blood Pressure Education Program Working Group, 2000).
   c. Diagnosed by presence of gestational hypertension plus proteinuria
   d. Preeclampsia may be superimposed on chronic hypertension, with a prognosis that is worse than either condition alone.
5. Eclampsia is the occurrence of seizure activity or coma in a woman with preeclampsia, which cannot be attributed to other causes.
6. HELLP syndrome is a severe sequela of preeclampsia.
7. Preeclampsia or eclampsia does not predispose a woman to chronic hypertension.
8. A sign of latent chronic hypertension may be recurring hypertension with subsequent pregnancies.
9. Implications of classification of hypertensive disorders
   a. Preeclampsia is a clinical syndrome that progresses on a continuum from mild to severe disease.
   b. Progression from mild to severe disease may occur slowly or may occur rapidly over a course of several days.
   c. Better to over-diagnose preeclampsia than to miss the diagnosis because of the potential for maternal and perinatal morbidity and mortality.
C. **Risk factors for preeclampsia**
   1. Primigravida (six to eight times greater risk)
      a. Previous pregnancy or second trimester abortion may have a protective effect.
      b. A multiparous woman with a change in paternity is at the same risk for development of preeclampsia as nulliparous woman (Dekker, 1999).
      c. Of interest, men who fathered a pregnancy complicated by preeclampsia are almost twice as likely to father a pregnancy complicated by preeclampsia in a different woman.
   2. Age extremes (under age 17 or over 35 years)
      a. 20% incidence among teens
      b. Two to three times greater risk for primigravida over 40 years of age
      c. However, age has not been shown to be independent of other risk factors, especially parity.
   3. Diabetes
   4. Preexisting hypertensive, vascular, or renal disease occurs in approximately 20% of superimposed preeclampsia.
   5. Multiple gestation (five times greater risk)
   6. Fetal hydrops (10 times greater risk)

7. Hydatidiform mole (10 times greater risk)
8. Preeclampsia in previous pregnancy
   a. Risk of recurrence is related to onset of preeclampsia in first pregnancy.
      (1) Recurrence in subsequent pregnancy is much higher (approximately 65%) if preeclampsia occurred before 30 weeks' gestation or is superimposed on chronic hypertension.
      (2) Recurrence is approximately 25% if preeclampsia occurred in the last trimester in previous pregnancy.
   b. Recurrence of HELLP syndrome appears to be much lower (< 4%) than previously believed.
9. Family history of preeclampsia or eclampsia
10. Obesity
11. Immunologic factors

D. **Although the precise origin of preeclampsia remains unknown, the underlying pathophysiology appears to be related to hypoperfusion, vasospasm, endothelial cell damage, and platelet aggregation;** several theories continue to be investigated.
   1. Altered pressor response to angiotensin II
      a. An increased sensitivity to the pressor effects of angiotensin II causes vasoconstriction and a subsequent rise in blood pressure.
      b. Sensitivity to angiotensin II is related to a decrease in the production of prostaglandin dilators (prostacyclin) and an increase in prostaglandin vasoconstrictors (thromboxane).
   2. Abnormal prostacyclin/thromboxane ratio
      a. Prostacyclin, produced by endothelial cells and the placenta, causes vasodilation, inhibits platelet aggregation, and encourages uterine relaxation.
      b. Thromboxane, produced by the platelets, renal cells, and the placenta, causes the opposite: vasoconstriction, platelet aggregation, and uterine contraction.
      c. Prostacyclin is increased with normal pregnancy and decreased with preeclampsia.
      d. Thromboxane is increased in both normal pregnancy and preeclampsia, but the decrease in prostacyclin allows thromboxane dominance with preeclampsia.
   3. Alteration in endothelin and endothelin-derived relaxing factor (EDRF)
      a. Endothelin-1, a peptide regulator, is increased in preeclampsia and may contribute to the pathology.
      b. Endothelin, a vasoconstrictor more potent than angiotensin II, is secreted in response to endothelial cell injury.
      c. Endothelial cell injury then decreases the production of potent vasodilators such as EDRF.
   4. Immunologic theory
      a. Presence of foreign protein, the placenta, the fetus, or any combination may trigger an adverse immunologic response.
      b. Immunologic theory is supported by the increased incidence of preeclampsia in primigravidas (first exposure to fetal tissue) and women who are pregnant by a new partner (different genetic material).
      c. Maternal antibody system is overwhelmed from excessive fetal antigens, especially when exposed to a large mass of trophoblastic tissue, as with multiple gestations and hydatidiform mole.
      d. Genetic predisposition may be another immunologic factor.

    5. Hemodynamic theory
       a. Endothelial cell damage may be caused by a high-output–low-resistance state in early pregnancy.
       b. Endothelial cell damage then triggers the opposite: decreased output and increased systemic vascular resistance.
       c. This hemodynamic model has limitations because many women with high cardiac output do not develop preeclampsia.
    6. Spiral artery erosion
       a. Initial defect of preeclampsia may be failure of the trophoblast to effectively erode the spiral arteries.
       b. Normally in early pregnancy the spiral arteries are invaded by the trophoblast, with the end result being dilated vessels that provide blood flow to the placenta and are incapable of constriction.
       c. If trophoblastic invasion does not occur, placental perfusion is decreased, and the spiral arteries remain responsive to vasoconstrictor substances.
  E. Differentiation of hypertensive disorders
    1. Gestational hypertension
       a. Preeclampsia
          (1) Hypertension
             (a) Gestational blood pressure elevation
             (b) At least two elevated values 4 to 6 hours apart or no more than 7 days apart
             (c) Hypertension is generally the first clinical sign of preeclampsia.
             (d) Elevation over prepregnancy or first trimester blood pressure (BP) baseline values is no longer considered diagnostic for preeclampsia.
               (i) Relative hypertension may be identified with an increase of 30 mmHg SBP or 15 mmHg DBP.
               (ii) Relative hypertension in the presence of proteinuria or hyperuricemia (uric acid of 6 mg/dl or more) warrants closer observation.
          (2) Proteinuria
             (a) 300 mg or more protein in 24-hour urine collection
             (b) 30 mg/dl (dipstick 1+) or more in the absence of a urinary tract infection (UTI)
             (c) Single random sample may not show significant proteinuria because proteinuria may fluctuate widely over a 24-hour period.
             (d) Proteinuria may be a late sign of preeclampsia.
             (e) It is recommended that diagnosis of proteinuria be based on a 24-hour urine or a timed collection for total protein excretion and creatinine clearance.
          (3) Edema
             (a) Pathologic edema associated with preeclampsia is more than the dependent edema common during a normal pregnancy.
             (b) Usually involves the face and hands, as well as the lower extremities.
             (c) Involves weight gain of 2 kg (5 lb) or more in 1 week.
             (d) Presence of edema, as the only finding, is not diagnostic for preeclampsia.
          (4) Classic triad of preeclampsia
             (a) Historically the classic triad of preeclampsia was hypertension, proteinuria, and edema or weight gain.

      (b) Current research disputes this triad and defines preeclampsia in relation to decreased organ perfusion (hypoperfusion), endothelial dysfunction (capillary leaking and proteinuria), and hypertension.

  b. Severe preeclampsia is defined as the presence of one or more of the following in the woman diagnosed with preeclampsia:

    (1) BP

      (a) SBP of at least 160 mmHg, or

      (b) DBP of at least 110 mmHg

    (2) Proteinuria of at least 2 g in 24-hour urine collection or 2+ to 3+ or greater on dipstick (National High Blood Pressure Education Program Working Group, 2000) or at least 5 g in 24-hour urine collection or 3+ or greater on dipstick (ACOG, 2002)

      (a) Proteinuria should occur for the first time in pregnancy and resolve after delivery; if preexisting, may indicate underlying renal disease.

      (b) Significant proteinuria in itself not indication for delivery if stable maternal-fetal status.

    (3) Oliguria of less than 400 to 500 ml/24 hr or persistent urine output of less than 30 ml/hr

    (4) Cerebral and visual disturbances: altered consciousness, headache, blurred vision, and scotomata

    (5) Pulmonary edema or cyanosis

    (6) Epigastric or right upper quadrant pain

    (7) Thrombocytopenia

    (8) Hepatic dysfunction

    (9) Fetal intrauterine growth restriction (IUGR)

    (10) Development of eclampsia or HELLP syndrome

  c. Eclampsia

    (1) Preeclampsia with seizures not attributed to other causes

      (a) Cause of seizures is unknown; theories include cerebral vasospasm, hemorrhage, ischemia, edema, and platelet and fibrin clots that occlude cerebral vasculature.

      (b) Periods of hypoxia may occur in mother and fetus.

      (c) Risk of aspiration resulting from relaxation of gastroesophageal sphincter during pregnancy.

      (d) Other risks include cerebrovascular accident (CVA), cerebral edema, anoxia, coma, and maternal death (0.4% to 14%).

    (2) Eclampsia may be preventable if preeclampsia is recognized in its early stages, surveillance is adequate, and therapy is appropriate.

    (3) Seizure may be initial sign of preeclampsia.

2. Chronic hypertension

  a. Hypertension before twentieth week of pregnancy and persisting after 12 weeks' postpartum

  b. The *Seventh Report of the Joint National Committee on Prevention, Detection, Evaluation, and Treatment of High Blood Pressure* (JNC, 2003) has revised the BP classification for adults over 18 years of age

    (1) Normal BP: SBP < 120 mmHg and DBP < 80 mmHg

    (2) Prehypertension: SBP 120 to 139 mmHg or DBP 80 to 89 mmHg

    (3) Stage 1 (mild) hypertension: SBP 140 to 159 mmHg or DBP 90 to 99 mmHg

    (4) Stage 2 (severe) hypertension: SBP ≥ 160 mmHg or DBP ≥ 100 mmHg

  c. Research is needed to know the significance of prehypertension BP values early in pregnancy and the relationship to preeclampsia.

3. Chronic hypertension with superimposed preeclampsia or eclampsia
   a. Chronic hypertension carries a 25% risk of developing superimposed preeclampsia.
   b. Morbidity is 25% to 35% higher than with preeclampsia alone; close observation is therefore required.
   c. Increased risk of intracranial bleeding and abruptio placentae
   d. May be related to renal or vascular disease.
   e. Superimposed preeclampsia is highly likely with the following findings:
      (1) New onset of proteinuria, defined as the urinary excretion of 0.3 g protein or greater in a 24-hour specimen in a woman with hypertension
      (2) Hypertension and proteinuria present before 20 weeks' gestation
      (3) Sudden increase in BP in a woman whose hypertension has previously been well controlled
      (4) Thrombocytopenia with a platelet count < 100,000 cells/mm^3
      (5) An increase in alanine aminotransferase (ALT) or aspartate aminotransferase (AST) to abnormal values
4. Transient (gestational) hypertension
   a. Development of elevated BP during pregnancy or in the first 24 hours' postpartum without other signs of preeclampsia or preexisting hypertension
   b. BP spontaneously returning to normal within 12 weeks' postpartum
5. HELLP syndrome
   a. Laboratory diagnosis for variant of severe preeclampsia with a primary presentation consistent with hepatic dysfunction
   b. Incidence with severe preeclampsia ranges from 2% to 12% (Stone, 1998).
   c. Occurs more often in older (age > 25 years), white, multiparous women.
   d. Acronym of HELLP was first described in 1982 by Dr. Louis Weinstein.
      (1) Hemolysis
         (a) Red blood cell (RBC) destruction as they travel through constricted vessels, causing microangiopathic hemolytic anemia and changes in RBC morphology
         (b) Reduced oxygen-carrying capacity
         (c) Peripheral blood smear confirms marked changes in RBC morphology; may show burr cells (contracted RBCs with spiny projections along the periphery), schistocytes (small, irregularly shaped RBCs), and polychromasia (variation in the hemoglobin content of RBCs).
         (d) Elevated lactic dehydrogenase (LDH) greater than 600 IU/L resulting from RBC injury (normal LDH is 90 to 200 IU/L)
         (e) Elevated bilirubin greater than 1.2 mg/dl and jaundice may also develop because of hemolysis of RBCs.
      (2) Elevated liver enzymes
         (a) Vasospasm decreases blood flow to the liver, resulting in tissue ischemia and hemorrhagic necrosis.
         (b) AST greater than 70 IU/L (laboratory test formerly called serum glutamic-oxaloacetic transaminase [SGOT])
         (c) Lactic dehydrogenase greater than 600 IU/L
         (d) Symptoms of hepatic damage include right upper quadrant or epigastric pain, nausea and vomiting, and tenderness when liver is palpated.

      (3) Low platelets
        (a) Platelets aggregate at the site of damaged vascular endothelium, causing platelet consumption and thrombocytopenia.
        (b) Thrombocytopenia is considered a platelet count less than 150,000/mm^3; however, the more clinically significant thrombocytopenia is a platelet count under 100,000/mm^3.
        (c) Signs and symptoms may include bleeding gums, bruising, petechiae, and bleeding from intravenous (IV) and other sites.
        (d) Platelet transfusions are considered when platelet counts are less than 20,000/mm^3.
        (e) If cesarean section is required, platelets are transfused to maintain count at greater than 50,000/mm^3 during surgery.
  e. Pathophysiology of HELLP syndrome
      (1) Arteriolar vasospasm damages the endothelial layer of small vessels, causing lesions.
        (a) These lesions allow formation of platelet aggregation and, in turn, a fibrin network.
        (b) As RBCs are forced through the network under high pressure, the cells are hemolyzed.
      (2) Maternal hepatic damage results from microemboli in the liver.
        (a) Ischemia and tissue damage result from the microemboli.
        (b) Obstruction to the hepatic blood flow and fibrin deposits cause hepatic distention.
        (c) Increasing intrahepatic pressure potentiates liver rupture, which is rare but often fatal.
      (3) Circulating volume of platelets decreases as a result of an increase in consumption.
        (a) Circulating platelets adhere to damaged endothelium.
        (b) As the platelets are consumed, thrombocytopenia results (Figure 21-1).
  f. Comparison of HELLP syndrome and DIC (see Chapter 23 for a complete discussion of DIC)
      (1) Causes of DIC in obstetrics
        (a) Abruptio placentae
        (b) Preeclampsia or eclampsia
        (c) Intrauterine fetal demise (IUFD)
        (d) Sepsis or systemic inflammatory response syndrome (SIRS)
        (e) Anaphylactoid syndrome of pregnancy (formerly known as amniotic fluid embolism [AFE])
        (f) Hemorrhage
      (2) Women with severe preeclampsia complicated by HELLP syndrome may also develop a consumptive DIC.
      (3) Coagulation factors (Table 21-1)
F. Potential complications of preeclampsia that may threaten maternal and fetal well being
  1. Maternal morbidity or mortality from:
    a. Abruptio placentae
    b. Seizures
    c. Acute renal failure
    d. Pulmonary edema or embolism
    e. Cardiac dysfunction, dysrhythmias, and left ventricular failure
    f. Cerebral hemorrhage

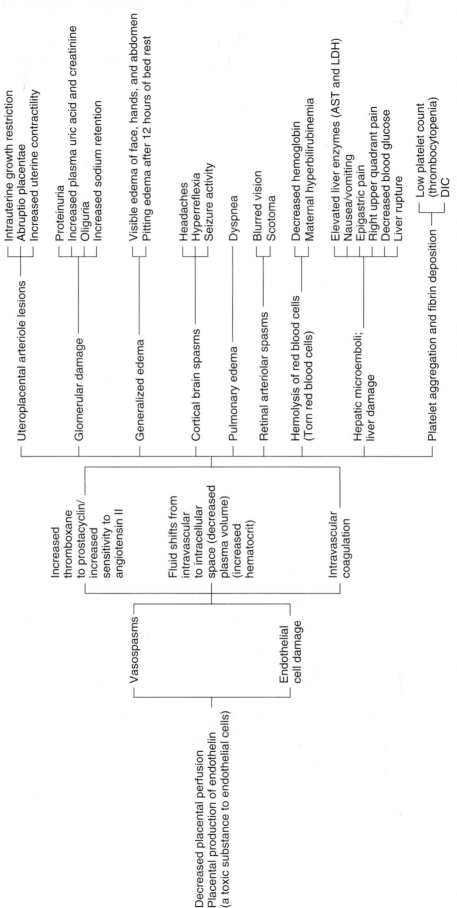

FIGURE 21-1 ■ Pathophysiologic changes of preeclampsia. *AST*, Aspartate transaminase; *LDH*, lactate dehydrogenase. (From Gilbert, E.S., & Harmon, J.S. [2003]. *Manual of high risk pregnancy & delivery* [3rd ed.]. St. Louis: Mosby.)

■ TABLE 21-1
■ ■ **Coagulation Factors**

	Normal Value	DIC	HELLP Syndrome
Platelets	150,000-400,000	Decreased	<100,000
Fibrinogen	300-500	Decreased	Unchanged
PT	11-13	Prolonged	Unchanged
PTT	25-45	Prolonged	Unchanged
Fibrin split products	< 10	> 40 U	Unchanged

DIC, Disseminated intravascular coagulation; *HELLP,* hemolysis, elevated liver enzymes, low platelets; *PT,* prothrombin time; *PTT,* partial thromboplastin time.

    g. DIC
    h. Hepatic failure, hypoglycemia, and coagulopathies
    i. Increased risk for cesarean birth secondary to worsening disease process or deterioration of fetal status
  2. Fetal or neonatal morbidity or mortality from:
    a. Fetal growth restriction
    b. Nonreassuring fetal heart rate pattern or antepartum testing
    c. Abruptio placentae
    d. Intrauterine fetal death
G. Generalized vasospasm and endothelial cell damage decrease oxygenation and perfusion throughout the body, causing widespread organ dysfunction; varying signs and symptoms of preeclampsia depend on the systems most affected.
  1. Cardiovascular system
    a. Hypertension is usually the first sign of preeclampsia.
    b. Hypertension is also the critical feature that should alert health care providers about possible preeclampsia; edema is the least valid sign, and proteinuria may be late in onset.
    c. BP rises and left ventricle work increases because of elevated systemic vascular resistance.
    d. BP may be labile because of intermittent vasospasm.
    e. Circulating plasma volume decreases as fluid shifts from the intravascular to extravascular space secondary to endothelial dysfunction and increased capillary permeability, causing hypovolemia, peripheral (and possibly pulmonary) edema, and hemoconcentration with a rise in hematocrit.
    f. Endothelial dysfunction allows for leaking of albumin and other plasma proteins causing a decrease in colloid osmotic pressure (COP), predisposing to pulmonary edema.
    g. The heart is generally unaffected unless preexisting cardiac disease is present.
  2. Renal system
    a. Intrarenal injury of endothelial cells causes a decrease in the production of prostacyclin and EDRF, allowing unopposed vasoconstriction by angiotensin II and endothelin-1.
    b. Vasospasm causes a decrease in blood flow (renal hypoperfusion) and glomerular filtration rate (GFR).

(1) Normally in pregnancy, GFR increases because of a 50% increase in blood flow to the kidneys; increase in GFR then causes a decrease in serum blood urea nitrogen (BUN), creatinine, and uric acid levels.

(2) The opposite occurs with preeclampsia—a decrease in GFR occurs because of a decrease in effective renal blood flow.

c. Uric acid, BUN, and serum creatinine levels all increase because of the decrease in renal clearance.

(1) Fractional urate clearance decreases, resulting in hyperuricemia; an important marker for preeclampsia.

(2) Serum creatinine levels > 1 mg/dl prevent adequate renal filtration, including excretion of magnesium sulfate and other renally excreted drugs.

d. Glomerular membrane is damaged from vasoconstriction, increasing permeability to proteins.

e. Significant proteinuria causes a decrease in serum albumin, which further decreases COP and results in severe interstitial edema in the kidneys.

f. Proteinuria is routinely checked at every prenatal visit; however, the most accurate method to assess total protein excretion is with a 24-hour collection.

g. Sodium excretion may be impaired; in the severest forms of preeclampsia there may be no edema.

h. Oliguria and hematuria may develop as gestational hypertension worsens.

(1) Oliguria may be the result of intravascular fluid volume depletion or renal vasospasms; increasing IV fluids or administering a crystalloid fluid bolus of 500 to 750 ml may increase the urine output.

(2) Oliguria may also result from decreased cardiac output when intense vasospasm and increased systemic vascular resistance (SVR) lead to depressed left ventricular function; IV fluids should then be restricted.

(3) Persistent oliguria is an indication for invasive hemodynamic monitoring if delivery not imminent.

i. Renal ischemia increases renal medullary lactic acid.

j. Urine-concentrating ability is decreased in hypertensive women.

(1) Specific gravity is normally 1.010 to 1.025.

(2) Specific gravity may decrease as kidneys lose ability to concentrate the urine (low specific gravity indicates dilute urine).

(3) High specific gravity indicates concentrated urine.

(4) Specific gravity may be an unreliable measure of osmolality; urine osmolality test can be performed (normal urine osmolality is 25 to 88 mOsm/kg).

(5) Urine color is not an accurate indicator of urine concentration as a result of sloughing by the kidney.

3. Pulmonary system

a. Pulmonary complications may be caused by dramatic changes in COP

(1) During pregnancy the plasma volume increases 30% to 50% while the RBCs increase by 10% to 20%, causing a physiologic dilution of the blood, including plasma proteins, as evidenced by a decrease in hematocrit and a decrease in COP.

(2) COP decreases during pregnancy; thus, hydrostatic pressure pushing fluid out of the capillaries may become greater than COP pulling fluid into the capillaries, increasing the risk of pulmonary edema.

(3) Colloids (albumin, globulin, and fibrinogen) are large protein molecules that normally do not cross capillary membranes; rather, they work as magnets, pulling fluid toward them.

(4) In women with preeclampsia, COP drops because of loss of protein (albumin) across damaged systemic vessels and renal vasculature (Table 21-2).

(5) Administration of IV fluids changes COP.

    (a) Crystalloid solutions (e.g., D_5W, normal saline [NS], Ringer's lactate) decrease COP and increase hydrostatic pressure, therefore pushing fluid into interstitial spaces.

    (b) Colloid solutions (e.g., albumin, blood products) increase COP and pull fluid into the vessels.

    (c) Colloid infusions are not recommended with preeclampsia because the infused colloid molecules can leak across damaged capillaries into interstitial space, pulling fluids with them and further depleting intravascular volume and increasing the risk for pulmonary edema.

(6) After delivery, autotransfusion and extravascular to intravascular fluid shifts cause a dramatic drop in COP caused by dilution; during the period 6 to 24 hours after delivery, a woman is at greater risk for pulmonary edema; this is also the time of lowest cardiac contractility.

(7) Pulmonary edema can be cardiogenic, noncardiogenic, or both

    (a) Cardiogenic pulmonary edema results from left ventricular dysfunction caused by increased systemic vascular resistance.

    (b) Noncardiogenic pulmonary edema results from a reduction in colloid osmotic pressure and increased pulmonary permeability (can also be caused by fluid overload).

4. Central nervous system

  a. Any time a pregnant patient presents with a persistent headache, it should be considered a potentially serious situation and may be the result of cerebral vasoconstriction, which can lead to cerebral ischemia, seizures, and hemorrhage.

  b. Visual changes may be caused by retinal arteriolar spasms, petechial hemorrhages, or retinal edema.

    (1) Although visual changes may last for many days postpartum, in most cases, the prognosis is excellent for complete recovery.

    (2) Retinal detachment is a more serious complication and can result in permanent blindness.

■ TABLE 21-2
■ ■ Colloid Osmotic Pressure (COP) Values (in mmHg)

Nonpregnant	28
Antepartum	22-23
Intrapartum	19-23
Postpartum	13-17
GH (antepartum)	17-18.5
GH (postpartum)	13-14

GH, Gestational hypertension.

  c. Eclamptic seizures
    (1) Result from excess discharge of neurotransmitter cells in the brain.
    (2) May have origin in focal area of the brain but spread rapidly, leading to generalized tonic-clonic seizures.
    (3) May occur before, during, or after delivery.
      (a) 71% of seizures occur before delivery.
      (b) 29% occur postpartum.
    (4) Magnesium sulfate is the preferred drug in the United States for preventing and treating eclamptic seizures.
      (a) Improves cerebral circulation and perfusion and decreases plasma levels of endothelin-1.
      (b) Interferes with platelet aggregation (predisposes to bleeding) and changes serum osmolality (may increase risk for pulmonary and cerebral edema).
      (c) May cause a transient decrease in BP because of the relaxant effect on smooth muscle; BP return to preinfusion values within several hours after infusion initiation; antihypertensive agents should be used for BP control to prevent maternal vascular damage and cerebral hemorrhage.
      (d) Contraindicated in women with myasthenia gravis because magnesium sulfate reduces transmission of acetylcholine at the synaptic junction and can result in respiratory failure.
      (e) Contraindicated in women with heart block, myocardial insufficiency, and possibly renal disease.
      (f) Excreted via the kidneys; decreased urine output or elevated serum creatinine levels (> 1 mg/dl) may lead to dangerously high magnesium levels.
      (g) Cardiac monitoring is recommended when administering IV labetalol concomitantly with magnesium sulfate; at increased risk for potential life-threatening dysrhythmias and bradycardia.
    (5) If seizure occurs:
      (a) Provide for patient safety.
        (i) Assess for airway, breathing, and pulse.
        (ii) Anticipate the need for suctioning to minimize risk for aspiration.
      (b) Assess maternal and fetal status.
        (i) Uterine hyperstimulation and fetal bradycardia are common responses in postictal state.
        (ii) Provide measures for intrauterine resuscitation (oxygen, IV fluids, and lateral position).
        (iii) Assess for abruptio placentae or precipitous birth.
        (iv) Document time of onset, associated symptoms, and duration of seizure.
      (c) Prepare for delivery as indicated.
        (i) Stabilization of maternal and fetal status comes first.
        (ii) Timing and route of delivery is determined by individual patient (maternal or fetal) status.
    (6) Best predictors of eclampsia
      (a) Extreme hypertension
      (b) Headache, with or without visual disturbances
      (c) Epigastric pain
      (d) Proteinuria may be absent.

(7) Cerebral hemorrhage is a common cause of maternal death.
   (a) Cerebral blood flow approximately 50 ml/min/100 g of brain tissue
   (b) Cerebral blood flow regulated to maintain a constant cerebral perfusion pressure
   (c) In previously normotensive patient, the process of cerebral blood flow autoregulation is not reliably maintained at levels of MAP greater than 140 mmHg.
   (d) Life-threatening complications from uncontrolled hypertension should be suspected with the following clinical assessment findings:
      (i) Progressive decrease in the patient's level of consciousness or stupor
      (ii) Complaints of flashes of light
      (iii) Focal neurologic deficits (e.g., nuchal rigidity, seizures, slurring of speech, local or unilateral motor weakness)
      (iv) New onset of vomiting
      (v) Sudden increase in BP may be a sign of, rather than cause of, intracranial bleeding.

5. Uteroplacental system
   a. Maternal blood is carried via spiral arterioles to the intervillous space, where maternal blood bathes the chorionic villi and oxygen, nutrients, carbon dioxide, and waste products are exchanged across the placental membrane.
   b. Spiral arterioles in a normotensive pregnancy transform and remodel from thick-walled, muscular vessels to dilated vessels, which can accommodate a tenfold increase in uterine blood flow; this change does not occur with preeclampsia.
   c. Fetal complications caused by reduced blood flow may include:
      (1) IUGR
      (2) Oligohydramnios (decreased amniotic fluid from decreased fetal urine output)
      (3) Hypoxia and metabolic acidosis
      (4) Intolerance to intrauterine stressors and labor; places woman at higher risk for cesarean birth.
      (5) Intrauterine fetal demise
   d. Hypertension increases the risk of abruptio placentae.
      (1) Incidence of abruptio placentae is less than 1% in normal pregnancy and approximately 10% in preeclampsia.
      (2) A tense, tender, irritable uterus should be considered an abruption.
   e. Must consider other factors that alter uterine blood flow.
      (1) Antihypertensive therapy
         (a) Lowering DBP below 90 mmHg decreases uteroplacental perfusion.
         (b) Be aware of potential for rebound hypotension resulting from constricted intravascular volume.
      (2) Regional anesthesia: generally improves uteroplacental perfusion if hypotension is avoided.
      (3) Uterine contractions
      (4) Maternal position
   f. Major concern with antihypertensive medications is that, along with reducing maternal BP, uteroplacental perfusion will be reduced below the level necessary for fetal oxygenation and growth.

    g. Steroids (e.g., betamethasone) may be given to enhance fetal lung maturity when preeclampsia is diagnosed remote from term and preterm delivery is anticipated.

6. Hematologic system

    a. Changes in the hematologic and hepatic systems are the main criteria for HELLP syndrome, but hematologic changes may occur in preeclampsia without an actual diagnosis of HELLP syndrome.

    b. Be aware of platelet counts and liver function studies in all pregnant women with hypertension.

    c. Hemoconcentration

        (1) Pregnant women normally experience a drop in hematocrit resulting from the dilution of RBCs from plasma volume expansion.

        (2) Hemoconcentration may occur as fluid shifts from the intravascular to extravascular space; therefore hematocrit rises.

            (a) Hematocrit drops when fluid is mobilized from extravascular space back to the vessels, as occurs with bed rest, lateral positioning, and especially diuresis after delivery.

            (b) Differentiate a physiologic drop in hematocrit from a decrease in hemoglobin and hematocrit caused by excess blood loss during delivery.

    d. Thrombocytopenia is common because of platelet consumption, when platelets adhere to damaged vessel walls.

        (1) Platelets decrease to a mild degree in almost 50% of women with preeclampsia.

        (2) Assess bleeding at any site.

            (a) Urine (hematuria)

            (b) Gums

            (c) IV site

            (d) Skin (petechiae); assess skin under automatic BP cuffs.

        (3) Platelet counts usually return to normal within 72 hours postpartum; the more severe the preeclampsia is, the longer the recovery will be.

        (4) Hepatic dysfunction also contributes to thrombocytopenia.

        (5) Platelet number may be normal, but platelet function secondary to drug therapy can be abnormal (e.g., magnesium sulfate, low-dose aspirin, steroid therapy).

    e. Activation of fibrinogen and blood coagulation may increase the risk of deep vein thrombosis.

CLINICAL PRACTICE

A. Assessment

Gestational Hypertension

1. History

    a. Estimated date of confinement (EDC)

    b. Risk factors

        (1) Primigravida or new partner

        (2) Multiple gestation

        (3) Diagnosis of preeclampsia in previous pregnancy

        (4) Preexisting hypertension, vascular or renal disease

        (5) Age under 17 or over 35 years

(6) Diabetes
(7) Family history of preeclampsia (mother or sister)
c. Nutritional assessment
(1) Weight gain
(2) Exercise: amount and frequency
(3) Drug, tobacco, and alcohol use
(a) Tobacco use may decrease risk of preeclampsia, but it increases risk of low birth weight, abruption, IUGR, and preterm birth.
(b) Vasoconstriction and hypertension secondary to illicit drug use can mimic severe preeclampsia thus the entire clinical picture must be considered.
(4) Intake: protein, calcium, daily calories, and fluids
(5) No dietary deficiencies (e.g., protein, calcium, zinc, magnesium) have been proven to cause or prevent preeclampsia; thus it is no longer considered a "disease of malnutrition and low socioeconomic status."
(6) Women should eat a nutritious, balanced diet as per recommendations for pregnancy (see Chapter 5 for a complete discussion of nutrition in pregnancy).
(7) Encourage women to consume at least the recommended daily allowance (RDA) of 1200 mg/day of calcium and to use a supplement if this amount cannot be met from diet alone; calcium helps regulate BP through its role in:
(a) Membrane receptor and ion transport
(b) Angiotensin II stimulation of aldosterone secretion
(c) Modulating prostaglandin synthesis (refer to research studies about calcium supplementation)
(8) No sodium restriction because women need sodium for maintenance of blood volume and placental perfusion; exception may be with chronic hypertension or cardiac disease when a low-salt diet is being used for management of preexisting condition.
(9) Women should drink 8 to 10 glasses of water each day; adequate fluid intake helps to maintain optimal fluid volume and renal perfusion.
2. Physical findings
a. EDC established
(1) Maternal history is taken.
(2) Fundal height is measured with tape measure is taken.
(3) Ultrasonography is used to assess gestational age, fetal growth, and placental aging (see Chapter 8 for further discussion of antepartum testing).
b. Fetal assessment
(1) Heart rate is checked with Doppler or electronic fetal monitor (EFM); trends in baseline rate and presence or absence of accelerations or decelerations are important.
(2) Reasons for ultrasonography
(a) Possible intrauterine growth restriction
(b) Assess amniotic fluid index
(c) Perform biophysical profile
(3) Doppler flow studies assess uteroplacental perfusion by measuring the velocity of blood flow through the uterine and umbilical arteries; placental vascular resistance is determined by comparing systolic with diastolic waveforms (S/D ratio > 3.0 is abnormal).

(4) Nonstress test (NST): loss of variability or accelerations may indicate fetal compromise or may occur secondary to maternal drug therapy.

(5) Contraction stress test (CST)

(6) Biophysical profile; oligohydramnios is a marker of chronic fetal hypoxemia.

(7) Amniocentesis for pulmonary maturity if need for delivery is imminent (see Chapter 8 for a complete discussion of antepartum fetal assessment)

c. Maternal subjective reports

(1) Decreased fetal movements: consistent with ongoing fetal compromise

(2) Epigastric pain (reported as heartburn) or right upper quadrant pain

(3) Nausea, vomiting, or both, especially if new complaint or cannot be explained by other assessment findings

(4) Headache; generally described as the "worst headache I've ever had" or "feels like my head is going to explode"

(5) Visual disturbances

(6) Edema in face, hands, and feet

(7) Excessive thirst

d. BP values

(1) Correct for variables that affect accuracy.

(a) Use correct cuff size; small cuff results in elevated readings, and cuff that is too large results in falsely low readings.

(b) Same position and arm should be used for each measurement; consistency in the procedure and position enables BP changes to be recognized.

(c) BPs are lowest (by 10 to 20 mmHg) in a lateral recumbent position, highest when supine or standing, and intermediate when sitting.

(d) Sitting position is recommended for antenatal assessments and general practice; measurement should be obtained from the right arm, which is supported on a desk in a horizontal position at the level of the heart.

(e) Procedure for BP measurement

(i) After positioning the woman, allow for minimum of 5 minutes of quiet rest before taking measurement to avoid false elevation.

(ii) In an upright position the arm should be resting on a surface at the level of the heart; hydrostatic influence increases if arm not supported, and reading may be elevated.

(iii) Use arm with higher pressure in an upright position; if differences between two arms is greater than 20 mmHg for SBP and greater than 10 mmHg for DBP on three consecutive readings, cardiovascular consult is indicated.

(iv) In a lateral position, the lower arm should be positioned so the woman is not lying on the arm, and the BP is then taken in the dependent arm; more closely approximates the arterial pressure.

(v) In a woman whose upper arm is too large for standard-size cuff (cuff is too narrow), place cuff on forearm instead of using wider cuff.

(vi) Use Korotkoff phase V (disappearance of sound) for recording diastolic value.

(vii) If using noninvasive automatic BP monitoring devices be aware of equipment's cycle time and margin of error; the device can elevate SBP values and decrease DBP values.

e. Screening tests for preeclampsia are unreliable.

(1) Rollover test, first described in 1974, is inappropriate for clinical practice because of numerous false-positive results.

(2) Elevated MAP may be useful to note, but MAP is not a reliable predictor of preeclampsia.

(a) MAP is the average pressure throughout the cardiac cycle.

(b) To calculate MAP, add systolic pressure to twice diastolic pressure and divide the product by 3.

$$\text{MAP} = \frac{SP + (2 \times DP)}{3}$$

(c) MAP at least 90 in the second trimester, MAP at least 105 in the third trimester, or an increase of 20 mmHg is considered abnormal.

(3) Other predictive tests such as uric acid and fibronectin levels, isometric exercise, and Doppler studies have been proposed as predictors of hypertension or preeclampsia; however, their validity has not been proven; therefore diagnostic criteria of hypertensive disorders remain the focus of clinical practice.

f. Renal assessment

(1) Clean-catch urine specimen is assessed for protein using a dipstick (1+ to 2+ with mild preeclampsia, 3+ to 4+ with severe preeclampsia); dipstick readings identify the presence of proteinuria but are inaccurate to quantify the amount of protein excreted.

(2) 24-hour collection is more accurate (up to 300 mg may be normal during pregnancy, ≥ 300 mg considered proteinuria, ≥ 5 g considered severe).

(3) Oliguria (< 30 ml/hr) or hematuria may be present.

g. Edema and weight gain

(1) Weight gain can be an indicator of edema.

(2) Sudden, excessive weight gain of at least 5 lb (2.3 kg) per week

(3) Edema reduces tissue perfusion.

(4) Classification of edema

(a) Edema minimal at pedal and pretibial sites = 1+

(b) Edema of lower extremities is marked = 2+

(c) Edema evident in face, hands, lower abdominal wall, and sacrum = 3+

(d) Generalized massive edema, including ascites from the accumulation of fluid in the peritoneal cavity = 4+

(e) Can also describe edema by depth of indention left when depressing the area.

(i) 2 mm indention = 1+

(ii) 4 mm indention = 2+

(iii) 6 mm indention = 3+

(iv) 8 mm indention = 4+

    h. Assessment for signs and symptoms of pulmonary edema
       (1) Abnormal breath sounds; rales and wheezing
       (2) Shortness of breath
       (3) Decreased oxygen saturation
          (a) Assess capillary refill of extremity before placing sensor.
          (b) Desaturation is a later finding for pulmonary compromise; changes in vital signs and level of consciousness are earlier findings.
          (c) Falsely elevates saturation values in low perfusion states.
       (4) Tachypnea; increasing pulse and respiratory rate one of the earliest findings
       (5) Tachycardia
       (6) Lungs dull to percussion
       (7) Productive or nonproductive cough
       (8) Neck vein distention
       (9) Anxiety, apprehension and restlessness
    i. Neurologic assessment
       (1) Severe, continuous headaches or pressure in the head, often frontal or occipital
       (2) Alteration in level of consciousness, drowsiness, or dizziness
       (3) Tinnitus
       (4) Visual disturbances: diplopia, blurred vision, and scotomata
       (5) Nausea and vomiting; especially concerning if new onset is accompanied by hypertension or worsening neurologic status
       (6) Deep-tendon reflexes (DTRs); classification:

0 Absent
1 Decreased
2 Average
3 Brisker than average
4 Very brisk; may be associated with clonus

       (7) Clonus
          (a) Briskly dorsiflex the foot while slightly flexing the knee.
          (b) Involuntary oscillations may be seen between flexion and extension when continuous pressure is applied to the sole of the foot.
          (c) Recorded as number of beats (e.g., three beats clonus).
3. Psychosocial responses
    a. The additional crisis of high-risk pregnancy exacerbates the normal crisis situation, with concerns for herself, her fetus, and her family.
    b. Concerns
       (1) Need for long-term bed rest or hospitalization; strict bedrest no longer recommended because of hazards of immobility, including pulmonary embolism
          (a) Boredom
          (b) Need to be off from work
          (c) Family's need for "substitute" for household and family activities
       (2) Separation from family, friends, and other children when hospitalized
          (a) Need for satisfactory child care
          (b) Need for substitute interaction (e.g., telephone calls, letters)
    c. Behaviors
       (1) Expressed feelings of ambivalence
       (2) Crying or withdrawal; grief over loss of "perfect" pregnancy

  d. Stress responses
    (1) Crying, withdrawal, or silence
    (2) Fear
    (3) Anxiety
    (4) Hospital psychosis: aberrant behavior that occurs when hospitalized for long periods, especially when deprived of sunlight and time orientation
  4. Diagnostic procedures
    a. BP as determined in lateral position
    b. Laboratory tests (Table 21-3)
      (1) Complete blood count (CBC) with platelets
      (2) Type and screen or crossmatch for two units of packed RBCs
      (3) Urine for protein and specific gravity

■ TABLE 21-3
■ ■ **Laboratory Tests Affected by Gestational Hypertension and HELLP**

	Pregnancy	Preeclampsia
Hemoglobin	10-12 g/dl	Decreased in HELLP
Hematocrit	32%-40%	Increased
		Decreased in HELLP
Platelets	150,000-400,000/mm^3	Decreased
Fibrinogen	300-600 mg/dl	Decreased
Fibrin split products	Absent or minimal	Increased
PT	10-14 sec	Unchanged
PTT	20-31 sec	Unchanged
Bleeding time	1-3 min (Duke)	Unchanged
	2-4 min (Ivy)	Decreased
	2-8 min (Template)	Increased
Respiratory:		
Oxygen consumption	180-270 ml/min	Increased
FRC	1.41 L	Decreased
Carbon dioxide content	18-26 mmol/L	Increased
Factors VII, VIII, IX, X	Increased	Increased
Factors XI, XIII	Decreased	Decreased
Renal:		
Creatinine	0.4-1 mg/dl	Increased
BUN	5-10 g/dl	Increased
Uric acid	< 6 mg/dl	Increased in HELLP
Creatinine clearance	130-180 ml/min	Decreased in HELLP
Uric acid clearance	10% of creatinine clearance	
Hepatic:		
Alkaline phosphatase	60-480 IU/ml	Increased in HELLP
Albumin	2.8-3.7 g/dl	Decreased
Bilirubin	Slight elevation from 0.2-0.9 mg/dl	Increased in HELLP
AST (SGOT)	5-40 IU	Increased in HELLP
ALT (SGPT)	3-21 IU	Increased in HELLP
LDH	90-200 IU	Increased in HELLP

HELLP, Hemolysis, elevated liver enzymes, and low platelets; *PT,* prothrombin time; *PTT,* partial thromboplastin time; *FRC,* functional residual capacity; *BUN,* blood, urea, and nitrogen; *AST,* aspartate aminotransferase; *SGOT,* serum glutamic-oxaloacetic transaminase; *ALT,* alanine aminotransferase; *SGPT,* serum glutamic-pyruvic transaminase; *LDH,* lactic dehydrogenase.

(4) Additional tests for women with severe preeclampsia
    (a) Electrolytes
    (b) Fibrinogen, fibrin split products, and D-dimer
    (c) Clot observation: a tube of blood is drawn to observe for clot formation and potential clot degradation.
    (d) Serum uric acid, BUN, creatinine, and creatinine clearance
    (e) Liver function tests
    (f) Kleihauer-Betke analysis to detect fetal red cells in maternal circulation in cases of suspected abruptio placentae; serial platelet counts may provide faster information.
(5) Serial real-time ultrasound evaluation for amniotic fluid index and volume and fetal growth
5. Invasive hemodynamic monitoring with pulmonary artery (Swan-Ganz) catheter
  a. Indications to guide therapy
    (1) Pulmonary edema
    (2) Persistent oliguria (unresponsive to fluid challenge)
    (3) BP greater than 160/110 mmHg despite treatment with antihypertensives
  b. Normal values in pregnancy (Table 21-4)
  c. Goal is to maintain intravascular volume status to optimize pulmonary capillary wedge pressures (PCWP) and cardiac output.
  d. Expect increase in PCWP with cardiogenic pulmonary edema and decrease in PCWP with hypovolemia.

Chronic Hypertension

1. History
  a. Risks depend on:
    (1) Maternal age
    (2) Duration of hypertension
    (3) Presence of medical complications
    (4) Severity of hypertension early in pregnancy
  b. Maternal mortality is usually caused by a critical rise in BP with subsequent congestive heart failure or CVA.
  c. Detailed evaluation to determine severity and nature of hypertension
  d. Review
    (1) Current medications; angiotensin-converting enzyme (ACE) inhibitors and angiotensin II antagonists are contraindicated for use during pregnancy.

■ TABLE 21-4
■ ■ **Normal Swan-Ganz Catheter Values in Pregnancy**

Right atrial or central venous pressure (right preload)	1-7 mmHg
Pulmonary artery pressure (reflects right afterload)	Systolic 18-30 mmHg
	Diastolic 6-10 mmHg
	Mean 11-15 mmHg
Pulmonary capillary wedge pressure (PCWP) (left preload)	6-10 mmHg
Systemic vascular resistance (SVR) (left afterload)	1210 ± 266 dyne/cm/sec-5
Pulmonary vascular resistance (PVR) (true right afterload)	78 ± 22 dyne/cm/sec-5
Cardiac output	6-7 L/min at rest (expect 50% increase during labor)

      (2) History of diabetes or cardiac, renal, or thyroid disease

      (3) Outcome of previous pregnancies (superimposed preeclampsia, preterm delivery, abruptio placentae, perinatal outcomes, infant's birth weight, and appropriateness for gestational age)

2. Physical findings

   a. Hypertension diagnosed before the twentieth week of pregnancy

   b. Increased morbidity and mortality

   c. Increased incidence of superimposed preeclampsia

   d. Increased incidence of abruptio placentae

   e. Clients with labile or borderline hypertension have pathophysiologic alterations with:

      (1) Elevated cardiac output

      (2) Central redistribution of blood volume

      (3) Enhanced activity of autonomic nervous system

      (4) Increased left ventricular ejection rate

      (5) Normal total vascular resistance

   f. Vascular resistance and arterial pressure are elevated, with increased ventricular workload.

   g. Heart rate is increased but stroke volume and left ventricular ejection rate are normal.

   h. Danger of pulmonary edema or congestive heart failure; can be sudden in onset.

   i. Primary essential hypertension: cardiac strain is evident with moderate essential hypertension.

      (1) Stroke volume remains normal or starts to fall.

      (2) Myocardial contractility is normal.

3. Diagnostic procedures

   a. Electrocardiograph (ECG) studies show increased thickness in left ventricular wall.

4. Treatment: see the drugs listed in Table 21-5.

Secondary Hypertension

1. History

   a. The duration of hypertension is important to know.

   b. The client may have:

      (1) Essential or primary hypertension

      (2) Acute or chronic glomerulonephritis

      (3) Chronic pyelonephritis

      (4) Collagen vascular disease

      (5) Systemic lupus erythematosus

   c. Renal disorder is usually the main cause of other origins.

2. Physical findings

   a. Diastolic BP greater than 105 mmHg

   b. Involvement of systems

      (1) Renal conditions

         (a) Acute glomerulonephritis

         (b) Chronic nephritis

         (c) Lupus nephritis

         (d) Diabetic nephropathy

      (2) Endocrinologic conditions

         (a) Cushing's syndrome

         (b) Primary aldosteronism

TABLE 21-5
Drugs Used for Hypertensive Disorders in Pregnancy

Medication/Action	Dosage/Route	Potential Side Effects	Nursing Interventions
MAGNESIUM SULFATE: SEIZURE PROPHYLAXIS			
Decreases acetylcholine released by motor nerve impulse; thereby depresses CNS and provides anticonvulsant effect. Acts peripherally as a vasodilator with transient decrease in BP; however, decreased BP does not continue with prolonged infusion. Use with caution when impaired renal function. Contraindicated with myocardial damage, heart block, or myasthenia gravis.	IV loading dose 4-6 g over 20-30 min, followed by maintenance infusion of 2-4 g/hr. Dosing dependent on renal function.	**Maternal:** Flushing Diaphoresis Lethargy Blurred vision Nausea Hypocalcemia Depressed reflexes Decreased platelet aggregation Cardiac dysrhythmias Respiratory paralysis Circulatory collapse **Fetal/neonatal:** Decreased variability of fetal heart rate Hypotonia Respiratory depression Decreased suck reflex	Monitor strict intake and output. Because magnesium sulfate is excreted via the kidneys, patients with oliguria or renal disease are at risk for toxic levels of magnesium. Assess vital signs every 5-15 min during loading dose, then every 30-60 min (frequency determined by patient status). Assess reflexes every hr. Monitor for signs and symptoms of magnesium toxicity; antidote is calcium gluconate or calcium chloride 5-10 mEq given IV slowly over 5-10 min. Provide seizure precautions and resuscitation equipment at the bedside. If administering IV labetalol for BP control, maternal cardiac monitoring is indicated.

Serum Magnesium Levels	(mEq/L)
Normal	1.5-2
Therapeutic	4-7
ECG changes	5-10
Loss of reflexes	8-12
Respiratory distress	15
Cardiac arrest	25

HYDRALAZINE HYDROCHLORIDE (APRESOLINE): ANTIHYPERTENSIVE AGENT

Action	Dosage	Side Effects	Considerations
Antihypertensive; reduces BP by direct relaxation of vascular smooth muscle. Resultant vasodilation reduces peripheral vascular resistance and increases cerebral and renal blood flow and uteroplacental perfusion. May be contraindicated with cardiac disease because of side effects of tachycardia, increased cardiac output, and oxygen consumption.	For acute dosing: 5-10 mg IV slowly; may repeat every 20 min for max acute dose of 30 mg. Oral dose 10 mg qid.	Tachycardia Hypotension Headache Sodium retention	After IV bolus dose, assess BP every 3-5 min for 30 min. Goal is to maintain diastolic BP between 90 and 100 mmHg. Hypotension might decrease uteroplacental perfusion. Monitor fetal heart rate continuously. Assess intake and output. Use with caution if tachycardia is present. Effect of agent dependent on intravascular volume; rebound hypotension likely.

LABETALOL HYDROCHLORIDE (NORMODYNE, TRANDATE): ANTIHYPERTENSIVE

Action	Dosage	Side Effects	Considerations
Antihypertensive and nonselective beta blocker; produces drop in BP without decreasing maternal heart rate or cardiac output.	IV bolus doses: initial dose 10-20 mg over 2 min; may repeat 20 mg, 40 mg, up to 80 mg every 10 min to maximum dose of 300 mg IV push. IV infusion: 2 mg/min until desired effect; may repeat infusion every 6-8 hrs as needed. Oral dose 100-400 mg bid.	Hypotension Dizziness Nausea/vomiting Bradycardia (maternal and fetal) Rash Increased airway resistance Dysrhythmias Hypoglycemia (maternal and fetal)	After IV bolus dose, assess BP every 5 min for 30 min, then every 30 min for 2 hrs, then hourly for 6 hrs. More frequent assessments may be required according to patient status. With IV administration, continuous cardiac monitoring for dysrhythmias.

NIFEDIPINE (PROCARDIA): ANTIHYPERTENSIVE

Action	Dosage	Side Effects	Considerations
Calcium antagonist used for hypertension and preterm labor; dilates coronary arteries and decreases systemic vascular resistance by relaxing arterial smooth muscle; increases urine output by improving renal blood flow. Contraindicated with heart disease.	10 mg orally every 30 min for three doses, then every 4-8 hrs. Oral maintenance dose 10-30 mg qid to maximum of 180 mg/day.	Hypotension Headache Dizziness	Assess BP every 2-3 min for 30 min during acute treatment. Assess BP before every dose during maintenance therapy. Contraindicated with acute hypertension or with hypertensive crisis.

Continued

■ TABLE 21-5
■ **Drugs Used for Hypertensive Disorders in Pregnancy—cont'd**

Medication/Action	Dosage/Route	Potential Side Effects	Nursing Interventions
SODIUM NITROPRUSSIDE: ANTIHYPERTENSIVE			
Fast-acting antihypertensive by causing direct dilation of arterioles and veins; used for acute management of severe hypertension.	IV infusion: mix 100 mg in 250 ml D_5W for concentration of 400 mcg/ml. Start infusion at 0.25-0.50 mcg/kg/min. Increase every 5 min until desired BP is reached. Maximum dose of 10mcg/kg/min. Takes effect in ½-2 min and lasts 3-5 min.	Hypotension Concern is about cyanide toxicity in fetus caused by drug metabolite.	Assess BP frequently, in accordance with ICU guidelines. Requires invasive hemodynamic monitoring.
METHYLDOPA (ALDOMET): ANTIHYPERTENSIVE			
A slow-acting antihypertensive, methyldopa is not the drug of choice for acute hypertensive crisis; however, it may be used for chronic hypertension. By reducing antenatal BP, uterine blood flow and fetal growth may improve. Use with caution when pregnancy is complicated by liver disease. Metabolized in the liver and excreted in the urine.	Oral dose: 1 g initially, then 1-2 g/day in four divided doses.	Postural hypotension Drowsiness Fluid retention	Assist patient when ambulating if postural hypotension. Monitor fetal heart rate.
FUROSEMIDE (LASIX): DIURETIC			
Diuretics not recommended as adjunct to drug therapy unless pulmonary edema is present; may further deplete intravascular fluid volume, which is already compromised resulting from preeclampsia.	IV bolus for pulmonary edema: 10-40 mg (maximum dose 80 mg) given over several min; may repeat every hr until desired effect.	Maternal: Hypokalemia Hyponatremia Fetal or neonatal: Decreased placental perfusion Thrombocytopenia Hyperbilirubinemia Altered carbohydrate metabolism	Maintain strict intake and output. Assess pulmonary status. Assess hemodynamic values if patient has a Swan-Ganz catheter. Should not be used to treat oliguria or tissue edema.

        (c) Pheochromocytoma

        (d) Thyrotoxicosis

    (3) Neurologic conditions

        (a) CVA

        (b) Quadriplegia

        (c) Blindness

  c. Mortality increases twofold with BP above 160/90 mmHg versus BP below 140/90 mmHg.

3. Treatment

  a. Morbidity is lower in treated women.

  b. Thiazide diuretics are not used during pregnancy.

  c. See the drugs listed in Table 21-5.

Transient Hypertension

1. History

  a. Transient hypertension in the second half of pregnancy, during labor, or within 48 hours after delivery

  b. May be difficult to differentiate from preeclampsia.

  c. A postpartum diagnosis of exclusion

2. Physical findings

  a. Proteinuria of less than 300 mg/L

  b. Renal disease must be ruled out.

3. Treatment: although no treatment is required, the client is often placed on antihypertensive drugs (see Table 21-5).

B. Nursing Diagnoses

1. Risk for central nervous system (CNS) injury related to hypertension, cerebral edema, hemorrhage, or any combination

2. Ineffective tissue perfusion related to renal disturbances

3. Ineffective tissue perfusion related to cardiovascular disturbances and potential for hemorrhage

4. Risk for decreased respiratory function related to excess fluid volume (pulmonary edema)

5. Risk for hepatic injury related to hypertension and ischemia

6. Risk for impaired fetal well being related to altered uteroplacental perfusion and risk of abruptio placentae

7. Anxiety and fear related to risk of harm to self and fetus

C. Interventions/Outcomes

1. Risk for CNS injury related to hypertension, cerebral edema, hemorrhage, or any combination

  a. Interventions

    (1) Monitor BP every 15 to 30 minutes; frequency depends on type of monitoring device being used and patient status.

        (a) More frequently with values of at least 160/110 mmHg and during IV antihypertensive therapy

        (b) Less frequently may be acceptable with values below 160/100 mmHg, when other parameters are reassuring, and after delivery.

        (c) Convenient to use automated BP measurement such as Dinamap (i.e., device for indirect noninvasive automatic MAP); less accurate in high-flow or low-flow states

    (2) Maintain fluid balance and document intake and output (I&O).

        (a) May restrict fluids to 125 ml/hr of combined IV and oral fluids if so ordered.

(b) Monitor urine output.

(c) Measure and document any emesis.

(d) Invasive hemodynamic monitoring (CVP or PA catheter or arterial line) may be ordered with severe preeclampsia.

(3) Assess DTRs and clonus.

(4) Assess for subjective symptoms.

(a) Headaches or pressure

(b) Visual changes and disturbances

(c) Level of consciousness

(5) Maintain woman on bed rest in a lateral position (either left or right lateral is acceptable, as long as supine position is avoided) (Figure 21-2).

(6) Administer antihypertensives to maintain diastolic maternal BP between 90 and 104 mmHg.

(a) This action prevents adverse outcome of sustained hypertension and reduced organ perfusion in the mother.

(b) Avoid compromised uteroplacental perfusion from excessive reduction in BP.

(7) Administer magnesium sulfate or other anticonvulsant as ordered and continue therapy for at least 24 hours after delivery to prevent seizures (see Table 21-5 for drug information).

(8) Interpret laboratory test results of serum magnesium level.

(a) Normal magnesium levels: 1.5 to 2.0 mEq/L

(b) Therapeutic level: 4.0 to 7.0 mEq/L

(9) Maintain antidote for magnesium toxicity on hand: 10 to 20 ml of calcium chloride or calcium gluconate.

b. Outcomes

(1) BP remains within acceptable limits.

(2) Fluid balance is maintained, with urine output greater than 30 ml/hr.

(3) Deep tendon reflexes are within normal limits with no clonus.

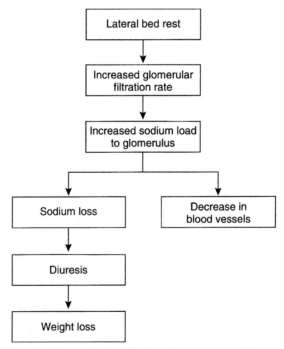

FIGURE 21-2 ■ Effects of lateral bed rest on patient with preeclampsia.

      (4) No symptoms of headaches or visual disturbances are reported.

      (5) Level of consciousness is appropriate.

      (6) No seizures or other CNS damage is evident.

      (7) Serum magnesium level is within therapeutic range.

2. Ineffective tissue perfusion related to renal disturbances

  a. Interventions

      (1) Assess for edema of face, hands, and lower extremities.

      (2) Document I&O.

         (a) Use urometer to measure hourly output with severe preeclampsia or decreased urine output.

         (b) Monitor urine protein and specific gravity.

      (3) Obtain daily weight.

      (4) Administer drugs to dilate vasculature (see Table 21-5 for complete drug information).

      (5) Interpret laboratory test results of renal function (BUN, uric acid, creatinine, creatinine clearance) and 24-hour urine collections.

  b. Outcomes

      (1) No excessive edema is observed.

      (2) I&O balance is maintained with urine output greater than 30 ml/hr.

      (3) Weight gain is within normal limits.

      (4) Laboratory tests of renal function are within normal limits or showing improvement.

3. Ineffective tissue perfusion related to cardiovascular disturbances and potential for hemorrhage

  a. Interventions

      (1) Take vital signs every 15 to 30 minutes or as determined by patient status.

      (2) Maintain continuous cardiorespiratory (pulse and respiratory rate, quality, rhythm) monitoring during IV magnesium sulfate therapy and as indicated per physician's orders.

      (3) Administer antihypertensive medications as ordered to maintain maternal diastolic BP less than 105 mmHg.

      (4) Observe for and report any cardiac irregularities, tachycardia, or chest pain.

      (5) Observe for neck vein distension.

      (6) Assess for generalized edema.

      (7) Instruct woman to remove rings and constrictive clothing.

      (8) Assess capillary refill time (< 3 seconds normal).

      (9) Assess temperature of extremities.

     (10) Assess peripheral pulses.

     (11) Interpret CBC for evidence of anemia, hemoconcentration, and thrombocytopenia.

     (12) Assess for bleeding at all sites.

     (13) When pulmonary artery catheter (Swan-Ganz) is placed for hemodynamic monitoring, interpret values and report to physician and follow institution's intensive care policies.

  b. Outcomes

      (1) Vital signs remaining within normal limits

      (2) No cardiac dysfunction or dysrhythmias observed

      (3) No neck vein distension observed

      (4) No signs of congestive heart failure (CHF) noted

      (5) Capillary refill within normal limits

        (6) Extremities neither cold nor excessively warm

        (7) Laboratory values within normal limits

        (8) No evidence of bleeding at any sites

        (9) Hemodynamic monitoring values within normal limits

4. Risk for decreased respiratory function related to excessive fluid volume (pulmonary edema)

  a. Interventions

     (1) Take vital signs, especially respiratory rate, every 15 to 30 minutes.

     (2) Auscultate breath sounds and evaluate for evidence of pulmonary edema.

     (3) Assess oxygen saturation with pulse oximeter as clinically indicated.

     (4) Assess for tachypnea, tachycardia, and shortness of breath.

     (5) Note presence of cough (dry or productive) and orthopnea.

     (6) Administer oxygen at 10 to 12 L/min as needed.

     (7) Interpret blood gases (Table 21-6 lists arterial blood gas values).

     (8) Assess for increased anxiety or irritability.

     (9) Note distended neck veins.

    (10) Maintain maternal position that optimizes maternal cardiac output and uteroplacental perfusion.

  b. Outcomes

     (1) Vital signs within normal limits

     (2) No signs and symptoms of pulmonary edema

     (3) No signs of respiratory distress

     (4) Oxygen saturation using pulse oximeter and arterial blood gases within normal limits

5. Risk for hepatic injury related to hypertension and ischemia

  a. Interventions

     (1) Assess epigastric pain, right upper quadrant pain, nausea and vomiting.

     (2) Assess jaundice, if present.

     (3) Interpret laboratory test results of liver function (AST, bilirubin, lactic dehydrogenase [LDH]).

     (4) Observe for signs of shock and be prepared for immediate intervention.

     (5) Avoid deep palpation of abdomen.

     (6) Assess for signs and symptoms of hypoglycemia, secondary to liver dysfunction.

  b. Outcomes

     (1) No signs of hepatic injury or rupture are observed.

     (2) Jaundice is documented.

     (3) Liver function studies are within normal limits or showing improvement.

■ TABLE 21-6
■ ■ **Arterial Blood Gas Values**

	Nonpregnant	**Pregnant**	**Fetus**
pH	7.35-7.45	7.40-7.45	7.25-7.35
PO_2	85-100 mmHg	101-108 mmHg	20-30 mmHg
PCO_2	36-44 mmHg	27-32 mmHg	40-50 mmHg
Bicarbonate	24-30 mEq/L	18-21 mEq/L	<10 mEq/L

6. Risk for impaired fetal well being related to altered uteroplacental perfusion and risk of abruptio placentae
   a. Interventions
      (1) Maintain woman on bed rest in a lateral position.
      (2) Antepartum fetal testing as ordered
         (a) Nonstress test
         (b) Contraction stress test
         (c) Biophysical profile with amniotic fluid index
         (d) Ultrasonography for possible IUGR
         (e) Doppler flow studies for impaired uterine artery perfusion
      (3) Instruct mother in technique for daily fetal movement counts (see Chapter 8 for a complete discussion of antepartum tests).
      (4) Continuous EFM while in labor
         (a) Observe for nonreassuring fetal heart rate patterns (see Chapter 12 for a complete discussion of fetal assessment during labor).
            (i) Tachycardia or bradycardia
            (ii) Severe variable decelerations, especially with documented oligohydramnios
            (iii) Late decelerations
            (iv) Decreased variability
            (v) Loss of accelerations
         (b) Report any nonreassuring signs to physician or certified nurse midwife (CNM).
         (c) Provide interventions for intrauterine resuscitation of fetus (e.g., IV fluids, oxygen, lateral position).
         (d) Prepare for delivery as indicated.
   b. Outcomes
      (1) Assessments of systemic and uteroplacental perfusion within normal limits
      (2) Antepartum tests within normal limits
      (3) Reassuring fetal heart rate pattern on EFM
7. Anxiety and fear related to risk of harm to self and fetus
   a. Interventions
      (1) Explain disease process appropriately for woman's and family's level of understanding.
      (2) Explain rationale for interventions and anticipate possible actions.
      (3) Clarify and interpret results of antepartum tests.
      (4) Reassure the woman and family about the fetal status.
      (5) Involve the family in care.
         (a) Explain the need for the woman to remain on bed rest.
         (b) Assist in mobilizing resources to take over the woman's usual functions.
         (c) Refer to social services if necessary for community and financial support.
      (6) Reassure woman and family that preeclampsia was not caused by her lifestyle or diet.
      (7) Before discharge, provide information about risk of recurrence and recommend preconceptual counseling before subsequent pregnancy.
   b. Outcomes
      (1) Woman reports a decrease in anxiety.
      (2) Woman and family members verbalize understanding of the disease process and treatment.

(3) Family members act as support system.

(4) Assistance is obtained from other resources as needed.

HEALTH EDUCATION

A. Provide the client and her family with the following information:

1. The effect of hypertension on all organ systems and the potential for harm resulting from altered tissue perfusion and edema

2. The effect of hypertension on the fetus: with reduction of blood flow to the uterus and resultant decrease in nutrients and oxygen, the fetus may be growth restricted and experience hypoxemia or hypoxia.

3. The importance of activity restriction and rest in a lateral position

4. The signs and symptoms of worsening of condition and when to report them to the health care provider

5. The side effects of magnesium sulfate therapy, including lethargy, nausea, and feeling flushed during the IV bolus

6. The prenatal monitoring that will be performed
   a. Antepartum tests for fetal well being
   b. Laboratory work
   c. Frequent visits to health care provider

7. Recurrence risk of preeclampsia, eclampsia, and HELLP syndrome in subsequent pregnancies and implications for future health

8. For women with chronic hypertension, lifestyle changes that will minimize long-term health risks such as smoking cessation, adequate rest, and weight control through exercise and diet

9. Breastfeeding is permitted while a mother is receiving IV magnesium sulfate and while receiving antihypertensive therapy.

10. Women who were self-monitoring their BP at home before delivery should be instructed to continue checking their BP at home until their postpartum follow-up visit with their health care provider.

B. Methods of teaching

1. Participate in one-to-one teaching, with diagrams of blood vessels, heart, and kidneys if the client has mild preeclampsia.

2. Meet with the family to discuss the requirements of care.

3. Arrange a meeting with the social worker to assess financial needs, emotional needs, and plan solutions.

4. Use interpreters (or other teaching aids) if the woman or family does not speak English.

5. Use videotapes, books, or pamphlets.

6. Review teaching as often as needed, because the client's perception may be altered because of her state of denial, anxiety, lack of comprehension, or general knowledge base.

7. Help the family to recognize the life-threatening potential of this condition.

8. Assist the woman with developing her support systems to help with her care and with child care if needed.

C. Ongoing research about prevention of preeclampsia

1. Often called the *disease of theories*, preeclampsia has been researched throughout the world in an effort to better understand the pathophysiology, predictability, and strategies for prevention.

2. Roles of calcium supplementation and low-dose aspirin are two areas that continue to be investigated.

3. Preliminary studies have supported the hypothesis that calcium supplementation reduces the incidence of preeclampsia and possibly preterm labor; more data have been presented, yet a proven benefit has not been demonstrated.

4. Initial studies of low-dose aspirin reported a reduction in the incidence of preeclampsia among women at risk; further studies have shown conflicting and less promising results.

5. More definitive research is needed to identify predictive risk factors for the development of preeclampsia so preventive interventions can target those at highest risk.

CASE STUDIES AND STUDY QUESTIONS

Ms. M, a 22-year-old, gravida 1, para 0 (G1, P0) black woman, is admitted with BP of 148/96 mmHg, which at her last two prenatal visits had been 130/80 and 140/90 mmHg. Her prepregnancy BP was 100/60 mmHg. She has been on bed rest for 1 week. Her weight gain in the last 2 weeks has been 3.2 kg (7 lb) and 3.6 kg (8 lb) each week. She has pedal edema and is spilling 3+ protein in her urine. She is given a 4-g loading dose of magnesium sulfate followed by a 2-g/hr maintenance dose. Her laboratory reports remain within normal limits, with the exception of the elevated urine protein. The decision is made to continue bed rest. Orders are written for BP checks every 30 minutes, I&O, daily weight, assessment of deep tendon reflexes, and a protein check with every voiding. Fetal surveillance with serial ultrasonography and nonstress tests is instituted.

1. Which of the following is the most common warning sign of preeclampsia?
   a. Edema
   b. Headache
   c. Hypertension
   d. Proteinuria

2. The nurse would suspect the diagnosis of preeclampsia if which of the following was found during assessment?
   a. Ankle edema and ketonuria
   b. Hypertension and hyporeflexia
   c. Proteinuria and hypertension
   d. Proteinuria and ketonuria

3. Which of the following physiologic changes may be present in Ms. M?
   a. Decreased mean arterial BP
   b. Decreased peripheral vascular resistance
   c. Increased plasma renin activity
   d. Increased pressor responsiveness to angiotensin II

4. Her condition has worsened to severe preeclampsia. What signs might you expect?
   a. BP of 152/100 mmHg
   b. Diminished reflexes
   c. Proteinuria 3+ to 4+, 5 g in 24-hour urine testing
   d. Weight loss of 2 lb or more

The client has an eclamptic seizure. She is turned to a lateral position. After the seizure, reflexes are 4+ and clonus is present. The fetus experienced an episode of bradycardia, and oxygen is administered to the mother at 10 L/min via facemask to assist the fetus with intrauterine resuscitation. Delivery is not attempted at this time so the patient can be stabilized.

5. Which of the following is the major complication from a seizure?
   a. Aspiration
   b. Blindness

   c. Pulmonary embolism
   d. Uremia

6. In eclampsia, what organ is particularly affected?
   a. Brain
   b. Heart
   c. Kidney
   d. Lungs

7. What renal lesion is most associated with eclampsia?
   a. Acute tubular necrosis
   b. Cortical necrosis
   c. Glomerular endothelial swelling
   d. Pyelonephritis

Ms. T, a 29-year-old, G2, P1 woman with chronic hypertension of 2 years' duration and superimposed preeclampsia, is at 34 weeks' gestation. Her baseline BP had been 130/90 mmHg; 1 week ago, her BP was 160/105 and today it is 170/110 mmHg. She had a 2.3-kg (5-lb) weight gain in 1 week, 3+ pitting edema, and 4+ proteinuria. Her usual hypertension medications are methyldopa (Aldomet) and hydralazine. She is managed with one-to-one nursing care, with precautions taken to prevent seizures, administration of IV magnesium sulfate, an indwelling catheter with a urometer, BP checks every 15 minutes, reflexes and clonus checks, IV fluid balance monitoring, hypertensive medications, and EFM. Laboratory work included a CBC, liver enzymes, and renal function studies. Induction of labor will be initiated once the client is stabilized.

8. What laboratory values would you expect with Ms. T?
   a. AST of 40 IU/L
   b. Creatinine of 0.6 mg/dl
   c. Platelets of 250,000/mm^3
   d. Uric acid of over 10 mg/dl

9. Clients with hypertension are at risk for damage to many organs during pregnancy. What change increases this risk?
   a. Poor renal function
   b. Cardiac enlargement
   c. Poor pulmonary function
   d. Preeclampsia superimposed on the hypertension

10. Magnesium sulfate should not be administered if which of the following is true?
   a. Respirations are 16/min.
   b. Reflexes are 2+.
   c. Irritability and nervousness are evident.
   d. Patient has myasthenia gravis.

Ms. E, a 37-year-old, G4, P3 woman, gave birth 1 hour ago. She had a normal spontaneous vaginal delivery of a female infant weighing 8 lb, 10 oz. (3912 g) with Apgar scores of 9 and 9. During recovery, Ms. E's BP was 147/90, 152/97, 160/96, and 160/90 mmHg. No edema is evident, and her urine is negative for protein. All laboratory values were normal. The following day, her BP remained elevated. The client and infant were discharged with office follow-up. Her BP remained elevated for 10 days.

11. When all laboratory values are returned normal, and the patient has only hypertension, one must suspect _____ hypertension.

Ms. D, a 32-year-old woman, G1, P0 at 33 weeks' gestation, has had an elevated BP of 140/90 mmHg for 2 weeks, with proteinuria and generalized edema, and has stayed at home on bed rest. She was hospitalized with severe epigastric pain. Laboratory values demonstrated hemolysis with an abnormal peripheral blood smear, an increased bilirubin exceeding 1.2 mg/dl, elevated liver enzymes (AST > 70 IU/L and LDH > 600 IU/L), and a platelet count of less than 100,000/mm^3.

12. The acronym of HELLP syndrome stands for which of the following?
   a. Hemolysis, eclampsia, and low platelets

    b. Hemolysis, elevated liver enzymes, and low platelets

    c. Hyperbilirubinemia, elevated liver enzymes, and low platelets

    d. Hyperbilirubinemia, eclampsia, and low platelets.

13. Ms. J is a 16-year-old woman at 37 weeks' gestation with a BP of 155/105 mmHg; 3+ proteinuria; edema of the face, hands, feet, and ankles; and no seizure activity. She probably has which of the following?
    a. Mild preeclampsia
    b. Severe preeclampsia
    c. Gestational hypertension
    d. Eclampsia

14. Which of the following is found in patients with severe preeclampsia?
    a. Decreased response to angiotensin II
    b. Reduced plasma volume and increased hematocrit
    c. Decrease in uric acid
    d. Increase in creatinine clearance

15. Which of the following are warning signals of preeclampsia that should alert the health care provider?
    a. Sudden excessive weight gain (> 2 or 3 lb/week [1 or 1.5 kg/week])
    b. Generalized skin rash
    c. Elevated diastolic BP greater than 90 mmHg

    d. Elevated systolic BP greater than 140 mmHg
    (1) a, b, c
    (2) a, b
    (3) b, c
    (4) a, c, d

16. A 40-year-old at 32 weeks' gestation has retinal changes and a BP of 180/120 mmHg, which has not changed during her pregnancy, but she has no edema or proteinuria. Which of the following is the correct diagnosis?
    a. Severe preeclampsia
    b. Chronic hypertension
    c. Superimposed preeclampsia
    d. Renal disease

17. Which of the following is a common side effect of magnesium sulfate?
    a. Decreased FH baseline rate
    b. Decreased uteroplacental blood flow
    c. Smooth muscle relaxation
    d. Sympathetic nervous system stimulation

18. A 30-year-old woman at 16 weeks' gestation with a BP of 144/95 mmHg, no edema, and no proteinuria probably has which of the following?
    a. Preeclampsia
    b. Preexisting hypertension
    c. Renal disease
    d. Diabetes

ANSWERS TO STUDY QUESTIONS

1. c	6. a	11. transient	16. b
2. c	7. c	12. b	17. c
3. d	8. d	13. b	18. b
4. c	9. d	14. b	
5. a	10. d	15. 4	

REFERENCES

American College of Obstetricians and Gynecologists (ACOG). (1992). *Invasive hemodynamic monitoring in obstetrics and gynecology.* ACOG Tech Bulletin 175. Washington, DC: ACOG.

American College of Obstetricians and Gynecologists. (2001). *Chronic hypertension in pregnancy.* Washington, DC: ACOG.

American College of Obstetricians and Gynecologists. (2002). *Diagnosis and management of preeclampsia and eclampsia.* Washington, DC: ACOG.

Beevers, G., Lip, G., & O'Brien, E. (2001). ABC of hypertension. BP measurement. Part I—Sphygmomanometry: Factors common to all techniques. *British Medical Journal, 322*(7292), 981-985.

Blackburn, S. (2003). *Maternal, fetal, and neonatal physiology: A clinical perspective* (2nd ed.). St. Louis: Saunders.

Caritis, S., Sibai, B., Hauth, J., Lindheimer, M., VanDorsten, P., Klebanoff, M., et al. (1998). Predictors of pre-eclampsia in women at high risk. National Institute of Child Health and Human Development Network of Maternal-Fetal Medicine Units. *American Journal of Obstetrics and Gynecology, 179*(4), 946-951.

Caritis, S., Sibai, B., Hauth, J., Lindheimer, M.D., Klebanoff, M., Thom, E., et al. (1998). Low-dose aspirin to prevent preeclampsia in women at high risk. National Institute of Child Health and Human Development Network of Maternal-Fetal Medicine Units. *New England Journal of Medicine, 338*(11), 701-705.

Chang, J., Elam-Evans, L., Berg, C., Herndon, J., Flowers, L., Seed, K., et al. (2003). Pregnancy-related mortality surveillance—United States, 1991-1999. *Surveillance Summaries, Morbidity and Mortality Weekly Report, 52*(No. SS-2), 1-8.

Chappell, L., Seed, P., Bailey, A., Kelly, F., Lee, R., Hunt, B., et al. (1999). Effect of antioxidants on the occurrence of preeclampsia in women at increased risk: A randomised trial. *Lancet, 354*(9181), 810-816.

Cunningham, E. (2001). Coping with bedrest. *AWHONN Lifelines, 5*(5), 50-55.

Dekker, G. (1999). Risk factors for preeclampsia. *Clinical Obstetrics and Gynecology, 42*(3), 422-435.

Dekker, G. (2001). Prevention of preeclampsia. In B. Sibai (Ed.), *Hypertensive disorders in women* (pp. 61-84). Philadelphia: Saunders.

Dekker, G.A., Robillard, P.Y., & Hulsey, T.C. (1998). Immune maladaptation in the etiology of preeclampsia: A review of corroborative epidemiologic studies. *Obstetric and Gynecologic Survey, 53*(6), 377-382.

Dekker, G.A., & Sibai, B.M. (1998). Etiology and pathogenesis of preeclampsia: Current concepts. *American Journal of Obstetrics and Gynecology, 179*(5), 1359-1375.

Dekker, G., & Sibai, B. (1999). The immunology of preeclampsia. *Seminars in Perinatology, 23*(1), 24-33.

Dekker, G., & Sibai, B. (2001). Primary, secondary, and tertiary prevention of pre-eclampsia. *Lancet, 357*(9251), 209-215.

Egerman, R., & Sibai, B. (1999a). HELLP Syndrome. *Clinical Obstetrics and Gynecology, 42*(2), 381-389.

Egerman, R., & Sibai, B. (1999b). Imitators of preeclampsia and eclampsia. *Clinical Obstetrics and Gynecology, 42*(3), 551-562.

Fairlie, F., & Sibai, B. (1999). Hypertensive diseases in pregnancy. In E. Reece et al. (Eds.), *Medicine of the fetus and mother* (2nd ed.). Philadelphia: Lippincott.

Feldman, D. (2001). Blood pressure monitoring during pregnancy. *Blood Pressure Monitoring, 6*(1), 1-7.

Ferrer, R., Sibai, B., Mulrow, C., Chiquette, E., Stevens, K., & Cornell, J. (2000). Management of mild chronic hypertension during pregnancy: A review. *Obstetrics & Gynecology, 96*(5, Pt 2), 849-860.

Gilbert, E.S., & Harmon, J.S. (2003). *Manual of high risk pregnancy & delivery* (3rd ed.). St. Louis: Mosby.

Joint National Committee (JNC). *Seventh Report of the Joint National Committee on Prevention, Detection, Evaluation, and Treatment of High Blood Pressure.* (2003). National Institutes of Health (NIH), National Heart, Lung, and Blood Institute. NIH Publication No. 03-5233. Washington, DC: NIH.

Kennedy, R., & French, R. (2003). The effect of the interval between blood pressure determinations on the delay in the detection of changes: A computer simulation. *Anesthesia & Analgesia, 96*(4), 944-948.

Koonin, L.M., MacKay, A.P., Berg, C.J., Atrash, H.K., & Smith, J.C. (1997). Pregnancy-related mortality surveillance—United States, 1987-1990. *Morbidity and Mortality Weekly Report CDC Surveillance Summary, 46*(4), 17-36.

Leicht, T., & Harvey, C. (1999). Hypertensive disorders in pregnancy. In L. Mandeville & N. Troiano (Eds.), *AHWONN's high risk and critical care intrapartum nursing* (2nd ed., pp.159-172). Philadelphia: Lippincott.

Li, D., & Wi, S. (2000). Changing paternity and the risk of preeclampsia/eclampsia in subsequent pregnancy. *American Journal of Epidemiology, 151*(1), 57-62.

Livingston, J., & Sibai, B. (2001). Chronic hypertension in pregnancy. *Obstetrics and Gynecology Clinics, 28*(3), 1-15.

Lowdermilk, D., & Grohar, J. (1998). *High-risk antepartal home care.* White Plains, NY: March of Dimes.

Magpie Trial Collaboration Group. (2002). Do women with preeclampsia, and their babies, benefit from magnesium sulphate? The Magpie Trial: A randomised placebo-controlled trial. *Lancet, 359*(9321), 1877-1890.

Maloni, J. (1998). *Antepartum bed rest: Case studies, research and nursing care.* Washington, DC: AWHONN.

Martin, J.A., Hamilton, B.E., Ventura, S.J., Menacker, F., & Park, M.M. (2002). *Births: Final data for 2000. National Vital Statistics Reports* (Vol. 50, No. 5).

Hyattsville, MD: National Center for Health Statistics.

Martin, J.A., Hamilton, B.E., Ventura, S.J., Menacker, F., Park, M.M., & Sutton, P. (2002). *Births: Final data for 2001.* Hyattsville, MD: National Center for Health Statistics.

Marx, G.F., Schwalbe, S.S., Cho, E., & Whitty, J.E. (1993). Automated blood pressure measurements in laboring women: Are they reliable? *American Journal of Obstetrics and Gynecology, 168*(3, Pt. 1), 796-798.

Mattar, F., & Sibai, B. (1999). Prevention of preeclampsia. *Seminars in Perinatology, 23*(1), 58-64.

Minino, A., Kochanek, K., Murphy, S., & Smith, B. (2002). Deaths: Final data for 2000. *National Vital Statistics Reports, 50*(15), 1-129.

National High Blood Pressure Education Program. (2000). *Working group report on high blood pressure in pregnancy.* (NIH Publication No. 00-3029). Bethesda, MD: National Institutes of Health, National Heart, Lung, and Blood Institute, National High Blood Pressure Education Program.

National High Blood Pressure Education Program Working Group on High Blood Pressure in Pregnancy. (2000). Report of the National High Blood Pressure Education Program Working Group on high blood pressure in pregnancy. *American Journal of Obstetrics and Gynecology, 183*(1), S1-S22.

Newman, M., Robichaux, A., Stedman, C., Jaekle, R., Fontenot, M., Dotson, T., et al. (2003). Perinatal outcomes in preeclampsia that is complicated by massive proteinuria. *American Journal of Obstetrics and Gynecology, 188*(1), 264-268.

O'Brien, E., Asmar, R., Beilin, L., Imai, Y., Mallion, J., Mancia, G., et al. (2003). European Society of Hypertension recommendations for conventional, ambulatory and home blood pressure measurement. *Journal of Hypertension, 21*(5), 821-848.

O'Brien, E., Beevers, G., & Lip, G. (2001). ABC of hypertension. Blood pressure measurement. Part III—Automated sphygmomanometry: Ambulatory blood pressure measurement. *British*

Medical Journal, 322(7294), 1110-1114.

Penny, J., Aidan, A., Shennan, A., Lambert, P., Jones, D., deSwiet, M., et al. (1998). Automated, ambulatory, or conventional blood pressure measurement in pregnancy: Which is the better predictor of severe hypertension? *American Journal of Obstetrics and Gynecology, 178*(3), 521-526.

Poole, J.H. (2004). Hypertensive disorders in pregnancy. In D.L. Lowdermilk & S.E. Perry (Eds.), *Maternity & women's health care* (8th ed., pp. 837-859). St. Louis: Mosby.

Portis, R., Jacobs, M.A., Skerman, J.H., & Skerman, E.B. (1997). HELLP syndrome (hemolysis, elevated liver enzymes, and low platelets) pathophysiology and anesthetic considerations. *American Association of Nurse Anesthetists Journal, 65*(1), 37-47.

Roberts, J. (1999). Pregnancy-related hypertension. In R. Creasy & R. Resnik (Eds.), *Maternal-fetal medicine* (4th ed., pp. 833-872). Philadelphia: Saunders.

Roberts, J., & Cooper, D. (2001). Pathogenesis and genetics of pre-eclampsia. *Lancet, 357*(9249), 53-56.

Robillard, P. (2002). Interest in preeclampsia for researchers in reproduction. *Journal of Reproductive Immunology, 53*(1-2), 279-287.

Scott, J., et al. (1999). *Danforth's obstetrics and gynecology* (8th ed.). Philadelphia: Lippincott.

Seidel, H., Ball, J., Dains, J., et al. (1999). *Mosby's guide to physical examination* (4th ed.). St. Louis: Mosby.

Sibai, B. (2002a). Chronic hypertension in pregnancy. *Obstetrics and Gynecology, 100*(2), 369-377.

Sibai, B. (2002b). Hypertension in pregnancy. In S. Gabbe, J. Niebyl, & J. Simpson (Eds.), *Obstetrics: Normal and problem pregnancies* (4th ed., pp. 945-1004). New York: Churchill Livingstone.

Sibai, B. (2002c). High-risk pregnancy series: An expert's view. Chronic hypertension in pregnancy. *Obstetrics & Gynecology, 100*(2), 369-377.

Sibai, B., & Rodrigues, J. (1999). Preeclampsia: Diagnosis and management. In E. Reece, et al. (Eds.), *Medicine of the fetus and mother.* Philadelphia: Lippincott.

Sibai, B.M. (1998). Prevention of preeclampsia: A big disappointment. *American Journal of Obstetrics and Gynecology, 179*(5), 1275-1278.

Sibai, B.M. (1999). Thrombophilias and adverse outcomes of pregnancy— What should a clinician do? *New England Journal of Medicine, 340*(1), 50-52.

Sibai, B.M., Lindheimer, M., Hauth, J., Caritis, S., VanDorsten, P., Klebanoff, M., et al. (1998). Risk factors for preeclampsia, abruptio placentae, and adverse neonatal outcomes among women with chronic hypertension. National Institute of Child Health and Human Development Network of Maternal-Fetal Medicine Units. *New England Journal of Medicine, 339*(10), 667-671.

Stone, J.H. (1998). HELLP syndrome: Hemolysis, elevated liver enzymes, and low platelets. *Journal of the American Medical Association, 280*(6), 559-562.

Thadhani, R., Ecker, J., Kettyle, E., Sandler, L., & Frigoletto, F. (2001). Pulse pressure and risk of preeclampsia: A prospective study. *Obstetrics & Gynecology, 97*(4), 515-520.

von Dadelszen, P., Ornstein, M., Bull, S., Logan, A., Koren, G., & Magee, L. (2000). Fall in mean arterial pressure and fetal growth restriction in pregnancy hypertension: A meta-analysis. *Lancet, 355*(9198), 87-92.

Walker, J.J. (1998). Antioxidants and inflammatory cell response in preeclampsia. *Seminars in Reproductive Endocrinology, 16*(1), 47-55.

Walker, S.P., Higgins, J.R., & Brennecke, S.P. (1998a). Ambulatory blood pressure monitoring in pregnancy. *Obstetrics and Gynecologic Survey, 53*(10), 636-644.

Walker, S.P., Higgins, J.R., & Brennecke, S.P. (1998b). The diastolic debate: Is it time to discard Korotkoff phase IV in favour of phase V for blood pressure measurements in pregnancy? *Medical Journal of Australia, 169*(4), 203-205.

Wong, D.L, & Perry, S.E. (1998). *Maternal child nursing care.* St. Louis: Mosby.

Yeo, S., & Davidge, S. (2001). Possible beneficial effect of exercise, by reducing oxidative stress, on the incidence of preeclampsia. *Journal of Women's Health and Gender Based Medicine, 10*(10), 983-989.

22 Maternal Infections

BARBARA A. MORAN

OBJECTIVES

1. Identify causative pathogens and describe primary signs and symptoms of perinatal infections.
2. Identify risk groups for acquired immunodeficiency syndrome (AIDS) and other sexually transmitted diseases (STDs).
3. Correlate history and physical findings with early indicators of maternal infection.
4. Recognize clinical signs and symptoms of perinatal infections.
5. Discuss potential fetal complications associated with maternal infections.
6. Formulate nursing interventions from information obtained in the history.
7. Define health-education strategies to prevent maternal infections.

INTRODUCTION

Infection is a common complication of pregnancy. Some infections affect only the mother, such as urinary tract infection (UTIs) and trichomonis. Other infections such as rubella, cytomegalovirus (CMV), and parvovirus infection have little effect on mother but cause significant fetal injury; and others such as gonorrhea culture (GC), syphilis, Toxoplasmosis, rubella, and human immunodeficiency virus (HIV) may cause serious problems for both mother and infant. Infections may be acquired transplacentally, may ascend in the birth canal, or be acquired during the passage through the vagina at the time of birth.

Torch (Table 22-1)

A. TORCH is an acronym for a group of five infectious diseases.
   1. Toxoplasmosis
   2. Other (hepatitis B)
   3. Rubella
   4. CMV
   5. Herpes simplex virus (HSV)

B. Each disease is teratogenic.
   1. Each crosses the placenta.
   2. Each may adversely affect the developing fetus.
   3. The effect of each varies, depending on developmental stage at time of exposure.

Clinical Practice

A. Assessment
   1. History
      a. Influenza-like illness
      b. Fever of unknown origin
      c. Exposure to sick children

Text continued on p. 598

Continued

TABLE 22-1
TORCH Disease

Infection	Agent	Mode of Transmission	Detection	Maternal Effects	Neonatal Effects	Treatment	Incidence and Prevention	High-Risk Potential
Toxoplasmosis	Single-celled protozoan parasite *Toxoplasma gondii*	Transplacental Eating raw meat, especially pork, lamb, or venison Touching your hands or your mouth after handling undercooked meat containing *T. gondii* Secreted in feces of infected cats Cyst is destroyed with heat	Serologic antibody testing IgM-specific antibody IgG seroconversion from negative to positive Most accurate confirmation of active infection is a rise in IgG titer in two appropriately spaced tests	Most infections in humans are asymptomatic However, may include fatigue, muscle pains, and sometimes lymphadenopathy In the immunocompetent person, toxoplasmosis can be a devastating infection	Severity varies with gestational age Congenital infection can occur if a woman develops acute toxoplasmosis during pregnancy (most likely in the third trimester) May have miscarriage if acquired early Fetal infections more virulent the earlier the infection is acquired but less frequent Sequela include low birth weight, hepatosplenomegaly, icterus, anemia, neurologic disease, and chorioretinitis Clinical significant congenital toxoplasmosis occurs in approximately 1 in 8000 pregnancies	Pyrimethamine and sulfadiazine may reduce incidence of congenital toxoplasmosis Treatment of the mother has shown to reduce the risk of congenital infection *Pyrimethamine is not recommended for use during the first trimester of pregnancy*	ACOG does not recommend routine screening except for pregnant women with HIV infection Incidence varies throughout world (1-4 infants per 1000 live births) 30% of U.S. women have been exposed Approximately 40%-50% of U.S. adults have antibody to this organism Frequency of seroconversion during pregnancy is ≤ 5%, and approximately 3 in 1000 infants show evidence of congenital infection Incidence on congenital toxoplasmosis infection in U.S. is 1 in 1000-8000 More than 60 million people in the U.S. carry the parasite Cook meat to a safe temperature Peel or thoroughly wash fruits and vegetables	Populations that consume raw or poorly cooked meat High-risk gestational age is 10-24 weeks Toxoplasmosis is more common in Western Europe, particularly France

TABLE 22-1
■ TORCH Disease—cont'd

Infection	Agent	Mode of Transmission	Detection	Maternal Effects	Neonatal Effects	Treatment	Incidence and Prevention	High-Risk Potential
							Clean cooking surfaces and utensils after contact with raw meat Pregnant women should avoid changing cat litter	
Hepatitis B	HBV Incubation usually 60-90 days	Direct contact with the blood or body fluids of an infected person Sexual Perinatal Percutaneous Transplacental Blood, stool, amniotic fluid, and saliva transmission Shared razors, toothbrushes, towels, and other personal items	HbsAg identified 7-14 days after exposure Hepatitis B surface antibody present with HbsAg indicates noninfectious HbcAg, HbeAg, and AntiHBc evaluate stage and progression of infection	Course of the disease is not altered during pregnancy Symptoms are seen in only 30%-50% of patients; these include low-grade fever, nausea, anorexia, jaundice, hepatomegaly, malaise, premature labor, and premature birth No specific treatment, but may include bed rest and a high-protein, low-fat diet Mother to child transmission of HBV occurs in 10%-20% of women who are seropositive for HbsAg and in 90% of women who are seropositive for both HBsAg and HBcAg	Infants infected at birth have a 90% risk of becoming chronically infected with HBV (carrier) and 25% risk of developing significant liver disease—yet if they receive prophylaxis at birth, 95% can be prevented Increased risk of transmission to infant if mother is HBeAg-positive (indicating acute infection) Stillbirth Clinical illness is relatively infrequent Most (90%-95%) of those infected are symptomatic and become chronic hepatitis B carriers Infants born to women who have hepatitis B infection during pregnancy should be given	Mother: rest Infant: vaccine If mother is carrier, infant receives HBIg HBV vaccine recommended (three doses)	Screen all pregnant women The incidence of hepatitis B in the U.S. declined by >60% from 1985 to 1995 Estimated that 1 to 1.25 million people in the U.S. are chronically infected with HBV Estimated that 300 million people worldwide are chronically infected with HBV Approximately 8000 acute HBV infections were reported to CDC HBV vaccine (available since 1982) Acute infection occurs in 1-2 per 1000 pregnancies Minimize exposure of close physical contact Heptavax-B	High-risk categories: Pregnant women from China, Southeast Asia, Africa, Philippines, and Indonesia Eskimos Prostitutes Homosexuals IV drug users Hemophiliacs Transfusion recipients People with other sexually transmitted diseases or multiple sex partners CDC recommends universal screening of all prenatal patients

Infection	Mode of transmission	Signs and symptoms	Diagnosis	Fetal/neonatal effects	Management/nursing considerations
	Transmission to the neonate appears to occur as a result of exposure to infected blood and genital secretions during delivery				HBIg within 12 hrs of delivery; (pregnancy does not contraindicate vaccination)
Rubella (German measles)	Nasopharyngeal secretions; Transplacental	Erythematous; Maculopapular rash on face, neck, arms, and legs lasting 3 days; Lymph node enlargement; Slight fever, malaise, headache, and arthralgia; History of exposure 3 weeks earlier	Virus isolated from throat; Rubella-specific IgM antibodies; Hemagglutination-inhibition antibodies; Complement-fixing antibodies; Rubella antibody titer of 1:8 or more indicates immune status	Overall risk of congenital rubella syndrome is approximately 20% for primary maternal infection in the first trimester; High incidence of congenital abnormalities in newborns whose mother contracted rubella within first 4 months of pregnancy; Approximately 50% of infants exposed to the virus within 4 weeks of conception will manifest signs of congenital infection; When infection occurs in second 4-week period after conception, approximately 25% of fetuses will be infected; when infection develops in third month, approximately 10% of fetuses will be infected; Spectrum anomalies: Deafness (60%-75%); Eye defects (10%-30%)	Women with rubella require no special therapy other than mild analgesics and rest; Infants born with congenital rubella may shed the virus for many months and thus be a threat to other infants, as well as to susceptible adults
Rubella virus; Incubation is 2-3 weeks					Last epidemic in 1965—since introduction of vaccine in late 1960s, rubella is rare; Absence of rubella antibody indicates susceptibility; Estimated that 6%-25% of women are susceptible; Occurs more commonly in springtime; Vaccinate immediately postpartum and use contraception for a minimum of 3 months after vaccination; Vaccine is contraindicated during pregnancy

Continued

TABLE 22-1
■ **TORCH Disease—cont'd**

Infection	Agent	Mode of Transmission	Detection	Maternal Effects	Neonatal Effects	Treatment	Incidence and Prevention	High-Risk Potential
					CNS anomalies (10%-25%) Cardiac malformation (10%-20%)			
Cytomegalovirus (CMV)	DNA virus of the herpesvirus group	Transmitted horizontally by droplet infection and contact with saliva and urine, vertically from mother to fetus-infant, and as a sexually transmitted disease Intimate contact with infected secretions (breast milk, cervical mucus, semen, saliva, tears, semen, and urine) Transplacental Organ transplantation	Isolation of virus from urine or endocervical secretions	Most infections are asymptomatic, but approximately 15% of adults have a mononucleosis-like syndrome characterized by fever, pharyngitis, lymphadenopathy, and polyarthritis	Risks appear to be almost exclusively associated with women who previously have not been infected with CMV Even in this case, ⅔ of infants will not become infected and, only 10%-15% of the remaining will have symptoms Infection is most likely to occur with primary maternal infection The timing of infection during pregnancy is major determinant of outcome (first and second trimester being more severely affected) CID includes low birthweight, IUGR, microcephaly CNS abnormalities, mental and motor retardation, intracranial calcifications, sensorineural	Mother: treat symptoms Infant: no satisfactory treatment is available Isolate infant Approximately 50% of females in the United States have antibodies Estimates are that approximately 2% of susceptible pregnant women acquire primary CMV infection during pregnancy in the United States	As with other herpesviruses, maternal immunity to CMV does not prevent recurrence Found in 0.5%-2.0% of all neonates Incidence of primary CMV infection in pregnant women in the United States varies from 1%-3% Rigorous personal hygiene throughout pregnancy	Day care centers are a common source of infection Prevalence depends on age, race, sex, class, sexual behavior, and occupational or institutional exposure Serologic screening is not recommended by ACOG Vaccine is experimental

Herpes simplex virus (HSV)	Transmission	Diagnosis	Signs and Symptoms	Fetal/Neonatal Effects	Prevention	Epidemiology	Risk Factors
Herpes virus type 1 (more common with oral lesions) and type 2 (more common in genital lesions) Incubation is 2-10 days	Ascending infection Intimate mucocutaneous exposure Transmission is more likely to occur from men to women Passage through an infected birth canal Transplacental (although rare) if initial infection occurs during pregnancy	Tissue culture (swab specimen from vesicles) and immunofluorescent staining of the cell can differentiate HSV-1 from HSV-2 Swelling, redness, and painful lesions	Painful genital, vesicle lesions Vesicles on cervix, vagina, or external genitalia area Primary infection is commonly associated with fever, malaise, and myalgia; numbness, tingling, burning, itching, and pain with lesions; lymphadenopathy; and urinary retention	deafness, blindness with chorioretinitis, mental retardation, hepatosplenomegaly, and jaundice Rare transplacental transmission have resulted in miscarriage Mortality of 50%-60% if neonatal exposure is with active primary infection Neurologic morbidity such as chorioretinitis, microcephaly, mental retardation, seizures, and apnea	Protect neonate from exposure at time of delivery Cultures are done when mother has active lesions Avoid routine sue of scalp electrodes If lesions are visible, delivery by cesarean section is the current standard of care Acyclovir has been used near delivery to suppress outbreak	Estimated 1 million Americans are newly infected with genital HSV annually Seroprevalence of HSV is approximately 25% Approximately 1%-2% of pregnancies 1 in 3000-20,000 live births for the development of neonatal herpes Up to 70% of women delivering infected infants have no history of genital herpes Prophylactic treatment with oral acyclovir may be appropriate in women with frequent recurrent infections in pregnancy If symptoms or lesions are present, cesarean delivery should be performed Avoid genital contact when male partner has penile lesions Use condoms	Risk factors include female sex, African-American, or Mexican-American ethnic background, older age, low educational level, poverty, cocaine use, and a greater number of lifetime sexual partners Unprotected sex and having a sexual partner with genital herpes

ACOG, American College of Obstetricians and Gynecologists; *AntiHBc*, antibody to hepatitis B core antigen; *CDC*, Centers for Disease Control and Prevention; *CID*, cytomegalic inclusion disease; *CNS*, central nervous system; *DNA*, deoxyribonucleic acid; *HBV*, hepatitis B virus; *HIV*, human immunodeficiency virus; *HbsAg*, surface antigen to HBC; *HbcAg*, core antigen to HBV; *HbeAg*, hepatitis B early antigen; *HBIg*, hepatitis B immunoglobulin; *IgG*, immunoglobulin G; *IgM*, immunoglobulin M; *IUGR*, intrauterine growth restriction; *IV*, intravenous.

      d. Rash

      e. Painful genital lesions

      f. Close contact with possibly infected cats (outside-dwelling cats)

      g. Chronic fatigue

      h. Blood or secretion exposure

      i. Raw meat ingestion

  2. Physical findings

      a. Lymphadenopathy: suboccipital, postauricular, cervical

      b. Rash: pink or red maculopapules

      c. Ulcerated, painful lesions on the cervix, vagina, and genital area

      d. Low-grade temperature

      e. Headache

      f. Malaise

      g. Anorexia

      h. Jaundice

      i. Hepatomegaly

      j. Arthralgias or arthritis

      k. Nausea and vomiting

      l. Clay-colored stool

  3. Psychosocial findings

      a. Anxiety

      b. Fear

      c. Apprehension

  4. Diagnostic tests and findings

      a. Complete blood count (CBC) (white blood cell [WBC] count increased to over 12,000)

      b. TORCH screen

      c. Immunoglobulin G (IgG)–specific antibody (i.e., rubella-specific IgG to document prior infection)

      d. IgM-specific antibody (i.e., rubella-specific IgM to confirm recent infection; it becomes detectable approximately 1 week after onset of illness and persists for approximately 1 month).

      e. Culture lesions

      f. Hepatitis B surface antigen (HBsAg) is present in blood 30 to 50 days after exposure and 7 to 21 days before the onset of jaundice.

      g. Hepatitis B e antigen (HBeAg): the presence of e antigen denotes a high degree of infectivity.

      h. Enzyme-linked immunosorbent assay (ELISA)

      i. Liver function

        (1) Elevated bilirubin levels

        (2) Elevated transaminase enzyme levels

      j. Serial sonography (to detect intrauterine growth restriction [IUGR])

B. Nursing Diagnoses

  1. Deficient knowledge related to infection and its treatment

  2. Anxiety and fear related to possible sequelae

  3. Risk for injury related to infection

C. Interventions/Outcomes

  1. Deficient knowledge related to infection and its treatment

      a. Interventions

        (1) Give factual information on the infection: mode of transmission and possible sequelae.

        (2) Give directions on any medication the client needs to take.

      (3) Provide written material that contains the same information at the client's level of understanding.

      (4) Review options in cases of known teratogenic effects.

    b. Outcomes

      (1) Client is able to verbalize knowledge about the infection and treatment needed.

      (2) Client is able to verbalize signs and symptoms that would indicate a need to seek further care.

      (3) Client is able to use self-care measures and to comply with recommended regimen.

2. Anxiety and fear related to possible sequelae

    a. Interventions

      (1) Provide information as previously described to increase the client's sense of control and decrease the client's anxiety by minimizing fear of unknown.

      (2) Develop trust and rapport by being nonjudgmental.

      (3) Give information in a calm and consistent manner.

      (4) Have client's significant other involved in counseling if she desires.

      (5) Encourage questions and verbalizations of fears.

    b. Outcomes

      (1) Client is able to verbalize decreased anxiety related to infection.

3. Risk for injury related to infection

    a. Interventions

      (1) Teach the importance of follow-up care.

      (2) Teach mode of transmission.

      (3) Breastfeeding is usually not discouraged.

    b. Outcomes

      (1) Client is able to minimize and prevent further risk factors.

ACQUIRED IMMUNODEFICIENCY SYNDROME (Table 22-2)

Introduction

A. Major public health issue: first recognized in 1981; by the end of 2000, over 450,000 deaths among persons with AIDS in the United States had been reported to the Centers for Disease Control and Prevention (CDC); the number of deaths in persons with AIDS increased each year from the beginning of the epidemic until 1995; the introduction of highly active antiretroviral therapy (HAART) in 1996 had a dramatic effect on the survival time of persons with HIV infection and AIDS, resulting in large increases in the number of persons living with HIV and AIDS; data from the National Vital Statistics System show that from 1992 to 1995, HIV infection was the eighth leading cause of death among all persons in the United States; in 2000, HIV infection was the eighteenth leading cause of death; an HIV-infected person receives a diagnosis of AIDS after developing one of the CDC-defined AIDS indicator illnesses.

B. HIV

  1. Agent: retrovirus (ribonucleic acid [RNA] virus)

    a. A virus containing RNA that has the ability to produce deoxyribonucleic acid (DNA) in its cellular host

    b. HIV destroys blood cells—CD4 T cells (helper cells) that are crucial to the normal function of the human immune system; loss of these cells in people with HIV is an extremely powerful predictor of the development of AIDS.

TABLE 22-2
Sexually Transmitted Diseases

Infection	Agent	Detection	Maternal Effects	Neonatal Effects	Treatment	Incidence
Acquired immunodeficiency syndrome (AIDS)	HIV retrovirus	EIA—if positive repeat; if the second test is positive, a confirmatory Western blot assay or IFA Decreased number of CD4 cells and inverted CD4:CD8 ratio	Studies have shown no effect of pregnancy on the progression of HIV disease Complications include preterm delivery, preterm PROM, intrauterine growth restriction, increased perinatal mortality and postpartum endometritis Fever, malaise, fatigue, anorexia, nausea, vomiting, diarrhea, weight loss, and generalized lymphadenopathy Opportunistic infections include *pneumocystis carinii* pneumonia, mycobacterium avium complex, pulmonary tuberculosis, toxoplasmosis, candidiasis, and CMV infection	Mother to child transmission accounts for vast majority of pediatric HIV infection 25%-30% chance on transmission from infected mother, unless she is treated Antiretroviral prophylaxis has reduced perinatal transmission to < 2% If HIV positive as newborn, repeat antibody testing at 6 months	All patients should be offered voluntary screening ZDV should be given orally starting at 14 weeks gestation and continued throughout pregnancy, intravenously during labor, and to the newborn for the first six wks of life—reduces the risk of perinatal transmission by 66% and is recommended Many drug combinations are now being used including Laminvudine, Zidovudine, and Nelfinavir	First recognized in 1981 and appears to have originated in Africa Increasing incidence in women An estimated 16.4 million women worldwide are living with HIV; 600,000 children are infected annually
Human papilloma virus (condyloma acuminatum)	Human papilloma virus (HPV) a heterogeneous group of DNA viruses; known to be the primary cause of cervical carcinoma and causative factor in cancers of the vulva, vagina, and anus Over 200 HPV genotypes have been identified Incubation: 3-9 mos	Cervical cytologic testing Colposcopy used as adjunct in equivocal situation Single or multiple, irregular, painless papules in the genital or perianal area	May enlarge during pregnancy If enlarged, may interfere with delivery; therefore, may need a cesarean section	Approximately 2%-5% of all births are at risk for neonatal HPV exposure Potential transmission of laryngeal papillomata Vaginal delivery is estimated to carry a 0.04% risk of laryngeal infection to the neonate	Small lesions: trichloroacetic acid, 80%-90% (TCA); cryotherapy; CO_2 laser therapy; electrocautery; podophyllin; or 5-FU *(which is contraindicated in pregnancy)* Large lesions: surgical excisions In pregnancy, small lesions do not require treatment, but larger lesions may be	Most common sexually transmitted infection in the United States, causing 5.5 million new cases each year Estimated 20 million Americans are currently infected with HPV Prevalence of Increasing incidence noted in STD clinics and private offices Risk factors: number of

Disease	Etiology/Diagnosis	Maternal Effects	Fetal/Neonatal Effects	Treatment	Comments
(continued from previous page)				treated with TCA or surgically removed by cryotherapy, laser, electrocautery, or excision	sexual partners, age of first intercourse < 16 considered greater risk), number sexual partners male partner has had, age of first male partner (older, greater risk) Peak occurrence at age 15-35
Chlamydia	Bacteria: *Chlamydia trachomatis* Endocervical and urethral culture Tissue culture	Approximately 75% of women are asymptomatic Mucopurulent cervicitis, bartholinitis, salpingitis, friable cervix, and postpartum endometritis May be associated with other STDs Up to 40% of women with untreated chlamydia will develop PID, 20% will become infertile, 18% will experience chronic pelvic pain, and 9% will experience tubal pregnancy Occasional effects include PROM, preterm labor, IUGR, and chorioamnionitis	Up to 50% of exposed infants develop conjunctivitis 10% of exposed infants develop pneumonia Nearly ⅔ of infants born vaginally to mothers with chlamydial infection become infected during delivery	Erythromycin or amoxicillin (when pregnant) Doxycycline (postpartum) Tetracycline (nonpregnant) Simultaneous treatment of partner Test of cure 2 weeks after therapy Erythromycin ophthalmic ointment for newborn	Associated with other STDs An estimated 3-4 million cases occur annually in the United States An estimated 30% of pregnant women are infected Increase in adolescent and young adult population, multiple sex partners, and nonbarrier contraceptive methods
Gonorrhea	Bacteria: *Neisseria gonorrhoease,* gram-negative diplodocus Incubation: 10 days Endocervical, oral, or rectal cultures Gram stain	Asymptomatic to mildly symptomatic localized infection of urethra, endocervix, rectum, or any combination Acute PID May cause severe disseminated infection: arthritis, dermatitis, pericarditis, endocarditis, and meningitis Dysuria, urinary frequency, PPROM, chorioamnionitis, and endometritis	Purulent conjunctivitis Sepsis or meningitis	Ceftriaxone (125 mg IM) and cefixime (400 mg PO) Treat sex partners Treat infant with either silver nitrate or tetracycline ophthalmic preparation	One of the most common STDs—second only to chlamydial infections Over 1 million cases are reported in United States each year Primarily seen in women with multiple sex partners and history of other STDs

Continued

■ TABLE 22-2
■ ■ **Sexually Transmitted Diseases—cont'd**

Infection	Agent	Detection	Maternal Effects	Neonatal Effects	Treatment	Incidence
Syphilis	Bacteria: spirochete—*Treponema pallidum* Incubation: 10-90 days (average 21 days)	VDRL RPR Positive screening needs to be confirmed with FTA-ABS Will have positive tests within 4 weeks of initial infection Secondary syphilis—increased liver enzymes	Primary chancre—painless ulcerative lesion Secondary syphilis—fever and malaise, red macules on palms or soles of feet Generalized lymphadenopathy Early latent positive serology <1 year's duration Late latent >1 year Cardiovascular syphilis and neurosyphilis	Transplacental transmission Effects vary on gestation Stillbirth IUGR Prematurity (caused by preterm labor) Frequency of vertical transmission varies with stage of maternal disease	Bicilin Erythromycin (if allergic to penicillin) Tetracycline (*not used during pregnancy*) Pregnant women receiving penicillin for treatment of syphilis may develop uterine contractions and decreased fetal movement that resolves within 24 hrs	Greatest increase in infection has been in women age 15-24 30,000 new cases annually primarily in persons ages 20-39 Congenital syphilis—92 cases per 100,000 live births Associated with other STDs
Trichomonas	Protozoan: *Trichomonas vaginalis*	"Wet prep" saline examination Papanicolaou smear Urinalysis	Malodorous, frothy, discolored vaginal discharge 75% have symptoms, including pruritus, vaginal bleeding, dysuria, and dyspareunia	Infant contact through infected vagina Usually asymptomatic or short lived	Metronidazole (Flagyl) for mother and sex partner (avoid during first trimester) Single dose of 2 g; 250 mg TID ×7 days; or 500 mg BID ×7 days Local therapy	Responsible for approximately 25% of cases of vaginitis Estimated 3 million cases per year More common in women with multiple sex partners Also nonvenereally acquired
Bacterial vaginosis	Polymicrobial massive overgrowth of anaerobic bacteria *Gardnerella vaginalis, Mobiluncus* species	Thin, gray, homogeneous, malodorous vaginal discharge "Wet prep" for Clue cells—vaginal epithelial cell covered with bacteria pH > 4.5 Fishy odor	Associated with preterm labor, PROM, chorioamnionitis, endometritis, and UTIs	No specific risks other than secondary to prematurity	Metronidazole (Flagyl) 250 mg TID ×7 days, for mother and sex partner (avoid during first trimester) Clindamycin, 300 mg TID ×7 days	Responsible for approximately 45% of cases of vaginitis

5-FU, 5-Fluorouracil; *BID*, two times daily; *CMV*, cytomegalovirus; *CO$_2$*, carbon dioxide; *DNA*, deoxyribonucleic acid; *EIA*, enzyme immunoassay; *FTA-ABS*, fluorescent treponema antibody absorption test; *HIV*, human immunodeficiency virus; *IFA*, immunofluorescent antibody assay; *IM*, intramuscular; *IUGR*, intrauterine growth restriction; *PID*, pelvic inflammatory disease; *PO*, by mouth; *PPROM*, preterm, premature rupture of membranes; *PROM*, premature rupture of membranes; *RPR*, rapid plasma reagin; *STD*, sexually transmitted disease; *TID*, three times daily; *UTI*, urinary tract infection; *VDRL*, Venereal Disease Research Laboratory; *ZDV*, zidovudine.

2. Transmission
   a. By exposure to blood and blood products or byproducts
      (1) Transfusions: this mode of transmission has dramatically decreased since screening of donated blood for HIV started in 1985.
      (2) Needle sharing among addicts
      (3) Accidental inoculation in health care workers
   b. Perinatal exposure
      (1) Transplacental
      (2) Intrapartal
      (3) Breast milk
   c. Sexual contact: factors that increase the rate of transmission include:
      (1) Lack of condoms
      (2) Sex during menses
      (3) Number of sexual contacts
      (4) Presence of genital sores
      (5) Advanced disease
   d. Highest concentrations of HIV have been isolated from blood, semen, and cerebrospinal fluid.
   e. HIV also is found in vaginal secretions, saliva, tears, breast milk, amniotic fluid, and urine; contact with saliva or tears have not been shown to result in infection.
   f. Not transmitted through casual contact (e.g., water, food, environmental services)
C. **Counseling and early diagnosis are recommended for the following:**
   1. Persons who consider themselves at risk for infection
   2. Women of childbearing age who are at risk for infection
   3. Persons attending STD clinics and drug abuse clinics
   4. Women seeking family planning services
   5. Tuberculosis patients and selected patients who received transfusions of blood and blood components between 1978 and 1985
   6. The CDC operates a free telephone service that is available 24 hours, 7 days a week (1-800-342-2437); services for Spanish-speaking audiences and the deaf are also available.
D. **Women and AIDS** (Table 22-3 and Figure 22-1)
   1. Total number of AIDS cases reported in the United States through December 2001 was 816,149.
   2. Total number of female AIDS cases reported in the United States through December 2001 was 145,461.
   3. AIDS is the fifth leading cause of death among women 25 to 44 years of age; among African-American women in this same age group, HIV-AIDS was the third leading cause of death in 1999.
   4. African-American and Hispanic women together represent less than one-fourth of all U.S. women, yet they account for more than three-fourths (78%) of AIDS cases reported to date among women in this country.
   5. Percentage of infected women is increasing
      a. 1981: women constituted 3% of total cases.
      b. 1985: women constituted 6.6% of total cases.
      c. 1989: women constituted 10.9% of total cases.
      d. 1994: women constituted 18% of total cases.
      e. 1999: women constituted 25% of total cases.
      f. 2001: women constituted 32% of total cases.

■ TABLE 22-3
■ ■ **Women with AIDS by Race/Ethnicity per 100,000 Women—United States (Reported in 2001)**

Race/Ethnicity	Number	Percentage
Black	84,681	57%
White	30,854	19%
Hispanic	28,554	18%
Asian/Pacific Islander	803	4%
American Indian/Alaska native	480	2%
Total	145,372	100%

    6. Heterosexual contact is now the greatest risk for women.
    7. States with the highest rates of AIDS among women are New York, Maryland, Delaware, and Florida, as well as the District of Columbia (Figure 22-2).
    8. Women are at a higher risk than men to contract HIV infection through heterosexual activity because of the vaginal mucus.
    9. Perinatal transmission has been decreasing because of the advent of drug therapies such as zidovudine (ZDU).
E. Treatment
    1. Prevention of several opportunistic infections affecting persons with HIV infection is available.
       a. Until recently, the main drug treatment for HIV infection was nucleoside analogs; recently, major advances in HIV therapy have been made; a significant number of investigations have shown that a combination of nucleoside analogs (zidovudine, didanosine, zalcitabine, or lamivudine) given with a protease inhibitor (indinavir, ritonavir, or saquinavir) is highly effective.
       b. Few studies have been conducted regarding this particular multidrug use in pregnancy; however, because of the mortality and morbidity associated with the disease, these may be recommended to pregnant women.

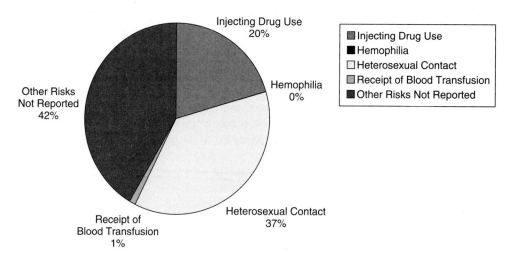

FIGURE 22-1 ■ Exposure category of female AIDS cases, reported through December 2001.

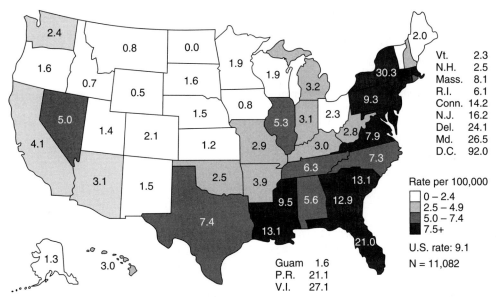

FIGURE 22-2 ■ Female adult-adolescent annual AIDS rates per 100,000 population, for cases reported in 2001 in the United States. (From Centers for Disease Control and Prevention, National Center for HIV, STD, and TB Prevention, Divisions of HIV/AIDS Prevention. [2002]. *HIV/AIDS surveillance report* [Vol. 13, No. 2]. Washington, DC: CDC.)

2. ZDU was formerly known as azidothymidine (AZT).
   a. The safety and efficacy of ZDU during pregnancy has been documented.
   b. The use of ZDU (Retrovir) can substantially reduce the risk of mother-to-child transmission of HIV in some patients to approximately < 8% from approximately 30%.
   c. Medical care of the HIV infected pregnant woman requires coordination and communication between the HIV specialist caring for the woman and her obstetrician.

Clinical Practice

A. Assessment
   1. History
      a. Fatigue
      b. Malaise
      c. Fever
      d. Night sweats
      e. Diarrhea
      f. Weight loss
      g. Anorexia
      h. Cognitive changes
      i. Neurologic disorders
      j. History of blood transfusion before 1985
      k. Oral or gingival lesions
      l. Nasal congestion
      m. Cough and shortness of breath
      n. Recurrent or persistent vaginal infections
      o. Lymphadenopathy

    p. Menstrual cycle disturbance (substance abuse and weight loss may cause oligomenorrhea and amenorrhea)

    q. Tuberculosis (TB); including association with persons with TB

    r. Intravenous (IV) drug abuse

    s. Prostitution

    t. Sexual behavior: number of sexual partners, sexual orientation, contraceptive use, and specific sexual practices

    u. Partner who is an IV drug user or is bisexual

2. Physical findings

    a. Elevated temperature

    b. Lymphadenopathy

    c. Oral or gingival lesions

    d. Vaginitis caused by *Candida, Trichomonas,* and bacterial vaginosis

    e. Presence of opportunistic infection

        (1) *Pneumocystis carinii* pneumonia

        (2) Kaposi's sarcoma; reddish-blue or purple lesions on hard palate; rare in women with AIDS

        (3) Candidiasis (thrush)

            (a) White patches on mucous membrane

            (b) Candida esophagitis; more common in women

        (4) Disseminated mycobacterial infections

        (5) Ulcerative herpes simplex

        (6) Salmonella

        (7) Hepatitis

        (8) CMV; may cause CMV retinitis ("floaters," blurring vision)

        (9) Toxoplasmosis

        (10) Human papillomavirus (HPV) condyloma

        (11) Syphilis

        (12) TB

        (13) *Staphylococcus aureus*; most common bacterial skin disease

3. Psychosocial findings

    a. Anxiety

    b. Fear

    c. Lack of social support and social isolation

    d. Stress

    e. Depression

    f. Emotional instability

    g. Denial

    h. Financial problems

    i. Possible lack of food, clothing, and basic child care or health care

    j. Transportation problems

4. Diagnostic procedures

    a. The enzyme immunoassay assay (EIA) is used as a screening test for HIV antibodies; a positive screening test has a sensitivity of over 99.5%; antibodies can be detected in 95% of patients within 6 months of infection.

    b. Diagnostic tests

        (1) CBC with differential and platelet count (to monitor anemia, leukocytopenia, and thrombocytopenia)

        (2) Type, Rh factor, and antibody screen

        (3) Rubella titer

        (4) HbsAg

        (5) Purified protein derivative (PPD) or radiograph (incidence of active TB is markedly elevated among HIV-infected patients).

      (6) Immunoglobulin levels are elevated.
      (7) Papanicolaou (Pap) smear: increased incidence of invasive cervical cancer
      (8) *Gonorrhea, Chlamydia* cultures, and TORCH screen
      (9) Ultrasonography every trimester for IUGR, congenital abnormalities, and placental problems
     (10) Venereal Disease Research Laboratory (VDRL) testing
     (11) Urinalysis: may reveal proteinuria resulting from AIDS nephropathy.
     (12) Blood chemistries
        (a) Elevated blood, urea, nitrogen (BUN) and creatinine levels may indicate presence of AIDS-related renal disease.
        (b) Abnormal liver enzymes may indicate liver infiltration by opportunistic infection.
        (c) Elevated total protein may indicate hypergammaglobulinemia.
        (d) Decreased albumin may indicate poor nutrition.
     (13) Antigen capture assay
     (14) Viral culture

B. Nursing Diagnoses
   1. Deficient knowledge related to HIV infection, other infections, treatment, and sequelae
   2. Fear related to risk for infection and deterioration of maternal condition
   3. Anticipatory grieving related to decreased quality of life for self and fetus
   4. Interrupted family processes related to pregnancy
   5. Imbalanced nutrition: less than body requirements related to infection
   6. Ineffective individual coping related to infection

C. Interventions/Outcomes
   1. Deficient knowledge related to infection, its treatment, and sequelae
    a. Interventions
      (1) Provide information about HIV antibody testing and benefits of early diagnosis.
        (a) Encourage all pregnant women to be tested.
        (b) Inform the client that antibodies generally appear within 3 months after infection with HIV but may take up to 6 months in some persons.
      (2) Provide information about the infection and how it is transmitted in an open and nonjudgmental manner; make safer sex a routine part of health teaching for all clients.
      (3) Discuss high-risk behaviors for HIV transmission.
      (4) Provide information on implications of HIV infection versus the disease of AIDS.
      (5) Counsel client about the risk to sexual partners and lack of risk to casual contacts at home and work; explain precautions regarding blood and body fluids.
      (6) Give written information on the foregoing at a level that the client can understand; refer to support groups and appropriate web sites.
      (7) Assure client of confidentiality; ask the client to consider if and to whom she wishes to disclose diagnosis (if she wants family or partner to know), and document this information.
      (8) Explain all procedures and treatments.
        (a) Counsel about risk of HIV transmission to infant.
        (b) Provide information on ZDU to reduce risk of perinatal infection.

(c) Discuss CDC guidelines for treatment during pregnancy; refer to the latest CDC guidelines on their website at *www.cdc.gov/hiv.*
(d) Emphasize adherence of taking medications as directed.
(9) Explain local and federal laws.
b. Outcomes
(1) Client verbalizes meaning of HIV antibody testing.
(2) Client understands implications of a positive result.
(3) Client expresses understanding of procedures.
(4) Client will use latex or polyurethane condoms correctly.
(5) Client understands rights related to confidentiality.
2. Fear related to risk for infection and deterioration of maternal condition
a. Interventions
(1) Acknowledge the client's fears.
(2) Encourage ventilation of feelings of anger and guilt in an emotionally supportive environment.
(3) Provide appropriate information to enable the client to make informed decisions.
(4) Assess coping mechanism in prior crises and history with illness.
(5) Encourage the client to use family and significant others for support if available.
(6) Assess available support (family, friends, religious group).
(7) Provide factual information and correct misconceptions.
(8) Assist significant others to provide needed support.
(9) Provide information on support groups.
(10) Give as many options as possible to maintain feeling of control.
b. Outcomes
(1) Client is able to express her concerns openly.
(2) Client identifies source of fear and concern.
(3) Client exercises control in decision making.
(4) Client is able to accept support.
3. Anticipatory grieving related to decreased quality of life for self and fetus
a. Interventions
(1) Acknowledge client's grief and anger.
(2) Assist in understanding grief process.
(3) Encourage expression of feelings of potential loss.
(4) Assist support people in adjusting to situation.
(5) Assess support systems within the client's life.
(6) Help the client identify potential loss.
(7) Encourage the client to identify strengths and positively reinforce them.
b. Outcomes
(1) Client is able to move through grieving process.
(2) Client identifies potential loss.
(3) Client communicates understanding of grieving process.
(4) Client seeks support groups.
4. Interrupted family processes related to pregnancy
a. Interventions
(1) Assess the client's perception of pregnancy and her role as mother.
(2) Assess significant others' support of the client and self.
(3) Refer the client for stress management techniques.
b. Outcomes
(1) Client is able to communicate with her family and significant others about her pregnancy and the potential of the disease process.

(2) Family is willing to meet emotional and physical needs of the client.
5. Imbalanced nutrition: less than body requirements related to infection
   a. Interventions
      (1) Supplemental vitamins
      (2) Ferrous sulfate
      (3) Folic acid (if low folate levels)
      (4) Provide nutritional information, emphasizing increased protein intake.
      (5) Refer the client to a nutritionist.
   b. Outcomes
      (1) Client prevents further nutritional decline.
      (2) Client has appropriate uterine growth for gestational age.
6. Ineffective individual coping related to infection
   a. Interventions
      (1) Assist the client in objectively viewing illness.
      (2) Provide accurate information of potential procedures.
      (3) Assist the client in developing appropriate coping skills.
      (4) Assist the client in identifying feelings such as anger and guilt.
      (5) Refer the client to health care workers who focus on AIDS.
      (6) Refer the client to mental health worker or support group.
   b. Outcomes
      (1) Client verbalizes threat of disease accurately.
      (2) Client appropriately expresses her feelings, including anger and guilt.
      (3) Client has ability to solve problems and make decisions.

SEXUALLY TRANSMITTED DISEASES

Introduction

A. **Other STDs include the following:**
   1. Gonorrhea
   2. Syphilis
   3. HPV
   4. Chlamydia
   5. Trichomonas
   6. Candida
B. **Definition**
   1. STDs are any diseases spread by sexual contact between partners.
   2. Transmission occurs through contact with the genitalia, mouth, or rectal area of an infected person.
C. **High-risk population**
   1. Adolescents
   2. Women with multiple sex partners
   3. Indigent women with no prenatal care
D. **Statistics**
   1. Approximately 3 to 4 million new infections with *Chlamydia*, 1 million new cases of gonorrhea, 30,000 new cases of syphilis, 5 million new cases of HPV, and 3 million new infections with *Trichomonas* occur each year; reasons may include:
      a. Age of sexual activity has declined.
      b. Number of sexual partners has increased.
      c. Most common method of birth control is oral contraceptives, which do not protect against STDs.

  d. Many avoid treatment and, if treated, do not inform partner.
 2. Most cases occur among persons under 25 years of age.

Clinical Practice

A. Assessment
 1. History: sexual history needs to be taken in a nonjudgmental manner.
  a. Previous STD infection for self or partner
  b. Multiple sexual partners
  c. Sex with new partner in the preceding 2 months
  d. Sexual partners with penile discharge, condyloma, or ulcer
  e. Dysuria
  f. Fever
  g. Dyspareunia
  h. Vaginal discharge, itching, or odor
  i. Exposure to infected sexual partner
  j. Recent use of antibiotics or other medications
  k. Allergy history (allergic reactions to soap or medications often mimic STD lesions).
 2. Physical findings
  a. Purulent urethral or cervical discharge
  b. Friable cervix
  c. Genital lesion that may or may not be painful
  d. Tender uterus, adnexal structures, or both
  e. Pain on motion of cervix
  f. Inguinal adenopathy
  g. Low-grade temperature
  h. Disseminated lymphadenopathy
  i. Rash on palms and soles of feet in secondary syphilis
  j. Papillomatous excrescences (genital warts)
  k. Poor personal hygiene
 3. Psychosocial findings
  a. Anxiety
  b. Fear
  c. Confusion
  d. Difficulty in communicating
  e. Guilt
 4. Diagnostic tests and findings
  a. Positive cervical, oral, or rectal culture for gonorrhea
  b. Positive cervical culture for *Chlamydia* or *Streptococcus*
  c. Gram stain showing gram-negative diplococci
  d. VDRL or rapid plasma reagin (RPR) test for general screening
  e. Fluorescent treponemal antibody absorption (FTA-Abs) test for specific testing
  f. Tissue cultures
  g. Potassium hydroxide (KOH) smear and wet prep (to identify *Trichomonas*, *Monilia*, and "clue cells")
  h. Culture of herpes lesions
  i. Microscopic darkfield examination for motile spirochetes
B. Nursing Diagnoses
 1. Deficient knowledge related to infection, its treatment, and sequelae
 2. Impaired comfort related to infection
 3. Anxiety and fear related to infection and its possible sequelae

C. Interventions/Outcomes

1. Deficient knowledge related to infection, its treatment, and sequelae
   a. Interventions
      (1) Provide factual information about cause, mode of transmission, and rationale for treatment of the related STD.
      (2) Explain importance of taking prescribed medication and completion of entire course, even if symptoms subside.
      (3) Provide written material for the client to take home.
      (4) Instruct client in warning signs of complications (e.g., fever, increased pain, bleeding).
      (5) Advise the client to abstain from intercourse until she and partner are free of infection.
      (6) Advise the client of possible side effects of medications.
      (7) Instruct the client in good hygiene to prevent secondary infection.
      (8) Advise the client of importance of having her sexual partners evaluated and treated.
   b. Outcomes
      (1) Client is able to verbalize understanding of the infection and its treatment.
      (2) Client is able to use self-care measures.
      (3) Client complies with medication treatment and returns for follow-up appointments.
      (4) Client has her partner examined and treated.
      (5) Client states the warning signs of complications and side effects of medications and ways to prevent reinfection.
2. Impaired comfort related to infection
   a. Interventions
      (1) Assess level of discomfort.
      (2) Administer analgesics as ordered (acetaminophen or aspirin).
      (3) Aid the client in taking warm sitz baths.
      (4) Advise the client to use a hair dryer to dry the genital area.
      (5) Advise the client to expose lesions to air.
   b. Outcomes
      (1) Client appears comfortable.
      (2) Client has fewer complaints of pain.
      (3) Client returns to an infection-free state.
3. Anxiety and fear related to infection and its possible sequelae
   a. Interventions: same as with other infections
   b. Outcomes: same as with other infections

URINARY TRACT INFECTION AND PYELONEPHRITIS

Introduction

A. Includes

1. Lower urinary tract disease; asymptomatic bacteriuria (ABS) during pregnancy and cystitis—most common bacterial infection encountered during pregnancy
2. Upper urinary tract disease (acute pyelonephritis)

B. Anatomic and physiologic changes

1. A change in urine composition occurs that supports bacterial growth.
2. Dilation of the upper part of ureter occurs—renal calyces and pelvis, as well as the ureters.

    3. Enlarging uterus compresses ureters.

    4. Smooth muscle relaxation effect of progesterone leads to stasis of urine and delayed emptying.

C. Predisposing history

    1. History of UTI before pregnancy

    2. History of childhood UTI

    3. Advanced maternal age

    4. Low socioeconomic status

    5. Underlying chronic diseases

    6. Hypertension: studies demonstrate mixed association.

    7. Risk factors include sickle cell trait, preeclampsia, diabetes, and poor hygiene.

D. Statistics

    1. Asymptomatic bacteriuria is found in 2% to 10% of pregnant women, depending on parity, race, and socioeconomic status; more common in women who are older, of higher parity, of lower socioeconomic status, and have a past history of UTI.

    2. Pyelonephritis in pregnancy is 1% to 2%; however, will develop in 25% to 30% of cases of bacteriuria, if untreated.

    3. Approximately 75% to 80% of cases of pyelonephritis occur on the right side.

    4. Acute pyelonephritis may cause premature labor and delivery and causes postpartum endometritis.

Clinical Practice

A. Assessment

    1. History

       a. Previous asymptomatic bacteriuria or UTIs, voiding habits, and urine continence

       b. Recent catheterization

       c. Frequent intercourse

       d. Presence of predisposing diseases such as hypertension, diabetes, sickle cell trait, or kidney disease

       e. Abdominal or pelvic surgery or trauma to the pelvis

    2. Physical findings

       a. Dysuria

       b. Frequency

       c. Hematuria

       d. Fever or chills

       e. Urgency

       f. Suprapubic pain

       g. Nocturia

       h. Malaise

       i. Malodorous urine

       j. Flank pain

       k. Low abdominal pain and tenderness: may be mistaken for labor, chorioamnionitis, appendicitis, placental abruption, or infarcted myoma.

       l. Nausea, vomiting, or diarrhea

       m. Tender urethra and trigone (bladder neck)

       n. Spiking or elevated temperature 37.2° to 38.9° C (99° to 102° F) (with pyelonephritis, may be above 38.9° C [102° F])

       o. Costovertebral angle (CVA) tenderness

       p. Decreased bowel sounds (with pyelonephritis)

3. Psychosocial findings: anxiety
4. Diagnostic findings
  a. Urine: midstream, clean-catch specimen
    (1) Pyuria (more than 5 WBCs per high-power field)
    (2) Hematuria
    (3) Bacteria: greater than 100,000 colonies/ml of a single organism
      (a) *Escherichia coli* can account for majority (80% to 90%) of UTIs.
      (b) A mixed culture suggests a specimen contamination.
      (c) Other organisms may include the following:
        (i) *Proteus*
        (ii) *Klebsiella*
        (iii) *Enterobacter*
        (iv) Group B streptococci
        (v) Staphylococci
  b. CBC with differential
    (1) Elevated WBC count (12,000 to 20,000 WBCs) and 80% polymor-phonuclear leukocytes (PMNs)
    (2) Anemia (from chronic bacteriuria)
    (3) Serum creatinine
  c. Fever and anatomical location of the pain and tenderness are the findings most commonly used to tentatively distinguish cystitis from pyelonephritis.
B. Nursing Diagnoses
  1. Deficient knowledge related to infection, its treatment, and possible sequelae
  2. Risk for injury related to infection
  3. Anxiety and fear related to possible sequelae
C. Interventions/Outcomes
  1. Deficient knowledge related to infection, its treatment, and possible sequelae
    a. Interventions: provide information related to the following:
      (1) Signs and symptoms of a UTI (pain with urination, urgency, frequency) and importance of reporting them to health care provider
      (2) Importance of adequate hydration: 8 to 10 glasses of water each day
      (3) Correct method of wiping perineal area
      (4) Prompt voiding
      (5) Possible effects of UTI on pregnancy (e.g., preterm labor)
    b. Outcomes
      (1) Client is able to state the signs and symptoms of a UTI and the importance of seeking treatment quickly.
  2. Risk for injury related to infection: acute pyelonephritis during pregnancy is associated with a significantly increased rate of prematurity; relationship of ASB to premature delivery is controversial.
    a. Interventions
      (1) Importance of completing treatment with antibiotics must be explained so client will take all of her medications; possible treatments include.
        (a) Amoxicillin, 500 mg 3 times a day for 3 days
        (b) Ampicillin 250 to 500 mg 4 times a day for 3 days
        (c) Cephalosporin, 250 mg 4 times a day for 3 days
        (d) Nitrofurantoin 50 to 100 mg 4 times a day; 100 mg twice daily for 3 days
        (e) Sulfonamide 500 mg 4 times a day for 3 days

             (f) For frequent bacteriuria recurrences, suppressive therapy for the remainder of pregnancy may be indicated; one regimen that has been successful is nitrofurantoin, 100 mg at bedtime.

             (g) Cephalosporins have replaced ampicillin as the choice for single-agent therapy for acute pyelonephritis in pregnancy.

        (2) Obtain follow-up urine cultures; continuous surveillance for recurrent bacteriuria by repeated urine cultures is essential.

        (3) Instruct the client on signs and symptoms of early labor, and tell her to report them promptly.

    b. Outcomes

        (1) Client returns to an infection-free state and remains free of infection throughout pregnancy.

  3. Anxiety and fear related to possible sequelae

    a. Interventions

        (1) Providing information as described earlier increases the client's sense of control.

        (2) Give information in a calm, consistent manner.

    b. Outcomes

        (1) Client verbalizes a decrease in her anxiety level.

OTHER INFECTIOUS DISEASES

Introduction

A. Other communicable diseases include the following:

  1. Measles

  2. Mumps

  3. Chickenpox

  4. Influenza

  5. Mononucleosis

  6. Upper respiratory infection (URI)

  7. Parvovirus

B. Effects

  1. Pregnant women are exposed to the same communicable diseases as the general population.

  2. Both mother and fetus must be considered.

  3. Effect of infection varies depending on disease and stage of pregnancy during which infection occurs.

Clinical Practice

See Table 22-4 for a complete discussion of the previously named communicable diseases: transmission, maternal and fetal effects, and treatment.

A. Assessment

  1. History

    a. Previous exposure

    b. Lack of immunization

  2. Physical findings

    a. Stuffy nose or nasal discharge

    b. Watery eyes

    c. Fever, chills, or low-grade fever

    d. Enlarged lymph nodes

    e. Fatigue, malaise

Text continued on p. 620

■ TABLE 22-4
■ ■ **Infectious Diseases**

Infection	Agent	Mode of Transmission	Maternal Effect	Neonatal Effect	Incidence and Prevention
Varicella (chickenpox) zoster (shingles)	Virus: VZU Member of herpes virus family Incubation: 10-21 days May be latent in dorsal root ganglia and reactivated years later to cause herpes zoster or shingles	Portal of entry is respiratory tract Transmitted via aerosolized reparatory droplets Transplacental Vesicular secretions are highly contagious Contagious from 1-2 days before the onset of the characteristic rash through the crusting over of all the lesions (4-5 days after onset of the rash)	No evidence that pregnancy specifically influences the spectrum of initial signs and symptoms Varicella is a febrile systemic illness associated with generalized pruritic rash Death per case ratio is 50 in 100,000 in adults compared with 2 in 100,000 in children Risk of premature labor caused by high temperature Risk of varicella pneumonia appears to be increased during pregnancy Postexposure prophylaxis is available through the use of VZIG, which is shown to reduce the maternal risks of varicella infection associated complications if administered within 72-96 hours after exposure	Congenital varicella syndrome (usually exposed before 20 wks) may cause congenital malformations by transplacental infection Chorioretinitis Cerebral cortical atrophy Hydronephrosis Leg defects Spontaneous abortion Intrauterine fetal demise Frequency of congenital infection was 0.4% when maternal infection occurred before 13 weeks' gestation Fetal exposure later in pregnancy is associated with congenital varicella lesions If mother contracts infection 5-7 days or less before delivery, administer VZIG to reduce the occurrence and severity of varicella	All women should be assessed for immunity High rate of seropositive women (93%-95%); therefore only approximately 5% of the childbearing women are susceptible Generally occurs during late winter or early spring Incidence estimated in 0.7 per 1000 pregnancies If seronegative, an attenuated live-virus (Varivax) before conception *Not recommended for pregnant women* Preconception vaccinations—delay pregnancy for 3 months Avoid exposure Passive immunization with VZIG—give within 96 hrs of exposure— safe during pregnancy

Continued

TABLE 22-4
■ Infectious Diseases—cont'd

Infection	Agent	Mode of Transmission	Maternal Effect	Neonatal Effect	Incidence and Prevention
Mumps	Paramyxovirus Incubation: 16-18 days	Respiratory secretions	Spontaneous abortion rate is increased twofold	Teratogenicity is unknown, but probably rare or nonexistent	Up to 80%-90% of adults are seropositive *Mumps vaccine is contraindicated during pregnancy*
Influenza	Virus: influenza virus Incubation: 24-72 hours	Respiratory secretions Spread from person to person when an infected person coughs or sneezes	Usually brief but incapacitating disease Pregnancy can increase the risk for complications of influenza Effects include fever, headache, extreme tiredness, dry cough, sore throat, runny or stuffy nose, and muscle aches Deaths occur from secondary bacteria pneumonia	No firm evidence exists that influenza virus causes congenital malformations	Approximately 10%-20% of U.S. residents get influenza Peak influenza season in the United States occurs from late December through March Vaccination against influenza is recommended by the CDC for all pregnant women after the first trimester Antiviral drugs to treat early influenza in adults not recommended for pregnant women Marked decline with improved vaccinations
Measles (rubeola)	RNA virus Incubation is 10-19 days	Highly contagious Respiratory secretions Airborne Transplacental	Prodromal period lasting 4 days before the appearance of the rash Fever, malaise, cough, and conjunctivitis Pulmonary complications	Does not appear to be teratogenic Increased mortality in preterm and term infants with neonatal measles Evaluate fetus (with sonogram) for microcephaly, growth restriction, and oligohydramnios	Second vaccination for older children and college students Vaccination contraindicated during pregnancy Susceptible women are

				If mother has had infection 7-10 days before birth, infant should receive IM immunoglobulin	vaccinated routinely postpartum
Tuberculosis (TB)	Tubercle bacillus	Respiratory secretions	5%-10% risk of contracting active, clinical disease if infected Need to be evaluated for treatment with IPT	Neonatal tuberculosis carried a high morbidity and mortality rate At birth, evaluate for congenital TB and have PPD	Approximately one third of world's population infected with TB 8 million new cases diagnosed annually and 3 million deaths annually worldwide
Group B Streptococcus	*Streptococcus agalactiae*— gram-positive organism	Colonizes the female genital track and anorectum Vertical transmission occurs both during pregnancy and labor Horizontal transmission occurs after birth	UTI, pyelonephritis, chorioamnionitis, preterm labor, GBS bacteriuria, vaginal discharge, postpartum endometritis, post-cesarean wound infection, and endocarditis	Most common cause of neonatal infectious morbidity and mortality in the United States The transmission rate from mother to baby at birth is 50%-75% EOD: before 7 days after birth (80%-85%)— pneumonia and sepsis, reparatory distress, apnea (mortality rate: 4.5)—vertical transmission LOD: after first week of life—3-4 months of age, not as severe as EOD, meningitis, fever, lethargy, vomiting, bulging fontanel— mortality rate 2% Risk factors include prematurity, maternal	Rx: Penicillin G antibiotic of choice Erythromycin or clindamycin for penicillin allergic women Estimated 50,000 women experience GBS infection Approximately 20%-25% of pregnant women harbor group B strep Prevalence of neonatal group B strep is 1-2 per 1000 live births Approximately 7000 to 8000 cases each year in the United States Either risk-based or screening-based approach to prevention: Risk-based—intrapartum antibiotic prophylaxis is given to women with

Continued

TABLE 22-4
■ **Infectious Diseases—cont'd**

Infection	Agent	Mode of Transmission	Maternal Effect	Neonatal Effect	Incidence and Prevention
				intrapartum fever (ROM > 12-18 hrs), previously infected infant with GBS, GBS bacteriuria in this pregnancy	preterm labor, PPROM, ROM 18 hours or longer or with intrapartum fever of 38° C or greater Screening-based: CDC recommends routine cultures on pregnant women at 35-37 weeks gestation and if positive, give antibiotics (penicillin G) during labor Ampicillin is an acceptable alternative
Parvovirus B19 (fifth disease)	DNA virus	Respiratory secretions Possible through infectious particles on surfaces Transplacental	Bright red macular rash and erythroderma that affects the face giving a "slapped face" appearance; elevated temperature; arthralgia affecting hands, wrists and knees; and malaise Associated with miscarriage	Most frequently cited frequencies of risk of transmission to fetus is 5%-15% Diagnose with ultrasound will show evidence of hydrops	Confirmation of infection is by parvovirus-specific IgM Typically occurs in elementary school and day care populations in the late winter and early spring Having children ages 6-7 years was associated with a fourfold rate of seroconversion Risk of women with primary infection during first 20 weeks of pregnancy is 15%-17%

Disease	Organism	Transmission/Characteristics	Clinical manifestations	Fetal/Neonatal effects	Notes/Treatment
					50% of adults in the United States have had a past infection
Listeriosis	*Listeria monocytogenes* gram-positive aerobic motile bacillus	Isolated from soil, water, and sewage. Foodborne transmission is important	May be asymptomatic or cause a febrile illness. Associated with preterm labor	Neonate is particularly susceptible to infection and mortality approaches 50%. Early onset: diffuse sepsis with multi-organ involvement. Associated with high stillbirth rate and high neonatal mortality rate. Late onset: meningitis, neurologic sequelae	CDC estimates that nearly 2500 individuals in the United States annually are ill with listeriosis and over 500 will die. From 1%-5% of adults carry Listeria in their feces. Penicillin G and ampicillin are effective
Lyme disease	*Borrelia burgdorferi*	Tick-borne infection	Multisystem illness characterized by a distinct lesion, erythema chronicum migrans. Neurologic, cardiac, or arthritic manifestations	Experience with pregnancy is limited. CDC identified five adverse outcomes: prematurity, cortical blindness, fetal demise, and syndactyly and rash in the neonate. No relationship demonstrated between congenital malformation and the presence of antibody to Lyme disease	Tetracycline is an effective agent for eradicating *B. burgdorferi* but is *contraindicated in pregnancy*

CDC, Centers for Disease Control and Prevention; *DNA*, deoxyribonucleic acid; *EOD*, early onset disease; *IgM*, immunoglobulin M; *IPT*, isoniazide prevention therapy; *IM*, intramuscular; *LOD*, late onset disease; *PPROM*, preterm, premature rupture of membranes; *RNA*, ribonucleic acid; *ROM*, rupture of membranes; *UTI*, urinary tract infection; *VZIG*, zoster immune globulin; *VZU*, varicella zoster virus.

     f. Myalgia (muscle aches)

     g. Skin rash (macules, papules, or vesicles)

     h. Sore throat and cough

     i. Adenopathy

     j. Parotitis (swollen salivary glands)

  3. Psychosocial findings

     a. Anxiety

     b. Fear

     c. Apprehension

  4. Diagnostic findings

     a. CBC (increased WBC count)

     b. Throat culture

     c. Mononucleosis spot test and heterophile test

     d. Disease-specific serology antibody tests of IgG and IgM

     e. Virus isolation

     f. Serological testing: ELISA or fluorescent antibody membrane antigen (FAMA)

B. Nursing Diagnoses

  1. Deficient knowledge related to infection, its causes, treatment, and possible sequelae

  2. Anxiety and fear related to infection, its treatment, and possible sequelae

C. Interventions/Outcomes

  1. Deficient knowledge related to infection, its causes, its treatment, and possible sequelae

     a. Interventions

       (1) Provide information about the signs and symptoms of the communicable disease, its mode of transmission and prevention, and the importance of reporting exposure to health care provider.

       (2) Provide written material containing information at appropriate level for the client.

       (3) Reinforce need for the client to take all of medication.

       (4) Provide information about the safety of vaccines during pregnancy.

     b. Outcomes

       (1) Client understands disease process.

       (2) Client is able to prevent or decrease occurrence of the disease.

       (3) Client will report any signs or symptoms.

  2. Anxiety and fear related to infection, its treatment, and possible sequelae

     a. Interventions

       (1) Provide information as described earlier to increase the client's sense of control and to decrease her uncertainty.

       (2) Give information in a calm, consistent manner.

     b. Outcomes

       (1) Client expresses concerns about communicable disease.

       (2) Client's anxiety about effect of disease process on her pregnancy is decreased.

CHORIOAMNIONITIS

Introduction

A. Definition

  1. Inflammation of the chorion and amnion occurs.

  2. Mononuclear leukocytes and PMNs infiltrate the membranes.

3. Organisms are usually present in vagina (most commonly *Streptococcus*).
4. Chorioamnionitis occurs in approximately 1% to 5% of term pregnancies.
B. **Chorioamnionitis is associated with the following:**
  1. Premature rupture of membranes
  2. Prolonged rupture of membranes
  3. In patients with preterm delivery, the frequency of infection may approach 25%.
  4. About 5% to 10% of infants born to mothers with chorioamnionitis have pneumonia or bacteremia.
C. **Management**
  1. Identification of the infecting organism
  2. Parenteral antibiotic therapy
  3. Delivery of the infant
  4. Vaginal delivery preferred, but cesarean section may be performed in presence of severe infection

Clinical Practice

A. **Assessment**
  1. History
    a. Premature rupture of membranes before the onset of labor
    b. Prolonged rupture of membranes during or before the onset of labor
    c. Prenatal infection
    d. Poor prenatal care
  2. Physical findings
    a. Maternal fever (39° C [102.2° F] in mild infection and 40° C [104° F] in severe infection)
    b. Maternal and fetal tachycardia (usually over 180 beats/minute)
    c. Fetal monitoring tracing consistent with hypoxia
    d. Chills
    e. Uterine pain and tenderness
    f. Foul-smelling vaginal discharge
    g. Hypotension
    h. Tachycardia
  3. Psychosocial findings
    a. Fear
    b. Anxiety
  4. Diagnostic findings
    a. Amniotic fluid (bacteria and neutrophils seen)
    b. Culture of amniotic fluid and cervix: possible pathogens include the following:
      (1) Group A and B streptococci
      (2) *Neisseria gonorrhea*
      (3) *Chlamydia*
      (4) *Staphylococcus aureus*
      (5) *Haemophilus influenzae*
      (6) *Escherichia coli*
      (7) Anaerobic gram-positive cocci
    c. CBC: increased WBC count (over 15,000 to 20,000/mm^3 with over 90% PMNs and bands)
    d. Urinalysis to rule out UTI
B. **Nursing Diagnoses**
  1. Deficient knowledge related to infection, its treatment, and sequelae
  2. Anxiety related to well being of self and infant

3. Ineffective individual coping related to stress of increased discomfort and illness

C. **Interventions/Outcomes**
1. Deficient knowledge related to infection, its treatment, and sequelae
   a. Interventions
      (1) Provide information on antibiotic treatment in a calm, reassuring manner.
      (2) Involve the client and her family or significant other in the learning process.
      (3) Reinforce information provided by the physician on the possible course of labor, including possibility of cesarean section.
   b. Outcomes
      (1) Client accurately verbalizes what chorioamnionitis is and how it is treated
2. Anxiety related to well being of self and infant
   a. Interventions
      (1) Develop trust and rapport by being nonjudgmental and interested in the client.
      (2) Facilitate client communication with the physician.
      (3) Provide information that will increase the client's sense of control and decrease her uncertainty.
      (4) Suggest to the client coping strategies that are distracting or relaxing or that change how the client perceives her situation.
   b. Outcomes
      (1) Client verbalizes sources of anxiety, concerns, and issues in a supportive environment.
      (2) Client verbalizes a decrease in anxiety.
      (3) Client uses coping skills effectively as evidenced by following instructions, solving problems, and using relaxation techniques.
      (4) Client appropriately expresses her feelings.
      (5) Client maintains communication with health care providers and her family or significant other.
3. Ineffective individual coping related to stress of increased discomfort and illness
   a. Interventions
      (1) Provide accurate information about chorioamnionitis and potential risks.
      (2) Assist the client in identifying feelings of anger, guilt, and frustration; refer to mental health professional as needed.
      (3) Include family member or significant other in discussion.
   b. Outcomes
      (1) Client is able to verbalize knowledge of infection and potential risks.
      (2) Client is able to verbalize feelings of anger, guilt, and frustration as needed.
      (3) Significant other is knowledgeable about situation and supportive of mother.

HEALTH EDUCATION
Torch

A. **Stress the need to vaccinate susceptible women before conception or immediately postpartum.**
B. **Instruct the client on good hand washing, especially after handling raw meat.**
C. **Instruct the client to wash all kitchen surfaces that come into contact with uncooked meat.**

D. Instruct the client to avoid eating insufficiently cooked meat.
E. Instruct the client to avoid contact with cat feces in litter boxes during pregnancy and avoid gardening in soil contaminated with cat feces.

Acquired Immunodeficiency Syndrome

A. **Testing: incorporate risk assessment for HIV into all health histories;** strongly encourage all pregnant women to be tested; the following populations need to undergo HIV testing:
1. IV drug users
2. Homosexual or bisexual males
3. Hemophiliacs
4. Clients being evaluated for STDs
5. Victims of sexual abuse
6. Clients who have had transfusions, tattoos, or acupuncture since 1977
7. Clients who are uncertain about the risk status of their partners

B. **Prevention**
1. Abstinence
2. Mutually monogamous sexual relationships minimize sexual transmission.
3. Avoid sex with multiple partners, partners with multiple partners, or prostitutes.
4. Avoid sexual contact with people with genital discharge, genital warts, or herpes lesions.
5. Use latex condoms in combination with spermicide (Nonoxynol 9) to avoid transmission of semen or vaginal secretions; use only water-based lubricants
6. Never share needles or syringes.
7. Avoid breastfeeding because it is associated with transmission.
8. Avoid alcohol and illicit drugs because they may impair the immune system and judgment.

C. **Resources**
- AIDS Hotline: (800) 342-AIDS (2437; 24 hour/day); Línea Nacional de SIDA (800) 344-7432 (Spanish 8:00 AM until 2:00 AM EST); TTY Deaf and Hard of Hearing (800) 243-7889 (Monday through Friday 10:00 AM until 10:00 PM EST)
- American Family Physician's Management of Newborns exposed to Maternal HIV: *www.aafp.org/afp/2002051/2049.html*
- American Liver Foundation: (800) 465-4837, *www.liverfoundation.org*
- American Social Health Association (ASHA): (919) 361-8400, (800) 783-9877, *www.ashastd.org*
- American Society for Colposcopy and Cervical Pathology: (800) 787-7227, *www.asccp.org*
- Centers for Disease Control and Prevention: Hepatitis Information Service: *www.cdc.gov/ncidod/diseases/hepatitis/*
- Centers for Disease Control and Prevention National AIDS Clearinghouse: (800) 458-5231
- Centers for Disease Control and Prevention National Prevention Information Network: (800) 458-5231
- Centers for Disease Control and Prevention, National STD and AIDS Hotline: (800) 227-8922, *www.ashastd.org/NSTD/index.html*
- Centers for Disease Control and Prevention, Perinatal HIV Prevention Program: *www.cdc.govlhiv/projects/perinatal/default.html*

- Foundation for Children With AIDS: (617) 783-7300
- Free HIV/AIDS Treatment Information: (800) 874-2572
- Hepatitis Foundation International: (800) 891-0707, *www.hepfi.org*
- Johns Hopkins AIDS Service Guidelines for Managing HIV in Pregnancy: *www.hopkins-aids.edu/publications/reprts/may01_1.html*
- MedlinePlus AIDS and Pregnancy: *www.nlm.nih.gov/medlineplus/aidsandpregnancy.html*
- National Digestive Diseases Information Clearinghouse: (301) 654-3819, *www.niddk.nih.gov*
- National Herpes Hotline: (919) 361-8488
- National HPV and Cervical Cancer Prevention Hotline: (919) 361-4848, *www.ashastd.org/hpvccrc/*
- National Institute of Allergy and Infectious Diseases National Institutes of Health: *www.niaid.hih.gov/factsheets/stdherp.htm*
- National Self-Help Clearinghouse: (212) 840-1258
- Office on Women's Health—CDC: (404) 639-7230
- Virtual Hospital's HIV/AIDS: Pregnancy in AIDS: *www.vh.org/Providers/CinRef/FPHandbook/Chapter11/12-11.htms*
- State or local health departments

D. **Provide information about self-help groups**
E. **Provide information about effective birth control after pregnancy**

Sexually Transmitted Diseases

A. **Provide information on prevention of STDs.**
   1. Limit number of sexual partners.
   2. Use condoms or diaphragms with spermicide Nonoxynol 9.
   3. Use cotton underwear and cotton-based clothing.
B. **Instruct the client on self-care measures.**
   1. Burrow's solution.
   2. Warm sitz baths.
   3. Dry heat from hair dryer.
C. **Provide information about hygiene measures, including wiping vulva from front to back after urination.**
D. **Encourage hand washing.**
E. **Educate the client about the importance of reporting symptoms to health care provider, especially in the last trimester.**
F. **Educate the client on the need to take all of medication prescribed for self and partners.**

Urinary Tract Infection and Pyelonephritis

A. **Provide information about hygiene measures, including wiping from front to back after urinating and washing hands frequently.**
B. **Instruct the client to void before and after sexual intercourse.**
C. **Instruct the client on the need to drink 8 to 10 glasses of water daily;** include cranberry juice to lower the pH of the urinary tract.
D. **Instruct the client to void frequently as the need arises;** holding urine increases time bacteria are in bladder.
E. **Suggest the use of lubrication such as K-Y jelly during sexual intercourse as needed.**
F. **Instruct the client in the importance of completing antibiotic therapy, even if she no longer has symptoms.**

Chorioamnionitis

A. Prevention
1. Adequate prenatal care
2. Treatment of prenatal vaginal infection
3. Notification of health care provider in case of premature rupture of membranes (PROM)

CASE STUDIES AND STUDY QUESTIONS

TORCH

Mrs. S, a health care worker in a day care setting, is a 27-year-old multigravida with her last menstrual period 11 weeks ago. Her 3-year-old daughter experienced a fever and rash 5 days earlier. Two days later, the pediatrician established a diagnosis of rubella. On examination, Mrs. S is found to be healthy, and her uterus is 10 to 11 weeks in size. She does not remember having had rubella. Her friend told her to be tested for TORCH. She wants to know what it is.

1. What does TORCH stand for?
   toxo other Hepa Rubella CMV herpes

2. What laboratory test might determine her susceptibility?
   a. CBC
   b. Rubella titer
   c. Nasopharyngeal swab

3. For what other TORCH disease might she be at risk?
   a. AIDS
   b. CMV
   c. Toxoplasmosis
   d. Rubeola

4. Which of the following will reduce her chances of exposure?
   a. Cooking chicken until it is well done
   b. Using a mask to protect her from airborne diseases
   c. Rigorous personal hygiene while at work and home
   d. Taking acyclovir
   e. Undergoing serial cervical cultures
   (1) a, c, d
   (2) b, d

(3) a, b, c
(4) None of the above

Acquired Immunodeficiency Syndrome

Ms. D is a 21-year-old primigravida (G1) woman with her last menstrual period 12 weeks ago. She is in for her initial prenatal visit. Her uterus is approximately 12 weeks in size and her blood pressure is 110/72 mmHg. During your discussion with Ms. D, she expresses some concern over the possibility of being exposed to AIDS. She states she has had only one sexual partner and they have been in a monogamous relationship for 2 years. When questioned, her concern stems from the fact that a colleague at work recently tested positive for HIV.

5. As part of your assessment, what other information do you need to know?
   a. Does she live with other people?
   b. Has she eaten at her colleague's home?
   c. Sexual history of her partner

6. In your discussion with Ms. D about AIDS, you may tell her (answer the following true or false):
   F a. AIDS is spread only through sexual contact.
   F b. The occurrence of AIDS in women has not been increasing.
   c. She may take ZDU prophylactically.
   d. Symptoms of AIDS include fatigue, night sweats, and lymphadenopathy.

7. If it is established that Ms. D's partner had previous partners, which of the following would you recommend for general screening?
   a. ELISA
   b. Western blot
   c. T-cell count

8. If this test result were positive, what test would confirm HIV infection?
   a. ELISA
   b. Western blot
   c. T-cell count

9. The HIV virus has been found in all of the following except:
   a. Saliva
   b. Tears
   c. Sweat
   d. Semen

Sexually Transmitted Diseases

Ms. G is a 17-year-old single primigravida (G1) woman who is seen for her first prenatal visit at 20 weeks' gestation. Her history is unremarkable with the exception of treatment for gonorrhea 1 year previously. Examination of the skin, head, ears, nose, and throat yields normal results. Ms. G is afebrile, her pulse is 88 beats/minute, and her blood pressure is 118/72 mmHg. The size of her uterus corresponds with gestational age by dates. There is a small amount of yellow discharge at the cervix. The vulva appears red and inflamed.

10. What is the causative agent of gonorrhea?
    a. Gram-negative diplococcus
    b. Gram-positive diplococcus
    c. Protozoa
    d. Spirochete

11. Determine whether the following statements are true or false.
    a. Because Ms. G does not appear to have symptoms, you need not worry about gonorrhea or chlamydia.
    b. Untreated gonorrhea may cause PROM.
    c. Gonorrhea has been on the decline for the last 5 years because of better hygiene.
    d. An allergic reaction to soap or medications can mimic STD symptoms.

Urinary Tract Infection and Pyelonephritis

Ms. A is a 23-year-old gravida 2, para 1 (G2, P1) woman whose last menstrual period was 24 weeks ago. She has had one prenatal visit. She now complains of increasing urinary frequency for 5 days and of burning on urination for 2 days. For the last 24 hours, she has had a constant aching pain in her back and right side, along with chills and fever. Her temperature is 38.9° C (102° F), her pulse is 110 beats/minute, and her blood pressure is 110/70 mmHg. There is marked costovertebral angle tenderness on the right. Her uterus measures 23 cm, the fetal heart rate is 146 beats/minute, and her cervix is long and closed. Based on urine laboratory values, she is diagnosed as having acute pyelonephritis.

12. Name three physiologic changes that occur during pregnancy that predispose women to UTI.
    a. Changes in urine composition
    b. Dilatation of the upper third of ureters
    c. Decreased frequency of urination
    d. Compression of ureters by enlarging uterus
    e. Increased intake of liquids
    (1) a, b, c
    (2) b, c, e
    (3) a, b, d
    (4) b, c, d

13. A history of which of the following places a pregnant woman at an increased risk for UTI?
    a. History of childhood UTIs

b. Chronic disease and hypertension
c. Prior UTIs
d. a, c
e. a, b, c

Mrs. V is a 24-year-old school teacher approximately 14 weeks' pregnant with her first pregnancy. She is concerned about many of the diseases she may be exposed to and asks many questions.

14. How is chickenpox transmitted?
a. Aerosolized droplets
b. Blood and mucus
c. Skin-to-skin contact

15. Mumps is caused by what agent?
a. Paramyxovirus
b. Protozoa
c. RNA virus

16. What is the incubation period for measles?
a. 5 to 9 days
b. 10 to 14 days
c. 15 to 20 days

Ms. R. is a 16-year-old single primigravida (G1) woman who is admitted at 36 weeks' gestation with a temperature of 39.4° C (103° F), uterine tenderness, chills, and a blood pressure of 102/72 mmHg. Fetal heart rate is 180 beats/ minute. Fetal monitoring tracing shows absent short-term variability but no decelerations. Catheterized urinaly-

sis is unremarkable. CBC shows hemoglobin values of 10.5 g/dl, hematocrit of 36%, and WBC count 22,000/mm^3 with 85% PMNs, 10% bands, and 5% lymphocytes.

17. All of the following are possible pathogens associated with chorioamnionitis except:
a. Escherichia coli
b. Group A and B streptococci
c. Toxoplasma gondii

18. All of the following are diagnostic for chorioamnionitis except:
a. Culture of cervix
b. Amniotic fluid smear
c. Vaginal smear

19. Chorioamnionitis is associated with premature rupture of membranes and what other factor?
a. Cerclage use
b. Prolonged rupture of membranes
c. Inadequate hydration

20. Determine whether the following statements are true or false.
a. Mononuclear leukocytes and PMNs infiltrate the chorion.
b. Teenage unwed pregnancy and poor nutrition are factors that predispose to chorioamnionitis.
c. A cesarean section is the preferred method of delivery in a client with chorioamnionitis.

ANSWERS TO STUDY QUESTIONS

1. Toxoplasmosis, other (hepatitis B), rubella, cytomegalovirus, herpes simplex
2. b
3. b
4. 3
5. c
6. a. False
   b. False
   c. False
   d. True
7. a
8. b
9. c
10. a
11. a. False
    b. True
    c. False
    d. True
12. 3
13. e
14. a
15. a
16. b
17. c
18. c
19. b
20. a. True
    b. True
    c. False

REFERENCES

Armstrong, G., Mast, E., Wojczynski, M., & Margolis, H. (2001). Childhood hepatitis B virus infections in the United States before hepatitis B immunization. *Pediatrics, 108*(5), 1123-1128.

Brown, Z., Hollier, L., & Whitley, R. (2002). Sexually transmitted infections: Herpes simplex virus. In S. Cox & F. Stewart (Eds.), *APOG educational series on women's health issues*. Crofton, MD: Association of Professors of Gynecology and Obstetrics.

Brucker, M., & Faucher, M. (1999). Antimicrobial agents: Pharmacology and clinical applications in obstetric, gynecologic, and perinatal infections. *Journal of Obstetric, Gynecologic, and Neonatal Nursing, 28*(6), 639-648.

Centers for Disease Control and Prevention. (2000a). *Preventing congenital toxoplasmosis*. Available online at *www.cdc.gov/mmwr/preview/mmwrhtml/rr4902a5.htm*.

Centers for Disease Control and Prevention. (2000b). *Neisseria gonorrhea*. Available online at *www.cdc.gov/ncidod/dastlr/gcdir.html*.

Centers for Disease Control and Prevention. (2001a). *Chlamydia in the United States*. Available online at *www.cdc.gov/nchstp/dstd/fact_sheets/chlamydia_facts.htm*.

Centers for Disease Control and Prevention. (2001b). *HIV/AIDS surveillance report*. Available online at *www.cdc.gov/hiv/stats/hasr1302.htm*.

Centers for Disease Control and Prevention. (2002a). *Recommendations for use of antiretroviral drugs in pregnant HIV-1-infected women for maternal health and interventions to reduce perinatal HIV-1 transmission in the United States*. Atlanta: CDC.

Centers for Disease Control and Prevention. (2002b). *Sexually transmitted diseases treatment guidelines—2002*. Available online at *www/cdc.gov/cdcrecommends.htm*.

Centers for Disease Control and Prevention. (2002c). *Some facts about syphilis*. Available online at *www.cdc.gov*.

Centers for Disease Control and Prevention. (2002d). *HIV/AIDS among US women: Minority and young women at continuing risk*. Available online at *www.cdc.gov/hiv/pubs/facts/women.htm*.

Centers for Disease Control and Prevention. (2002e). *Cytomegalovirus (CMV)*. Available online at *www.cdc.gov/ncidod/diseases/cmv.htm*.

Centers for Disease Control and Prevention. (2002f). *Commentary*. Available online at *www.cdc.gov/hiv/stats.htm*.

Centers for Disease Control and Prevention. (2002g). *HIV and its transmissions*. Available online at *www.cdc.gov/hiv/pubs/facts*.

Centers for Disease Control and Prevention. (2003a). *Viral hepatitis*. Available online at *www.cdc.gov/ncidod/diseases/hepatitis/resource.htm*.

Centers for Disease Control and Prevention. (2003b). *Toxoplasmosis*. Available online at *www.cdc.gov/ncidod/dpd/parasites/toxoplasmosis.htm*.

Centers for Disease Control and Prevention. (2003c). *The influenza (flu) viruses*. Available online at *www.cdc.gov/ncidod/diseases/flu/viruses.htm*.

Centers for Disease Control and Prevention. (2003d). *Varicella disease*. Available online at *www.cdc.gov/nip/diseases/varicella.htm*.

Cox, T., Gall, S., & Harper, D. (2002). *Sexually transmitted infections: Human papillomavirus*. Crofton, MD: Association of Professors of Gynecology and Obstetrics. APOG Series on Women's Health Issues.

Cunningham, F.G., Gant, N., Leveno, K., Gilstrap, L., Hauth, J., & Wenstrom, K. (2001a). Sexually transmitted diseases. In *Williams obstetrics* (21st ed., pp. 1485-1513). New York: McGraw-Hill.

Cunningham, F.G., Gant, N., Leveno, K., Gilstrap, L., Hauth, J., & Wenstrom, K. (2001b). Renal and urinary tract disorders. In *Williams obstetrics* (21st ed., pp. 1251-1271). New York: McGraw-Hill.

Cunningham, F.G., Gant, N., Leveno, K., Gilstrap, L., Hauth, J., & Wenstrom, K. (2001c). Infections. In *Williams obstetrics* (21st ed., pp. 1461-1483). New York: McGraw-Hill.

Duff, P. (2002). Maternal and perinatal infection. In S. Gabbe, J. Niebyl, & J. Simpson (Eds.), *Obstetrics: Normal and problem pregnancies* (4th ed., pp. 1293-1345). New York: Churchill Livingstone.

Duff, P., & Sheffield, J. (2002). Sexually transmitted infections: Hepatitis B and C: The Ob/Gyn's role. In S. Cox & F. Stewart (Eds.), *APGO education series of women's health issues*. Crofton, MD: Association of Professors of Gynecology and Obstetrics.

Fiore, A. (2002). Chronic maternal hepatitis B infection and premature rupture of membranes. *Pediatric Infectious Disease Journal, 21*(4), 357-358.

Frank, S., Esch, J., & Marageson, N. (1998). Mandatory HIV testing of newborns: The impact on women. *American Journal of Nursing, 98*(10), 49-51.

Gibbs, R., & Sweet, R. (1999). Maternal and fetal infectious disorders. In R. Creasy & R. Resnik (Eds.), *Maternal-fetal medicine* (4th ed., pp. 659-724). Philadelphia: Saunders.

Ickovics, J.R., Wilson, T.E., Royce, R.A., Minkoff, H.L., Fernandez, M.I., Fox-Tierney, R., et al. (2002). Prenatal and postpartum zidovudine adherence among pregnant women with HIV: Results of a MEMS substudy from the Perinatal Guidelines Evaluation Project. *Journal of Acquired Immune Deficiency Syndromes, 30*(3), 311-315.

Lackritz, E.M., Shaffer, N., & Luo, C. (2002). Prevention of mother-to-child HIV transmission in the context of a comprehensive AIDS agenda in resource-poor countries. *Journal of Acquired Immune Deficiency Syndromes, 30*(2), 196-199.

Litwin, C., & Hill, H. (1997). Serologic and DNA-based testing for congenital and perinatal infections. *Pediatric Infectious Disease Journal, 16*(12), 1166-1175.

Marsland, T., & King, V. (2002). Maternal screening strategy more effective than risk-based approaches for preventing group B streptococcal disease in neonates. *Journal of Family Practice, 51*(11), 926-929.

Maupin, R. (2002). Obstetric infectious disease emergencies. *Clinical Obstetrics and Gynecology 45*(2), 393-404.

Montgomery, K. (2002). Resource column: HIV and pregnancy web sites. *Journal of Perinatal Education, 11*(4), 41-43.

Petrova, A., Smulian, J., & Ananth, C. (2002). Obstetrician preferences for prenatal strategies to reduce early-onset group B streptococcal infection in neonates: A population-based survey. *American Journal of Obstetrics and Gynecology, 187*(30), 709-714.

Swyer, P., & O'Reilly, M. (2002). Recurrent urinary tract infection in the female. *Current Opinion in Obstetrics and Gynecology, 14*(5), 537-543.

Tuomala, R., Shapiro, D., Mofenson, L., Bryson, Y., Culnane, M., Hughes, M., et al. (2002). Antiretroviral therapy during pregnancy and the risk of an adverse outcome. *New England Journal of Medicine, 346*(24), 1863-1870.

U.S. Department of Health and Human Services (2002). *Guidelines for the use of antiretroviral agents in HIV-infected adults and adolescents*. Washington, DC: USDHHS.

U.S. Preventive Services Task Force. (2002). Screening for bacterial vaginosis in pregnancy: Recommendations and rationale. *American Journal of Nursing, 102*(8), 91-93.

Watts, H. (2002). Drug therapy: Management of human immunodeficiency virus infection in pregnancy. *New England Journal of Medicine, 346*(24), 1879-1891.

23 Hemorrhagic Disorders

JUDITH H. POOLE

OBJECTIVES

1. Define the hemorrhagic complications of placenta previa, abruptio placentae, disseminated intravascular coagulation (DIC), and gestational trophoblastic disease.
2. Recognize the common signs and symptoms of placenta previa, abruptio placentae, DIC, and trophoblastic disease.
3. State the appropriate initial nursing interventions.
4. Record client response to nursing treatment.
5. Associate less common signs and symptoms of placenta previa, abruptio placentae, and DIC with their respective conditions.
6. Correlate client response with desired response to treatment to anticipate subsequent care.
7. Assemble the appropriate healthcare provider team and coordinate the healthcare team as long as is necessary.

INTRODUCTION

A. **Hemorrhagic disorders are obstetric emergencies and significantly impact maternal morbidity and mortality** (Martin, Hamilton, Ventura, Menacker, & Park, 2002; Ventura, Martin, Curtin, Menacker, & Hamilton, 2001).
   1. Bleeding complicates one in five pregnancies.
   2. Incidence and type of bleeding varies by trimester.
      a. Most maternal deaths from obstetric hemorrhage after first trimester of pregnancy occur secondary to placental abruption.
      b. Risk of mortality related to maternal age and race, with highest rates among U.S. black women.
B. **From 1991 to 1999 the rate of maternal deaths related to obstetric hemorrhage was 12.7 per 100,000 live births** (Centers for Disease Control and Prevention [CDC], 2003).
   1. Specific causes of death after a live birth, in rank order, were uterine atony, complications from disseminated intravascular coagulation (DIC), and abruptio placentae.
   2. Specific causes of death after a stillbirth, in rank order, were abruptio placentae and uterine rupture.
   3. 68% of maternal deaths secondary to hemorrhage occur within 48 hours after the pregnancy ends.
C. **Obstetric hemorrhage is defined as a 10% decrease in hematocrit, total blood loss of more than 1000 ml, or need for transfusion therapy** (Benedetti, 2002).

PLACENTA PREVIA
Introduction
A. **Placenta previa is an implantation of the placenta in the lower uterine segment, near or over the internal cervical os.**
   1. Reported incidence varies widely in published research but averages approximately 0.5% to 1% (1 in 200) of births; among grand multiparous women it is 2% (Clark, 1999; Stables, 1999).
   2. Recurrence risk following one pregnancy complicated by a previa ranges from 4% to 8% (Konje & Taylor, 1999).
   3. There is a direct relationship between the number of previous cesarean births and risk of placenta previa, probably due to uterine scarring (Benedetti, 2002; Clark, 1999; Gilbert & Harmon, 2003; Konje & Taylor, 1999).
B. **Classification for placenta previa**
   1. Classification for placenta previa is based on the degree to which the internal cervical os is covered by the placenta.
   2. Low-lying placenta: reserved for those situations in which the exact relationship of placenta to the cervical os has not been determined.
   3. Marginal previa: edge of the placenta is within 2 to 3 cm of the internal cervical os but does not cover it.
   4. Placenta previa: placenta covers part or all of the internal cervical os in the third trimester.
C. **The degree of occlusion of internal cervical os may depend on the degree of cervical dilatation so what may appear to be low-lying or marginal on ultrasound exam prior to the onset of labor can become more serious as labor progresses.**

CLINICAL PRACTICE
A. **Assessment**
   1. History
      a. Presents with confirmed placenta previa or vaginal bleeding.
         (1) Is previously diagnosed by ultrasonogram.
             (a) About 12% to 25% of women might be diagnosed with placenta previa or low-lying placenta before 30 weeks' gestation.
             (b) Low-lying and placenta previa before 30 weeks usually resolves (up to 75%) or migrates.
             (c) If the placental edge is 15 mm or more over the internal os at 12 to 16 weeks' gestation, the incidence of third trimester previa becomes 5.1% (Taipale, Hiilesmaa, & Ylostalo, 1997).
         (2) Is documented on medical record.
         (3) Is common to have a history of one or more previous bleeding episodes.
             (a) Hallmark of placenta previa is sudden onset of painless vaginal bleeding in the second or third trimester.
             (b) Peak incidence for initial bleeding episode is early third trimester.
                 (i) 33% become symptomatic before 30 weeks' gestation.
                 (ii) 33% become symptomatic after 36 weeks.
         (4) Risk factors include:
             (a) Previous placenta previa; risk increased eight-fold
             (b) Short interval between pregnancies and multiparity (Cunningham, MacDonald, Gant, Leveno, Gilstrap, Hankins, et al., 1997)

        (c) Uterine scars.
            (i) Previous abortions with curettage; risk increased 1.3 times (VandeKerkhove & Johnson, 1998)
           (ii) Previous cesarean birth; 1.5 to 15 times increased risk (Clark, 1999)
           (iii) Previous endometritis or conditions that cause defective decidual vasculature, inflammation, or atrophic changes
           (iv) Previous molar pregnancy
        (d) Smoking might have a dose response with a 1.4- to 3-fold increased risk.
        (e) Multiparous women
        (f) Race; Asian women have a 1.9 times greater risk.
        (g) Age: older than 35, incidence 1 in 100; more than 40, 1 in 50
        (h) Large placenta related to multiple gestation, diabetes, or erythroblastosis fetalis (VandeKerkhove & Johnson, 1998)
      (5) Most risk factors involve a need for increased uteroplacental surface area.
  b. Presents with initial bleeding episode.
      (1) Classically, placenta previa is suspected when the woman presents with painless vaginal bleeding, especially during the late second or third trimester of pregnancy.
        (a) Bleeding is associated with a normal uterine resting tone and an absence of uterine tenderness; bleeding can be intermittent or continuous.
        (b) The absence of abdominal pain, with or without uterine contractions, is usually the distinguishing criterion between placenta previa and placental abruption. However, labor-induced uterine contractions might precipitate vaginal bleeding from placenta previa (Carter, 1999).
        (c) Approximately 10% of pregnancies complicated by placenta previa will be asymptomatic until the onset of labor triggers vaginal bleeding (Clark, 1999).
      (2) First bleeding is usually self-limiting.
        (a) Usually no fetal compromise occurs in the term fetus unless the mother suffers shock or severe hypovolemia.
        (b) However, if at a preterm gestation, neonatal morbidity and mortality are increased secondary to preterm birth, low birthweight, intrauterine growth restriction (IUGR), and fetal malformations occur (Clark, 1999; Konje & Taylor, 1999).
  c. Ultrasonography can aid in diagnosing placenta previa and helps exclude other causes of vaginal bleeding.
2. Physiologic response to blood loss
  a. Shock, defined as circulatory insufficiency, coexists with disordered metabolism, resulting in altered cellular metabolism (Franklin, Darovic, & Dan, 2002).
  b. With acute blood volume loss compensatory mechanisms attempt to correct the deficit to maintain organ perfusion and cellular function
  c. Rapid, acute loss of 1000 ml circulating blood volume results in vasoconstriction of both the arterial and venous beds to preserve perfusion of vital organs.
      (1) Due to expanded blood volume of pregnancy this loss is generally asymptomatic with vital signs remaining within normal parameters.

      (2) Maternal blood pressure is maintained secondary to increasing systemic vascular resistance; blood pressure is a poor indicator of blood volume deficit.

      (3) Organ perfusion and maternal cardiac output generation is maintained, but this compensatory mechanism is volume dependent. Once the total acute blood loss exceeds 20%, the ability to maintain adequate cardiac output and organ perfusion can no longer be met by increasing vascular resistance, and there is a parallel, progressive decrease in cardiac output and blood pressure (Benedetti, 2002; Franklin et al, 2002).

3. Physical findings

  a. Bleeding

      (1) Bleeding, with or without uterine contractions, due to placental separation from cervical os or lower uterine segment and the inability of the uterus to contract at the vessel sites; the initial bleed is rarely profuse and usually stops spontaneously; bleeding recurs later.

      (2) Presence of clots usually indicates normal coagulation process.

      (3) Absence of clots might indicate evolving coagulopathy, either hypofibrinogenemia or thrombocytopenia.

      (4) Painless bleeding is common in placenta previa (70% to 80%).

      (5) Painful bleeding can occur when the placenta abrupts away from the uterine tissue, even with a placenta previa.

  b. Risk associated with blood loss

      (1) Maternal blood loss results in decreased oxygen-carrying capacity, which directly affects oxygen delivery to maternal organ systems and indirectly affects oxygen delivery to the fetus.

         (a) Placental blood flow is directly proportional to uterine perfusion pressures; uterine perfusion pressures are proportional to maternal systemic blood pressure.

         (b) Maternal hemorrhage, if not identified and corrected, leads to a hypovolemic state, decreasing maternal cardiac output and systemic perfusion pressures (Benedetti, 2002).

         (c) Decreased maternal systemic blood pressure leads to decreased uterine perfusion pressures and fetal compromise.

         (d) Decreased oxygenation and hypoperfusion can set up cascade of events predisposing to multiorgan dysfunction syndrome (MODS) (Benedetti, 2002; Secor, 1996).

      (2) Maternal blood loss can occur rapidly; approximately 700 to 1000 ml/min (10%-15% of maternal cardiac output) of blood flow is directed to the uterine vasculature and placenta during pregnancy (Parer, 1997; Sosa, 2001).

      (3) Fetal oxygenation decreases proportionally to changes in maternal cardiac output generation and systemic perfusion pressures (Blackburn, 2003; Clark, Cotton, Hankins, & Phelan, 1997; Feinstein & Atterbury, 2003).

         (a) Fetal risks from maternal hemorrhage include blood loss, anemia, hypoxemia, hypoxia, anoxia, and preterm birth.

         (b) Fetal blood loss is always significant because of the small fetal blood volume (80–100 ml/kg).

         (c) Disruption of uteroplacental blood flow can result in a progressive deterioration of fetal status; the degree of fetal compromise is directly related to the total volume of blood loss and duration of the bleeding episode (Sosa, 2001).

   c. Shock with significant blood loss
     (1) Rising pulse rate: initially it will be full and easily palpable; as bleeding continues, pulse becomes weak and thready.
     (2) Increase in respiratory rate; desaturation of hemoglobin as measured by pulse oximetry is a later finding and might overestimate value if vasoconstriction is present in the extremity in which measurement is taken.
     (3) Systemic vasoconstriction to ensure perfusion to essential organs and as a result shunting from skin; mottling, pallor, and clammy skin.
     (4) Falling blood pressure; hypotension is a later finding.
     (5) Air hunger
     (6) Decreasing urinary output secondary to acute left ventricular dysfunction and renal hypoperfusion
     (7) Decreasing level of consciousness with increasing anxiety, apprehension and restlessness
     (8) Changes in laboratory findings consistent with acute blood loss
   d. Fetal heart rate (FHR) response to maternal bleeding or shock
     (1) Loss of variability and accelerations
     (2) Abnormal FHR and loss of variability
       (a) Initial compensatory tachycardia
       (b) Subsequent bradycardia; fetal cardiac output is rate dependent, and, therefore, when baseline rate decreases by 50%, fetal cardiac output decreases by 50%.
       (c) Sinusoidal pattern, indicating fetal anemia, hypoxia, and acidemia
       (d) Persistent late decelerations indicating impaired uteroplacental perfusion
     (3) If maternal status remains unstable, and bleeding is allowed to continue, intrauterine demise is possible.
   e. Complications associated with placenta previa
     (1) Coagulopathy is rare (Wing, Paul, & Millar, 1996).
     (2) Placenta accreta is an abnormality of implantation defined by degree of invasion into uterine wall of trophoblast.
       (a) Classification of placenta accreta (see Chapter 3 for complete discussion of placental development)
         (i) Placenta accreta: invasion of trophoblast is beyond normal boundary of the Nitabuch's fibrinoid layer.
         (ii) Placenta increta: invasion of trophoblast extends into the myometrium.
         (iii) Placenta percreta: invasion of trophoblast extends beyond the serosa.
       (b) Placenta accreta occurs in 5% to 10% of pregnancies with a previa (Lockwood & Funai, 1999).
         (i) Prevalence of accreta is increasing and is closely correlated with number of cesarean births a woman has undergone (Benedetti, 2002; Gilbert & Harmon, 2003).
         (ii) One prior cesarean: risk of accreta is 10% to 25%; risk is greater than 50% with two or more cesarean births.
         (iii) Presence of accreta significantly increases risk of severe hemorrhage and peripartal hysterectomy (Flamm, 2001).
     (3) Postpartum hemorrhage due to placental implantation in the less muscular, lower uterine segment, which contracts poorly and lacerates easily during delivery and manual removal of placenta.

      (4) Uterine rupture

      (5) Abnormal placental development and abnormal cord insertion are rare but significant causes of fetal bleeding (see Chapter 11 for complete discussion of placental variations).

         (a) Vasa previa: fetal vessels cross the placental membranes in the lower uterine segment and cover the cervical os.

         (b) Velamentous cord insertion: fetal vessels run across chorion and amnion without protective Wharton's jelly before entering the placental surface.

         (c) Succenturiate placenta: one or more small accessory lobes of placental vascular tissue in membranes that are attached to main placenta by fetal vessels

         (d) Classic presentation of vasa previa, velamentous cord insertion, or succenturiate placenta is vaginal bleeding with rupture of membranes, followed quickly by abrupt change in fetal heart rate and fetal death.

         (e) Increased fetal mortality rate

         (f) Greater risk of compression, rupture, or both, when velamentous vessels are close to cervix

   f. Fetal malpresentation in third trimester (Neilson, 2001)

      (1) Nonpolar fetal lie is common; includes transverse lie, breech, and unengaged vertex.

      (2) With placenta implanted in lower uterine segment, fetal presenting part remains at high station late in pregnancy.

4. Psychosocial findings

   a. Maternal stress factors

      (1) Anxiety

      (2) Fear of pregnancy loss

      (3) Fear for self

      (4) Confusion and panic

   b. Maternal behavioral factors

      (1) Difficulty in making decisions

      (2) Loss of pregnancy and loss of own life and health questioned

      (3) Tense body posture and expression

      (4) Feelings of helplessness

5. Diagnostic procedures

   a. Ultrasonography accuracy 93% to 98% by combination of abdominal, transperineal, and transvaginal techniques.

      (1) Need more than one view to locate placenta, including lateral uterine walls, to diagnose placenta previa.

      (2) Differentiate placenta previa from abruptio placentae or other causes of bleeding.

      (3) Determine if placenta previa and abruptio placentae coexist.

      (4) Approximately 7% to 10% of women are asymptomatic when placenta previa is found on routine ultrasonogram.

      (5) Magnetic resonance imaging (MRI) is occasionally used to diagnose placenta previa; especially useful for posterior uterine wall placenta.

      (6) Doppler color flow aids diagnosis of placental vessel abnormalities associated with placenta previa, such as velamentous insertion of cord.

   b. Avoid speculum and digital vaginal examinations to diagnose placenta previa.

    (1) Speculum examination might be performed after placenta previa has been ruled out by ultrasonography.

    (2) Digital examination risks perforation or abruption of placenta previa.

  c. If there is significant blood loss, clotting problems develop; therefore, evaluate baseline clotting values.

  d. Clotting studies (e.g., prothrombin time [PT], partial thromboplastin time [PTT], platelets, D-dimer, complete blood count [CBC], fibrinogen, fibrin split products [FSP], or fibrin degradation products) or clotting screen such as CBC, platelets, and D-dimer.

  e. Test for presence of fetal RBCs in maternal blood sampling or vaginal blood using rapid tests (4 to 7 minutes): Ogita (most sensitive at 20% fetal blood), APT (sensitive at 60%), Loendersloot (sensitive at 60%), or more lengthy tests (1 hour): Kleihauer-Betke stain or hemoglobin electrophoresis.

B. Nursing Diagnoses

 1. Ineffective tissue perfusion related to blood loss

 2. Ineffective fetal perfusion and oxygenation related to maternal blood loss

 3. Maternal anxiety related to threat to self and fetus

C. Interventions/Outcomes

 1. Ineffective tissue perfusion related to blood loss

  a. Interventions

    (1) Draw blood and send for clotting studies, as ordered.

    (2) Establish intravenous (IV) line with large-bore intracatheter (16 gauge preferable, or 18 gauge).

    (3) Type and crossmatch at least two units of blood products.

    (4) Rapidly administer nondextrose crystalloids, such as Ringer's lactate or normal saline to increase blood volume.

     (a) Measure urine output.

     (b) Measure urine specific gravity.

     (c) Obtain electrolyte values periodically, as ordered.

     (d) Obtain hematocrit as ordered.

    (5) Avoid vaginal examinations.

    (6) Administer oxygen at 8 L per mask (10 to 12 L if rebreather bag used).

    (7) Monitor maternal pulse and blood pressure.

     (a) Assess trends in vital signs: hemodynamic status is stable or further fluid resuscitation is needed.

     (b) Use electrocardiogram (ECG) monitor or maternal rate mode on electronic fetal monitor (EFM), as needed.

     (c) Monitor central venous pressure (CVP) or pulmonary pressures with Swan-Ganz catheter.

    (8) Observe for clotting of blood.

    (9) Measure or estimate blood loss.

     (a) Metric scale: 1 g = 1 ml

     (b) Nonmetric scale: 1 oz = 29 ml

    (10) Tocolysis indicated if client is not in active labor with bleeding; long-term tocolysis might offer advantages.

     (a) Increased birth weight

     (b) Increased gestational age

    (11) If initial stabilization measures fail, or bleeding cannot be stopped, anticipate need for emergency cesarean and mobilize appropriate resources.

    (12) Postdelivery blood loss and retained tissue due to accreta or increta tissue might be treated with plain or thrombin-soaked uterine pack, methotrexate, hypogastric artery ligation, hysterectomy.

   b. Expectant management usually includes the following (Gilbert & Harmon, 2003):
   - (1) Initial hospitalization for evaluation of maternal and fetal status
   - (2) Activity restriction might be ordered with some cases, requiring bedrest with bathroom privileges; as maternal and fetal status allows, the client may be allowed limited periods of ambulation.
   - (3) Assessment for active vaginal bleeding
   - (4) Venous access with active bleeding
   - (5) Laboratory testing to monitor hemoglobin/hematocrit levels, blood type/Rh, and possibly coagulation profile; maternal status determines need to hold blood in blood bank for possible type and cross-match.
   - (6) Continuous electronic fetal monitoring initially and during bleeding episodes
   - (7) Biophysical profile (BPP) or nonstress test (NST) with amniotic fluid index (AFI), followed by a weekly modified biophysical profile
   - (8) Antenatal corticosteroids to enhance fetal pulmonary maturity between 24 and 34 weeks' gestation
   - (9) Monitor for signs and symptoms of preterm labor and intrauterine infection; uterine irritability or preterm labor can be treated with tocolytics, such as magnesium sulfate, if client is otherwise stable (Baron & Hill, 2002).
   - (10) Amniocentesis can be done between 34 and 36 weeks' gestation to determine fetal lung maturity.
   c. Outcomes: improved tissue perfusion shown by the following:
   - (1) Clotting of blood
   - (2) Improved vital signs
   - (3) Decreased blood loss
   - (4) Improved or stable color and warmth of skin and hemodynamic parameters
   - (5) Improved or stable clotting studies
   - (6) Respiratory rate normal and breathing unlabored
   - (7) Few or no uterine contractions
2. Ineffective fetal perfusion and oxygenation related to maternal blood loss
   a. Interventions
   - (1) Continuously monitor FHR, preferably with EFM, to evaluate variability.
   - (2) Observe for abnormal FHR patterns (see Chapter 12 for further discussion of FHR patterns).
     - (a) Loss of variability; accelerations
     - (b) Sinusoidal pattern
     - (c) Tachycardia
     - (d) Persistent late decelerations
     - (e) Terminal bradycardia
   - (3) Place client in lateral position or wedge to left.
   - (4) Treat client for alteration in tissue perfusion (as needed).
     - (a) Oxygen therapy
     - (b) Fluids and blood products
     - (c) Position change
     - (d) Tocolysis
   - (5) Anticipate cesarean delivery and close observation for postpartum hemorrhage.
   - (6) Provide home care instructions and preparation.

    b. Outcomes

        (1) Normal or improved FHR patterns

        (2) Normal or improved FHR variability

        (3) Home care instructions and preparation provided

  3. Maternal anxiety related to threat to self and fetus

    a. Interventions

        (1) Speak calmly to client and support persons.

        (2) Explain interventions and why they are being performed.

           (a) Observation while waiting for fetus to mature and grow

           (b) Administration of tocolysis to treat and prevent uterine contractions

           (c) Responses for profuse bleeding or fetal compromise

           (d) Reassurances and instructions for home care

        (3) Reassure client regarding type of care selected.

    b. Antepartum home care

        (1) Focus on accurate assessments and appropriate referral.

        (2) Criteria for home care management vary with primary perinatal provider and home care agency. To be considered for home care referral, the client must be in stable condition with no evidence of bleeding for at least 72 hours before discharge, with no signs of preterm labor, and with evidence of fetal well-being. The client also must be able to return to the hospital immediately if active bleeding resumes (Baron & Hill, 2002; Gilbert & Harmon, 2003; Simpson & Creehan, 2001).

        (3) Ongoing assessments include: assessment of vaginal bleeding; evaluation of fetal well-being and uterine activity; warning signs of preterm labor, including possible home uterine monitoring; daily or at least twice weekly home visits for comprehensive maternal-fetal evaluation; timing of appropriate laboratory assessment; fetal kick counts (after 24 weeks gestation), vaginal bleeding, uterine activity, maternal activity level, and adherence to prescribed nursing care plan (Simpson & Creehan, 2001).

    c. Outcomes

        (1) Client reports less anxiety.

        (2) Client's body posture and expressions are less tense.

        (3) Client describes home care plans, recognition of signs and symptoms needing attention or transport, preparations for immediate hospitalization.

ABRUPTIO PLACENTAE

A. Abruptio placentae is the premature separation of a normally implanted placenta from the decidual lining of the uterus after 20 weeks' gestation.

  1. Separation can be either partial or complete.

  2. The resultant loss of blood can be either revealed (external) or concealed (internal) depending on the dissection of membrane edges away from the uterine wall.

B. Incidence is reported as ranging from 0.3% to 1.6% (Ananth, Smulian, & Vintzileos, 1999; Baumann, Blackwell, Schild, Berry, & Friedrich, 2000).

  1. Average rate of abruption is 1 case per 120 births (0.83%) (Clark, 1999; Sosa, 2001).

  2. In pregnancies complicated by abruption, approximately 1 out of 420 births are severe enough to threaten fetal viability (Clark, 1999).

CLINICAL PRACTICE

A. Assessment

1. History
   a. Classically, presents with vaginal bleeding, abdominal pain, uterine tenderness, and contractions; vaginal bleeding is present in up to 70% to 80% of women presenting with abruption (Benedetti, 2002).
   b. Presents with signs and symptoms of bleeding; external bleeding, or enlarging uterus (without external bleeding).
   c. Might present with painful abdomen or tense, tender uterus, and uterine contractions; increased uterine tone and tenderness might be absent unless the abruption is a grade 2 or grade 3 (Benedetti, 2002).
   d. Occurs in 1 in 150 deliveries; extent of abruption varies and might be expressed in a grading system.
      (1) Recurrence rate ranges from 5% to 17%, which yields a relative risk of 30 times higher than general population (Clark, 1999; Konje & Taylor, 1999).
      (2) Perinatal mortality rate is 20%.
      (3) Overall, 12% of stillbirths are due to abruptio placentae.
      (4) Racial incidence: black 1 in 595, white 1 in 876, Latino 1 in 1473
   e. Possible etiologic factors contribute to degeneration of spiral arterioles, causing necrosis of decidual basalis; process leads to rupture of these vessels and bleeding.
      (1) Maternal hypertension, whether chronic, gestational, or preeclampsia/eclampsia: five times more likely to have abruption
      (2) Cigarette smoking: maternal cigarette smoking also significantly increases the risk for placental abruption, along with related fetal compromise, including low birth weight and death. Ananth et al. (1999) report an overall 90% increase in the risk of abruption with maternal smoking (random-effects pooled odds ratio 1.9, 95% confidence interval, 1.8-2.0).
         (a) Decidual necrosis found
         (b) Dose-related effects on birth weight
         (c) Worse if over 40 years of age (compared with teen years) (Cnattingius, 1997)
      (3) Multiparity, especially women under 30 years of age
      (4) Abortions, spontaneous and elective
      (5) Cocaine use: reported incidence is 10%.
      (6) Methamphetamine use
      (7) Short umbilical cord
      (8) Abdominal trauma: symptomatic response might be delayed.
         (a) Blunt abdominal trauma places a woman at increased risk for abruption.
            (i) 5% incidence with minor trauma
            (ii) Up to 50% incidence with major injuries
            (iii) Because of the increased risk of placental abruption following maternal trauma continuous fetal heart rate monitoring is recommended until the woman is stabilized. The American College of Obstetricians and Gynecologists (ACOG, 2000) recommends a minimum of 2 to 6 hours of fetal monitoring after maternal abdominal trauma.
         (b) Fetomaternal bleed is of concern if blood type is Rh D^u negative.
         (c) Trauma includes amniocentesis, uterine catheter, accidents, and assaults.

(9) Rupture of membranes
  (a) Premature and prolonged risk increases 5 to 10 times; fetal distress is increased if rupture preceded by bleeding.
  (b) Sudden uterine decompression as with second twin or in polyhydramnios
  (c) Chorioamnionitis (Kramer et al., 1997)
(10) Uterine leiomyoma located behind placenta (Cunningham et al., 1997)
(11) Controversial etiology
  (a) Folic acid deficiency
  (b) Hyperhomocysteinemia (Goddijn-Wessel, Wouters, Van de Molen, Spuijbroek, Steegers-Thunissen, Blom, et al., 1996)
  (c) Vena caval compression

2. Physical findings: common, not absolute
  a. Blood loss, painful abdomen, or both, and firm, tender uterus
    (1) Grading for placental abruption (Konje & Taylor, 1999):
      Grade 0 = asymptomatic; small retroplacental clot noted after birth; normal maternal/fetal assessment findings; normal laboratory findings
      Grade I = minimal vaginal bleeding; minimal uterine tenderness and mild tetany; no coagulopathy; maternal/fetal hemodynamic status stable
      Grade II = external vaginal bleeding might or might not be present; tetanic contractions; maternal hemodynamic stability with tachycardia; nonreassuring fetal heart rate pattern; hypofibrinogenemia (150-250 mg/dl)
      Grade III = Heavy vaginal bleeding; bleeding may be concealed; tetanic, painful uterus; persistent abdominal pain; maternal/fetal hemodynamic instability; hypofibrinogenemia (< 150 mg/dl); coagulopathy present
    (2) Prediction of an abruptio placentae is difficult; grade I is subtle and difficult to diagnose.
    (3) Antepartum testing results tend to be normal until placenta significantly abrupts.
    (4) Continuous dull back pain and abdominal pain might occur.
    (5) Intermittent abdominal cramping might occur.
    (6) Ultrasonography used to rule out placenta previa; however, it is not diagnostic during acute phase of abruptio.
  b. Uterine contractions: frequent and mild; tonus might be elevated; must be differentiated from preterm labor.
  c. Symptoms of significant bleeding from abruptio placentae
    (1) Rising pulse rate with falling blood pressure; hypotension with tachycardia is a late finding.
      (a) Blood pressure drops to normal range with hypertensive clients.
      (b) True blood pressure returns after intravascular volume replaced.
      (c) Noninvasive automatic blood pressure/pulse monitoring less accurate in hypotensive state; verify values.
    (2) Pale, clammy skin
    (3) Increasing uterine distention
      (a) Abdominal girth and fundal height might increase.
      (b) More common with concealed bleeding
    (4) Concealed (internal) bleeding in 10% of clients
      (a) Bleeding is behind placenta with margins adherent or membranes attached to uterine wall.
      (b) Blood might break through membranes into amniotic cavity.

  (c) When fetal head is in the lower uterine segment, external bleeding might be obstructed.
  (d) Can be self-limiting and not expand during pregnancy.
  (5) Nausea and vomiting
  (6) Shock
  (7) Renal output decreases until hypovolemia treated.
  d. FHR changes
  (1) Increased baseline rate initially
  (2) Decreased baseline variability
  (3) Late deceleration pattern
  (4) Decreased baseline rate
  (5) Absence of heart rate; fetal death occurs when 50% or more of blood volume from placenta is lost.
3. Psychosocial findings
  a. Maternal stress factors (Nichols & Zwelling, 1997)
  (1) Anxiety
  (2) Fear of loss or injury of pregnancy
  (3) Fear for self
  (4) Confusion
  (5) Pain
  b. Maternal behavioral factors
  (1) Client has difficulty in communicating facts and concerns.
  (2) Client expresses pain verbally, by body posture, or both.
  (3) Client expresses fear of events and situation.
4. Diagnostic procedures
  a. Observe for coagulation abnormalities with clotting studies (PT, PTT, platelet count, D-dimer, fibrinogen, FSP).
  b. Obtain results of alkaline denaturation tests that mark presence of fetal blood: Ogita, APT, or Loendersloot (Odunsi, Bullough, Henzel, & Polanska, 1996); D-dimer level is twice as high and useful in diagnosing abruptio placentae; thrombomodulin and CA125 markers are under study and might prove helpful (Cunningham et al., 1997).
  c. Consider ultrasonography for placental condition, if possible, and to differentiate from placenta previa.
  (1) Ultrasonography for diagnosis of abruptio placentae can be unreliable; 25% of cases are confirmed; false-positive results can occur if lacunae or normal lakes of placental blood are viewed.
  (2) Several minutes after delivery, placenta begins to reveal—clotted blood over an area of depression.
  d. Palpation of abdomen might reveal:
  (1) Tenderness
  (2) Rigidity
  (3) Elevated tonus
  (4) Frequent uterine contractions
5. Complications
  a. Couvelaire uterus
  (1) Bleeds into and sometimes through the myometrium beneath serosa into the tube, broad ligament, and ovaries and across the serosa into the peritoneum.
  (2) Abrupts in center of placenta; blood is trapped.
  (3) Immediate blood loss is concealed.
  (4) Unclotted blood flows into the amniotic sac; amniotic fluid becomes a port-wine color.

   (5) Actual versus observed blood loss estimates are disparate, and, therefore, actual loss is underestimated.
 b. Fetal growth restriction
 c. Fetal anoxia and demise
 d. Fetal exsanguination
 e. Prematurity
 f. Maternal shock
 g. Maternal or neonatal coagulopathy (or both)
   (1) Hypofibrinoginemia (less than 150 mg/dl)
   (2) Elevated FSP (greater than 100 mg/ml)
   (3) Positive D-dimer levels
   (4) Thrombocytopenia
 h. Maternal renal failure; usually reversible; proteinuria resolves.
 i. Hypoxic damage to liver, adrenal glands, and anterior pituitary (Sheehan syndrome)
 j. Postpartum hemorrhage

B. Nursing Diagnoses
 1. Ineffective maternal tissue perfusion related to blood loss
 2. Ineffective fetal oxygenation and tissue perfusion related to maternal blood loss
 3. Anxiety related to fear for self and fetus
 4. Impaired comfort: abdominal pain

C. Interventions/Outcomes
 1. Ineffective maternal tissue perfusion related to blood loss
  a. Interventions
   (1) Ensure laboratory studies are performed.
     (a) CBC
     (b) Electrolyte values
     (c) Urinalysis
     (d) Type and crossmatch for blood products
     (e) Clotting studies
   (2) Establish one or more IV lines with 18-gauge or larger intracatheter.
   (3) Rapidly administer parenteral crystalloids or colloids as ordered (e.g., Ringer's lactate or plasmanate).
   (4) Avoid vaginal examinations until placenta previa has been ruled out; specific order advised.
   (5) Administer oxygen via face mask at 8 to 10 L/min.
   (6) Assist with CVP or insertion of Swan-Ganz catheter as needed; recommended ranges vary.
     (a) CVP 5 to 12 mmHg
     (b) Pulmonary arterial pressure (PAP) 10 to 20 mmHg
     (c) Pulmonary wedge pressure (PWP) less than 6 to 8 mmHg
   (7) Insert Foley catheter: 30 to 60 ml/hour output is desired.
   (8) Prepare for immediate cesarean delivery based on the following:
     (a) Gestational age, viability of fetus, and status of fetus
     (b) Maternal condition (e.g., anemia, hypoxia)
   (9) Prepare for amniotomy if vaginal delivery anticipated.
     (a) Might hasten delivery of a fetus of adequate size.
     (b) Might decrease bleeding.
   (10) Observe labor progress.
     (a) Uterine contractions often stronger
     (b) Oxytocin used if contractions are inadequate or absent
   (11) Type and crossmatch for 2 to 4 units of packed red blood cells (PRBCs); administer blood products as necessary and ordered.

(a) More than 10 units is considered to be a massive transfusion.

(b) After administration of 4 to 6 units, reevaluate clotting studies and potassium level for replacement of clotting factors.

(12) Monitor maternal pulse and blood pressure.

(13) Treat or prevent shock (e.g., ensure that body is warm and dry).

(14) Measure and estimate blood loss.

(a) Weigh blood loss on metric scale (1 g = 1 ml) or on nonmetric scale (1 oz = 29 ml).

(b) Measure and mark height of fundus on the abdomen, especially if bleeding is concealed.

(15) Position for comfort (analgesics might be contraindicated during signs of maternal or fetal compromise).

b. Outcomes: improved tissue perfusion shown by the following:

(1) Improved vital signs

(2) Improved or stable clotting studies; improved or no anemia

(3) Improved or stable color and warmth of skin

(4) Decreased blood loss; no hypovolemia

(5) Normal respiratory rate and unlabored breathing; no hypoxia

(6) Improved comfort level

2. Ineffective fetal oxygenation and tissue perfusion related to maternal blood loss

a. Interventions

(1) Continuously monitor fetal heart for the following:

(a) Baseline rate changes

(b) Variability

(c) Late deceleration pattern

(d) Sinusoidal pattern

(e) Absence of fetal heart rate; rule out demise when rate is bradycardic with variability or when maternal heart rate appears similar to fetal rate, even with electrode mode.

(2) Avoid supine hypotension by positioning client laterally or wedged to left.

(3) Treat client for alteration in tissue perfusion (e.g., oxygen therapy, ventilator-assisted respirations).

b. Outcome: normal or improved FHR and variability

3. Anxiety related to fear for self and fetus

a. Interventions

(1) Speak calmly to client and support persons.

(2) Reassure with information about events and efforts of team.

(3) Explain status of problem and plan.

(a) Imminent delivery

(b) Observation

(4) Answer questions directly.

b. Outcomes

(1) Client expresses fewer concerns and fears.

(2) Client's body posture and facial expression are less tense.

4. Impaired comfort: abdominal pain

a. Interventions

(1) Position for comfort (except not supine).

(2) Medicate or assist with regional anesthesia, as ordered.

(3) Assist with supportive strategies used in labor, especially for the medicated client.

(4) Explain rationale for avoiding medication.

b. Outcomes
  (1) Client reports increased comfort.
  (2) No side effects from analgesia or regional anesthesia in mother or fetus.

DISSEMINATED INTRAVASCULAR COAGULATION

A. Disseminated intravascular coagulation (DIC, defibrination syndrome, defibrination coagulopathy, consumption coagulopathy) is a pathologic form of clotting that is diffuse and consumes large amounts of clotting factors, causing widespread external or internal bleeding or both (Benedetti, 2002; Gonik, 1999; Horn, Davies, & Kean, 2000; Kilpatrick & Laros, 1999; Maresh, James, & Neales, 2000).
  1. Overactivation of clotting cascade and the fibrinolytic system
  2. Depletion of soluble clotting factors and platelets; lysis, or breakdown, of fibrinogen, which creates low fibrinogen levels and elevated FSP (or FDP, fibrin degradation products).
B. Not a primary disease process, but it is a secondary process activated by a number of serious illnesses.
C. Pathophysiology is dependent upon inciting event and represents a failure of normal hemostatic function.
  1. Activation of intravascular coagulation and fibrinolytic pathway results in simultaneous fibrin clot formation and clot lysis.
  2. Microthrombi occlude small vessels, which results in tissue ischemia.
D. Possible clinical consequences of DIC:
  1. Hemorrhage secondary to platelet consumption and depletion of clotting factors with potentiation by the anticoagulant effects of FDP or FSP
  2. Tissue hypoxia and ischemic necrosis secondary to obstruction of the microvasculature by fibrin plugs
  3. Microangiopathic hemolysis due to destruction of erythrocytes within the microvasculature

CLINICAL PRACTICE

A. Assessment
  1. History
    a. Client presents with previous obstetric complications such as the following:
      (1) Abruptio placentae
      (2) Intrauterine fetal death
      (3) Preeclampsia/eclampsia and HELLP (*h*emolysis, *e*levated *l*iver [enzymes], *l*ow *p*latelets) syndrome
      (4) Sepsis/SIRS (systemic inflammatory response syndrome)
      (5) Anaphylactoid syndrome of pregnancy (formerly called amniotic fluid embolism [AFE])
      (6) Gestational trophoblastic disease
      (7) Placenta accreta
      (8) Couvelaire uterus with concealed (internal) abruptio placentae
      (9) Hypovolemic shock after obstetric hemorrhage
        (a) Large blood loss with treatment of crystalloid and 5 to 10 units of PRBCs
        (b) Platelets and clotting factors depleted
      (10) Cardiopulmonary arrest

   b. Client presents with medical complication during pregnancy, such as the
     following:
     (1) Thrombocytopenia
     (2) Vascular disorders
     (3) Acid-base imbalance
     (4) Malignancy
     (5) Hemolytic transfusion reaction; intravascular hemolysis
2. Physical findings: diagnosis is based on clinical findings and laboratory markers.
  a. Bleeding
     (1) Might occur from gums, nose, puncture sites, bladder, uterus,
        incision sites, episiotomy; might continuously ooze.
     (2) Is usually without clots.
     (3) Might distend abdomen after cesarean section.
     (4) Increases the risks of thrombosis or hemorrhage, especially if
        low-grade DIC is present.
     (5) Causes petechia or purpura.
  b. Signs and symptoms of shock
     (1) Pale, clammy skin
     (2) Rising thready pulse rate and falling blood pressure
     (3) Altered level of response and consciousness
     (4) Organ hypoperfusion and tissue ischemia (e.g., respiratory distress,
        renal failure)
  c. Abnormal clotting study results (some, but not all, might be abnormal);
     platelets and activated partial thromboplastin time (aPTT) are cost-
     effective screenings, especially for preeclampsia.
     (1) Fibrinogen level less than 100 mg/dl; normal is 300 to 600 mg/dl
        during pregnancy.
     (2) Platelet count less than 50,000; normal is 150,000 to 400,000 mm^3;
        symptomatic when less than 100,000 mm^3.
     (3) FSP present, elevated, or both; normal is 10 fg/ml.
     (4) D-dimer is positive in 34% of cases and is a specific diagnostic
        test.
     (5) Plasma antithrombin III (AT III) consumption
     (6) Elevated fibrinopeptide A
     (7) Abnormal PT and PTT (values might vary with method).
        (a) Thrombin time (TT) is 15 seconds.
        (b) PT is 11 sec and at least 60%.
        (c) Whole blood clotting time (WBCT) is 4 to 12 minutes.
        (d) Activated coagulation time (ACT) by hand is 75 to 90 seconds.
        (e) aPTT is 26 to 39 seconds.
     (8) Blood vessel and RBC damage
        (a) Arteriolar vasospasms damage the endothelial layer of small
           blood vessels, forming lesions that allow platelet aggregation
           and formation of a fibrin network.
        (b) When RBCs are forced through the fibrin network under high
           pressure, the cell membrane is morphologically damaged,
           causing schistocytes or abnormally shaped RBCs and
           hemolysis.
     (9) Leukocytosis
    (10) Positive result on protamine sulfate test, a coagulation test based
        upon FSP
    (11) Abnormal clot retraction

    d. FHR patterns indicative of fetal distress
      (1) Loss of variability
      (2) Tachycardia or bradycardia
      (3) Late decelerations
      (4) Occasional sinusoidal pattern
  3. Psychosocial findings
    a. Maternal anxiety
      (1) Related to self
      (2) Related to infant
    b. Maternal sense of impending doom
    c. Maternal altered consciousness and response
  4. Diagnostic procedures
    a. Complete clotting studies
    b. Liver studies
    c. Arterial blood gas studies
    d. Type and crossmatching for blood products
    e. Measurement of fundal height as appropriate (see Physical Findings)
    f. Palpation for uterine tone and contractions

B. Nursing Diagnoses
  1. Ineffective maternal tissue perfusion related to blood loss
  2. Ineffective fetal tissue perfusion (if undelivered) related to maternal blood loss
  3. Altered respiratory function, decreased, related to blood loss
  4. Maternal anxiety related to threat to self and fetus
  5. Risk for altered consciousness related to altered respiratory function

C. Interventions/Outcomes
  1. Ineffective maternal tissue perfusion related to blood loss
    a. Interventions
      (1) Draw blood for clotting studies and send to laboratory.
        (a) Serial levels might be helpful in diagnosis.
        (b) Studies might be repeated as needed.
      (2) Cultures if sepsis is suspected
      (3) Establish IV line with large-bore intracatheter (16- or 18-gauge).
      (4) Administer fluid volume and blood products as ordered to replace and maintain circulating blood volume and clotting factors.
        (a) Anticipate aggressive fluid therapy.
        (b) Crystalloids, colloids, albumin, plasmanate, cryoprecipitate, platelets, fresh frozen plasma, prothrombin, and packed erythrocytes might be used.
      (5) Monitor vital signs, including quality of respiratory rate and baseline characteristics.
      (6) Administer oxygen via face mask at 8 L/min; support cardiorespiratory system as needed.
      (7) Position client for comfort.
      (8) Administer medications ordered.
        (a) Heparin use is rare and controversial; it is given to normalize PTT and prevent thrombosis.
          (i) Heparin effectiveness improves when AT III is over 70%.
          (ii) Usual heparin dose is 2500 to 5000 U every 4 to 12 hours.
        (b) Other medications: AT III concentrates and antiplatelet drugs
    b. Outcomes: improved tissue perfusion shown by the following:
      (1) Decreased blood loss

        (2) Improved results in clotting studies

        (3) Improved vital signs

        (4) Normal or improved respirations

        (5) Improved color and warmth of skin

  2. Ineffective fetal perfusion (if undelivered) related to maternal blood loss

    a. Interventions

        (1) Continuously monitor fetal heart for rate, variability, and sinusoidal pattern.

        (2) Avoid supine position when positioning client for comfort.

        (3) Treat mother for alteration in tissue perfusion.

    b. Outcomes

        (1) Normal or improved FHR and variability

  3. Altered respiratory function, decreased, related to blood loss

    a. Interventions

        (1) Administer oxygen as needed.

        (2) Position for improvement in respiration.

        (3) Observe rate and quality of respirations.

    b. Outcomes: stable or improved respiratory status as evidenced by the following:

        (1) Adequate oxygenation maintained as confirmed by blood gas studies

        (2) Respiration within normal limits

  4. Maternal anxiety related to threat to self and fetus

    a. Interventions

        (1) Speak calmly to client and support persons.

        (2) Reassure regarding care for mother and fetus.

        (3) Explain interventions and their rationale.

        (4) Provide comfort measures and pain medication when needed.

    b. Outcomes

        (1) Client reports less anxiety and increased comfort.

  5. Risk for altered consciousness related to altered respiratory function

    a. Interventions

        (1) Assess level of consciousness in client.

           (a) Is oriented to place, person, and time.

           (b) Answers questions appropriately.

           (c) Responds to stimuli.

           (d) Follows commands.

        (2) Explain ongoing and future events; provide information.

    b. Outcomes

        (1) Level of consciousness remains within normal limits.

GESTATIONAL TROPHOBLASTIC DISEASE

A. Gestational trophoblastic disease describes a spectrum of trophoblastic diseases that have common clinical findings, such as abnormal proliferative tissues and abnormally high human chorionic gonadotropin (hCG) levels.

B. Classifications have varied over the years, but the symptoms are unchanged for the hydatidiform mole and neoplasia.

C. Molar pregnancy is characterized by chronic or acute bleeding and a uterus that is large for gestational age after all other causes have been ruled out, such as:

1. Myoma
2. Hydramnios
3. Multiple fetuses
4. Inaccurate gestational dating

CLINICAL PRACTICE

A. Assessment
  1. History
     a. Hydatidiform mole (molar pregnancy)
        (1) Complete (classic)
            (a) Absence of maternal genetic tissue: no nucleus in fertilized egg
            (b) No fetal tissue
            (c) Neoplasia rate, 20%
            (d) Other microscopic differences from incomplete type occur.
        (2) Incomplete (atypical)
            (a) Fetal tissue noted: amniotic sac, fetus, or both
            (b) Triploid karyotype: 69 chromosomes often present with extra paternal haploid set.
            (c) Neoplasia rate, 5%
        (3) Incidence
            (a) In 1 of 200 pregnancies in United States and Europe; rate doubles in Japan.
            (b) Is higher in countries outside United States and Europe.
            (c) Is 10 times higher if mother is older than 45 years.
            (d) Has four to five times increased risk of recurrence.
            (e) Genetic predisposition of gene translocation error has been shown.
            (f) Risk of recurrence is 1% to 2%.
     b. Invasive mole (chorioadenoma destruens)
        (1) Severity is intermediate between mole and choriocarcinoma: usually a locally invasive lesion.
        (2) Occurs when trophoblastic tissue continues to grow.
        (3) Trophoblastic tissue locally invades:
            (a) Uterine myometrium
            (b) Pelvic blood vessels
            (c) Vagina (occasionally)
        (4) Occurrence rate is 15% after hyatidiform mole.
     c. Choriocarcinoma
        (1) Is highly malignant, with widespread metastasis.
        (2) Spreads to:
            (a) Lungs
            (b) Brain
            (c) Liver
            (d) Kidneys
            (e) Intestines
            (f) Spleen
            (g) Vagina
        (3) Is not always preceded by mole.
            (a) About 25% of diagnosed choriocarcinoma is preceded by spontaneous abortion.
            (b) About 20% of cases of diagnosed choriocarcinoma occur after normal pregnancy when abnormal tissue proliferates.

      (4) About 5% of molar pregnancies turn into choriocarcinoma—
         normal value of serum interleukin-2 (SIL-2R) assay excludes
         choriocarcinoma.

      (5) High levels of human chorionic gonadotropin (hCG) persist after
         delivery, and serum granulocyte macrophage colony stimulating
         factor (GM-CSF) elevates when malignant.

2. Physical findings

  a. Hydatidiform mole (molar pregnancy)

    (1) Trophoblast proliferates.

      (a) Villi become edematous because of lack of fetal circulation.

      (b) In classic type, villi become mass of clear vesicles hanging in
         clusters.

      (c) Can be located in uterus, oviduct, or ovary.

    (2) Chronic or acute bleeding occurs by 12 weeks' gestation.

      (a) Overt or concealed bleeding

      (b) Brown or bright-red blood

    (3) Signs and symptoms might include dilutional anemia, hypervolemia,
      pulmonary edema, nausea, hyperemesis after first trimester,
      abdominal cramping, and expulsion of vesicles.

    (4) Uterus rapidly enlarges.

      (a) Palpation is difficult because of soft tissue.

      (b) Ovaries might be enlarged and tender.

    (5) Fetal heart rate is absent or a single heartbeat is detected when the
      molar pregnancy affects only one twin.

    (6) In multiple pregnancies with normal fetuses, diagnosis is often
      delayed; beta-hCG levels are higher; and persistent tumors are more
      likely to develop.

    (7) Ultrasonograph shows molar pregnancy as numerous disorganized
      echoes or as abnormal gestational sacs.

  b. Neoplasia: chorioadenoma destruens or choriocarcinoma

    (1) Prognosis can be good or poor, depending on the extent of disease.

    (2) Condition often develops early as a bloodborne trophoblast.

    (3) Lungs are invaded in 75% of metastases.

      (a) Cough and bloody sputum are present.

      (b) Evidence of original lesion might disappear.

    (4) Also invades vagina (50%), vulva, kidney, liver, brain, ovaries, and
      bowel.

    (5) Good prognosis

      (a) Detected and therapy started within 4 months of onset

      (b) hCG levels less than 40,000 (1 U/L)

      (c) No prior chemotherapy

      (d) Cure rate of 90% to 100% when the foregoing are present

    (6) Poor prognosis

      (a) Detected at more than 4 months duration

      (b) hCG levels of greater than 40,000 (1 U/L) or rising indicate
         extensive disease.

      (c) Prior chemotherapy failure

      (d) Metastasis to brain and liver (irradiation might be useful)

      (e) Occurs after a term pregnancy.

      (f) Remission rate is 45% to 65% when the above listed factors
         (*a* through *e*) are present.

      (g) Death is usually a result of hemorrhage.

    c. Other placental trophoblastic tumors
      (1) Chorioangioma or hemangioma
        (a) Small tumors: asymptomatic
        (b) Large tumors: might lead to antepartum hemorrhage, hydramnios, fetal anemia, or fetal death.
      (2) Metastatic placental tumors
        (a) Any bloodborne metastasis might involve placenta.
        (b) Leukemias and lymphoma account for 30% of cases.
        (c) Malignant melanoma accounts for 30% of cases.
3. Complications
  a. Acute respiratory distress syndrome (2% to 11%)
    (1) Pulmonary edema
    (2) Pulmonary emboli
  b. Preeclampsia at less than 24 weeks' gestation
  c. Hyperthyroidism; thyrotoxicosis
  d. Theca-lutein cysts
  e. Sepsis (20% to 50%)

B. Nursing Diagnoses
1. Risk for deficient fluid volume related to evacuation of hydatidiform mole
2. Grieving related to loss of pregnancy
3. Risk for ineffective health maintenance related to insufficient knowledge of trophoblastic disease
4. Anxiety related to fear of carcinoma secondary to trophoblastic disease

C. Interventions/Outcomes
1. Risk for deficient fluid volume related to evacuation of hydatidiform mole
  a. Interventions
    (1) Monitor vital signs and blood pressure.
    (2) Monitor amount of bleeding by pad count and/or weight.
    (3) Obtain preoperative laboratory work ordered.
      (a) CBC
      (b) Quantitative beta-hCG
      (c) Clotting studies; PT, PTT, platelets, fibrinogen
      (d) Type and crossmatch 2 to 4 units PRBCs prn.
      (e) Urinalysis
      (f) Chest radiograph
    (4) Begin or maintain IV line with 18-gauge or larger intracatheter.
    (5) Administer ordered IV fluids for volume expansion without overloading.
    (6) Careful intake and output.
    (7) Assist with curettage and use of uterine stimulants prn or assist with hysterectomy (especially if future fertility is not an issue).
  b. Outcomes
    (1) Vital signs are within normal limits.
    (2) Vaginal bleeding is absent or minimal.
2. Grieving related to loss of pregnancy (see Chapter 29 for a complete discussion of perinatal grief)
3. Risk for ineffective health maintenance related to insufficient knowledge of trophoblastic disease
  a. Interventions
    (1) Encourage compliance with a close follow-up regimen (see Health Education for specifics of follow-up).
    (2) Discuss contraceptive options to prevent pregnancy for 1 year (see Chapter 15 for a complete discussion of contraception).

b. Outcomes
   (1) Client agrees to comply with follow-up plan.
   (2) Client has made plans for contraception.
4. Anxiety related to fear of carcinoma secondary to trophoblastic disease
   a. Interventions
      (1) Encourage client to verbalize concerns.
      (2) Clarify the relatively low risk of conversion to carcinoma.
      (3) Reiterate the importance of follow-up care.
   b. Outcomes
      (1) Client's anxiety is decreased.
      (2) Client verbalizes concerns, fear, and frustrations related to trophoblastic disease.

HEALTH EDUCATION

A. Second-trimester placenta previa
   1. Client may be prepared for discharge:
      a. If transportation is immediately available
      b. If located within reasonable distance of hospital
   2. Explain diagnosis, using pictures.
   3. Review symptoms that will necessitate a return to hospital.
      a. Bleeding
         (1) Describe amounts in metric or nonmetric units (e.g., 2 cups).
         (2) Describe appearance of clots (e.g., dark red, falls apart).
         (3) Describe feeling of dizziness, difficulty breathing, and pallor.
      b. Uterine and abdominal pain
      c. Uterine contractions
      d. Rupture of membranes
      e. Reassure that home-care outcomes are similar to hospital outcomes.
   4. Review risk of intrauterine growth restriction.
      a. Importance of good nutrition
      b. Avoidance of smoking
      c. Importance of rest
      d. Avoidance of supine hypotension
         (1) Tilt to side, even with semi-Fowler position.
         (2) Side-lying positions
         (3) Upright positions if possible
   5. Explain importance of follow-up.
      a. Ultrasound tests often are repeated, especially if bleeding recurs.
         (1) Placental status and position
         (2) Fetal growth
         (3) Techniques might involve transvaginal probe or transperineal scan for improved visualization, diagnosis, follow-up; client is often asked to insert probe for improved comfort and a sense of control.
      b. Other antepartum testing
      c. Maternal status
         (1) Hypovolemia
         (2) Anemia
         (3) Coagulopathy
         (4) Fatigue
         (5) Signs of labor
         (6) Avoidance of coitus

B. Late third-trimester placenta previa
    1. Explain reasons for hospitalization.
        a. Cervical changes occurring near delivery
        b. Bleeding
            (1) Need for transfusion
            (2) Need for observation and/or blood testing
        c. Viability of fetus
            (1) Neonatal resuscitation anticipated
            (2) Immediate neonatal care needed, especially if preterm
        d. Need to observe labor status
            (1) Tocolytics, as needed
            (2) Likelihood of cesarean section
        e. Need for fetal observation and testing
            (1) FHR monitoring
            (2) Fetal lung maturity
            (3) Ultrasound testing
        f. Provide educational videotapes and reading materials regarding the following:
            (1) Labor and delivery
            (2) Infant care
            (3) Nutrition
            (4) Postpartum self-care

C. Abruptio placentae
    1. Explain problem of placental separation before delivery.
        a. Risk to fetus
        b. Risk to mother
        c. Symptoms to report to caregivers:
            (1) Increased blood loss
            (2) Increased pain and contractions
            (3) Difficulty in breathing and dizziness
            (4) Rupture of membranes
    2. Explain plan of care.
        a. Fluid replacement
        b. Blood product replacement, as needed
        c. Need to monitor FHR and maternal status or changes
        d. Reason for ultrasound scan
        e. Preoperative preparation for possible cesarean section
        f. Close observation of both mother and infant after delivery

D. Chronic DIC
    1. Explain that blood is not clotting properly.
    2. Explain necessity for observation and tests.
        a. Fetal monitoring
        b. Coagulation factors
        c. Signs of increased bleeding
        d. Signs of other complications
    3. Prepare for events related to changing status.
        a. Explain present plan of care.
        b. Explain plans if condition worsens.

E. Acute DIC
    1. Explain that blood is not clotting properly.
    2. Explain immediate actions in progress.
        a. Fluid replacement

    b. Laboratory testing and blood product replacement
    c. Use of Foley catheter
    d. Use of CVP or Swan-Ganz catheter to evaluate response to interventions and status
  3. Reassure client regarding interventions in progress.
  4. Prepare client for possible imminent events, such as:
    a. Cesarean section
    b. Postdelivery surgery
    c. Critical care equipment and personnel

F. Gestational trophoblastic disease
  1. Provide information on condition, symptoms, and cause; explain the following:
    a. Abnormal formation of a pregnancy
    b. Cause unknown
    c. Presence of placental tissue and absence of fetal tissue
    d. Symptoms of nausea, vomiting, cramping, and bleeding
  2. Describe events to expect during evacuation procedures.
    a. Vacuum curettage is usually the preferred procedure.
      (1) Medication for pain
      (2) Cramping and bleeding
      (3) Environment and equipment to be used
    b. Hysterectomy procedure is performed:
      (1) If excessive bleeding is present
      (2) If mother is over 40 to 45 years of age
  3. Provide information regarding need for follow-up of 1 year, which might consist of the following:
    a. hCG levels
      (1) Weekly for 3 weeks
      (2) Monthly for 6 months
      (3) Every 2 months for 6 months
    b. No pregnancy for 1 year
    c. Chest radiograph
  4. Acknowledge family concerns and provide information about resources for support and additional understanding.

CASE STUDIES AND STUDY QUESTIONS

Ms. A, a 29-year-old, gravida 6, para 1 (G6, P1), has been admitted to a local level-I hospital at 26 or 27 weeks' gestation complaining of bleeding without pain. Vital signs are stable, hematocrit is 30.5%, and an ultrasound scan reveals a complete placenta previa. She is given IV magnesium sulfate and oral terbutaline for mild uterine contractions and transferred to a level-III (tertiary) regional hospital. After 12 days hospitalization, no further bleeding is noted and Ms. A is discharged to home on bed rest. She lives within 15 minutes of the hospital.

Upon readmission for bleeding at 29 weeks, about 200 ml of vaginal blood is noted. Ms. A is started on a graduated-dose regimen of magnesium sulfate, 5 g the first hour, 4 g the second hour, 3 g the next hour, and then a maintenance dose. At this time, an ultrasound scan reveals a complete previa, grade II placenta, and transverse fetal lie.

On the 10th day of admission, uterine contractions and increased amounts of bleeding begin. Her hematocrit is 25.9%, hemoglobin value is 8.5 g/dl, vital signs are stable, and a nonstress test (NST) is reactive. On day 14, she experiences spontaneous rupture of membranes (SROM) with clear amniotic fluid, increasing uterine contractions, persistent bloody drainage; ultrasonography shows an oblique lie. A cesarean section is performed, and the placenta previa is noted to have abrupted free of the internal os. The combined blood loss before and during surgery is estimated at 2000 ml.

In the recovery room, lochia rubra is light to moderate, the fundus is firm at the umbilicus, and oxygen saturation (SaO$_2$) is 98% to 99%. Ms. A receives a continuous infusion of Ringer's lactate with 20 U of oxytocin, morphine sulfate for pain, an additional two units of PRBCs, and prophylactic ampicillin.

1. As Ms. A's nurse, you should know that a transverse lie:
   a. Is an isolated condition.
   b. Indicates an occiput presentation of either left occipitotransverse (LOT) or right occipitotransverse (ROT).
   c. Is more common with a placenta previa.
   d. Will be rotated by her physician to a normal presentation.

2. Measuring her hematocrit periodically:
   a. Will prevent undue blood loss.
   b. Reflects the normal hemodilution of her pregnancy.
   c. Reflects the need for cryoprecipitate.
   d. Serially reflects her blood loss from placenta previa.

3. In providing intrapartum and recovery care to Ms. A, your observations and care are influenced by the knowledge that with a placenta previa:
   a. The risk of postpartum hemorrhage is the same as that for any cesarean delivery.
   b. The risk of an accreta placenta is greater.

   c. A history of smoking is a noncontributory factor.
   d. Coagulopathy is an unlikely occurrence.

4. As Ms. A's high-risk antepartum nurse, which of the following actions would you try to initiate?
   a. Enrollment in hospital preterm infant care program
   b. Instruction before discharge to home about the danger signs of bleeding and cramping
   c. Chain-of-command process to deny discharge to home order
   d. Enrollment in hospital childbirth exercise program

Ms. P is a 21-year-old Laotian Hmong, G4, P3, with a history of one cesarean section followed by two vaginal births after cesarean (VBAC) who appears at the hospital complaining of vaginal bleeding. She is uncertain of her estimated date of confinement, and an ultrasound scan places her at 27 to 28 weeks' gestation with an anterior fundal placenta and breech presentation. Her vital signs are stable, hematocrit is 34.1%, hemoglobin value is 11.5 g/dl, and during the next 2 weeks, Ms. P experiences small amounts of dark, bloody discharge with occasional scant, bright-red, mucus-like bleeding.

Ms. P remains hospitalized and receives a tapering magnesium sulfate regimen; oral terbutaline, 2.5 mg every 3 hours; oral indomethacin, 25 mg every 6 hours; and steroids for stimulating fetal lung maturity.

On day 14, she has increased mucous and bloody discharge, low back pain, and cramps, and she seems tense. She refuses lunch. Now the uterine tone is palpable and cervical changes are noted; the FHR is 160 with decreased long-term variability, and variable decelerations occur with uterine contractions.

A decision is made to perform a cesarean section. Ms. P is now at 29 to 30 weeks' gestation. During the surgery, a 20% to 25% abruption is noted with a 200-g retroplacental clot; estimated blood loss at delivery is 800 ml. A 1360-g (3 lb) girl with Apgar scores of 5 and 6 is delivered, and no immediate fetal respiratory distress is noted.

Although Ms. P recovers well. Her second-day hematocrit is 22%, and her hemoglobin value is 7.3 g/dl; two units of PRBCs are administered. On postpartum day 3, she is discharged in stable condition with a hematocrit of 30% and a hemoglobin value of 9.7 g/dl.

5. As her intrapartum nurse you
a. Recognize the potential of abruptio placentae and request an ultrasound scan.
b. Reassure her that her infant is fine right now.
c. Request a Kleihauer-Betke blood test.
d. Recognize the symptoms of uterine rupture and request an emergency cesarean section.

6. At delivery, a retroplacental clot was noted near the center of the placenta. If Ms. P continued to bleed from the clot site, she would have been likely to develop which of the following?
a. Iatrogenic thrombocytopenia
b. Revealed bleeding
c. Couvelaire uterus
d. Uterine rupture

7. If Ms. P had not undergone a cesarean, and was in labor, the following scenario might have occurred. At 9 cm, she suddenly loses consciousness; she becomes cyanotic; she has shallow, irregular respirations and a rapid, thready pulse; and the FHR decreased to 50 bpm. These are symptoms of which of the following?
a. Precipitous delivery
b. Abruptio placentae
c. Impending cardiac arrest
d. Supine hypotension

8. This situation:
a. Is associated with consumptive coagulopathy.
b. Is associated with abruptio placentae.
c. Occurs frequently with abruptio placentae.
d. Describes an unrealistic event.

Ms. R is a 23-year-old G4, P1, 167.6-cm, 73.5-kg (5 ft, 6 in, 162-lb) woman who is at 27 to 28 weeks gestation by ultrasonography and at 30.5 weeks' gestation by dates. She presents to her local level-I hospital when she notes vaginal spotting of bright-red blood and is transferred to a level-III tertiary hospital for preterm labor and partial separation of the placenta. Her total blood loss is 400 to 500 ml, and 4 days later her hematocrit is 32.7%. Ms. R tests positive for amphetamine and methamphetamine and negative for cocaine. She smokes one pack of cigarettes daily and drinks five to eight cups of coffee per day. Ms. R begins a regimen of magnesium sulfate, oral indomethacin, prophylactic ampicillin, and steroids. After 5 days of bed rest, she is stable, and, therefore, weaned from her tocolytics to return home under the care of her local provider.

9. Her bleeding was potentially caused by which of the following?
a. Polydrug use
b. Fetal growth restriction
c. Increased physical exertion
d. Cocaine use

10. In her situation, it is most important that the following be evaluated:
a. Her source of amphetamines
b. Her awareness of the harm caused to her infant
c. Local contact with a drug treatment center for pregnant women
d. Her interest in utilizing local resources for health evaluation and promotion

11. Ms. R is returned to her local level-I hospital because of which of the following?
    a. She has no insurance.
    b. She uses drugs.
    c. There is no medical problem.
    d. Her condition is stable.

12. Discharge teaching includes her risk of the following potential problems:

    a. Recurrence of preterm labor and bleeding
    b. Underestimation of blood loss when partially concealed
    c. Fetal compromise following decreased fetal movements
    d. Maternal coagulopathy and shock

ANSWERS TO STUDY QUESTIONS

1. c	4. b	7. c	10. d
2. d	5. a	8. b	11. d
3. b	6. c	9. a	12. a

REFERENCES

American College of Obstetricians and Gynecologists (Ed.). (1998). *Postpartum Hemorrhage.* (Educational Bulletin No. 243). Washington, DC: ACOG.

American College of Obstetricians and Gynecologists (Ed.). (1999). *Prevention of Rh D Alloimmunization.* (Practice Bulletin No. 4). Washington, DC: ACOG.

American College of Obstetricians and Gynecologists (Ed.). (2000). *Obstetric Aspects of Trauma Management.* (Practice Bulletin No. 251). Washington, DC: ACOG.

Amiel-Tison, C., Sureau, C., & Shnider, S.M. (1988). Cerebral handicap in full-term neonates related to the mechanical forces of labour. *Baillieres Clinical Obstetrics and Gynaecology, 2*(1), 145-165.

Ananth, C.V., Smulian, J.C., & Vintzileos, A.M. (1999). Incidence of placental abruption in relation to cigarette smoking and hypertensive disorders during pregnancy: A meta-anaylsis of observational studies. *Obstetrics and Gynecology, 93*(4), 622-628.

Baron, F. & Hill, W.C. (2002). Managing placenta previa and abruptio placentae on an outpatient basis. In W.C. Hill (Ed.), *Ambulatory Obstetrics* (pp. 65-72). Philadelphia: Lippincott Williams & Wilkins.

Baumann, P., Blackwell, S.C., Schild, C., Berry, S.M., & Friedrich, H.J. (2000). Mathematic modeling to predict abruptio placentae. *American Journal of Obstetrics and Gynecology, 183*(4), 815-822.

Benedetti, T.J. (2002). Obstetric hemorrhage. In S.G. Gabbe, J.R. Niebyl, & J.L. Simpson (Eds.), *Obstetrics: Normal and problem pregnancies* (pp. 503-538). New York: Churchill Livingstone.

Berman, M., DiSaia, P., & Brewster W. (1999). Pelvic malignancy, gestational trophoblastic neoplasm, and nonpelvic malignancies. In R. Creasy & R. Resnik (Eds.), *Maternal-fetal medicine* (4th ed.). Philadelphia: Saunders.

Blackburn, S.T. (2003). *Maternal, fetal, & neonatal physiology: A clinical perspective* (2nd ed.). St. Louis: Saunders.

Carter, S. (1999). Overview of common obstetric bleeding disorders. *Nurse Practitioner, 24*(3), 50-51, 54, 57-58.

Centers for Disease Control and Prevention. (1999). State-specific maternal mortality among black and white women-United States, 1987–1996. *Morbidity and Mortality Weekly Report, 48*(23), 492-496.

Centers for Disease Control and Prevention. (2003). Pregnancy-related mortality surveillance_United States, 1991-1999. CDC Surveillance Summaries, February 21, 2003. *Morbidity and Mortality Weekly Report, 52*(SS02), 1-8.

Chichakli, L.O., Atrash, H.K., MacKay, A.P., Musani, A.S., & Berg, C.J. (1999).

Pregnancy-related mortality in the United States due to hemorrhage: 1979-1992. *Obstetrics and Gynecology, 94*(5, Pt 1), 721-725.

Clark, S.L. (1999). Placenta previa and abruptio placenta. In R. Creasy & R. Resnik (Ed.), *Maternal fetal medicine* (4th ed., pp. 616-631). Philadelphia: Saunders.

Clark, S.L., Cotton, D.B., Hankins, G.D.V., & Phelan, J.P. (1997). *Critical care obstetrics* (3rd. ed.). Malden, MA: Blackwell Science.

Cnattingius, S. (1997). Maternal age modifies the effect of maternal smoking on intrauterine growth retardation but not on late fetal death and placental abruption. *American Journal of Epidemiology, 145*(4), 319-323.

Conklin, K.A., & Backus, A.M. (1999). In D.H. Chestnut (Ed.), *Obstetric anesthesia: Principles and practice* (2nd ed., pp. 17-42). St. Louis: Mosby.

Connolly, A.M., Katz, V.L., & Bash, K.L., et al. (1997). Trauma and pregnancy. *American Journal of Perinatology, 14*(6), 331-336.

Copeland, L., & Landon, M. (2002). Malignant diseases and pregnancy. In S. Gabbe, J. Niebyl, & J. Simpson (Eds.), *Obstetrics: Normal and problem pregnancies* (4th ed.). New York: Churchill Livingstone.

Coppens, M., & James, D.K. (1999). Organization of prenatal care and identification of risk. In D.K. James, P.J. Steer, C.P. Weiner, & B. Gonik (Ed.), *High risk pregnancy: Management options* (2nd ed., pp. 11-22). Philadelphia: Saunders.

Cunningham, F., MacDonald, P., Gant, N., Leveno, K., Gilstrap, L., Hankins, G., et al. (1997). *Williams obstetrics* (20th ed.). Stamford, CT: Appleton & Lange.

Curet, M.J., Schermer, C.R., & Demarest, G.B., et al. (2000). Predictors of outcome in trauma during pregnancy: Identification of patients who can be monitored for less than 6 hours. *Journal of Trauma, 49*(1), 18-25.

Daddario, J.B. (1999). Trauma in pregnancy. In L.K. Mandeville & N.H. Troiano (Ed.), *High-risk and critical care intrapartum nursing* (2nd ed). Philadelphia: Lippincott.

Davies, S. (1999). Amniotic fluid embolism and isolated disseminated intravascular coagulation. *Canadian Journal of Anesthesia, 46*(5, Pt 1), 456-459.

Davies, S. (2001). Amniotic fluid embolus: A review of the literature. *Canadian Journal of Anesthesia, 48*(1), 88-98.

Dildy, G.A. III (2002). Postpartum hemorrhage: New management options. *Clinical Obstetrics and Gynecology, 45*(2), 330-344.

Feinstein, N., & Atterbury, J.L. (2003). Intrinsic influences on the fetal heart rate. In N. Feinstein, K.L. Torgersen, & J.L. Atterbury (Eds.), *AWHONN fetal heart monitoring principles and practices* (3rd ed.). Dubuque, Iowa: Kendall/ Hunt Publishing Company.

Flamm, B.L. (2001). Vaginal birth after cesarean: Reducing medical and legal risks. *Clinical Obstetrics and Gynecology, 44*(3), 622-629.

Franklin, C.M., Darovic, G.O., & Dan, B.B. (2002). Monitoring the patient in shock. In G.O. Darovic (Ed.), *Hemodynamic monitoring: Invasive and noninvasive clinical application* (3rd ed.). Philadelphia: Saunders.

Gilbert, E.S., & Harmon, J.S. (2003). *Manual of high risk pregnancy & delivery* (3rd ed.). St. Louis: Mosby.

Goddijn-Wessel, T.A., Wouters, M.G., Van de Molen, E.S., Spuijbroek, M.D., Steegers-Theunissen, R.P., Blom, H.J., et al. (1996). Hyperhomocysteinemia: A risk factor for placental abruption or infarction. *European Journal of Obstetrics, Gynecology, and Reproductive Biology, 66*(1), 23-29.

Gonik, B. (1999). Intensive care monitoring of the critically ill pregnant patient. In R. Creasy & R. Resnik (Ed.), *Maternal-fetal medicine* (4th ed). Philadelphia: Saunders.

Hankins, G.D.V., & O'Day, M.P. (1997). Disseminated intravascular coagulation. In S.L. Clark, D.B. Cotton, G.D.V. Hankins, & J.P. Phelan (Ed.), *Critical care obstetrics* (3rd ed.; pp. 551-563). Boston: Blackwell Scientific.

Horn, E., Davies, J., & Kean, L. (2000). Other hematologic conditions. In D.K. James, P.J. Steer, C.P. Weiner, & B. Gonik (Ed.), *High risk pregnancy: Management options* (2nd. ed.). Philadelphia: Saunders.

Jackson, M., & Branch, D.W. (2003). Alloimmunization in pregnancy. In S.G. Gabbe, J.R. Niebyl, & J.L. Simpson (Ed.), *Pocket companion to accompany Obstetrics: Normal and problem pregnancies* (pp. 545-569). Philadelphia: Churchill Livingstone.

Kilpatrick, S., & Laros, R. (1999). Maternal hematologic disorders. In R. Creasy & R. Resnick (Ed.), *Maternal-fetal medicine* (4th ed). Philadelphia: Saunders.

Konje, J.C., & Taylor, D.J. (1999). Bleeding in late pregnancy. In D.K. James, P.J. Steer, C.P. Weiner, & B. Gonik (Ed.), *High risk pregnancy: Management options* (2nd. ed, pp. 111-128). Philadelphia: Saunders.

Koonin, L.M., MacKay, A.P., Berg, C.J., Atrash, H.K., & Smith, J.C. (1997). Pregnancy-related mortality surveillance—United States, 1987-1990. CDC surveillance summaries, August 8, 1997. *Morbidity and Mortality Weekly Report, 46*(SS04), 17-36.

Kramer, M.S., Usher, R.H., Pollak, R., et al. (1997). Etiologic determinants of abruptio placentae. *Obstetrics and Gynecology, 89*(2), 221-226.

Lanni, S.M., & Seeds, J.W. (2001). Malpresentations. In S.G. Gabbe, J.R. Niebyl, & J.L. Simpson (Ed.), *Obstetrics: Normal and problem pregnancies* (4th ed., pp. 493). New York: Churchill Livingstone.

Lockwood, C.J., & Funai, E.F. (1999). In J.T. Queenan (Ed.), *Management of high-risk pregnancy* (4th ed., pp. 466-474). Malden, MA: Blackwell Science.

Maresh, M., James, D., & Neales, K. (2000). Critical care of the obstetric patent. In D.K. James, P.J. Steer, C.P. Weiner, & B. Gonik (Ed.), *High risk pregnancy: Management options* (2nd. ed.). Philadelphia: Saunders.

Martin, J.A., Hamilton, B.E., Ventura, S.J., Menacker, F., & Park, M.M. (2002). Births: Final data for 2000. *National vital statistics reports, 50*(5). Hyattsville, Maryland: National Center for Health Statistics.

Murphy, S.L. (2000). Deaths: Final Data for 1998. *National vital statistics reports, 48*(11). Hyattsville, Maryland: National Center for Health Statistics.

Neilson, J. (2001). Interventions for suspected placenta previa (Cochrane Review). In *The Cochrane Library*, Issue 2, Oxford, Update Software.

Nichols, F., & Zwelling, E. (1997). *Maternal-newborn nursing theory and practice*. Philadelphia: Saunders.

Odunsi, K., Bullough, C.H., Henzel, J., & Polanska, A. (1996). Evaluation of chemical tests for fetal bleeding from vasa previa. *International Journal of Gynacology and Obstetrics, 55*(3), 207-212.

Pak, L.L., Reece, E.A., & Chan, L. (1998). Is adverse pregnancy outcome predictable after blunt abdominal trauma? *American Journal of Obstetrics and Gynecology, 179*(5), 1140-1144.

Parer, J.T. (1997). *Handbook of fetal heart rate monitoring* (2nd ed.). Philadelphia: Saunders.

Penning, D. (2001). Trauma in pregnancy. *Canadian Journal of Anesthesia, 48*, R7.

Samuels, P. (1997). Acute care of thrombocytopenia and disseminated intravascular coagulation complicating pregnancy. In M. Foley & T. Strong (Eds.), *Obstetric intensive care*. Philadelphia: Saunders.

Secor, V.H. (1996). *Multiple organ dysfunction & failure: Pathophysiology and clinical implications.* (2nd. ed.). St. Louis: Mosby.

Seeds, J.W., & Walsh, M. (2002). Malpresentations. In S.G. Gabbe, J.R. Niebyl, & J.L. Simpson (Eds.), *Obstetrics: Normal and problem pregnancies* (4th ed.). New York: Churchill Livingstone.

Silver, L.E., Hobel, C.J., Lagasse, L., Luttrull, J., & Platt, L. (1997). Placenta previa percreta with bladder involvement: New considerations and review of the literature. *Ultrasound in Obstetrics and Gynecology, 9*(2), 131-138.

Simpson, K.R., & Creehan, P.A. (2001). Guidelines for home care management of high-risk pregnancy conditions. In K.R. Simpson & P.A. Creehan (Ed.), *Perinatal nursing* (2nd ed.; pp. 292-296). Philadelphia: Lippincott Williams & Wilkins.

Sosa, M.E.B. (2001). High risk pregnancy, bleeding disorders. In K.R. Simpson & P.A. Creehan (Ed.), *Perinatal nursing* (2nd ed.; pp. 190-206). Philadelphia: Lippincott Williams & Wilkins.

Stables, D. (1999). *Physiology in childbearing: With anatomy and related biosciences.* Edinburgh: Bailliere Tindall.

Taipale, P., Hiilesmaa, V., & Ylostalo, P. (1997). Diagnosis of placenta previa by transvaginal sonographic screening at 12-16 weeks in a nonselected population. *Obstetrics and Gynecology, 89*(3), 364-367.

VandeKerkhove, K., & Johnson, T. (1998). Chapter 9. In M. Pearlman & J. Tintinalli (Eds.), *Emergency care of the woman*. New York: McGraw-Hill Health Professions Division.

Ventura, S.J., Martin, J.A., Curtin, S.C., Menacker, F., & Hamilton, B.E. (2001). Births: Final data for 1999. *National Vital Statistics reports, 49*(1). Hyattsville, Maryland: National Center for Health Statistics.

Wing, D., Paul, R., & Millar, L. (1996). Management of the symptomatic placenta previa: A randomized, controlled trial of inpatient versus outpatient expectant management. *American Journal of Obstetrics and Gynecology, 175*(4, Pt 1), 806-811.

Yap, O.W., Kim, E.S., & Laros, R.K. Jr. (2001). Maternal and neonatal outcomes after uterine rupture in labor. *American Journal of Obstetrics and Gynecology, 184*(7), 1576-1581.

24 Endocrine and Metabolic Disorders

CHERYL WALLERSTEDT AND DIANA E. CLOKEY

OBJECTIVES

1. Describe maternal and fetal complications associated with endocrine and metabolic disorders in pregnancy.
2. Recognize alterations in pregnancy associated with various endocrine and metabolic disorders.
3. Identify signs and symptoms associated with endocrine and metabolic disorders diagnosed prior to conception or during pregnancy that require specific nursing interventions and care for the childbearing woman and her fetus.
4. Evaluate significant clinical signs and symptoms characterized by various endocrine and metabolic disorders during the childbearing period.
5. Plan nursing assessments and interventions essential in caring for the childbearing woman with an endocrine or metabolic disorder.
6. Implement specific educational content and strategies to empower the childbearing woman with an endocrine or metabolic disorder to knowledgeably participate in her plan of care throughout the childbearing experience.

DIABETES MELLITUS

A. Definition
   1. Chronic, systemic endocrine disorder of insulin production or of the body's response to insulin
   2. Caused by absent or inadequate insulin secretion or increased cellular resistance to insulin, resulting in its impaired utilization.
   3. Characterized by an abnormal metabolism of carbohydrates, proteins, fats, and electrolytes, resulting in hyperglycemia and other systemic metabolic disturbances.
   4. Might be associated with severe neurologic, cardiovascular, ocular, renal, and microvascular complications.
   5. Classified according to cause rather than treatment.
   6. Complicates more than 200,000 pregnancies per year in the United States (American Diabetes Association [ADA], 2003).
B. Symptoms
   1. Excessive thirst and hunger
   2. Frequent urination
   3. Fatigue
   4. Blurred vision
   5. Weight loss
   6. Recurrent infections
   7. Often asymptomatic in its early stages

C. Classification

1. Type 1 diabetes mellitus (formerly IDDM)
   a. Cause is an absolute deficiency of insulin secretion by the pancreatic beta cells.
   b. Might occur by an autoimmune process involved in beta-cell destruction, genetic defects, and disease of the pancreas, endocrinopathies, and use of certain drugs.
   c. Usually appears before the age of 30 years.
   d. Has an abrupt onset of symptoms requiring prompt medical treatment.
   e. Approximately 10% of those diagnosed with diabetes have type 1 diabetes.
2. Type 2 diabetes mellitus (formerly NIDDM)
   a. Cause is a combination of resistance to insulin action and an inadequate compensatory insulin secretory response.
   b. Type 2 diabetes is diagnosed primarily in adults older than 30 years of age, but is now seen more frequently in children.
   c. Disease is typically symptom-free for many years, with slow onset and gradual progression of symptoms.
   d. Type 2 diabetes increases with age, accounting for approximately 90% of all diagnosed cases of diabetes.
   e. Disease is managed with diet and exercise: the use of oral hypoglycemic medications and/or insulin might also be indicated when hyperglycemia persists.
3. Gestational diabetes mellitus (GDM)
   a. Defined as any degree of glucose intolerance with onset or first recognition during pregnancy (Metzger & Coustan, 1998).
   b. Estimated to occur in approximately 7% of pregnancies; however, prevalence might range from 1% to 14%, depending on the population studied and diagnostic test used (ADA, 2003).
   c. Women diagnosed with GDM are at increased risk for developing diabetes later in life.
   d. Symptoms are generally mild and not life-threatening in the pregnant woman.
   e. Maternal hyperglycemia is associated with increased fetal morbidity secondary to fetal hyperinsulinemia, which potentates fetal size (large for gestational age or macrosomia > 4000 g); therefore, maintenance of normal glucose levels is required for optimal perinatal outcome (Table 24-1).
4. Impaired fasting glucose (IFG) and impaired glucose tolerance (IGT)
   a. Characterized by hyperglycemia at a level lower than what qualifies as a diagnosis of diabetes.

■ TABLE 24-1
■ ■ **Blood Glucose Values in Pregnancy**

	Ideal*	Goal
Fasting blood glucose	55-60 mg/dl	< 90 mg/dl
1 hour postprandial	120-140 mg/dl	< 140 mg/dl
Mean blood glucose	84 mg/dl	< 100 mg/dl
Hemoglobin A1c	2%-5%	< 7%

*These values are demonstrated in women with neither diabetes nor carbohydrate intolerance during pregnancy.

     b. Symptoms of diabetes are absent.

     c. Infants born to women with IGT are at increased risk for being large for gestational age (LGA).

D. Maternal metabolism and pathophysiology in pregnancy

    1. Changes in carbohydrate, protein, and fat metabolism in normal pregnancy are profound, mediated in part by the developing fetus and production of placental hormones.

    2. First half of pregnancy is considered an anabolic phase (protein and fat storage).

      a. In pregnant women without diabetes, this is associated with increased estrogen and progesterone secretion, leading to pancreatic beta-cell hyperplasia and hyperinsulinemia.

      b. Increased insulin production leads to an increased tissue response to insulin and increased uptake and storage of glycogen and fat in the liver and other tissues.

    3. Second half of pregnancy is characterized by a catabolic phase (protein and fat breakdown) with increased insulin resistance due to the production of placental hormones (insulinase, human placental lactogen), cortisol, and growth hormones, which are diabetogenic and act as insulin antagonists; in women who cannot meet the increasing demands for insulin production, this leads to altered carbohydrate metabolism and progressive hyperglycemia; characteristics of this catabolic phase include:

      a. Increased production of human placental lactogen (HPL)

      b. Elevated levels of estrogen, progesterone, blood triglycerides, free fatty acids, and serum cortisol

      c. Tendency for decreased glycogenesis and increased lipolysis, gluconeogenesis, and ketone production; maternal lipolysis provides maternal fuel needs while sparing glucose for fetal use, creating a starvation-like state in the mother (accelerated starvation of pregnancy).

    4. The developing fetus continuously removes glucose and amino acids from the maternal circulation.

      a. Glucose and amino acids are readily transported across the placenta to the developing fetus; insulin is not.

      b. Maternal hyperglycemia leads to fetal beta-cell hyperplasia and fetal hyperinsulinemia.

        (1) Fetal hyperinsulinism functions as a growth hormone for the developing fetus.

        (2) Fetal hyperinsulinism contributes to increased fetal size and leads to a decrease in surfactant production, with potential development of respiratory distress syndrome in the neonate.

    5. The constant transport of maternal glucose levels across the placenta leads to lowered blood glucose levels (hypoglycemia) and explains the lower fasting blood glucose levels observed during normal pregnancy. *Note:* Fasting blood glucose levels decline 10% to 20% in the first trimester when fetal demands for glucose are low.

E. Primary goals in the treatment of diabetes and pregnancy

    1. Achieve and maintain normal maternal glucose levels. *Note:* normal blood glucose levels are lower during pregnancy than in the nonpregnant state.

    2. Promptly identify and manage complications associated with diabetes and pregnancy in the childbearing woman, fetus, and neonate.

CLINICAL PRACTICE

Pregestational Diabetes (Type 1 and Type 2 Diabetes)

A. Assessment

1. Definition and prognosis
   a. Type 1 diabetes is primarily a chronic autoimmune disorder resulting from the destruction of the pancreatic beta-cells, which usually leads to absolute insulin deficiency.
   b. Type 2 diabetes arises because of insulin resistance, sometimes combined with relative insulin deficiency.
   c. Predisposition is genetically determined
2. Incidence
   a. Incidence of pregestational diabetes is approximately 0.2% to 0.3% of all pregnancies and affects 10,000 to 14,000 women annually.
   b. Pregestational diabetes accounts for 10% of all diabetic pregnancies.
3. Prognosis
   a. Pregnant women with pregestational diabetes might be categorized prognostically according to the classic system of White, with some minor modifications (Table 24-2).
   b. The quality of metabolic regulation (diabetic control) throughout pregnancy and the presence or absence of serious complications of diabetes, especially nephropathy, hypertension, and heart disease, account for most of the risks associated with diabetes in pregnancy rather than the genetic characteristics of the maternal diabetes.
   c. Observe for complications associated with diabetes: ketoacidosis, preeclampsia, and pyelonephritis.
      (1) Diabetic ketoacidosis (DKA) affects about 1% of diabetic pregnancies; it is usually associated with:
         (a) Poor glycemic control
         (b) Hyperemesis gravidarum contributing to dehydration
         (c) Tocolytic therapy (beta-sympathomimetic agents)
         (d) Infections (most common)
         (e) Insulin pump failure
      (2) Risk of preeclampsia increases with diabetes; complicates 10% to 15% of diabetic pregnancies versus 5% of nondiabetic pregnancies.
      (3) Maternal infections occur more frequently in diabetic pregnancies than in nondiabetic pregnancies.
4. History
   a. Preconceptual assessments for preexisting diabetics
      (1) Classification of diabetes in pregnancy
      (2) Blood glucose control, Hgb A1c (glycosylated hemoglobin), and frequency of self-blood glucose monitoring (SBGM)
      (3) Presence of vascular complications and current vascular status; evaluation of renal, retinal, and cardiac status is recommended if duration of diabetes is longer than 5 years.
      (4) Thyroid panel (type 1 diabetic women only)
      (5) Neuropathy testing if indicated
      (6) Adequacy of current diet and plans for dietary adjustments in pregnancy
         (a) Recommended total calorie intake is 30 kcal/kg prepregnant weight of nonobese individuals given as three meals and three snacks (ADA 2003; American College of Obstetricians and

■ TABLE 24-2
■ ■ **Modified White's Classification of Diabetes in Pregnancy**

Class	Age of Onset		Duration	Vascular Disease	Treatment
A	Any		Any	None	Diet alone
A1	During pregnancy			None	Diet alone
A2	During pregnancy			None	Insulin
B	≥ 20		< 10	None	Insulin
C	10-19	or	10-19	None	Insulin
D	≤ 10	or	> 20	Benign (hypertension, background retinopathy)	Insulin
F	Any		Any	Nephropathy	Insulin
R	Any		Any	Proliferative retinopathy	Insulin
H	Any		Any	Cardiac disease	Insulin
T	Any		Any	Renal transplant	Insulin

Gynecologists [ACOG], 2001). For obese women with a body mass index (BMI) greater than 30, a calorie restriction to approximately 25 kcal/kg actual weight per day (ADA, 2003).
   (b) Recommended dietary composition is 40% to 50% carbohydrate, 20% protein, and 30% to 40% fat (ADA, 2003).
(7) Current insulin regimen: might need to be adjusted to attain euglycemia. *Note:* women with type 2 diabetes on oral hypoglycemic agents might need to be controlled on insulin prior to conception (contributing to an increase in weight prior to pregnancy); oral agents in pregnancy are controversial. Further studies are needed for safety and efficacy of the newer oral hypoglycemic agents.
(8) Understanding of self-care responsibilities and comprehensive collaborative management of diabetes in pregnancy to promote optimal perinatal outcomes
(9) Current lifestyle and related health habits
   (a) Exercise
   (b) Current method of family planning
 b. Prenatal assessments
   (1) Adequacy of dietary intake; pattern and composition of intake
   (2) SBGM
      (a) Frequency and method of testing
      (b) Pattern and recorded results of SBGM
      (c) Ability to adjust insulin requirements based on changing pattern of blood glucose levels
      (d) Hgb A1c, usually each trimester
   (3) Insulin administration and intensified insulin therapies
      (a) Multiple injections
         (i) The Diabetes Control and Complications Trial (DCCT) recommends tight control in type 1 diabetes. The documented methods to achieve tight control include multiple (three or more) daily injections or treatment with an insulin pump (DCCT, 1993).
         (ii) Multiple injections of regular or lispro (rapid-acting) insulin before meals. Intermediate-acting insulin administered with the evening meal or at bedtime. Lispro has a more rapid

onset, an earlier peak, and a shorter duration than regular insulin (ACOG, 2001).
- (b) Continuous subcutaneous insulin infusion using an insulin pump with administration of basal rate and bolus doses
- (c) Dosage adjustments according to changing insulin requirements during pregnancy to maintain euglycemia; typically, insulin requirements increase by two to three times beginning at approximately 18 weeks, peaking at 36 weeks' gestation.
- (d) Human forms of insulin recommended; less likely to result in insulin antigenicity
- (4) Episodes of maternal hypoglycemia and hyperglycemia
  - (a) Might experience increase in episodes of hypoglycemia; signs of hypoglycemia might be altered and not as readily perceived in pregnancy because the release of normal counter-regulatory hormones can be suppressed.
  - (b) Assessment of ketones in the urine is recommended:
    - (i) In the morning (first morning specimen)
    - (ii) When blood glucose levels are greater than 200 mg/dl
    - (iii) During illness
- (5) Urinalysis (UA) and urine culture (UC) are usually obtained each trimester, or if symptoms are present.
- (6) Evaluation of fetal status
  - (a) Ultrasound testing
    - (i) Pregnancy dating (estimation of gestational age)
    - (ii) Fetal growth and development; assess for:
      - Intrauterine growth restriction (IUGR)
      - Polyhydramnios
      - Fetal macrosomia
    - (iii) Assessment for congenital anomalies: increased risk of neural tube defects and congenital heart disease
  - (b) Maternal serum alpha-fetoprotein (AFP)
  - (c) Biophysical profile (BPP)
  - (d) Nonstress testing (NST)
  - (e) Maternal assessment of fetal activity and fetal movement counts
  - (f) Amniocentesis for lecithin/sphingomyelin (L/S) ratio and phospholipid phosphatidylglycerol (PG) to assess fetal lung maturity and optimize timing of delivery; indicated if induction is planned before 38.5 weeks' gestation.
  - (g) Doppler studies using Doppler umbilical and uterine artery velocimetry to assess pregnancies at risk for placental vascular disease; might be particularly helpful in the early detection of fetal growth restriction in women with diabetes and vasculopathy.
5. Physical findings
  a. Maternal effects and complications
  - (1) Altered insulin requirements
  - (2) Metabolic disturbances related to hyperemesis, nausea and vomiting of pregnancy, and diabetogenic effects of pregnancy
    - (a) Increased risk of hypoglycemia, especially in first trimester
    - (b) Increased risk of ketoacidosis, especially in second trimester
  - (3) Increased risk of maternal infection related to hyperglycemia
    - (a) Urinary tract infection
    - (b) Chorioamnionitis
    - (c) Postpartum endometritis

(4) Progression and possible acceleration of vascular disease secondary to alterations in diabetic control, including retinopathy, nephropathy, and neuropathy
(5) Polyhydramnios; related to fetal anomalies and fetal hyperglycemia
(6) Preeclampsia or gestational hypertension
(7) Increased maternal mortality, associated with the following:
  (a) Ischemic heart disease
  (b) Advanced vascular disease
  (c) Ketoacidosis
  (d) Hypoglycemia
  (e) Labor disturbances and dystocia; related to fetal increased size and shoulder dystocia
  (f) Complications of cesarean birth
  (g) Postpartum hemorrhage and subsequent anemia; related to:
    (i) Birth trauma
    (ii) Uterine atony secondary to prolonged labor
    (iii) Fetal macrosomia
    (iv) Polyhydramnios
    (v) Infection

b. Fetal effects and complications
(1) Increased incidence of congenital malformations and anomalies, including cardiac, skeletal, neurologic, genitourinary, and gastrointestinal; related to maternal hyperglycemia during organogenesis (first 6 to 8 weeks of pregnancy)
  (a) The incidence of anomalies can be correlated with HgbA1c levels in the mother.
  (b) It is suggested that levels be kept below 7% to reduce the incidence of anomalies (Cefalo & Moos, 1994).
(2) Growth disturbances
  (a) Large fetal size; related to fetal hyperinsulinemia (increased risk in mothers without vascular disease; White's classes A to C (see Table 24-2)
    (i) Unlike other LGA neonates, the organs of the infant of a diabetic mother (IDM) are affected by the macrosomia (organomegaly), and body fat is increased (Behrman, 1995).
    (ii) A cesarean section might be warranted if the fetus is estimated to weigh more than 4200 to 4300 g (9 lb, 4 oz to 9 lb, 8 oz), to avoid traumatic injury from a vaginal birth.
  (b) IUGR; related to maternal vasculopathy and decreased placental perfusion (increased risk in mothers with vascular disease; White's classes D to T (see Table 24-2) (see Chapter 18 for further discussion of risks associated with size and age)
(3) Fetal asphyxia; related to fetal hyperglycemia and fetal hyperinsulinemia
(4) Birth trauma; related to fetal macrosomia and shoulder dystocia (see earlier comment about possible cesarean section)
(5) Stillbirth, especially after 36 weeks' gestation in pregnancies complicated by:
  (a) Poor blood glucose control
  (b) Large fetal size
  (c) Maternal vascular disease
  (d) Ketoacidosis

c. Neonatal effects and complications
  (1) Prematurity; related to preterm birth associated with maternal complications
  (2) Respiratory distress syndrome; related to delayed fetal lung maturity and preterm birth
    (a) Excess insulin produced by the pancreas of the fetus results in delayed surfactant production, probably by interfering with the lung's ability to use phospholipids by blocking receptor sites.
      (i) This delay in surfactant production is found primarily in classes A-C of diabetic amniotic fluid.
      (ii) Classes D-T diabetic infants might have accelerated lung maturation because the incidence of respiratory distress syndrome (RDS) is less in the presence of intrauterine stress often found in these pregnancies.
    (b) To avoid iatrogenic RDS, it is suggested that the usual parameters of lung maturity be adjusted for IDMs.
      (i) An amniotic fluid L/S ratio of two or greater does not always ensure that lung maturity has been achieved (Tyrala, 1996).
      (ii) The presence of PG is reassuring. (See Chapter 19 for a complete discussion of respiratory distress.)
  (3) Metabolic and hematologic disturbances; related to maternal hyperglycemia
    (a) Hypoglycemia
      (i) Glucose molecules readily cross the placenta, but insulin does not; fetal blood sugars are 70% to 80% of maternal levels.
      (ii) The fetus responds by producing large quantities of insulin, leading to hyperinsulinemia.
      (iii) When the umbilical cord is cut after delivery, the supply of glucose rapidly diminishes, yet the level of insulin remains constant, leading to neonatal hypoglycemia.
      (iv) Glucose levels should be monitored frequently in the newborn (as per agency protocol); levels should be above 40 mg/dl. If below, offer glucose, breast milk, or formula, or, if necessary, IV glucose infusion.
    (b) Hypocalcemia
      (i) Defined as serum calcium below 7 mg/dl.
      (ii) Is usually manifested in first 2 to 3 days of life.
      (iii) Might occur as result of birth injury or decreased magnesium level, which suppresses parathyroid hormone production, thus decreasing calcium levels (Tyrala, 1996).
    (c) Hypomagnesemia
    (d) Polycythemia and hyperbilirubinemia
      (i) Polycythemia occurs in 15% to 30% of IDMs, subsequent breakdown of increased RBCs predisposes to hyperbilirubinemia.
      (ii) Might result from fetal hypoxia, increase in fetal erythropoietin, sequestered blood from birth injuries, and/or impairment of hepatic function by neonatal hypoglycemia that interferes with bilirubin conjugation. (See Chapter 19 for a complete discussion of hyperbilirubinemia.)
  (4) Cardiomyopathy and anomalies; related to maternal hyperglycemia. (See the previous discussion and Chapter 17 for more information about congenital anomalies.)

     6. Psychosocial considerations
       a. Adaptation to presence of chronic illness
       b. Presence and adequacy of support systems: partner, family, significant others
       c. Adequacy of coping responses associated with diagnosis of high-risk pregnancy
       d. Occupation and employment status
       e. Financial concerns related to need for more intensive monitoring of pregnancy
       f. Planned or unplanned pregnancy
       g. Family's response to pregnancy
       h. Feelings regarding high-risk status of pregnancy
       i. Availability of specialized health care team for management of pregnancy
     7. Diagnostic procedures
       a. Hgb A1c (blood test that reflects mean blood glucose levels during the previous 4 to 8 weeks)
       b. Renal evaluation
       c. Ophthalmologic evaluation
       d. Cardiovascular assessment

B. Nursing Diagnoses
   1. Altered metabolism of carbohydrates, proteins, fats, and electrolytes related to preexisting diabetes and pregnancy
   2. Anxiety related to risk for exacerbation of maternal vascular complications; anxiety related to pregnancy and its outcome
   3. Powerlessness related to fetal outcome
   4. Deficient knowledge related to altered plan of diabetes self-care and obstetrical management of diabetes during pregnancy
   5. Risk for fetal injury related to fetal dependence on maternal blood glucose levels
   6. Interrupted family processes related to demands of recommended diabetes and obstetric care during pregnancy

C. Interventions/Outcomes
   1. Altered metabolism of carbohydrates, proteins, fats, and electrolytes related to preexisting diabetes and pregnancy
     a. Interventions
       (1) Encourage monitoring blood glucose levels and recording results of testing at least four to seven times daily (before and after meals and at bedtime). *Note:* abnormal glucose results are most frequently caused by:
         (a) Improper user technique
         (b) Anemia; might falsely elevate results.
         (c) Erythemia; might falsely lower results of blood glucose testing.
       (2) Assist with regulation of insulin dosage according to changing physiologic needs and blood glucose levels throughout pregnancy.
         (a) Might switch to human forms of insulin.
         (b) Intensify insulin regimen with multiple injections three to four (or more) times daily.
         (c) Might initiate insulin pump therapy.
       (3) Encourage urine testing for ketones to assist with identification of starvation ketosis or developing ketoacidosis:
         (a) On first morning specimen
         (b) For blood glucose levels greater than 200 mg/dl

(c) During maternal illness
(d) When glucose control is altered. *Note:* persistent ketonuria might indicate the need for an additional snack or change in insulin regimen.
(4) Review signs and symptoms for maternal hypoglycemia, which might be altered during pregnancy; and the prevention and management of hypoglycemic episodes (clients should be instructed to have a source of fast-acting carbohydrate with them at all times, such as six to eight Lifesavers, 4 oz (120 ml) of fruit juice, or 2 tablespoons of raisins).
  (a) Mild
    (i) Tremors
    (ii) Tachycardia
    (iii) Diaphoresis
    (iv) Paresthesia
    (v) Excessive hunger
    (vi) Pallor
    (vii) Shakiness (associated with adrenergic system response)
  (b) Moderate
    (i) Headache
    (ii) Mood change
    (iii) Irritability
    (iv) Inability to concentrate
    (v) Drowsiness
    (vi) Confusion
    (vii) Impaired judgment
    (viii) Slurred speech
    (ix) Staggering gait
    (x) Double or blurred vision (associated with adrenergic plus neuroglycopenic symptoms)
  (c) Severe
    (i) Disorientation
    (ii) Unconsciousness
    (iii) Seizures
  b. Outcomes
  (1) Blood glucose levels remain within individualized goals determined for optimal maternal and fetal outcome.
  (2) Insulin dosages are regulated according to changing physiologic needs and maternal blood glucose levels throughout pregnancy.
  (3) Urine is tested for ketones in the morning, when blood glucose levels are 200 mg/dl or higher, during maternal illness, and when blood glucose control is altered.
  (4) Signs and symptoms of maternal hypoglycemia and ketoacidosis are recognized promptly and managed appropriately during pregnancy.
2. Anxiety related to risk for exacerbation of maternal vascular complications; anxiety related to pregnancy and its outcome
  a. Interventions
  (1) Clinical assessments
    (a) Blood-pressure monitoring
    (b) Presence of visual disturbances
    (c) Signs and symptoms of preeclampsia and urinary tract infections (UTIs)

      (2) Prompt identification of alterations in clinical assessments and referral for appropriate medical and obstetrical management

   b. Outcomes

      (1) Alterations in blood pressure, presence of visual disturbances, and signs and symptoms of preeclampsia and UTIs are promptly assessed.

      (2) Appropriate referrals for medical and obstetric management of clinical alterations in pregnancy are obtained to minimize potential maternal, fetal, and neonatal complications.

3. Powerlessness related to fetal outcome

   a. Interventions

      (1) Discuss strategies for maintenance of optimal glycemic control during pregnancy.

      (2) Provide information about tests and procedures for fetal assessment and surveillance.

      (3) Encourage active participation in decision making and planning for medical and obstetric care throughout pregnancy.

      (4) Discuss feelings about pregnancy and self-monitoring practices for management of diabetes during pregnancy.

   b. Outcomes

      (1) Client maintains optimal blood glucose control during pregnancy.

      (2) Client receives information about tests and procedures for fetal assessment.

      (3) Client actively participates in decision making and planning for medical and obstetric care throughout pregnancy.

      (4) Client expresses her feelings about her pregnancy and self-monitoring practices for management of diabetes during pregnancy.

4. Deficient knowledge related to altered plan of diabetes self-care and obstetric management of diabetes during pregnancy

   a. Interventions

      (1) Discuss the rationale for blood glucose control and importance of euglycemia before conception and during pregnancy.

      (2) Review self-care practices.

         (a) Blood glucose monitoring and frequency of testing

         (b) Insulin administration

         (c) Adjustment of insulin dosages based on blood glucose determinations

         (d) Dietary adjustments and management during pregnancy

      (3) Refer for dietary counseling to ensure optimal diet for glycemic control and fetal growth and development.

      (4) Discuss plan of care for obstetric management and fetal surveillance.

   b. Outcomes

      (1) Client verbalizes rationale for blood glucose control and importance of euglycemia before conception and during pregnancy.

      (2) Client demonstrates proper techniques and frequency for blood glucose monitoring and insulin administration, adjusts insulin dosages based on blood glucose determinations, and modifies dietary intake during pregnancy.

      (3) Client receives dietary counseling to ensure optimal diet for glycemic control and fetal growth and development.

      (4) Client verbalizes recommended plan of care for obstetric management and fetal surveillance.

    5. Risk for fetal injury related to fetal dependence on maternal blood glucose levels
      a. Interventions
        (1) Monitor maternal glycemia.
        (2) Assess fetal well-being, including results of NST, AFP, BPP, Doppler studies, and ultrasound testing.
        (3) Encourage maternal assessment of fetal movement using daily fetal movement counts.
      b. Outcomes
        (1) Client demonstrates dietary management, blood glucose monitoring, and insulin dosage adjustments to maintain euglycemia.
        (2) Fetal status and well-being are monitored via NST, BPP, Doppler studies, and ultrasound testing.
        (3) Client participates in assessment of fetal well-being using daily movement counts and records, and reports changes in the pattern of fetal activity.
    6. Interrupted family processes related to demands of recommended diabetes and obstetric care during pregnancy
      a. Interventions
        (1) Assess maternal support systems and the presence and involvement of significant others in assisting the client with self-care behaviors and practices.
        (2) Assess alterations in maternal work or employment status and potential economic impact of pregnancy, including financial concerns and expenses.
        (3) Encourage active participation of significant others in prenatal care and testing.
        (4) Discuss family's responses to pregnancy.
      b. Outcomes
        (1) Client describes support systems and the presence and involvement of significant others in the performance of self-care behaviors and practices during pregnancy.
        (2) Client expresses financial concerns related to alterations in maternal work or employment status during pregnancy.
        (3) Client's significant others will actively participate in prenatal care and testing.
        (4) Client discusses family's responses to pregnancy.

GESTATIONAL DIABETES MELLITUS

A. Definition
    1. Carbohydrate intolerance of variable severity with onset or first recognition during the current pregnancy
    2. Client might require an oral hypoglycemic agent/insulin.
    3. Diabetes mellitus might persist after pregnancy.
    4. Glucose intolerance might have antedated the pregnancy.
B. Incidence
    1. Occurs in approximately 7% of all pregnant women.
    2. Affects 200,000 women per year (ADA, 2003).
    3. Accounts for 90% of diabetic pregnancies.
    4. Blacks, Hispanics, Southeast Asians, and American Indians are at increased risk for GDM (ACOG, 2001)

CLINICAL PRACTICE

A. Assessment

1. History (preconceptual risk factors associated with GDM)
   a. Previous infant larger than 9 lb (4000 g)
   b. Previous infant with congenital anomaly
   c. Previous unexplained intrauterine fetal demise (IUFD) or neonatal death
   d. History of GDM in previous pregnancy
   e. History of polyhydramnios in prior pregnancy
   f. Poor reproductive history (i.e., history of preterm birth or recurrent) spontaneous abortions
   g. Family history of diabetes (i.e., parent or sibling with diabetes)
   h. Age 35 years or over
   i. Body mass index (BMI) > 30 (maternal obesity)
   j. Hypertension
   k. Ethnic background: Black, Asian, Hispanic, and American Indian
2. Physical findings and associated risk factors in current pregnancy
   a. Maternal effects
      (1) Development of polyhydramnios, suspected large fetal size, or increased fundal height relative to dating of pregnancy
      (2) Persistent glycosuria on two successive prenatal visits
      (3) Proteinuria
      (4) Urinary frequency after first trimester
      (5) Recurrent monilial infections
      (6) Reported feelings or behaviors of excessive thirst or hunger
   b. Fetal and neonatal effects
      (1) Increased fetal size; associated with operative delivery, birth trauma, and shoulder dystocia.
      (2) Neonatal hypoglycemia
      (3) Neonatal hypocalcemia
      (4) Neonatal polycythemia
      (5) Neonatal hyperbilirubinemia
      (6) Respiratory distress syndrome
      (7) Infants of mothers with fasting and postprandial hyperglycemia are at greatest risk for intrauterine death or neonatal mortality.
      (8) Overall perinatal mortality has been reported to be 6.4% when GDM is untreated; studies suggest that there is no increase in perinatal mortality when GDM is managed appropriately and maternal glucose levels are normal.
      (9) Increased risk of childhood obesity
3. Psychosocial considerations
   a. Adaptation to diagnosis and management of GDM (see Pregestational Diabetes, Psychosocial Considerations)
4. Diagnostic procedures
   a. Glucose screening
      (1) ACOG recommends universal screening (ACOG, 2001); however, published data indicate that universal screening is not cost effective. Current recommendation by ADA is for selective screening for GDM of pregnant women with one or more of the following criteria:
         (a) Age > 25 years
         (b) Obesity
         (c) Family history of type 2 diabetes (first-degree relative)

    (d) Ethnic group with a high prevalence of type 2 diabetes
    (e) History of abnormal glucose tolerance
    (f) History of poor obstetric outcome
  (2) Testing protocol
    (a) Women meeting the criteria should undergo a glucose challenge test between the 24th and 28th week of gestation; an earlier screen should be performed on those women with identified risk factors.
    (b) Administer 50 g of oral glucose, given without regard to time of day or interval since the last meal.
    (c) Measure venous plasma glucose 1 hour later; level should be below 140 mg/dl (the recommended test threshold); any value equal to or greater than 140 mg/dl requires a full 3-hour diagnostic oral glucose tolerance test (OGTT). A glucose threshold of 140 identifies approximately 80% of GDM, and using a threshold value of 130 results in about 10% more abnormal screens.
 b. OGTT
  (1) Diagnosis of GDM is based on results of the 100-g OGTT during pregnancy.
  (2) There are currently two diagnostic criteria sets for GDM. The Expert Committee on the Diagnosis and Classification of Diabetes Mellitus (ACOG, 2001) accepts both criteria until clinical trials can determine which is superior. Criteria set by the American Diabetes Association (Carpenter/Coustan) and the National Diabetes Data Group (NDDG) are as follows:

Status	ADA (Plasma)	NDDG (Plasma)
Fasting	95 mg/dl	105 mg/dl
1 hour	180 mg/dl	195 mg/dl
2 hour	155 mg/dl	165 mg/dl
3 hour	140 mg/dl	145 mg/dl

  (3) Definitive diagnosis requires that two or more of the venous plasma (or serum) glucose concentrations be met or exceeded.
  (4) Current studies suggest that a single abnormal test value should be regarded as a pathologic finding, and, therefore, patients should be treated similarly to the patient with GDM (Langer, Brustman, Anyaegbunam, & Mazze, 1987).
B. Nursing Diagnoses
  1. Altered metabolism of carbohydrates, proteins, fats, and electrolytes related to pregnancy
  2. Anxiety related to maternal diagnosis and implications for neonatal outcome
  3. Altered self-concept related to diagnosis of high-risk pregnancy
  4. Risk for fetal injury related to macrosomia associated with fetal dependence on maternal blood glucose levels
  5. Deficient knowledge related to altered management plan and self-care activities required for control of blood glucose levels during pregnancy
  6. Risk for imbalanced nutrition: more than body requirements related to maintaining normal blood glucose levels and providing adequate dietary intake for maternal and fetal needs without causing excessive maternal weight gain
  7. Interrupted family processes related to demands of optimal diabetes and obstetric care during pregnancy

C. Interventions/Outcomes

1. Altered metabolism of carbohydrates, proteins, fats, and electrolytes related to pregnancy
   a. Interventions
      (1) Review normal changes in carbohydrate metabolism during pregnancy and significance of impaired glucose tolerance to developing fetus.
      (2) Discuss rationale for normalizing blood glucose levels during pregnancy, and review the effects of elevated blood glucose levels on fetal growth and development and neonatal outcome.
      (3) Monitor fasting and postprandial blood glucose levels. *Note:* the recommended frequency of monitoring blood glucose levels varies in women with GDM.
      (4) Instruct client in self-monitoring of blood glucose levels and recording results; review instructions and monitoring techniques. *Note:* the decision to initiate SBGM for women with GDM might vary according to maternal age, gestational age, degree of metabolic abnormality on the OGTT, whether the administration of insulin is required, and other risk factors.
      (5) If indicated, instruct client in proper technique for administration of insulin and how to record insulin dose and time of injection.
   b. Outcomes
      (1) Client states normal changes in carbohydrate metabolism during pregnancy and significance of impaired glucose tolerance to developing fetus.
      (2) Client verbalizes rationale for normalization of blood glucose levels during pregnancy and describes the effects of elevated blood glucose levels on fetal growth and development and neonatal outcomes.
      (3) Alterations in fasting and postprandial blood glucose levels are recognized and managed with dietary modifications, exercise, and insulin administration.
      (4) Client demonstrates proper technique in SBGM and records results accurately.
      (5) If indicated, client demonstrates proper technique in administration of insulin and records insulin dose and time of injection.
2. Anxiety related to maternal diagnosis and implications for neonatal outcome
   a. Interventions
      (1) Provide information regarding effects of elevated blood glucose levels on developing fetus and rationale for normalizing maternal glucose levels.
      (2) Discuss dietary modifications, exercise, and SBGM to promote normalization of blood glucose levels.
      (3) Encourage active participation in self-monitoring practices and decision making about plan for managing GDM.
      (4) Discuss results of fetal assessment tests and procedures for evaluation of fetal status and well-being.
   b. Outcomes
      (1) Client states effects of elevated blood glucose levels on developing fetus and rationale for normalizing maternal glucose levels.
      (2) Client modifies her dietary intake, adopts a regular exercise plan, and self-monitors blood glucose levels to promote normalization of blood glucose levels.

         (3) Client actively participates in self-monitoring practices and decision making regarding the plan for managing GDM.

         (4) Client is informed of results of fetal assessment tests and procedures for evaluation of fetal status and well-being.

3. Altered self-concept related to diagnosis of high-risk pregnancy

  a. Interventions

      (1) Encourage maternal expression of feelings and concerns related to diagnosis of GDM.

      (2) Discuss alterations in anticipated plan for obstetric care, and provide support to minimize potential complications related to unexpected interventions necessitated in pregnancy.

  b. Outcomes

      (1) Client expresses her feelings and concerns about the diagnosis of GDM.

      (2) Client describes alterations in anticipated plan for obstetric care and identifies sources of support to minimize potential complications related to unexpected interventions necessitated in pregnancy.

4. Risk for fetal injury related to macrosomia associated with fetal dependence on maternal blood glucose levels

  a. Interventions

      (1) Monitor blood glucose levels.

      (2) Monitor fetal status and development using NST, BPP, and ultrasound testing. *Note:* twice-weekly NSTs, weekly BPPs, or weekly NST alternated with BPP may be initiated as early as 32 weeks.

      (3) Encourage maternal assessment of fetal movement using daily fetal movement counts.

  b. Outcomes

      (1) Client participates in monitoring of blood glucose levels.

      (2) Fetal status and development are monitored using NST, BPP, and ultrasound testing.

      (3) Client participates in the assessment of fetal well-being using daily fetal movement counts and reports changes in the pattern of fetal activity.

5. Deficient knowledge related to altered management plan and self-care activities required for blood glucose levels during pregnancy

  a. Interventions

      (1) Review rationale for normal blood glucose levels in pregnancy.

      (2) Discuss plan for normalizing blood glucose levels, including dietary management, exercise, blood glucose monitoring, and possible insulin administration.

        (a) Recommended calorie intake is 30 kcal/kg ideal body weight.

          (i) Typically provides additional 300 to 400 calories per day.

          (ii) Calorie restrictions might be recommended for the overweight woman with GDM to minimize the likelihood of fetal macrosomia and prevent or decrease exogenous insulin requirements.

          (iii) Weight loss and ketonuria should be avoided.

        (b) Exercise assists in glucose normalization in women with type 2 diabetes, women with GDM, and obese women with carbohydrate intolerance; benefits include improved insulin sensitivity and glucose utilization with potential prevention of need for insulin or reduction in insulin requirements.

      (c) Recommendations for the initiation and frequency of SBGM for women with GDM vary; generally, all women with GDM requiring insulin require SBGM.

      (d) Insulin is usually prescribed if fasting or postprandial blood glucose levels are persistently elevated despite dietary modifications.

         (i) Insulin is prescribed if fasting glucose is greater than 105 mg/dl on one occasion or postprandial glucose is greater than 120 mg/dl on two or more occasions within a 2-week interval.

         (ii) Insulin might also be recommended for women with an elevated fasting blood glucose level on the 3-hour OGTT.

b. Outcomes

  (1) Client verbalizes rationale for normal blood glucose levels in pregnancy.

  (2) Client demonstrates normalization of blood glucose levels through dietary management, exercise, blood-glucose monitoring, and possible administration of insulin, if prescribed.

6. Risk for imbalanced nutrition: more than body requirements related to maintaining normal blood glucose levels and providing adequate dietary intake for maternal and fetal needs without causing excessive maternal weight gain

a. Interventions

  (1) Refer client for dietary counseling to ensure proper diet for normalization of blood glucose levels and optimal fetal growth and development.

  (2) Encourage client to record dietary intake and blood glucose results.

b. Outcomes

  (1) Client receives dietary counseling to ensure proper diet for normalization of blood glucose levels and optimal fetal growth and development.

  (2) Client records dietary intake and blood glucose levels.

7. Interrupted family processes related to demands of optimal diabetes and obstetric care during pregnancy

a. Interventions

  (1) Encourage client to express concerns related to plan for management of GDM and presence of family support to encourage adherence to dietary recommendations and maintain blood glucose control.

  (2) Provide anticipatory guidance about the frequency of prenatal appointments and testing for evaluation of maternal glycemic status and the need for additional fetal assessment tests and surveillance.

  (3) Assess impact of the diagnosis of GDM on the family.

b. Outcomes

  (1) Client expresses her concerns about the plan for diabetes management during pregnancy and describes presence of family support to encourage adherence to dietary recommendations and maintenance of blood glucose control.

  (2) Client receives anticipatory guidance about the frequency of prenatal appointments and testing for evaluation of maternal glycemic status and the need for additional fetal assessment tests and surveillance.

  (3) Appropriate resources and support are available to the family to minimize the impact of the diagnosis of GDM and its management on the family.

HYPERTHYROIDISM

A. **Hyperthyroidism is caused by hyperfunctioning of thyroid gland, so that the thyroid gland produces excessive amounts of thyroid hormone.** An overactivity of hypothalamus, pituitary, or thyroid gland can cause hyperthryoidism (ACOG, 2002).

B. **Graves' disease (an autoimmune process) is the most common cause of hyperthryoidism during pregnancy.** It is typified by "production of thyroid stimulating immunoglobulin (TSI) and thyroid stimulating hormone binding inhibitory immunoglobulin (TBII) and acts on thyroid stimulating hormone (TSH) receptor to inhibit thyroid stimulation" (ACOG, 2002; p. 537).

C. **Diagnosis and management of thyroid disease in pregnancy is complicated by the normal physiologic changes of pregnancy that mimic hyperthyroidism and a hypermetabolic state.** Hyperdynamic symptoms are characteristic of both normal pregnancy and hyperthyroidism.
1. Increased metabolic rate
2. Increased protein-bound iodine values
3. Increased iodine uptake; plasma iodine decreases during pregnancy.
4. Increased thyroid binding globulin (TBG) due to reduced hepatic clearance and estrogen stimulation of TBG synthesis
5. Increased size of thyroid gland
6. Increased total thyroxine (TT_4) and total triiodothyronine (TT_3) (most significant thyroid hormones)

D. **Various metabolic and hormonal changes that occur in pregnancy affect the thyroid gland.**
1. Presence of placental estrogen alters thyroid function studies, such as the total thyroxine (T_4) and triiodothyronine resin uptake (T_3RU).
2. TSH testing is used for initial screening and evaluation of symptomatic cases in men and women.
3. Other metabolic changes can be seen in thyroid function tests during pregnancy (Table 24-3).

E. **Incidence of hyperthyroidism in pregnancy is approximately 0.2%.** In Grave's disease, there is an increase in levels of free thyroxine (FT_4) or free thyroxine index (FTI) (see Table 24-3). Other causes of hyperthyroidism include increased

---

■ TABLE 24-3
■ ■ **Changes in Thyroid Function Test Results in Normal Pregnancy and in Thyroid Disease**

Maternal Status	TSH	FT_4	FTI	TT_4	TT_3	RT_3U
Pregnancy	No change	No change	No change	Increase	Increase	Decrease
Hyperthyroidism	Decrease	Increase	Increase	Increase	Increase or no change	Increase
Hypothyroidism	Increase	Decrease	Decrease	Decrease	Decrease or no change	Decrease

From American College of Obstetricians and Gynecologists. (2002). Thyroid disease in pregnancy. *Practice Bulletin*, 387-396.
FT_4, Free thyroxine; *FTI*, free thyroxine index; RT_3U, resin T3 uptake; *TSH*, thyroid-stimulating hormone; TT_3, total tri-iodothyronine; TT_4, total thyroxine.

TSH, gestational trophoblastic neoplasia, hyperfunctioning thyroid adenoma, goiter, and subacute thyroiditis (ACOG, 2002).

F. **Fetal synthesis of thyroid hormones**
   1. Synthesis begins at 10 to 12 weeks and is controlled by pituitary TSH by 20 weeks' gestation.
   2. Fetal serum levels of TSH, TBG, FT_4, and FT_3 increase during pregnancy.

G. **Treatment of hyperthyroidism is complicated by the presence of the fetus.**
   1. Inadequate treatment is associated with risk for preterm deliveries, low birth weight, and fetal loss.
   2. The fetus might be jeopardized by surgery or antithyroid medications. If maternal drug treatment is not effective or if drug intolerance exists, partial thyroidectomy or total resection of the maternal thyroid gland might be indicated. If indicated, maternal surgery is usually recommended after the first trimester to decrease the risk of spontaneous abortion. Postoperative hypothyroidism is common, affecting at least 20% of women with hyperthyroidism.
   3. Patients with Grave's disease can have TSI or TBII that can stimulate or inhibit fetal thyroid, possibly resulting in either neonatal hypothyroidism or hyperthyroidism. Also, fetal thyrotoxicosis should be considered in maternal Grave's disease (ACOG, 2002).
   4. Hyperthyroidism in pregnancy is treated with thioamides. Drugs that inhibit synthesis of thyroid hormones such as propylthiouracil (PTU) or methimazole can be used to decrease thyroid synthesis (ACOG, 2002).
      a. The dosage of PTU is gradually tapered to the smallest effective dosage to prevent unnecessary fetal hypothyroidism.
      b. Maintain FT_4 or FTI in upper limits of normal range.
      c. PTU is usually well tolerated by the mothers, but infrequent side effects might occur.
         (1) Rash
         (2) Nausea
         (3) Pruritus
         (4) Hepatitis
         (5) Arthralgias
         (6) Vasculitis
         (7) Thrombocytopenia
         (8) Agranulocytosis
      d. Can breastfeed while taking PTU (ACOG, 2002).

H. **Associated with increased incidence of postpartum hemorrhage if poorly controlled.**

I. **When diagnosed during pregnancy, hyperthyroidism might be transient or permanent; spontaneous remissions might occur during pregnancy.**

J. **Thyroid storm is an extreme hypermetabolic state that has a high risk of maternal heart failure occurring in 1% of patients with hyperthyroidism during pregnancy.**
   1. Signs and symptoms include fever, extreme tachycardia, changes in mental status, nervousness, seizures, vomiting, and cardiac arrhythmia.
   2. If untreated, thyroid storm can result in shock, coma, or maternal heart failure.
   3. Pharmacologic treatment includes drugs that will suppress thyroid function.
      a. PTU
      b. Saturated solution of potassium iodide and sodium iodide
      c. Dexamethasone

    d. Propranolol (beta-blockers)

    e. Phenobarbital (for extreme restlessness)

  4. Supportive treatment would include:

    a. Oxygen

    b. Intravenous solutions

    c. Use of antipyretics

    d. Fetal monitoring

    e. Continuous maternal cardiac monitoring (ACOG, 2002)

K. Thyroid nodules in pregnancy should be investigated to rule out malignancy due to increased risk for malignancy during pregnancy.

CLINICAL PRACTICE

A. Assessment

  1. History

    a. Clinical symptoms

      (1) Weakness

      (2) Muscle tremors

      (3) Heat intolerance and sensitivity

      (4) Increased appetite

      (5) Failure to gain weight or actual weight loss

      (6) Fatigue

      (7) Insomnia

      (8) Frequent stools

      (9) Nervousness and hyperactivity

     (10) Excessive perspiration

     (11) Exophthalmos

     (12) Enlargement of the thyroid gland (goiter)

    b. Infertility

      (1) Anovulation and amenorrhea might occur if hyperthyroidism is not treated.

      (2) When treated, hyperthyroidism is not usually associated with infertility.

  2. Physical findings

    a. Maternal effects

      (1) Resting pulse greater than 100 beats/min

      (2) Proximal muscle wasting

      (3) Separation of the distal nail from the nailbed

      (4) Eye signs

        (a) Stare with exophthalmos

        (b) Lid lag

        (c) Lid retraction

        (d) Chemosis

      (5) Goiter: diffusely enlarged, soft gland

      (6) Soft skin with fine hair

      (7) Increased skin warmth

      (8) Development of thyroid storm or thyrotoxic crisis

        (a) Medical emergency that presents clinically with:

          (i) High fever

         (ii) Tachycardia

        (iii) Severe dehydration

        (iv) Profuse sweating

(v) Restlessness

(vi) Nausea and vomiting associated with abdominal pain

(vii) Possible pulmonary edema or congestive heart failure

(viii) Hypotension

(ix) Stupor

(b) Most commonly occurs in pregnant women when hyperthyroidism has not been detected or is poorly controlled.

(c) Precipitating factors include:

(i) Infection

(ii) Labor

(iii) Cesarean birth

(d) Requires prompt treatment with IV fluids, oxygen, and pharmacologic treatment.

(9) Increased incidence of preeclampsia if poorly controlled

(10) Side effects associated with antithyroid medications

b. Fetal and neonatal effects

(1) Increased incidence of preterm labor and delivery

(2) Increased risk of small-for-gestational-age (SGA) or low birth weight (LBW) infants

(3) Small increase in perinatal mortality

(4) Maternal use of antithyroid medication might impair fetal thyroid function and cause hypothyroidism, goiter, or mental deficiencies.

(5) If hyperthyroidism is untreated, rates of spontaneous abortion, intrauterine death, and stillbirth increase.

(6) Rare occurrence of fetal thyrotoxicosis in presence of maternal thyroid storm

(7) If untreated, iodine-deficient hypothyroidism increases risk of congenital cretinism.

3. Psychosocial considerations (see Pregestational Diabetes, Psychosocial Considerations)

4. Diagnostic procedures

a. Laboratory findings: elevated FTI, elevated FT_4, elevated TT_4, and decreased RT_3 U resin T_3 uptake (see Table 24-3)

b. Maintaining the fetus in an euthyroid state, especially in the last trimester, is recognized as essential for brain development; the FTI is a useful index of fetal thyroid status.

c. Neonates born to mothers with hyperthyroidism undergo serum thyroxine determinations at birth and are observed closely during the first 2 weeks of life for signs and symptoms of hyperthyroidism.

d. Most cases of neonatal hyperthyroidism are transient, lasting 3 to 12 weeks after birth and treated with propanolol (Lowdermilk & Perry, 2004)

B. **Nursing Diagnoses**

1. Anxiety related to maternal diagnosis, pregnancy, and its outcome

2. Altered metabolism related to excessive thyroid hormone

3. Deficient knowledge related to therapeutic regimen to optimize maternal and fetal outcomes in pregnancy complicated by hyperthyroidism

4. Risk for injury to fetus or neonate related to medical management with antithyroid drugs

C. **Interventions/Outcomes**

1. Anxiety related to maternal diagnosis, pregnancy, and its outcome

a. Interventions

(1) Assess maternal anxiety level, including behavioral and physiologic changes.

(2) Encourage maternal expression of feelings and concerns.

(3) Inform the client of all procedures and expectations, presenting accurate information and answering her questions.

(4) Encourage active participation in decision making about the therapeutic regimen.

b. Outcomes

(1) Behavioral and physiologic changes associated with maternal anxiety do not compromise the client's ability to participate in the therapeutic regimen prescribed during pregnancy.

(2) Client expresses feelings and concerns about pregnancy and its outcome.

(3) Client describes accurate information about procedures and expectations during pregnancy.

(4) Client actively participates in decision-making process concerning implementation of the therapeutic regimen.

2. Altered metabolism related to excessive thyroid hormone

a. Interventions

(1) Perform head to toe assessment.

(2) Monitor for cardiovascular signs and symptoms.

(a) Vital signs

(b) ECG

(c) Arterial blood gases

(d) Arterial oxygen saturation

(3) Assess for signs and symptoms of pulmonary edema.

(a) Dyspnea

(b) Rales

(c) Persistent cough

(d) Mechanical ventilation might be needed

(4) Assess for hyperthermia.

(a) If maternal fever increases, treat immediately.

b. Outcomes

(1) Cardiovascular/respiratory systems are stable.

(2) Maternal temperature remains normal.

(3) Reassuring fetal heart rate pattern is noted.

3. Deficient knowledge related to therapeutic regimen to optimize maternal and fetal outcomes in pregnancy complicated by hyperthyroidism

a. Interventions

(1) Assess understanding of effects of hyperthyroidism on pregnancy and fetal development, including possible fetal goiter and hypothyroidism.

(2) Discuss plan for frequent monitoring of FTI and TT_4 to ensure that lowest possible amount of antithyroid medication is administered for control of client's symptoms while minimizing fetal exposure to antithyroid medications.

(3) Perform clinical assessment to determine adequacy of maternal response to antithyroid medications.

(a) Pulse below 100

(b) Reflexes 2+ to 3+

(c) Loss of tremor

(d) Normal weight gain

(e) Normal fetal growth

(4) Review complications of antithyroid therapy.
  (a) Purpuric skin rash
  (b) Pruritus
  (c) Fever
  (d) Nausea
  (e) Rarely, agranulocytosis (usually after 1 to 2 months of therapy)
(5) Instruct the client to report fever, sore throat, or other symptoms of infection.
(6) Provide accurate information about all procedures, tests, and interventions planned during pregnancy and after birth of the infant.
(7) Inform the client of the results of laboratory tests and provide information about fetal status and well-being.
(8) Review dietary requirements in pregnancy to reinforce adequate nutritional intake and facilitate fetal growth and development. *Note:* increased metabolic state requires increased calories and protein intake.
(9) Instruct the client about the signs and symptoms of preterm labor.
(10) Review the signs and symptoms of hyperthyroidism, the use of self-monitoring diaries, and self-assessment records.
b. Outcomes
(1) Client verbalizes understanding of effects of hyperthyroidism on pregnancy and fetal development, including possible fetal goiter and hypothyroidism.
(2) Client verbalizes plan for frequent monitoring of total free T_4 levels to ensure lowest possible amount of antithyroid medication is administered for control of her symptoms while minimizing fetal exposure to antithyroid medications.
(3) Client demonstrates therapeutic response to antithyroid medications.
(4) Client states possible complications of antithyroid therapy, including skin rash, pruritus, fever, and nausea.
(5) Client reports fever, sore throat, or other symptoms of infection.
(6) Client receives accurate information about all procedures, tests, and interventions planned during pregnancy and after birth of infant.
(7) Client is informed of fetal status and well-being throughout pregnancy and at birth.
(8) Client reports adequate nutritional intake during pregnancy.
(9) Client verbalizes signs and symptoms of preterm labor.
(10) Client actively participates in monitoring and recording signs and symptoms of hyperthyroidism during pregnancy.
4. Risk for injury to fetus or neonate related to medical management with antithyroid drugs
  a. Interventions
  (1) Monitor fetal growth and development through ultrasound testing and fundal height measurement.
  (2) Fetal heart rate (FHR) monitored in utero as metabolic guide for the following:
    (a) Fetal hyperthyroidism (FHR above 160)
    (b) Fetal hypothyroidism (FHR below 120)
  (3) Assess maternal serum for FTI and TT_4 levels for possible adjustment of dosage for thiourias therapy.

(a) The lowest possible amount is used to control symptoms; the client is kept mildly hyperthyroid or within the high end of the normal range of pregnancy to minimize potential detrimental effects to the fetus.

(b) Keeping the fetus in euthyroid state, especially near term, is recognized as essential for brain and neurologic development.

(4) Assess client for signs and symptoms of preterm labor.

(5) Perform fetal movement counts to assess fetal well-being.

(6) Assess for fetal hydrops.

(7) Assess fetal heart rate for sinusoidal patterns or tachycardia.

b. Outcomes

(1) Fetal growth and development and FHR are within normal parameters.

(2) Maternal total free T_4 levels are maintained in the prescribed range to control symptoms (the client might be mildly hyperthyroid).

(3) Signs and symptoms of preterm labor are promptly reported and managed to minimize incidence of preterm birth.

(4) Fetal activity and movement indicate fetal well-being.

HYPOTHYROIDISM

A. Definition

1. This is a rare condition in pregnancy because women with hypothyroidism ovulate irregularly and frequently are infertile, and they experience menstrual dysfunction or amenorrhea.

2. Hypothyroidism is caused by inadequate thyroid hormone production.

3. Increased likelihood of having another autoimmune disease; 5% to 8% of patients with hypothyroidism have type 1 diabetes.

B. Etiology

1. Primary hypothyroidism is due to the following:

   a. Hashimoto's thyroiditis; production of antithyroid antibodies including thyroid antimicrosomal and antithyroglobulin antibodies (ACOG, 2002)

   b. Therapy with antithyroid drugs

   c. Iodine deficiency associated with goiters (most common cause of hypothyroidism worldwide)

   d. Destruction of the thyroid gland (by radiation or previous surgery)

2. Secondary hypothyroidism is from pituitary-hypothalamic disease.

C. Prognosis for the mother and fetus is favorable with successful hormone replacement.

1. Levothyroxine (Synthroid) is most often prescribed in pregnancy.

2. Dosage is gradually increased until normal levels of TSH and thyroxine are reached.

3. Thyroid hormones cross placenta in small amounts early in gestation. The fetus is dependent on maternal thyroid hormones until 12 weeks' gestation, when fetal production begins.

D. High fetal mortality and morbidity are characteristics of the hypothyroid state when replacement therapy is inadequate or not instituted during pregnancy.

E. Thyroidectomy for women who fail thioamide treatment can be performed during pregnancy.

F. Iodine[131] is contraindicated in pregnancy.

G. Avoid breastfeeding for at least 120 days after I[131] treatment.

CLINICAL PRACTICE

A. Assessment
   1. History
      a. Fatigue and malaise; lack of energy
      b. Cold intolerance
      c. Lethargy
      d. Headache
      e. Constipation
      f. Paresthesias
      g. Mental impairment
      h. Infertility, if thyroid function is significantly impaired
      i. Increased incidence of spontaneous abortion (risk doubled if maternal hypothyroidism is untreated), preeclampsia, anemia, abruptio placentae, postpartum hemorrhage, and stillbirth
   2. Physical findings
      a. Maternal effects
         (1) Dry, scaly skin
         (2) Thin, brittle nails
         (3) Alopecia or hair loss
         (4) Poor skin turgor
         (5) Delayed deep tendon reflexes (slow relaxation phase)
         (6) Carpal tunnel syndrome
         (7) Enlarged thyroid gland (goiter)
         (8) Can progress to increased weight gain, mental impairment, voice changes, and insomnia.
         (9) Thyroid nodules should be further evaluated for possible thyroid cancer as malignancy during pregnancy occurs in 40% of these nodules.
      b. Fetal and neonatal effects
         (1) If mother is treated, infants might be low birth weight, but usually without evidence of hypothyroidism.
         (2) If mother is untreated, fetal loss is 50%.
         (3) Increased risk of congenital goiter
         (4) Increased risk of true cretinism
         (5) Increased incidence of congenital anomalies (risk tripled if maternal hypothyroidism is untreated)
   3. Psychosocial considerations (see Pregestational Diabetes, Psychosocial Considerations)
   4. Diagnostic procedures
      a. Diagnosis is confirmed by the presence of low total T_4, free T_4, and T_3RU.
      b. TSH is above normal (see Table 24-3).
      c. Monitor levels of TSH or FT_4/FI during pregnancy for thyroid disease.
      d. Screen newborn for T_4 levels.

B. **Nursing Diagnoses**
   1. Anxiety related to maternal diagnosis, pregnancy, and its outcome
   2. Altered metabolism related to inadequate thyroid hormone production
   3. Deficient knowledge related to therapeutic regimen to optimize maternal and fetal outcomes in pregnancy complicated by hypothyroidism
   4. Risk for injury to fetus or neonate related to inadequate thyroid replacement therapy

C. Interventions/Outcomes
   1. Anxiety related to maternal diagnosis, pregnancy, and its outcome
      a. Interventions: see Hyperthyroidism, Nursing Diagnoses, Anxiety
      b. Outcomes: see Hyperthyroidism, Nursing Diagnoses, Anxiety
   2. Altered metabolism related to inadequate thyroid hormone production
      a. Interventions
         (1) Assess for temperature stabilization and regulation.
         (2) Assess for activity level due to decrease metabolic rate.
      b. Outcomes
         (1) Temperature is stable.
         (2) Maternal response to levothyroxine will be therapeutic.
         (3) Fetal heart rate is reassuring.
   3. Deficient knowledge related to therapeutic regimen to optimize maternal and fetal outcomes in pregnancy complicated by hypothyroidism
      a. Interventions
         (1) Assess the client's understanding of the effects of hypothyroidism on pregnancy and fetal development.
         (2) Provide accurate information about all procedures, tests, and interventions planned during pregnancy and after birth of the infant. *Note:* thyroid hormones administered endogenously or exogenously do not cross the placenta in significant amounts.
         (3) Inform the client of fetal status and well-being, including plans for monitoring the neonate's thyroid status to detect any abnormalities after birth.
         (4) Instruct the client in self-monitoring fetal activity via daily fetal movement counts.
      b. Outcomes
         (1) Client verbalizes an understanding of pregnancy and normal growth and development of the fetus.
         (2) Client receives accurate information about all procedures, tests, and interventions planned during pregnancy and after birth of the infant.
         (3) Client is informed of fetal and neonatal status and well-being throughout pregnancy and during and after birth.
         (4) Client participates in assessment of fetal well-being by performing daily fetal movement counts.
   4. Risk for injury to fetus or neonate related to inadequate thyroid replacement therapy
      a. Interventions
         (1) Monitor fetal growth and development by ultrasound screening.
         (2) Assess maternal serum total T_4 and T_3RU levels for possible adjustment of dosage to keep within the normal range during pregnancy and to minimize detrimental effects to fetus.
      b. Outcomes
         (1) Fetal growth and development are within normal parameters.
         (2) Maternal serum free T_4 levels are maintained in the prescribed range to ensure a euthyroid state throughout pregnancy.

ADRENAL DISORDERS

Hyperadrenocorticism (Cushing Syndrome)

A. General overview
   1. Many parameters of adrenal function are altered during pregnancy.

     2. Normal physiologic changes in pregnancy mimic adrenal disease.
       a. Abdominal striae
       b. Edema
       c. Increased pigmentation
       d. Decreased glucose tolerance
     3. Physiologic hypercortisolism occurs in normal pregnancy and is associated with the following:
       a. Progressive rise in circulating levels of adrenocorticotropic hormone (ACTH) (does not cross the placenta)
       b. Dexamethasone suppressibility
       c. Increased plasma cortisol levels by two to three times in pregnancy (can cross the placenta)

B. Definition
     1. Adrenal hyperfunction occurs most commonly as Cushing syndrome, a rare disorder of steroid overproduction, primarily corticotrophin, that occurs with pituitary or adrenal tumors or adenomas or with adrenal hyperplasia secondary to elevated ACTH secretion.
     2. Adrenal hyperfunction also occurs with exogenous steroid administration (women with this syndrome are generally infertile because of ovulatory failure; this condition is extremely rare in pregnancy).
     3. In most cases, Cushing syndrome is rare during pregnancy with just under 100 cases of Cushing syndrome during pregnancy; usually adenoma is the underlying cause (Molitch, 2000).

C. Etiology due to long-term overabundance of glucocorticoid
     1. Abnormality of pituitary gland-adenomas, producing excess amounts of ACTH, the hormone that stimulates adrenal glands to produce cortisol
     2. Adrenal hyperplasia
     3. Large doses of glucocorticoids given for asthma, rheumatoid arthrititis, or other chronic diseases

D. Diagnosis
     1. Radiographs to locate any tumors
     2. 24-hour urinary tests to measure corticosteroid hormones
     3. Computer tomography scan
     4. Magnetic resonance imaging
     5. Dexamethasone-suppression test
     6. Corticotropin-releasing hormone stimulation test

E. Effects on pregnancy: data are limited regarding maternal prognosis in pregnancy because most women with this condition are infertile.
     1. Maternal effects/complications
       1. Abnormal glucose tolerance test (GTT)
       2. Pulmonary edema
       3. Hypertension in most patients
       4. Myopathy
       5. Increased risk for postoperative wound infection or dehiscence
     2. Fetal and neonatal effects
       a. Increased incidence of spontaneous abortions
       b. Increased stillbirths and neonatal mortality
       d. Premature births (50%) (Molitch, 2000)
       e. Suppression of fetal/neonatal adrenals
       f. Patients with poorly controlled hyperplasia have increased production of androgens; fetus is at risk for adrenogenital syndrome.

CLINICAL PRACTICE

A. **Assessment**
   1. History
      a. Emotional lability
      b. Psychiatric disorders
      c. Glucose intolerance
      d. Excessive weight gain, primarily in face, neck, trunk, and abdomen
      e. Menstrual irregularities
      f. Infertility
   2. Physical findings
      a. Centripetal obesity with muscle wasting and proximal myopathy
      b. Acne
      c. Striae
      d. Hirsutism
      e. Moon face, facial rounding
      f. "Buffalo hump" (increased fat over the dorsal vertebrae)
      g. Hypertension
      h. Muscle loss and weakness
      i. Glucose intolerance; increased blood glucose in diabetes
   3. Psychosocial considerations
      a. Emotional lability, depression, panic attacks, and paranoia
      b. Insomnia
      c. Psychiatric disorders (see Pregestational Diabetes, Psychosocial Considerations)
   4. Fetal/neonatal effects
      a. Increased prematurity by 50%
      b. Increased abortions, stillbirths, and neonatal mortality
      c. Possible suppression of fetal adrenals
   5. Diagnostic procedures
      a. Plasma cortisol level is elevated.
      b. Dexamethasone suppression test result is abnormal.
      c. Ultrasonography might indicate adrenal tumors of the adrenal glands.

B. **Nursing Diagnoses**
   1. Anxiety related to maternal diagnosis, pregnancy, and its outcome
   2. Deficient knowledge related to therapeutic regimen to optimize maternal and fetal outcomes in pregnancy complicated by hyperadrenocorticism
   3. Risk for injury to fetus or neonate related to suppression of adrenal function and maternal hypertension

C. **Interventions/Outcomes**
   1. Anxiety related to maternal diagnosis, pregnancy, and its outcome
      a. Interventions: see Hyperthyroidism, Nursing Diagnoses, Anxiety
      b. Outcomes: see Hyperthyroidism, Nursing Diagnoses, Anxiety
   2. Deficient knowledge related to therapeutic regimen to optimize maternal and fetal outcomes in pregnancy complicated by hyperadrenocorticism
      a. Interventions
         (1) Assess client's understanding of effects of adrenal hyperfunction on pregnancy and fetal development.
         (2) Provide accurate information about all procedures, tests, and interventions planned during pregnancy and after birth of the infant.
         (3) Inform client of fetal status and well-being.

(4) Instruct client regarding the signs and symptoms of preterm labor and self-monitoring of fetal activity with daily fetal movement counts.
  b. Outcomes
    (1) Client verbalizes understanding of the effects on pregnancy and normal growth and development of the fetus.
    (2) Client receives accurate information about all procedures, tests, and interventions planned during pregnancy and after birth of the infant.
    (3) Client is informed of fetal status and well-being throughout pregnancy and at birth.
    (4) Client reports any signs or symptoms of preterm labor and any decrease or significant change in fetal movement patterns.
3. Risk for injury to fetus or neonate related to suppression of adrenal function and maternal hypertension
  a. Interventions
    (1) Monitor fetal growth and development.
    (2) Monitor signs and symptoms of preterm labor.
  b. Outcomes
    (1) Fetal growth and development are within normal parameters.
    (2) Preterm labor will be recognized early, and management will be instituted promptly to minimize incidence of preterm birth.

ADRENAL INSUFFICIENCY

A. Definition
1. Classified as either primary or secondary adrenal insufficiency; further classified as congenital or acquired.
2. Primary adrenal insufficiency occurs when the adrenal gland itself is dysfunctional and is uncommon in pregnancy. Secondary adrenal insufficiency is seen with pituitary lesions. There is lack of corticotrophin-releasing hormone (CRH) from hypothalamus or lack of ACTH secretion from pituitary.
3. Acquired occurs with autoimmune destruction of the adrenals usually caused by diseases such as tuberculosis, fungal diseases or, more rarely, metastatic cancer. Any severe sepsis might precipitate adrenal insufficiency. Congenital causes might include congenital adrenal hypoplasia or hyperplasia or defects in ACTH receptor.
4. Diagnosis is usually established before pregnancy, and the woman is on maintenance steroid replacement when conception occurs.
5. Long-term use of glucocorticoids might precipitate adrenal insufficiency due to chronic suppression of CRH-ACTH-adrenal axis.

B. Effects on pregnancy
1. Maternal effects
  a. Mild cases might go undetected during pregnancy, and client might go on to adrenal crisis with stress of labor or illness.
  b. Risk of adrenal crisis is increased in the postpartum period because of the inability to mount an adrenal response to the stress of delivery.
  c. Hyperkalemia, hyponatremia, and hypoglycemia
2. Fetal and neonatal effects
  a. Increased incidence of small for gestational age infants
  b. Depressed adrenal function related to maternal therapy with steroids
  c. IUGR

CLINICAL PRACTICE

A. **Assessment**
   1. History
      a. Weakness
      b. Fatigue
      c. Nausea and vomiting, diarrhea
      d. Anorexia
      e. Apathy
      f. Altered mental status
   2. Physical findings (*Note:* some of these signs and symptoms might occur in normal pregnancy; suspect adrenal insufficiency if the symptoms are unusually severe or persistent.)
      a. Weight loss
      b. Hypotension
      c. Hyperpigmentation
      d. Fever
      e. Fatigue and depression
      f. Salt craving with chronic primary adrenal insufficiency
      g. Acute dehydration
      h. Hypoglycemia
   3. Psychosocial considerations (see Pregestational Diabetes, Psychosocial Considerations)
   4. Diagnostic and therapeutic procedures
      a. For previous diagnosis, stabilize on glucocorticoids and increase for labor and delivery, surgery, or other severe stress.
      b. Diagnosis is confirmed by serum cortisol concentration less than 18 mcg/dl with increased serum ACTH and plasma renin activity, or a concentration lower than the level obtained 60 minutes following cosyntropin administration. Because plasma cortisol increases during gestation, this value might be in the normal, nonpregnant range and still represent a deficiency. Cosyntropin administration is controversial but might be specified. The standard CRH-stimulation test is reliable in diagnosis and differential diagnosis of adrenal insufficiency. If serum cortisol is low with elevated ACTH, antiadrenal antibodies can confirm an autoimmune cause for the disorder (Wilson, 2002).
      c. Laboratory studies
         (1) Electrolytes
         (2) Fasting blood sugar
         (3) Serum ACTH
         (4) Plasma renin activity
         (5) Serum cortisol
         (6) Serum aldosterone
      d. Imagining studies
         (1) Computed tomography scan
         (2) Abdominal radiographs
      e. Glucocorticoid replacement therapy recommended; use of mineralocorticoids might be suggested for replacement of aldosterone deficiency.
      f. Increase dose of steroids before delivery and 24-hour postpartum with patients on chronic therapy.

B. Nursing Diagnoses
1. Anxiety related to maternal diagnosis, pregnancy, and its outcome
2. Deficient knowledge related to therapeutic regimen to optimize maternal and fetal outcomes in pregnancy complicated by hypoadrenocorticism
3. Risk for injury to fetus or neonate related to maternal steroid replacement therapy

C. Interventions/Outcomes
1. Anxiety related to maternal diagnosis, pregnancy, and its outcome
   a. Interventions: see Hyperthyroidism, Nursing Diagnoses, Anxiety
   b. Outcomes: see Hyperthyroidism, Nursing Diagnoses, Anxiety
2. Deficient knowledge related to therapeutic regimen to optimize maternal and fetal outcomes in pregnancy complicated by hypoadrenocorticism
   a. Interventions
      (1) Assess understanding of effects of adrenal hypofunction on pregnancy and fetal development.
      (2) Provide explanations regarding possible needs for altering or increasing dosage of adrenocortical hormones during pregnancy.
         (a) Minor illnesses
         (b) Acute adrenal crisis
         (c) At time of delivery (either vaginal or cesarean birth)
         (d) In the postpartum period
      (3) Review signs and symptoms of acute adrenal crisis
         (a) Nausea and vomiting
         (b) Abdominal pain
         (c) Fever
         (d) Hypotension
         (e) Shock
      (4) Provide accurate information about all procedures, tests, and interventions planned during pregnancy and after birth of the infant.
      (5) Inform client of fetal status and well-being.
      (6) Review dietary requirements for adequate nutritional intake and to promote normal fetal growth and development during pregnancy.
   b. Outcomes
      (1) Client verbalizes understanding of risks associated with adrenal hypofunction to self and fetus.
      (2) Client states rationale and management plan for alterations in adrenocortical hormone therapy during pregnancy and childbirth.
      (3) Client verbalizes the signs and symptoms of acute adrenal crisis.
      (4) Client receives accurate information about all procedures, tests, and interventions planned during pregnancy and after birth of the infant.
      (5) Client is informed of fetal status and well being throughout pregnancy and at birth.
      (6) Client verbalizes adequate nutritional intake during pregnancy.
3. Risk for injury to fetus or neonate related to maternal steroid replacement therapy
   a. Interventions
      (1) Monitor fetal growth and development.
      (2) Assess adrenal function at birth.
   b. Outcomes
      (1) Fetal growth and development are within normal parameters.
      (2) Neonatal adrenal function is assessed at birth.

MATERNAL PHENYLKETONURIA

A. **Definition**

1. Phenylketonuria (PKU) (also known as hyperphenylalaninemia) is a rare metabolic disorder resulting from a deficiency of the liver enzyme phenylalanine (Phe) hydroxylase.

2. PKU is a genetic disease with an autosomal recessive genetic trait (defect). There is an inborn error of metabolism, in which the body's ability to efficiently metabolize Phe is impaired because of an enzyme hepatic deficiency (Phe hydroxylase).

3. Phenylalanine is an essential amino acid found in all protein foods; deficiency of Phe hydroxylase prevents metabolization of Phe and causes Phe to rise in blood stream. The enzyme deficiency keeps this essential amino acid from being synthesized and converted to tyrosine (Kirby, 1999).

4. In classic PKU, the absence of Phe hydroxylase results in the accumulation of Phe and its metabolites in the blood and urine, inhibiting normal brain development. Excessive levels of Phe lead to severe and irreversible mental retardation.

5. When untreated, children normal at birth become severely mentally retarded, exhibit a variety of behavioral disabilities, and are at increased risk for congenital heart disease and low birth weight (Kirby, 1999).

6. Clinical manifestations of PKU besides mental retardation might include irritability, vomiting, "musty odor," skin rashes, hyperactivity, schizoid like behavioral patterns, convulsions (Purnell, 2001).

7. Children with PKU commonly have blond hair, blue eyes, and fair skin.

B. **Incidence and screening**

1. Incidence of PKU is reported to be 1 in 10,000 to 15,000 live births in the United States (National Institutes of Health [NIH] Consensus Development Panel, 2001).

2. Approximately 300 to 400 infants with PKU are born each year in the United States.

3. Approximately 3000 women of childbearing age in the United States have been successfully treated for PKU.

4. Guthrie test is the most common and inexpensive screening test. A few drops of newborn blood is placed on filter paper. The test is considered positive when Phe rises above 120 μMoL/L.

C. **Management of classic PKU**

1. "Diet for life" approach: Phe levels >10 mg/dl should be treated before the neonate is 7 days old. Medical nutritional therapy for newborns with levels between 7 to 10 mg/dl. No consensus concerning optimal levels of blood Phe. Most common in the United States are 2 to 6 mg/dl for patients younger than 12 years of age and 2 to 10 mg/dl for those older than 12 years of age.

2. Infants can be breastfed: initially infants are placed on a Phe-restricted diet limiting infant formula and breast milk. The infant is fed a special milk preparation such as Lofenalac or Albumaid XP until Phe levels are at acceptable ranges. Then precalculated amounts of breast milk or formula can be added to diet while observing the Phe levels. Breast milk has lower levels of Phe than formulas, allowing for greater intake of breast milk and still remain in the therapeutic Phe range (Kirby, 1999; Purnell, 2001).

3. Monitor monthly or more frequently if needed.

4. Diet has been highly successful in preventing mental retardation.

D. Maternal PKU
1. Because women identified as newborns with PKU have been successfully treated with dietary management and have reached childbearing age, the emergence of maternal PKU has been recognized as another form of PKU.
2. Associated fetal and neonatal effects are caused when elevated maternal serum Phe levels cross the placenta and overwhelm the fetus' ability to metabolize Phe. *Note:* this occurs even in the presence of a normal genetic make-up in the fetus; however, there is also a higher incidence of hyperphenylalaninemic infants born to mothers with PKU. Placenta aids in maintaining higher levels of amnio acids (NIH Consensus Development Panel, 2001).
3. Maternal PKU prevents the normal expression of liver Phe hydroxylase during fetal development, creating phenotypic hyperphenylalaninemia.
4. Management of maternal PKU
   a. Key to successful management of maternal PKU is the institution of the specific low-Phe diet before conception. Patients are advised to continue to maintain a restricted Phe diet.
      (1) Ideally, the program of dietary therapy is coordinated in collaboration with a PKU clinic.
      (2) In the past, it was believed to be safe to discontinue the Phe diet after age 6; however, because of the effects of increased Phe on intellectual and neurologic function and effects on fetuses, the Phe diet is recommended throughout life.
      (3) The recommended low-Phe diet is highly restrictive, allowing only measured amounts of low protein cereals, fruits, vegetables, fats, and grains and requiring the consumption of a special formula that is unpalatable to many women. Dairy products, meats, nuts, and aspartame must be avoided, and prescribed supplements must be taken. Vitamin B_{12} and folic acid are recommended prior to conception (NIH Consensus Development Panel, 2001); Waisbren et al., 1995).
   b. Poor adherence to dietary restrictions and medical recommendations to stop the Phe diet continue to contribute to adverse effects on children born to mothers with PKU. Further, serious consequences to fetus exposed to elevated Phe can occur.
   c. Acceptable suggested range in the United States is 2 to 6 mg/dl; British and German standards are even lower (NIH Consensus Development Panel, 2001).
   d. Suggested frequency of monitoring by NIH Consensus Development Panel (2001):
      (1) Once a week during first year
      (2) Twice monthly ages 1 through 12
      (3) Monthly after age 12
      (4) Twice weekly during pregnancy
E. Effects on pregnancy
1. Maternal effects
   a. None specific to pregnancy
   b. Requirements of low-Phe diet and careful dietary management during pregnancy
2. Fetal and neonatal effects
   a. Women with classic PKU and other forms of PKU classified with Phe concentrations exceeding 20 mg/dl are at increased risk of having infants with:
      (1) Mental retardation or cognitive impairment
      (2) Intrauterine and postnatal growth restriction

(3) Low birth weight
(4) Microcephaly
(5) Congenital heart defects
(6) Other malformations
(7) Spontaneous abortions
   b. Fetal Phe levels are about 50% higher than maternal levels.
   c. Incidence of hyperphenylalaninemia among infants born to mothers with PKU is increased as a result of impaired expression of liver Phe hydroxylase during fetal development.
   d. Depending on the zygosity of the father for PKU, the infant either inherits the disease or is a carrier.

CLINICAL PRACTICE

A. Assessment
   1. History
      a. Identification of childhood PKU, ideally prior to conception
      b. Dietary assessment and counseling: a low-Phe diet is mandatory before conception and metabolic control is necessary across the life span.
   2. Physical findings: none is specific to maternal PKU, although serum Phe levels might be elevated if diet is not restricted.
   3. Psychosocial considerations
      a. Feelings regarding high-risk status of pregnancy due to maternal condition that might affect fetal growth and development
      b. Concerns about low-Phe diet and adhering to it during pregnancy
      c. Access to clinic or health care provider specializing in care and support of women with maternal PKU (see Pregestational Diabetes, Psychosocial Considerations)
   4. Diagnostic procedures
      a. Serum Phe levels are carefully monitored twice weekly during pregnancy.
      b. The goal of dietary management is to maintain levels between 2 to 6 mg/dl.
   5. Assess option to breastfeed. Breastfeeding was once discouraged for women with PKU. Breast milk contains 40 mg/dl of phenylalanine compared with infant formula of 85 mg/dl. Can pump and bottle-feed premeasured amounts and give with prescribed special formula, or can weigh infant before and after breastfeeding and supplement with Phe-free metabolic formula.

B. Nursing Diagnoses
   1. Risk for fetal injury related to dependence on maternal Phe levels
   2. Anxiety related to maternal diagnosis, pregnancy, and its outcome
   3. Deficient knowledge related to therapeutic regimen to minimize potential effects of PKU on developing fetus
   4. Imbalanced nutrition: less than body requirements related to low-Phe diet required before conception and during pregnancy

C. Interventions/Outcomes
   1. Risk for fetal injury related to dependence on maternal Phe levels.
      a. Interventions
         (1) Monitor fetal growth and development.
         (2) Assess maternal serum Phe levels.
            (a) The level recommended is 2 to 6 mg/dl.
            (b) Ideally, this level is achieved at least 3 months before conception.
         (3) Refer client for genetic counseling.

    (4) Encourage compliance with low-Phe diet.

    (5) Prenatal vitamins are not recommended.

    (6) Monitor plasma levels of tyrosine, and other amino acids, zinc, iron, selenium levels once a month.

  b. Outcomes

    (1) Fetal growth and development are within normal parameters.

    (2) Maternal serum Phe levels are maintained in the prescribed range throughout pregnancy.

    (3) Client receives information relevant to fetal outcome and genetic inheritance through genetic counseling.

    (4) Client adheres to low-Phe diet.

2. Anxiety related to maternal diagnosis, pregnancy, and its outcome

  a. Interventions: see Hyperthyroidism, Nursing Diagnoses, Anxiety

  b. Outcomes: see Hyperthyroidism, Nursing Diagnoses, Anxiety

3. Deficient knowledge related to therapeutic regimen to minimize potential effects of PKU on developing fetus

  a. Interventions

    (1) Assess understanding of low-Phe diet and food-exchange lists.

    (2) Refer for dietary counseling and adaptation of diet to ensure adequate dietary intake for pregnancy and normal growth and development of fetus.

    (3) Provide accurate information about all procedures, tests, and interventions planned during pregnancy and after birth of the infant.

    (4) Inform client of fetal status and well-being.

    (5) Assess and inform option to breastfeed.

  b. Outcomes

    (1) Client verbalizes understanding of low-Phe diet and food-exchange lists.

    (2) Client receives information about adequate dietary intake for pregnancy and normal growth and development of the fetus.

    (3) Client receives accurate information about all procedures, tests, and interventions planned during pregnancy and after birth of the infant.

    (4) Client is informed of fetal status and well being throughout pregnancy and at birth.

4. Imbalanced nutrition: less than body requirements related to low-Phe diet required before conception and during pregnancy

  a. Interventions

    (1) Assess understanding of low-Phe diet and food-exchange lists.

    (2) Refer client for dietary counseling and adaptation of diet to ensure adequate dietary intake for pregnancy and normal growth and development of fetus.

      (a) Diet combines low-protein foods (primarily fruits and vegetables) with special formulas containing all amino acids except Phe.

      (b) Prenatal vitamins should not be prescribed because all except folic acid are provided in special dietary formulas used to treat PKU.

      (c) Folic acid supplements should be provided separately.

    (3) Monitor client's ability to follow dietary requirements and reported intake.

    (4) Monitor maternal weight gain and fetal growth during pregnancy.

  b. Outcomes

    (1) Client verbalizes understanding of low-Phe diet and food-exchange lists.

(2) Client's dietary intake is adequate for pregnancy and normal growth and development of the fetus.

(3) Client verbalizes her ability to follow dietary requirements and reports actual dietary intake as prescribed.

(4) Client demonstrates adequate weight gain with appropriate fetal growth during pregnancy.

HEALTH EDUCATION
Pregestational Diabetes Mellitus
A. **Preconceptual**
1. Discussion of potential maternal and fetal risks associated with diabetes and pregnancy, effects of diabetes on pregnancy, and pregnancy on diabetes
2. Discussion of financial expenses and other demands related to the increased surveillance of maternal and fetal status during pregnancy
3. Discussion of rationale for interdisciplinary team approach and role of each team member in the management of diabetes and pregnancy
4. Discussion of rationale for optimal blood glucose control before conception to ensure optimal timing of conception and early diagnosis of pregnancy. *Note:* research has demonstrated that near-normal blood glucose levels at the time of conception and in the early weeks of gestation might significantly reduce the increased incidence of congenital anomalies associated with infants of mothers with diabetes (Kitzmiller, Combs, Buchanan, Ratner, & Kjos, 1996).
5. Review of self-care practices and self-monitoring expectations during pregnancy, including diet, intensification of insulin regimen, and multidisciplinary plan for medical and obstetric management

B. **Prenatal**
1. Reinforcement of multidisciplinary plan for medical and obstetric management during pregnancy
2. Ongoing assessment of blood glucose levels and adjustment of insulin requirements to ensure euglycemia
3. Minimization and prompt recognition of potential maternal and fetal complications associated with diabetes and pregnancy

C. **Postpartum**
1. A precipitous decrease in insulin requirements in the immediate postpartum period is related to delivery of placenta and cessation of contra-insulin hormones associated with pregnancy; usually persists for at least 72 hours after birth.
2. Breastfeeding is usually encouraged in women with diabetes.
   a. Improves glucose metabolism and promotes high-density lipoprotein (HDL) cholesterol.
   b. Might be associated with decreased insulin requirements (up to 27%).
   c. Necessitates increased calories and continued dietary modifications to ensure adequate nutrition during lactation and milk production.
   d. Might experience increased incidence of mastitis, sore nipples secondary to candidiasis, and hypoglycemic episodes. *Note:* maternal hypoglycemia is most likely to occur 1 hour after breastfeeding, and women with pre-existing diabetes should be encouraged to eat a small snack just before breastfeeding.
   e. Hypoglycemia decreases milk production and might lead to problems with establishing milk supply and maintaining lactation.

    f. Maternal hyperglycemia sweetens the breast milk and might result in infant hyperinsulinemia; therefore, lactating mothers with diabetes are encouraged to maintain normal blood glucose levels.

    g. Insulin secreted in breast milk is digested by the infant and does not affect the infant's blood glucose levels.

Gestational Diabetes—Postpartum

A. Breastfeeding should be encouraged in women with GDM because breastfeeding improves glucose utilization and promotes HDL cholesterol.

B. Women diagnosed with GDM should be closely observed postpartum to detect diabetes early in its course.

    1. Reclassification of maternal glycemic status should be performed at 6 weeks' postpartum (ADA, 2003). If glucose levels are normal, reassessment of glycemia should be undertaken every 3 years. Women with IFG or IGT should be tested annually for diabetes.

    2. Initially, evaluation should occur at the first 6-week postpartum visit with a 2-hour OGTT with a 75 g glucose load.

    3. The incidence of abnormal glucose tolerance at 6 to 8 weeks' postpartum in women with previous GDM varies between 20% and 65%, depending on the population.

    4. Criteria for the diagnosis of diabetes mellitus in the nonpregnant state (Table 24-4)

C. Preventive health measures emphasizing the importance of weight management through diet and regular exercise should be promoted. *Note:* women with GDM and their children are at increased risk for developing hypertension, obesity, and overt diabetes; weight reduction can reduce these risks.

D. The history of GDM confers a 60% to 70% chance of GDM in subsequent pregnancies.

E. Approximately 40% of women diagnosed with GDM develop overt diabetes within 20 years of index pregnancy; maintaining ideal body weight, eating a healthful diet, and regular exercise might decrease the likelihood of developing overt diabetes or delay its onset.

■ **TABLE 24-4**
■ ■ **Criteria for Diagnosis for Diabetes Mellitus**

Normal	IFG or IGT	Diabetes Mellitus
FPG < 110 mg/dl	FPG 110-125	FPG ≥ 126 mg/dl
75-g 2h OGTT	75-g 2h OGGT	75-g 2h OGTT
2hPG <140 mg/dl	2hPG 140-199	2hPG ≥ 200 mg/dl
		or
		Symptoms of DM and PG
		≥ 200 mg/dl (no regard to last meal)

From American Diabetes Association. (2003). Position statement: Gestational diabetes mellitus. *Diabetes Care, 26*(1), 103-105.
DM, Diabetes mellitus; *FPG,* fasting plasma glucose; *IFG,* impaired fasting glucose; *IGT,* impaired glucose tolerance.

Hyperthyroidism

A. Preconceptual
1. Assessment of adequacy of antithyroid medications with baseline laboratory values
2. Discussion of potential maternal and fetal complications associated with hyperthyroidism in pregnancy, including thyroid storm

B. Prenatal
1. Careful history-taking and physical assessment of the client's symptoms at each prenatal visit
2. Treatment with antithyroid drugs in pregnancy and close monitoring to determine minimal dosage required to control symptoms
3. Discussion of information regarding fetal status and potential maternal and fetal complications associated with hyperthyroidism in pregnancy
4. Explanation and discussion of the presence of congenital goiter or signs of airway obstruction necessitating intubations at birth; evaluation of thyroid function of the newborn
5. Nutritional counseling to meet additional calorie requirements

C. Postpartum
1. Clients taking antithyroid medications such as PTU may breastfeed if the infant's thyroid status is closely monitored (every 2 to 4 weeks).
2. Infants exposed to small amounts of antithyroid medications do not usually become hypothyroid.

Hypothyroidism

A. Preconceptual
1. Assessment of adequacy of thyroid replacement as indicated by the free T_4 index (plasma free T_4 index) and achievement of clinical and biochemical euthyroidism
2. Assessment of fertility and ovulation
3. Discussion of potential maternal and neonatal complications associated with hypothyroidism in pregnancy; with adequate hormonal replacement, outcomes for the mother and fetus are improved.

B. Prenatal
1. Careful history-taking and physical assessment of the client's symptoms at each prenatal visit
2. Treatment should begin as soon as possible with thyroid replacement medication.
   a. During pregnancy, thyroid replacement must be adequate for maternal needs and for adequate fetal growth and development.
   b. The plasma-free T_4 index is used to monitor the adequacy of replacement therapy during pregnancy.
   c. Placental transfer of thyroid hormone replacement is negligible.
   d. Long-term T_4 replacement therapy during pregnancy usually continues at the same dosage prescribed before pregnancy.
3. Information about fetal status and potential maternal and fetal complications associated with hypothyroidism in pregnancy should be discussed.
4. Tests and procedures indicated during pregnancy and used for assessment of the neonate at birth should be explained and discussed with the client.
   a. Monitoring the plasma T_4 index
   b. Adjusting dosage of thyroid medication

C. Postpartum

1. Long-term T_4 replacement therapy after birth is usually resumed at the same dosage prescribed before pregnancy.
2. Results of tests and procedures performed to assess the neonate should be discussed with the client.

Hyperadrenocorticism (Cushing Syndrome)

A. Preconceptual

1. Assessment of fertility and ovulation
2. Discussion of potential maternal and neonatal complications associated with adrenal hyperfunction in pregnancy

B. Prenatal

1. Careful history-taking and physical assessment of the client's symptoms at each prenatal visit
2. Endocrine consultation to determine the cause of syndrome
3. Information regarding fetal status and potential maternal and fetal complications associated with adrenal hyperfunction in pregnancy, including increased risk of preterm labor and stillbirth

Hypoadrenocorticism (Addison's Disease)

A. Preconceptual

1. Assessment of adequacy of adrenocortical hormone replacement as indicated by serum cortisol levels
2. Assessment of fertility and ovulation
3. Discussion of potential maternal and neonatal complications associated with adrenal hypofunction in pregnancy; with adequate steroid replacement, outcomes for the mother and neonate are improved.

B. Prenatal

1. Careful history-taking and physical assessment of the client's symptoms at each prenatal visit are important in the diagnosis of adrenal hypofunction (Addison's disease).
2. Treatment with steroid replacement should begin as soon as possible.
3. Information regarding potential maternal and neonatal complications associated with adrenal hypofunction in pregnancy should be discussed, as well as alterations in dosage of prescribed adrenocortical hormones to minimize potential complications of acute adrenal crisis and to provide adequate glucocorticoid coverage during birth and in the postpartum period.

Maternal Phenylketonuria

A. Preconceptual

1. Counseling regarding the potential risks associated with maternal PKU, including the genetic assessment of risk to potential children of the inheritance of PKU and the effects of elevated Phe levels on fetal development
2. Discussion of information regarding the potential dangers to the developing fetus from untreated maternal PKU as well as the fetal protection offered by dietary treatment beginning before conception and maintained throughout pregnancy
3. Counseling regarding the need for family planning so that a low-Phe diet can be initiated prior to conception. *Note:* it is particularly important that this

information is also presented to adolescents with childhood PKU so that unintentional pregnancy might be prevented and appropriate dietary requirements can be instituted prior to conception.

4. Discussion of the importance of early identification of pregnancy and information regarding the specific dietary treatment and therapeutic regimen prescribed before conception and during pregnancy
5. Ideally, preconceptual referral to a PKU clinic for genetic counseling, biochemical analysis, nutritional formulas, and support for comprehensive and multidisciplinary management of maternal PKU

B. **Prenatal**
1. Counseling regarding the importance of maintaining a prescribed low-Phe diet to optimize pregnancy and neonatal outcomes
2. Ongoing explanations and education regarding rationale for prescribed tests and procedures to assess fetal growth and well-being

C. **Postpartum**
1. Assessment and screening of neonate to evaluate PKU status
2. Institution of low-Phe diet for neonate with PKU (usually recommended to be initiated before 3 weeks of age)
3. May breastfeed along with low-Phe diet.
4. Counseling regarding the need for family planning to prevent unintended pregnancy and to encourage return to low-Phe diet before conception; many centers specializing in the care of persons with PKU recommend indefinite continuation of the PKU diet for women with PKU throughout their childbearing years and lifetime.

CASE STUDY AND STUDY QUESTIONS

Ms. G is a 28-year-old, gravida 1, para 0 (G1, P0) woman with preexisting diabetes of 18 years' duration. She is hospitalized at 9 weeks' gestation to evaluate her blood glucose levels and to assess the adequacy of her current diabetes regimen. She describes this pregnancy as unplanned, but states she is very excited and wants to "get my blood sugars in a normal range again as soon as possible." Ms. G is currently taking regular and neutral protamine Hagedorn (NPH) insulin before breakfast and before her evening meal. She self-monitors her blood glucose levels two or three times a day. She reports two nighttime episodes of hypoglycemia during the past week. She states that she has had laser treatments in both eyes for proliferative retinopathy and was hospitalized 10 years ago for management of diabetic ketoacidosis.

1. The nurse assesses Ms. G's anxiety about the possible effects of

diabetes on pregnancy and tells her that the most important factor in achieving a successful pregnancy with minimal complications is which of the following?
   a. The number of years that she has had diabetes and the age at which she was diagnosed
   b. The absence of vascular complications
   c. Maintenance of near-normal blood glucose levels throughout pregnancy
   d. Frequency of self-monitoring of blood glucose levels

2. According to the information initially obtained by the nurse, how is Ms. G classified using White's classification of diabetes in pregnancy?
   a. Class C diabetes
   b. Class D diabetes
   c. Class F diabetes
   d. Class R diabetes

3. The nurse prepares Ms. G for the laboratory work, clinical assessments, and consults that will be obtained during her care. These additional tests and referrals will include all of the following except:
   a. Biophysical profile
   b. Dietary counseling
   c. Urinalysis and urine culture
   d. Glycosylated hemoglobin (Hgb A1c)

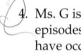

4. Ms. G is concerned about the episodes of hypoglycemia that have occurred at night during the previous week. The nurse explains that this commonly occurs early in pregnancy for what reason?
   a. The fetus produces insulin that crosses the placenta and decreases maternal insulin requirements.
   b. The fetus is constantly using maternal glucose for its growth and development.
   c. The placenta produces hormones that decrease maternal insulin requirements during pregnancy.
   d. The metabolic changes associated with pregnancy predispose women with preexisting diabetes to experience decreased needs for insulin during pregnancy.

5. Strategies that Ms. G and the nurse discuss during Ms. G's hospitalization to normalize blood glucose levels include all of the following except:
   a. Increasing the frequency of self-monitoring of blood glucose levels to at least six times daily, before and after meals and at bedtime.
   b. Adding additional protein for her bedtime snack to decrease the likelihood of nocturnal hypoglycemia.
   c. Reviewing the plan for adjusting insulin dosages based on blood

glucose levels and changing insulin requirements throughout pregnancy.
   d. Decreasing exercise and physical activity to minimize energy expenditures that alter insulin requirements.

6. Risk factors associated with gestational diabetes include all of the following except:
   a. Previous history of a low birth weight infant
   b. Family history of diabetes
   c. Obesity
   d. Maternal age older than 35 years

7. Infants born to women with gestational diabetes are at increased risk for which of the following?
   a. Fetal macrosomia
   b. Neonatal hyperglycemia
   c. Neonatal seizures
   d. Congenital anomalies

8. Ms. W presents to labor and delivery at 36 weeks' gestation with the possible diagnosis of thyroid storm. Which of the following signs and symptoms are characteristic of thyroid storm?
   a. Fatigue, sudden weight loss, heat intolerance, extreme weakness
   b. Low blood pressure, bradycardia, lethargy, generalized interstitial edema
   c. Blurred vision, hypertension, epigastric pain, severe headache
   d. High fever, tachycardia, dehydration, profuse sweating, restlessness

9. Ms. O was diagnosed with Addison's disease 3 years ago. Since that time, she has been managed with prednisone for maintenance steroid replacement. She is admitted to labor and delivery at 40 weeks' gestation and is in labor. In addition to monitoring Ms. O's progress in

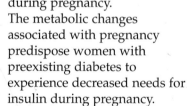

labor and fetal status, what following clinical signs and symptoms should be closely monitored during labor, during delivery, and in the immediate postpartum period?

a. Nausea and vomiting, abdominal pain, fever, hypotension, shock

b. Hyperventilation, dehydration, odor of acetone on breath, impaired mental status

c. High fever, tachycardia, dehydration, congestive heart failure

d. Hypertension, central nervous system irritability, edema, proteinuria

10. Why is the institution of a low-Phe diet indicated before conception and during pregnancy in a woman with PKU?

a. To prevent the inheritance of this disease by the developing fetus.

b. To minimize the incidence of mental retardation, microcephaly, congenital heart defects, and growth restriction in the developing fetus.

c. To promote the fetus' ability to metabolize Phe in utero.

d. To prevent the expression of liver Phe hydroxylase during fetal development.

ANSWERS TO STUDY QUESTIONS

1. c	4. b	7. a	10. b
2. d	5. d	8. d	
3. a	6. a	9. a	

REFERENCES

American College of Obstetricians and Gynecologists: ACOG Practice Bulletin. (2001). *Gestational Diabetes, 30,* 525-538.

American College of Obstetricians and Gynecologists: ACOG Practice Bulletin. (2002). *Thyroid disease in pregnancy,* 387-396.

American Diabetes Association. (1995). *Medical management of pregnancy complicated by diabetes* (2nd ed.; pp. 47-56.)

American Diabetes Association (ADA). (2003). Position statement: Gestational diabetes mellitus. *Diabetes Care, 26*(1), 15, 103-105.

Bailey, B.K., & Cardwell, M.S. (1996). A team approach to managing preexisting diabetes complicated by pregnancy. *The Diabetes Educator, 22*(2), 111-115.

Behrman, R. (Ed). 1995. *Nelson textbook of pediatrics* (15th ed.). Philadelphia: Saunders.

Cefalo, R., & Moos, M. (1994). *Preconceptual health care—A practical guide.* St. Louis: Mosby.

Coustan, D.R. (1993). Methods of screening for and diagnosing of gestational diabetes. *Clinics in Perinatology, 20*(3), 593-602.

Diabetes Control and Complications Trial (DCCT) Research Group. (1993). The effect of intensive treatment of diabetes on the development and progression of long-term complications in insulin-dependent diabetes mellitus. *New England Journal of Medicine, 329*(14), 977-986.

Kirby, R. (1999). Maternal phenylketonuria: A new cause for concern. *Journal of Obstetric, Gynecologic, and Neonatal Nursing, 28*(3), 227-234.

Kitzmiller, J.L., Combs, C.A., Buchanan, T.A., Ratner, R.E., & Kjos, S. (1996). Preconception care of diabetes, congenital malformations, and spontaneous abortions. *Diabetes Care, 19*(5), 514-541.

Landon, M. B., & Gabbe, S.G. (1993). Fetal surveillance in the pregnancy complicated by diabetes mellitus. *Clinics in Perinatology, 20*(3), 549-560.

Langer, O., Brustman, L., Anyaegbunam, A., & Mazze, R. (1987). The significance of one abnormal glucose tolerance test value on adverse outcome in pregnancy. *American Journal of Obstetrics and Gynecology, 157*(3), 758-763.

Langer, O. (1993). Management of gestational diabetes. *Clinics in Perinatology, 20*(3), 603-617.

Lowdermilk, D.L., & Perry, S.E. (2004). *Maternity & women's health care* (8th ed.). St. Louis: Mosby.

Mandeville, L., & Trioiano, N. (1999). *High risk and critical care intrapartum nursing.* Philadelphia: Lippincott Williams & Wilkins.

Metzger, B.E., & Coustan, D.R. (1998). Proceedings of the Fourth International workshop conference on gestational diabetes mellitus. *Diabetes Care, 21* (Suppl 2), B1-B167.

Molitch, M. (2000). Pituitary, thyroid, adrenal, and parathyroid disorders. In Barron W., & Lindheimer, M. (Eds.), *Medical disorders during pregnancy* (pp. 101-146). Philadelphia: Mosby.

National Institutes of Health (NIH) Consensus Development Panel (2001). Phenylketonuria screening and management. *Pediatrics, 108(4),* 972-982.

Purnell, H. (2001). Phenylketonuria and maternal phenylketonuria. *Breastfeeding Review, 9*(2), 19-21.

Tyrala, E. (1996). The infant of the diabetic mother. *Obstetrics and Gynecology Clinics of North America, 23*(1), 221-242.

Waisbren, S.E., Hamilton, B.D., St. James, P.J., Shiloh, C.L., & Levy, H.L. (1995). Psychosocial factors in maternal phenylketonuria: Women's adherence to medical recommendations. *American Journal of Public Health, 85*(12), 1636-1641.

Wilson, T. (2002). *Adrenal insufficiency.* Available online at *www.emedicine.com/PED/topic47.htm.*

York, R., Brown, L.P., Miovech, S., & Armstrong, C.L. (1995). Pregnant women with diabetes: Antepartum and postpartum morbidity. *The Diabetes Educator, 21*(3), 211-213.

25 Trauma in Pregnancy

STARRE HANEY

OBJECTIVES

1. State the normal physiologic changes that potentially affect the evaluation of a pregnant trauma patient.
2. Identify the major mechanisms of injury that affect the pregnant trauma patient.
3. Describe the components of the primary and secondary survey for a pregnant trauma patient.
4. List interventions to prevent maternal and fetal mortality resulting from trauma.
5. Develop a plan of care for a pregnant patient experiencing blunt or penetrating trauma.
6. Demonstrate knowledge of the physiologic changes of pregnancy and the specific mechanisms of injury in the assessment, diagnosis, planning, intervention, and evaluation of a pregnant trauma patient and her fetus.
7. Interpret physiologic assessment and diagnostic findings to establish priorities for the care of the pregnant trauma patient and her fetus.
8. Identify health promotion needs, and promote behavioral changes that produce healthy outcomes of pregnancy.

INTRODUCTION

A. Incidence and epidemiology
   1. Trauma is the fourth leading cause of death worldwide and the leading cause of maternal death during pregnancy.
      a. In the United States, 6% to 7% of all pregnant women experience some sort of trauma, with the greatest frequency in the last trimester (Chang, 2001).
      b. Trauma is more likely to cause maternal death than any other medical complication of pregnancy (Newton, 2002).
      c. The most common cause of maternal death by trauma is serious abdominal injury (Shah et al., 1998) leading to hemorrhagic shock and head injury (Rita & Reed, 2003).
      d. Shah and colleagues (1998) found that the most common cause of fetal death is maternal death, high maternal injury severity score (ISS), maternal abdominal injury, and maternal hemorrhagic shock, and in the study by Ali, Yeo, Gana, and McLellan (1997), ISS, blood transfusion, incidence of disseminated intravascular coagulation (DIC), and length of stay were significant among causes of fetal mortality.
   2. Injury to the pregnant patient can result from forces causing blunt or penetrating trauma (Emergency Nurses Association, 2000c).
      a. Blunt trauma is the most frequent cause of maternal and fetal injury (Emergency Nurses Association, 2000c).
      b. The most common causes of blunt trauma are motor-vehicle collisions, falls, and assaults.
         (1) Blunt trauma might result from force applied to the abdomen from direct impact or as a result of secondary injury from abdominal organ

            displacement and hemorrhage from a coup-contre-coup event (Rita & Reed, 2003).

            (2) Rapid compression, deceleration, or shearing forces can also result in abruptio placentae (American College of Surgeons, 1997).

            (3) Blunt abdominal trauma can lead to retroperitoneal bleeding as well as abruption or premature onset of labor (Colburn, 1999).

      c. Penetrating trauma occurs most frequently from gunshot or stab wounds with gunshot wounds being more common.

      d. Fetal injury is more common during the third trimester when the head is relatively fixed in the pelvis and less amniotic fluid is present to buffer energy transfer (Emergency Nurses Association, 2000b, 2000c).

      e. The incidence of intentional injury from domestic violence rises during pregnancy (Emergency Nurses Association, 2000c).

            (1) Women who claim fall injuries but whose patterns of injuries do not correlate might have been abused.

            (2) Screening for abuse assessment should be done privately.

B. Important concepts for trauma in pregnancy

    1. The initial goal in trauma evaluation is maternal stabilization.

      a. Resuscitation during pregnancy proceeds as in any other trauma patient.

      b. The primary assessment includes the ABCs: airway, breathing, circulation, and cervical spinal precautions, as well any emergent interventions needed to support the ABCs.

      c. The secondary assessment includes a full set of vital signs (including fetal heart rate [FHR]), brief head-to-toe examination (maternal and fetal), and important historical data; further injury-focused assessments are completed once all of the injuries are identified.

    2. Trauma in pregnancy involves two patients: mother and fetus.

      a. Minor injuries to the mother might cause significant or fatal injury to the fetus.

      b. Maternal outcome in trauma corresponds to the injury, whereas fetal outcome depends on the injury and the maternal physiologic response.

      c. Early recognition of pregnancy assists in identification of pregnancy-related changes that might alter assessment findings and mask signs of shock (Smith, 2002).

    3. Proper seat belt usage prevents ejection during motor-vehicle collisions; ejection from vehicles frequently results in head trauma with high maternal and fetal death rates.

    4. Risk factors predictive of fetal death include ejection, motorcycle and pedestrian collisions, maternal death, maternal tachycardia, abnormal fetal heart rate, lack of restraints, and injury severity score > 9 (Curet, Schermer, Demarest, Bieneik, & Curet, 2000).

    5. Frequently, trauma cases involve litigation; accurate, well-documented records protect both patients and the health care system.

C. Important physiologic considerations for trauma in pregnancy (altered physiologic state of the pregnant patient alters the patients' response to trauma) (Baerga-Varela, Zietlow, Bannon, Harmsen, & Ilstrup, 2000).

    1. Cardiovascular changes

      a. Blood volume increases 50%; and of this plasma volume increases 30% to 40% and red blood cell volume only increases 10% to 30%, leading to a physiologic anemia in pregnancy (Henderson & Mallon, 1998; Moise & Belfort, 1997).

(1) By the third trimester, maternal cardiac output peaks at 50% above non-regnant values and is indicated by an increase in baseline normal heart rates of 10 to 15 bpm.

(2) Blood pressure change also occurs with a 2 to 4 mmHg drop in the systolic reading and 5 to 15 mmHg drop in the diastolic reading (Neufeld, 1998).

(3) Uterine blood flow increases from a baseline of 60 ml/min to 600 ml/min during the third trimester (Rita & Reed, 2003); maternal perfusion pressure is needed to maintain uterine blood flow.

b. Pregnant women in shock might not have cool, clammy skin typical of shock because of maternal vasodilation in the first and second trimester (Rita & Reed, 2003).

(1) The physiologic changes in pregnancy might delay the usual vital sign changes of hypovolemia; blood loss of up to 1500 ml can occur without change in maternal vital signs.

(2) A 15% to 30% reduction of uterine blood flow can occur without change in maternal blood pressure; fetal compromise can occur before there are any changes in maternal vital signs.

c. Compression of the inferior vena cava, from the fetus, when the mother is in a supine position (after 20 weeks' gestation) can result in a systolic blood pressure drop of up to 30 mmHg and a 28% cardiac output decrease (Rita & Reed, 2003); therefore, by displacing the uterus to the left when a supine position or spinal immobilization is required, the compression can be relieved (Figure 25-1).

d. Because the fetal heart rate is often the first vital sign to change, all pregnant trauma patients need continuous fetal heart rate monitoring.

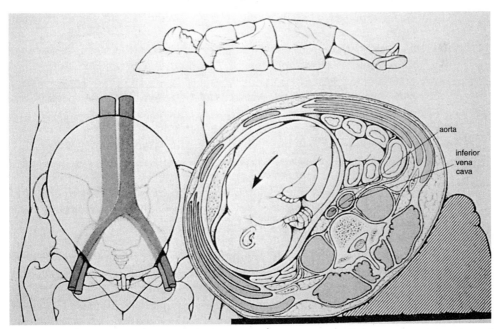

aorta

inferior
vena
cava

FIGURE 25-1 ■ Left lateral positioning displaces the uterus and decreases compression of major abdominal vessels. (From McQuillan, K.A., Von Rueden, K.T., Hartsock, R.L., Flynn, M.B., & Whalen, E. [2002]. *Trauma nursing: From resuscitation through rehabilitation* [3rd ed.]. Philadelphia: Saunders.)

2. Respiratory changes affect both maternal and fetal outcome when trauma occurs.
   a. Hormonal and mechanical (enlarging uterus) changes combine to produce hyperventilation (Newton, 2002).
      (1) The elevation of the diaphragm by the gravid uterus results in a 20% decrease in functional residual capacity (FRC); increased maternal oxygen consumption, and diminished oxygen reserves occur, increasing susceptibility to hypoxia (Rita & Reed, 2003).
      (2) Minute ventilation and tidal volume are increased 50% and 40%, respectively (Newton, 2002), and respiratory rate will increase, leading to a predisposition to rapid hypoxemia with apnea (Foley, 2003).
   b. PaO_2 is normal or slightly increased, but the $PaCO_2$ decreases to 30 to 32 mmHg; a compensated respiratory alkalosis occurs with the pH remaining in the normal range due to increased excretion of bicarbonate by the kidneys (Moise & Belfort, 1997).
      (1) The pregnant patient does not tolerate changes in $PaCO_2$; even a 5-minute episode of hyperventilation that drops the maternal $PaCO_2$ by 6 mm can drop the fetal $PaCO_2$ by 4 mm and the fetal PaO_2 by 3.5 mmHg (Newton, 2002).
      (2) Anxiety and pain can cause respiratory rate increases that result in hypocapnia and can lead to faintness and perioral numbness.
   c. Maternal hypoxia (diminished oxygen reserve) affects fetal oxygenation; therefore, fetal heart rate changes might indicate maternal hypoxia; arterial blood gas measurement is the best indicator of maternal status (Rita & Reed, 2003).
3. Gastrointestinal changes occur during pregnancy.
   a. The small bowel is pushed up by the uterus, and the large bowel moves posteriorly; penetrating trauma might injure multiple loops of bowel (Henderson & Mallon, 1998).
      (1) Diminished bowel sounds might be normal or indicate intraperitoneal injury (Rita & Reed, 2003).
      (2) Chronic distention of the parietal peritoneum by the uterus reduces the symptoms of intraperitoneal bleeding, such as rigidity and guarding (Moise & Belfort, 1997).
   b. Progesterone causes smooth muscle relaxation, and lower esophageal sphincter tone is decreased (Newton, 2002), increasing the need for a nasal gastric tube in the trauma patient.
   c. The enlarged uterus is vulnerable to injury but can protect the maternal abdominal organs (spleen, liver, kidneys, bowel).
4. The genitourinary system changes in pregnancy increase the risk of injury.
   a. The bladder moves from the pelvis area to the abdominal area by 12 weeks' gestation, increasing the risk of traumatic injury (Colburn, 1999; Rita & Reed, 2003). Figure 25-2 shows uterine size and location, reflecting gestational age.
   b. Renal blood flow increases in pregnancy, the serum creatinine and blood urea nitrogen values are lower, and hydronephrosis is common due to the smooth muscle relaxing properties of progesterone.
5. The hematologic changes that occur in pregnancy put the pregnant trauma patient at risk for disseminated intravascular coagulopathy.
   a. Platelet levels might be normal or slightly lower.
   b. Fibrinogen levels are doubled by the third trimester.
   c. There is an increase in clotting factors VII, VIII, IX, and X resulting in hypercoagulopathy and increased thromboembolic risk (Emergency Nurses Association, 2000c; Rita & Reed, 2003).

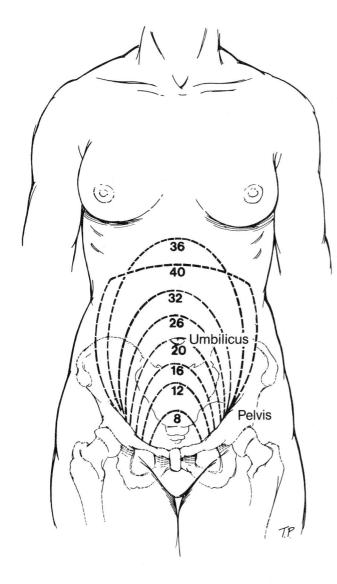

FIGURE 25-2 ■ Uterine size and location, reflecting gestational age. (From McQuillan, K.A., Von Rueden, K.T., Hartsock, R.L., Flynn, M.B., & Whalen, E. [2002]. *Trauma nursing: From resuscitation through rehabilitation* [3rd ed.]. Philadelphia: Saunders.)

6. The pelvis becomes more flexible during pregnancy, and a widening occurs,
   a. An unsteady gait caused by the widening pelvis and increased abdomen might predispose the pregnant patient to falls (Rita & Reed, 2003).
   b. A widened symphysis pubis by the third trimester decreases the risk for pelvic fractures (Emergency Nurses Association, 2000c).
D. **Types of trauma injuries**
   1. Maternal injuries
      a. Head injuries
      b. Chest injuries
      c. Abdominal and pelvic injuries
      d. Spinal trauma
      e. Burns and inhalation injuries
      f. Fracture/sprain/dislocation
      g. Soft tissue injuries
   2. Fetal injuries
      a. Skull fractures
      b. Other direct fetal injury
      c. Fetal death

E. Cause or mechanism of injury

1. Motor-vehicle crashes (MVCs)
   a. MVCs account for most traumas and are the leading cause of more serious maternal injury (66%-67%) (Chang, 2001; Pak, Reece, & Chan, 1998).
   b. Lack of seat belt use contributes to increased morbidity and mortality (Shah et al., 1998) by increasing the number of patients who have been ejected from the vehicle as well as the number receiving blunt head and abdominal trauma.
   c. Head and blunt abdominal injuries are the most common causes of maternal death.
   d. Maternal death is the most common cause of fetal death.
   e. MVCs are the most frequent cause of blunt injury, which can result in abruptio placentae, uterine rupture, and preterm labor.
   f. Pelvic fracture occurs most often with an MVC and can cause massive bleeding as well as fetal skull fracture.

2. Falls
   a. Falls are the second most common cause of blunt trauma in pregnancy (26%) (ACEP News: Annals of Emergency Medicine, 1999).
   b. Head and spinal cord injuries, and fractures of the pelvis and lower extremities are common as the pregnant women is likely to fall on her buttock or side (Smith, 2002).
   c. Observation for abruptio placentae is important.
   d. Details of the fall, such as the height of the fall and landing surface material, can be important factors to consider when assessing for injuries.

3. Assaults
   a. Assaults are rapidly edging out falls as the second leading cause of injury to pregnant women, especially in urban areas; assaults cause blunt and penetrating injuries.
   b. Assaults might cause death, direct maternal or fetal injury, preterm labor, and abruptio placentae.
   c. Domestic violence occurs often (22.3%) (Connolly, Katz, Bash, McMahon, & Hansen, 1997); domestic violence is rarely an isolated event and often escalates in pregnancy (see Chapter 20 for a complete discussion of domestic violence in pregnancy); any nonvehicular trauma in pregnancy warrants domestic violence screening (Henderson & Mallon, 1998).
   d. Younger pregnant women (ages 15 to 24) are more likely to be hospitalized for assault than older pregnant women (ACEP News: Annals of Emergency Medicine, 1999).

4. Burns/inhalation
   a. The incidence of burns is low, but burns are detrimental to fetal survival (Smith, 2002).
      (1) Burns are generally caused from flames or hot liquids.
      (2) Fetal survival is influenced by gestational age and maternal survival as well as the total body surface area (TBSA) burned.
   b. Inhalation injuries and carbon monoxide intoxication should always be suspected in the burn victim.
      (1) Carbon monoxide poisoning impairs the release of oxygen from the mother to the fetus and from the fetal hemoglobin to fetal tissue (Smith, 2002).
      (2) Concentration of carboxyhemoglobin is 10% to 15% higher in the fetus than in the mother, and the fetal half life of carbon monoxide is twice as long as the maternal half life (Smith, 2002).

(3) Automobile exhaust and faulty heating systems are also major causes of carbon monoxide poisoning (the leading cause of all poisoning deaths).

5. Gunshot and stab wounds
   a. Gunshot wounds are the most common and usually require surgical exploration and repair.
   b. The uterine muscle absorbs energy from penetrating bullets, which decreases the velocity and lessens the likelihood of visceral injury (American College of Surgeons, 1997).
   c. Penetrating wounds to the uterus can cause significant injury to the fetus (70%) (Chang, 2001), but they generally have a good maternal outcome.
   d. With penetrating injury above the umbilicus after the second half of pregnancy, there is an increased likelihood of injury to the bowel.

F. **Complications**
   1. Premature labor
   2. Abruptio placentae
      a. Occurs in as many as 50% of patients with major injuries (Chang, 2001).
      b. Occurs in as many as 5% of patients with minor injuries (Chang, 2001).
   3. Uterine rupture
   4. Maternal cardiopulmonary arrest/fetal delivery

CLINICAL PRACTICE

A. **Assessment**
   1. History
      a. A brief history is obtained if possible, including chief complaint, mechanism of injury, previous assessment, and treatment.
      b. Mechanism of injury
         (1) Blunt injury
            (a) Motor-vehicle crash
               (i) Position in vehicle (driver, passenger, front, rear)
               (ii) Restraints used (shoulder harness, lap belt, three-point restraint, helmet)
               (iii) Speed of all vehicles involved in collision
               (iv) Point of impact: head on, rear, or side collision (T-bone) and amount of intrusion into the passenger compartment
               (v) Airbag deployment
               (vi) Ejection from vehicle versus extrication required
            (b) Assault
               (i) Blunt trauma versus penetrating instrument
               (ii) Single or multiple assaults
               (iii) Area of injury
            (c) Fall
               (i) Height of fall
               (ii) Landing surface
               (iii) Body part impacted
               (iv) Was fall broken or straight impact
         (2) Penetrating injury
            (a) Stab wound
               (i) Offending object, type
               (ii) Length and width of object

           (iii) Direction of assault
           (iv) Depth of penetration
        (b) Ballistic or gunshot wound
           (i) Type and caliber of weapon
           (ii) Low or high velocity
           (iii) Distance from weapon to victim-range
           (iv) Trajectory
    (3) Burns
        (a) Causative agent (direct flame, hot liquid, chemical, electric, radiation)
        (b) Extent of burn (total body surface area burned)
        (c) Depth of burn (partial or full thickness)
        (d) Carbon monoxide exposure
        (e) Inhalation damage/hoarseness of voice

2. Primary maternal assessment: rapid, brief assessment of the patient to identify any life-threatening problem requiring immediate intervention per Trauma Nursing Core Course guidelines (Emergency Nurses Association, 2000a) (Figure 25-3).
    a. A—airway
        (1) Open and clear
           (a) Patient able to speak
           (b) No stridor
           (c) No visible foreign matter in the upper airway

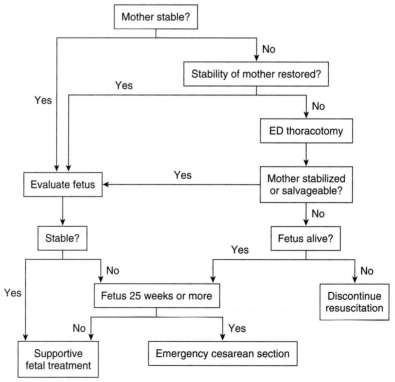

FIGURE 25-3 ■ Algorithm for decision making in emergency obstetric care. (From Rosen, P., & Barkin, R. [1998]. *Emergency medicine: Concepts and clinical practice* [4th ed.]. St. Louis: Mosby.)

(2) Obstructed
  (a) Patient unable to speak
  (b) Stridor, noisy, or absent respirations
  (c) Vomitus, teeth, blood, secretions, or debris in upper airway
  (d) Substernal and intercostal retractions
  (e) Decreased level of consciousness
  (f) Soft tissue damage to the face and neck
  (g) Cyanosis and dusky mucous membranes and nail beds
(3) Interventions if airway obstruction
  (a) Jaw thrust maneuver to open airway
  (b) Gentle oral suction to remove vomitus, blood, secretions, and so on
  (c) Insertion of oral or nasal airway to maintain airway if needed
(4) Cervical spine precautions
  (a) Maintain cervical spine precautions or initiate them if not previously done.
  (b) Cervical collar, head block, back board, and straps in correct placement needed
b. B—breathing
(1) Effective
  (a) Spontaneous rise and fall of chest
  (b) Unlabored respirations
  (c) Equal chest expansion
  (d) No accessory muscle use
(2) Ineffective
  (a) Apnea or agonal respirations less than 10/min
  (b) Shallow, ineffective respirations
  (c) Unequal or absent breath sounds
  (d) Asymmetry of chest wall expansion, severe retractions
  (e) Tracheal shift or distended neck veins
  (f) Obvious chest wounds, such as an open pneumothorax; impaled object in chest; multiple rib fractures
  (g) Decreased level of consciousness
  (h) Cyanosis and dusky mucous membranes and nail beds
(3) Interventions if breathing ineffective
  (a) 100% oxygen with nonrebreather mask
  (b) Bag-valve mask with 100% oxygen
  (c) Assist with needle thoracostomy or chest tube insertion if pneumothorax or tension pneumothorax is suspected.
  (d) Cover open wound with three-sided dressing.
  (e) Stabilize impaled object (but do not remove).
  (f) Assist with intubation if needed.
c. C—circulation
(1) Effective
  (a) Palpable radial pulse between 60 and 100 beats/min
  (b) Normal capillary refill time (less than 2 seconds)
  (c) Pink, warm, and dry skin
  (d) Patient alert and oriented
(2) Ineffective
  (a) Unable to palpate peripheral pulses
  (b) Obvious external hemorrhage
  (c) Delayed capillary refill (more than 2 seconds)
  (d) Decreased level of consciousness
  (e) Pale, cool, moist skin

        (3) Interventions if circulation is ineffective
           (a) Stop any obvious external sources of bleeding.
           (b) Start two large-bore (14- to 16-gauge) intravenous (IV) lines and run warmed fluid (lactated ringers or normal saline) in rapidly.
           (c) Transfuse blood products as ordered, O-negative, until type-specific blood is available.
           (d) Administer volume expanders such as Hespan as ordered.
           (e) Assist with emergency thoracotomy if needed.
           (f) Cardiopulmonary resuscitation if needed for circulatory support.
    d. D—deficit (brief neurologic examination)
        (1) AVPU assessment method
           (a) A: alert
           (b) V: responds to verbal stimuli
           (c) P: responds to painful stimuli
           (d) U: unresponsive
        (2) Can follow commands; moves all extremities; note any numbness or tingling noted by patient.
        (3) Brief pupil examination looking for pupil size, symmetry, and reaction to light.
3. Secondary maternal assessment: brief, complete head-to-toe survey is performed to determine all injuries, both obvious and hidden.
    a. E—expose and environmental controls
        (1) Remove all clothing for examination.
           (a) Clothes should be cut off in the interest of time.
           (b) If the client is unstable, particularly with a suspected spinal injury, cut clothing off.
        (2) Keep patient warm with blankets, warmed IV fluids, and warming lights.
    b. F—five interventions, full set of vital signs, facilitate family presence
        (1) Obtain vital signs: BP—auscultated blood pressures (both arms if chest injuries are suspected); heart rate (HR), respiratory rate, and temperature; include FHR.
        (2) Obtain pulse oximetry.
        (3) Apply cardiac monitor.
        (4) Draw blood for type and crossmatch and other lab tests.
        (5) Consider indwelling urinary catheter.
        (6) Consider oral or nasal gastric tube.
        (7) Facilitate family presence (i.e., notification of family or significant other).
    c. G—give comfort measures
        (1) Pain medications as ordered
        (2) Verbal assurances/psychosocial support
        (3) Touch/repositioning
    d. H—history and head-to-toe examination focused on identifying all injuries per Emergency Nurses Association's *Trauma Nursing Core Course* guidelines (2000a)
        (1) Any pertinent maternal history
           (a) Medications and allergies
           (b) Maternal history: gravida, parity, abortion, living children
           (c) Additional data regarding the details and mechanism of injury
        (2) Any pertinent fetal history
           (a) Fetal movement since incident
           (b) Any problems with pregnancy

(3) Head-to-toe brief examination to identify all injuries using inspection, palpation, percussion, and auscultation skills
    (a) General appearance of patient: abnormal posturing, other unusual body positioning or alignment, and unusual odors
    (b) Head and face:
        (i) Surface wounds, ecchymosis, edema, deformity, and tenderness
        (ii) Pupils: size, equality, and reactivity
        (iii) Raccoon eyes (periorbital ecchymosis caused by dissection of blood from a basilar skull fracture)
        (iv) Drainage (clear or bloody) from nose or ears
        (v) Battle sign (ecchymosis over mastoid process behind the ear)
        (vi) Nasal deformity or tenderness
        (vii) Neck, surface wounds and edema, tracheal deviation, and distended neck veins
    (c) Neck
        (i) Surface wounds and edema
        (ii) Trachea position
        (iii) Distended neck veins
        (iv) Subcutaneous emphysema
        (v) Tenderness and crepitus (especially posteriorly)
    (d) Chest
        (i) Subcutaneous emphysema
        (ii) Surface wounds and ecchymosis
        (iii) Impaled objects
        (iv) Bilateral and symmetric chest rise
        (v) Accessory muscle use
        (vi) Breath sounds and heart sounds
        (vii) Pain on palpation, crepitus, and deformity
    (e) Abdomen and flanks
        (i) Note the shape of the abdomen (deformity or irregular size might indicate uterine rupture).
        (ii) Bowel signs auscultated (before palpation of abdomen to prevent false-positive findings)
        (iii) Surface wounds, ecchymosis, seat belt marks; any injuries from airbag deployment
        (iv) Impaled objects
        (v) Distention, rigidity, and tenderness
        (vi) Uterine tenderness or increased uterine tone on palpation
    (f) Pelvis and genitalia
        (i) Surface wounds, ecchymosis, and edema of perineum or genitalia
        (ii) Instability or tenderness on gentle squeeze of anterior iliac crests and/or symphysis pubis
        (iii) Bleeding from the urinary meatus, vagina, or rectum
        (iv) Pain and/or urge to void
    (g) Extremities
        (i) Surface wounds, edema, and/or ecchymosis
        (ii) Deformities: open or closed fractures
        (iii) Bony crepitus on palpation
        (iv) Skin color, temperature, and presence of distal pulses
        (v) Spontaneous motor function of all extremities
        (vi) Gross sensory function of all extremities

(h) Posterior surface
  (i) Observe cervical spine precautions, and log-roll client to assess for presence of injuries on posterior body.
  (ii) Surface wounds of back, flanks, buttocks, or thighs
  (iii) Pain or deformity on palpation of entire spinal column
4. Fetal assessment (should occur simultaneously with maternal secondary assessment).
   a. Fetal heart rate is the best indicator of fetal and maternal condition source.
      (1) Assess fetal heart rate (Doppler or ultrasound); 120 to 160 is normal.
      (2) Continuous electronic fetal monitoring is ideal for essential ongoing fetal assessment.
   b. Fundal height (to assess gestational age)
   c. Fetal movement
5. Focused obstetric assessment
   a. Spontaneous rupture of membranes
   b. Vaginal bleeding
      (1) Assess vaginal fluid for amniotic fluid by testing the ph (7.0 to 7.5).
      (2) Place fluid on slide and observe for fern effect when dried.
   c. Labor status
      (1) Contractions
      (2) Cervical dilatation, effacement, station, and presenting part
   d. Abruptio placentae-abdominal trauma in 1.5% to 9.4% of all cases (Gaufberg, 2001)
   e. Uterine rupture
   f. Fetal distress
6. Focused obstetric history
   a. Present pregnancy
      (1) Gestational age (last menstrual period [LMP]) and expected date of confinement (EDC)
      (2) Complications of current pregnancy
   b. Past obstetric history
   c. Events preceding injury (suspected domestic abuse)
7. Glasgow Coma Scale Score (Table 25-1)
8. Psychosocial findings
   a. Anxiety or fear about life of fetus
   b. Anxiety or fear about own well-being and ability to care for infant
   c. Guilt about being injured and causing potential harm to fetus
   d. Injuries inconsistent with reported history, anxiety regarding abusive significant other
B. **Diagnostic procedures**
1. Laboratory
   a. Complete blood count (CBC), differential, and platelet count
   b. Blood type and crossmatch
   c. Sodium, potassium, and chloride
   d. Glucose, blood urea nitrogen (BUN), and creatinine
   e. Clotting factors: prothrombin time (PT), partial thromboplastin time (PTT), fibrinogen, and fibrin split products
   f. D-dimer
   g. Amylase and liver function tests
   h. Urinalysis

■ TABLE 25-1	
■ ■ Glasgow Coma Scale	
Finding	**Score**
EYE OPENING	
Spontaneous	4
To voice	3
To pain	2
None	1
BEST VERBAL RESPONSE	
Oriented	5
Confused	4
Inappropriate words	3
Incomprehensible sounds	2
None	1
BEST MOTOR RESPONSE	
Obey commands	6
Purposeful movement (pain)	5
Withdrawal (pain)	4
Flexion (pain)	3
Extension (pain)	2
None	1

Total score from each section equals the Glasgow Coma Scale Score.

       i. Arterial blood gases, serum bicarbonate (altered levels correlate with fetal outcome) (Emergency Nurses Association, 2000c).

       j. Blood alcohol and/or toxicology studies

      k. Urine or serum beta-hCG

       l. Tests for presence of fetal erythrocytes in maternal blood sampling or in vaginal blood (indicates fetal-maternal hemorrhage)

          (1) Kleihauer-Betke (KB) stain or hemoglobin electrophoresis takes 1 hour (not needed in minor trauma [Chang, 2001], but should be completed in major trauma).

          (2) More rapid tests (4 to 7 minutes) might be more useful in the emergency room.

             (a) Ogita (most sensitive at 20% fetal blood)

             (b) Apt (sensitive at 60%)

             (c) Loendersloot (sensitive at 60%)

  2. Radiology

     a. Perform studies as indicated; radiation risk to fetus should not interfere with life-saving interventions for mother.

     b. Avoid duplicate films.

     c. Uterus should be shielded with lead apron whenever possible.

     d. IV pyelogram (IVP) dye does not cross placenta.

  3. Computed tomography (CT) scan

     a. Using sequential slices of tissue with small gaps between cuts decreases radiation exposure.

     b. Shield for nonabdominal scans.

     c. Assess for bleeding and solid organ injury, occult fracture diagnosis.

4. Magnetic resonance imaging (MRI) (might be used because of its advantages over CT).
   a. MRI uses no ionizing radiation.
   b. Vascular structures can be evaluated without the need to inject iodinated contrast medium.
   c. Imaging of deep pelvic structures does not depend on a urine-filled bladder.
   d. Ability to identify flowing blood and distinguish blood from other fluid collections (Neufeld, 1998).
   e. Takes longer than CT scan; patient must be relatively stable.
5. Ultrasonography
   a. Triage tool for the pregnant patient with blunt abdominal trauma (Goodwin, Holmes, & Wisner, 2001)
   b. A safe, noninvasive bedside study for both maternal and fetal assessment (Henderson & Mallon, 1998)
   c. Detects uterine rupture (Goodwin, Holmes, and Wisner, 2001) as well as detects free fluid in the blunt abdominal trauma patient (Nordenholz, Rubin, Gularte, & Liang, 1997).
   d. Can identify fetal activity, determine fetal heart rate, and diagnose fetal death.
   e. Determines:
      (1) Gestational age (accuracy varies with trimester)
      (2) Fetal position
      (3) Amount of amniotic fluid
      (4) Multiple gestations
      (5) Fetal weight
      (6) Placental location and possible placental abruption (not 100% accurate)
6. Electronic fetal monitor and uterine monitoring (for more than 20 to 24 weeks' gestational age)
   a. Note baseline heart rate and variability (variability is a sign of fetal well being) (Henderson & Mallon, 1998).
   b. Monitor uterine contractions (observe for trauma induced pre-term labor).
   c. Monitoring fetal heart rates detects trends such as bradycardia (ominous sign) and prolonged tachycardia, which might indicate fetal distress.
   d. Assists in diagnosing abruptio placentae.
   e. Fetal distress might be a sign of occult maternal distress (Neufeld, 1998).
   f. Is recommended for all pregnant patients with viable pregnancies after trauma, regardless of physiologic status and location or severity of injury (Theodorou et al., 2000).
   g. Fetal monitoring for a minimum of 4 hours if no FHR abnormality or maternal complications or 24 hours until fetal well being is established (Pearlman, 1997; Rita & Reed, 2003).
7. Diagnostic peritoneal lavage (DPL) surgical technique to diagnose intraperitoneal bleeding
   a. Indications include:
      (1) Altered level of consciousness
      (2) Unexplained shock
      (3) Major chest injuries
      (4) Signs and symptoms of intraabdominal bleeding
   b. Will not assess retroperitoneal or intrauterine injuries.
   c. Insert an indwelling urinary catheter and nasal/oral gastric tube before the procedure.

    d. Procedure

        (1) Peritoneal catheter is inserted with direct visualization using the open technique to avoid the gravid uterus (Rita & Reed, 2003) with the insertion site above the umbilicus.

        (2) Aspiration of gross blood is considered positive.

            (a) If aspiration is negative, 1 L of warmed lactated Ringer's solution or normal saline solution is infused over 10 to 15 minutes into the peritoneal cavity.

            (b) The solution bag is lowered to gravity drainage, and the return fluid is analyzed for the presence of blood cells, amylase, bile, food fiber, or feces.

        (3) Surgical intervention is needed for positive results.

C. Nursing Diagnoses

    1. Ineffective airway clearance related to chest injury

    2. Impaired gas exchange related to chest injury

    3. Ineffective breathing pattern related to chest injury

    4. Ineffective cardiovascular tissue perfusion related to severe blood loss

    5. Decreased cardiac output related to severe blood loss

    6. Deficient fluid volume related to severe blood loss

    7. Anticipatory grieving related to actual or potential loss of fetus

    8. Ineffective fetal tissue perfusion related to maternal blood loss and abdominal injury

D. Interventions/Outcomes

    1. Ineffective airway clearance related to chest injury

      a. Interventions

        (1) Position patient in supine position and immobilize the cervical spine if not done.

            (a) Manual stabilization (Figure 25-4)

            (b) Rigid cervical collar

            (c) Apply rolled blankets to side of neck; place patient on backboard and secure with straps and tape.

        (2) Open airway with jaw thrust or chin lift, keeping head in neutral, midline position.

        (3) Remove loose objects, and suction gently if needed to clear airway.

        (4) Maintain open airway with appropriate adjunct (oropharyngeal or nasopharyngeal airway); consider endotracheal intubation.

        (5) Consider insertion of nasogastric tube for gastric decompression and airway protection.

      b. Outcomes

        (1) Airway is open and clear; patient is able to speak.

        (2) Patient exhibits no stridor.

        (3) No foreign matter is visible in the upper airway.

        (4) Cervical spine precautions are maintained.

    2. Impaired gas exchange related to chest injury

    3. Ineffective breathing pattern related to chest injury

      a. Interventions

        (1) If client is not breathing:

            (a) Provide positive-pressure ventilation with bag-valve-mask device and 100% oxygen.

            (b) Assist with endotracheal intubation.

        (2) If breathing is present but ineffective:

            (a) Administer oxygen by nonrebreather mask at 12 to 15 L/min to keep reservoir bag inflated.

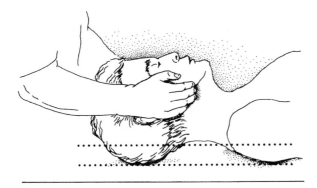

FIGURE 25-4 ■ Manual stabilization of the cervical spine.

    (b) Assist ventilations with bag valve mask device with 100% oxygen as necessary.

    (c) Identify and intervene for specific life-threatening injuries.

        (i) Tension pneumothorax
- Severe respiratory distress
- Restlessness; agitation
- Tracheal shift
- Distended neck veins
- Absent breath sounds
- Immediate needle thoracostomy on affected side

        (ii) Open pneumothorax
- Sucking or gurgling chest wound
- Severe respiratory distress
- Cyanosis
- Apply three-sided sterile occlusive dressing; monitor for development of tension pneumothorax.

        (iii) Flail chest
- Severe respiratory distress
- Cyanosis
- Paradoxical chest wall movement
- Assist with intubation and mechanical ventilation.
- Prevent IV fluid overload.

        (iv) Massive hemothorax
- Severe respiratory distress
- Signs of hypovolemic shock (previous conditions ruled out)
- Assist with insertion of large-bore chest tube on affected side at fifth or sixth intercostal space.

    (3) Monitor arterial blood gas and pulse oximetry readings.

  b. Outcomes

    (1) Rise and fall of chest is spontaneous.

    (2) Respirations are not labored.

    (3) Chest wall expansion is equal and symmetric.

    (4) Trachea is midline.

    (5) No accessory muscle is used.

    (6) Skin is pink, warm, and dry.

    (7) Patient is alert and oriented.

    (8) Pulse oximetry readings are at 100% on oxygen and blood gas results within normal pregnancy range.

4. Ineffective cardiovascular tissue perfusion related to severe blood loss
5. Decreased cardiac output related to severe blood loss
6. Deficient fluid volume related to severe blood loss
  a. Interventions
   (1) If pulse is absent:
     (a) Begin cardiopulmonary resuscitation.
     (b) Initiate advanced life support measures.
     (c) Prepare for emergency open thoracotomy to control intrathoracic hemorrhage.
     (d) Administer blood as ordered; prepare for autotransfusion.
     (e) Prepare for surgery after open thoracotomy.
   (2) If pulse is present but ineffective:
     (a) Control obvious external bleeding by direct pressure, elevation of extremities, application of pressure on arterial pressure points, and tourniquet only as a last resort.
     (b) Establish two 14- to 16-gauge IV lines with Y-type blood administration tubing, and administer warmed normal saline or lactated Ringer's solution.
       (i) Assist with possible placement of central line.
       (ii) Rapid transfusion device or pressurized IV bags
       (iii) Fluids titrated to hemodynamic status
       (iv) Burn injury fluid resuscitation
         ■ 4 ml of crystalloid solution × the percentage of body surface area burned × patient weight in kg given over first 24 hours
         ■ Half of the total volume given in first 8 hours after burn injury
     (c) Draw blood for hemoglobin/hematocrit, type and crossmatching, and other studies.
     (d) Administer uncrossmatched, O-negative blood as ordered.
     (e) Administer typed and crossmatched blood as soon as possible.
     (f) Initiate continuous cardiac monitoring (heart rate increases 15 to 20 bpm during pregnancy).
     (g) Place client in left lateral position to prevent supine hypotension syndrome; might need to manually displace uterus or place supports under client's right hip to tilt client 30 degrees to the left side. See Figure 25-1 for left lateral positioning.
     (h) Replacement of clotting factors must be considered when packed cells are given.
     (i) Anticipate autotransfusion if hemothorax is present.
     (j) Consider using pneumatic antishock garment (legs only). See Figure 25-5 for application.
     (k) Insert indwelling urinary catheter to monitor hourly output; urinary output is a sensitive indicator of tissue perfusion status and of the adequacy of fluid replacement.
  b. Outcomes
   (1) Patient has improved level of consciousness.
   (2) Skin is pink, warm, and dry.
   (3) Urinary output is more than 30 ml/hr.
   (4) Distal pulses are present and strong.
   (5) Capillary refill time is less than 2 seconds.
   (6) Heart rate and blood pressure are within normal pregnancy range.

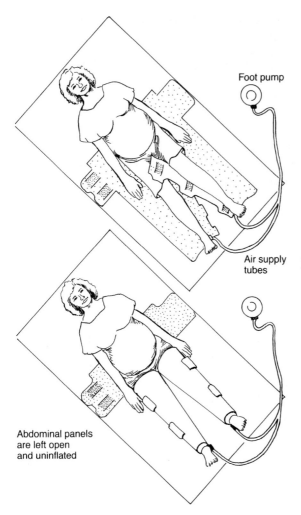

Foot pump

Air supply tubes

FIGURE 25-5 ■ Application of the MAST suit during pregnancy.

Abdominal panels are left open and uninflated

7. Anticipatory grieving related to actual or potential loss of fetus
   a. Interventions
      (1) Establish trusting relationship by being nonjudgmental; stay with patient and explain all procedures and interventions.
      (2) Provide updates on both maternal and fetal status and encouragement when appropriate.
      (3) Actively listen to patient's questions and responses.
      (4) Involve significant others.
      (5) Involve pastoral care service if patient/family requests, social worker, mental health nurse, or other support available in the hospital.
      (6) Answer questions regarding fetus honestly and realistically.
   b. Outcomes
      (1) Exhibits appropriate grieving behavior.
      (2) Verbalizes feelings and fears.
      (3) Patient is able to participate in decision making.
      (4) Physiologic symptoms of fear, such as increased heart rate, blood pressure, diaphoresis, hyperventilation, and complaints of heart palpitations are absent.

8. Ineffective fetal tissue perfusion related to maternal blood loss and abdominal injury
    a. Interventions
        (1) Aggressive maternal resuscitation (leading cause of fetal death is maternal death).
        (2) Emergency (crash) cesarean section for a fetus of viable gestational age
            (a) Indications
                (i) Fetal distress
                    ■ Late and ominous decelerations of fetal heart rate; severe bradycardia or tachycardia
                    ■ Blood on amniocentesis
                    ■ Positive fetal erythrocytes in maternal blood
                (ii) Development of DIC
                (iii) Fetal malpresentation during premature labor (Neufeld, 1998)
                (iv) Improving surgical access to save the mother
                (v) Placental abruption
                (vi) Uterine rupture
                (vii) Uncontrolled hemorrhage
                (viii) Maternal arrest (postmortem cesarean section)
            (b) Factors affecting fetal survival of postmortem cesarean section
                (i) Time interval between maternal arrest and fetal delivery is the most important factor (Rita & Reed, 2003).
                (ii) Fetal condition
                (iii) Maternal cause of death (e.g., severe hemorrhage)
                (iv) Fetal gestational age
            (c) Newborn resuscitation required (see Chapter 16 on newborn resuscitation)
        (3) Admit all pregnant patients with viable fetuses and with major injuries to the hospital for continuous fetal monitoring after resuscitation and stabilization for 24 to 48 hours; in particular, all abdominal injuries must be observed for 48 hours to rule out abruptio placentae; Rogers et al. (1999) concluded that fetal monitoring is underutilized in injured pregnant patients admitted to major trauma centers.
    b. Outcomes
        (1) Fetal perfusion is improved.

HEALTH EDUCATION

A. Prevention

1. Wearing a three-point seat belt properly during pregnancy might prevent ejection or serious injury from collision with steering wheel or dashboard (see Figure 25-6 for seatbelt positioning).
    a. Seat belt should be worn with the shoulder strap positioned between breasts and above dome of uterus.
        (1) Lap belt is worn under the uterus and across the anterior spines of the pelvis.
        (2) Padding the seatbelt for comfort is discouraged because the belt can shift upward on impact, causing injury to the thinner portion of the fundus (Smith, 2002).
    b. Three-point restraints help prevent rapid deceleration, forward-flexion injuries that can cause shearing forces on the uterus.

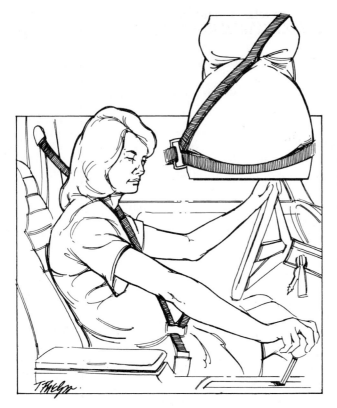

FIGURE 25-6 ■ Proper use of a seat belt during pregnancy. (From McQuillan, K.A., Von Rueden, K.T., Hartsock, R.L., Flynn, M.B., & Whalen, E. [2002]. *Trauma nursing: From resuscitation through rehabilitation* [3rd ed.]. Philadelphia: Saunders.)

    c. Lap belts used alone might cause injury to enlarged gravid uterus.
       (1) A pregnant patient should be advised that use of only a lap belt is preferable to using no restraint.
       (2) It is then preferable that she rides in the back seat, however.
    d. If one is driving a car with an airbag, one should direct a tilting steering wheel away from the abdomen, move the front seat backward as far as possible, have the airbag disconnected, or sit in the back seat as a passenger.
  2. Referral to public education programs regarding danger to mother and fetus when seat belt is not worn; omission of seat belt for all persons increases chance of ejection, which increases chance of death by 20 times; referral to programs for automotive infant restraint devices as needed.
  3. Support enforcement of current laws that require seat belt use.
  4. Educate providers on risk factors, assessment for domestic violence injuries and illnesses, and referral resources for women identified in need of intervention and/or resources (see Chapter 20).

B. Education
  1. Prenatal care should include information about normal anatomical changes that predispose pregnant women to accidents.
  2. Encourage frequent rest breaks.
  3. Safety measures in the home and workplace, such as avoiding climbing on chairs and ladders, should be instituted.
  4. Counseling regarding possibility of spousal or partner abuse during pregnancy in confidential, supportive settings should be offered.
  5. Provide information at an appropriate reading level and in a cultural context, with illustrations to clarify information and instructions.

CASE STUDIES AND STUDY QUESTIONS

1. In trauma, the most common cause of fetal death is:
   a. Death of the mother
   b. Placental abruption
   c. Uterine rupture
   d. Penetrating injury to the fetus

2. The primary survey in trauma focuses on:
   a. In-depth management and definitive care interventions
   b. Life-threatening priorities
   c. A thorough head-to-toe assessment
   d. Chief complaint, past medical history, and allergies

3. Of the following IV solutions, which is preferred in the initial resuscitation of a pregnant trauma client?
   a. D5½ normal saline at 100 ml/hr
   b. Warm normal saline or lactated Ringer's solution titrated to the hemodynamic status of the client
   c. 500 ml of colloid solution over 2 hours
   d. Two to four units of packed erythrocytes

4. Tissue perfusion is considered adequate if all of the following are present except:
   a. Client is alert and oriented.
   b. Capillary refill time is less than 2 seconds.
   c. Skin is pink, warm, and dry.
   d. Urinary output is less than 20 ml/hr.

5. The best overall indicator for maternal well-being is:
   a. Maternal blood pressure
   b. Fetal heart rate within normal limits
   c. Maternal self-reporting
   d. Lack of uterine contractions

Ms. M, 26 years old and 36 weeks' pregnant, was involved in a motor-vehicle accident. She was driving a compact car that was broadsided on the driver's side by a delivery van. Damage to her car was moderate. She was wearing a seat belt that included a shoulder harness and lap belt in the proper position. The paramedics found her to be alert, but she continued to ask, "What happened?" The field primary survey revealed a patent airway, no respiratory distress, and slightly pale, diaphoretic skin. Her chief complaint was abdominal pain "all over." She had what appeared to be a seat-belt contusion across the lower abdomen. Her vital signs were: heart rate, 92 bpm; respirations, 24/min; and blood pressure, 92/64. Oxygen was applied at 15 L/min by mask as full spinal immobilization was instituted. En route to the nearest trauma center, two 16-gauge IV lines were established in each forearm.

On arrival at the emergency department, she was evaluated by the trauma team with the assistance of the obstetric and neonatal intensive care unit (NICU) teams. She remained alert, but confused about the circumstances of the accident and the date.

After it had been determined that Ms. M's airway, breathing, and circulation were intact, the secondary survey was performed with her completely undressed and covered with warm blankets. The assessment revealed only a small laceration on the left parietal area of the head, abdominal contusions, pain on palpation of the anterior iliac crests, and superficial abrasions to both anterior knees.

Baseline laboratory studies were performed, and diagnostic radiographs were negative. Continuous electronic fetal monitoring revealed regular uterine contractions every 2 to 3 minutes, and a fetal heart rate of 136 bpm. A Foley catheter was inserted, and urine was negative for blood. A nasal gastric tube was inserted without complications.

Soon after the initial evaluation of Ms. M, the fetal heart rate was noted to be 180 to 200 bpm. Ms. M's vital signs were now heart rate, 134 bpm; respirations, 28/min; blood pressure, 88 and palpable. An emergency cesarean section and exploratory laparotomy were performed immediately. The operation revealed both a ruptured spleen and partial placental detachment from the uterine wall. A boy was delivered without evidence of distress, and a splenectomy was performed.

Ms. M was discharged home on postoperative day 6 without complications. Her son had not been injured in the accident and had been discharged to the maternal grandmother on day 3 in good condition.

6. Ongoing assessment of the adequacy of resuscitation efforts includes:
   a. Vital signs every 5 to 15 minutes until stable
   b. Urinary output every 30 to 60 minutes
   c. Frequent level-of-consciousness evaluations
   d. All of the above

7. Because of Ms. M's mechanism of injury, a complete neurologic examination must be completed. This evaluation includes assessment of her
   a. Level of consciousness
   b. Motor and sensory responses
   c. Pupil size, equality, and reactivity to light
   d. All of the above

8. Additional information regarding the mechanism of injury in the described accident might include all of the following except:
   a. The need for extrication
   b. The speed at which the vehicles were traveling
   c. The intersection at which the accident occurred
   d. Passenger space intrusion

9. The most appropriate position for Ms. M to be placed in, especially once her cervical spine has been cleared, is:
   a. Flat with her legs elevated and her uterus displaced to the left
   b. Semi-Fowler's position to facilitate breathing
   c. Head down, left lateral position to prevent vomiting and possible aspiration
   d. Trendelenburg position to improve blood flow to the brain

Ms. S was brought by private car to the emergency department after being involved in a drive-by gang-related shooting in front of her home. She was 17 years old and 32 weeks' pregnant with her second child. She had received no prenatal care for this pregnancy.

The emergency department staff removed her from the back seat of the car. She had no pulse and was not breathing. She had an obvious gunshot wound to the upper back between the shoulder blades, and no exit wound was apparent. Cardiopulmonary resuscitation was begun, and the trauma team was assembled immediately.

On arrival in the trauma room, she underwent immediate open thoracotomy to identify the extent of her internal injuries, to perform internal cardiac massage, and to crossclamp the aorta. A pericardiocentesis was performed, and no blood was found. The heart was in ventricular fibrillation. A simultaneous emergency cesarean section was performed. A boy was delivered, and the development of some palpable pulse was noted before transfer to the NICU.

Despite vigorous volume resuscitation and manual cardiac compression, Ms. S died in the emergency department. Her baby remained in the NICU in critical condition because of respiratory failure and probable cerebral anoxia.

10. In addition to the emergency trauma staff, who else should the nurse immediately notify?
    a. Labor and delivery staff
    b. Obstetric and NICU physician and nurses
    c. Blood bank staff
    d. All of the above

11. Factors affecting fetal survival of a postmortem cesarean section include which of the following?
    a. Time interval between maternal death and fetal delivery
    b. Fetal gestational age
    c. Cause of maternal death
    d. All of the above

12. Priorities in the initial care of Ms. S include:
    a. Applying the pneumatic antishock garment and inflating the legs and abdominal compartments.
    b. Establishing a patent airway and ventilating the client by endotracheal intubation and administration of 100% oxygen.
    c. Amniocentesis to determine fetal lung maturity.

    d. Administration of crystalloid solution at 125 ml per hour.

13. In addition to maternal death, indications for a crash cesarean section include all of the following *except:*
    a. All pelvic fractures
    b. Uterine rupture
    c. Severe placental abruption
    d. Late and ominous decelerations of fetal heart rate

14. The best choice of volume resuscitation for Ms. S is:
    a. Infusion of 100 ml of crystalloid solution for each 100 ml of estimated blood loss
    b. Rapid transfusion of uncrossmatched, O-negative blood and crystalloid solution until maternal hemodynamics are normal
    c. Administration of 250 ml of colloid solution to improve volume expansion rapidly
    d. Rapid crystalloid solution infusion until complete type and crossmatch are completed to avoid possible transfusion reaction

ANSWERS TO STUDY QUESTIONS

1. a	5. b	9. a	13. a
2. b	6. d	10. d	14. b
3. b	7. d	11. d	
4. d	8. c	12. b	

REFERENCES

ACEP News: Annals of Emergency Medicine. (1999). *Pregnant women more likely to be hospitalized for assault.* Retrieved February 8, 2003 from *www. merginet.com/tgp/literature/acep/acep9911. shtml.*

Ali, J., Yeo, A., Gana, T.J., & McLellan, B.A. (1997). Predictors of fetal mortality in pregnant trauma patients. *Journal of Trauma: Injury, Infection and Critical Care, 42*(5), 782-785.

American College of Obstetricians and Gynecologists. (1999). Obstetric aspects of trauma management, Educational Bulletin 251, *International Journal of Gynaecology and Obstetrics, 64*(1), 87-94.

American College of Surgeons. (1997). Trauma in women. In *Advanced Trauma Life Support for Doctors Instructor Course Manual* (6th ed.; pp. 379-387). Chicago: First Impression.

Baerga-Varela, Y., Zietlow, S.P., Bannon, M.P., Harmsen, W.S., & Ilstrup, D.M. (2000). Trauma in pregnancy. *Mayo Clinic Proceeding, 75*(12), 1243-1248.

Chang, A.K. (2001). Pregnancy, trauma. Retrieved February 8, 2003 from *www.emedicine.com/emerg/topic484.htm.*

Colburn, V. (1999). Trauma in pregnancy. *Journal of Perinatal and Neonatal Nursing, 13*(3), 21-32.

Connolly, A., Katz, V.L., Bash, K.L., McMahon, M.J., & Hansen, W.F. (1997). Trauma and pregnancy. *American Journal of Perinatology, 14*(6), 331-336.

Curet, M.J., Schermer, C.R., Demarest, G.B., Bieneik, E.J. III, & Curet, L.B. (2000). Predictors of outcome in trauma during pregnancy: Identification of patients who can be monitored for less than 6 hours. *Journal of Trauma: Injury, Infection, and Critical Care, 49*(1), 18-25.

Emergency Nurses Association. (2000a). Initial assessment. In *Trauma nursing core course* (5th ed.). Des Plaines, IL: Emergency Nurses Association.

Emergency Nurses Association. (2000b). Obstetrical and gynecological emergencies. In *Orientation to emergency nursing: Concepts, competencies, and critical thinking* (2nd ed.). Des Plaines, IL: Emergency Nurses Association.

Emergency Nurses Association. (2000c). Trauma and pregnancy. In *Trauma nursing core course* (5th ed.). Des Plaines, IL: Emergency Nurses Association.

Foley, M. (2003). *When all else fails: Perimortem cesarean delivery.* Paper presented at Scottsdale Health Care-Shea, February 14, Scottsdale, Arizona.

Gaufberg, S.V. (2001). Abruptio placentae. Retrieved February 8, 2003 from *www.emedicine.com/EMERG/topic12.htm.*

Goodwin, H., Holmes, J.F., & Wisner, D.H. (2001). Abdominal ultrasound examination in pregnant blunt trauma patients. *Journal of Trauma: Injury, Infection, and Critical Care, 50*(4), 689-694.

Henderson, S.O., & Mallon, W.K. (1998). Trauma in pregnancy. *Emergency Medicine Clinics of North America, 16*(1), 209-228.

Moise, K.J., & Belfort, M.A. (1997). Damage control for the obstetric patient. *Surgical Clinics of North America, 77*(4), 835-852.

Neufeld, J. (1998). Trauma in pregnancy. In Rosen, P., & Barkin, R. (Eds.), *Emergency medicine: Concepts and clinical practice* (4th ed.; Vol. 1; pp. 368-381). St. Louis: Mosby.

Newton, E.R. (2002). Trauma and pregnancy. Retrieved February 8, 2003 from *www.emedicine.com/med/topic3268.htm.*

Nordenholz, K.E., Rubin, M.A., Gularte, G.G., & Liang, H.K. (1997). Ultrasound in the evaluation and management of blunt abdominal trauma. *Annals of Emergency Medicine, 29*(3), 357-366.

Pak, L.L., Reece, E.A., & Chan, L. (1998). Is adverse pregnancy outcome predictable after blunt abdominal trauma? *American Journal of Obstetrics and Gynecology, 179*(5), 1140-1144.

Pearlman, M.D. (1997). Motor vehicle crashes, pregnancy loss and preterm labor. *International Journal of Gynaecology and Obstetrics, 57*(2), 127-132.

Rita, S. & Reed, B.A. (2003). Obstetric trauma. In L. Newberry (Ed.), *Sheehy's emergency nursing: Principles and practice* (5th ed.; pp. 410-420). St. Louis: Mosby.

Rogers, F.B., Rozycki, G.S., Osler, T.M., Shackford S.R., Jalbert, J., Kirton, O., et al. (1999). A multi-institutional study of factors associated with fetal death in injured pregnant patients. *Archives of Surgery, 134*(11), 1274-1277.

Shah, K.H., Simons, R.K., Holbrook, T., Fortlage, D., Winchell, R.J., & Hoyt, D.B. (1998). Trauma in pregnancy: maternal and fetal outcomes. *Journal of Trauma: Injury, Infection and Critical Care, 45*(1), 83-86.

Smith, L. (2002). The pregnant trauma patient. In McQuillan, K.A. et al. *Trauma nursing: From resuscitation through rehabilitation* (3rd ed.; pp. 718-746). Philadelphia: Saunders.

Theodorou, D.A., Velmahos, G.C., Souter, I., Chan, L.S., Vassiliu, P., Tatevossian, R., et al. (2000). *Fetal death after trauma.* Paper presented at Annual Meeting of the Southern California Chapter, American College of Surgeons, January 21-23, Huntington Beach, California.

26 Surgery in Pregnancy

LINDA CALLAHAN

OBJECTIVES

1. Describe the incidence of nonobstetric surgery performed during pregnancy in the United States.
2. Analyze alterations in the pregnant client's physiology and the risks associated with anesthesia.
3. Discuss optimal timing for nonobstetric surgery when performed during pregnancy.
4. Describe potential complications of nonobstetric surgery for the pregnant client.
5. Describe the potential effects of nonobstetric surgery and anesthesia on the fetus.
6. Assess the client's response to surgery and the potential for preterm labor.
7. Outline important parameters of general maternal preoperative assessment.
8. Discuss basic and specific considerations in anesthetic choices for the pregnant client requiring nonobstetric surgery.
9. Describe assessment of symptoms of the pregnant client with acute cholecystitis.
10. Describe assessment of symptoms of appendicitis in the pregnant client.
11. Describe assessment of symptoms of the pregnant client with ovarian cyst/tumor requiring surgical intervention.
12. Discuss the use of laparoscopy as a surgical technique in pregnant clients in need of cholecystectomy or appendectomy.
13. Describe the client at risk for cervical incompetence.
14. Define the function and types of surgical approaches to cervical cerclage.
15. Discuss procedure-specific assessment of the pregnant client in need of cervical cerclage.
16. Discuss indications for endoscopic gastrointestinal procedures that might be present in the pregnant patient.
17. Discuss the risks that might be present for pregnant clients undergoing esophagogastroduodenoscopy (EGD) or endoscopic retrograde cholangiopancreatography (ERCP).
18. Outline methods for risk reduction in pregnant clients undergoing endoscopic gastrointestinal procedures.
19. Describe the potential maternal complications associated with intrauterine fetal surgery.
20. Discuss specific life-threatening fetal anomalies that might be amenable to treatment by intrauterine fetal surgery.
21. Describe the utility of intrauterine fetal surgery in correction of nonfatal fetal anomalies such as myelomeningocele or obstructive uropathy.
22. Select appropriate nursing actions based on acquired knowledge of the alterations in the pregnant client's physiology, and integrate that knowledge into preoperative, intraoperative, and postoperative care.
23. Define psychosocial stressors affecting the pregnant client undergoing surgery.
24. Describe the care of the pregnant surgical client and her family based on analysis of the client's needs in this emotionally and physically stressful situation.
25. Formulate nursing interventions to prevent postoperative surgical complications in the pregnant surgical client.

INTRODUCTION

A. Incidence of nonobstetric surgery performed during pregnancy ranges from 1% to 2%, or as many as 75,000 women per year in the United States (Rosen & Weiskopf, 1999).
1. Incidence is probably underestimated because pregnancy might be unrecognized at time of surgery.
2. A Swedish study indicated that 42% underwent surgery in the first trimester, 35% during the second trimester, and 23% during the third trimester.

B. Types of procedures
1. Laparoscopy for appendicitis is the most common first-trimester procedure (Rosen & Weiskopf, 1999).
2. Other situations that might lead to surgery during pregnancy include:
   a. Nongynecologic: acute cholecystitis, intestinal obstruction, trauma with visceral injury, vascular accidents (ruptured aneurysms), peptic ulcer, rectal cancer, breast tumors or other malignancies; rarely, maternal cardiac or neurosurgical conditions
   b. Gynecologic: cervical incompetence, ovarian cyst, torsion of fallopian tube, tuboovarian abscess, uterine myoma with degeneration or torsion
   c. Intrauterine fetal surgery as an intervention for certain prenatal congenital defects

CLINICAL PRACTICE

Anesthetic Considerations

A. Concepts essential to planning and management
1. Anesthetic management priorities
   a. Possibility of increased maternal morbidity
      (1) Risk of preterm delivery after surgery during pregnancy is approximately 8.8% (Ludmir & Stubblefield, 2002).
      (2) Risk of spontaneous abortion after surgery is approximately 8% in the first trimester and 6.9% in the second trimester.
   b. Possibility of increased fetal risk from:
      (1) Effects of maternal disease or treatment modalities
      (2) Possible teratogenicity of anesthetic agents
      (3) Intraoperative decrease in uteroplacental flow: fetal hypoxia; uterine flow is not autoregulated and represents approximately 10% of maternal cardiac output by full term (Rosen & Weiskopf, 1999).
      (4) Increased risk of preterm delivery
2. Pregnancy-induced changes in maternal physiology of importance during anesthesia and surgery
   a. Pregnancy-induced changes result from:
      (1) Increases in human chorionic gonadotropin, progesterone, and estrogen; responsible for most first-trimester changes
      (2) Mechanical effects of the gravid uterus
      (3) Increased metabolic demand
      (4) Hemodynamic changes due to presence of low-pressure placental circulation (Gordon, 2002)
   b. Cardiovascular changes
      (1) Increased pulse rate and stroke volume result in cardiac output increases of 30% to 50% during pregnancy.

(2) By 8 weeks' gestation, 57% of the overall increase in cardiac output and 78% of the total increase in stroke volume have occurred (Gordon, 2002).

(3) 90% of overall decrease in peripheral resistance has occurred by 24th week.

(4) During the second trimester, the weight of the uterus compresses the inferior vena cava when mother is supine (25% to 30% decrease in venous return and cardiac output), which can produce supine hypotensive syndrome, especially in the face of anesthetics that abolish compensatory mechanisms.

(5) A gravid uterus can also compress the aorta in a supine client (leading to decreased uteroplacental blood flow and fetal compromise).

(6) Combined hypotensive effect of general or regional anesthesia and aortocaval compression, leading to fetal asphyxia.

(7) Chronic vena caval obstruction in the third trimester predisposes to venous stasis, phlebitis, and lower-extremity edema (Gordon, 2002).

(8) Distention of epidural venous plexus due to vena caval compression contributes to wide spread of smaller amounts of local anesthetics administered epidurally during pregnancy.

c. Respiratory changes

(1) Alveolar ventilation is increased by 25% by 20 weeks' gestation; increased 45% to 70% by term, leading to chronic respiratory alkalosis ($PaCO_2$ is 28 to 32 mmHg; slightly alkaline pH).

(2) Functional residual capacity (FRC) decreases 20%, leading to decreased oxygen reserve.

(3) Decreased FRC, increased oxygen consumption, and decreased buffering capacity cause rapid hypoxemia and acidosis if stressed by hypoventilation or apnea.

(4) Capillary engorgement of nasal and pharyngeal mucosa predisposes to bleeding, trauma, and obstruction.

d. Hematologic changes

(1) Blood volume expansion begins in first trimester, increases to 30% to 45% by term; increased plasma volume causes dilutional anemia. Moderate blood loss is well tolerated, but reserve is decreased when significant hemorrhage occurs.

(2) Pregnancy-induced leukocytosis makes white blood cell (WBC) count an unreliable indicator of infection; might be as high as 12,000/μL during pregnancy with increases up to 20,000/μL during labor.

(3) Hypercoagulable state of pregnancy (increased fibrinogen, factors II, VII, VIII, X, and XII) leads to high postoperative risk of thromboembolic events.

e. Gastrointestinal changes

(1) Lower esophageal sphincter incompetence and distortion of gastric and pyloric anatomy increases risk of esophageal reflux with possible aspiration and resultant pneumonia.

(2) All pregnant patients, after 18 to 20 weeks' gestation, are considered to be at increased risk for aspiration.

3. Potential effects of surgery and anesthesia on the fetus

a. Greatest risk to fetus is intrauterine asphyxia.

(1) Transient decrease in maternal PaO_2 is well tolerated because of increased affinity of fetal hemoglobin for oxygen.

(2) Maternal hypercarbia leads to fetal acidosis, which might cause fetal myocardial depression and hypotension (Gordon, 2002).

(3) Maternal hypocarbia from stress-induced or positive-pressure hyperventilation might produce decreased fetal oxygenation due to resultant umbilical artery constriction and shift of the maternal oxygen/hemoglobin dissociation curve to the left (acidosis); administration of 100% oxygen to mother will result in oxygen tension in fetus of approximately 65 mmHg, which is the maximal possible (Rosen & Weiskopf, 1999).

(4) Uteroplacental perfusion might be reduced as a result of maternal hypotension, which might occur in response to deep general anesthesia, sympathetic blockade from high spinal or epidural blockade, aortocaval compression, hemorrhage, or hypovolemia.

(5) The administration of alpha-adrenergic vasopressor agents, preoperative anxiety, and/or very light levels of general anesthesia might produce increased maternal circulating catecholamines, which can lead to decreased uterine blood flow.

b. Risk of teratogenicity
  (1) Drug-related factors
    (a) Greatest risk of structural abnormalities occurs with drug exposure from approximately day 31 to day 71 after the first day of the last menstrual period.
    (b) Currently administered inhaled or local anesthetics, narcotics, and skeletal muscle relaxants in clinical concentration are not deemed to be teratogenetic or carcinogenic (Rosen & Weiskopf, 1999).
    (c) Long-standing relative contraindication and concern over first-trimester use of benzodiazepine agents has been removed. Research failed to demonstrate link with increased incidence of cleft lip/palate (Koran, Pastuszak, & Ito, 1998).
  (2) Non–drug-related factors
    (a) No congenital defects have been noted after brief periods of hypoxia, hypercarbia, or hypoglycemia.
    (b) Effect of maternal stress and anxiety is questionable because of the lack of supportive research.
    (c) Central nervous system congenital anomalies are associated with maternal fever (>39° C) during the first half of pregnancy.
    (d) Ionizing radiation: no congenital defects from exposure below 10 rads (average chest radiograph exposure = 8 millirads).
    (e) The increased incidence of abortion, early delivery, and perinatal mortality associated with anesthesia and surgery might be attributed to the surgical site and/or underlying conditions; no clear relationship between outcome and type of anesthesia has been demonstrated.

B. General maternal preoperative assessment
  1. History and physical examination
   a. Gestational age
    (1) By date of last menstrual period (LMP) or ultrasound test
    (2) Palpation of uterine size; fundal height
   b. Urgency of need for surgery
   c. Presence of underlying chronic or acute illness
   d. Known drug allergies
   e. Current medications (prescription, over-the-counter, herbal, and recreational)
   f. Surgical history: previous procedures and responses to anesthesia
   g. Previous obstetric history

     h. Pain evaluation: location, intensity, characteristics, duration, and client tolerance

     i. Vital signs

       (1) Temperature

       (2) Pulse

       (3) Respiration

       (4) Blood pressure

     j. Evaluation of fetal heart rate (FHR) by Doppler or continuous fetal monitoring

     k. Evaluation of uterine activity

       (1) Palpation and client reported

       (2) Continuous fetal monitoring

     l. Respiratory status: dyspnea, evidence of distress, history of recent fever, or congestion, asthma, inhalant allergies, or smoking

     m. Cardiovascular status: presence of pregnancy-induced hypertension (PIH), history of rheumatic fever, or mitral valve dysfunction

     n. Hepatic status: history of hepatitis and alcohol consumption

     o. Renal status: history of bladder or kidney infection

  2. Psychosocial response

     a. Stress factors producing anxiety

       (1) Fear of loss or harm to fetus

       (2) Fear of harm to self

       (3) Lack of understanding of planned procedure, anesthesia options, and possible outcomes

     b. Behavioral factors

       (1) Desire to meet cultural expectation

       (2) Variable response to pain

       (3) Difficulty with open expression of fears and anxieties

  3. Laboratory/diagnostic procedures

     a. Ultrasonography

     b. Fetal monitoring

     c. Preoperative laboratory evaluation: complete blood count (CBC), urinalysis (UA), and type and crossmatch of blood products as indicated

     d. Electrocardiogram (ECG); chest radiograph (shielded), if indicated because of preexisting cardiovascular or pulmonary disease (e.g., floppy mitral valve, questionable aspiration pneumonitis, history of rheumatic fever)

C. Surgical choices: open laparotomy versus laparoscopic approach

  1. Overall safety of laparoscopy during the first half of pregnancy has been confirmed (Reedy, Kallen, & Kuehl, 1997).

  2. Laparoscopy is safest during the second trimester when there is less risk of spontaneous abortion or premature labor due to manipulation. There is increased risk of uterine puncture during the third trimester due to large size of the uterus (Malangoni, 2003).

  3. Risk might be lessened during laparoscopy if:

     a. Intraperitoneal pressure is maintained at 10 to 15 mmHg or lower to protect uterine perfusion (Cappell, 2003; Malangoni, 2003; Affleck, Handrahan, Egger, Wallace, & Lu, 1999).

     b. Carbon dioxide should be used for production of pneumoperitoneum.

     c. Client should be placed in reverse Trendelenburg in the left-side-down position, if possible.

     d. Intraoperative fetal monitoring is performed, if possible.

    4. Advantages of laparoscopy include better visualization, smaller incision, less pain, less operative time, decreased recovery time, earlier ambulation, decreased risk of thromoembolic disease.

    5. Open laparotomy is required when sufficient access is not possible with laparoscopy or when profound uterine relaxation is required to facilitate the planned procedure.

D. Anesthetic choices

  1. Preoperative medication

    a. Low-dose benzodiazepine and/or narcotic to allay maternal anxiety

    b. H_2 receptor antagonist and 30 ml of clear antacid as a precaution against acid aspiration

  2. Choice of anesthetic technique

    a. Basic considerations

      (1) No studies correlate improved maternal or fetal outcome with any specific anesthetic technique.

      (2) Local and regional techniques are useful for cervical cerclage, urologic, or lower-extremity procedures.

      (3) General anesthesia is required for most abdominal procedures.

    b. Specific considerations

      (1) After 18 to 20 weeks, left displacement of uterus is necessary when client is positioned on the operating table to avoid supine hypotensive syndrome and aortocaval compression.

      (2) Basic perioperative monitoring: blood pressure, ECG, and pulse oximetry; general anesthesia requires the addition of capnography, temperature monitor, and nerve stimulator to assess skeletal muscle relaxation.

      (3) General anesthetic choices

        (a) High concentration oxygen plus a potent opioid (fentanyl or sufentanil) and/or a moderate concentration of a volatile agent (e.g., isoflurane, enflurane, sevoflurane), and a skeletal muscle relaxant

        (b) N_2O might be safely chosen, especially after the sixth week of gestation.

      (4) Regional anesthesia

        (a) Epidural/spinal anesthesia

          (i) Fetal hypoxia occurs if maternal systolic blood pressure drops below 100 mmHg; in healthy pregnant women; 1 to 2 L of crystalloid fluid might be infused to prevent maternal hypotension.

          (ii) Clients with PIH experience decreased placental flow at higher systolic pressures than do normal pregnant women.

        (b) Increased vascularity and sensitivity to local anesthetics present during pregnancy; observe for signs of toxicity after injection (e.g., tingling, tinnitus, shivering, unexplained confusion or drowsiness).

  3. Other intraoperative considerations

    a. FHR monitoring

      (1) If feasible, with external tocodynamometer intraoperatively and in immediate postoperative period to detect any need for administration of tocolytic agents.

      (2) Unexplained change in FHR: evaluate maternal position, blood pressure, oxygenation, acid-base balance, whether surgeon or retractor placement is impairing uterine perfusion.

    (3) Maternal hypothermia can cause a decrease in baseline fetal heart rate, as well as beat to beat variability, but it does not cause spontaneous decelerations (Rosen & Weiskopf, 1999).

    (4) Management plan must be in place regarding what to do in the face of persistent fetal distress (i.e., feasibility of cesarean section).

  b. Prevention of aortocaval compression

  c. Prevention of preterm labor

    (1) Procedures with minimal uterine manipulation occurring after the first trimester of pregnancy carry the lowest risk for preterm labor.

    (2) Prophylactic use of tocolytic agents is not without complications but has been suggested for clients at greatest risk (e.g., for cervical cerclage); if unsuccessful, beta$_2$-agonist tocolytic agents might complicate anesthesia because of production of tachycardia (Ludmir & Stubblefield, 2002).

E. Nursing Diagnoses

  1. Altered maternal physiologic dynamics related to surgery and anesthesia

  2. Altered fetal physiologic dynamics related to surgery and anesthesia

  3. Pain and anxiety related to risk for altered client and fetal health

F. Interventions/Outcomes

  1. Altered maternal physiologic dynamics related to surgery and anesthesia

  2. Altered fetal physiologic dynamics related to surgery and anesthesia

  a. Interventions: preoperative

    (1) Monitor and record vital signs.

    (2) Provide intravenous (IV) hydration.

      (a) Maintenance by 16- or 18-gauge intracatheter infusion of nondextrose crystalloid solution (Ringer's lactate or normal saline)

      (b) 1 to 2 L might be ordered for volume expansion before administration of epidural or spinal anesthetic or if patient is fluid depleted due to illness.

    (3) Utilize left lateral positioning in the second and third trimesters to prevent aortocaval compression, which might result in decreased uteroplacental blood flow; if left lateral position is not possible, place a wedge (pillow or rolled blanket) under right hip to displace uterus to the left.

    (4) Utilize FHR monitoring: Doppler or external fetal monitor.

    (5) Assess preoperative laboratory test results for abnormalities that might alter or complicate perioperative care.

    (6) Communicate findings to other members of the care team.

  b. Interventions: postoperative (in addition to those just mentioned)

    (1) Monitor vital signs frequently within the first 1 to 2 postoperative hours.

      (a) Overall, general anesthetics produce varying degrees of vasodilatation and impair compensatory mechanisms, thereby increasing the potential for postoperative hypotension.

      (b) A major side effect of regional anesthesia (spinal or epidural) is hypotension due to sympathetic paralysis and resultant peripheral vasodilatation; increased fluid and lateral positioning might stabilize this transient event.

    (2) Administer humidified oxygen via face mask (8 to 10 L/min).

(a) Presence of general anesthetic agents that might depress respiration.

(b) Pregnancy-induced increased mucosal vascularity of nose and throat predisposes client to hoarseness and laryngeal edema following endotracheal intubation during general anesthesia.

(3) Monitor and record intake and output (I&O).

(4) Assess for thrombosis/phlebitis (Homans' sign) and apply antiembolic stockings.

(5) FHR and uterine activity should be monitored to assess any alteration in fetal tissue perfusion.

(6) Adequate analgesics to manage pain should be administered systemically or by spinal/epidural injection, as appropriate.

(a) Client receiving analgesics might be unaware of onset of uterine contractions.

(b) Apply comfort measures (e.g., positioning, use of pillows for support).

(c) After cervical cerclage, position client in slight Trendelenburg position to decrease cervical pressure.

(d) Provide and instruct client in incentive spirometry and coughing/deep breathing exercises.

(7) Avoid vasoconstrictors (might decrease uteroplacental blood flow).

  c. Outcomes

(1) Client's vital signs remain stable.

(2) Client maintains adequate oxygenation and circulation throughout the perioperative period.

(3) Client maintains adequate intake and output.

(4) Client avoids thromboembolic phenomenon.

(5) Client experiences adequate pain control.

(6) FHR remains within normal range.

(7) Signs of impending preterm labor are recognized and treated properly.

3. Pain and anxiety related to risk for altered client and fetal health

  a. Interventions

(1) During the preoperative and postoperative periods:

(a) Assess client's response and ability to cope with current situation.

(b) Assess presence of social support systems and plan integration into client care.

(c) Provide opportunity for verbalization of fears, anxieties, and concerns.

(d) Facilitate ability of surgeon, anesthesia provider, client, and family to discuss surgical and anesthetic options.

(e) Teach stress reduction techniques, and reinforce client's ability to implement techniques.

(f) Integrate mental health care team into client care, if needed.

  b. Outcomes

(1) Client demonstrates positive coping strategies.

(2) Social support system is involved with client care.

(3) Client demonstrates stress reduction techniques.

(4) Client demonstrates knowledge of anesthetic choices, risks and benefits, and recommendations.

SPECIFIC SURGICAL PROCEDURES

Cholecystectomy

A. Introduction

1. Incidence of acute cholecystitis during pregnancy is 1 per 1000 to 1600 gestations; is the cause of more than 90% of cholecystectomies performed during pregnancy (Winstrom & Malee, 1999).

   a. Risk of gallstone development during pregnancy is 2% to 10% due to decreased motility and resultant increased biliary sludge (Winstrom & Malee, 1999).

   b. Glasgow and colleagues (1998) indicated that conservative treatment failed in 36% of cases in a study, including summary case data from 1980 to 1996, whereas Ghumman, Barry, & Grace (1997) reported that in 90% of patients, an acute process resolves with conservative treatment.

2. Previous pregnancies predispose to cholecystitis.

3. Surgical management is used only if medical management is unsuccessful or if rupture of gallbladder or pancreatitis is evident.

4. Optimal timing of surgery is during second trimester (after highest risk of spontaneous abortion and organogenesis has passed and before enlarging, uterus impairs surgical exposure).

5. Maternal mortality (15%) and fetal loss (60%) have been associated with secondary pancreatitis; gallstone pancreatitis can be managed with an endoscopic retrograde cholangiogram (Barone, Bears, Chen, Tasi, & Russell, 1999; Barthel, Chowdhury, & Miedema, 1998).

6. Surgery should not be delayed if urgently indicated, such as in gallstone pancreatitis or unresolved cholecystitis.

7. Primary second-trimester risk of surgery is preterm labor.

8. A laparoscopic surgical approach might be selected for cholecystectomy or appendectomy in the first trimester of pregnancy (LeMaire & van Erp, 1997). This approach has been reported to significantly reduce the time of hospitalization, decrease the need for narcotic analgesics, and produce quicker return to regular diet compared with open laparotomy in pregnant women. Open laparotomy is the chosen approach later in pregnancy (Affleck et al., 1999).

9. Specific considerations of laparoscopic approach include:

   a. Additional risk of gastric reflux and aspiration due to upward pressure of pneumoperitoneum during surgery

   b. During immediate postoperative period, client experiencing shoulder or back pain from irritation by CO_2 used to produce pneumoperitoneum

B. Procedure-specific client assessment (in addition to general maternal preoperative assessment)

1. History

   a. Assessment of pain: stabbing, colicky, or steady midepigastric pain that radiates to the right upper quadrant, right flank, or right shoulder

   b. Excessive flatulence, heartburn, or fatty-food intolerance

   c. Increased discomfort after meals

   d. Nausea or vomiting

   e. Medical and surgical history

   f. Obstetric history

   g. Gestational age by LMP or ultrasonography

2. Physical examination

   a. Abdominal examination

      (1) Palpation: rebound tenderness, rigidity, and uterine contractions
      (2) Auscultation
        (a) Presence of bowel sounds
        (b) Peristaltic rushes (borborygmi) might indicate an intestinal obstruction.
  b. Vaginal examination
      (1) Presence or absence of vaginal bleeding: the client should not experience bleeding with a diagnosis of cholecystitis.
      (2) Cervical examination to differentiate pain from preterm labor contractions
  c. Inspiratory effort often accentuates pain (Murphy's sign).
  d. Evaluate for volume deficit due to decreased oral intake, vomiting, or nasogastric suction.
 3. Laboratory/diagnostic procedures
  a. Laboratory tests
      (1) CBC with differential
        (a) WBC of 15,000 to 20,000 mm^3 might be normal in pregnancy.
        (b) Hemoglobin level should be stable (greater than 10.0 g/dl).
      (2) UA and urine culture to differentiate cholecystitis from pyelonephritis or cystitis
      (3) Electrolytes, liver function tests, and bilirubin
        (a) Hyperamylasemia is usually indicative of gallstone pancreatitis.
        (b) Serum alkaline phosphatase value might be increased to twice that of nonpregnant values (even higher values might occur in cholecystitis).
        (c) Severely elevated bilirubin predisposes to pancreatitis.
        (d) Jaundice and abnormal hepatic transaminase levels suggest choledocholithiasis (Mayer & Hussain, 1998).
  b. Ultrasonography: fetal viability; if cholelithiasis is present, dilated common bile duct and biliary tree will be present.
  c. Fetal monitoring to rule out preterm labor (see Chapter 12 for further discussion)

Ovarian Tumors: Ovarian Cystectomy or Oophorectomy

A. Introduction
 1. Hazards related to ovarian tumors
  a. Possibility of malignancy
  b. Torsion
  c. Rupture with hemorrhage
  d. Infection
 2. Corpus luteum cysts
  a. Corpus luteum cysts are most common during the first trimester; support pregnancy during that time.
  b. After first trimester, there is a decreased risk of spontaneous abortion from removal (Ludmir & Stubblefield, 2002).
 3. Benign ovarian tumors
  a. Dermoids
  b. Serous cystadenomas
  c. Mucinous cystadenomas
 4. Malignant ovarian tumors
  a. Dysgerminomas

   b. Granulosa cell tumors
  5. Ultrasound test is the most useful tool for diagnosis and evaluation.
  6. Surgical intervention indicated if tumor is:
    a. Solid
    b. Bilateral
    c. Hormonally active
    d. Symptomatic
    e. Increasing in size
B. Procedure-specific client assessment (in addition to general maternal preoperative assessment)
  1. History
    a. Pain: onset, location, and quality
    b. Presence of vaginal bleeding
    c. Gestational age by date of LMP or ultrasound test
    d. Presence of adnexal mass by palpation or ultrasound test
    e. Medical and surgical history, especially previous gynecologic surgery
    f. Obstetric history: previous pregnancies or complications
    g. Ability to urinate: as tumor enlarges, might cause urinary obstruction.
  2. Physical examination
    a. Presence of adnexal mass confirmed by pelvic examination, ultrasound test, or both
    b. Palpation of uterine contractions
    c. Presence of vaginal bleeding
    d. Cervical status: presence of dilation
    e. Fundal height: approximate for gestational age or increasing as tumor enlarging
    f. Abdominal examination: presence of ascites and distended bladder
  3. Diagnostic procedures
    a. Ultrasound test: fetal and adnexal mass evaluation (solid or cystic and estimation of size)
    b. Fetal monitoring to assess FHR and rule out preterm labor preoperatively and postoperatively

Appendectomy

A. Introduction
  1. Incidence
    a. Is the most common surgical complication of pregnancy.
    b. Surgery to remove the appendix occurs in approximately 1 in every 500 to 1000 pregnancies (Winstrom & Malee, 1999).
    c. Occurs most often in first and second trimester (Visser, Glasgow, Mulvihill, & Mulvihill, 2001).
    d. Misdiagnosis is estimated to occur in 36% of all cases, with a rate of approximately 23% during the first trimester and 43% during the last two trimesters.
  2. Symptoms
    a. Enlarged uterus makes interpretation of physical signs difficult.
    b. Right flank pain is present rather than right lower quadrant pain, because during pregnancy the appendix rotates counterclockwise as the uterus enlarges; near term, the appendiceal tip lies over the right kidney, well above McBurney's point; the tip can also be anchored in the pelvis by adhesions (Winstrom & Malee, 1999; Tracey & Fletcher, 2000; Visser et al., 2001) (Figure 26-1).

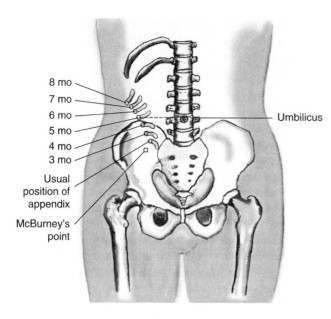

8 mo
7 mo
6 mo
5 mo
4 mo
3 mo
Usual
position of
appendix
McBurney's
point

Umbilicus

FIGURE 26-1 ■ Relative position of appendix during progression of pregnancy. (From Lowdermilk, D.L., & Perry, S.E. [2004]. *Maternity & women's health care* [8th ed.]. St. Louis: Mosby.)

 c. Rebound tenderness has been noted to be less in late pregnancy; abdominal guarding is a less reliable symptom late in pregnancy due to the laxity of the abdominal wall muscles (Tracey & Fletcher, 2000; Visser et al., 2001).

 d. Symptoms might be confused with:

  (1) Preterm labor

  (2) Pyelonephritis

 e. No cervical change should be present.

3. Peritonitis increases the incidence of preterm labor.

 a. Symptoms of perforation with peritonitis might be masked during pregnancy because of increased steroid levels, which decrease the normal inflammatory response.

 b. If perforation is present, client must be evaluated for administration of tocolytic agents.

 c. Perinatal outcome is worst if acute appendicitis occurs in the second trimester, although maternal morbidity appears to be the same across the entire gestational period.

 d. If perforation and peritonitis are absent, a laparoscopic approach might be chosen during the first trimester; an open laparotomy will be chosen later in gestation or in complicated cases (for laparoscopic considerations, see discussion of cholecystectomy).

B. Procedure-specific client assessment (in addition to general maternal preoperative assessment)

 1. History

  a. Gestational age by date of LMP or ultrasonography

  b. Symptoms

   (1) Nausea and vomiting

   (2) Fever

   (3) Periumbilical pain

   (4) Right flank pain

   (5) Anorexia

   (6) Constipation

   (7) Diarrhea

    c. Assessment of pain: location, duration, quality, and aggravating or alleviating factors

2. Physical examination
   a. Abdominal examination
     (1) Rebound tenderness: less prevalent in late pregnancy
     (2) Uterine contractions
   b. Evidence of vaginal bleeding
   c. Cervical examination for labor status

3. Diagnostic procedures
   a. Laboratory tests
     (1) CBC with differential
       (a) Hemoglobin level should be greater than 10.
       (b) WBC might not be helpful because values of 15,000 to 20,000 mm^3 occur in pregnancy and labor; however, a shift to the left (differential count of greater than 80% polymorphonuclear leukocytes) is a significant finding (Tracey & Fletcher, 2000; Visser et al., 2001).
     (2) UA and urine culture
       (a) Help to differentiate urinary tract infection from the clinical picture.
       (b) In the second half of pregnancy, pyuria has been found in 20% of patients with appendicitis; sterile pyuria might result from the proximity of the appendix to the ureter or renal pelvis.
   b. Ultrasonography: to assess fetal well-being as well as signs of placental abruption

Cervical Cerclage
A. **Introduction**
1. Cervical incompetence (Benifla et al., 1997).
   a. Painless dilation of cervix during second trimester
   b. Repeated second-trimester abortion in absence of contractions
   c. Short cervical length as assessed by vaginal sonography
2. Surgical technique that closes or supports cervix at level of internal os is done to support pregnancy to viability.
   a. McDonald's suture: Mersilene suture placed at cervicovaginal junction and removed for labor.
   b. Shirodkar procedure: Mersilene tape encircles the cervix, is passed under the mucosa; might be removed for labor or to perform cesarean section.
   c. Laparoscopic placement and removal of a transabdominal cerclage has been reported as a promising therapeutic option for clients with history of failed cerclage (Lesser, Childers, & Surwit, 1998).
3. Optimal timing
   a. After first trimester, most practitioners choose between 14 and 18 weeks' gestation.
   b. After 20 weeks' gestation, preliminary research indicates a significant negative linear relationship between term at time of cerclage and prolongation of pregnancy.
   c. Suture usually removed electively at 37 weeks.
4. Tocolytic therapy as an adjunctive therapy might be considered to treat preterm labor or uterine irritability.

B. **Procedure-specific client assessment** (in addition to general maternal preoperative assessment)
   1. History
      a. Gestational age by date of LMP or ultrasound test
      b. Obstetric history of second-trimester cervical dilation or fetal losses
      c. Previous gynecologic surgery and cervical laceration
      d. History of premature rupture of membranes (PROM) in previous pregnancies
      e. History of vaginal bleeding
      f. Diethylstilbestrol (DES) exposure
   2. Physical examination
      a. Pelvic examination
         (1) Cervical dilation (less than or equal to 3 to 4 cm to be candidate for cerclage)
         (2) Evidence of infection (treatment of infection before cerclage)
         (3) Status of membranes (must be intact for cerclage)
      b. FHR: presence (viability)
   3. Diagnostic procedures
      a. Ultrasonography: gestation, cervical length, and internal os dilation
      b. Palpation of uterus to assess uterine activity and/or use of external fetal monitor to determine presence of distress

ENDOSCOPIC GASTROINTESTINAL PROCEDURES

A. **Introduction**
   1. Incidence
      a. Approximately 12,000 pregnant women each year in the United States have strong indications for EGD; indications for sigmoidoscopy or colonoscopy exist in an additional 6000 pregnancies (Cappell, 2003).
      b. Approximately 1000 pregnant women each year demonstrate the need for therapeutic ERCP (Cappell, 2003).
   2. Risks of endoscopy during pregnancy include:
      a. Premature labor
      b. Potential teratogenesis from medications administered during the procedure
      c. Placental abruption or fetal trauma during placement of the endoscope in certain procedures
      d. Systemic hypotension/hypertension
      e. Transient maternal or fetal hypoxia
   3. Cholelithiasis occurs in approximately 8% of pregnancies.
      a. Cholecystectomy might be delayed until the postpartum period for uncomplicated cholelithiasis that responds to conservative medical treatment.
      b. Choledocholithiasis usually requires urgent therapy due to the potential for cholangitis or gallstone pancreatitis that might be life-threatening. In this situation, therapeutic ERCP is an alternative to biliary surgery but carries more risk than EGD due to longer procedure time, needs for greater exposure to medications, and radiation exposure.
   4. Gastrointestinal bleeding is the primary indication for EGD during pregnancy.
      a. Increased incidence in susceptible clients might be due to increased variceal bleeding from portal hypertension secondary to gestational increases in plasma volume.
      b. Other indications for EGD include undiagnosed abdominal pain and prolonged vomiting (Cappell, 2003).

5. Sigmoidoscopy does not induce labor or produce congenital abnormalities in medically stable pregnant women with indications, such as lower gastrointestinal bleeding, rectal mass, or rectal obstruction.
6. Few safety data are available on colonoscopy during pregnancy, but it might be considered for confirmation of suspected colonic cancer, for severe colonic bleeding, or prior to urgent colonic surgery (Cappell, 2003).
7. Colorectal and gastric cancer are the most common malignancies found during pregnancy. Incidence might be increasing, owing to a trend toward delaying pregnancy until later in life when the overall prevalence of cancer is higher (Visser et al., 2001).
8. Most cancer of the large bowel found during pregnancy is in the rectal area. This differs from nonpregnant women of the same age; the reason is unknown.

B. **Procedure-specific client assessment** (in addition to general maternal preoperative assessment)
   1. Risks to the mother/fetus
      a. EDG or ERCP can produce maternal respiratory compromise and resultant hypoxia from:
         (1) Medications administered
         (2) Vagally mediated bronchospasm due to stretching of the viscera
         (3) Laryngeal impingement during esophageal intubation with resultant pulmonary aspiration (Cappell, 2003)
      b. Sigmoidoscopy/colonoscopy can produce hypoxia due to:
         (1) IV sedation medications administered
         (2) Circulatory changes due to vagal responses to colonic distension (Cappell, 2003)
   2. Methods of risk management (Cappell, 2003)
      a. Defer endoscopy until after the first trimester if possible.
      b. Defer endoscopy until postpartum if possible.
      c. Administer smallest effective dose of all required medications during procedure.
      d. Involve client in decisions about use of potentially fetotoxic drugs; always use drugs with greatest fetal safety, if possible.
      e. Consider use of qualified anesthesia provider (physician anesthesiologist or Certified Registered Nurse Anesthetist) to provide sedation during procedure.
      f. If bipolar cautery is used for hemostasis, biopsy, polypectomy, or papillotomy, be sure grounding pad is positioned so uterus is not directly between the cautery and the grounding pad to minimize fetal exposure.
   3. Laboratory/diagnostic procedures
      a. Endorectal ultrasound is useful to stage rectal carcinomas.
      b. Magnetic resonance imaging (MRI) is preferred to abdominal computed tomography scan (CT) to evaluate metastatic or regional disease.
      c. Serum carcinoembryonic antigen (CEA) levels remain reliable diagnostic indicators and should be measured, because this value is not affected by pregnancy.

INTRAUTERINE FETAL SURGERY

A. **Introduction**
   1. Birth defects account for more than 21% of all infant deaths; first intrauterine fetal surgery to repair a congenital defect took place in 1981 (Hamid & Newfield, 2001).

    2. Was initially considered only for treatment of life-threatening defects; now considered for repair of nonlethal defects as well (Farmer, 2003).

    3. Decision requires balancing risk to mother and fetus against potential benefit to only the fetus.

    4. Maternal safety increased by use of fetoscopic approach over open hysterotomy.

    5. Potential maternal complications associated with fetal surgery include (Farmer, 2003; Hamid & Newfield, 2001; Ranzini, 1999):

      a. Oligohydramnios: should prompt search for uterine rupture (Ranzini, 1999).

      b. Premature separation of membranes: incidence is as high as 47% following hysterotomy (Sydorak, 2002).

      c. Preterm labor

      d. Earlier gestational age at delivery

      e. Increased life-long risk of uterine rupture following hysterotomy

    6. Defects in which fetal surgery has made a positive impact on fetal outcomes (Flake, 2003; Holmes, Harrison, & Baskin, 2001; Wilson, 2002):

      a. Congenital diaphragmatic hernia

      b. Twin-twin transfusion syndrome

      c. Certain pulmonary lesions

      d. As use of fetal surgery in nonfatal defects increases, it has been suggested that prenatal correction of cleft lip/palate might be attempted because fetal wound healing leaves no scars up to a certain point in gestation (Wagner & Harrison, 2002).

    7. Defects in which fetal surgery risks and outcomes have been more controversial include (Holmes et al., 2001):

      a. Spina bifida/hydrocephalus

      b. Obstructive uropathy

    8. Survey of Society for Maternal-Fetal Medicine members indicated that (Lyerly, Cefalo, Socol, Fogarty, & Sugarman, 2001):

      a. 47% refer clients for open fetal surgery for nonlethal conditions.

      b. 69% believe it is the physician's responsibility to inform client of this option.

      c. 87% believe fetal surgical procedures should be done only under institutional review board approved management protocols.

B. Specific anomalies amenable to fetal surgery

    1. Severe congenital diaphragmatic hernia (with liver herniated into the chest)

      a. Initially treatment was by open hysterotomy with full anatomic repair; newer approach is the use of minimally invasive fetoscopic repair by temporary tracheal occlusion by Fetendo balloon. Tracheal occlusion prevents lung fluid from leaving and increases the transpulmonic pressure, thereby distending the hypoplastic lungs (Flake et al., 2002; Harrison et al., 2001). The overall efficacy of this procedure is currently under study.

      b. Fetoscopic procedure produces survival rate of 75%; treatment after birth yields 40% to 50% survival of the fetus (Farmer, 2003)

      c. Candidates for procedure must be identified before 24 weeks gestation and the ratio of lung to head is less than 1.4 (Cauldwell, 2002; Farmer, 2003)

      d. Tracheal balloon is removed at time of delivery by cesarean section under deep general anesthesia. Deep anesthesia is necessary to produce maximal uterine relaxation while maintaining optimal fetal-placental circulation (Harrison et al., 2001; Schwartz et al., 2001).

2. Twin-twin transfusion syndrome (Cauldwell, 2002)
   a. Results from unbalanced intertwin transfusion between monochorionic twins, which leads to:
      (1) A recipient twin with polyhydramnios and hydrops, and
      (2) A donor twin who develops oligohydramnios, growth restriction, and increased mortality
   b. A similar pathology is twin reversal arterial perfusion syndrome in which:
      (1) One twin is acardiac/anencephalic and nonviable with a vascular anastomosis.
      (2) A normal twin develops heart failure due to the stress of providing cardiac output for both fetuses.
   c. 80% fetal mortality if diagnosed in mid-trimester
   d. Trials underway comparing fetoscopic laser ablation of abnormal placental vessels with amnioreduction to treat this abnormality (Farmer, 2003)
3. Central nervous system lesions
   a. Spina bifida/hydrocephalus
      (1) Neural tube defects are among most common congenital abnormalities
         (a) Anencephaly and encephalocele account for 50% of all neural tube defects.
         (b) The remainder occurs along the spine with myelomeningocele being most prevalent (4.4-4.6 cases per 10,000 live births; approximately 2000 infants/year in the United States) (Bruner, Boehm, & Tulipan, 1999; Hamid & Newfield, 2001).
      (2) Myelomeningoceles occur at end of the fourth week of gestation if the neural tube fails to close spontaneously. Early diagnosis is aided by measuring maternal alpha-fetoprotein levels with follow-up use of sonography in the second trimester (Hamid & Newfield, 2001).
      (3) The "two-hit hypothesis" for the pathology: primary defect in closure of the neural tube plus secondary injury to exposed neural tissue from chronic mechanical trauma and amniotic fluid–induced chemical injury. In utero repair might decrease this damage (Bannister, 2000; Hamid & Newfield, 2001).
      (4) Hydroureteronephrosis and vesicoureteral reflux present in 10% to 30% of fetuses with myelomeningocele. If untreated, 40% to 90% suffer significant upper urinary tract deterioration (Hamid & Newfield, 2001).
      (5) Fetal surgery at 23 weeks gestation for a lesion extending from T11 to S1 level with associated Arnold-Chiari type malformation and borderline hydrocephalus has been reported to be successful in reducing hydrocephalus (Adzick, Sutton, Crombleholme, & Flake, 1998).
      (6) Nonfatal lesion; more than 100 have been repaired by fetal surgery; most show no change in level of paralysis, but up to 33% have improvement in Chiari formation, thus decreasing the need for ventriculoperitoneal shunting. It has been noted that lesions above L3 in fetuses older than 25 weeks gestation might not benefit in terms of decreasing hydrocephalus (Farmer, 2003; Tulipan et al., 2003).
   b. Sacrococcygeal teratoma (Paek et al., 2001; Farmer, 2003)
      (1) Solid, highly vascular tumor identified by ultrasonograph can lead to fetal demise due to vascular steal syndrome. Substantial arteriovenous shunting through the tumor might result in heart failure and hydrops fetalis.
      (2) In a small study by Paek and colleagues (2001), a noninvasive radiofrequency needle probe ablation of vessels feeding the tumor

decreased blood flow sufficiently to reverse high output fetal heart failure.

(3) Fetus with a cystic, avascular tumor will survive neonatal period regardless of tumor size; can be treated postnatally.

4. Obstructive uropathy

a. First done with open fetal surgery at University of California, San Francisco in 1981; now performed via percutaneous insertion of vesicoamniotic shunts in office setting. Efficacy of procedure currently under study (Farmer, 2003; Holmes et al., 2001).

b. Indication for surgery is presence of bilateral hydronephrosis with oligohydramnios.

c. Posterior urethral valves are thin membranes of obstructive tissue; most common cause of lower urinary tract obstruction in male infants (1 in 8000 to 1 in 25,000 births). Laser ablation of valves via fetal endoscopy can be done; mean gestational age at intervention is 22.5 weeks (Holmes et al., 2001).

d. Removal of obstruction allows restoration of amniotic fluid levels necessary for normal pulmonary maturation. Lung development takes place between 16 and 28 weeks; without adequate fluid, bronchi never develop, pulmonary hypoplasia appears, and death from respiratory failure occurs at birth.

e. Overall efficacy in preserving lung and kidney function is currently under study.

C. Approaches and concerns in fetal surgery

1. Surgical approaches

a. Minimal access fetal surgery is performed endoscopically with one small uterine trocar for placement (Bruner et al., 1999).

(1) Can be performed under general or regional anesthesia.

(2) Study by Aaronson (2002) indicated potential for future use of robot-assisted, minimally invasive endoscopic systems to decrease the associated risks of fetal surgery.

b. Hysterotomy is a procedure in which the uterus is opened to allow direct operation on the fetus.

(1) Always requires general anesthesia to produce maximal uterine relaxation.

(2) Might open the uterus using electrocautery following assessment of placental location and fetal lie by ultrasonography.

c. Intraoperative management

(1) Maternal safety

(2) Avoidance of teratogenic anesthetic and ancillary drugs

(3) Avoidance of fetal and maternal asphyxia

(4) Adequate fetal anesthesia and monitoring

(5) Adequate uterine relaxation

(6) Prevention of premature labor (Cauldwell, 2002)

d. Trends during past 10 years in fetal surgery (Fowler, 2002)

(1) Shorter operative times

(2) Use of less numerous and smaller entry ports to the uterus

(3) Decreased blood loss

(4) Type of cases centered on twin-twin transfusion syndrome and congenital diaphragmatic hernia treatment

D. **Procedure-specific client assessment** (in addition to general maternal preoperative assessment): following determination of the surgical approach same as endoscopic considerations and perioperative nursing interventions.

HEALTH EDUCATION

Client Education and Preparation for Perioperative Experience

A. **Involve client in planned care.**
   1. Surgical options
   2. Anesthetic options
   3. Methods of pain control
   4. Postoperative care
B. **Teach signs and symptoms of preterm labor** (see Chapter 29 for further information).
C. **Discharge instructions should include:**
   1. Follow-up care as ordered by physician
   2. Report signs and symptoms of:
      a. Infection
      b. Fever
      c. Vaginal bleeding
      d. Excessive pain
   3. Report signs and symptoms of preterm labor.
   4. Discussion of importance of client's awareness of and cooperation with the following:
      a. Antiembolic or support stockings
      b. Progressive ambulation and activity (or restrictions)
      c. Diet and fluid intake
      d. Adequate rest
      e. Avoidance of heavy lifting (including lifting children)
      f. Avoidance of constipation
   5. Review medications: dose, route, frequency, and potential side effects.
D. **Emphasize importance of social support and increased assistance at home during immediate postoperative period.**

SUMMARY

A. **The greatest risk to the fetus during nonobstetric surgery is intrauterine asphyxia.**
B. **No anesthetic technique or agent has been shown to make a significant difference in maternal or fetal outcome after nonobstetric surgery in the pregnant client.**
C. **Management of the pregnant surgical client should focus on prevention of hypoxemia, acidosis, hypotension, and hyperventilation.**

CASE STUDIES AND STUDY QUESTIONS

A 25-year-old gravida 1, para 0 (G1, P0) patient at 18 weeks of gestation arrives in the emergency room with a 2-day history of right flank pain, nausea and vomiting, and anorexia. She denies urinary frequency, urgency, or burning and states that her last bowel movement was 24 hours prior to admission. On examination, pain is elicited with deep palpation at the right flank and right lower abdominal quadrant. The uterus is soft and nontender. The pelvic examination reveals a long cervix without dilation, and the adnexa are not palpable.

Vital signs: oral temperature, 38.3° C (101° F); pulse of 92/min; respiratory rate of 16 breaths/min; blood pressure, 124/72; FHR, 140/min.

Admission laboratory values: hemoglobin, 12.4 g/dl; WBC, 24,000 mm³; UA, clear. Client is sent for an ultrasound test that reveals a viable singleton pregnancy at 18 weeks' gestation, with no evidence of separation of the placenta. A laparoscopic appendectomy is performed, and the postoperative course is without complication. A healthy infant is delivered without complication at term.

1. During surgery the *greatest* risk to the viability of the infant would be:
   a. Administration of beta-adrenergic vasopressors
   b. Severe maternal hypotension
   c. Exposure to general anesthetic agents
   d. Maternal hypothermia

2. During perioperative management of this client:
   a. Therapy with tocolytic agents is essential.
   b. Dehydration is not a consideration because of her expanded blood volume.
   c. Left lateral uterine displacement should be applied to protect fetal blood flow.
   d. Steroids should be administered to prevent laryngeal edema.

3. In the immediate postoperative period the client complains of right shoulder and chest pain; this is most likely due to:
   a. Irritation from retained abdominal CO_2
   b. Referred pain from onset of uterine contractions
   c. Right upper lobe aspiration
   d. Pneumothorax

4. In the immediate postoperative period, the client complains of a scratchy throat and mild hoarseness. This is due to:
   a. Intraoperative damage to the vocal cords
   b. Normal, hormone-induced edema
   c. Mild, transient irritation from endotracheal tube placement during surgery
   d. Right upper-lobe pulmonary aspiration

5. Immediately after surgery, the client receives narcotics for pain control. During this period of time, it is important to:
   a. Give as little as possible to avoid damage to the fetus.
   b. Get the client to take oral medications as quickly as possible.
   c. Begin tocolytic therapy.
   d. Monitor carefully for unrecognized uterine contractions.

6. Immediately after the laparoscopic appendectomy, the client's lungs sound slightly congested and it is reported to you that she vomited upon emergence from anesthesia and there is a possibility of aspiration of a small amount of gastric contents into her lungs. This event is probably due to:
   a. Carelessness by the anesthesia provider
   b. Increased pressure on the stomach and diaphragm during laparoscopy
   c. Failure of the patient to relate preoperative fluid intake accurately
   d. Fear and anxiety of the patient

7. Had this client's appendix perforated, symptoms of the resultant peritonitis might have been blunted by:
   a. Pregnancy-induced rotation of the appendix with referred pain
   b. Lack of inflammatory response due to pregnancy-induced increases in steroid levels
   c. Prophylactic administration of tocolytic agents

    d. An increased tendency to wall off abscesses that exist during pregnancy

A 30-year-old G4 P1 client at 18 weeks' gestation has arrived for evaluation at the antenatal clinical. She relates an obstetric history of a preterm birth at 32 weeks' gestation and two midtrimester losses at 18 and 22 weeks, respectively. Pelvic examination reveals a cervix that is 25% effaced and 1 cm dilated. The membranes are intact.

Vital signs: oral temperature, 37° C (98.6° F); pulse rate of 90/min; respiratory rate of 20/min; blood pressure, 120/68; FHR, 132/min.

Diagnostic ultrasound test reveals a singleton, 18-week viable uterine pregnancy. The client is scheduled for surgical placement of cervical cerclage in 2 days.

8. The criteria that make this client an excellent candidate for immediate cerclage are:
    a. She is young and healthy.
    b. She has a positive history of cervical incompetence, and her membranes are intact.
    c. Once the membrane ruptures, it is more difficult to complete the procedure.
    d. She is not a good candidate because no labor contractions have begun.

9. The optimal time for cervical cerclage to be attempted is:
    a. 4 to 8 weeks
    b. 10 to 14 weeks
    c. 14 to 18 weeks
    d. 18 to 22 weeks

10. Throughout the entire perioperative period, tocolytic agents will be administered to this client:
    a. Continuously
    b. If the membranes rupture
    c. Only if uterine irritability is demonstrated
    d. Adjunctively with narcotics to prevent pain

11. To eliminate pressure on the cervix in the immediate postoperative period, the client:
    a. Should be placed in Trendelenburg position in bed.
    b. Should be positioned on her side in reverse Trendelenburg position.
    c. Should be catheterized for 48 hours.
    d. Should be kept sedated for 24 hours.

12. In preparation for discharge, it is most important that this client be counseled to:
    a. Resume sexual activity immediately.
    b. Remain bedridden as much as possible.
    c. Take no medication of any kind.
    d. Avoid heavy lifting for any reason.

13. Cervical cerclage in this client will be accomplished under spinal anesthesia. During the anesthesia and surgery, if the maternal blood pressure drops below 100 mmHg, the *most* important factor to consider is:
    a. Administration of alpha-adrenergic vasopressors will be necessary.
    b. The increased risk of fetal hypoxia.
    c. Too much local anesthetic has been injected by the anesthesia provider.
    d. The client received inadequate preoperative fluid preparation.

14. During spinal or epidural anesthesia, maternal hypotension is due to:
    a. Transient anesthesia-induced paralysis of sympathetic outflow
    b. Transient anesthesia-induced paralysis of parasympathetic outflow
    c. Concurrent intraoperative administration of tocolytic agents
    d. Pregnancy-induced changes in peripheral resistance

ANSWERS TO STUDY QUESTIONS

1. b	5. d	9. c	13. b
2. c	6. b	10. c	14. a
3. a	7. b	11. a	
4. c	8. b	12. d	

REFERENCES

Aaronson, O.S. (2002). Robot-assisted endoscopic intrauterine myelomeningocele repair: A feasibility study. *Pediatric Neurosurgery, 36*(2), 85-89.

Adzick, N.S., Sutton, L.N., Crombleholme, T.M., & Flake, A.W. (1998). Successful fetal surgery for spina bifida. *Lancet, 352*(9141), 1675-1676.

Affleck, D.D., Handrahan, D.L., Egger, M.J., Wallace, D.O., & Lu, C. (1999). The laparoscopic management of appendicitis and cholelithiasis during pregnancy. *American Journal of Surgery, 178*(6), 523-529.

Bannister, C.M. (2000). The case for and against intrauterine surgery for myelomeningocele. *European Journal of Obstetrics, Gynecology, and Reproductive Biology, 92*(1), 109-113.

Barone, J.E., Bears, J., Chen, S., Tasi, J., & Russell, J.C. (1999). Outcome study of cholecystectomy during pregnancy. *American Journal of Surgery, 177*(3), 232-236.

Barthel, J.S., Chowdhury, T., & Miedema, B.W. (1998). Endoscopic sphincterotomy for the treatment of gallstone pancreatitis during pregnancy. *Surgical Endoscopy, 12*(5), 394-399.

Benifla, J.L., Goffinet, F., Darai, E., Proust, A., DeCrepy, A., & Mandelenat, P. (1997). Emergency cervical cerclage after 20 weeks' gestation: A retrospective study of 6 years practice in 34 cases. *Fetal Diagnostic Therapeutics, 12*(5), 274-278.

Bruner, J.P., Boehm, F.H., & Tulipan, N. (1999). The Tulipan-Bruner trocar for uterine entry during fetal surgery. *American Journal of Obstetrics and Gynecology, 181*(5), 1188-1191.

Cappell, M.S. (2003). The fetal safety and clinical efficacy of gastrointestinal endoscopy during pregnancy. *Gastroenterology Clinics of North America, 32*(1), 123-179.

Cauldwell, C.B. (2002). Anesthesia for fetal surgery. *Anesthesiology Clinics of North America, 20*(1), 211-226.

Farmer, D. (2003) Fetal surgery. *British Medical Journal, 326*, 461-462.

Flake, A.W., Crombleholm, T.E., Johnson, M.P., Howell, L.J., & Adzick, N.S. (2002). Treatment of severe congenital diaphragmatic hernia by fetal tracheal occlusion: Clinical experience with fifteen cases. *American Journal of Obstetrics and Gynecology, 183*(5), 1059-1066.

Flake, A.W. (2003). Surgery in the human fetus: The future. *Journal of Physiology, 547*(Pt 1), 45-51.

Fowler, S.F. (2002). Chorioamniotic membrane separation following fetal surgery. *Journal of Perinatology, 22*(5), 407-410.

Ghumman, E., Barry, M., & Grace, P.A. (1997). Management of gallstones in pregnancy. *British Journal of Surgery, 84*(12), 1646-1650.

Glasgow, R.E., Visser, B.C., Harris, H.W., Patti, M.G., Kilpatrick, S.J., & Mulvihill, S.J. (1998). Changing management of gallstone disease during pregnancy. *Surgical Endoscopy, 12*(3), 241-246.

Gordon, M.C. (2002). Maternal physiology in pregnancy. In S.G. Gabbe, J.R. Niebyl, & J.L. Simpson (Eds.), *Obstetrics: Normal and problem pregnancies* (pp. 63-89). Philadelphia: Churchill Livingstone.

Hamid, R.K.A., & Newfield, P. (2001). Pediatric neurosurgery-neural tube defects. *Anesthesiology Clinics of North America, 19*(2), 219-228.

Harrison, M.R., Albanese, C.T., Hawgood, S.B., Farmwe, D.L., Farrell, J.A., Sandberg, P.L., et al. (2001). Fetoscopic temporary tracheal occlusion by means of detachable balloon for congenital diaphragmatic hernia. *American Journal of Obstetrics and Gynecology, 185*(3), 730-733.

Holmes, N., Harrison, M.R., & Baskin, L.S. (2001). Fetal surgery for posterior urethral valves: Long-term postnatal outcomes. *Pediatrics, 108*(1), E7.

Koran, G., Pastuszak, A., & Ito, S. (1998). Drugs in pregnancy. *New England Journal of Medicine, 338*(16), 1128-1137.

LeMaire, B.M., & van Erp, W.F. (1997). Laparoscopic surgery during pregnancy. *Surgical Endoscopy, 11*(1), 15-18.

Lesser, K.B., Childers, J.M., & Surwit, E.A. (1998). Transabdominal cerclage: A laparoscopic approach. *Obstetrics and Gynecology, 91*(5, Pt 2), 855-856.

Ludmir, J., & Stubblefield, P.G. (2002). Surgical procedures in pregnancy. In S.G. Gabbe, J.R. Niebyl, & J.L. Simpson (Eds.), *Obstetrics: Normal and problem pregnancies* (pp. 607-620). Philadelphia: Churchill Livingstone.

Lylerly, A.D., Cefalo, R.C., Socol, M., Fogarty, L., & Sugarman, J. (2001). Attitudes of maternal-fetal specialists concerning maternal-fetal surgery. *American Journal of Obstetrics and Gynecology, 185*(5), 1052-1058.

Malangoni, M.A. (2003). Gastrointestinal surgery and pregnancy. *Gastroenterology Clinics of North America, 32*(1), 181-200.

Mayer, I.E., & Hussain, H. (1998). Abdominal pain during pregnancy. *Gastroenterology Clinics of North America, 27*(1), 1-36.

Paek, B.W., Jennings, R.W., Harrison, M.R., Filly, R.A., Tacy, T.A., Farmer, D.L., et al. (2001). Radiofrequency ablation of human fetal sacrococcygeal teratoma. *American Journal of Obstetrics and Gynecology, 184*(3), 503-507.

Ranzini, A.C. (1999). Prenatal sonographic diagnosis of uterine rupture following open fetal surgery. *Obstetrics and Gynecology, 93*(5, Pt 2), 826-827.

Reedy, M.B., Kallen, B., & Kuehl, T.J. (1997). Laparoscopy during pregnancy: A study of five fetal outcome parameters with use of the Swedish health registry.

American Journal of Obstetrics and Gynecology, 177(3), 673-679.

Rosen, M.A., & Weiskopf, R.B. (1999). Management of anesthesia for the pregnant surgical patient. *Anesthesiology, 91*(4), 1159-1163.

Schwartz, D.A., Moriarity, K.P., Tashjian, D.B., Wool, R.S., Parker, R.K., Markenson, G.R., et al. (2001). Anesthetic management of the exit (ex utero intrapartum treatment) procedure. *Journal of Clinical Anesthesia, 13*(5), 387-391.

Sydorak, R.M. (2002). Chorioamniotic membrane separation following fetal surgery. *Journal of Perinatology, 22*(5), 407-410.

Tracey, M., & Fletcher, H.S. (2000). Appendicitis in pregnancy. *The American Surgeon, 660*(6), 555-559.

Tulipan, N., Sutton, L.N., Bruner, J.P., Cohen, B.M., Johnson, M., & Adzick, N.S. (2003). The effect of intrauterine myelomeningocele repair on the incidence of shunt-dependent hydrocephalus. *Pediatric Neurosurgery, 38*(1), 27-33.

Visser, B.C., Glasgow, R.E., Mulvihill, K.K., & Mulvihill, S.J. (2001). Safety and timing of nonobstetric abdominal surgery in pregnancy. *Digestive Surgery, 18*(5), 409-417.

Wagner, W., & Harrison, M.R. (2002). Fetal operations in the head and neck: Current state. *Head and Neck, 24*(5), 482-490.

Wilson, R.D. (2002). Prenatal evaluation for fetal surgery. *Current Opinions in Obstetrics and Gynecology, 14*(2), 187-193.

Winstrom, K.D., & Malee, M.P. (1999). Medical and surgical complications of pregnancy. In J.R. Scott, P.J. DiSaia, C.B. Hammond, & W.N. Spellacy (Eds.), *Danforth's obstetrics and gynecology* (8th ed.; pp. 333-334, 356-357). Philadelphia: Lippincott Williams & Wilkins.

27 Substance Abuse in Pregnancy

BARBARA A. MORAN

OBJECTIVES

1. Discuss the scope of substance abuse in pregnancy.
2. Recognize signs of substance abuse.
3. Describe the effects of drug use during pregnancy on the developing fetus.
4. Elicit appropriate history and pertinent information from the client.
5. Describe the special needs of the drug-dependent pregnant woman.
6. Recognize the teaching needs and appropriate referrals for the pregnant substance abuser.
7. Formulate a plan of care based on a client's history of substance abuse.

SUBSTANCE ABUSE

A. **Major public health issue**
   1. Drug use in pregnancy and its associated problems has become a major public health issue.
   2. Polydrug use, such as alcohol and tobacco with marijuana or cocaine, has become more common.
B. **Statistics**
   1. Illegal drugs are used by 9 million women in the United States.
   2. Half of women of childbearing age in the United States, ages 18 to 44, have taken illegal drugs at least once in their lifetime.
   3. Incidence of substance abuse during pregnancy is estimated at 5% to 15%
   4. The use of drugs during pregnancy occurs in women of all ages, races, ethnicities, and social groups.
   5. The National Institute on Drug Abuse (NIDA) Household Survey (2003b) revealed that 14% of pregnant women reported that they drank some alcohol, 1.3% engaged in binge drinking, and 2.5% used some kind of illicit drug. In addition, this survey reported that 1.5% of pregnant women used marijuana, 0.2% used cocaine or crack, and 0.2% used heroin.
   6. Disproportionately high incidence of teen pregnancy associated with substance abuse is especially prevalent among those who live in poverty.
C. **Outcomes relate to the following:**
   1. Molecular weight influences whether or not the drug crosses the placenta.
   2. The first 8 weeks of pregnancy are the most critical time in terms of embryonic development. During the third trimester, drug use has the greatest potential for impairing fetal growth.
   3. Route of ingestion
      a. Drugs taken orally might reduce the drug's ability to cross the placenta.

      b. Drugs taken intravenously and intranasally more readily cross the placenta.

      c. Intravenous (IV) drug use increases maternal and fetal exposure to HIV.

  4. Adequacy of prenatal care

  5. Presence of obstetric or maternal complications

  6. Multiple drug use

  7. Lifestyle of mother, including poverty, homelessness or inadequate housing, lack of education, domestic violence, and social and emotional problems

  8. Nutritional status

  9. Acute cessation might lead to withdrawal symptoms, abruptio placenta, and premature labor.

10. Many medical conditions, including anemia, bacteremia/septicemia, cardiac disease, cellulitis, depression, diabetes, edema, hepatitis B and C, tuberculosis (TB), hypertension, phlebitis, sexually transmitted diseases (STDs), urinary tract infections, and vitamin deficiency compromise many drug-involved pregnancies.

11. Obstetric complications include abruptio placenta, placenta previa, intrauterine death, spontaneous abortion, premature labor and delivery, premature rupture of membranes, and intrauterine growth retardation (IUGR) and polyhydramnios.

D. Effects on fetus

  1. Generalized growth restriction and its associated complications

  2. Increase in the frequency of sudden infant death syndrome (SIDS)

  3. Signs of withdrawal, which can occur from birth to 6 days of life, include:

      a. High-pitched or shrill cry

      b. Gastrointestinal disturbances

         (1) Vomiting

         (2) Diarrhea

         (3) Excessive sucking

      c. Tremulousness

      d. Excoriation of knees and elbows from increased restlessness and sleeplessness

      e. Perianal excoriation (chemical dermatitis due to acidic stool)

      f. Respiratory disturbances

         (1) Tachypnea

         (2) Nasal congestion

         (3) Frequent yawning

         (4) Sneezing

      g. Seizure activity

  4. Many of the signs of drug withdrawal in the neonate are similar to other neonatal problems, such as sepsis, hypoglycemia, and central nervous system (CNS) disorders; therefore, testing to rule out these conditions should be considered in addition to drug screening.

E. Cocaine

  1. Is found in the leaves of the *Erythroxylon* coca plant of Peru, Ecuador, and Bolivia.

  2. Cocaine use is second only to marijuana in pregnant women who used an illicit drug during pregnancy.

  3. Incidence of cocaine exposure in utero is 1 to 10 per 1000 live births.

  4. Crosses the placenta by diffusion.

5. Cocaine blocks the reuptake of catecholamines at nerve terminals, which increases circulating concentrations of catecholamines in the blood, resulting in vasoconstriction, tachycardia, hypertension, and uterine contractions.
6. Cardiovascular and neurologic complications, such as hypertension, myocardial ischemia, sudden death, dysrhythmias, subarachnoid hemorrhage, and seizures have been described among parturients who abuse cocaine.
7. Acute cocaine use during the third trimester might result in preterm labor, abruptio placenta, a greater incidence of premature membrane rupture, and an increased risk of meconium staining and precipitous delivery.
8. Fetal anomalies involving the upper limbs, neurologic (myelomeningocele, microcephaly, growth retardation, increased flow velocity in cerebral artery), cardiovascular (congenital heart defects), genitourinary (prune belly syndrome, hydronephrosis, ambiguous genitalia), and gastrointestinal systems (ilea atresia, necrotizing enterocolitis) have been attributed to cocaine use early in pregnancy.

F. **Heroin**
1. Derived from seeds of the poppy *Papaver somniferum*; an off white or pale brown powder that can be sniffed, smoked, or injected parenterally, that is approximately 25 times stronger than morphine and crosses the placenta readily, appearing in fetal tissue within 1 hour of maternal consumption.
2. Primary effects are analgesia, sedation, feeling of well-being, and euphoria.
3. Signs and symptoms of early pregnancy might be confused with heroin use (i.e., fatigue, nausea/vomiting, pelvic cramping).
4. Heroin is not generally thought to be a teratogen capable of producing congenital malformation.
   a. Easily crosses the placenta via simple diffusion.
   b. Hazards of heroin to the fetus are thought to be the direct effects of the drug on the fetus and the maternal lifestyle associated with heroin use.
      (1) The woman typically does not seek early prenatal care—this is related to fear of detection of heroin use and to an absence or irregularity of menses caused by heroin that makes amenorrhea a norm in her life.
      (2) There is an increased maternal and fetal exposure to serious infection such as:
         (a) STDs
         (b) Hepatitis
         (c) HIV
5. Neonatal effects of prenatal heroin exposure include the following:
   a. Neonatal abstinence syndrome
      (1) Causes severe neonatal withdrawal symptoms.
      (2) Has an average onset of symptoms between 6 and 12 hours after birth, with an average peak of symptoms between 48 and 72 hours.
   b. Withdrawal symptoms might persist in a subacute form for 4 to 6 months after birth.
   c. Increased incidence of meconium aspiration at birth
   d. Increased incidence of neonatal sepsis
   e. Symmetric IUGR
      (1) Low birth weight
      (2) Decreased length
      (3) Small head circumference

     f. Neurodevelopmental behavioral problems
       (1) Tremulous and irritable
       (2) Poor organizational responses to environmental stimuli
       (3) Poor motor control
       (4) Difficult to console
       (5) Poor suck and swallow coordination, which leads to poor feeding tolerance

G. Marijuana

1. Most commonly used illicit drug: more than 83 million Americans (37%) age 12 and older have tried marijuana at least once.
2. Often called pot, grass, reefer, weed, herb, Mary Jane, or MJ.
3. Is a greenish-gray mixture of the dried, shredded leaves, stems, seeds, and flowers of *Cannabis sativa*, the hemp plant.
4. Causes tachycardia and decreased blood pressure, resulting in orthostatic hypotension.
5. Research has shown that babies born to women who used marijuana during pregnancy display altered responses to visual stimuli, increased tremulousness, and a high-pitched cry, which might indicate problems with neurologic development.

H. Methadone hydrochloride

1. Developed as a substitute for morphine and heroin. Frequently used to treat pregnant heroin-dependent women to prevent repeated episodes of heroin withdrawal in the fetus.
2. Blocks the craving of withdrawal.
3. Is longer-acting and, therefore, is thought to stabilize the environment for the fetus, sustaining the addict and avoiding withdrawal, thus:
     a. Decreasing maternal complications
     b. Decreasing prematurity and low birthweight
4. Methadone maintenance requires enrollment in a drug-treatment program, therefore increasing the likelihood of prenatal care.
5. Mother may breastfeed infant if not infected with HIV, hepatitis, or TB; long-term effects on the neonate have not been determined.

CLINICAL PRACTICE

A. Assessment

1. History
     a. Menstrual history: irregular menses in 60% to 90% of addicted women
     b. Obstetric/gynecologic history
       (1) Little or no prenatal care
       (2) Number of pregnancies and method of delivery, miscarriages, abortions, and living children
       (3) Gynecologic infections
       (4) STDs
       (5) Method of contraception
     c. Medical history
       (1) Preexisting medical conditions, and treatments; the most common comorbid diagnoses for women are affective disorders, such as chronic or acute depression, and anxiety disorders.
       (2) Hospitalizations
       (3) Surgeries
       (4) History of physical or sexual abuse or family violence

       (5) Weight less than the 50th percentile and little or no weight gain
         during pregnancy
   d. Drug abuse history
       (1) Drugs currently used
       (2) Length of use
       (3) Age of onset
       (4) Duration
       (5) Frequency and route of administration
       (6) Date of last use
       (7) Any previous treatment
       (8) Family history of substance abuse
   e. Erratic appetite
   f. Poor nutrition
   g. Deterioration in personal hygiene
   h. Allergies
   i. Hepatitis
   j. AIDS
   k. History of child abuse, neglect, and/or sexual abuse
2. Physical findings
   a. Bloodshot eyes, conjunctivitis, and yellow sclera
   b. Slurred speech
   c. Dilated or constricted pupils
   d. Restlessness or fatigue
   e. Shortness of breath
   f. Poor dental hygiene, abscesses, and gum disease
   g. Rhinitis, nasal or sinus irritation, septal erosion, and loss of sense of smell
   h. Hepatomegaly, jaundice, or distended neck veins secondary to liver failure
   i. Scars from injuries or surgery
   j. Subcutaneous abscesses or cellulitis, and rashes
   k. Needle marks and ecchymotic spots or scars
   l. Unsteady walk and impaired coordination
   m. Slowed reflexes
   n. Elevated blood pressure
   o. Tachycardia
   p. Altered moods and perceptions/inappropriate behavior
   q. Nausea
   r. Dizziness
   s. Odor of substance on clothing
   t. Burns on fingertips or singed eyebrows or eyelashes
   u. Phlebitis
   v. Placental abruption
3. Psychosocial findings
   a. Low self-esteem
   b. Depression
   c. Chronic anxiety
   d. Inability to maintain close relationships
   e. Family disorganization
   f. Manipulative
   g. Hostility or anger
   h. Homelessness
   i. Unplanned pregnancy
   j. Denial

      k. Late prenatal care, missed appointments, or late for appointments

      l. Difficulty following through on referrals

      m. Intimate partner violence

  4. Diagnostic studies

      a. Complete blood count (CBC), differential, and urinalysis (UA)

      b. Toxicologic urine screening (detects cocaine ingestion within past 24 hours).

      c. Venereal Diseases Research Laboratory (VDRL) test

      d. Cervical culture for gonorrhea and chlamydia

      e. Papanicolaou test (Pap smear)

      f. Hepatitis profile

      g. HIV testing

      h. Sonography (to detect IUGR)

      i. TB skin test

      j. Rubella titer

      k. Sickle cell screening (when appropriate)

      l. Blood type and antibody screen

      m. Alpha-fetoprotein (if between 16 and 20 weeks' gestation)

      n. Hepatitis panel (Hep B core antibody, Hep B surface antibody, Hep B surface antigen, Hep A antibody profile, Hep C antibody)

      o. Baseline liver and renal function tests

      p. Group B strep culture

      q. Toxoplasmosis, cytomegalovirus, and herpes cultures

B. Nursing Diagnoses

  1. Deficient knowledge related to substance abuse and its effect on self and pregnancy

  2. Imbalanced nutrition: less than body requirements related to pregnancy and drug abuse

  3. Interrupted family processes related to developmental transition of pregnancy

  4. Anxiety related to drug use during pregnancy

  5. Noncompliance related to difficulty in following prenatal recommendations

  6. Risk for injury to self and fetus related to drug use during pregnancy

  7. Ineffective health maintenance related to lack of prenatal care

  8. Risk for impaired parenting related to effects of drugs

  9. Situational low self-esteem related to need for drugs

C. Interventions/Outcomes

  1. Deficient knowledge related to substance abuse and its effect on self and pregnancy (Box 27-1)

      a. Interventions

        (1) Give accurate and specific information on complications associated with drug use and the increase in morbidity and mortality in a nonjudgmental way.

        (2) Explain that quitting or decreasing drugs at any time in pregnancy improves obstetric outcome.

        (3) Explain dangers of operating vehicles or machinery while under the influence of drugs.

        (4) Reinforce client's understanding with printed material at a level she can understand.

      b. Outcomes

        (1) Client verbalizes effects of substance abuse on self and developing fetus.

        (2) Client avoids substance abusive behavior.

■ BOX 27-1
■ **OBSTETRIC COMPLICATIONS ASSOCIATED WITH THE ADDICTED PATIENT**

Complications of Mother	Difficult to console
Abruptio placenta	Exaggerated startle response
Anemia	Generalized growth restriction
Cellulites	High-pitched cry
Cesarean sections	Hyperactivity
Chorioamnionitis	Hypoactivity
Gestational diabetes	Hypoglycemia
Maternal hypertension	Increased frequency of sudden
Placental insufficiency	infant death syndrome
Postpartum hemorrhage	Intracranial hemorrhage
Precipitous delivery	Intrauterine growth restriction
Preeclampsia/eclampsia	Gastrointestinal disturbances
Premature rupture of membranes	Low birth weight
Preterm labor/delivery	Meconium aspiration
Septic thrombophlebitis	Neurobehavioral abnormalities
Sexually transmitted diseases	(altered sleep patterns, irritability,
Spontaneous miscarriage	jitteriness, tremors, depressed sucking)
Stillbirths	Pneumonia
Urinary tract infection	Poor feeding
Uterine rupture	Possible seizures
	Respiratory distress syndrome
Complications of Newborn	Small head circumference
Apnea	Tachycardia
Bradycardia	Tachypnea
Detrimental maternal-infant bonding	

2. Imbalanced nutrition: less than body requirements related to pregnancy and drug abuse
   a. Interventions: maternal
      (1) Provide supplemental vitamins.
      (2) Provide ferrous sulfate.
      (3) Provide folic acid if folate levels are low.
      (4) Provide nutritional counseling, emphasizing protein intake.
      (5) Reinforce information with printed material to take home.
      (6) Use a variety of teaching methods to reinforce education.
      (7) Discourage breastfeeding if the mother is using a substance that might pass through the breast milk.
   b. Interventions: infant
      (1) Assess daily nutritional intake for volume and calories.
      (2) Assess daily weight.
      (3) Assess hydration, daily output, urine, stool, and insensible water loss.
      (4) Assess oxygenation by pulse oximeter and capillary refill time.
      (5) Assess suck, swallow, breathing, and coordination; provide pacifier to meet increased sucking need.
   c. Outcomes: maternal
      (1) Client avoids further nutritional decline.
      (2) Client has appropriate uterine growth for gestational age.
      (3) Client goes to a nutritionist on referral.
   d. Outcomes: infant

      (1) Neonate shows adequate signs of hydration.

      (2) Neonate gains adequate daily weight after initial normal birth weight loss.

      (3) Incident of diarrhea or vomiting is incidental or absent.

3. Interrupted family processes related to developmental transition of pregnancy

   a. Interventions

      (1) Assess client's perception of her pregnancy and her role as a new mother.

      (2) Assist client in identifying support systems and identifying needs for food, clothing, shelter, and legal aid as needed.

      (3) Use an interdisciplinary team approach in a nonjudgmental and sensitive manner.

      (4) Assist family in supporting patient in a nonjudgmental and supportive fashion.

      (5) Help client identify stresses in her family life.

      (6) Promote attachment by recommending attendance at childbirth preparation and parenting classes.

      (7) Provide reading material on pregnancy, parenting, and newborn care.

      (8) Encourage verbalization of fears and concerns.

   b. Outcomes

      (1) Client identifies support system.

      (2) Client verbalizes acceptance of pregnancy.

      (3) Client maintains support from significant others.

      (4) Client expresses her feelings freely and appropriately.

      (5) Client and her family express understanding of pregnancy and role transition.

4. Anxiety related to drug use during pregnancy

   a. Interventions

      (1) Establish trusting relationship by providing consistent care.

      (2) Present as many options as possible for increased control over situation.

      (3) Involve significant others in prenatal care.

      (4) Be patient, be concrete, and repeat explanations.

      (5) Phrase questions positively to elicit honest responses (i.e., "To care for you and your baby, I need to know" or "I noticed track marks and I'm concerned for you and your baby and need to know").

   b. Outcomes

      (1) Client verbalizes concerns and issues in the supportive environment.

5. Noncompliance related to difficulty in following prenatal recommendations

   a. Interventions

      (1) Provide information on effects of drugs on self and infant repeatedly and in a variety of teaching methods.

      (2) Educate the client and her family or support person regarding importance of follow-up prenatal visits.

      (3) Refer the client to social services and other supportive agencies.

      (4) Explore with the client ways to reduce barriers to noncompliance.

      (5) Encourage continued prenatal care.

   b. Outcomes

      (1) Client acknowledges the need and importance of prenatal care.

      (2) Client keeps appointments.

      (3) Client participates actively in health care maintenance.

6. Risk for injury to self and fetus related to drug use during pregnancy (Figure 27-1).

   a. Interventions

   (1) Identify substance abuse in client. Watch for:

   (a) Unexplained late first obstetric visit or no prenatal care

   (b) Multiple missed visits

   (c) History of unexplained miscarriages, fetal growth restriction, stillbirths, abruptio placentae, and precipitous birth

   (d) Children with developmental problems

   (e) History of drug- or alcohol-related medical problems

   (f) History of physical or sexual abuse

   (2) Teach, review, and reinforce information on a level the client understands.

   (3) Monitor maternal and fetal withdrawal.

   (4) Instruct the client to monitor fetal activity.

   (5) Help family members or significant other develop skills necessary to support the client.

   (6) Refer the client to appropriate counseling or rehabilitation.

   b. Outcomes

   (1) Client minimizes potential for further injury by decreasing substance abuse.

   (2) Family or significant other supports the client.

7. Ineffective health maintenance related to lack of prenatal care

   a. Interventions

   (1) Determine the client's capability for maintaining health.

   (2) Provide anticipatory guidance on common concerns of pregnancy.

   (3) Encourage self-care measures (i.e., sleep, nutrition, exercise).

   b. Outcomes

   (1) Client recognizes normal physiologic pregnancy changes.

   (2) Client maintains or improves current health status.

8. Risk for impaired parenting related to effects of drugs

   a. Interventions

   (1) Encourage verbalization of the client's feelings about her pregnancy.

   (2) Involve significant others in prenatal care and discussion.

   (3) Encourage listening to fetal heart rate by the mother and significant other at each visit.

   (4) Show sonogram to the client so she can visualize the fetus.

   (5) Provide information on fetal growth and development.

   (6) Help the client to identify major areas in her life that will be affected by the new infant.

   (7) Encourage and document parental visits and telephone calls.

   (8) During visits, encourage parents' active participation in the infant's care while protecting infant from any potentially harmful handling.

   (9) Develop and implement a teaching strategy that gives parents or guardians anticipatory guidance, knowledge, and specific techniques for dealing with a drug-exposed infant.

   (10) Give parents or guardians counseling regarding available resources and necessary follow-up care for the infant.

   (11) Facilitate referral to child protective services, welfare, adoption, community health, or charity agencies as needed.

   b. Outcomes

   (1) Client accepts pregnancy.

   (2) Client begins attachment behaviors.

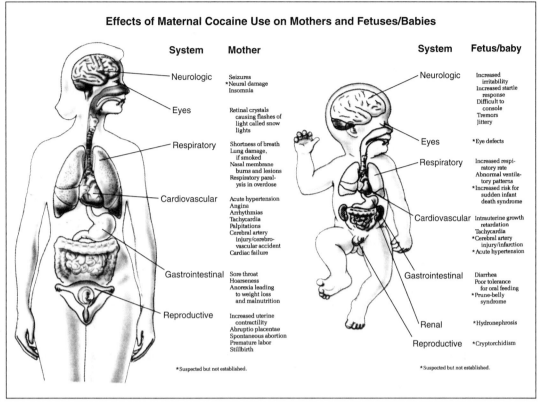

FIGURE 27-1 ■ Effects of maternal cocaine use on mothers and fetuses/infants. (From Smith, J. [1988]. The dangers of prenatal cocaine use. *MCN: The American Journal of Maternal Child Nursing, 13*[3], 174-179. By permission of Network Graphics.)

    (3) Client develops role identity as a parent.
    (4) Client has a knowledge base for effective parenting.
    (5) Parents/guardians demonstrate effective ways of handling and feeding the neonate; demonstrate attachment behaviors.
    (6) Parents/guardians demonstrate effective ways of comforting the neonate and initiate an active role in determining infant's safe care.
    (7) Parents/guardians express and cope with their frustrations about the infant and begin to use outside resources as sources of support.
    (8) Parents/guardians freely express any feelings of guilt about their contribution to the infant's physical withdrawal and distress.
  9. Situational low self-esteem related to need for drugs
    a. Interventions
      (1) Provide a nonjudgmental, concerned, and empathetic environment.
      (2) Encourage the client to express her feelings and concerns about herself, her drug use, and her unborn child.
      (3) Assist the client in identifying factors that decrease her self-esteem.
      (4) Assist the client in identifying ways that will restore her self-esteem.
    b. Outcomes
      (1) Client verbalizes positive and realistic statements about herself.
      (2) Client verbalizes factors that decrease her self-esteem.
      (3) Client actively participates in restorative activities.

TOBACCO

A. **Introduction**
   1. Smoking is the chief, single avoidable cause of death.
   2. Several reports have established that maternal tobacco smoking during pregnancy adversely affects:
      a. Prenatal and postnatal growth
      b. Increased risk of fetal mortality and morbidity
      c. Cognitive development
      d. Spontaneous abortion
      e. Sudden infant death syndrome
      f. Long-term neurobehavioral effects
   3. Indirect effects
      a. Poor nutritional status of the mother associated with the anorexigenic effect of nicotine, carbon monoxide exposure
      b. Blood flow restriction to the placenta due to the vasoconstrictive effects of catecholamines released from the adrenals and nerve cells after nicotine activation
   4. Direct effects
      a. Interactions of nicotine with nicotinic acetylcholine receptors, which are present very early in the fetal brain
      b. Products of cigarette smoke can directly affect the fetal brain.
B. **Tobacco use occurs in approximately 25% of all pregnancies in the United States.**
C. **Compounds in cigarettes are readily absorbed, causing maternal vaso-constriction and reduced oxygen availability.**
   1. Carbon monoxide: binds available hemoglobin, thereby decreasing oxygen to tissue and fetus.
   2. Nicotine: linked to dependency; is a powerful vasoconstrictor that causes increased maternal heart rate and blood pressure.
   3. Cyanide

CLINICAL PRACTICE

A. **Assessment**
   1. History
      a. Prior tobacco use
      b. Current use
      c. Quantity of cigarettes smoked daily
      d. Family members who smoke
   2. Physical findings
      a. Cough
      b. Congestion
      c. Tobacco air (smell) surrounding patient
   3. Psychosocial findings
      a. Anxiety
      b. Guilt
      c. Denial
      d. Hostility or anger
      e. Depression
   4. Diagnostic procedure: ultrasonography (to detect IUGR)

B. Nursing Diagnoses
   1. Deficient knowledge related to effects of smoking on self and pregnancy
   2. Imbalanced nutrition: less than body requirements related to smoking during pregnancy
   3. Risk for injury related to smoking during pregnancy
   4. Ineffective individual coping related to smoking
C. Interventions/Outcomes
   1. Deficient knowledge related to effects of smoking on self and family
     a. Interventions
       (1) Provide the client with factual information about the health hazard of smoking to herself.
         (a) Hemorrhage (from abruptio placentae and placenta previa)
         (b) Sepsis (from ruptured membranes)
         (c) Bronchitis
         (d) Lung cancer
         (e) Hypertension and cardiovascular disease
         (f) Spontaneous abortion
         (g) Depletion of vitamin C level, which is needed to produce collagen and enhances absorption of iron
       (2) Provide the client with factual information about the health hazard of smoking to the unborn child.
         (a) Reduction in uteroplacental flow that might impair oxygen exchange across the placenta
         (b) Abortion, stillbirth, and prematurity
         (c) IUGR
         (d) Low birthweight (200 to 400 g [7 to 14 oz] or smaller)
         (e) SIDS: occurs twice as frequently in children of smokers.
         (f) Low Apgar scores
         (g) Neurobehavioral effects
         (h) Increased frequency of apnea
       (3) Emphasize that the earlier a pregnant woman gives up smoking, the lower her risk of having a low birth weight infant.
       (4) Use a variety of teaching techniques to meet learning needs.
       (5) Provide written information at appropriate level for the client to take home.
       (6) Involve the client's family and friends in the learning process.
     b. Outcomes
       (1) Client verbalizes the effects of smoking on herself and her unborn child.
       (2) Client expresses a desire to quit smoking.
   2. Imbalanced nutrition: less than body requirements related to smoking during pregnancy
     a. Interventions
       (1) Provide supplemental vitamins.
       (2) Provide ferrous sulfate.
       (3) Provide folic acid.
       (4) Provide vitamin C.
       (5) Provide nutritional counseling on foods enriched with iron and vitamin C.
     b. Outcomes
       (1) Client avoids further nutritional decline.
       (2) Client experiences appropriate uterine growth for gestational age.

3. Risk for injury related to smoking during pregnancy
   a. Interventions
      (1) Teach, review, and reinforce information.
      (2) Provide specific suggestions for decreasing cigarette use.
         (a) Assess when the client is smoking (i.e., with meals, at social occasions, when bored).
         (b) Support decreasing client's intake by one cigarette per day.
         (c) Substitute a healthy behavior for a cigarette (i.e., a walk, a nutritious snack).
   b. Outcomes
      (1) Client reduces the potential for further injury by decreasing the number of cigarettes smoked per day.
4. Ineffective individual coping related to smoking
   a. Interventions
      (1) Assist the client in identifying stressors that trigger smoking.
      (2) Help the client identify alternative ways of coping (i.e., relaxation or substitution of fruits or vegetables in place of cigarettes).
      (3) Refer the client to appropriate programs for stress reduction and smoking cessation.
      (4) Refer for comprehensive approach to effective parenting.
   b. Outcomes
      (1) Client uses other coping mechanisms appropriately.
      (2) Client develops skills to reduce stress and anxiety.
      (3) Client identifies stressors that trigger smoking.

ALCOHOL

A. **Major public health problem**
   1. Most commonly used drug; it is estimated that 18 million Americans, including women of childbearing age, are chronic consumers of alcohol. Drug of choice for most teenagers.
   2. Prenatal exposure to alcohol is one of the leading preventable causes of birth defects, mental retardation, and neurodevelopment disorders.
   3. A cluster of birth defects resulting from prenatal alcohol exposure was recognized in 1973 and called fetal alcohol syndrome. Recently, alcohol exposure in utero has been linked to a variety of other neurodevelopment problems, and the term alcohol-related neurodevelopment disorder (ARND) and alcohol-related birth defects (ARBD) have been proposed to identify infants affected.
   4. Alcohol in a pregnant woman's bloodstream circulates to the fetus by crossing the placenta and interferes with the ability of the fetus to receive sufficient oxygen and nourishment for normal cell development in the brain and other body organs.
   5. According to the 1999 Behavioral Risk Factor Surveillance System, 12.8% of women reported drinking alcohol during pregnancy.
   6. Birth defects associated with prenatal alcohol exposure can occur in the first 3 to 8 weeks of pregnancy, before a woman even knows she is pregnant.
B. **Statistics**
   1. FAS is estimated to occur at the rate of 1 to 2 in 1000 live births in the United States and 4 in 1000 for fetal alcohol effects (FAE).
   2. Higher rates are reported among selected subgroups (e.g., 30 in 10,000 among American Indians).

3. Annual cost estimates for the United States range from $75 million to $9.7 billion.
4. The total lifetime cost of caring for a typical child with FAS might be as high as $1.4 million.
5. The consumption of one or more drinks (a drink is defined as 1.5 oz distilled spirits, 5 oz of wine, or 12 oz of beer) per day was associated with increased risk of giving birth to an infant with growth retardation. Current data do not support the concept of a "safe level" of alcohol consumption by pregnant women below which no damage to a fetus will occur. The American Academy of Pediatrics recommends that all pregnant women and women who are planning to become pregnant not drink alcohol.

C. **Fetal alcohol syndrome**
1. FAS refers to a constellation of physical, behavioral, and cognitive abnormalities. The exact mechanism by which alcohol damages the fetus and critical times of exposure are not known. However, exposure during the first trimester results in the structural defects (i.e., facial changes) characteristic of FAS, whereas the growth and CNS disturbances could occur from alcohol use during any time in pregnancy.
2. Pattern of mental, physical, and behavioral defects in children (Box 27-2)
   a. Prenatal and postnatal growth deficiency
   b. Facial malformations (Figures 27-2 and 27-3)
      (1) Microcephaly
      (2) Flattened midfacies
      (3) Broad nasal bridge
      (4) Flattened and elongated philtrum (groove between the nose and upper lip)
      (5) Short palpebral fissures (the opening between the margins of the upper and lower lids)
      (6) Epicanthal folds (vertical fold of skin over the angle of the inner canthus of eye)
      (7) Abnormal palmar creases
   c. CNS handicaps: small brain, mental retardation, learning disabilities, short attention span, irritability in infancy, hyperactivity in childhood, poor body, hand, and finger coordination

■ BOX 27-2
■ **POSSIBLE FETAL ALCOHOL SYNDROME MANIFESTATIONS**

Attention deficits	Microcephaly
Cardiac defects	Mild-to-moderate mental retardation
Cleft lip or palate	Poor coordination
Delayed motor and language development	Poor suck
Flat midface (hypoplasia of midface)	Prenatal and postnatal growth restriction
Fusion of cervical vertebrae	Retarded bone growth
Hyperactive	Short palpebral fissures (small eye openings)
Increased infections	Sleep disturbances
Increased irritability	Small in size, height, and/or weight
Indistinct philtrum (groove above the upper lip)	Strabismus, ptosis, myopia
Kidney defects	Thin upper lip
Learning disabilities	

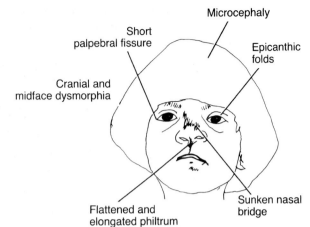

FIGURE 27-2 ■ Fetal alcohol syndrome.

Microcephaly

Short palpebral fissure

Epicanthic folds

Cranial and midface dysmorphia

Sunken nasal bridge

Flattened and elongated philtrum

D. **Fetal alcohol effects**
   1. Growth deficiency
   2. Behavioral mannerisms
   3. Delays in motor and speech performance
E. **Alcohol related neurodevelopmental disorder (ARND):** Children with ARND have CNS abnormalities and behavior and cognitive abnormalities. They do not have the facial features and growth retardation that can be caused by FAE. ARND can occur either along or in combination with FAS or FAE.
F. **Alcohol-related birth defects (ARBD):** Alcohol might cause one or more birth defects of the eyes, ears, heart, kidneys, and bones. ARBD can occur either alone or in combination with FAS or FAE.
   1. Factors contributing to different teratogenic effects might include:
      a. Genetic makeup
      b. Type, amount, and duration of alcohol consumption

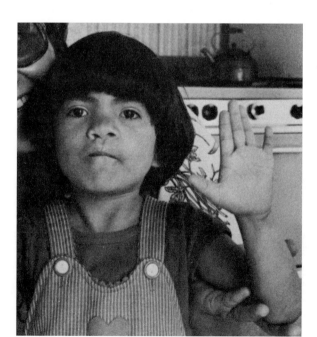

FIGURE 27-3 ■ Fetal alcohol syndrome. (Courtesy March of Dimes Birth Defects Foundation, White Plains, NY.)

   c. Access to prenatal care, education, and support services
   d. Maternal age, parity and health

CLINICAL PRACTICE

A. **Assessment**
   1. History
      a. Alcohol history of client to include:
         (1) Type
         (2) Amount of daily intake
         (3) Polysubstance use, especially use of cocaine
      b. Disorientation
      c. Clumsiness
      d. Hepatic disease
      e. Family history of alcohol abuse
      f. Allergies
   2. Physical findings
      a. Poor nutritional and hygiene status
      b. Hepatomegaly
      c. Tremors
      d. Edema
      e. Agitated behavior
      f. Memory difficulty
   3. Psychosocial findings
      a. Low self-esteem
      b. Anxiety and fear
      c. Depression
      d. Family disorganization
      e. Hostility or anger
      f. Denial
      g. Possibly unplanned pregnancy
   4. Diagnostic studies
      a. Blood alcohol level (to establish presence of alcohol in system); a blood alcohol level of 0.10 is legally defined as intoxication in most of the United States.
      b. CBC
      c. Serum electrolytes
      d. Serial sonograms to detect IUGR
      e. VDRL and other STD testing
      f. Hepatitis profile
      g. HIV testing
B. **Nursing Diagnoses**
   1. Deficient knowledge related to alcohol use and its effect on pregnancy
   2. Imbalanced nutrition: less than bodily requirements related to pregnancy and alcohol use
   3. Anxiety related to alcohol effects on pregnancy and self
   4. Interrupted family processes related to developmental transition of pregnancy
   5. Noncompliance related to difficulty in following prenatal recommendations
   6. Risk for injury related to use of alcohol during pregnancy
   7. Risk for impaired parenting related to alcohol use

C. Interventions/Outcomes
  1. Deficient knowledge related to alcohol use and its effect on pregnancy
    a. Interventions
      (1) Provide factual information about health hazards of alcohol to women and developing fetus.
        (a) Fetal risk factors
            (i) CNS involvement (including mental retardation)
            (ii) Facial dysmorphia
            (iii) Growth restriction (before and after birth)
            (iv) Spontaneous abortion
            (v) Stillbirth
        (b) Maternal risk factors
            (i) Cirrhosis
            (ii) Increased obstetric complications
            (iii) Infertility
            (iv) Malnutrition
            (v) Withdrawal
            (vi) Major factor in the spread of HIV and other STDs
            (vii) Unwanted pregnancy
      (2) Inform the client that decreasing and stopping alcohol intake at any point during pregnancy will improve the outcome.
      (3) Give written information at a level the woman will understand.
    b. Outcomes
      (1) Client verbalizes the effects of alcohol on the developing fetus.
      (2) Client decreases or eliminates alcohol intake.
  2. Imbalanced nutrition: less than body requirements related to pregnancy and alcohol use
    a. Interventions
      (1) Provide supplemental vitamins, ferrous sulfate, folic acid, as with other substance abuse patients.
    b. Outcomes
      (1) Same as with other substance abuse patients
  3. Anxiety related to alcohol effects on pregnancy and self
    a. Interventions
      (1) Same as with other substance abuse patients
    b. Outcomes
      (1) Same as with other substance abuse patients
  4. Interrupted family processes related to developmental transition of pregnancy
    a. Interventions
      (1) Assess family's ability to support the client in a nonjudgmental and supportive fashion and involve them in counseling, referral, and treatment.
      (2) Use interdisciplinary team approach in a nonjudgmental and sensitive manner.
      (3) Recommend attendance at childbirth preparation and parenting classes.
      (4) Provide written material about pregnancy, parenting, and newborn care.
      (5) Assess for physical, sexual, and emotional abuse.
    b. Outcomes
      (1) Client identifies support systems.
      (2) Significant other is involved in a supportive manner.
      (3) Client is referred for appropriate treatment.
      (4) Client verbalizes impact of alcoholism on herself and her family.

5. Noncompliance related to difficulty in following prenatal recommendations
   a. Interventions
      (1) Same as with other substance abuse patients
   b. Outcomes
      (1) Same as with other substance abuse patients
6. Risk for injury related to use of alcohol during pregnancy
   a. Interventions
      (1) Identify alcohol use and its severity.
      (2) Teach, review, and reinforce information.
      (3) Give specific suggestions for controlling alcohol intake.
         (a) Measure alcohol.
         (b) Avoid two-liquor mixes.
         (c) Never gulp down drinks.
         (d) Learn to refuse a drink and substitute an alternative, such as juice.
      (4) Help family members and significant others develop skills necessary to support the client.
      (5) Refer the client to appropriate counseling and rehabilitation.
      (6) Develop high-quality educational programs about the deleterious consequences of alcohol for the unborn child, and integrate into drug prevention education at all school age levels.
   b. Outcomes
      (1) Client minimizes potential for further injury by decreasing alcohol intake.
7. Risk for impaired parenting related to alcohol use
   a. Interventions
      (1) Same as with other substance abuse patients
   b. Outcomes
      (1) Same as with other substance abuse patients

HEALTH EDUCATION

A. Prevention
1. Dispel myths that drugs, alcohol, and smoking are harmless; educate client on the potential dangers of their use to both mother and baby.
2. Inform client of contraindication of drug use while breastfeeding (include alcohol, amphetamines, cocaine, heroin, marijuana, and nicotine).

B. Referral to community
1. Refer pregnant women to specialized programs that address the medical, obstetric, psychological, neonatal, and pediatric needs of women and their babies.
2. Resources
   a. Center on Addiction and Substance Abuse at Columbia University: *www.casacolumbia.org*
   b. Centers for Disease Control and Prevention (CDC): *www.cdc.gov*
   c. Cocaine hotline: (800) 662-HELP
   d. March of Dimes Birth Defects Foundation: (914) 428-7100
   e. National Clearinghouse for Alcohol and Drug Information (NCADI): (301) 468-2600; *www.health.org*
   f. National Institute of Child Health and Human Development (NICHD): (301) 496-5133
   g. National Institute on Drug Abuse: (800) 662-HELP, (301) 443-1124; *www.nida.nih.gov*
   h. Substance Abuse and Mental Health Services Administration: *www.samhsa.gov*

CASE STUDIES AND STUDY QUESTIONS

SUBSTANCE ABUSE

Mrs. G is a 29-year-old gravida 2, para 0 (G2, P0) who is 18 weeks pregnant. She is married and very excited about the pregnancy. On her third prenatal visit, you notice that she has nasal congestion and slightly slurred speech. There is no odor of alcohol. You suspect she might be using cocaine.

1. A toxicologic urine screen can detect cocaine ingestion within the past:
   a. 10 hours
   b. 24 hours
   c. 1 week
   d. 2 hours

2. A possible result of cocaine use would be:
   a. IUGR
   b. Polyhydramnios
   c. Polydipsia
   d. Postterm pregnancy

3. It is probable that Mrs. G is using cocaine intranasally. What is the significance of this?
   a. It might reduce its ability to cross the placenta.
   b. It more readily crosses the placenta.
   c. It does not reach the placenta because it is exhaled immediately.

4. Answer the following true or false.
   a. Stillbirths are associated with the addicted patient. T
   b. Both premature rupture of membranes (PROM) and abruptio placenta are associated with drug abuse during pregnancy. T
   c. Cocaine will not cause ill effects to the fetus if used only in the second trimester. F
   d. Maternal-infant bonding might be enhanced by some drug use because of the relaxation effect. F

   e. SIDS is not associated with addiction. F

SMOKING

Ms. U is an 18-year-old G1 whose last menstrual period was 21 weeks earlier. Her history is unremarkable except for the fact that she smokes a pack of cigarettes a day. She believes smoking helps her control her weight and also helps her relax. She has been told that smoking will not harm the baby. On examination, Ms. U has gained 908 g (2 lb) since the beginning of her pregnancy. Her blood pressure is 118/72, the fetal heart rate is 140. She has not noticed fetal movement.

5. What three detrimental compounds are found in cigarettes?
   a. Carbon monoxide
   b. Nicotine
   c. Cyanide
   d. Tar
   e. Tannic acid

6. All of the following are major effects of smoking on pregnancy except:
   a. Maternal vasoconstriction and reduced oxygen availability
   b. Reduced oxygen-carrying capacity of erythrocytes
   c. Fetal bradycardia

7. Which of the following are maternal risks due to smoking?
   a. Abruptio placenta
   b. Vitamin C depletion
   c. Excessive weight gain
   d. Bronchitis

8. Answer the following true or false.
   a. Impaired uteroplacental blood flow decreases oxygen exchange across the placenta. T
   b. Babies born to mothers who smoke will not have weight problems. F

c. SIDS occurs less frequently in babies of mothers who smoke. *F*

d. It is not important if a mother quits smoking in the second trimester, because the damage is already done. *F*

ALCOHOL

Mrs. J, 29 years old, delivered a 3203-g (7 lb, 1 oz) baby boy 24 hours earlier. She says that she had been concerned during her pregnancy because she drank heavily in her first trimester before knowing she was pregnant. She begins to ask questions.

9. Answer the following true or false.
   a. Growth restriction might result from alcohol ingestion. *T*

b. Spontaneous abortions occur more frequently in mothers who drink heavily. *T*

c. Drinking after the first trimester is acceptable. *F*

10. Features of fetal alcohol syndrome are all the following *except:*
    a. CNS damage
    b. Flattened philtrum
    c. Cardiac defects
    d. Short fingers

11. When counseling a woman who is pregnant, what should you tell her?
    a. Alcohol in the third trimester will not affect the fetus.
    b. One glass of wine is considered safe.
    c. There is no safe limit of alcohol during pregnancy.

ANSWERS TO STUDY QUESTIONS

1. b
2. a
3. b
4. a. True; b. True; c. False; d. False; e. False
5. a,b,c
6. c
7. a,b,d
8. a. True; b. False; c. False; d. False
9. a. True; b. True; c. False;
10. d
11. c

REFERENCES

American Society of Addiction Medicine. (1998). *Principles of addiction medicine.* Chevy Chase, MD: American Society of Addiction Medicine.

Baldwin, J., Rawlings, A., Marshall, E., Conger, C., & Abbott, K. (1999). Mom empowerment, too: A program for young mothers involved in substance abuse. *Public Health Nursing, 16*(6), 376-383.

Bragg, E. (1997). Pregnant adolescents with addictions. *Journal of Obstetric, Gynecologic, and Neonatal Nursing, 26*(5), 577-584.

Centers for Disease Control and Prevention (2002). *Alcohol use among women of childbearing age—United States, 1991-1999.* Available online at *www.cdc.gov/mmwr/review/mmwrhtml/mm5113a3.htm.*

Centers for Disease Control and Prevention. (2002). *National task force on fetal alcohol syndrome and fetal alcohol effect.* Available online at *www.cdc.gov/ mmwr/preview/mmwrhtml/rr5114a2.htm.*

Centers for Disease Control and Prevention. (2003). *Fetal alcohol syndrome.* Available online at *www.cdc.gov/ncbddd/fas.*

Corrarino, J., Williams, C., Campbell, W., Amrhein, E., LoPiano, L., & Kalachik, D. (2000). Linking substance-abusing pregnant women to drug treatment services: A pilot program. *Journal of Obstetric, Gynecologic, and Neonatal Nursing, 29*(4), 369-376.

Davis, S. Comprehensive interventions for affecting the parenting effectiveness of chemically dependent women. (1997). *Journal of Obstetric, Gynecologic, and Neonatal Nursing, 26*(5), 604-610.

Ernst, M., Moolchan, E., & Robinson, M. (2001). Behavioral and neural consequences of prenatal exposure to nicotine. *Journal of the American Academy of Child and Adolescent Psychiatry, 40*(6), 630-641.

Jacobs, E., Joffe, A., Kulig, J., McDonald, C., Rogers, P., & Shah, R. (2000). Fetal alcohol syndrome and alcohol-related neurodevelomental disorders. *Pediatrics, 106*(2), 358-361.

Kaltenbach, K., & Finnegan, L. (1998, June 21). Prevention and treatment issues for pregnant cocaine-dependent women and their infants. *Annals of the New York Academy of Sciences, 846*, 329-334.

Lindenberg, C. (1998). Risk and resilience: Building protective factors. An intervention for preventing substance abuse and sexual risk-taking and for promoting strength and protection among young, low-income Hispanic women. *MCN: The American Journal of Maternal Child Nursing, 23*(2), 99-104.

National Institute on Drug Abuse (NIDA). (1999). *Pregnancy and drug use trends.* Available online at *www.drugabuse.gov/Infofax/pregnancytrends.html.*

National Institute on Drug Abuse (NIDA). (2003a). *Research report series—Marijuana abuse.* Available online at *www.nida.hih.gov/ResearchReports/Marijuana/Marijuana4.html.*

National Institute on Drug Abuse (NIDA). (2003b). *Women and drug abuse.* Available online at *www.nida.nih.gov.*

Substance Abuse and Mental Health Services Administration. (1998). *Substance abuse and mental health statistics source book.* Rockville, MD: U.S. Department of Health and Human Services.

Weissman, M., Warner, V., Wickramaratne, P., & Kandel, D. (1999). Maternal smoking during pregnancy and psychopathology in offspring followed to adulthood. *Journal of the American Academy of Child and Adolescent Psychiatry, 38*(7), 892-899.

28 Other Medical Complications

MARGARET YANCY

OBJECTIVES

1. Describe the data to be documented in obtaining a history from pregnant clients with cardiac, respiratory, renal, hematologic, gastrointestinal, and hepatic complications.

2. Select nursing diagnoses appropriate for pregnant clients with cardiac, respiratory, renal, hematologic, gastrointestinal, and hepatic complications.

3. Describe the fetal implications for pregnant clients with medical complications.

4. Describe the signs and symptoms and laboratory data that indicate cardiac, respiratory, renal, hematologic, gastrointestinal, and hepatic complications of pregnancy.

5. Formulate a plan of care (consisting of nursing diagnoses, interventions, and outcome measures based on nursing history and assessments) for the pregnant client with cardiovascular, respiratory, renal, hematologic, gastrointestinal, and hepatic complications.

6. Design a plan to teach principles necessary for maintenance of health for pregnant clients with cardiac, respiratory, renal, hematologic, gastrointestinal, and hepatic complications.

INTRODUCTION

A. **Women who enter pregnancy with a preexisting disease or a chronic condition are at risk for complications;** the disease can complicate the course of pregnancy or, alternatively, the pregnancy might worsen the disease process.

B. **Women with medical complications of pregnancy often experience anxiety regarding the impact of the complication on the outcome of the pregnancy.**

CLINICAL PRACTICE

A. **Assessment**
   1. History
      a. Duration and course of disease
      b. Treatment and medications
      c. Medical complications affecting previous pregnancies
   2. Physical findings
      a. Refer to specific disease or condition.
   3. Diagnostic procedures and laboratory tests
      a. Refer to specific disease or condition.
B. **Nursing Diagnoses**
   1. Anxiety and fear related to complicated pregnancy
   2. Risk for interrupted family processes related to maternal complications of pregnancy and hospitalization
   3. Deficient knowledge related to disease complicating pregnancy
C. **Interventions/Outcomes**
   1. Anxiety and fear related to complicated pregnancy
      a. Interventions

    (1) Discuss client's fears and concerns about her pregnancy and its outcome.

    (2) Provide reassurance and comfort.

    (3) Obtain and begin involvement of social worker and other health team members.

    (4) Encourage client to ask questions about tests, medications, treatments, and physician orders.

    (5) Explain all procedures and their purpose.

    (6) Acknowledge client's feelings and respond appropriately to her needs.

    (7) Maintain clean, orderly, quiet, and stress-free environment.

    (8) Assess family members' level of anxiety and knowledge of disease process; assess them as a support system for client.

    (9) Arrange for a tour of special care nursery or for infant special care staff to visit with client/family as appropriate; orient client to realistic expectations for newborn.

    (10) Encourage client's interest in diversional activities (e.g., crafts, books, music).

    (11) Encourage client to use visualization exercises, music, and crafts for relaxation.

  b. Outcomes

    (1) Client verbalizes her fears and concerns about her pregnancy.

    (2) Client feels supported.

    (3) Client is able to relax and sleep.

2. Risk for interrupted family processes related to maternal complications of pregnancy and hospitalization

  a. Interventions

    (1) Allow client and her family members to ventilate fears about pregnancy outcome.

    (2) Assess client and family members' responses to complicated pregnancy.

      (a) Presence of unresolved guilt, blame, hostility, or jealousy

      (b) Inability to problem solve adequately

      (c) Ineffective patterns of communication

    (3) Assess level of financial burden on family.

    (4) Discuss effects of prolonged hospitalization on the family process.

    (5) If client is hospitalized, encourage client's friends and family to visit frequently; instruct them about visiting hours.

    (6) Encourage client and her family to participate in support groups and education programs.

    (7) Utilize additional resources as appropriate.

      (a) Social worker

      (b) Clinical nurse specialist

      (c) Clinical psychologist

      (d) Lay support and self-help groups

      (e) Home health care

      (f) Financial assistance programs

    (8) Assist family in reorganizing roles at home and setting priorities to maintain family integrity and to reduce stress.

    (9) Aid family members in changing their expectations of the client realistically.

    (10) Prepare client and her family members for signs of depression, anxiety, and dependency.

(11) Assess the client and family's spiritual needs and help them to meet those needs.

    b. Outcomes: client and family demonstrate a functional system of mutual support for each other as evidenced by the following:

        (1) Seeking appropriate external resources when needed

        (2) Engaging in open communication with the health team

        (3) Participating in care of the hospitalized family member

3. Deficient knowledge related to disease complicating pregnancy

    a. Interventions

        (1) Assess client and family members' readiness and ability to learn.

        (2) Determine clients knowledge of her illness, its treatment, and preventive measures.

        (3) Assess clients adherence to prescribed treatment regimen and its effect on her lifestyle.

        (4) Begin client and family education regarding the disease and its effects on the mother and fetus.

        (5) Discuss signs and symptoms to report.

        (6) Explain the purpose of treatments, interventions, and tests.

        (7) Teach client behavioral interventions as appropriate to her condition.

            (a) Bed rest in lateral position (explain physiologic rationale).

            (b) Observance of prescribed medication regimen

            (c) Maintenance of as quiet and stress-free an environment as possible

        (8) Explain to client the rationale and procedure for fetal assessment tests such as:

            (a) Nonstress test (NST)

            (b) Biophysical profile

            (c) Amniocentesis

    b. Outcomes

        (1) Client verbalizes an understanding of her disease and its effect on the fetus.

        (2) Client can describe the disease process, causes, signs and symptoms, and interventions for disease control.

CARDIAC COMPLICATIONS

A. Cardiac disease of varying severity occurs in approximately 1% of all pregnancies and is the leading nonobstetric cause of maternal mortality (Cunningham et al., 2001).

B. Pregnancy causes significant alterations in maternal cardiovascular physiology; these hemodynamic changes have a profound effect on pregnant patients with cardiac disease; each of these changes increases cardiac work and might exceed the functional capacity of a diseased heart, resulting in pulmonary hypertension, pulmonary edema, congestive heart failure, or maternal death (Gei & Hankins, 2001); these changes include:

1. Increased heart rate

2. Increased stroke volume

3. Increased cardiac output

4. Expanding blood volume

5. Decreased peripheral vascular resistance

6. Decreased pulmonary vascular resistance

7. Decreased colloid oncotic pressure

C. **The risk of maternal mortality associated with specific cardiac lesions is outlined in Box 28-1;** the potential for a successful pregnancy is also determined by the functional limitation with which the patient enters pregnancy; those patients entering pregnancy at New York Heart Association (NYHA) functional class I or II usually do well during pregnancy (Cunningham et al., 2001) (Table 28-1); the risk of perinatal and maternal morbidity and mortality associated with cardiac disease during pregnancy depends on:
1. The specific cardiac lesion
2. The functional abnormality produced by the lesion
3. Development of pregnancy-related complications, such as infection, hemorrhage, or preeclampsia
D. **Cardiac disease during pregnancy may be categorized as congenital, acquired (rheumatic), or ischemic** (Gei & Hankins, 2001; Wenstrom & Malee, 1999).
1. Congenital cardiac disease
   a. Is more common because with improvements in diagnosis and treatment, more women with congenital heart defects are surviving to reproductive age.
   b. Includes atrial septal defect, ventricular septal defect, pulmonic stenosis, congenital aortic stenosis, coarctation of the aorta, tetralogy of Fallot, and Eisenmenger syndrome.
2. Acquired cardiac disease
   a. Is mainly rheumatic in origin.
   b. Frequency of rheumatic heart disease has been decreasing.
   c. Includes valvular lesions such as mitral stenosis and aortic stenosis.

■ BOX 28-1
■ **MORTALITY RISK ASSOCIATED WITH PREGNANCY**

Group I: Mortality < 1%
Atrial septal defect, uncomplicated
Ventricular septal defect, uncomplicated
Patent ductus arteriosus, uncomplicated
Pulmonic/tricuspid disease
Corrected tetralogy of Fallot
Porcine valve
Mitral stenosis, NYHA classes I and II

Group II: Mortality 5%-15%
Mitral stenosis with atrial fibrillation
Artificial valve
Mitral stenosis, NYHA classes III and IV
Aortic stenosis
Coarctation of aorta, uncomplicated
Uncorrected tetralogy of Fallot
Previous myocardial infarction
Marfan's syndrome with normal aorta

Group III: Mortality 25%-50%
Pulmonary hypertension
Coarctation of aorta, complicated
Marfan's syndrome with aortic involvement

From Clark, S., Cotton, D., Hankin, G., & Phelan J. (1994). *Handbook of critical care obstetrics.* Boston: Blackwell Scientific Publications.

■ TABLE 28-1
■ ■ **New York Heart Association Cardiac Disease Classification**

Class	Description
I	Clients with cardiac disease and no limitation of physical activity. Clients in this class do not have symptoms of cardiac insufficiency, nor do they experience pain.
II	Clients with cardiac disease and slight limitation of physical activity. They are comfortable at rest, but if ordinary physical activity is undertaken, discomfort results in the form of excessive fatigue, palpitation, dyspnea, or anginal pain.
III	Clients with cardiac disease and marked limitation of physical activity. They are comfortable at rest, but less-than-ordinary activity causes discomfort in the form of excessive fatigue, palpitation, dyspnea, or anginal pain.
IV	Clients with cardiac disease and inability to perform any physical activity without discomfort. Symptoms of cardiac insufficiency or of the anginal syndrome might occur even at rest, and if any physical activity is undertaken, discomfort is increased.

   3. Ischemic cardiac disease
      a. Coronary artery disease (rare in pregnancy)
      b. Myocardial infarction (rare in pregnancy)
   E. **Fetus is at increased risk.**
      1. The fetus is at risk for hypoxia because of maternal hypoxemia.
      2. The incidence of prematurity, intrauterine growth restriction (IUGR), spontaneous abortion, and stillbirth is increased because of maternal hypoxemia.
      3. If the woman has congenital heart disease, there is an increased incidence of fetal congenital cardiac anomalies.

CLINICAL PRACTICE

A. **Assessment**
   1. History
      a. Category of heart disease: congenital, acquired, or ischemic
      b. Duration and course of disease
      c. NYHA Functional Classification of Cardiac Disease: degree of limitation of physical activity
      d. Previous surgeries
      e. Response to previous pregnancies
      f. Prescribed medications
   2. Physical findings
      a. Vital signs: blood pressure and apical/radial pulse
      b. Signs and symptoms of heart disease; Table 28-2 lists the signs and symptoms common to normal pregnancy compared with those of actual heart disease.
      c. Signs and symptoms of cardiac decompensation (Gilbert & Harmon, 2003)
         (1) Dyspnea severe enough to limit usual activity
         (2) Progressive orthopnea
         (3) Paroxysmal nocturnal dyspnea
         (4) Syncope during or immediately following exertion
         (5) Chest pain associated with activity

■ TABLE 28-2
■ ■ **Signs and Symptoms Common to Normal Pregnancy Compared with Signs and Symptoms of Actual Cardiac Disease**

Normal Pregnancy	Actual Heart Disease
Chest discomfort	Chest discomfort with myocardial ischemia
Dyspnea	Severe dyspnea that limits activity; paroxysmal nocturnal dyspnea
Orthopnea	Progressive orthopnea
Palpitations	Cardiac arrhythmia
Easy fatigability	Fatigue with chest pain and syncope
Dizzy spells	Dizzy spells plus other actual signs and symptoms
Syncope	Syncope with exertion
Systolic murmurs	Loud, harsh, systolic murmurs: grade III intensity, diastolic murmurs
Dependent edema	Dependent plus nondependent edema
Rales in lower lung fields	Rales that do not clear with deep inspiration; hemoptysis
Visible neck veins	Persistent neck vein distention
Cardiomegaly	Cardiomegaly plus hepatomegaly and ascites

     d. Signs and symptoms of congestive heart failure
        (1) Right-sided congestive heart failure (CHF)
           (a) Neck vein distension
           (b) Hepatomegaly
           (c) Dependent and nondependent edema
           (d) Weight gain
        (2) Left-sided CHF
           (a) Dyspnea
           (b) Orthopnea
           (c) Rales
           (d) Cough
           (e) Extreme fatigue
           (f) Chest pain
           (g) Syncope
           (h) Pallor
           (i) Cyanosis
           (j) Cardiac arrhythmias
     e. Laboratory and diagnostic studies
           (a) Arterial blood gas values or pulse oximetry, as indicated
           (b) Coagulation studies
           (c) Serum electrolytes
           (d) White blood cell count
           (e) Hemoglobin and hematocrit
           (f) Cardiac enzymes as indicated
           (g) Electrocardiogram
           (h) Cardiac ultrasonography
           (i) Echocardiogram
           (j) Chest radiograph
     f. Fetal assessment tests
  B. Nursing Diagnoses
     1. Risk for decreased cardiac output related to structural defects, CHF, or pulmonary edema
     2. Activity intolerance related to decreased cardiac output and tissue malnutrition

3. Risk for infection related to bacterial invasion, pulmonary congestion, or invasive procedures
4. Ineffective protection related to thromboembolism secondary to valvular defects, decreased venous return, or hypercoagulability of pregnancy
5. Risk for fetal injury related to decreased uteroplacental blood flow secondary to decreased cardiac output

C. **Interventions/Outcomes**

1. Risk for decreased cardiac output related to structural defects, CHF, or pulmonary edema

   a. Interventions

      (1) Monitor for signs and symptoms of decreased cardiac output (Carpenito, 1997).
         (a) Decreased and/or irregular pulse rate
         (b) Increased respiratory rate
         (c) Decreased blood pressure
         (d) Abnormal heart sounds
         (e) Decreased urine output (less than 30 ml/hr)
         (f) Changes in mentation
         (g) Abnormal lung sounds (crackles)
         (h) Cool, moist, cyanotic, mottled skin
         (i) Delayed capillary refill time
         (j) Neck vein distention
         (k) Weak peripheral pulses
         (l) Electrocardiogram (ECG) changes
         (m) Dysrhythmias
         (n) Decreased oxygen saturation
      (2) Teach client to avoid stress and anxiety.
      (3) Instruct the client in following a low-sodium diet to prevent fluid retention.
      (4) Monitor weight gain; encourage client to avoid excessive weight gain, which causes increased cardiac workload.
      (5) Counsel client to avoid physical exertion and encourage frequent rest periods in left lateral recumbent position.
      (6) Administer cardiovascular medications as ordered; evaluate the client's response to medication (Table 28-3 lists cardiovascular drugs during pregnancy).
      (7) Provide nutritional counseling, encourage high-iron foods, and administer iron and vitamin supplements as ordered to prevent anemia.
      (8) Encourage patient to labor in lateral position; avoid lithotomy position during second stage of labor.
      (9) Provide effective pain control during labor and delivery to decrease cardiac workload.
      (10) Encourage gentle pushing to avoid erratic venous return associated with Valsalva.
      (11) Assess hemodynamic function and cardiac output during the intrapartum period and after delivery by implementing hemodynamic monitoring as ordered (e.g., cardiac monitor, arterial line, central venous pressure catheter, pulmonary artery catheter).
      (12) Monitor intake and output carefully, and regulate intravenous (IV) fluids with an infusion pump to prevent fluid overload and possible pulmonary edema.
      (13) Minimize postpartum blood loss to prevent hypovolemia.

    b. Outcomes

        (1) Client maintains adequate cardiac output to meet maternal demand.

        (2) Client maintains optimal hemodynamic parameters.

2. Activity intolerance related to decreased cardiac output and tissue malnutrition

    a. Interventions

        (1) Assess activity tolerance.

        (2) Assist client in modifying schedule and spacing activities to allow for more rest.

        (3) Maintain client's activity level short of fatigue.

        (4) Encourage client to obtain 8 to 10 hours of sleep per night and to take frequent rest periods during the day.

        (5) Iron and folic acid supplements are frequently needed, and hemoglobin and hematocrit levels should be carefully monitored.

        (6) Assist client with activities of daily living (ADLs) and ambulation as necessary, or refer to appropriate social services for help with household responsibilities, as needed.

    b. Outcomes

        (1) Client tolerates mild activity with no functional limitation.

        (2) Vital signs and other parameters remain normal.

3. Risk for infection related to bacterial invasion, pulmonary congestion, or invasive procedures

    a. Interventions

        (1) Teach the client to recognize the signs and symptoms of infection.

        (2) Caution the client to avoid exposure to infection.

        (3) Antibiotic prophylaxis is frequently used to prevent bacterial endocarditis.

        (4) Use strict aseptic technique during invasive procedures.

        (5) Monitor for leukocytosis.

        (6) Assess vital signs.

    b. Outcomes

        (1) Client does not exhibit signs or symptoms of infection.

        (2) Vital signs and other parameters are normal.

4. Ineffective protection related to thromboembolism secondary to valvular defects, decreased venous return, or hypercoagulability of pregnancy

    a. Interventions

        (1) Assess for signs and symptoms of thromboembolism (Carpenito, 1997).

            (a) Diminished or absent peripheral pulses

            (b) Unusual warmth and redness or coolness and cyanosis

            (c) Increasing leg pain

            (d) Sudden severe chest pain, increased dyspnea, and tachypnea

            (e) Positive Homans' sign

        (2) Antiembolic stockings as ordered

        (3) Anticoagulant therapy (usually heparin) and monitoring of blood coagulation laboratory results to detect any preliminary indications or risk of abnormal bleeding

            (a) Hematuria

            (b) Bleeding gums

            (c) Ecchymoses

            (d) Petechiae (Carpenito, 1997)

■ TABLE 28-3
■ ■ **Cardiovascular Drugs during Pregnancy**

Drug Group	Use during Pregnancy	Adverse Effects
Diuretics	Use as in nonpregnant women. Should not be used prophylactically or to treat pedal edema unless there is associated pulmonary vascular congestion.	Might exacerbate preeclampsia by reducing uterine blood flow.
Inotropic agent	Pregnancy does not alter the indications for digitalis therapy. An increased dose might be required to achieve acceptable serum levels. Digitalis crosses the placenta and is excreted in breast milk, but fetal or infant toxicity is unusual. Beta-stimulating or dopaminergic agents should be reserved for life-threatening situations.	Labor potentially earlier and shorter in women on digitalis. Might decrease uterine blood flow.
Vasodilators	Afterload-reducing agents; adverse fetal effect not reported with hydralazine. Avoid angiotensin-converting enzyme (ACE) inhibitors. Preload-reducing agents; nitrates indicated as in nonpregnant state. Nitroprusside justified in life-threatening situations. Little experience with pregnancy.	Hypotension may jeopardize uterine blood flow. Fetal renal development abnormalities with ACE inhibitors. Concern about, but no documentation of, cyanide toxicity with nitroprusside.
Antiarrhythmic agents	Indications for use as in nonpregnant state. Greatest experience with quinidine, but procainamide and disopyramide not clearly inferior. Lidocaine crosses the placenta, but no teratogenic effects have been reported.	Potential fetal dysrhythmias. Phenytoin can cause fetal abnormalities and should be avoided.
Beta-blocking agents	May be used to treat hypertension, angina and supraventricular tachyarrhythmias when there are no reasonable alternatives. Close fetal and newborn monitoring required. Selective beta-blockers may result in fewer adverse fetal effects.	Can depress intrauterine growth. Newborn bradycardia, hypotension, hypoglycemia, and respiratory depression occur.

Continued

TABLE 28-3
Cardiovascular Drugs during Pregnancy—cont'd

Drug Group	Use during Pregnancy	Adverse Effects
Calcium channel blockers	Verapamil and nifedipine can be used as blockers in nonpregnant state. Little information on diltiazem and almost none on newly introduced agents.	Might cause uterine relaxation.
Anticoagulants	Warfarin *contraindicated* at time of conception and during pregnancy because of teratogenic effect and because placental and fetal bleeding.	Teratogenic effect 10%-20% in first trimester.
	When anticoagulation required, heparin via subcutaneous administration at home is preferred. It does not cross the placenta.	Maternal and placental bleeding.
	Acetylsalicylic acid can be used, but there is some increased risk of bleeding. No reported experience with dipyridamole or sulfinpyrazone.	Maternal and fetal bleeding. Potential premature closure of ductus arteriosus by prostaglandin inhibition.

From Burrow, G., & Ferris, T. (1995). *Medical complications during pregnancy* (4th ed.; p. 134). Philadelphia: Sanders.

b. Outcomes
  (1) Client does not exhibit signs or symptoms of thromboembolism.
  (2) Client does not show any indications of abnormal bleeding problems or thromboembolism.
  5. Risk for fetal injury related to decreased uteroplacental blood flow secondary to decreased cardiac output: see Chapters 8 and 12 for a discussion of decreased uteroplacental blood flow interventions and outcomes.

HEALTH EDUCATION

A. Preconceptual counseling
  1. Discuss the risk of pregnancy to the mother and the risks to the fetus.
  2. Discuss potentially teratogenic cardiovascular drugs.
    a. Warfarin
    b. Propranolol
    c. Thiazide diuretics
    d. Angiotensin-converting enzyme (ACE) inhibitors
  3. Discuss the advances that have improved the outcome for women with cardiac disease in:
    a. Medical and surgical therapy
    b. Fetal surveillance
    c. Neonatal care
B. Discuss the importance of regular and frequent medical supervision and encourage client to be in the care of an obstetrician and a cardiologist.
C. Discuss the importance of a multidisciplinary team including nursing, dietary, and social service.
D. Teach client about rationale for modifying her diet and activities and for taking prescribed medications.
E. Teach client to limit exposure to infection.
F. Discuss the importance of obtaining antibiotic prophylaxis before dental and surgical procedures.
G. Teach client to get adequate rest with frequent rest periods and to restrict activity to that which is just short of fatigue.
H. Teach client to modify diet; no added salt or about 2 g/day (more stringent with CHF).
I. Teach client to avoid excessive weight gain.
J. Teach client to maintain normal hemoglobin levels by eating increased amounts of high-iron and folic-acid–containing foods and taking supplements if needed.
K. Teach client to report signs and symptoms of cardiac decompensation.

RENAL COMPLICATIONS

A. Anatomic and physiologic changes that occur in the kidney during pregnancy include:
  1. Marked dilation of the collecting system
  2. Stasis of urine in the upper part of the collecting system
  3. Delayed emptying
  4. Increase in renal plasma flow
  5. Increase in glomerular filtration rate (GFR)
  6. Changes in tubular reabsorption of glucose and amino acids so glycosuria and aminoaciduria are normal in pregnancy
  7. Decrease in blood urea nitrogen (BUN) and serum creatinine

8. Decreased serum osmolality
9. Increased uric acid filtration and secretion, leading to decreased levels of uric acid (Thorsen, 2002)

B. **Renal disease during pregnancy falls into two categories:** new onset of renal disease during pregnancy and chronic renal disease.
   1. New onset of renal disease during pregnancy
      a. Acute pyelonephritis
         (1) Approximately 4% to 10% of all pregnant women have asymptomatic bacteriuria, and, if untreated, 25% to 40% of them will experience pyelonephritis; acute pyelonephritis effects 1% to 3% of pregnancies (Cunningham et al., 2001; Wenstrom & Malee, 1999).
         (2) *Escherichia coli* is responsible for more than 80% of infections.
      b. Acute nephrolithiasis (renal stones): occurs in 1 of every 1000 deliveries.
      c. Acute renal failure
         (1) Incidence of 1 in 10,000 pregnancies
         (2) Multiple causes are categorized as:
            (a) Women with preexisting renal disease.
            (b) Consequences of pregnancy associated event.
            (c) Consequences of a nonpregnant event (i.e., trauma) (Thorsen, 2002).
         (3) Most common cause is severe preeclampsia or following hemorrhagic shock.
      d. Nephrotic syndrome
         (1) Proteinuria greater than 3 g/day
         (2) Serum albumin less than 3 g/dl
         (3) Edema
         (4) Hyperlipidemia
   2. Chronic renal disease
      a. In patients with mildly impaired renal function, pregnancy does not usually accelerate renal damage (Cunningham et al., 2001).
      b. Preexisting hypertension along with the degree of renal insufficiency are predictive of pregnancy outcome.
      c. Patients with renal transplants can sustain a pregnancy; pregnancy should not be considered for 2 years following implantation of a cadaver kidney, or 1 year after a live donor kidney; with the understanding that continuation of immunosuppressive therapy is essential (Thorsen, 2002).

C. **Adverse consequences of pregnancy in renal disease**
   1. Maternal consequences
      a. Hypertension
         (1) New onset
         (2) Increased severity
         (3) Superimposed preeclampsia
      b. Proteinuria
         (1) Worsens
         (2) Nephrotic syndrome can develop
      c. Decreased renal function
         (1) New onset
         (2) Accelerated rate of decline
   2. Fetal consequences
      a. Fetal loss
         (1) Spontaneous abortion
         (2) Stillbirth
         (3) Neonatal death

b. Preterm birth

c. Intrauterine growth restriction (IUGR)

CLINICAL PRACTICE

A. Assessment

  1. History

    a. Incidence of urinary tract infections (UTIs)

      (1) Pregnant women are at greater risk for UTI because of the physiologic changes of pregnancy.

        (a) Decreased bladder tone can cause stasis of urine.

        (b) Delayed or incomplete emptying of bladder

    b. Incidence and duration of acute and/or chronic renal disease

    c. History of medical conditions associated with acute renal failure

  2. Physical findings

    a. Signs and symptoms of UTI

      (1) Dysuria

      (2) Frequency

      (3) Urgency of urination

      (4) Lower abdominal pain

    b. Signs and symptoms of pyelonephritis

      (1) Fever

      (2) Chills

      (3) Flank pain: sometimes reported as lower back pain

      (4) Costovertebral angle (CVA) tenderness

      (5) Urgency

      (6) Frequency

      (7) Nausea

      (8) Vomiting

      (9) Malaise

      (10) Dehydration

    c. Signs and symptoms or fluid overload and systemic vascular resistance

      (1) Vital signs

      (2) Peripheral edema

      (3) Distended neck veins

      (4) Breath sounds

    d. Neurologic signs and symptoms of rapid onset acute renal failure

      (1) Fatigue

      (2) Lethargy

      (3) Somnolence

      (4) Irritability

      (5) Disorientation

      (6) Tonic-clonic seizures

    e. Laboratory and diagnostic tests for renal disease

      (1) Urinalysis

        (a) Proteinuria: indicates glomerular damage.

        (b) Hematuria: if with red cell casts, indicates glomerular inflammation and injury.

        (c) Pyuria: indicates inflammation/infection.

      (2) Urine culture and sensitivity

      (3) Serum creatinine

      (4) Creatinine clearance

      (5) 24-hour urine protein

      (6) BUN

      (7) Uric acid

      (8) Electrolytes

      (9) Intravenous pyelography (IVP)

      (10) Renal ultrasonography

      (11) Arterial blood gases as indicated

      (12) ECG as indicated

      (13) Pulse oximetry as indicated

   f. Fetal assessment

      (1) Because of the strong association of renal disease with IUGR, fetal surveillance is important.

      (2) Fetal heart rate monitoring, biophysical profile (BPP), ultrasonography, and fetal lung maturity if severity of maternal disease warrants early delivery

B. Nursing Diagnoses

  1. Risk for infection related to anatomic and physiologic changes of the renal system in pregnancy

  2. Excess or deficient fluid volume related to inability of kidney to regulate fluid balance

  3. Risk for renal insufficiency related to chronic renal disease

  4. Impaired comfort related to bladder spasm or renal colic; risk for renal calculi

C. Interventions/Outcomes

  1. Risk for infection related to anatomic and physiologic changes of the renal system in pregnancy

    a. Interventions

      (1) Monitor signs and symptoms of infection (UTI or pyelonephritis).

      (2) Administer antibiotics as ordered.

      (3) Maintain adequate hydration; encourage oral intake, and, if necessary, administer IV fluids as ordered.

      (4) Assess for maternal bacteremia via blood culture.

      (5) Assess for maternal septic shock by monitoring vital signs for tachycardia and hypotension.

      (6) Monitor for contractions and other signs and symptoms of preterm labor.

      (7) Obtain follow-up urine culture.

    b. Outcomes

      (1) Client exhibits no fever, chills, dysuria, frequency, or abdominal or CVA pain.

      (2) Clean-catch urine specimen has a bacteria count below 100,000 colonies/ml.

  2. Excess or deficient fluid volume related to inability of the kidney to regulate fluid balance

  3. Risk for renal insufficiency related to chronic renal disease

    a. Interventions

      (1) Monitor for signs and symptoms of improvement or deterioration in renal status by observing the following parameters:

        (a) Urinalysis reports

        (b) Kidney function tests: serum creatinine, BUN, uric acid, and creatinine clearance

        (c) Complete blood count (CBC)

        (d) Electrolytes

        (e) Intake and output

        (f) Proteinuria

  (g) Blood pressure values
  (h) Dependent edema and sacral edema
  (i) Daily weight
  (j) Skin turgor, color, and temperature
  (k) Color, odor, and appearance of urine
(2) Position in left lateral position when on bed rest.
(3) Administer prescribed medications (e.g., antihypertensives).
(4) Maintain prescribed sodium restrictions.
(5) Adjust the client's daily fluid intake as ordered, and distribute fluid intake fairly evenly throughout the day.
(6) Observe for signs and symptoms of superimposed preeclampsia.
(7) Observe for signs and symptoms of renal insufficiency (Carpenito, 1997).
  (a) Increased BUN
  (b) Increased serum creatinine; decreased creatinine clearance
  (c) Nausea and vomiting
  (d) Systemic edema
  (e) Urticaria
  (f) Anemia
  (g) Elevated blood pressure
  (h) Fatigue and lethargy
  (i) Headache
  (j) Electrolyte imbalance (sodium, potassium, calcium, phosphorus, magnesium)
  (k) Mental confusion or apathy
  (l) Urine output less than 30 ml/hr
  (m) Metabolic acidosis
(8) Monitor for signs and symptoms of metabolic acidosis.
  (a) Rapid, shallow respirations
  (b) Headaches
  (c) Nausea and vomiting
  (d) Low plasma pH
  (e) Behavioral changes, drowsiness, and lethargy
(9) Consult with dietician for an appropriate diet.
b. Outcomes
(1) No evidence of excess or deficient fluid volume, renal failure, hypertension, or superimposed preeclampsia.
  (a) Urinalysis within normal limits
  (b) BUN, creatinine, uric acid, CBC, and electrolytes within normal limits
  (c) Urine output 30 to 60 ml/hr
  (d) Vital signs, especially blood pressure, within normal limits for client
  (e) Absence of edema, hyperreflexia, and clonus
  (f) 24-hour urinary protein not more than 300 mg/24 hr
  (g) Good skin turgor
4. Impaired comfort related to bladder spasm or renal colic; risk for renal calculi
  a. Interventions
  (1) Monitor for signs and symptoms of calculi.
    (a) Sediment in urine
    (b) Flank or loin pain
    (c) Hematuria
    (d) Abdominal pain, distention, nausea, and diarrhea (Carpenito, 1997)
  (2) Strain urine for calculi as indicated.

(3) Instruct the client to increase fluid intake, if not contraindicated.
(4) Assess pain-precipitating factors, and document deviation from baseline.
    (a) Quality
    (b) Region radiation
    (c) Severity
    (d) Duration
    (e) Relieving factors
(5) Have client evaluate pain intensity on a 1 to 10 scale (10 being most severe).
(6) Observe, report, and record verbal and nonverbal expressions of pain, fear, and anxiety.
(7) Provide and encourage rest periods and a restful environment.
(8) Medicate client with analgesics, antispasmodics, and antibiotics as ordered.
(9) Assess effectiveness of pain medications.
(10) Provide comfort measures.
(11) Teach client and her family about factors that contribute to pain experience.
(12) Assess client's urgency and frequency of urination and nocturia.
(13) Palpate client's bladder for distention.
(14) Provide preoperative and postoperative care if surgery is required for ureteral obstruction.

b. Outcomes
(1) Client verbalizes decreased pain intensity (using a scale of 1 to 10) in response to analgesics or other interventions within 1 hour of administration.
(2) Client maintains pain control or absence of pain as evidenced by the following:
    (a) Client's statement
    (b) Decreased use of analgesics
    (c) Increased activity
(3) Client does not develop renal calculi.

HEALTH EDUCATION

A. Preconceptual counseling
  1. Discuss increased risk of fetal loss and preeclampsia with clients already demonstrating proteinuria and hypertension.
  2. Discuss increased incidence of anovulation, menstrual irregularities, loss of libido, and decreased fertility among clients with underlying chronic renal disease.
  3. Discuss effects of pregnancy on chronic renal disease.
B. Teach client self-monitoring of weight gain, edema, and blood pressure.
C. Teach client to avoid exposure to infection.
D. Educate regarding prophylactic antibiotic therapy.
E. Discuss importance of adequate nutrition and compliance with prescribed diet and fluid intake.
F. Teach client to recognize and report signs of fluid and electrolyte imbalance and superimposed preeclampsia.
G. Stress importance of keeping appointments with her nephrologist and obstetrician.
H. Teach proper front to back perineal hygiene.

I. Teach all women to recognize and report the symptoms of UTI.
J. Teach signs and symptoms of premature labor and increased uterine irritability and when to report.

RESPIRATORY COMPLICATIONS

Pulmonary diseases have become more prevalent in the general population and, therefore, in pregnant women. Normal physiologic changes of pregnancy can cause a woman with a history of compromised respirations to decompensate. The outcome of a pregnant woman with respiratory complications depends on the adequacy of ventilation and oxygenation as well as early detection of decompensation. Hypoxia is the major fetal threat.

A. **Asthma**
1. Asthma is the most common form of lung disease that can impact pregnancy and affects approximately 4% of pregnancies (Murdock, 2002).
2. Asthma is a reversible syndrome characterized by varying degrees of airway obstruction, bronchial hyperresponsiveness, and bronchial edema (Wendel, 2001).
3. Well-controlled asthma during pregnancy allows women to continue a normal pregnancy with little or no increased risk to their health or that of their fetuses (Murdock, 2002).
4. Pregnancy has variable effects on the course of asthma with a third each becoming worse, improving, or remaining unchanged; the course of asthma in a previous pregnancy predicts the course in a subsequent pregnancy in approximately 60% of women; typically the more severe the disease, the more likely it is to worsen (Cunningham et al., 2001; Murdock, 2002; Wenstrom & Malee, 1999).
5. If asthma is poorly controlled, it can lead to hypoxia caused by severe bronchoconstriction; in pregnancy, this can be particularly threatening to fetal well-being.
6. Arterial blood gases should be interpreted according to normal values for pregnancy.
   a. pH 7.40-7.45
   b. PO_2 100-108
   c. PCO_2 28-31 (Murdock, 2002)
7. Asthma should be as aggressively treated during pregnancy as at any other time because the benefits of asthma control far outweigh the risks of medication usage.
8. Virtually all of the commonly used asthma medications are considered safe during pregnancy (De Swiet, 1999).
9. Asthma in pregnancy is associated with an increase in:
   a. Perinatal mortality
   b. Preterm birth
   c. Low birth weight
   d. IUGR
   e. Neonatal hypoxia (National Asthma Education Program, 1993)
10. According to the National Institutes of Health (NIH) guidelines for diagnosis and management of asthma, there are four management components.
    a. Ongoing monitoring of signs and symptoms, pulmonary function studies with a spirometer and peak expiratory meter
    b. Avoidance of triggers and other factors contributing to asthma severity

    c. Pharmacologic therapy using the stepwise approach

    d. Education to promote self management

  11. Goals of therapy include:

    a. Control symptoms, including nocturnal symptoms.

    b. Maintain normal or near normal pulmonary function.

    c. Prevent acute exacerbations.

    d. Avoid adverse effects from asthma medications.

    e. Deliver a healthy infant.

  12. Refer to National Asthma Education Program (1993) for a comprehensive discussion of management of patients with asthma during pregnancy.

B. Tuberculosis

  1. Tuberculosis (TB) is caused by infection with the acid-fast bacillus *Mycobacterium tuberculosis;* the bacillus is carried on droplet nuclei and spread by airborne transmission. TB remains a major health problem and has undergone a resurgence related to influx of women from Asia, Africa, Mexico, and Central America; homelessness; drug abuse; poverty; and HIV (Cunningham et al., 2001).

  2. Pregnancy is not altered by the patient's tuberculosis, and pregnancy itself is not a risk factor for tuberculosis. With the advent of effective chemotherapy treatment for active TB, pregnant women have the same good prognosis as their nonpregnant counterparts.

  3. Screening is recommended for pregnant women who fall into a high-risk group (Cunningham et al., 2001).

    a. Foreign-born persons from high-prevalence countries

    b. Medically underserved, low-income populations; high-risk racial/ethnic minorities

    c. Persons with HIV infection

    d. Alcoholics and IV drug users

    e. Those with close contact to infectious cases

    f. Persons with medical conditions that increase the risk of TB

  4. The method of screening is the tuberculin skin test using purified protein derivative (PPD); the antituberculous drugs recommended for use in pregnancy are isoniazid (INH), ethambutol, and rifampin (Cunningham et al., 2001; Lake, 2001).

    a. If the induration is more than 5 mm, and if any of the following risk factors are present, the test is positive.

      (1) HIV infection

      (2) Recent contact with person who has infectious TB

      (3) Abnormal chest radiograph typical of old TB infection

      (4) Recipients of organ transplants on immunosuppressant therapy

      (5) Other immunosuppressed individuals receiving the equivalent of more than 15 mg/day of prednisone for more than 1 month

    b. If the induration is more than 10 mm and any of the following risk factors are present, the test is positive.

      (1) Immigrants who have arrived within the last 5 years from countries with high prevalence

      (2) Injection drug use

      (3) High risk medical conditions

      (4) Residents or employees of hospitals, shelters, correctional facilities

      (5) Children younger than 4 years old

      (6) Adolescents, infants or children exposed to adults in high risk categories

    c. If the person has no risk factors, the induration must be more than 15 mm for the test to be positive.

5. The cornerstone of treatment for tuberculosis is maintaining and completing treatment (Lake, 2001).
6. Congenital tuberculosis remains relatively rare; neonatal tuberculosis might reflect acquisition of infection in utero (i.e., congenital) or during the first few weeks of life from a contagious mother or other person. Neonatal tuberculosis has a high morbidity and mortality rate (Simpkins , Hench, & Bhatia, 1996), Newborns born to mothers with TB should be evaluated and treated per the guidelines of the American Thoracic Society and the Centers for Disease Control and Prevention (1994).
7. Breast feeding can begin and can continue during treatment. The mother with active tuberculosis must be separated from her baby until she is bacteriologically negative and the baby has undergone appropriate prophylaxis (Lake, 2001).

CLINICAL PRACTICE

A. **Assessment**
   1. History
      a. Specific form of respiratory disease
      b. Duration and course of disease
      c. For women with asthma: history of status asthmaticus, hospitalization, and endotracheal intubation
      d. Duration and severity of shortness of breath and dyspnea
      e. Degree of exercise and activity limitations
      f. Type of cough
      g. Amount of hemoptysis
      h. Amount, color, and consistency of sputum
      i. Duration and severity of wheezing and chest tightness
      j. Duration and severity of fever, chills, and night sweats
      k. Medication use (prescribed and over-the-counter)
      l. Smoking history (amount, length of time)
      m. Exposure to respiratory infections
   2. Physical findings
      a. Rate, rhythm, and depth of respirations
      b. Auscultation of the lungs
      c. Skin color
      d. Blood pressure and pulse
      e. Level of consciousness
      f. Intake and output (I&O)
   3. Diagnostic procedures
      a. Arterial blood gases; pulse oximetry
      b. Chest radiograph (with abdominal shield)
      c. CBC
      d. Pulmonary function tests
         (1) Forced expiratory volume in 1 second (FEV_1) by spirometry
         (2) Peak expiratory flow rate (PEFR) by peak flow meter
      e. Sputum smear and culture
   4. Fetal assessment for signs and symptoms of fetal hypoxia
B. **Nursing Diagnoses**
   1. Altered respiratory function related to the pathophysiology of the respiratory structure

2. Impaired gas exchange related to the pathophysiology of respiratory structures or functions
3. Ineffective airway clearance related to thickened mucous secretions
4. Activity intolerance related to hypoxia
5. Risk for infection transmission related to airborne transmission of tuberculosis
6. Risk for fetal injury related to decreased uteroplacental blood flow secondary to altered respiratory function and maternal hypoxia

C. **Interventions/Outcomes**
1. Altered respiratory function related to the pathophysiology of the respiratory structures
2. Impaired gas exchange related to the pathophysiology of respiratory structures or functions
3. Ineffective airway clearance related to thickened mucous secretions
   a. Interventions
      (1) Administer supplemental oxygen as indicated.
      (2) Position in semi- or high-Fowler's position with lateral tilt and supported arms for adequate breathing and decreased dyspnea.
      (3) Auscultate lung fields for baseline, and monitor frequently.
      (4) Observe respiration for rate, rhythm, and regularity.
      (5) Administer prescribed medications and respiratory treatments.
         (a) Bronchodilators
         (b) Antibiotics
         (c) Antiinflammatory agents
         (d) Antituberculosis drugs (refer to Table 28-4 for drugs and dosages for antituberculosis drugs).
      (6) Monitor and trend:
         (a) Arterial blood gas analysis
         (b) Pulse oximetry
         (c) PEFR

■ TABLE 28-4
■ ■ **Commonly Used Antituberculosis Drugs**

Drug	Daily Dose (Adults) (mg/kg/day)	Major Toxicity
Isoniazid	5 (maximum 300 mg)	Hepatitis Peripheral neuropathy
Rifampin	10 (maximum 600 mg)	Hepatitis Flu-like syndrome Thrombocytopenia Orange discoloration of secretions Alteration of other drug levels (e.g., OCP)
Ethambutol	15-25	Optic neuritis*
Pyrazinamide†	15-30 (maximum 2 g)	Hepatitis Arthralgias Hyperuricemia
Streptomycin†	15 (maximum 1 g)	Ototoxicity‡ Nephrotoxicity‡

From Simpkins, S., Hench, C., & Bhatia, G. (1996). Management of the obstetric patient with tuberculosis. *Journal of Obstetric, Gynecologic, and Neonatal Nursing, 25*(4), 309.
*Conduct baseline and monthly monitoring of visual acuity and color vision.
†Do not use in pregnancy.
‡Perform baseline audiometry and renal function studies.

    (7) Assess for productive and nonproductive cough.

    (8) Teach the client effective coughing technique.

    (9) Assist in coughing and deep breathing, administer incentive spirometer, and note effectiveness of treatment.

  (10) Maintain adequate hydration to help liquefy secretions.

  (11) Assess fluid volume status by:

    (a) Orthostatic vital signs

    (b) Capillary refill time

    (c) Thirst

    (d) Skin turgor and mucous membranes

  (12) Provide steroid supplementation for 24 to 48 hours prior to delivery, as indicated, in asthmatic women who have undergone recent steroid therapy.

  (13) Prevent increased oxygen consumption related to painful contractions by medicating the woman adequately during labor.

  (14) Prevent client from hyperventilating during labor by providing coaching and support.

b. Outcomes: client maintains adequate respiratory function and gas exchange as reflected by:

    (1) Normal arterial blood gas values, CBC, and chest radiograph

    (2) Respirations of normal rate, rhythm, and depth

    (3) No adventitious breath sounds

    (4) No fatigue with normal activity

    (5) Normal skin color and pulses

    (6) Orientation to person, place, and time

4. Activity intolerance related to hypoxia

a. Interventions

    (1) Assess activity tolerance.

    (2) Assist client in modifying her schedule and spacing her activities to allow time for more rest.

    (3) Maintain client's activity level just short of fatigue.

    (4) Provide long periods for sleep at night and frequent rest periods during the day.

    (5) Assist client with activities of daily living (ADLs) and ambulation as required.

b. Outcomes

    (1) Client tolerates progressive activities as evidenced by:

    (a) Normal vital signs with both rest and activity

    (b) Normal depth and clarity of respirations

5. Risk for infection transmission related to airborne transmission of tuberculosis

a. Interventions

    (1) Implement respiratory isolation while client is considered infectious; clients with TB are not considered infectious if they meet all the following criteria:

    (a) Adequate therapy received for 2 to 3 weeks

    (b) Favorable clinical response to therapy

    (c) Three consecutive negative sputum smear results from sputum collected on different days (Carpenito, 1997)

    (2) Instruct the client to cough and expectorate into disposable tissues to prevent disease transmission.

    (3) Provide support and counseling for the new mother who is isolated at delivery and separated from her neonate.

(4) Consult social services as needed to arrange temporary care of the infant outside the home until the infant and the mother have received adequate treatment.
  b. Outcomes
    (1) TB is not transmitted to the newborn.
    (2) TB is not transmitted to other individuals.
  6. Risk for fetal injury related to decreased uteroplacental blood flow secondary to altered respiratory function and maternal hypoxia: see Chapters 8 and 12 for a discussion of decreased uteroplacental blood flow interventions and outcomes.

HEALTH EDUCATION

Asthma (Box 28-2)

A. Explain disease and therapy goals.
B. Teach client to avoid exposure to allergens and infection.
C. Teach how to use a peak flow meter to manage symptoms.
D. Clarify when primary provider should be contacted (Carpenito, 1997).
  1. When medications have to be increased to control symptoms
  2. Persistent cough; difficulty breathing, with or without wheezing
  3. Peak flows less than 80% of normal
E. Discuss signs and symptoms to report.
  1. Shortness of breath
  2. Dyspnea
  3. Rapid respirations
  4. Cough and congestion
  5. Fever and chills
  6. Decreased ability to perform activities
  7. Extreme fatigue

■ BOX 28-2
■ **PATIENT SELF-CARE STRATEGIES FOR ASTHMA**

- Know own patterns of asthma symptoms (e.g., dyspnea, wheezing, tightness in the chest, recurrent cough persisting more than 1 week).
- Evaluate severity of symptoms on a scale of 1 to 10.
- Monitor daily PEFR.
- Monitor daily symptoms in relation to peak expiratory flow rate, weather patterns, activity level, and medications.
- Practice relaxation and breathing techniques.
- Identify and avoid precipitating factors including bronchial irritants (e.g., active and passive smoking, personal use of scented cosmetics, aerosols).
- Adjust activity patterns according to climatic conditions.
- Take medications as prescribed.
- Use metered-dose inhaler medications properly and with a spacer if appropriate.
- Learn what triggers asthma by keeping a symptom diary.
- Identify and prioritize strategies that work best.
- Develop a crisis-management plan.
- Maintain a daily exercise program.
- Place reasonable limits on activity to avoid hypoxemia.
- Receive annual influenza vaccine in the fall if after the third trimester.
- Control weight gain during and following pregnancy.

From Geiger-Bronsky, M. (1992). Asthma and pregnancy: Opportunities for enhancing outcomes. *Journal of Perinatal & Neonatal Nursing, 6*(2), 43.

Tuberculosis

A. Teach medication regimen and importance of adherence to treatment.
B. Explain mechanism of transmission for tuberculosis.

Systemic Lupus Erythematosus and Antiphospholipid Antibody Syndrome

A. **Systemic lupus erythematosus (SLE) is a chronic multisystem inflammatory disorder characterized by autoimmune antibody production resulting in inflammation of connective tissue in various organs or systems in the body.** Development of antibody to autologous DNA and other cell components leads to the deposition of antigen-antibody complexes and resultant inflammatory responses in target tissues (Cunningham et al., 2001; De Swiet, 1999).

   1. Incidence of SLE is approximately 1 per 1000; 90% of cases occur in women during their childbearing years; incidence is higher among U.S. blacks, Asian Americans, and American Indians (Cunningham et al., 2001; De Swiet, 1999).
   2. SLE is characterized by remissions and exacerbations.
   3. Etiology is unknown, but evidence suggests genetic, environmental, hormonal, and immunologic factors (Cunningham et al., 2001; De Swiet, 1999; Wenstrom & Malee, 1999).
   4. SLE is considered a syndrome, and diagnosis is usually based on symptoms. The American College of Rheumatology has proposed a list of 11 criteria for diagnosis; four or more of these clinical manifestations should be present for one to confirm the diagnosis of SLE (Cunningham et al., 2001; Ramsey-Goldman, 2001).
      a. Malar rash (butterfly rash)
      b. Discoid rash
      c. Photosensitivity
      d. Oral ulcers (usually painless)
      e. Arthritis (involving two or more peripheral joints)
      f. Serositis (pleuritis or pericarditis)
      g. Renal disorder (persistent proteinuria over 0.5 g or cellular casts)
      h. Neurologic disorder (seizure or psychosis)
      i. Hematologic disorder (hemolytic anemia, leukopenia, lymphopenia, or thrombocytopenia)
      j. Immunologic disorder (positive lupus erythematosus cell preparation, anti-DNA, anti-Sm, or false-positive serologic test result for syphilis)
      k. Antinuclear antibody (ANA)
   5. SLE and pregnancy
      a. Lupus can be life-threatening to mother and fetus; the pregnancy outcome is better if (Cunningham et al., 2001):
         (1) SLE has been in remission for at least 6 months.
         (2) There is no active renal involvement.
         (3) Superimposed preeclampsia does not develop.
         (4) There is no evidence of antiphospholipid antibody activity.
      b. There is an increased risk of the following adverse outcomes:
         (1) Spontaneous abortion
         (2) Stillbirth
         (3) Preterm labor and potential preterm birth
         (4) Neonatal death
         (5) IUGR (Cunningham et al., 2001; De Swiet, 1999)

6. Neonatal lupus erythematosus (NLE) is a rare and often transient syndrome caused by passage of maternal autoantibodies across the placenta to the fetus; manifested by dermatologic lesions and cardiac abnormalities such as congenital heart block (Cunningham et al., 2001; De Swiet, 1999; Wenstrom & Malee, 1999).

B. Antiphospholipid (APS) is an autoimmune disorder characterized by the presence of specific clinical features and specified levels of circulating antiphospholipid antibodies (aPL); several aPL have been identified, but the lupus anticoagulant (LA) and anticardiolipin antibody (aCL) are the most widely accepted for clinical use (Cunningham et al., 2001; Silver & Branch, 1999; Wenstrom & Malee, 1999).

1. The information on APS is new and evolving and there remains some controversy and uncertainty.
2. The most frequent medical problems include arterial and venous thrombosis, autoimmune thrombocytopenia, and pregnancy loss (Silver & Branch, 1999; Wenstrom & Malee, 1999).
3. APS can coexist with other autoimmune conditions, especially SLE; the prevalence of aPL in patients with SLE is 30% to 40%.
4. The fetal loss rate in SLE patients with aPL is 73% compared with 19% in SLE patients without aPL (Scott & Branch, 1999).
5. Clinical and laboratory criteria for APS are listed below; one clinical and one laboratory finding are needed for clinical diagnosis (Cunningham et al., 2001; Silver & Branch, 1999; Wenstrom & Malee, 1999).
   a. Recurrent early pregnancy loss
   b. Fetal death (second and third trimester)
   c. Venous thrombosis
   d. Arterial thrombosis including stroke
   e. Autoimmune thrombocytopenia
   f. Autoimmune hemolytic anemia
   g. Livedo reticularis
   h. False-positive serologic test for syphilis
   i. Lupus anticoagulant
   j. Anticardiolipin antibody
6. Obstetric disorders associated with APS
   a. Preeclampsia
   b. IUGR
   c. Placental insufficiency
   d. Preterm delivery

CLINICAL PRACTICE

A. **Assessment**
1. History
   a. Duration and presence of signs and symptoms listed by the American College of Rheumatology
   b. Race: higher incidence among blacks, Asian Americans, and American Indians
   c. Family history of SLE or other connective tissue disorder
   d. Obstetric history
      (1) Stillbirth
      (2) Miscarriage
      (3) Neonatal death

       (4) IUGR

       (5) Preterm labor and/or preterm birth

   e. Duration of exacerbations and remissions

2. Physical findings (Cunningham et al., 2001; Ramsey-Goldman, 2001; Silver & Branch, 1999)

   a. Constitutional symptoms

       (1) Fatigue

       (2) Fever

       (3) Weight loss

       (4) Malaise

   b. Musculoskeletal

       (1) Arthralgia

       (2) Polyarthritis

       (3) Myalgia

       (4) Myopathy

   c. Mucocutaneous

       (1) Butterfly rash

       (2) Discoid rash

       (3) Oral/nasal ulcers

       (4) Photosensitivity

   d. Gastrointestinal

       (1) Anorexia

       (2) Nausea/vomiting

       (3) Abdominal pain

       (4) Diarrhea

       (5) Constipation

   e. Liver

       (1) Hepatomegaly

       (2) Enzyme elevation

       (3) Chronic hepatitis

   f. Cardiac disease

       (1) Pericarditis

       (2) Myocarditis

       (3) Endocarditis

       (4) Ischemia

       (5) Hypertension

       (6) Tachycardia

   g. Pulmonary

       (1) Pleuritis

       (2) Pleural effusion

       (3) Pneumonitis

       (4) Dyspnea

   h. Hematologic

       (1) Anemia

       (2) Leukopenia

       (3) Thrombocytopenia

   i. Renal

       (1) Nephritis

       (2) Nephrotic syndrome

       (3) Urinary tract infection

       (4) Glomerular nephritis

    j. Nervous system
       (1) Seizures
       (2) Headaches
       (3) Irritability
       (4) Depression
       (5) Cognitive dysfunction
       (6) Psychosis
3. Laboratory and diagnostic studies
   a. Laboratory value abnormalities found in clients with SLE
     (1) Anemia
     (2) Leukopenia
     (3) Thrombocytopenia
     (4) Positive direct Coombs' test result
     (5) Positive antinuclear antibody (ANA) test result
     (6) Lupus erythematosus cells
     (7) Decreased complement levels
     (8) Increase in gamma-globulin
     (9) Positive rheumatoid factor
     (10) False-positive serologic test for syphilis
     (11) Positive lupus anticoagulant
     (12) Prolonged prothrombin and thrombin time
     (13) Positive anticardiolipin antibody
     (14) Anti-DNA and anti-Sm antibodies
   b. Critical laboratory tests to be performed are
     (1) CBC
     (2) Platelet count
     (3) Electrolytes
     (4) BUN
     (5) 24-hour urine for protein and creatinine clearance
     (6) Urinalysis
     (7) Urine culture
     (8) Serum glutamate pyruvate transaminase (SGPT)
     (9) Serum glutamic-oxalo-acetic transaminase (SGOT)
     (10) Bilirubin
     (11) Erythrocyte sedimentation rate (ESR)
     (12) Total serum complement for C3 and C4
     (13) Fluorescent antinuclear antibodies
     (14) ECG
B. Nursing Diagnoses
  1. Risk for infection related to corticosteroid therapy
  2. Fatigue related to chronic inflammatory process secondary to SLE
  3. Impaired comfort related to joint and systemic pain secondary to disease process
  4. Ineffective individual coping related to unpredictable course of physical and emotional condition
  5. Risk for complications: pregnancy complicated by SLE and APS
C. Interventions/Outcomes
  1. Risk for infection related to corticosteroid therapy
   a. Interventions
     (1) Use aseptic technique for all potential sites of infection.
     (2) Perform and instruct client in proper handwashing.
     (3) Maintain client's hydration with fluids.

  (4) Observe skin, joints, and extremities for areas of redness and swelling.

  (5) Encourage client to maintain caloric and protein intake.

  (6) Observe type, amount, and odor of discharge or drainage.

  (7) Assess client for:

   (a) Fundal tenderness

   (b) Pain, burning, and frequency of urination

   (c) Flank pain

  (8) Assess for fever and chills.

  (9) Monitor vital signs, especially temperature, every 4 hours and as needed.

  (10) Monitor laboratory results, especially white blood cell count.

 b. Outcomes

  (1) Client has no signs and symptoms of infection and remains afebrile.

  (2) Client identifies signs and symptoms of infection in a timely manner.

  (3) Client obtains appropriate medical and nursing intervention for infection.

2. Fatigue related to chronic inflammatory process secondary to SLE

 a. Interventions

  (1) Assess fatigue levels and activity tolerance.

  (2) Assist client in modifying her schedule and spacing her activities to allow time for more rest.

  (3) Teach energy conservation techniques.

  (4) Allow expression of feelings regarding effects of fatigue on life.

  (5) Assist client with ADL and ambulation as necessary.

 b. Outcomes

  (1) Client establishes priorities for activities and schedules activities in keeping with energy patterns.

3. Impaired comfort related to joint and systemic pain secondary to disease process

 a. Interventions

  (1) Assess pain-precipitating factors, quality, region radiation, severity, duration, and relieving factors; document deviation from baseline.

  (2) Have client evaluate pain intensity on a 1 to 10 scale (10 being most severe).

  (3) Observe, report, and record verbal and nonverbal expressions of pain, fear, and anxiety.

  (4) Provide and encourage rest periods and a restful environment.

  (5) Medicate client with analgesics as ordered.

  (6) Assess effectiveness of pain medications.

  (7) Teach client and family about factors that contribute to pain experience.

 b. Outcomes

  (1) Client verbalizes decreased pain intensity (using a scale of 1 to 10) in response to analgesics or other interventions within 1 hour of administration.

  (2) Client maintains pain control or absence of pain as evidenced by the following:

   (a) Client's statement

   (b) Decreased use of analgesics

   (c) Increased activity

4. Ineffective individual coping related to unpredictable course of physical and emotional condition

    a. Interventions
- (1) Assist client in improving her self-esteem.
- (2) Discuss the illness as a pathologic process.
- (3) Maintain a positive attitude to communicate that the client can overcome her physical and emotional problems.
- (4) Refer client to self-help groups and local and national SLE organizations.
- (5) Assist client in using alternative coping strategies: relaxation techniques, meditation.
- (6) Set short-term coping goals with client.

    b. Outcomes
- (1) Client verbalizes the need for continued treatment.
- (2) Client expresses a sense of hope in dealing with the disease process and her future.
- (3) Client uses alternative coping mechanisms to deal with stress.

5. Risk for complications: pregnancy complicated by SLE and APS

    a. Interventions
- (1) Monitor the client for placental competency and fetal well-being.
- (2) Observe for varied signs and symptoms indicating exacerbation of SLE.
- (3) Distinguish between the symptoms of SLE and preeclampsia.
- (4) Monitor client closely for preeclampsia; assess BP, edema, proteinuria, deep tendon reflexes, and clonus.
- (5) Administer prescribed medications and observe for side effects of:
  - (a) Corticosteroids
  - (b) Salicylates
  - (c) Nonsteroidal antiinflammatory agents
  - (d) Analgesics
  - (e) Antipyretics
  - (f) Immunosuppressants
  - (g) Antimalarials
  - (h) Heparin
- (6) Protect client from infection.
- (7) Observe client for signs and symptoms of glucose intolerance due to steroids.
- (8) Observe client for signs and symptoms of deteriorating cardiovascular and renal status.
- (9) Observe client for signs and symptoms of thrombosis formation.
- (10) Observe client for signs and symptoms of arterial occlusion, including stroke.
- (11) Observe client closely for worsening condition in the postpartum period; might need intensive nursing observation for the first 24 to 48 hours after delivery.
- (12) Observe client for early signs and symptoms of psychosis.
  - (a) Restlessness
  - (b) Distractibility
  - (c) Emotional sensitivity
  - (d) Confusion
  - (e) Vague personality changes
  - (f) Disorientation

    b. Outcomes
- (1) Client has remission or absence of signs and symptoms of SLE.

(2) Client does not develop complications of pregnancy secondary to SLE or APS or, if complications develop, they are detected promptly and managed effectively.

HEALTH EDUCATION

A. Preconceptual counseling
  1. Advise to postpone conception until at least 1 to 2 years after the diagnosis of SLE, when the disease is in good control and doses of corticosteroids are low.
  2. Provide reassurance that SLE patients with mild to moderate renal disease who are in remission before conception have a successful live birth rate of 80% to 90%.
B. Discuss the increased incidence of spontaneous abortions, stillbirths, IUGR, and premature birth.
C. Discuss the increased incidence of maternal nephritis, placental insufficiency, preeclampsia, and venous and arterial thrombosis.
D. Discuss the need for close monitoring of client's condition during pregnancy.
E. Discuss the need for close monitoring of fetal well-being.
F. Encourage client to keep appointments with her internist or rheumatologist and her obstetrician or perinatologist.
G. Teach client importance of frequent monitoring of creatinine clearance, proteinuria, and hematologic parameters.
H. Teach self-monitoring of weight gain, edema, and blood pressure.
I. Teach client about signs and symptoms to report.
  1. Chest pain
  2. Bleeding
  3. Confusion
  4. Decreased ability to perform activities
  5. Fever
  6. Extreme fatigue
  7. Edema
  8. Anorexia
  9. Vomiting
  10. Abdominal pain
  11. Weight loss
  12. Leg pain, tenderness, color change, or edema
J. Educate client about prescribed medications and side effects.
K. Inform the client that corticosteroids, a strong immunosuppressant, can mask the symptoms of infection.
L. Teach client to avoid exposure to infection, including persons with known infectious processes.
M. Plan with client how she can avoid periods of fatigue or stress.
N. Teach client to take 1200 mg of calcium and vitamin D to decrease the risk of osteoporosis if she is receiving corticosteroids or heparin.

HEMATOLOGIC COMPLICATIONS

A. Anemias
  1. Anemia complicates 15% to 25% of all pregnancies (Wenstrom & Malee, 1999).
  2. Pregnancy results in an intravascular volume expansion, with the increase in plasma volume larger than the rise in erythrocyte volume, resulting in

hemodilution of pregnancy; the net result is a physiologic drop in the hemoglobin and hematocrit; in pregnant women, anemia is present if the hemoglobin concentration drops below 10 g/dl or the hematocrit falls below 30% (Arias, 1993).

3. Iron-deficiency anemia
   a. Approximately 80% of all anemias in pregnancy result from iron deficiency, related to suboptimal iron content of the average U.S. diet and insufficient iron stores in women of reproductive years (Long, 1995; Wenstrom & Malee, 1999).
   b. Signs and symptoms
      (1) Pallor
      (2) Fatigue
      (3) Reduced exercise tolerance
      (4) Anorexia
      (5) Weakness
      (6) Malaise
      (7) Dyspnea
      (8) Edema
      (9) Pica
   c. Might be prevented by iron supplementation during pregnancy of 60 mg of elemental iron per day, the amount contained in 300 mg of ferrous sulfate (Wenstrom & Malee, 1999).
   d. Is treated by oral administration of iron sulfate.
   e. Oral iron therapy might be associated with gastrointestinal intolerance requiring a reduction in dose to a tolerable level.
4. Megaloblastic anemia
   a. Occurs in up to 1% of pregnant women; usually the result of folic acid deficiency and occasionally the result of vitamin B_{12} deficiency.
   b. Is often found in combination with iron deficiency.
   c. Is treated with 0.5 to 1 mg/day of folic acid, or parenteral cyanocobalamin every month (Wenstrom & Malee, 1999).
5. Sickle cell anemia (Cunningham et al., 2001; Wenstrom & Malee, 1999)
   a. Recessive inheritance: sickle cell trait is the heterozygous form of the condition, whereas sickle cell disease or anemia is the homozygous form of the condition (occurs when the gene for the production of S hemoglobin is inherited from both parents).
   b. When deoxygenated, the sickle cell hemoglobin molecule becomes rigid and dehydrated and assumes an abnormal sickled shape; these sickled erythrocytes are not deformable and cannot squeeze through the microcirculation; obstruction results in local hypoxia causing progressive tissue and organ damage (especially kidneys, lungs, and bone), painful vasoocclusive crises, and increased susceptibility to infection (Cunningham et al., 2001; Wenstrom & Malee, 1999).
   c. Pregnancy is associated with more severe anemia and more common vasoocclusive crises, and increased maternal and perinatal morbidity and mortality.
   d. Management during pregnancy includes:
      (1) Frequent prenatal visits
      (2) Careful screening for infections
      (3) Folic acid supplementation
      (4) Hospitalization at the earliest signs of crisis, and treatment with analgesics, oxygen, and hydration

        (5) Intensive fetal surveillance

        (6) Transfusion therapy for severe maternal anemia

    6. Thalassemia

        a. This hemoglobinopathy is characterized by a defect in the ability to synthesize alpha or beta globin chains at a normal rate.

        b. Alpha thalassemia minor is characterized by hypochromic microcytic erythrocytes but little or no anemia; pregnancy usually is uncomplicated; incidence is highest in Southeast Asians.

        c. Beta thalassemia minor is characterized by a mild hypochromic microcytic anemia, with hematocrit between 32% and 35% (Wenstrom & Malee, 1999).

B. Thrombocytopenia

    1. Thrombocytopenia can be a consequence of the following:

        a. Inadequate production of platelets

        b. Increased peripheral consumption of platelets

        c. Destruction of platelets

    2. The body can develop an antiplatelet antibody that is responsible for destruction of platelets; this immune process is called idiopathic thrombocytopenic purpura (ITP).

    3. The most common causes of thrombocytopenia in pregnancy are preeclampsia or eclampsia, SLE, and ITP.

    4. Therapy of choice for pregnant women with ITP is glucocorticoids or IV immunoglobulin (American Society of Hematology ITP Practice Guideline Panel, 1997).

    5. The signs and symptoms of thrombocytopenia include the signs and symptoms of bleeding.

        a. Petechiae

        b. Oozing from IV site or wound

        c. Hematuria

        d. Hematemesis

        e. Hemoptysis

        f. Signs of cerebral hemorrhage

C. Thromboembolic disease

    1. During pregnancy, there is an increased potential for thromboses resulting from increased levels of coagulation factors and decreased fibrinolysis, venous dilation, and obstruction of venous system by gravid uterus.

    2. Thromboembolic diseases occurring most frequently during pregnancy include deep vein thrombosis (DVT) of the lower extremities and pulmonary embolism.

    3. Thromboembolism is reported to occur during pregnancy at a rate of approximately 0.5 to 3 in 1000; events occur with equal frequency during antepartum and postpartum (Laros, 1999).

    4. Clients at high risk for thromboembolic disease during pregnancy include those with the following:

        a. Previous venous thromboembolism

        b. Advanced maternal age

        c. Increased parity

        d. Artificial heart valves

        e. Thrombophilia syndrome

        f. Obesity

        g. Cesarean delivery

        h. Prolonged immobilization or bedrest

        i. Dehydration

     5. Anticoagulation therapy with heparin is the mainstay of therapy for DVT, with or without pulmonary embolism (Laros, 1999).

D. Fetal implications

    1. Chronic anemia limits the amount of oxygen available for fetal oxygenation and increases the risk for the following:

       a. Abortion

       b. Premature birth

       c. Small-for-gestational-age neonates

    2. With ITP, the fetus is at risk for hemorrhage in utero or after birth because the antiplatelet antibodies are actively transported across the placenta, causing thrombocytopenia.

CLINICAL PRACTICE

A. Assessment

    1. History

       a. Iron-deficiency anemia

         (1) Evidence of decreased dietary iron intake

         (2) Risk factors, such as a history of poor nutritional status, close spacing of pregnancies, multiple gestation, excessive bleeding, adolescence, eating disorders, and personal or family history of anemia

       b. Sickle cell anemia

         (1) Family history

         (2) Black or Mediterranean ancestry

       c. Thrombocytopenia: family history

       d. Thromboembolic disease

         (1) DVT

         (2) Pulmonary embolus

         (3) Artificial heart valve

         (4) Hypercoagulable disorder

         (5) Prolonged immobilization

         (6) Obesity

    2. Physical findings: signs and symptoms specific to the diagnosed hematologic disorder

       a. Iron-deficiency anemia

         (1) Pallor

         (2) Fatigue

         (3) Decreased exercise tolerance

         (4) Anorexia

         (5) Weakness

         (6) Malaise

         (7) Dyspnea

         (7) Edema

         (8) Pica

       b. Sickle cell anemia or sickle cell crisis

         (1) Pain in the abdomen, chest, vertebrae, joints, or extremities

         (2) Sudden anemia

         (3) Marked pallor

         (4) Cardiac failure

       c. Thalassemia: mild persistent anemia with no unusual systemic problems

       d. Thrombocytopenia: signs and symptoms of bleeding

         (1) Petechiae

    (2) Oozing from IV site or wound
    (3) Hematuria
    (4) Hemoptysis
    (5) Signs of cerebral hemorrhage
  e. DVT
    (1) Pain
    (2) Tenderness
    (3) Edema (difference between leg circumference of > 2 cm)
    (4) Change in limb color
    (5) Calf pain with dorsiflexion (Homans' sign)
3. Diagnostic and laboratory studies: evaluate laboratory data for indicators or presence of specific disorder (Table 28-5).
  a. Iron-deficiency anemia
    (1) Hemoglobin below 10 g/dl
    (2) Hematocrit less than 30%
  b. Megaloblastic anemia
    (1) Elevated mean cell volume
    (2) Reduced serum levels of folate or vitamin B_{12}
  c. Sickle cell anemia; hemoglobin electrophoresis
  d. Thalassemia
    (1) Mild persistent anemia
    (2) Hypochromic microcytic RBCs
    (3) Elevated hemoglobin A_2 concentrations with normal serum iron and ferritin levels (Wenstrom & Malee, 1999)
  e. Thrombocytopenia
    (1) Low platelet count (less than $150/mm^3$)
    (2) Prolonged bleeding time
    (3) ITP is diagnosed by presence of antiplatelet antibodies in maternal serum.
  f. DVT
    (1) Doppler ultrasonography
    (2) Impedance plethysmography (IPG)
    (3) Contrast venography

■ TABLE 28-5
■ ■ Indices of Iron Homeostasis

	Normal Nonpregnant	Normal Pregnant	Iron-Deficiency Anemia in Pregnancy
Hemoglobin (g/dl)	12.5-14	11.5-12.5	< 10
Hematocrit (%)	37-45	33-38	< 30
Mean corpuscular hemoglobin concentration	32-36	32-36	< 30
Mean corpuscular volume (cubic micrometers)	80-100	70-90	
Mean corpuscular hemoglobin (pg/cell)	27-34	23-31	
Serum iron (μg/dl)	50-110	35-100	< 30
Unsaturated iron-binding capacity (μg/dl)	250-300	280-400	> 400
Transferrin saturation (%)	25-35	16-30	< 16
Serum ferritin (μg/l)	75-100	55-70	< 10

From Scott, J., DiSaia, P., Hammond, C., & Spellacy, W. (1994). *Danforth's obstetrics and gynecology.* (7th ed.; p. 384). Philadelphia: Lippincott Williams and Wilkins.

   B. **Nursing Diagnoses**
     1. Fatigue related to inadequate tissue oxygenation secondary to anemia
     2. Ineffective tissue perfusion related to DVT or thrombophlebitis
     3. Risk for sickling crisis related to precipitating event
     4. Risk for hemorrhage related to altered clotting factors secondary to heparin therapy or thrombocytopenia
   C. **Interventions/Outcomes**
     1. Fatigue related to inadequate tissue oxygenation secondary to anemia
       a. Interventions (Carpenito, 1997)
         (1) Treat causative or contributing factors (anemia) as ordered.
         (2) Refer to dietician for nutritional counseling.
         (3) Assess fatigue levels: onset, precipitating factors, pattern, and whether relieved by rest.
         (4) Allow expression of feelings regarding the effects of fatigue on life.
         (5) Assist client to identify energy patterns and the need to schedule activities.
         (6) Assist client to identify what tasks can be delegated.
         (7) Teach energy conservation techniques.
         (8) Assist client with ADL and ambulation as required.
       b. Outcomes
         (1) Client will establish priorities for activities and adapt to the fatigue state.
     2. Ineffective tissue perfusion related to DVT or thrombophlebitis
       a. Interventions
         (1) Assess extremity.
           (a) Temperature
           (b) Color
           (c) Pulses
           (d) Capillary refill
           (e) Swelling sensation
           (f) Movement
           (g) Strength
         (2) Elevate or position leg on pillows or use foot cradle as indicated.
         (3) Reduce or remove external compression that impedes flow: pillows, leg crossing, and so on.
         (4) Change client's position every 2 hours while she is on bed rest.
         (5) Measure and record calf and thigh circumference.
         (6) Assess skin integrity.
         (7) Assess for complications of DVT (i.e., pulmonary embolism).
           (a) Sudden chest pain
           (b) Cough
           (c) Dyspnea
           (d) Change in level of consciousness
         (8) Administer anticoagulant medications as ordered.
         (9) Give instructions to client concerning medications and side effects of bleeding.
        (10) Assess for signs and symptoms of bleeding if client is on anticoagulants.
           (a) Petechiae
           (b) Hematemesis
           (c) Hematuria
           (d) Epistaxis

          (e) Blood in stool
          (f) Bleeding from gums
          (g) Vaginal bleeding

  b. Outcomes
     (1) Adequate circulation to lower extremities is maintained.
         (a) Warmth
         (b) Pink color
         (c) Palpable pulses
         (d) No swelling
         (e) Immediate capillary refill
         (f) Movement
         (g) Sensation
         (h) Strength
         (i) Tone intact
         (j) Skin integrity
     (2) Client has no symptoms of bleeding.
     (3) Client has no evidence of complications of DVT.

3. Risk for sickling crisis related to precipitating event
  a. Interventions (Carpenito, 1997)
     (1) Monitor for signs and symptoms of anemia.
     (2) Monitor laboratory values, including CBC with reticulocyte count.
     (3) Monitor for signs and symptoms of infection.
         (a) Fever
         (b) Pain
         (c) Chills
         (d) Increased WBCs
     (4) Teach client to avoid factors that can initiate a vasoocclusive crisis.
         (a) Viral and bacterial infections
         (b) Fever
         (c) Acid-base imbalance
         (d) Dehydration
         (e) Severe emotional disturbance
         (f) Strenuous physical activity
         (g) Exposure to cold
         (h) Alcohol intoxication
         (i) Extreme fatigue
         (j) Air travel
         (k) Drug overdose
         (l) Anesthesia
        (m) Trauma or blood loss
     (5) Instruct client to report symptoms of vasoocclusion.
         (a) Any acute illness
         (b) Severe joint or bone pain
         (c) Chest pain
         (d) Abdominal pain
         (e) Headaches, dizziness
         (f) Gastric distress
     (6) Initiate therapy per physician order (e.g., antisickling agents, analgesics, oxygen, hydration, transfusions, antibiotics).
     (7) Avoid events that might precipitate a sickle cell crisis during the intrapartum period.

       (a) Promote rest and relaxation to reduce oxygen demands extraneous to the labor process.

       (b) Provide a calm, quiet atmosphere.

       (c) Control environmental temperature to prevent hypothermia.

    b. Outcomes

      (1) Client avoids sickling crisis.

      (2) Client seeks prompt treatment if sickling crisis occurs.

4. Risk for hemorrhage related to altered clotting factors secondary to heparin therapy or thrombocytopenia

    a. Interventions (Carpenito, 1997)

      (1) Monitor CBC, coagulation tests, and platelet counts.

      (2) Monitor for signs and symptoms of spontaneous or excessive bleeding.

        (a) Petechiae, ecchymoses, hematomas

        (b) Bleeding from nose or gums

        (c) Prolonged bleeding from venipuncture or IV sites

        (d) Hemoptysis

        (e) Hematemesis or coffee-ground emesis

        (f) Hematuria

        (g) Vaginal or rectal bleeding

        (h) Change in vital signs

      (3) Teach client to report signs and symptoms of bleeding.

      (4) Observe color, consistency, and amount of stool and urine.

      (5) Administer blood products per physician order following hospital protocol.

    b. Outcomes

      (1) Client demonstrates no evidence of bleeding.

      (2) Client verbalizes signs and symptoms of bleeding to report.

      (3) Client has a return to optimal blood levels of CBC, platelets, and bleeding time.

HEALTH EDUCATION

A. Preconceptual counseling: inheritance patterns for sickle cell trait/disease; implications for offspring.

B. Encourage client to keep appointments with her internist or hematologist and obstetrician.

C. Teach client how to prevent conditions that cause sickling and other exacerbations of hematologic disorders.

D. Ensure adequate nutrition with prescribed diet and iron supplements as appropriate.

E. Teach subcutaneous administration of heparin as required.

F. Teach client signs and symptoms of bleeding.

GASTROINTESTINAL COMPLICATIONS OF PREGNANCY

A. Hyperemesis gravidarum

    1. Hyperemesis gravidarum occurs in 3.3 to 10 in 1000 pregnancies and is defined as persistent vomiting unresponsive to outpatient treatment and severe enough to cause weight loss and disturbed nutritional status; it is associated with altered electrolyte balance, dehydration, weight loss, acidosis from starvation, alkalosis from loss of hydrochloric acid, ketonuria, and hypokalemia (Cunningham et al., 2001; Heppard & Garite, 2002; Scott, 1999).

2. The cause of hyperemesis gravidarum remains unclear and is most likely multifactorial; theories include hormonal, endocrine, psychologic, or metabolic.

3. Pregnancy outcome in hyperemesis gravidarum depends on the severity and duration of the nutritional deficit; significant weight loss might be associated with intrauterine growth restriction of the fetus (Scott, 1999).

4. Interventions might begin with dietary and lifestyle alterations, proceed to oral nutritional supplementation or pharmacologic preparations, and continue on to IV vitamin-mineral therapy and either parenteral nutrition or enteral tube feedings; supportive psychotherapy might be indicated (Cunningham et al., 2001; Scott, 1999).

5. In severe cases, persistent dehydration, acetonuria, and ketosis might occur with potential neurologic, hepatic, and renal damage.

B. **Inflammatory bowel disease (IBD)**

1. Chronic IBD, either Crohn's disease or ulcerative colitis, is relatively common in women of childbearing age.

2. If IBD is quiescent at the time of conception, the pregnancy outcome is essentially normal; active disease at conception has a worse prognosis (Cunningham et al., 2001; Wenstrom & Malee, 1999).

3. Pregnancy does not increase the likelihood of an attack of IBD; if the disease is quiescent in early pregnancy, flares are uncommon, but if they do occur, they might be severe (Cunningham et al., 2001).

4. When disease is active, aggressive management is essential (Wenstrom & Malee, 1999).

5. Diagnostic evaluations, including radiologic studies, should not be postponed if their results are likely to affect management.

6. Many of the usual treatment regimens, including corticosteroids and sulfasalazine might be continued during pregnancy, and, if indicated, surgery should be performed (Cunningham et al., 2001; Wenstrom & Malee, 1999).

CLINICAL PRACTICE

A. **Assessment**

1. History
   a. Duration and course of IBD or hyperemesis gravidarum
   b. Prescribed medications
   c. Any contributing or precipitating factors

2. Physical findings
   a. Signs and symptoms of gastrointestinal disturbances
      (1) Anorexia
      (2) Nausea and vomiting
      (3) Indigestion
      (4) Abdominal pain or distension
      (5) Diarrhea
      (6) Weight loss
      (7) Passage of blood or mucus per rectum
   b. Signs and symptoms of fluid and electrolyte imbalance and nutritional deficiencies
      (1) Dry mucous membranes
      (2) Poor skin turgor
      (3) Malaise
      (4) Low blood pressure

      c. Symptoms of severe fluid and electrolyte imbalance and nutritional deficiency
        (1) Weight loss
        (2) Acetonuria
        (3) Ketosis
   3. Laboratory and diagnostic studies
      a. Serum electrolytes
      b. Renal and liver function studies
      c. Acid base and pH
      d. Hemoglobin and hematocrit
      e. Urine dipstick for specific gravity, ketones, and glucose
      f. Serum glucose
      g. Abdominal ultrasonography
      h. Colonoscopy
   4. Nutrition-related factors (Carpenito, 1997)
      a. Pre-pregnancy weight and height; current weight
      b. Diet recall for 24 hours
      c. Appetite: usual and any changes
      d. Dietary patterns
        (1) Food/fluid likes/dislikes, preferences, food allergies, and taboos
        (2) Religious dietary practices
      e. Activity level
        (1) Occupation
        (2) Exercise: type and frequency
      f. Food procurement/preparation (and by whom)
        (1) Functional ability
        (2) Kitchen facilities
        (3) Income adequate for food needs
      g. Knowledge of nutrition
        (1) Basic four food groups
      h. Nutrition supplements
        (1) Folic acid
        (2) Vitamins
        (3) Iron

B. Nursing Diagnoses
   1. Deficient fluid volume related to abnormal fluid loss by vomiting or diarrhea
   2. Diarrhea related to malabsorption or inflammation secondary to IBD
   3. Imbalanced nutrition: less than body requirements related to anorexia, nausea, vomiting, or diarrhea
   4. Impaired comfort related to abdominal pain or nausea and vomiting
   5. Activity intolerance related to nutritional, fluid, and electrolyte imbalance

C. Interventions/Outcomes
   1. Deficient fluid volume related to abnormal fluid loss by vomiting or diarrhea
   2. Diarrhea related to malabsorption or inflammation secondary to IBD
      a. Interventions
        (1) Monitor client's vital signs.
        (2) Hydrate client adequately.
        (3) Monitor client's intake and output.
        (4) Assess client's skin turgor, color, and temperature.
        (5) Observe client's urine for color and amount.
        (6) Assess amount, color, and consistency of client's vomitus and stool.

(7) Assess client's oral mucous membranes.
(8) Assess level of consciousness.
(9) Weigh client daily, noting loss or gain.
(10) Assess client for edema of the legs, arms, hands, or sacral region.
(11) Auscultate client's lungs every shift and as needed.
(12) Observe client for cough, dyspnea, tachypnea, and sputum.
(13) Monitor serum electrolytes, BUN, creatinine, urine osmolality, hematocrit, and hemoglobin.
(14) Administer parenteral fluids, electrolytes, antiemetics, and supplements as prescribed and as needed.
(15) Administer prednisone and sulfasalazine as ordered for management of IBD.

b. Outcomes
(1) Client reports less diarrhea; client responds to treatment to correct alteration in fluid volume as evidenced by:
(a) Balanced I&O
(b) Maintenance of normal weight
(c) Absence of edema
(d) Clear lungs on auscultation
(e) Vital signs within normal limits
(f) Normal laboratory values
(g) Good skin turgor
(h) Normal level of consciousness
(i) Moist mucous membranes

3. Imbalanced nutrition: less than body requirements related to anorexia, nausea, vomiting, or diarrhea
a. Interventions
(1) Assess client's nutritional status by monitoring the following:
(a) Weight
(b) 24-hour diet recall
(c) Calorie counts
(d) Intake and output
(e) Appetite
(f) Nausea and vomiting
(g) Diarrhea
(2) Explain the physiologic changes and nutritional needs during pregnancy.
(3) Discuss signs and symptoms of hypoglycemia.
(4) Maintain an odor-free, well-ventilated room.
(5) Reduce or eliminate factors that contribute to anorexia, nausea, vomiting, and diarrhea.
(6) Consult with nutritionist and dietician to establish appropriate daily caloric and food-type requirements for the client.
(7) Determine the client's food preferences and arrange to have these foods provided, as appropriate.
(8) Administer progressive diets according to the client's tolerance.
(a) Provide small, frequent feedings.
(b) Restrict liquids with meals and avoid fluids 1 hour before and after meals.
(9) Help client maintain good oral hygiene before and after ingestion of food.
(10) Give client instructions according to proper diet.
(a) Foods and liquids to avoid

             (b) Specific times to eat specific foods

             (c) Alternative sources of foods

       (11) Provide oral nutrient supplementation as ordered.

       (12) Administer IV vitamin-mineral therapy and enteral tube feedings or parenteral nutrition as required and as prescribed.

       (13) Assess the client's affect and response to her family, environment, and pregnancy.

       (14) Initiate health teaching and referrals as indicated.

   b. Outcomes

      (1) Client maintains adequate nutrition as evidenced by the following:

          (a) Adequate weight gain

          (b) Eating a well-balanced diet

          (c) Ability to choose a proper diet

4. Impaired comfort related to abdominal pain or nausea and vomiting

   a. Interventions

      (1) Assess pain-precipitating factors, quality, region radiation, severity, duration, and relieving factors; document any deviation from baseline.

      (2) Have client evaluate pain intensity on a 1 to 10 scale (10 being the most severe).

      (3) Observe, report, and record verbal and nonverbal expressions of pain, fear, and anxiety.

      (4) Provide and encourage rest periods and a restful environment.

      (5) Medicate client with analgesics or antiemetics as ordered.

      (6) Assess effectiveness of pain medications and antiemetics.

      (7) Teach client and her family about factors that contribute to the pain experience.

   b. Outcomes

      (1) Client verbalizes decreased pain intensity (using a scale of 1 to 10) in response to analgesics or other interventions within 1 hour of administration.

      (2) Client maintains pain control or absence of abdominal pain and nausea and vomiting as evidenced by the following:

          (a) Client's statement

          (b) Decreased use of analgesics

          (c) Increased activity

5. Activity intolerance related to nutritional, fluid, and electrolyte imbalance

   a. Interventions

      (1) Assess client's activity tolerance.

      (2) Assist client in modifying her schedule and spacing her activities to allow for more rest.

      (3) Maintain client's activity level just short of fatigue.

      (4) Provide long periods for sleep at night and frequent rest periods during the day.

      (5) Assist client with ADLs and ambulation as required.

   b. Outcomes

      (1) Client tolerates progressive activities as evidenced by:

          (a) Normal vital signs

          (b) Decreased dizziness, light-headedness, and weakness

HEALTH EDUCATION

A. Preconceptual counseling: client with IBD should be advised to avoid pregnancy until disease is quiescent; discuss increased risk of developing IBD in offspring.

B. **Give specific diet and nutritional information and directions: amount, type, and time for food and liquid.**

C. Teach signs and symptoms to report.
1. Anorexia
2. Nausea
3. Vomiting
4. Weight loss
5. Abdominal pain or distension
6. Diarrhea
7. Decreased ability to perform activities
8. Extreme fatigue
9. Decreased urine output
10. Dry mucous membranes
11. Poor skin turgor

D. **Plan with the client how she can get adequate sleep and take frequent rests.**

E. **Teach client to avoid fatigue or stress.**

HEPATIC COMPLICATIONS—HEPATITIS

A. **Viral hepatitis occurs in at least five distinct forms (A, B, C, D, and E).**
1. "All are characterized by an incubation period, followed by anorexia, nausea, and weight loss with variable jaundice and laboratory evidence of hepatocellular dysfunction lasting for weeks or months" (Varner, 1994, p. 439) (Table 28-6).
2. The clinical course of viral hepatitis is not affected by pregnancy, but risk of transmission of the virus to the fetus or newborn is of concern.
3. Viral hepatitis is the most common cause of jaundice in pregnancy (Heppard & Garite, 2002).

B. **Hepatitis A**
1. Accounts for 30% to 35% of cases of acute hepatitis in the United States; course and management is the same as in nongravid patients.
2. There is no evidence that hepatitis A is teratogenic (Cunningham et al., 2001).
3. Spread by fecal-oral route; associated with poor hygiene and poor sanitation.
4. Perinatal transmission has not been documented.
5. Treatment with immune globulin appears to be safe during pregnancy (Heppard & Garite, 2002).

C. **Hepatitis B** (Cunningham et al., 2001; Freitag-Koontz, 1996; Heppard & Garite, 2002)
1. Accounts for 40% to 45% of all cases of hepatitis in the United States; acute hepatitis B occurs in 1 to 2 of 1000 pregnancies, and chronic infection occurs in 5 to 15 of 1000 pregnancies.
2. Transmitted primarily through direct contact with the blood or sexual fluid of an infected person.
3. Hepatitis B infections "are readily transmitted from an infected mother to her infant. Infants infected at birth have a 90% risk of becoming chronically infected with HBV (carrier) and an approximately 25% risk of developing significant liver disease or cancer as an adult. If these infants receive postexposure prophylaxis at birth and complete the series of HBV vaccinations, more than 95% of these HBV infections can be prevented. Key to the prevention of perinatal HBV infection is the screening of all pregnant women, because approximately 50% of the women thus identified do not fall into established high-risk groups" (Freitag-Koontz, 1996).

TABLE 28-6
■ Forms of Viral Hepatitis

Characteristics	Hepatitis A	Hepatitis B	Hepatitis C
Older name	Infectious hepatitis	Serum hepatitis	Non-A, Non-B
Virus type	RNA	DNA	RNA
Virus size	27 nm	42 nm	30-60 nm
Incubation period	15-50 days	30-180 days	30-160 days
Transmission	Fecal-oral	Parenteral or body fluids	Parenteral, sporadic
Vertical transmission to fetus	Not observed	Common	Uncommon
Immunologic diagnosis	HA antibody, IgM and IgG types	HBsAg; HBcAb HbsAb; HBeAg, Ab	HC antibody
Maximum infectivity	Prodrome	Prodrome or HBeAg positive, HbsAg carriers	Probably prodrome and carriers
Carrier state	None	5%-10%	50%
Acute clinical forms	Asymptomatic to fulminant	Asymptomatic to fulminant	Asymptomatic to fulminant; relapsing
Chronic clinical forms	None	Chronic persistent hepatitis; chronic active hepatitis	Chronic persistent hepatitis; chronic active hepatitis

From Burrow, G., & Ferris, T. (1995). *Medical complications during pregnancy* (4th ed.; p. 322). Philadelphia: Saunders.

4. The Centers for Disease Control and Prevention (CDC) recommends screening of all pregnant women for hepatitis B surface antigen (HBsAg), immunoprophylaxis of all infants born to women identified as HBsAg-positive with hepatitis B immune globulin (HBIG), and routine immunization of all infants against HBV.
5. There is no evidence that breastfeeding increases the risk of HBV transmission in infants, provided they have received HBIG prophylaxis at birth and completed their HBV immunizations on schedule.

D. **Hepatitis C**
   1. Accounts for 5% of all cases of hepatitis (Heppard & Garite, 2002).
   2. The greatest risk factor is a history of blood exposure.
   3. Perinatal outcome is not adversely affected in hepatitis C virus–positive women (Cunningham et al., 2001).
   4. Perinatal transmission of HCV is relatively rare, except in women who are immunocompromised, such as those co-infected with HIV.
   5. There is no recommendation at present to test pregnant women routinely for HCV because the risk of perinatal transmission is small, and there is no effective postexposure prophylaxis against HCV.
   6. Of all acute infection, 50% progress to chronic liver disease (Heppard & Garite, 2002).

CLINICAL PRACTICE

A. **Assessment**
   1. History
      a. Exposure to contaminated food or water
      b. Travel to high-prevalence areas for hepatitis A
      c. Risk factors for HBV infection
         (1) Sexual or household exposure to an HBV-infected person
         (2) Homosexual activity
         (3) Illicit parenteral drug use
         (4) Occupational exposure to blood
         (5) Heterosexual activity with multiple partners
      d. Long-term sequelae of hepatitis: chronic hepatitis, cirrhosis, primary hepatocellular carcinoma
   2. Signs and symptoms of hepatic dysfunction
      a. Jaundice
      b. Anorexia, indigestion, nausea, and vomiting
      c. Petechiae, ecchymoses
      d. Clay-colored stools
      e. Malaise
   3. Diagnostic and laboratory tests
      a. Elevated liver function test results
      b. Prolonged prothrombin time
      c. Hepatitis A: IgM antibody levels
      d. Hepatitis B (Cunningham et al., 2001)
         (1) Hepatitis B surface antigen (HBsAg)
         (2) Hepatitis B e antigen (HBeAg)
         (3) Antibody to viral core antigen (Anti-HBc)
         (4) Antibody to e antigen (Anti-HBe)
         (5) Antibody to HB surface antigen (Anti-HBs)
      e. Hepatitis C: IgG antibody levels

B. Nursing Diagnoses
  1. Risk for infection transmission to infant related to exposure during perinatal period to hepatitis through mother
  2. Risk for hepatic dysfunction related to hepatitis
C. Interventions/Outcomes
  1. Risk for infection transmission to infant related to exposure during perinatal period to hepatitis through mother
    a. Interventions
      (1) Identify susceptible newborns through prenatal screening of mother for HBsAg.
      (2) Implement universal precautions for blood and body fluids when caring for mother or newborn.
      (3) Bathe newborns of HbsAg-positive mothers as soon as possible after delivery to remove maternal blood and bodily fluids; after bathing, newborns can be managed without special precautions while in the nursery.
      (4) Administer HBIG immunoprophylaxis and hepatitis B vaccine to newborn as ordered.
      (5) Monitor for any adverse reactions to vaccine and teach parents about potential adverse reactions.
      (6) Teach parents about the importance of completing the series of three vaccines and where to obtain the vaccine after discharge from hospital.
    b. Outcomes
      (1) Transmission of HBV to infant and to other persons is prevented.
  2. Risk for hepatic dysfunction related to hepatitis
    a. Interventions (Carpenito, 1997)
      (1) Monitor for signs and symptoms of hepatic dysfunction.
      (2) Monitor for hemorrhage.
      (3) Teach the client to report any unusual bleeding.
      (4) Monitor for electrolyte and acid-base disturbances.
    b. Outcomes
      (1) Any complications of hepatic dysfunction will be managed and minimized.

CASE STUDIES AND STUDY QUESTIONS

Ms. M is a 30-year-old G3, P2002 woman admitted to labor and delivery for preterm labor at 32 weeks' gestation. Her pregnancy had been normal, with the exception of increasing dyspnea and easy fatigability. Her past medical history includes surgery to repair a ventricular septal defect in infancy. Her vital signs at admission are temperature 37° C, pulse 84, respirations 20, and blood pressure 110/64. Her assessment reveals the following: 1+ bilateral pedal edema, no proteinuria, and breath sounds clear to auscultation.

1. Which of the following would you include in obtaining a history from Ms. M?
  a. Previous pregnancy history
  b. Course of heart disease
  c. Prescribed medications
  d. Chest pain or syncope with fatigue
  e. All of the above

2. According to the New York Heart Association Cardiac Disease Classification, she would be

categorized as which of the following?

a. Class I
b. Class II
c. Class III
d. Class IV

Ms. S is a 21-year-old G1, P0 woman at 20 weeks' gestation. She calls your office at 1 PM with complaints of pain on her right side, fever, chills, nausea, and vomiting.

3. Your recommendation to her is:
   a. Drink plenty of fluids and the physician will call at the end of the day.
   b. Have her come to the office as soon as possible.
   c. Make an appointment first thing the next morning.
   d. Go to the nearest emergency room.

4. The most common cause of pyelonephritis is:
   a. *Klebsiella pneumoniae*
   b. *Proteus mirabilis*
   c. *Escherichia coli*
   d. *Staphylococcus saprophyticus*

5. Pyelonephritis might cause further complications, which include all of the following except:
   a. Preterm labor
   b. Renal insufficiency
   c. Septicemia
   d. Chorioamnionitis

Ms. B is a 28-year-old G1, P0 woman at 6 weeks' gestation, based on her last menstrual period. She presents to the clinic today for a new obstetric visit. She has a history of asthma since childhood and is very concerned about the effect this will have on her baby. She has considered stopping her medications. She is currently under good control and has not had an exacerbation in 4 months. Her vital signs are temperature 37° C, pulse 68, respirations 16, and blood pressure 96/68.

6. Education for Ms. B. should include the following except:

a. Well controlled asthma during pregnancy allows women to continue a normal pregnancy.
b. Pregnancy has variable effects on the course of asthma.
c. Most of the commonly used asthma medications are considered safe during pregnancy.
d. Asthma is not treated as aggressively in the pregnant woman.

7. Poorly controlled asthma during pregnancy is associated with an increase in all of the following except:
   a. Preterm birth
   b. Intrauterine growth restriction
   c. Neonatal hypoxia
   d. Postdate pregnancy

Ms. G is a G4, P0 woman at 28 weeks' gestation. Her pregnancy history includes two first-trimester and one second-trimester pregnancy losses. She has been diagnosed with antiphospholipid antibody syndrome and is currently receiving subcutaneous heparin. She is admitted to labor and delivery for decreased fetal movement.

8. The most frequent medical problem associated with antiphospholipid antibody syndrome is:
   a. Polyarthritis
   b. Photosensitivity
   c. Malar rash
   d. Arterial or venous thrombosis

9. Patient teaching for Ms. G should include all of the following except:
   a. Signs and symptoms to report, including bleeding and leg pain or edema.
   b. The need for 1200 mg of calcium and vitamin D.
   c. Antiphospholipid antibody syndrome will not affect all of her pregnancies.
   d. The importance of continued daily fetal movement counting.

Ms. P is a 17-year-old G1, P0 at 28 weeks' gestation. She is in obstetrics triage for preterm labor. Her vital signs are temperature 37° C, pulse 88, respirations 16, and blood pressure 100/64. She has a weight gain this pregnancy of 25 pounds and states she is not very hungry. You notice that she frequently chews ice. Her hemoglobin count is 9.6 g/dl.

10. Which of the above objective data in her history is indicative of iron deficiency anemia?
    a. Temperature of 37° C and her age
    b. Her age and chewing ice
    c. Poor weight gain and elevated blood pressure

d. Preterm labor and her poor weight gain

11. Which of the following is the best intervention to assess nutritional status?
    a. Current weight
    b. 24-hour diet recall
    c. Good skin turgor
    d. Ability of client to eat three meals and two snacks

12. All of the following require long-term follow-up due to the high rate of chronic hepatitis except:
    a. Hepatitis A
    b. Hepatitis B
    c. Hepatitis C
    d. Hepatitis D

ANSWERS TO STUDY QUESTIONS

1. e	4. c	7. d	10. b
2. a	5. d	8. d	11. b
3. b	6. d	9. c	12. a

REFERENCES

American Society of Hematology ITP Practice Guideline Panel. (1997). Diagnosis and treatment of idiopathic thrombocytopenic purpura: Recommendations of the American Society of Hematology. *Annals of Internal Medicine, 126*(4), 319-326.

American Thoracic Society and The Centers for Disease Control & Prevention. (1994). Treatment of tuberculosis and tuberculosis infection in adults and children. *American Journal of Respiratory and Critical Care Medicine, 149*(5), 1359-1374.

Arias, F. (1993). *Practical guide to high-pregnancy and delivery* (2nd ed.). St. Louis: Mosby.

Carpenito, L. (1997). *Nursing diagnosis: Application to clinical practice* (7th ed.). Philadelphia: Lippincott Williams and Wilkins.

Cruickshank, D. (1994). Cardiovascular, pulmonary, renal, and hematologic diseases in pregnancy. In R. Scott, P. DiSaia, C. Hammond, & W. Spellacy (Eds.),

Danforth's obstetrics and gynecology (7th ed.) (pp. 367-392). Philadelphia: Lippincott Williams and Wilkins.

Cunningham, F.G., Gant, N.F., Leveno, K.J., Gilstrap, L.C. III, Hauth, J.C., & Wenstrom, K.D. (2001). *Williams obstetrics* (21st ed.). New York: McGraw Hill.

De Swiet, M. (1999). Pulmonary disorders. In R.K. Creasy & R. Resnick (Eds.), *Maternal-fetal medicine* (4th ed.; pp. 921-934). Philadelphia: Saunders.

De Swiet, M. (1999). Rheumalogic and connective tissue disorders. In R.K. Creasy & R. Resnick (Eds.), *Maternal-fetal medicine* (4th ed.; pp. 1082-1090). Philadelphia: Saunders.

Freitag-Koontz, M. (1996). Prevention of hepatitis B and C transmission during pregnancy and the first year of life. *Journal of Perinatal and Neonatal Nursing, 10*(2), 40-55.

Gei, A., & Hankins, G. (2001). Cardiac disease in pregnancy. *Obstetrics and*

Gynecology Clinics of North America, 28(3), 465-512.

Gilbert, E.S., & Harmon, J.S. (2003). *Manual of high risk pregnancy & delivery* (3rd ed.). St. Louis: Mosby.

Heppard, M.C., & Garite, T.J. (2002). *Acute obstetrics* (3rd ed.) St. Louis: Mosby.

Lake, M.F. (2001). Tuberculosis in pregnancy. *Lifelines,* 5(5), 35-40.

Laros, R.K. (1999). Thromboembolic disease. In R.K. Creasy, & R. Resnick (Eds.), *Maternal-fetal medicine* (4th ed.; pp. 821-831). Philadelphia: Saunders.

Long, P. (1995). Rethinking iron supplementation during pregnancy. *Journal of Nurse-Midwifery,* 40(1), 36-40.

Luskin, A.T., & Lipkowitz, M.A. (2000). The diagnosis and management of asthma during pregnancy. *Immunology and Allergy Clinics of North America,* 20(4), 745-761.

Murdock, M.P. (2002). Asthma in pregnancy. *Journal of Perinatal and Neonatal Nursing,* 15(4), 27-36.

National Asthma Education and Prevention Program. (1997). *Guidelines for the diagnosis and management of asthma.* (NIH Publication no. 97-4051.) Bethesda, MD: National Institutes of Health.

National Asthma Education Program. (1993). *Report of the Working Group on Asthma and Pregnancy. Management of asthma during pregnancy* (NIH Publication no. 93-3279A.). Bethesda, MD: National Institutes of Health.

Ramsey-Goldman, R. (2001). Connective tissue disorders. In L. Robbins, C. Burckhardt, M. Hannan, & R. De Horatius (Eds.), *Clinical care in the rheumatic diseases* (pp. 97-103). Atlanta: Association of Rheumatology Health Professionals.

Scott, L. (1999). Gastrointestinal disease in pregnancy. In R.K. Creasy, & R. Resnick (Eds.). *Maternal-fetal medicine* (4th ed.; pp. 1038-1053). Philadelphia: Saunders.

Scott, J., & Branch, D. (1999). Immunologic disorder in pregnancy. In J.R. Scott, P. J. DiSaia, C.B. Hammond, & W.N. Spellacy (Eds.), *Danforth's obstetrics and gynecology* (8th ed.; pp. 363-391). Philadelphia: Lippincott Williams & Wilkins.

Shabetai, R. (1999). Cardiac diseases. In R.K. Creasy & R. Resnick (Eds.), *Maternal-fetal medicine* (pp. 793-819). Philadelphia: Saunders.

Silver, R., & Branch, D.W. (1999). Immunologic disorders. In R.K. Creasy, & R. Resnick (Eds.), *Maternal-fetal medicine* (4th ed.; pp. 465-483). Philadelphia: Saunders.

Simpkins, S., Hench, C., & Bhatia, G. (1996). Management of the obstetric patient with tuberculosis. *Journal of Obstetric, Gynecologic and Neonatal Nursing,* 25(4), 305-312.

Thorsen, M.S. (2002). Renal disease in pregnancy. *Journal of Perinatal and Neonatal Nursing,* 15(4), 13-26.

Varner, M. (1994). General medical and surgical diseases in pregnancy. In J. Scott, P. DiSaia, C. Hammond, & W. Spellacy (Eds.), *Danforth's obstetrics and gynecology* (7th ed.; pp. 427-463). Philadelphia: Lippincott Williams & Wilkins.

Wendel, P. (2001). Asthma in pregnancy. *Obstetrics and Gynecology Clinics of North America,* 28(3), 537-551.

Wenstrom, K., & Malee, M. (1999). Medical and surgical complications of pregnancy. In J.R. Scott, P.J. DiSaia, C.B. Hammond, & W.N. Spellacy, (Eds.), *Danforth's obstetrics and gynecology* (8th ed.; pp. 327-361). Philadelphia: Lippincott Williams & Wilkins.

29 Labor and Delivery at Risk

ELIZABETH GILBERT

OBJECTIVES

1. Identify factors in a client's prenatal history that put her at risk for preterm labor.
2. Describe important assessment parameters for clients who are at high risk for preterm labor.
3. Summarize treatments for the client in preterm labor.
4. Discuss side effects of tocolytic therapy.
5. Describe methods commonly used for pregnancy dating.
6. Define postterm pregnancy.
7. Differentiate between the postterm pregnancy and the postmature infant.
8. Identify early signs and symptoms of chorioamnionitis.
9. List potential complications for the client with premature rupture of the membranes.
10. Identify risk factors associated with multiple gestation.
11. Describe delivery room preparation and added precautions for a multiple birth.
12. Discuss physical findings that lead to a diagnosis of intrauterine fetal demise.
13. Describe the stages of grief.
14. Differentiate between perinatal grief and other grieving responses.
15. List potential bleeding or coagulation complications associated with intrauterine fetal demise.
16. Explain the pathophysiology of amniotic fluid embolism.
17. Describe the signs and symptoms that lead to a diagnosis of amniotic fluid embolism.
18. Discuss the mortality and morbidity associated with amniotic fluid embolism.
19. Identify clients at high risk for uterine rupture.
20. Discuss life-threatening complications that may result from uterine rupture.
21. Classify the types of uterine rupture.
22. Rank emergency actions in order of priority for a client presenting with traumatic uterine rupture.

PRETERM LABOR

Introduction

A. Preterm labor is defined as regular uterine contractions and cervical dilation before completion of the thirty-sixth week of gestation.
B. Factors such as stress, uterine anomalies, multiple gestation, polyhydramnios, and urinary tract infections (UTIs) are associated with a higher incidence of preterm labor.
C. Familiarity with risk factors and prudent client education are key to early diagnosis and successful treatment.

Clinical Practice

A. Assessment

1. History
   a. Signs and symptoms of uterine contractions, low back pain, or pelvic pressure
   b. Increased vaginal discharge or bloody show
   c. Presence of risk factors associated with preterm labor
      (1) Prior preterm birth
      (2) Prior episodes of preterm labor in this or previous pregnancy
      (3) Premature rupture of the membranes
      (4) Chorioamnionitis
      (5) Placental hemorrhage
      (6) Hypertensive disease
      (7) Diabetes
      (8) Uterine anomalies
      (9) Fetal anomalies
      (10) Hydramnios
      (11) Multiple gestation
      (12) Poor nutrition
      (13) Smoking
      (14) Drug or alcohol use
      (15) Low socioeconomic status
      (16) Domestic violence
      (17) Maternal age extremes (younger than 16 or older than 40 years)
      (18) Vaginal infections
   d. Signs and symptoms of UTI
      (1) Urinary frequency
      (2) Urgency
      (3) Dysuria
      (4) Flank pain
   e. Asymptomatic bacteruria
   f. Gastrointestinal (GI) upset
      (1) Nausea
      (2) Vomiting
      (3) Diarrhea
2. Physical findings
   a. Uterine contractions (painful or painless) palpable or evident on external fetal monitor
   b. Cervical changes: softening, effacement, dilation, or shortening of cervical length
   c. Engagement of fetal presenting part
   d. Elevated temperature or tachycardia (may indicate dehydration or infection)
   e. Costovertebral angle tenderness (CVAT)
   f. Evidence of nitrites, leukocytes or white blood cells (WBCs), and/or red blood cells (RBCs) in urine
   g. Presence of fetal fibronectin in cervicovaginal secretions
   h. Fetal heart rate (FHR): tachycardia (may indicate maternal infection)
3. Psychosocial findings
   a. Stress factors
      (1) Anxiety
      (2) Fear of pregnancy loss
      (3) Fear of unknown

    b. Behavioral response

      (1) Confusion, restlessness, disorganization, and/or difficulty communicating

      (2) Expresses fears

  4. Diagnostic procedures

    a. Complete blood count (CBC): elevated WBC count may indicate infection. (WBC count is normally elevated in pregnancy and in labor, but a WBC count above 18,000 is considered significant for infection).

    b. Urinalysis: note presence of WBCs, RBCs, bacteria, nitrites, or leukocytes.

    c. Urine culture and sensitivity testing

    d. Amniotic fluid

      (1) Gram stain

      (2) Culture and sensitivity

      (3) Amniotic fluid for lecithin-sphingomyelin (L/S) ratio to assess fetal lung maturity

    e. Cervical cultures

      (1) Group B streptococcus

      (2) Chlamydia

      (3) Gonorrhea

    f. Wet mount; assess for bacterial vaginosis or trichomonas vaginalis.

    g. Ultrasound examination to assess:

      (1) Gestational age

      (2) Presenting part

      (3) Cervical length

      (4) Multiple gestation

      (5) Placenta location

      (6) Evidence of fetal or uterine anomalies

      (7) Amniotic fluid volume

B. Nursing Diagnoses

  1. Risk for preterm birth related to signs and symptoms of uterine contractions and cervical changes prior to 36 weeks' gestation

  2. Fear related to unknown pregnancy outcome

  3. Anticipatory grieving related to threatened pregnancy loss

  4. Ineffective health maintenance related to insufficient knowledge to prevent preterm labor

C. Interventions/Outcomes

  1. Risk for preterm birth related to signs and symptoms of uterine contractions and cervical changes prior to 36 weeks' gestation

    a. Interventions

      (1) Hydrate client with oral (PO) or intravenous (IV) fluids (uterine contractions or irritability may result from dehydration).

      (2) Maximize uterine blood flow by placing client on bed rest in the lateral position.

      (3) Continuous external fetal monitoring for:

        (a) FHR pattern

        (b) Frequency, duration, and approximate intensity of uterine contractions

      (4) Palpate client's abdomen to assess strength of uterine contractions.

      (5) Administer tocolytic agents as ordered.

        (a) Magnesium sulfate ($MgSO_4$): smooth muscle relaxer

          (i) Dosage and administration

           ■ Loading dose: 4 to 6 g/hr IV piggyback (IVPB) over 20 to 30 minutes

- Maintenance dose: 1 to 3 g/hr IVPB
- Medication should be administered by infusion pump.
  (ii) Side effects
- Sweating
- Flushing
- Nausea and vomiting
- Depressed deep tendon reflexes (DTRs)
- Flaccid paralysis
- Hypocalcemia
- Depressed cardiac function
- Respiratory depression
  (iii) Nursing actions
- Monitor vital signs.
- Monitor DTRs (generally graded on a scale of 0 to 4): 4+: very brisk, hyperactive; associated with clonus (clonus is the series of rhythmic contractions or convulsive movements of the ankle when the foot is sharply dorsiflexed; it is measured in beats [e.g., "two beats of clonus"]); 3+: brisker than average; 2+: average; normal reflex response; 1+: diminished; 0: absent (Seidel, 2003); the patellar tendon is most commonly used to assess reflexes because it is easiest to elicit, but biceps or triceps reflexes may also be used.
- Monitor serum magnesium levels.
- Although laboratory values may vary slightly from one institution to another, approximate values are as follows: 4 to 7 mEq/L = therapeutic; 10 mEq/L = loss of DTRs; 15 mEq/L = respiratory depression; 25 mEq/L = cardiac arrest.
- Discontinue magnesium sulfate in the presence of elevated serum levels or of signs and symptoms of central nervous system (CNS) or cardiovascular depression.
- Administer antidote (calcium gluconate) if necessary.
  (b) Terbutaline sulfate: beta-adrenergic agonist
  (i) Dosage and administration
- IV dosage: 2.5 mg/min titrated according to uterine activity; increase by 2.5 mg/min every 10 to 30 minutes.
- IV medication must be given by infusion pump.
- Subcutaneous (SC) dosage: 0.25 to 0.5 mg
- PO dosage: 2.5 to 5 mg every 2 to 8 hours
  (ii) Side effects
- Elevated heart rate
- Nervousness
- Tremors
- Nausea and vomiting
- Transient elevation in blood and urine glucose levels
- Decrease in serum potassium level
- Cardiac dysrhythmias
- Pulmonary edema
  (iii) Contraindications
- Placental abruption
- Chorioamnionitis
- Pre-viable gestation
- Fetal demise
- Fetal anomalies incompatible with life

    (iv) Relative contraindications
- Maternal diabetes
- Severe pregnancy-induced hypertension (PIH)
- Intrauterine growth restriction (IUGR)
- Maternal cardiac disease
- Hyperthyroidism
- History of migraine headaches

    (v) Nursing actions
- Baseline electrocardiogram (ECG) is recommended.
- Monitor pulse rate: hold medication for resting pulse rate above 120 beats/min.

(c) Indomethacin: prostaglandin synthetase inhibitors

    (i) Dosage and administration
- Initial dose: 50 to 100 mg PO or by rectal suppository
- Maintenance dose: 25 to 50 mg every 4 to 6 hours

    (ii) Side effects
- Maternal: increased bleeding time; potential to exacerbate hypertensive disorders
- Fetal: oligohydramnios, premature closure of the ductus arteriosus, increased risk of necrotizing enterocolitis (NEC), increased risk of intraventricular hemorrhage (IVH) and renal dysfunction

    (iii) Contraindications (maternal)
- Poorly controlled maternal hypertension
- Renal disease
- Active peptic ulcer disease
- Vaginal bleeding
- Coagulation disorder
- Liver disease

    (iv) Contraindications (fetal)
- IUGR
- Oligohydramnios
- Chorioamnionitis
- Ductal dependent cardiac defect
- Twin-twin transfusion syndrome

    (v) Additional recommendations for use
- Limit to use in women with preterm labor at less than 32 weeks with no oligohydramnios.
- Limit use to 2 to 3 days.
- If needed for more than 3 days, monitor amniotic fluid index (AFI) and evaluate fetus by Doppler echo-cardiography to check for ductal flow and to assess for tricuspid regurgitation.

(d) Nifedipine: calcium channel blocker that works primarily by blocking the flow of calcium ions through the cell membrane, thereby decreasing the activation of smooth muscle contractile proteins.

    (i) Dosage and administration
- Initial loading dose: 30 mg PO or 30 mg then followed by additional 20 mg after 90 minutes *or* 10 mg SC every 20 minutes × 4; followed by 20 mg PO every 4 to 8 hours
- Maintenance dose: 10 to 30 mg PO every 6 to 12 hours

(ii) Side effects
- Insignificant decrease in blood pressure (no change in heart rate)
- Facial flushing
- Headache
- Nausea
- Dizziness
- Palpitations
- Tachycardia
- Fetal effects: decreased uteroplacental blood flow and fetal bradycardia, which can lead to fetal hypoxia

(iii) Clinical trials are limited to date, but increasing evidence continues to suggest that nifedipine is as effective as terbutaline for tocolysis, with significantly fewer adverse side effects; nifedipine, as well as other calcium channel blockers, will likely gain in popularity as tocolytic agents.

(6) Explain side effects of tocolytic agent to client (as noted earlier).
(7) Monitor vital signs and FHR.
(8) Monitor intake and output (I&O); avoid volume overload.

b. Outcomes
(1) Decreased uterine activity; pain eliminated or decreased as evidenced by the following:
  (a) Absence of uterine activity on external fetal monitor
  (b) Absence or decreased abdominal cramping as perceived by client
  (c) No further cervical dilation or effacement
(2) If cervix changes or uterine activity continues, reevaluate tocolytic agent and dose.

2. Fear related to unknown pregnancy outcome
a. Interventions
(1) Encourage client to verbalize her feelings and assist her in identifying specific concerns.
(2) Provide information about preterm labor and delivery.
(3) Provide information about premature infants; be as detailed as possible, giving information related to her specific gestational age.
(4) Visit neonatal intensive care unit (NICU) with client to familiarize her with that environment.
b. Outcomes
(1) Client demonstrates decreased signs of anxiety.
(2) Client's questions and concerns are appropriate and realistic.

3. Anticipatory grieving related to threatened pregnancy loss
a. Interventions
(1) Encourage verbalization of client's feelings.
(2) Assist client and family in identifying coping mechanisms.
(3) Be realistic with information given.
(4) Allow client and family to participate in plan of care whenever possible.
b. Outcomes
(1) Client and family continue to exhibit bonding behaviors.
(2) Client and family do not express unrealistic expectations.

4. Ineffective health maintenance related to insufficient knowledge to prevent preterm labor
a. Interventions

    (1) Identify and explain to client her particular risk factors for preterm labor.
    (2) Teach client all signs and symptoms of preterm labor.
    (3) Demonstrate palpation of uterine contractions to client.
    (4) Explain how to accurately assess and record the frequency and duration of uterine contractions.
    (5) Provide client with written instructions for follow-up care should uterine activity occur; provide emergency telephone numbers.
  b. Outcomes
    (1) Client is able to describe risk factors and signs and symptoms of preterm labor.
    (2) Client demonstrates proper technique of abdominal palpation of uterine contractions.
    (3) Client can discuss plan of action in the event of significant uterine activity.

Health Education

A. Teach client to recognize signs and symptoms of preterm labor.
  1. Uterine contractions, cramping, and low back pain
  2. Feeling of pelvic pressure or fullness
  3. Change in amount or character of vaginal discharge
  4. Bloody show; discharge of mucus plug
  5. GI upset: nausea, vomiting, and diarrhea
  6. General sense of discomfort or unease

B. Teach client how to palpate uterine contractions.
  1. Tell client to sit up from a reclining position and to palpate her abdomen immediately. (This action will usually induce a uterine contraction.)
  2. Client may also palpate the sensation of a muscular contraction by placing her hand over her biceps and flexing her arm.
  3. Describe contraction intensity; compare the feeling of firmness to the following:
    a. Tip of nose: mild
    b. Tip of chin: moderate
    c. Forehead: strong
  4. If any preterm labor symptoms occur, teach patient to:
    a. Empty bladder.
    b. Lie down on side.
    c. Drink two to three glasses of fluid.
    d. Palpate for uterine contractions.
    e. Notify her health care provider if symptoms persist or she experiences four or more contractions in 1 hour.

C. Review timing of contractions with the client; time contractions from onset to onset.

D. Client should call health care provider or come to the hospital if contractions are coming regularly.

E. Discuss treatment routines with the client.
  1. Try bed rest in the lateral position. (Mild uterine activity may subside with increased uterine blood flow.)
  2. Maintain adequate hydration. (Uterine activity or irritability may result from dehydration.)

3. If uterine activity persists, the client should call her health care provider or come to the hospital for further evaluation; hospitalization for IV tocolytic therapy may be required.

POSTTERM PREGNANCY
Introduction
A. **Definitions**
   1. Term pregnancy: 37 to 42 completed weeks from the last menses or 35 to 40 weeks from the time of conception
   2. Postterm pregnancy (prolonged pregnancy): exceeds 42 completed weeks of menstrual age
   3. Postmaturity: a diagnosis that cannot be made in the antepartal period but is made by recognizable clinical findings in the infant that are associated with dysmaturity
B. **Decreased amniotic fluid after 42 weeks' gestation is the most frequently associated factor, reducing the cushioning effect and increasing the risk for umbilical cord compression.**

Clinical Practice
A. **Assessment**
   1. History: pregnancy dating
      a. Nägele's rule: add 7 days to the first day of the last menstrual period (LMP) and count back 3 months (assumes regular 28-day menstrual cycle).
      b. Timing of positive pregnancy test result
      c. Timing of quickening
      d. When fetal heart tones can be auscultated
      e. Ultrasound examination: pregnancy can also be dated by ultrasound examination; by measuring crown-rump length, fetal biparietal diameter, femur length, abdominal circumference, or chest circumference; or by using a formula involving the ratio of these values; ultrasound dating is most accurate when done in the first trimester of pregnancy.
   2. Physical findings
      a. Gestational age by ultrasound examination
      b. Fundal height
         (1) Measurement from symphysis to top of fundus correlates approximately with the number of weeks of gestation (e.g., 28 cm indicates approximately 28 weeks' gestation).
         (2) If fetal presenting part is engaged, the fundal height is less accurate.
      c. Decreased amniotic fluid volume (AFV) occurs most commonly and can cause fetal distress related to cord compression.
      d. Macrosomia, another common finding, can lead to shoulder dystocia and birth trauma.
      e. Dysmaturity syndrome in response to uteroplacental insufficiency occurs in only 1% to 2% of the cases and is characterized by:
         (1) Long, lean bodies
         (2) Long fingernails
         (3) Abundant hair growth
         (4) Parchmentlike skin (dry, peeling)
      f. Higher incidence of meconium aspiration and asphyxia

    3. Psychosocial findings

      a. Stress factors

        (1) Anxiety

        (2) Fear of unknown: expectations of delivery by estimated date of confinement (EDC) have not been fulfilled.

      b. Behavioral response: impatience with normal discomforts of pregnancy

    4. Diagnostic procedures: antepartum testing (see Chapter 8 on antepartum testing)

      a. Amniotic fluid volume or index (AFV or AFI)

      b. Nonstress test (NST)

      c. Contraction stress test (CST)

      d. Biophysical profile

      e. Fetal movement counts

B. Nursing Diagnoses

    1. Fear related to unknown pregnancy outcome

    2. Risk for ineffective tissue perfusion related to umbilical cord compression or decreased placental function

C. Interventions/Outcomes

    1. Fear related to unknown pregnancy outcome

      a. Interventions

        (1) Provide information to client on postterm pregnancy.

        (2) Explain effects of prolonged pregnancy on the fetus.

        (3) Encourage verbalization of feelings and help client to identify specific concerns and questions.

        (4) Assist client in identifying her own best coping mechanism for dealing with stress.

        (5) Allow client to participate in her plan of care whenever possible.

      b. Outcomes

        (1) Client does not demonstrate high level of anxiety.

        (2) Client demonstrates understanding of her plan of care and is coping effectively.

        (3) Client can explain why she and the fetus are at risk with postterm pregnancy.

    2. Risk for ineffective tissue perfusion related to umbilical cord compression or decreased placental function

      a. Interventions

        (1) Antepartum

          (a) Antepartum testing protocols (NST, AFI, fetal movement counts, CST, biophysical profiles)

          (b) Prepare client for possibility of induction of labor.

          (c) Prostaglandin gel may be used for cervical ripening.

            (i) Explain methods of induction to client.

            (ii) Discuss indications and risks.

            (iii) Assist with insertion of prostaglandin gel intracervically.

            (iv) Continuous fetal monitoring should be performed after client receives prostaglandin gel to observe for uterine contractions and to monitor FHR pattern.

        (2) Intrapartum

          (a) Perform continuous fetal monitoring during labor and delivery.

          (b) Maintain client in the lateral position as much as possible to maximize placental blood flow.

          (c) Keep client well hydrated to maximize placental perfusion.

(d) Administer amnioinfusion to relieve variable decelerations secondary to low fluid volume or to dilute thick meconium.

    b. Outcomes

        (1) FHR tracing shows no evidence of uteroplacental insufficiency such as late decelerations or loss of variability.

        (2) FHR tracing shows no evidence of variable decelerations related to decreased AFV.

        (3) Client demonstrates understanding of labor induction process.

Health Education

A. Define terms of normal gestation.

B. Explain function of amniotic fluid.

  1. Delivery of oxygen

  2. Cushioning effect to umbilical cord

  3. Normal levels at term 800 to 1000 ml

  4. Gradual decreasing levels after 40 weeks

C. Explain function of placenta.

  1. Delivery of oxygen and gas exchange

  2. Delivery of nutrients for fetal growth

  3. Efficiency may decrease after fortieth week.

D. Review fetal growth and development.

  1. Organ development and maturation are complete by the thirty-sixth week.

  2. Last 4 weeks of gestation are primarily for weight gain.

  3. Vernix caseosa, the oily substance that protects the fetal skin in utero, begins to disappear after the thirty-sixth week, making the infant's skin appear dry and peeling.

E. Discuss physiology of labor.

  1. Precise mechanism for initiation of labor is unknown.

  2. Cervix may require ripening with prostaglandin gel.

    a. Gel is inserted intracervically to induce softening and effacement.

    b. Continuous fetal monitoring is recommended after the insertion of prostaglandin gel because it may induce uterine contractions; assess for uterine activity and FHR patterns.

  3. Induction or augmentation of labor may be necessary and is commonly done with oxytocin (Pitocin); it should not be done without continuous FHR monitoring.

F. Discuss effect of postterm pregnancy on the fetus.

  1. Meconium passage into the amniotic fluid occurs with higher frequency in postterm pregnancy.

  2. Meconium aspiration at delivery causes a chemical pneumonitis and alveolar obstruction in newborn lungs.

    a. Infant will be aggressively suctioned at delivery.

    b. Infant will most likely be intubated and suctioned after delivery to make every attempt to avoid aspiration of meconium into lungs.

    c. Amnioinfusion may be used to decrease the viscosity of the amniotic fluid in the event of thick meconium.

PREMATURE RUPTURE OF THE MEMBRANES

Introduction

A. Premature rupture of the membranes (PROM) refers to the spontaneous rupture of the amniotic membrane before the onset of labor; this may occur at or before term.

B. **Gestational age usually determines the plan and intervention.**
C. **The client at or near term generally benefits from expedited delivery if fetal pulmonary maturity is documented;** clients with PROM remote from term are at much greater risk for increased neonatal morbidity related to gestational age.
D. **Induction or augmentation of labor may be necessary.**
E. **For the purpose of this section, PROM refers to the rupture of membranes (ROM) before term;** often called PPROM.
F. **Strong clinical evidence links PROM to intrauterine infection;** clinical trials with antibiotic therapy have demonstrated a delay in the onset of infection, as well as a delay in delivery, decrease postpartum maternal endometritis, and decrease infant morbidity related to sepsis, pneumonia, respiratory distress syndrome (RDS), and NEC (ACOG, 1998).

Clinical Practice

A. **Assessment**
  1. History
     a. Gestational age
        (1) By last normal menstrual period (LNMP)
        (2) By ultrasound dating
     b. Date and time of ROM
     c. Associated labor symptoms, cramping, or feeling of pelvic pressure or back pain
     d. Any event that immediately preceded ROM (e.g., trauma)
     e. History of UTI: signs and symptoms of urinary frequency, urgency, dysuria, or flank pain
     f. History of vaginal or pelvic infection; signs and symptoms of change in vaginal discharge; pelvic pain
  2. Physical findings
     a. Sterile speculum examination findings
        (1) Evidence of fluid pooling in vaginal vault
        (2) Nitrazine test result positive
        (3) Ferning positive
        (4) Appearance of cervix
        (5) Any discharge
        (6) Inflammation or lesions
        (7) Protrusion of membranes
        (8) Presenting part visible
        (9) Umbilical cord prolapse
     b. Amount, color, and consistency of fluid
        (1) Odor
        (2) Presence of vernix, blood, or meconium in fluid
     c. Vital signs: elevated temperature or tachycardia may indicate presence of infection.
     d. CBC: elevated WBC count above 18,000 may indicate presence of infection.
     e. External fetal monitoring
        (1) Uterine contractions
        (2) Uterine irritability
        (3) FHR tachycardia: may be an early indication of infection.
  3. Psychosocial findings
     a. Stress factors
        (1) Anxiety
        (2) Fear of pregnancy loss

   (3) Feeling unprepared for delivery
   (4) Guilt
  b. Behavioral factors
   (1) Difficulty communicating
   (2) Expression of fears
   (3) Coping mechanisms
 4. Diagnostic procedures
  a. Aseptic speculum vaginal examination to check for evidence of fluid pooling in the posterior fornix
  b. Nitrazine test: paper turns blue in the presence of amniotic fluid (alkaline).
  c. Ferning: amniotic fluid on a slide crystallizes into a characteristic fern pattern as it dries, which can be readily identified under a microscope.
  d. AFV: as measured by ultrasound examination, AFV may help to confirm a questionable diagnosis of ROM (decreased if membranes are ruptured).
  e. Amniocentesis
   (1) Gram stain: positive result indicates infection.
   (2) Culture and sensitivity testing to identify specific organisms
   (3) Fetal maturity studies
    (a) L/S ratio
    (b) Phosphatidylglycerol (PG), if found in the pooled fluid, provides considerable reassurance of fetal pulmonary maturity.
    (c) If tests indicate fetal pulmonary maturity, delivery should be considered.
B. Nursing Diagnoses
 1. Risk for infection related to break in amniotic membrane barrier and proximity to vaginal and enteric flora
 2. Ineffective tissue perfusion related to umbilical cord compression caused by decreased amniotic fluid volume
 3. Fear related to possible preterm delivery
 4. Effective therapeutic regimen management related to PROM
C. Interventions/Outcomes
 1. Risk for infection related to break in amniotic membrane barrier and proximity to vaginal and enteric flora
  a. Interventions
   (1) Monitor maternal vital signs: elevated temperature or increased pulse rate may indicate infection.
   (2) Monitor CBC values: elevation in WBC count (above 18,000) may indicate infection.
   (3) Observe amniotic fluid for purulence or odor.
   (4) Observe vaginal discharge: purulence or foul odor may indicate infection.
   (5) Monitor FHR: observe for fetal tachycardia, which may develop with maternal infection.
   (6) Monitor uterine activity; note contractions or uterine irritability.
   (7) Palpate abdomen to assess for uterine tenderness.
   (8) Do not perform any vaginal examinations.
   (9) Administer antibiotics as ordered.
  b. Outcomes
   (1) Client remains afebrile, with no tachycardia.
   (2) WBC count is within normal limits.
   (3) Client is free from malodorous vaginal discharge or amniotic fluid drainage.

    (4) FHR pattern is within normal limits, and fetus remains active with accompanying FHR accelerations.

    (5) Client remains free of uterine contractions, irritability, or uterine tenderness.

2. Ineffective tissue perfusion related to umbilical cord compression caused by decreased amniotic fluid volume

    a. Interventions

       (1) Initiate bed rest with FHR monitoring.

          (a) Recommend continuous fetal monitoring for the first 48 hours.

          (b) Follow with bed rest with fetal heart check every 4 hours and daily NST and AFV.

       (2) Evaluate fetal presenting part by Leopold's maneuver or ultrasound examination.

          (a) Nonvertex presentations are at higher risk for umbilical cord prolapse.

          (b) Client with nonvertex presentations may be put in a slight Trendelenburg's position to decrease the chance of umbilical cord prolapse.

       (3) Observe for evidence of cord compression: variable decelerations visible on fetal monitor.

       (4) If severe variables are observed, amnioinfusion may be ordered according to institutional protocol.

    b. Outcomes

       (1) FHR patterns remain within normal limits with no variable decelerations.

       (2) Client does not experience prolapse of umbilical cord.

3. Fear related to possible preterm delivery

    a. Interventions

       (1) Provide client with as much information as possible about PROM.

       (2) Discuss fetal growth and development and focus on gestational age of this fetus.

       (3) Visit NICU if possible to prepare client for intensive care environment.

       (4) Include client in plan of care and decision making whenever possible.

       (5) Encourage verbalization of client's feelings and help her identify specific concerns.

       (6) Identify coping mechanisms most helpful during times of stress.

       (7) Identify client's support system.

       (8) Contact social service if necessary to assist client.

    b. Outcomes

       (1) Client demonstrates knowledge of fetal stages of development.

       (2) Client has realistic expectations for infant delivered at this gestational age.

       (3) Client understands possible need for delivery before term.

       (4) Client demonstrates effective coping mechanisms and appropriate use of support persons.

       (5) Lessening degree of anxiety accompanies client's increase in knowledge and use of support systems.

4. Effective therapeutic regimen management related to PROM

    a. Interventions

       (1) Review anatomy and physiology with client; describe fetal membranes.

(2) Discuss potential complications and their treatments.
    (a) Development of infection usually necessitates delivery.
    (b) FHR variable decelerations warrant continuous fetal monitoring, possible amnioinfusion, and possible delivery for fetal distress.
    (c) Prolapse of umbilical cord requires emergency cesarean section.
    (d) Developmental anomalies such as skeletal compression deformities, amniotic band syndrome, and pulmonary hypoplasia can result if PROM occurs before 26 to 28 weeks.
b. Outcomes
  (1) Client can discuss gestational age of fetus and related fetal development.
  (2) Client can list signs and symptoms of infection.
  (3) Client demonstrates awareness of potential complications related to PROM and discusses their treatments.

Health Education

A. Review anatomy and physiology of pregnancy.
  1. Enlarging uterus: appropriate for gestational age
  2. Function of placenta: to provide oxygen and nutrients to the fetus
  3. Umbilical cord: attaches fetal placental unit to mother.
  4. Fetal membranes:
    a. Provide protective barrier to fetus.
    b. Contain amniotic fluid to provide cushioning and flotation for fetus.
    c. Eliminate compression of any fetal part, including the umbilical cord.
B. Review fetal growth and development
  1. Use growth charts to give client a realistic idea of fetal size.
  2. Focus on key landmarks of fetal development.
    a. 28 weeks: fetal anatomic development complete; maturity needed
    b. 34 weeks: approaching pulmonary maturity
  3. Discuss care in the NICU.
C. Teach client signs and symptoms of infection; instruct her to report any of the following symptoms:
  1. Elevated temperature
  2. Foul-smelling amniotic fluid
  3. Significant increase in vaginal discharge
  4. Abdominal pain or tenderness
  5. Onset of uterine contractions
D. Instruct client to come to the hospital immediately for prolapse of umbilical cord; explain significance of such and the need for emergency cesarean section.

MULTIPLE GESTATION
Introduction

A. Multiple-gestation pregnancies are more common now because of the increased use of ovulation-stimulating drugs.
B. Approximately one-third of twins are monozygotic, and two-thirds are dizygotic (resulting from the fertilization of two eggs).
C. Pregnancy risk factors, such as discordant growth and twin-to-twin transfusion syndromes, arise from carrying more than one fetus and sharing the placenta.

D. The client with a multiple gestation is also at higher risk for many of the complications of pregnancy such as preterm labor, IUGR, PIH, and antepartum hemorrhage.

Clinical Practice

A. **Assessment**
  1. History
     a. Pregnancy dating: diagnosis is often preceded by the observation that size is greater than dates.
     b. Fertility enhancement: use of ovulation-stimulating drugs
     c. Family history of twins
  2. Physical findings
     a. Fundal height measurement greater than number of weeks of gestation
     b. Leopold's maneuver may distinguish more than one fetus.
     c. Auscultation of more than one fetal heartbeat
     d. Ultrasound examination gives evidence of more than one fetus or gestational sac.
     e. Laboratory data
        (1) Beta-human chorionic gonadotropin (hCG) greatly elevated
        (2) Maternal serum alpha-fetoprotein (AFP) elevated
     f. Once the diagnosis of multiple gestation is made, the client should be considered as high risk; assessment for pregnancy complications should include the following:
        (1) Congenital anomalies
        (2) Preterm labor
        (3) IUGR
        (4) Maternal anemia
        (5) PIH
        (6) Hydramnios
        (7) Antepartum hemorrhage, such as abruptio placentae
        (8) Intrauterine fetal demise
     g. Assessment for complications specific to multiple gestation
        (1) Discordant growth
        (2) Twin-to-twin transfusion syndrome
        (3) Vanishing twin syndrome; the prognosis for the one remaining twin is good.
  3. Psychosocial responses
     a. Stress factors
        (1) Fear related to high-risk pregnancy
        (2) Fear of pregnancy loss
        (3) Anxiety related to parenting more than one infant
     b. Behavioral factors
        (1) Fear of upcoming events
        (2) Compulsiveness in preparing for children
  4. Diagnostic procedures
     a. Ultrasound examination
        (1) Most reliable test for making diagnosis
        (2) Can identify separate placenta sites, dividing membranes, relationship, and gender.
        (3) Assessment of congenital anomalies
        (4) Serial ultrasound scans to follow fetal growth curves

(5) Used to estimate fetal weight and to diagnose discordance.

(6) Assessment of AFV: hydramnios more common in multiple-gestation pregnancies

  b. Amniocentesis to diagnose chromosomal anomalies

  c. Antepartum surveillance for early detection of risks

(1) NST and AFI

(2) CST

(3) Biophysical profile

B. Nursing Diagnoses

1. Ineffective health maintenance related to multiple-gestation pregnancy
2. Fear related to high-risk pregnancy and delivery
3. Impaired parenting related to delivery of more than one infant

C. Interventions/Outcomes

1. Ineffective health maintenance related to multiple-gestation pregnancy

  a. Interventions

(1) Increase client's caloric intake, iron, calcium, magnesium, and zinc to support growth and development of multiple gestation.

(2) Provide nutritional consultation to evaluate specific dietary needs and assist client in planning to meet these needs.

(3) Monitor hemoglobin levels and hematocrit for maternal anemia.

(4) Discuss importance of additional rest; ideally in 1- to 2-hour segments in the morning, afternoon, and evening.

(5) Observe for signs and symptoms of preterm labor.

  (a) Premature contractions

  (b) Uterine cramping

  (c) Pelvic pain and pressure

  (d) Change in vaginal discharge

  (e) Bloody show; discharge of mucus plug

  (f) GI upset; nausea, vomiting, or diarrhea

(6) Observe for signs and symptoms related to pregnancy complications.

  (a) Excessive weight gain

  (b) Proteinuria

  (c) Nondependent edema

  (d) Vaginal bleeding

  b. Outcomes

(1) Weight gain is appropriate throughout pregnancy.

(2) Fetal growth remains on normal growth curve for each fetus.

(3) Maternal hemoglobin levels and hematocrit remain within normal limits: hemoglobin above 11 mg/dl and hematocrit above 33%.

(4) Client does not exhibit signs and symptoms of excessive fatigue.

(5) Client does not demonstrate signs and symptoms of preterm labor.

(6) Client is free from other complications of pregnancy (as noted earlier).

2. Fear related to high-risk pregnancy and delivery

  a. Interventions

(1) Explain reasons for risk factors to client.

  (a) Increased placental demands for two or more developing fetuses

  (b) Overdistention of uterus, which may lead to uterine irritability or premature contractions

(2) List signs and symptoms of which the client should be aware and report immediately.

(3) Review delivery room practices and added precautions for multiple gestation.

      (a) On admission, an IV line is placed for administering fluids and treatment in the event of hemorrhage or the need for emergency delivery and anesthesia.

      (b) Prophylactic antacids may be given to reduce gastric pH and volume.

      (c) Continuous or simultaneous FHR monitoring

      (d) Ultrasound scan on admission to assess the presentation and estimated fetal weight of each infant

      (e) Double set-up: having equipment for cesarean section available and ready in the room at the time of delivery

      (f) Extra personnel are likely to be present at delivery to attend to needs of each newborn (especially if preterm).

      (g) Many times, cesarean delivery is standard practice for multiple-gestation pregnancies greater than two (i.e., triplets, quadruplets) and may be necessary for twins.

      (h) Cesarean delivery may be necessary for the second twin even after successful vaginal delivery of the first.

      (i) Ultrasound examination is often performed after the delivery of twin A to reassess position of twin B, as well as to guide external version if needed to facilitate vaginal delivery.

      (j) Oxytocin administration may be necessary to augment uterine activity and to enhance descent of the second twin.

      (k) Twin B is at considerably higher risk for delivery-related complications such as umbilical cord prolapse, malpresentation, and abruptio placentae; therefore intensive monitoring must be continued until twin B is delivered.

      (l) Each infant is individually stabilized, resuscitated as necessary, and identified; cord blood or other laboratory work is ordered as needed.

   (4) Visit NICU before births if possible to prepare client for intensive care environment.

   (5) Encourage verbalization and assist client in identifying specific concerns.

   (6) Assist client in identifying support system and other resources available.

  b. Outcomes

   (1) Client can list signs and symptoms of preterm labor.

   (2) Client identifies significant signs and symptoms of pregnancy complications that need to be reported immediately.

   (3) Client can discuss interventions specifically relating to multiple gestation that may be made either during pregnancy or during delivery.

   (4) Client has a realistic expectation of vaginal delivery.

   (5) Client can discuss components of NICU care as appropriate.

   (6) Client has developed a plan to use available resources and support services as needed.

3. Impaired parenting related to delivery of more than one infant

  a. Interventions

   (1) Provide a list of resources and services available (e.g., Mothers of Twins support group, lactation consultants).

   (2) Discuss aspects of normal newborn infant care; assess learning needs.

   (3) Explore client's specific concerns.

    b. Outcomes

        (1) Client can identify available resources.

        (2) Client demonstrates appropriate techniques for infant bathing and feeding.

        (3) Client can discuss her specific concerns relating to the parenting role.

Health Education

A. Twins

    1. Monozygotic: identical twins; originate from one zygote that divided around the end of the first week of pregnancy.

        a. Accounts for one-third of all twins.

        b. Genetically identical: very similar in appearance

    2. Dizygotic: fraternal twins; result from the fertilization of two ova.

        a. Accounts for two-thirds of all twins.

        b. Tends to repeat in families

        c. Increased risk with advancing maternal age

        d. May result from induction of ovulation by fertility drugs and procedures.

B. Other multiple births

    1. Triplets occur once in every 6900 pregnancies.

    2. Multiple births of more than three babies are rare.

C. Nutritional requirements

    1. Caloric intake must be greatly increased to support the growth of multiple fetuses.

    2. Outline a dietary plan for client.

D. Inform client of high-risk status.

E. Instruct client to be aware of any developing symptoms of complications.

    1. Preterm labor

        a. Uterine contractions, cramping, or low back pain

        b. Feeling of pelvic pressure or fullness

        c. Change in amount or character of vaginal discharge

        d. GI upset: nausea, vomiting, or diarrhea

    2. PROM: report any leaking of fluid.

    3. Precautionary measures

        a. Increase client's rest periods.

        b. Have client lie in the lateral position to maximize blood flow to the uterus.

        c. Teach client to palpate uterine contractions (see discussion of health education under Preterm Labor).

INTRAUTERINE FETAL DEMISE

Introduction

A. Perinatal death, whether it occurs before delivery as an intrauterine fetal demise or after delivery as a neonatal death, presents a unique set of physical and psychosocial problems.

B. The developmental task of attachment and preparing for parenthood is abruptly interrupted; parents are shocked and confused, and they suddenly find themselves faced with issues of grief and mourning.

C. The physical process of labor and delivery, as well as the handling of the infant after delivery, requires extreme sensitivity on the part of the nurse.

Clinical Practice

A. Assessment
  1. History
     a. Loss of fetal movement
     b. Diminishing signs of pregnancy
        (1) Maternal weight gain ceases.
        (2) Mother may even lose weight.
        (3) Breast changes begin to reverse.
     c. Associated high-risk factors
        (1) Advanced diabetes in pregnancy
        (2) Systemic vascular disease
        (3) Collagen vascular disease
        (4) Previous unexplained loss of fetus
  2. Physical findings
     a. Cessation or decrease in uterine growth
     b. Absence of fetal heart tones by auscultation or Doppler
     c. Ultrasound findings
        (1) Lack of cardiac activity
        (2) Spalding's sign: overlapping of the fetal skull bones
     d. Vaginal examination: observe for the following:
        (1) Bleeding
        (2) Umbilical cord prolapse
        (3) ROM: amniotic fluid often appears cloudy and brownish red if the fetus has been dead for several days.
        (4) Note any cervical dilation or effacement.
        (5) Note fetal presenting part or presence of any softening or overlapping of skull bones.
  3. Psychosocial findings
     a. Stress factors
        (1) Fear for self
        (2) Anxiety related to labor and delivery process
        (3) Confusion
     b. Behavioral factors
        (1) Difficulty in communicating
        (2) Shock and numbness (first stage of grief)
        (3) Demonstration of some attachment behaviors
        (4) Expression of significance of this pregnancy
        (5) Expression of significance of this loss
        (6) Expression of guilt
  4. Diagnostic procedures
     a. Ultrasound examination: most accurate to identify absence of fetal cardiac activity
     b. Radiologic signs of fetal death
        (1) Significant overlap of skull bones (process takes several days to develop)
        (2) Exaggerated curvature of the fetal spine (depends on the degree of maceration of sacral ligaments)
        (3) Evidence of gas in the fetus (uncommon but reliable sign)
     c. Palpation of collapsed fetal skull through the cervix
     d. Disseminated intravascular coagulopathy (DIC) screen: look for coagulation abnormalities because DIC is a complication related to intrauterine fetal demise.

B. **Nursing Diagnoses**
   1. Grieving related to fetal demise
   2. Risk for ineffective tissue perfusion related to DIC
C. **Interventions/Outcomes**
   1. Grieving related to fetal demise
      a. Interventions
         (1) Encourage client and her family to verbalize feelings.
         (2) Discuss the grieving process with the client and her family (see Health Education).
         (3) Allow client choices relating to labor and delivery (e.g., induction of labor immediately after diagnosis is made or waiting until the spontaneous onset of labor; clients often benefit from having a few days to deal with this issue before going through delivery).
         (4) Discuss the use of oxytocin or prostaglandin.
            (a) Induction with oxytocin is most often used for fetuses at 28 weeks' gestation or beyond.
            (b) Prostaglandin suppositories are often preferred for fetuses at earlier gestational stages.
            (c) Discuss side effects of prostaglandin.
               (i) Nausea
               (ii) Vomiting
               (iii) Diarrhea
         (5) Analgesia or anesthesia
            (a) More liberal use is possible when the drug effect on the fetus is not considered.
            (b) Avoid oversedation because it may interfere with the grieving process.
         (6) Offer client and family the opportunity to see, touch, and hold the infant.
         (7) Provide tangible remembrances (e.g., photographs, footprints, infant identification bands, locks of hair).
         (8) Offer support from clergy members.
         (9) Offer baptism or blessing.
         (10) Discuss autopsy with client and her family; explain its benefits.
         (11) Discuss plans for funeral or memorial services.
         (12) Prepare client and her family for appearance of the infant.
         (13) Provide client and her family with information about support groups.
         (14) Provide reading materials to the client and her family to take home because information may be overwhelming during hospitalization.
         (15) Provide materials or references to address specific areas of grieving, such as siblings' responses, grandparents' responses, and so forth.
         (16) Follow-up after delivery may be performed by a bereavement counselor, a social worker, or the nurse who cared for the client; follow-up should assess the progress of the client and her family in the grieving process after discharge and should continue to provide support.
      b. Outcomes
         (1) Client and family are able to verbalize their feelings and can identify specific areas of concern.
         (2) Client and family can discuss steps in the grieving process.

    (3) Client and family participate in plan of care whenever possible and feel a part of the decision-making process.

    (4) Client is as comfortable as possible during labor and delivery.

    (5) Client and family see, touch, and hold the infant if they desire.

    (6) Client and family have tangible memories of the infant.

    (7) Client and family are aware of available clergy support, as well as options such as baptism and blessing.

    (8) Client and family demonstrate understanding of autopsy.

    (9) Client and family are aware of options for funeral or memorial services.

    (10) Client and family have information on support groups and services available.

    (11) Client and family demonstrate appropriate grief response.

2. Risk for ineffective tissue perfusion related to DIC (see Chapter 23)

  a. Interventions

    (1) Assess client for signs and symptoms of DIC.

      (a) Bleeding from puncture sites

      (b) Oozing through surgical incision (if one is present)

      (c) Bleeding from gums

      (d) Hematuria

    (2) Check laboratory values (or obtain order from physician to have coagulation studies done).

      (a) Hemoglobin and hematocrit: may be low, reflecting blood loss.

      (b) Platelet count: may be low in DIC.

      (c) Prothrombin time (PT) and activated partial thromboplastin time (APTT): elevation indicates clotting dysfunction.

      (d) Clotting time: prolonged in DIC

      (e) Bleeding time: prolonged in DIC

      (f) Serum fibrinogen: elevated in DIC

      (g) Fibrin split products: elevated in DIC

    (3) Assess vital signs to estimate blood loss and its effect.

    (4) Administer blood and blood products as ordered.

  b. Outcomes

    (1) Client has no signs or symptoms of DIC.

    (2) Client's vital signs remain within normal limits.

Health Education

A. Stages of grief

  1. Shock, numbness, and yearning

  2. Searching (includes anger)

  3. Disorientation and depression

  4. Reorganization

B. Normal grief responses

  1. Preoccupation with the dead infant

  2. Guilt and self-blame

  3. Anger and hostility

  4. Parents may grieve at a different pace, and therefore parents may seem not to be available to each other for support.

  5. Strange dreams related to the infant

  6. Aching arms

  7. Hearing an infant cry

  8. Still feeling the infant move

C. **Appearance of dead infant**
1. Maceration (peeling) of the skin
2. Discoloration of areas that had pressure on them, which look grossly ecchymotic
3. Areas of swelling and fluid retention
4. Discussion of any specific abnormalities
5. Amniotic fluid often reddish brown and more viscous than normal
6. Delivery may cause trauma more readily (e.g., skull bones may collapse and cause unusual facial appearance).

AMNIOTIC FLUID EMBOLISM

Introduction

A. **Entry of amniotic fluid into the maternal circulatory system is a rare but extremely dangerous obstetrical complication;** the exact incidence is unknown; the complication is unpreventable and unpredictable; clinically a tumultuous labor is followed by an acute onset of maternal dyspnea and hypotension, followed shortly by cardiopulmonary collapse; of clients who survive the acute event, 40% develop adult respiratory distress syndrome (ARDS), left sided heart failure, as well as severe DIC.

B. **The mortality rate for this complication has been reported to be as high as 80%.**

Clinical Practice

A. **Assessment**
1. History
   a. Rapid, vigorous labor
   b. Evidence of abruptio placentae
2. Physical findings
   a. Acute onset of respiratory distress, often during delivery process
      (1) Dyspnea
      (2) Chest pain
      (3) Cyanosis
      (4) Loss of consciousness
      (5) Pulmonary edema
   b. Acute onset of circulatory collapse
      (1) Severe hypoxia
      (2) Severe hypotension
      (3) If client does not die from the initial respiratory insult, she needs to overcome the severe hemorrhage and coagulopathy that follow.
   c. Acute onset of coagulopathy
      (1) Uterine bleeding at delivery is not easily controlled.
      (2) Oozing may begin from puncture sites.
3. Psychosocial findings
   a. Fear of death
   b. Fear on the part of the family in response to the rapid onset of life-threatening complications
4. Diagnostic procedures
   a. The diagnosis of amniotic fluid embolism must be made from the clinical picture.

     b. A definitive diagnosis is made only on autopsy by the identification of amniotic fluid and particulate debris (e.g., meconium, vernix, lanugo, mucin) obstructing the pulmonary vasculature.

     c. Blood aspirated from a central venous or a pulmonary artery line has shown fetal squamous cells and other debris of presumed fetal origin in living patients who have apparently survived an amniotic fluid embolism.

     d. Sputum samples have also shown the presence of fetal squamous cells.

B. Nursing Diagnoses

    1. Ineffective tissue perfusion related to pulmonary obstruction by particulate amniotic fluid

    2. Fear related to life-threatening emergency

C. Interventions/Outcomes

    1. Ineffective tissue perfusion related to pulmonary obstruction by particulate amniotic fluid

     a. Interventions

      (1) Recognize life-threatening diagnosis.

      (2) Ensure IV access; if client does not have an IV line, start one immediately because a delay of even a few minutes may result in circulatory collapse and make IV access more difficult; consider having two IV lines in place.

      (3) Initiate cardiopulmonary resuscitation (CPR) if indicated.

      (4) Administer oxygen at a rate of at least 8 L/min.

      (5) Prepare for and assist with intubation and ventilation with 100% of the fractions of inspired oxygen (FiO_2) if client loses consciousness.

      (6) Administer crystalloid IV fluids rapidly if client is hypotensive; if blood pressure is maintained, do not overload with fluids because it can result in pulmonary edema resulting from developing ARDS

      (7) Monitor vital signs frequently.

      (8) Have emergency medications such as dopamine to assist in client stabilization.

      (9) Chest radiograph and 12-lead ECG can assist in hemodynamic management.

     (10) Observe for signs and symptoms of shock.

     (11) Observe for signs and symptoms of coagulopathy (inability to control intrapartum or immediate postpartum vaginal bleeding or bleeding from IV site or puncture or trauma sites).

     (12) Send laboratory work.

      (a) CBC

      (b) Platelet count

      (c) Arterial blood gases

      (d) Fibrinogen

      (e) Fibrin split products

      (f) PT and APTT

     (13) Prepare for and assist with placement of central line (a pulmonary artery catheter may be useful for further hemodynamic management).

     (14) Administer blood or volume expanders as ordered.

     b. Outcomes

      (1) Client survives incident.

      (2) Client survives resulting complications.

      (a) Client is hemodynamically stable.

      (b) CBC is within normal limits.

      (c) Coagulation studies are within normal limits.
      (d) Oxygen saturation is within normal limits.
    (3) Client does not experience ARDS.
  2. Fear related to life-threatening emergency
    a. Interventions
      (1) Inform and reassure client and family as much as possible during crisis.
      (2) After life-threatening emergency has resolved, allow client to verbalize her feelings.
    b. Outcomes
      (1) Client does not experience panic during episode.
      (2) Client resolves her fear once the crisis has passed.

Health Education

A. Amniotic fluid embolism is so rare an obstetrical complication that preparing a client for its possibility is not needed.
B. After a client has survived such an incident, the nurse may explain to her what is known about amniotic fluid embolism.
  1. Composition of amniotic fluid
    a. Particulate matter leads to embolism.
      (1) Fetal squamous cells (from exfoliation of skin)
      (2) Vernix caseosa
      (3) Lanugo
      (4) Meconium
        (a) When amniotic fluid embolism accompanies other complications, such as abruptio placentae, the incidence of fetal distress and resultant passage of meconium is much higher.
  2. Access to the maternal circulation
    a. Amniotic fluid is usually contained within the uterine cavity and is separated from the maternal circulatory system.
    b. Introduction of amniotic fluid into the maternal circulation may occur in the following instances:
      (1) The amnion and the chorion are open, such as occurs with rupture of the amniotic sac.
      (2) Uterine or cervical veins are open, such as occurs with placental separation.
      (3) A pressure gradient that is high enough to force the amniotic fluid into the maternal circulation, such as occurs in a highly vigorous labor or with the tetanic contractions that result from abruptio placentae.
  3. Emboli: obstruction of the pulmonary vessels and interruption of the gas exchange is the same mechanism that occurs in any embolism.

UTERINE RUPTURE
Introduction

A. Uterine rupture is rare; the incidence ranges from 1 in 6673 (0.02%) to 1 in 1230 pregnancies (0.08%) and is considered an obstetric emergency.
B. Clinical conditions associated with uterine rupture are uterine scar, uterine or fetal anomalies, prior invasive molar pregnancy, excessive uterine stimulation, history of placenta percreta or increta, obstructed labor, midforcep delivery, and malpresentation.

C. Sudden fetal distress is the most common sign and symptom even before the onset of abdominal pain or vaginal bleeding.

D. A normal uterus with no prior surgery contracting spontaneously is unlikely to rupture unless significant trauma exists.

E. Because a trial of labor after a previous cesarean delivery is now the standard of care, the nurse must be familiar with the signs and symptoms of uterine rupture.

Clinical Practice

A. **Assessment**
  1. History
     a. Pregnancies, viable pregnancies, and EDC
     b. Previous cesarean delivery and indication
     c. Types of uterine incision
        (1) Low transverse: considered to be the safest for subsequent stress of uterine contractions
        (2) Classic: considered to be at the highest risk for rupture with the stress of uterine contractions
     d. Type of uterine activity: contraction frequency, duration, and intensity
     e. Pain
     f. Uterine anomalies
     g. Abdominal trauma: sharp or blunt
     h. Previous uterine trauma, such as perforation at the time of dilatation and curettage (D&C) or instrumented abortion
     i. Intrauterine administration of hypertonic saline
     j. Aggressive administration of oxytocin or prostaglandin
  2. Physical findings
     a. Abdominal examination: observe for any pain or rigidity.
     b. Leopold's maneuver (position of fetus): observe for any unusual feeling of fetal parts because fetus can be outside of the uterus.
     c. Sudden fetal distress, especially the appearance of variable decelerations at a time in labor when they are usually unlikely to occur
     d. Vaginal bleeding
  3. Psychosocial findings
     a. Stress factors
        (1) Anxiety
        (2) Fear related to pain
        (3) Fear of the unknown
     b. Behavioral responses
        (1) Expression of fear
        (2) Difficulty in communicating
B. **Nursing Diagnoses**
  1. Risk for maternal injury (shock) related to blood loss secondary to uterine rupture
  2. Risk for fetal injury (distress) related to impaired uteroplacental blood flow
  3. Pain related to uterine rupture
  4. Fear related to life-threatening complication
  5. Fear related to threatened loss of infant
C. **Interventions/Outcomes**
  1. Risk for maternal injury (shock) related to blood loss secondary to uterine rupture

   a. Interventions

     (1) Monitor maternal vital signs: observe for hypotension and tachycardia, which may indicate hypovolemic shock.

     (2) Observe any blood loss and estimate amount as accurately as possible.

     (3) Maintain IV access with large bore.

     (4) Prepare for emergency cesarean delivery if any evidence of uterine rupture is present.

       (a) Alert operating room and anesthesia provider.

       (b) Alert client's physician.

       (c) Alert neonatal team, pediatrician, or both.

       (d) Perform abdominal shave and skin preparation.

       (e) Insert Foley catheter.

       (f) Have client sign consent forms.

     (5) Monitor hemoglobin and hematocrit levels.

     (6) Administer blood and blood products as ordered.

   b. Outcome

     (1) Client shows no evidence of hypovolemic shock.

2. Risk for fetal injury (distress) related to impaired uteroplacental blood flow

   a. Interventions

     (1) Maintain continuous FHR monitoring: observe for any indications of fetal distress, especially late decelerations or prolonged bradycardia.

     (2) Maintain client on her side to maximize uterine blood flow.

   b. Outcomes

     (1) Client delivers a viable infant with no irreversible damage.

3. Pain related to uterine rupture

   a. Interventions

     (1) Continuous monitoring in labor for FHR and to record uterine activity; it is preferable to have an intrauterine pressure catheter in place to document intensity of uterine contractions accurately.

     (2) Analgesics or anesthesia may be used for pain control if no evidence of abnormal uterine activity indicating rupture is present.

       (a) If the client has had analgesics or anesthesia, the pain associated with rupture may be masked.

       (b) The nurse must therefore be acutely aware of any changes in uterine activity patterns.

   b. Outcomes

     (1) Client does not experience intolerable pain during labor.

     (2) Analgesics are not given when evidence of uterine rupture is present.

4. Fear related to life-threatening complication

   a. Interventions

     (1) Inform client that this condition is serious and that hospital staff will be working quickly to ensure her health and that of her infant.

     (2) Encourage client and family to verbalize feelings and to identify specific concerns.

     (3) Provide as much information as possible to client and family.

     (4) Reassure client and family as often as possible during any emergency procedures.

   b. Outcomes

     (1) Client and family do not have unreasonable fears.

5. Fear related to threatened loss of fetus

    a. Interventions: if uterine rupture occurs, every effort is made to perform cesarean delivery immediately; a client's fear of losing the fetus at this point is valid.
      (1) Perform all tasks as quickly as possible.
      (2) Solicit help to minimize the time required to prepare client for delivery.
      (3) Stay calm and reassure client that health care team is doing everything possible to save the fetus.
    b. Outcomes
      (1) Client does not become uncooperative or hysterical as a result of fear.

Health Education

A. Definitions
    1. Uterine rupture is classified as complete or incomplete.
    2. According to *William's Obstetrics* (Cunningham, MacDonald, & Gant, 2001):
      a. Complete uterine rupture: laceration communicates directly with the peritoneal cavity.
      b. Incomplete uterine rupture: laceration is separated from the peritoneal cavity by the visceral peritoneum.
      c. Uterine scar dehiscence: previous scar begins to separate; this condition usually happens gradually, and if the fetal membranes are intact, no protrusion of fetal parts into the peritoneal cavity occurs.

B. Types of scar
    1. Low transverse
      a. Transverse or horizontal incision into the lower uterine segment
      b. Because of the way the muscle fibers are arranged, low transverse scars are under relatively little tension when the uterus contracts.
    2. Classical incision
      a. Uterine scar vertically placed on the body of the uterus and may extend up as far as the fundus
      b. This area is under a great deal of stress with contractions.
      c. Classical incisions are used if cesarean delivery is indicated before term because the lower uterine segment is not yet well enough developed, but they may also be used for an urgent cesarean delivery; this is why it is important to ask the reason for any previous cesarean delivery.

CASE STUDIES AND STUDY QUESTIONS

Mrs. C is a 22-year-old gravida 3, para 2 (G3, P2) woman. She delivered her first child spontaneously at 34 weeks' gestation, and the child has subsequently done well. Her second child underwent cesarean delivery at 29 weeks and died 10 days later from complications of prematurity.

    Mrs. C is currently at 25 weeks' gestation and has been feeling pelvic pressure and a vague sense of cramping since this morning at 7:00 AM. It is now 11:00 AM, and she has called the labor and delivery unit because of concerns about her cramping.

  1. Which of the following is your best response to her?
    a. Maintain bed rest in the lateral position and drink plenty of fluids.
    b. Come to the hospital immediately for further evaluation.
    c. Do not be concerned because the cramping is probably Braxton

Hicks contractions and is normal at this gestational stage.

2. Mrs. C is at risk for preterm labor because of which of the following?
   a. She is a young multipara.
   b. She has previously undergone cesarean delivery.
   c. She has had previous preterm labors and births.
   d. She is not at risk for preterm labor.

POSTTERM PREGNANCY

Ms. H is a 26-year-old G1, P0 woman. She has had no prenatal care, but her last menstrual period puts her at 42 weeks' gestation. She came into the hospital with possible rupture of membranes. She is not sure whether her membranes have ruptured because, although she felt a gush, she saw only a small amount of brownish fluid.

3. The labor and delivery nurse is concerned about Ms. H because of which of the following?
   a. She is probably in preterm labor.
   b. Her history indicates the risk for oligohydramnios and the probable presence of meconium.
   c. She is at risk because she is an elderly primipara.
   d. She is in active labor at this time.

After Ms. H has been on the external fetal monitor for 40 minutes, the tracing shows minimal FHR variability but no evidence of decelerations. No fetal movement and no spontaneous FHR accelerations are present.

4. Appropriate nursing interventions at this time include which of the following?
   a. Preparing her for emergency cesarean delivery
   b. Allowing her to ambulate to stimulate the onset of contractions

   c. Maintaining her on bed rest in lateral position, starting an IV, and continuing the FHR monitoring
   d. Discharging her home to return when contractions are 5 minutes apart

PREMATURE RUPTURE OF MEMBRANES

Mrs. L is a 30-year-old G3, P2 woman at 31 weeks' gestation. She presents to the labor and delivery suite complaining of leaking fluid for the last couple of hours. Her vital signs are blood pressure 108/60 mm Hg, pulse 70 beats/min, respirations 20, and a 97.6° F (36.4° C) temperature. She is monitored for 1 hour, and the FHR tracing is in the range of 130 to 145, reactive with no decelerations. No uterine contractions are perceived by Mrs. L or recorded on the monitor.

5. Mrs. L is a candidate for expectant management because of which of the following?
   a. She is afebrile and has no other symptoms of infection.
   b. Her fetus is in the vertex position.
   c. A normal amount of amniotic fluid by ultrasound examination is present.
   d. She is not a candidate for expectant management.

6. In your initial assessment of Mrs. L, you note that she is nitrazine-negative but positive for vaginal pooling and ferning. These findings would lead you to believe that she is which of the following?
   a. Probably not ruptured because nitrazine is the most accurate test
   b. Most likely ruptured because many factors may interfere with nitrazine testing

c. Definitely ruptured because ferning is 100% accurate
d. Most likely infected because that causes a positive fern test result

MULTIPLE GESTATION

Mrs. D is a 30-year-old G1, P0 woman. She has a history of infertility for 4 years and conceived while taking fertility drugs. She is carrying twins at 33 weeks' gestation and presents to the labor and delivery unit with complaints of cramping and a feeling of pelvic pressure. After 30 minutes on the fetal monitor, you note that Mrs. D has mild uterine contractions every 5 to 6 minutes. Her cervical examination reveals a long, closed posterior cervix.

7. Uterine activity at 33 weeks is particularly significant for Mrs. D because of which of the following?
   a. She is at high risk for preterm labor.
   b. She has been contracting and her cervix has not changed.
   c. She is at high risk for chorioamnionitis.
   d. No reason for concern exists; uterine contractions are common at this gestational age.

8. Mrs D. is also at high risk for which other pregnancy complications?
   a. PIH
   b. Antepartum hemorrhage
   c. PROM
   d. All of the above

INTRAUTERINE FETAL DEMISE

Ms. T is a 34-year-old G3, P1 woman with class C diabetes. She had a previous stillborn at 36 weeks' gestation with an undetermined cause of fetal death. She is currently at 35 weeks' gestation. She has had an uneventful pregnancy so far but now calls the labor and delivery unit because she has not felt the infant move since early this morning. It is now 1:00 PM.

9. Your best response to Ms. T is to tell her which of the following?
   a. Come in to labor and delivery as soon as possible for further evaluation.
   b. Wait at least 10 to 12 hours, then call her physician if she still has not felt movement.
   c. Her anxiety is most likely related to her previous loss at this gestation and therefore no need for concern exists.
   d. Maintain bed rest in the left lateral position.

10. When Ms. T arrives in the labor and delivery unit, you are unable to auscultate fetal heart tones. You suspect she may have experienced intrauterine fetal demise. The most definitive way to confirm this diagnosis is to do which of the following?
    a. Document the absence of fetal cardiac activity by ultrasonography.
    b. Send her for pelvic radiographs.
    c. Find an elevation in serum fibrinogen.
    d. Obtain an L/S ratio.

AMNIOTIC FLUID EMBOLISM

Ms. N is a 25-year-old G1, P0 woman at term who arrives in the labor and delivery unit at 2:00 AM. Her contractions started at midnight, and their frequency and intensity increased so rapidly that she was no longer able to tolerate the pain and came into the hospital. On examination, her cervix is 6 cm dilated and completely effaced. The presenting part is at zero station. She continues in very active labor with uterine contractions every 1 to 2 minutes over the next

30 minutes, at the end of which she is completely dilated and effaced. She pushes for 10 minutes and is prepared for delivery.

11. Immediately after the delivery of the infant, Ms. N complains of dyspnea and shortness of breath. Within minutes, she becomes cyanotic and lethargic and seems to be losing consciousness. Recognizing this clinical picture as most likely an amniotic fluid embolism, appropriate nursing actions are to do which of the following?
    a. Prepare a loading dose of $MgSO_4$ for seizure precaution.
    b. Open her IV line and administer oxygen at high concentrations.
    c. Notify the NICU and prepare for possible neonatal transfer because the newborn is at great risk for RDS.
    d. Perform an abdominal shave and skin preparation to get Ms. N ready for emergency surgery.

12. Ms. N is intubated and ventilated by the anesthesiologist for 10 minutes. She is fighting the endotracheal tube and breathing on her own. Blood for laboratory work is drawn, and her arterial blood gas values are within normal limits. She is extubated and resumes spontaneous respirations. Her color is good, but nasal oxygen is kept on at 10 L/min. Her oxygen saturation is 96% to 97%. She has survived the initial insult of an amniotic fluid embolism. Ms. N is still at great risk for which

subsequent complications?
    a. Preeclampsia
    b. ARDS
    c. Postpartum endometritis
    d. Deep vein thromboembolism

UTERINE RUPTURE

Mrs. P is a 30-year-old G2, P1 woman with class B diabetes who is at term. She had a previous cesarean delivery at 27 weeks' gestation for an abruptio placentae 6 years earlier.

13. Mrs. P is not a candidate for trial of labor because of which of the following?
    a. This infant is likely to be much bigger than her previous one.
    b. She has diabetes and therefore requires another cesarean delivery.
    c. A cesarean delivery at 28 weeks' gestation was likely to have involved a classical incision.
    d. She is a good candidate for trial of labor.

14. If Mrs. P arrived in the labor and delivery unit and told you she had been having contractions for the last 8 hours, and now the pain "just won't go away," you might consider the possibility of uterine rupture. Other assessment parameters consistent with uterine rupture are which of the following?
    a. Systolic hypertension
    b. Bleeding
    c. Fetal distress
    d. Excess fetal movement

ANSWERS TO STUDY QUESTIONS

1. b   5. a   9. a   13. c
2. c   6. b   10. a   14. c
3. b   7. a   11. b
4. c   8. d   12. b

REFERENCES

Agency for Healthcare Research and Quality. (2002). Management of prolonged pregnancy, *Evidence report/technology assessment, no. 23,* Durham, NC: Duke Evidence Based Practice Center.

American College of Obstetricians and Gynecologists. (2000). *Management of postterm pregnancy. ACOG practice bulletin, no. 6,* Washington, DC: American College of Obstetricians and Gynecologists.

American College of Obstetricians and Gynecologists. (1998). *Premature rupture of membranes: Clinical management guidelines for obstetrician-gynecologists. ACOG practice bulletin, no. 1,* Washington, DC: American College of Obstetricians and Gynecologists.

American College of Obstetricians and Gynecologists. (1998). *Special problems of multiple gestation. ACOG educational bulletin 253,* Washington, DC: American College of Obstetricians and Gynecologists.

Brown, J.E., & Carlson, M. (2000). Nutrition and multifetal pregnancy. *Journal of the American Dietetic Association, 100*(3), 343-348.

Cunningham, F.G., MacDonald, P.C., & Gant, N.F. (2001). *William's obstetrics* (21st ed.). Stanford: Appleton & Lange.

Elliott, J. (2000). *Multiple gestation.* Maternal-fetal medicine, Phoenix, AZ: Good Samaritan Regional Medical Center. *Available online at www.bestdoctors.com/en/conditions/g/gestation/gestation_100200.htm.*

Colombo, D. F., & Iams, J. D. (2000). Cervical length and preterm labor. *Clinical Obstetrics and Gynecology, 43*(4), 735-745.

Crowley, P. (2003). Interventions for preventing or improving the outcome of delivery at or beyond term (Cochrane review). In *The Cochrane Library,* issue 1, Oxford: Update Software.

Crowther, C. (2003). Hospitalization and bedrest for multiple pregnancy. In *The Cochrane Library,* issue 1, Oxford: Update Software.

Freda, M.C., & Patterson, E. (2001). *Preterm labor: Prevention, and nursing management* (2nd ed.). White Plains, NY: March of Dimes.

Gilbert, E.S., & Harmon, J.S. (2003). *Manual of high-risk pregnancy & delivery* (3rd ed.). St. Louis: Mosby.

Guyetvai, K., Hannah, M.E., Hodnett, E.D., & Ohlsson, A. (1999). Tocolytics for preterm labor: a systematic review. *Obstetrics and Gynecology, 94*(5, Pt 2):869-877.

Hearne, A.E., & Nagey, D.A. (2000). Therapeutic agents in preterm labor: Tocolytic agents. *Clinical Obstetrics and Gynecology, 43*(4), 787-801.

Hofmeyr, G. (2003). Prophylactic versus therapeutic amnioinfusion for oligohydramnios in labour (Cochrane review). In *The Cochrane Library,* issue 1, Oxford: Update Software.

Kenyon, S., Boulvain, M., & Neilson, J. (2003). Antibiotics for preterm premature rupture of membranes (Cochrane review). In *The Cochrane Library,* issue 1, Oxford: Update Software.

Limbo, R., & Wheeler, S. (1995). *When a baby dies: A handbook for healing and helping.* LaCrosse, WI: Resolve Through Sharing.

Luke, B., & Eberlein, T. (1999). *When you're expecting twins, triplets, and quads.* New York: Harper & Row.

Maloni, J.A. (2000). Preventing preterm birth: Evidence based interventions shift toward prevention, *AWHONN Lifelines, 4*(4), 26-33.

Mercer, B.M., Miodovnik, M., Thurnau, G.R., Goldenberg, R.L., Das, A.F., Ramsey, R.D., et al. (1997). Antibiotic therapy for reduction of infant morbidity after preterm premature of the membranes: A randomized controlled trial. *Journal of the American Medical Association, 278*(12), 989-995.

Robinson, J., & Abuhamad, A. (2002). Determining chorionicity and amnionicity in multiple pregnancies. *Contemporary OB/GYN, 6,* 94-108.

Schmidt, J. (1997). Fluid check: Making the case for intrapartum amnioinfusion. *AWHONN Lifelines, 1*(5), 46-51.

Seidel, H.M., Ball, J.W., Dains, J.E., & Benedict G.W. (2003). *Mosby's guide to physical examination* (5th ed.). St. Louis: Mosby.

Toppenberg, K.S., & Block, W.A. (2002). Uterine rupture: What family physicians need to know. *American Family Physician, 66*(5), 823-828.

U.S. Department of Health and Human Services. (2000). *Healthy People 2010: Understanding and improving health.* Washington, DC: USDHHS.

Weitz, B.W. (2001). Premature rupture of the fetal membranes: An update for advanced practice nurses. *MCN: The American Journal of Maternal Child Nursing, 26*(2), 86-92.

30 Postpartum Complications

PATRICIA GRANT HIGGINS

OBJECTIVES

1. Identify four different types of postpartum complications.

2. Recognize the causes of postpartum complications.

3. Select appropriate nursing actions to reduce postpartum complications.

4. Define specific treatments for postpartum complications.

5. Assess risk factors for women who are prone to postpartum complications.

6. Design health education strategies to prevent postpartum complications.

7. Appraise postpartum complications based on selected case studies.

8. Analyze assessment data for postpartum complications based on risk factors presented by women.

9. Interpret alterations in adaptation to maternal illness in the puerperium.

10. Analyze alterations in maternal psychologic adaptation in the puerperium.

11. Formulate nursing interventions to prevent disequilibrium in transition to parenthood and implement the nursing process to promote a healthy outcome.

12. Apply the nursing process to provide care to the high-risk postpartum client and her family based on analysis and synthesis of the client's needs in her particular situation.

POSTPARTUM HEMORRHAGE

Introduction

A. Approximately one-third of maternal deaths are related to postpartum hemorrhage (Scott, Hamond, & Gordon, 2003), which is defined as a blood loss greater than 500 ml in the first 24 hours after delivery.

1. Immediate postpartum hemorrhage occurs in the first 24 hours after delivery, and late postpartum hemorrhage occurs after the first 24 hours after delivery, usually at 7 to 14 days of the postpartum period.

2. The major causes of postpartum hemorrhage are:

    a. Uterine atony

        (1) The most frequent cause of bleeding in the puerperium arises from interference with involution of the uterus.

        (2) Uterine atony occurs early after delivery in 75% to 85% of the postpartum cases.

    b. Lacerations of the genital tract

    c. Hematomas

    d. Retained placental fragments; late postpartum hemorrhage is often caused by retained placental fragments.

   e. Uterine inversion
   f. Blood coagulation disorders
  3. The overall incidence of postpartum hemorrhage is 4% of deliveries.
B. Hematoma, a cause of postpartum hemorrhage, is a collection of blood in the pelvic tissue resulting from damage to a vessel wall without laceration of the tissue.
  1. This trauma can result from:
   a. Forceps manipulation
   b. Pressure of the presenting part on pelvic structures
   c. Large infant size
   d. Prolonged second stage
   e. Epidural regional anesthesia
   f. Excessive fundal pressure on the uterus
  2. May involve the vulva, vaginal, or subperitoneal area.
C. Disseminated intravascular coagulation (DIC) can cause postpartum hemorrhage by altering the blood clotting mechanism; abruptio placentae, fetal demise, or amniotic fluid embolism may be the underlying cause of DIC (see Chapter 23 for a complete discussion of hemorrhagic disorders).

Clinical Practice

A. Assessment
  1. History
   a. Precipitous or prolonged first or second stages of labor or both
   b. Overstretching of the uterus (which suggests a large fetus, hydramnios, or multiple gestation)
   c. Drugs (general anesthesia, oxytocin, and magnesium sulfate)
   d. Toxins (amnionitis and intrauterine fetal demise)
   e. Trauma through the use of midforceps or other intravaginal manipulations, such as internal podalic version or forceps rotation
   f. Previous postpartum hemorrhage, uterine rupture, or uterine surgery (cesarean section or dilatation and curettage)
   g. Past placenta previa, placenta increta, or placenta percreta
   h. Uterine malformation
   i. Maternal exhaustion, malnutrition, anemia, or pregnancy-induced hypertension (PIH)
   j. Defects in the decidua (outer layer of the endometrium that sloughs off as lochia)
   k. Manipulation of the placenta that occurs when the placenta is not delivered intact and manual extraction is necessary
   l. Rapid fetal descent
   m. Coagulation disorders, such as idiopathic thrombocytopenia, purpura, or von Willebrand's disease
   n. Grand multiparity
   o. Uterine infection
  2. Physical findings
   a. Uterine atony
    (1) Boggy, large uterus
    (2) Expelled clots
    (3) Bleeding (bright-red blood) visible and evident
    (4) Bleeding may be slow and steady or sudden and massive.
    (5) Bleeding may be caused by blood coagulation problems.

        b. Lacerations
          (1) Firm uterus with bright-red blood
          (2) Steady stream or trickle of unclotted blood
        c. Hematoma
          (1) Firm uterus with bright-red blood
          (2) Extreme perineal or pelvic pain
          (3) Bluish bulging area just under the skin surface
          (4) Difficulty in voiding
          (5) Unexplained tachycardia
          (6) Hypotension
          (7) Anemia
        d. Retained placental fragments
          (1) Placenta partially delivered and not intact
          (2) Fundal massage before placenta separates
          (3) Uterus remains large.
          (4) Bleeding is painless and blood is bright red.
        e. DIC
          (1) Petechiae
          (2) Ecchymosis
          (3) Prolonged bleeding from gums and venipuncture sites
          (4) Uncontrolled bleeding during childbirth
          (5) Tachycardia
          (6) Oliguria
          (7) Signs of acute renal failure
          (8) Convulsions
          (9) Coma
        f. Decreased systolic blood pressure
        g. Reduced pulse pressure and delayed capillary filling time
        h. Cold, clammy skin
        i. Profound hypotension
        j. Signs of metabolic acidosis
        k. Signs of shock do not appear until hemorrhage is advanced because of increased fluid and blood volume of pregnancy.
    3. Psychosocial response
        a. Fear
        b. Anxiety and restlessness
        c. Fatigue
    4. Diagnostic procedures
        a. Complete blood count (CBC)
        b. Type and cross-matching of blood products for transfusion
        c. Blood work-up to determine reduced platelets, prolonged prothrombin time, fibrinogen depression, normal clotting time, and prolonged partial thromboplastin time

B. Nursing Diagnoses
    1. Deficient fluid volume: risk for complications related to postpartum hemorrhage
    2. Fatigue related to blood loss
    3. Fear related to acute hemorrhage

C. Interventions/Outcomes
    1. Deficient fluid volume: risk for complications related to postpartum hemorrhage
        a. Interventions

(1) After initial postdelivery assessment, assess the height and midline position of the fundus at least each shift.

    (a) If uterus is soft and boggy, perform manual uterine massage.

    (b) For mild uterine bogginess, put infant to breast if mother is breastfeeding.

(2) Monitor lochia for color, odor, amount, consistency, clots, count or weight of used pads (1 g equals 1 ml).

(3) Keep accurate intake and output (I&O).

(4) Monitor and record vital signs.

(5) Turn client when assessing postpartal bleeding so blood does not pool unnoticed underneath her.

(6) Keep client flat to supply blood to heart and brain.

(7) Set up for intravenous (IV) infusion of Ringer's lactate or saline solution.

(8) Catheterization of distended bladder may assist uterine contraction and descent.

(9) Check that cross-matching is completed for blood replacement through volume expanders, blood products, or both.

(10) Administer oxytocin in 500 to 1000 ml of solution.

(11) If uterus remains atonic, give ergonovine maleate (Ergotrate) or methylergonovine (Methergine) IV or intramuscularly (IM), if ordered.

(12) If bleeding persists, ask physician to consider prostaglandin therapy.

(13) Antibiotics are given to prevent infection.

(14) Have physician check for retained placental fragments.

(15) Surgical intervention is last resort.

(16) Provide bimanual compression if physician is not available or no standing orders for oxytocin have been given.

(17) Provide explanations to the client of all procedures.

b. Outcomes

(1) Fundus is firm, midline, and at the level of the umbilicus or below.

(2) Lochia is red, odorless, moderate in amount, and unclotted.

(3) Vital signs are normal.

(4) I&O is adequate.

2. Fatigue related to blood loss

  a. Interventions

(1) Allow and schedule client rest periods that are undisturbed.

(2) Assist client with activities of daily living.

(3) Encourage client to monitor appropriate nutritional intake.

(4) Work around client's schedule to conserve energy.

(5) Organize work habits and tasks.

(6) Encourage client to take vitamins and iron tablets.

(7) Prevent orthostatic hypotension when getting client up.

(8) Mobilize support system or resources.

  b. Outcomes

(1) Client has enough energy to care for self and infant.

(2) Client has support from family and friends to help with household tasks.

(3) Client maintains optimal nutritional status.

(4) Client has adequate sleep and rest.

3. Fear related to acute hemorrhage

  a. Interventions

        (1) Stay with client and use physical touch if appropriate.
        (2) Offer client reassurance and support.
        (3) Give information to client in clear, brief statements.
        (4) Keep client's family informed.
    b. Outcomes
        (1) Client has positive support during a crisis situation.
        (2) Family is informed of client's progress and status.

POSTPARTUM INFECTIONS

Introduction

A. Defined as an infection accompanied by a temperature of 38° C (100.4° F) or higher after the first 24 hours after delivery
    1. Temperature remains elevated on two or more occasions for longer than 24 hours.
    2. There is no other defined cause for the fever.
B. Postpartum infection occurs after approximately 6% of births in the United States (Normand & Damato, 2001).
C. Other perinatal events that can cause an elevated temperature:
    1. Dehydration from fluid loss during labor and delivery
    2. Breast engorgement if temperature elevation occurs 48 to 72 hours after delivery
    3. Postoperative elevation after a cesarean birth
D. The most common type of postpartum infection is endometritis, which occurs secondary to chorioamnionitis before birth.
E. Cesarean section wound infection:
    1. Occurs after the third or fourth postoperative day.
    2. Can be masked by early postoperative fever.
F. The most common causative agents of postpartum infections are the following:
    1. Anaerobic streptococcus
    2. Clostridium
    3. Group A- or B-hemolytic streptococcus
    4. *Escherichia coli*
    5. *Klebsiella*
    6. *Gardnerella vaginalis*
    7. *Chlamydia trachomatis*
G. The three categories of postpartum infections are those involving:
    1. The reproductive or genital tract
    2. The urinary tract
    3. The breasts

Clinical Practice

A. Assessment
    1. History
        a. Long labor (longer than 24 hours, with fatigue and exhaustion that result in trauma or decrease the perception of the need to void)
        b. Anemia
        c. Traumatic delivery
        d. Postpartum hemorrhage
        e. Premature rupture of the membranes (PROM)

     f. Cesarean birth

     g. Malnutrition

     h. General debilitation

     i. Diabetes

     j. Intrauterine manipulation

     k. Many vaginal examinations during labor, especially after rupture of membranes (ROM)

     l. Hematoma

     m. Droplet infection from personnel

     n. Breaks in aseptic technique

     o. Frequent catheterization

     p. Poor personal care of client

     q. Laceration (third or fourth degree)

     r. Prolonged rupture of membranes

     s. Internal monitoring

2. Physical findings

     a. Genital tract infections involving the perineum, vulva, vagina, or cervix

          (1) Temperature: low grade fever of 38° to 38.5° C (100.4° to 101° F)

          (2) Site of infection is red and warm to the touch.

          (3) Drainage may or may not be present.

          (4) Dysuria (burning on urination)

          (5) Localized pain

          (6) Edema

          (7) White blood cell (WBC) count greater than $30,000/mm^3$ after the first day

     b. Genital tract infections involving the muscle of the uterus (metritis), at the placental site (endometritis), pelvic connective tissue (parametritis), tubes (salpingitis), or ovaries (oophoritis)

          (1) Temperature: 38.5° to 39.5° C (101° to 103° F)

          (2) Large, tender uterus and fundus on third postpartum day (subinvolution)

          (3) Lower abdominal pain

          (4) Malaise

          (5) Anorexia

          (6) Extreme lethargy

          (7) Chills

          (8) Headache

          (9) Backache

          (10) Increased pulse rate (100 to 140 bpm)

          (11) Foul-smelling lochia that can be normal, scant, or profuse in amount

          (12) Color of lochia from serosanguineous to brownish

          (13) Diaphoresis

     c. Urinary tract infections and cystitis

          (1) Small voiding volume or inability to void

          (2) Pain with urination

          (3) Low-grade fever 38.5° C (101° F)

          (4) Hematuria

          (5) Overdistended bladder

          (6) Increased vaginal bleeding

          (7) Boggy fundus

          (8) Backache

          (9) Restlessness

    d. Infections of the breast: mastitis
- (1) Temperature elevated to 40° C (104.1° F)
- (2) Chills
- (3) Malaise
- (4) Hard, red, and tender irregular mass in one or both breasts
- (5) Severe to acute pain and tenderness in one or both breasts
- (6) Cracked nipples
- (7) Engorgement
- (8) Lack of proper breast support

    e. Wound infections from cesarean section or dehiscence
- (1) Elevated temperature on third or fourth postpartum day
- (2) Drainage of pus or blood from the wound
- (3) Red and inflamed appearance of repaired edges
- (4) Presence of cellulitis
- (5) Wound opened and abdominal contents exposed to air

3. Psychosocial findings
- **a.** Anxiety
- **b.** Stress
- **c.** Pain

4. Diagnostic procedures
- **a.** Urinalysis
- **b.** Culture and sensitivity tests as necessary, for lochia, urine, breast milk, blood, wound, vagina, and vulva; obtain cultures before starting antibiotic therapy.
- **c.** Blood count: WBC count and hemoglobin and hematocrit

B. Nursing Diagnoses
- **1.** Acute pain related to infectious process
- **2.** Risk for infection (genital, urinary, or breast, or wound dehiscence) related to bacterial invasion
- **3.** Risk for imbalanced body temperature related to perineal or wound infections
- **4.** Impaired social interaction related to extended hospitalization for perineal or wound infection
- **5.** Risk for impaired parent and infant attachment related to postpartum infection

C. Interventions/Outcomes
- **1.** Acute pain related to infectious process
  - **a.** Interventions: provide the following (see Chapter 14 for a complete discussion of mastitis and lactation):
    - (1) Adequate nutrition
    - (2) Adequate fluids
    - (3) Adequate rest and sleep
    - (4) Frequent linen change
    - (5) Breast and perineal care
    - (6) Breast binder or brassiere
    - (7) Administration of analgesics
    - (8) Heat or cold treatment
    - (9) Breasts kept empty
    - (10) Facilitation of complete bladder emptying
    - (11) Bed bath with back rub
  - **b.** Outcomes
    - (1) Client is comfortable.
    - (2) Client is free of pain.

        (3) Client has no complaints.

        (4) Client is resting well.

2. Risk for infection (genital, urinary, or breast, or wound dehiscence) related to bacterial invasion

   a. Interventions

        (1) Perform culture and sensitivity tests.

        (2) Provide antibiotics.

        (3) Administer antipyretics.

        (4) Ensure isolation.

        (5) Use aseptic technique.

        (6) Use good hand washing.

        (7) Use semi-Fowler's position to facilitate drainage.

        (8) Assess fundus for involution.

        (9) Assess vital signs.

      (10) Assess pain symptoms and administer medications on time.

      (11) Monitor and record I&O.

      (12) Provide frequent rest periods.

      (13) Measure and record amount of redness and drainage.

      (14) Maintain an intact wound.

      (15) If wound opens:

          (a) Pack and repack the wound so it can heal by secondary intention.

          (b) If dehiscence occurs, apply normal saline solution to sterile cloth, cover the protruding organs, and return client to the operating room.

   b. Outcomes

        (1) Infection does not result in more serious complications.

        (2) Signs and symptoms of infection are recognized promptly, with treatment protocols followed.

        (3) No dehiscence occurs.

3. Risk for imbalanced body temperature related to perineal or wound infections

   a. Interventions

        (1) Assess vital signs every 4 hours.

        (2) Change bed linen when damp.

        (3) Offer client bed bath or shower.

        (4) Administer antipyretics.

        (5) Force 2000 ml of fluid per shift.

        (6) Record I&O.

        (7) Offer client back rub or application of cool cloth to forehead.

        (8) Change client's gown frequently.

   b. Outcomes

        (1) Body temperature remains normal for longer than 24 hours.

4. Impaired social interaction related to extended hospitalization for perineal or wound infection

   a. Interventions

        (1) Allow client's family and friends to visit or telephone if client has sufficient energy.

        (2) Keep client's family informed at all times.

        (3) Have same nurse care for client whenever possible.

        (4) Explain care measures to client.

        (5) Allow client time to discuss feelings and concerns.

   b. Outcomes

        (1) Client has support.

      (2) Client maintains family contact and interaction.

      (3) Client and family feel informed of client's condition.

      (4) Client discusses problems with nurse.

  5. Risk for impaired parent and infant attachment related to postpartum infection

    a. Interventions

      (1) Arrange for adequate rest and sleep.

      (2) Bring infant to client after she is rested.

      (3) Allow client to offer care and comfort to her infant if she has the energy to do so.

      (4) Explain positive aspects of infant to client.

      (5) Give client positive reinforcement for tasks achieved.

      (6) Allow other caregivers to care for the infant so client can rest and recover.

      (7) Encourage client to take care of herself first before she takes care of her infant.

    b. Outcomes

      (1) Client has minimal delay in bonding with infant.

      (2) Client expresses positive feelings toward infant.

      (3) Client feels comfortable with new skills learned to care for her infant's needs.

      (4) Client is able to care for infant after she is well rested.

      (5) Client allows others to care for infant.

      (6) Client has help when she goes home so she can focus on getting to know her infant.

THROMBOPHLEBITIS

Introduction

A. Thrombophlebitis is an infection of the lining of a vessel in which a clot attaches to the vessel wall.

B. This condition may involve the veins in the legs or the pelvis.

C. This condition occurs in less than 1% of all postpartum women (Olds, London, & Ladewig, 2000).

  1. Early ambulation after delivery decreases incidence.

  2. It still remains a concern because of the increased blood clotting factors in the postpartum period.

D. Onset is usually between the tenth and twentieth postpartum days.

E. Thrombophlebitis puts the new mother at risk for a pulmonary embolism and death related to obstruction of the circulation to the lung.

F. Superficial thrombophlebitis

  1. Involves the saphenous (surface) venous system.

  2. May be caused in some women by the lithotomy position during delivery.

G. Deep-vein thrombophlebitis

  1. Changes that take place in the deep veins of the calf, thighs, or pelvis predispose postpartum women to deep-vein thrombophlebitis.

  2. One cause may be pressure from the fetal head during delivery, which traumatizes the pelvic veins.

  3. Involves an increased risk of embolism.

Clinical Practice

A. Assessment

  1. History

    a. Use of oral contraceptives before pregnancy

       b. Employment that requires prolonged sitting
       c. Obesity
       d. Hemorrhage
       e. Operative delivery
       f. Heart disease
       g. Anemia
       h. Long labor
       i. Postdelivery pelvic infection
       j. Increased parity
       k. Advanced age
       l. Noted between tenth and twentieth postpartum days
       m. History of thrombophlebitis
       n. Endometritis
       o. Varicosities
  2. Physical findings
       a. Positive Homans' sign
          (1) Extend leg, support it under the knee, and apply pressure to the foot (forced dorsiflexion).
          (2) Pain is experienced behind calf or in calf when thrombosis is present.
          (3) A positive Homans' sign indicates the possibility of a deep-vein thrombosis (Kobler, Waterman, & DuMenil, 1997).
       b. Elevated body temperature: up to 40.5° C (105° F)
       c. Chills
       d. Pain experienced in leg
       e. Leg hot to touch
       f. Swelling and tenderness in leg
       g. Redness along vein affected in leg
       h. Pain in groin
       i. Leg looking white or pale in light-skinned women (which may suggest femoral thrombophlebitis [Kobler, et al., 1997])
       j. Elevated pulse rate
       k. Hypotension
       l. Pain experienced in leg when walking
  3. Psychosocial findings
       a. Change in pain perception
       b. Anxiety
       c. Inability to care for infant
       d. Discouragement
       e. Unwell feeling
  4. Diagnostic procedures
       a. Hemoglobin level and hematocrit values
       b. Phlebography (impedance plethysmograph [IPG])
       c. Doppler ultrasonography
       d. Contrast venography
B. Nursing Diagnoses
  1. Ineffective tissue perfusion related to thrombophlebitis
  2. Acute pain related to thrombophlebitis
  3. Anxiety related to changes in activities of daily living, inability to care for newborn, and thrombophlebitis
C. Interventions/Outcomes
  1. Ineffective tissue perfusion related to thrombophlebitis
       a. Interventions

(1) Ensure bed rest at all times.

(2) Administer anticoagulants (administration of IV heparin and warfarin to prevent embolus).

    (a) Because heparin is not excreted in breast milk, it is considered safe for breastfeeding mothers.

    (b) Therapeutic anticoagulation is achieved when the activated partial thromboplastin time is 1.5 to 2.5 times normal (Kobler et al., 1997).

(3) Elevate legs above heart level to empty the superficial veins and increase venous return.

(4) Administer oxygen as necessary.

(5) Administer sedatives as necessary.

(6) Force fluids each shift (2000 ml).

(7) Provide elastic bandages to mid-thigh or elastic stockings.

(8) Observe for signs and symptoms of embolism.

(9) Administer antibiotics if infectious process persists (a fever is usually indicative of deep-vein thrombosis) (Kobler et al., 1997).

(10) Ensure frequent rest periods.

(11) Assess infection site for pain, tenderness, temperature, and swelling.

(12) Assess vital signs at each shift.

(13) Instruct client to avoid oral contraceptives because of the increased risk of clot formation.

  b. Outcomes

    (1) Maintain bed rest, with legs elevated.

    (2) No signs or symptoms of embolism are noted.

    (3) Vital signs remain stable.

2. Acute pain related to thrombophlebitis

  a. Interventions

    (1) Apply continuous, moist heat to extremity to relieve pain and promote circulation.

    (2) Explain the importance of treatment.

    (3) Avoid pillows behind knees or raising the knee gatch of the bed.

    (4) Teach relaxation or distraction techniques.

    (5) Elevate extremities on pillows for relief of venous aching.

    (6) Avoid crossing of legs.

    (7) Change position whenever necessary.

    (8) Administer sedatives as necessary.

    (9) Use a bed cradle to keep linens and blankets off of extremities.

    (10) Administer pain relief medication, as needed (inflammation and arterial spasm contribute to the pain).

  b. Outcomes

    (1) Decreased pain reported by client

    (2) Effective use of relaxation techniques reported by client

3. Anxiety related to changes in activities of daily living, inability to care for newborn, and thrombophlebitis

  a. Interventions

    (1) Provide emotional support as necessary.

    (2) Stay with the client when she is anxious.

    (3) Provide occupational therapy or diversion.

    (4) Assure client that infant has appropriate care.

    (5) Allow infant's siblings to visit client.

    (6) Explain thrombophlebitis to the family.

    (7) Refer client to a social worker if necessary.

    b. Outcomes
      (1) Client is free to discuss concerns with nursing staff.
      (2) Nurse provides time with client to offer reassurance, explain procedures, or talk.
      (3) Infant is well cared for by a caregiver of the client's choice.
      (4) Client has a low level of anxiety.

DEPRESSION
Introduction

A. Postpartum depression, also called chronic depressive syndrome and postpartum psychosis, is a maladaptation to the stress and conflicts of the postpartum period (Kruckman, 2002).

B. "Baby blues" or adjusted reaction with depressed mood:
  1. Is the mildest form of postpartum depression.
  2. Occurs usually at home because of early postpartum discharge.
  3. Occurs on the third to eighth postpartum day.
  4. Has an incidence of 60% to 80% of all postpartum women (Beck, 2002).
  5. Predominant characteristics of a woman with this disorder:
    a. Mood swings
    b. Weepiness
    c. Anorexia
    d. Difficulty sleeping
    e. Fatigue
    f. Discomfort
    g. Overstimulation
  6. Symptoms disappear naturally by the second postpartum week with support and understanding.

C. Postpartum depression is a major mood disorder.
  1. Has an incidence of approximately 10% to 20% of all postpartum women (Kruckman, 2002)
  2. Greatest risk occurs around fourth postpartum week.
  3. Can occur at any time during the first postpartum year (60% to 70% in the first 3 weeks to 3 to 6 months (Beck, 2002; Kruckman, 2003).
  4. Depressed postpartum women:
    a. Are tearful and despondent.
    b. Have feelings of inadequacy, guilt, and irritability.
    c. Feel unable to cope and fatigued.
    d. Have difficulty concentrating and sleeping.
    e. Have a lack of interest in activities, appearance, and coitus.
  5. Is disabling.
  6. Can last up to 3 years postpartum.
  7. Biggest predictor is prenatal depression, with child care and life stress next (Beck, 2002).

D. Postpartum psychosis
  1. Includes hallucinations, delusions, and phobias.
  2. Has an incidence of 0.2% or 1 to 2 per 1000 postpartum women (U.S. Department of Health & Human Services, The National Women's Health Information Center, Office of Women's Health, 2003).
  3. Onset usually occurs within the first 3 postpartum months in primiparas.
  4. Etiologic theories
    a. Personal history

    b. Social and environmental factors

    c. Hormonal fluctuation during pregnancy and throughout the menstrual cycle

  5. Predominant characteristics of a woman with this disorder:

    a. Has a favorable attitude toward pregnancy.

      (1) Welcomes pregnancy

      (2) Elated during pregnancy

      (3) Free from discomforts of pregnancy

      (4) Eager to breastfeed and usually quite successful at breastfeeding

    b. Has labile emotions.

      (1) Initially anxious

      (2) Elated during later pregnancy

      (3) Depressed during postpartum period

      (4) Manic depressive history

      (5) Prenatal stressor

      (6) Obsessive personality

      (7) Poor relationship with parents or partner

  6. Hormonal basis

    a. A high level of elation is noted during pregnancy when the placental steroid levels are at high levels.

    b. Subsequent depression is noted during the postpartum period when a sudden loss of the placental steroid output occurs.

    c. Controversy exists in the literature about the effects of the high prolactin levels in breastfeeding women, which inhibit progesterone release, and their relation to an increased risk for postpartum depression or psychosis.

Clinical Practice

A. Assessment

  1. History: symptoms include:

    a. Previous psychologic problems

    b. Diagnosis of neurosis or psychosis (schizophrenia)

    c. Poor coping skills

    d. Low self-esteem

    e. Sleep disturbances

    f. Mood swings and emotional distress

    g. Irritability

    h. Restlessness

    i. Tearfulness

    j. Extreme anxiety about infant's feeding, sleeping, or crying

    k. Guilt

    l. Anorexia

    m. Helplessness

    n. Inability to complete activities of daily living

    o. Family history of psychiatric disorders

    p. Many life stressors

    q. Substance use

    r. Metabolic disorders

    s. Sexually transmitted diseases (if not treated, can manifest as signs and symptoms of depression and psychosis).

    t. Overwhelmed feelings

    u. Oversensitiveness

   2. Physical findings
      a. Serious hormonal disorders
      b. Dehydration related to inadequate intake of nutrition and fluids
      c. Fatigue, irritability, and exhaustion
      d. Anxiety behaviors
      e. Speech and behavior may not make sense
      f. Trouble concentrating or maintaining attention
      g. May be breastfeeding
      h. Difficulty in breathing
      i. Heart palpitations
      j. Tremors
   3. Psychosocial findings
      a. Mood changes
      b. Poor self-esteem
      c. Poor social support networks
      d. Expression of concern about difficult labor and delivery
      e. Single, separated, or divorced status
      f. Marital problems
      g. Unplanned pregnancy
      h. Unwanted pregnancy
      i. Feelings of being unloved
      j. Poor relationship with mother
      k. Detachment from reality
      l. Disturbances in thinking, feeling, and behavior
      m. Poor interactions with infant, family, and staff
      n. Inability to relax
      o. Poor coping skills
   4. Diagnostic procedures
      a. Hormonal level determinations, including thyroid
      b. Blood tests for drugs and alcohol
      c. Psychologic profile
B. Nursing Diagnoses
   1. Impaired parenting related to postpartum depression
   2. Risk for other-directed violence related to maternal depression
C. Interventions/Outcomes
   1. Impaired parenting related to postpartum depression
      a. Interventions
        (1) Observe client with infant, by herself, and with family and friends.
        (2) Discuss client's plans for her infant and for herself.
        (3) Assess sleeping, eating, resting, and coping behaviors.
        (4) Assess skin turgor, lips, mucous membranes, and urinary output for symptoms of dehydration.
        (5) Provide psychologic support for depression; nurses can provide or refer to prenatal and postpartum support groups.
        (6) Initiate psychiatric consultation, which may result in:
          (a) Psychopharmacologic use of antidepressants
          (b) Transfer to psychiatric inpatient service
          (c) Psychotherapy: individual, group, or both
      b. Outcomes
        (1) Client uses appropriate coping strategies to care for self and infant.
        (2) Client has realistic expectations for self and infant.
        (3) Client perceives that she is receiving the support she needs.

2. Risk for other-directed violence related to maternal depression
   a. Interventions
     (1) Assess psychosocial factors, mood, and support systems.
     (2) Determine when significant others can be present to learn about infant's needs and infant care.
     (3) Teach significant others signs and symptoms of depression.
     (4) Allow client time for self and encourage her to have time away from infant.
     (5) If client is breastfeeding, consider suggesting bottle-feeding to lower prolactin levels.
     (6) Reinforce client's self-care activities.
     (7) Encourage mothering behaviors and maternal role.
     (8) Assist client with learning parenting skills.
     (9) Arrange for social worker to visit client.
     (10) Praise client's positive actions of mothering.
     (11) Arrange for someone to be at home to help client.
     (12) Allow client to ventilate her feelings.
     (13) Accept client's feelings.
     (14) Provide reality orientation.
     (15) Listen to family's concerns and take very seriously.
     (16) Follow through with resources to help family.
     (17) Explain psychologic changes during the postpartum period.
     (18) Document client's learning needs.
     (19) Assist family in crisis.
     (20) Keep environment safe.
     (21) Remove potentially harmful objects and weapons.
     (22) Watch behavior of client: transfer to psychiatric inpatient service may be necessary or scheduled psychotherapy.
     (23) Ensure client takes all her medications.
     (24) Facilitate parental attachment.
     (25) Encourage family support for client.
     (26) Be aware that clients with depression or psychosis may harm their babies or commit suicide: take all clients' behaviors seriously.
   b. Outcomes
     (1) Home is a safe environment for client and infant.
     (2) Client has support to handle depressive episodes.
     (3) Client and family share feelings and concerns openly.
     (4) Infant is safe.
     (5) Appropriate bonding is observed.

HEALTH EDUCATION

Hemorrhage

A. Teach client about involution process (where the fundus should be and when she can no longer feel it).
B. Teach client about lochia changes (when bleeding should stop and how lochia should appear).
C. Teach client about perineal care (how to apply and change menstrual pads).
D. Teach client how to massage fundus as indicated by tone.
E. Teach client about other self-care such as nutrition, signs of infection, breast care, elimination, activity, and rest.

Infection

A. Teach client about perineal care and how to wipe after voiding and defecation.
B. Teach client about transmission of infection and ways to prevent complications and further infections.
C. Arrange for household help for client if necessary.
D. Teach client about importance of rest, nutrition, and fluids.

Thrombophlebitis

A. Teach client to avoid dehydration in warm weather.
B. Teach client to wear warm clothes during cold weather to maintain adequate circulation.
C. Teach client to avoid foods high in fat and cholesterol.
D. Teach client to avoid periods of prolonged sitting at work, while traveling, or while watching television; getting up to walk around every 30 minutes or every hour prevents venous pooling in the legs by increasing circulatory return to the heart.
E. Teach client to avoid pressure under the knees when propping up legs with pillows.
F. Teach client to elevate the foot of the bed to promote venous drainage.
G. Teach client to avoid crossing the legs while seated, which decreases circulation to the legs because of pressure on the popliteal space behind the knee.
H. Teach client to elevate the legs when sitting whenever possible.
I. Teach client to reduce gastric distress caused by daily dose of anticoagulant by dividing it or taking with food.
J. Teach client to avoid possible sodium warfarin (Coumadin) interaction with over-the-counter preparations, such as those containing acetylsalicylic acid formulations (aspirin-based products), and check with physician about the interactive effects of other prescribed drugs.
K. Teach client to use an electric razor to avoid nicks or scrapes, or depilatories.
L. Client should begin an exercise or daily walking program.
M. Client should avoid garters and knee-high stockings.
N. Client should practice relaxation techniques.
O. Discuss with client risks of oral contraceptive use related to thrombophlebitis.

Depression

A. Instruct family about how to provide safe and secure environment for client and infant.
B. Discuss benefits of contraception during the period of depression.
C. Instruct client about how to avoid crisis situations and develop coping skills.
D. Instruct client in stress reduction techniques.
E. Promote family awareness that postpartum depression and psychosis need professional intervention.

CASE STUDIES AND STUDY QUESTIONS

Ms. H is a 34-year-old woman who is a gravida 5, para 5 (G5, P5) and who delivered a healthy boy weighing 4800 g (10 lb, 9.5 oz) after 16 hours of labor. She is breastfeeding her infant in the recovery room when she is assigned to your care. Her vital signs are stable. Her lochia is bright red and heavy, and it has a clot approximately 2 cm (0.79 inches) in diameter.

1. Which of the following is the most important assessment that needs to be performed?
   a. Checking her vital signs every 5 to 15 minutes for the first hour after delivery.
   b. Checking location and firmness of the fundus.
   c. Charting the amount and saturation of menstrual pads every hour.
   d. Continuing to support her breastfeeding efforts.

2. Ms. H is considered to be at high risk for uterine atony because of which of the following?
   a. She is a grand multipara.
   b. The size of her infant
   c. The length of her labor
   d. All of the above

3. You notice that Ms. H has saturated four menstrual pads with bright-red blood during a 1-hour period. Her vital signs are stable. You assess her bleeding to be which of the following?
   a. Subinvolution related to retained placental fragments
   b. Related to a ruptured hematoma
   c. Uterine atony
   d. Related to a lacerated cervix

4. The first nursing action you perform is to do which of the following?
   a. Chart your findings.
   b. Open the IV to increase her level of oxytocin.
   c. Turn her on her left side.
   d. Massage the fundus.

5. The main cause of early postpartum hemorrhage is which of the following?
   a. Uterine atony
   b. DIC
   c. Retained placental fragments
   d. Hematomas and lacerations

6. The main cause of late postpartum hemorrhage is which of the following?
   a. Uterine atony
   b. DIC
   c. Retained placental fragments
   d. Hematomas and lacerations

7. The nursing actions to control bleeding and stabilize a mother's condition in hemorrhage related to atony are to do which of the following?
   a. Massage the fundus.
   b. Perform bimanual compression of the uterus if a physician is not available.
   c. Prepare an IV infusion of oxytocin.
   d. All of the above are correct.

8. A hematoma is a collection of blood in the pelvic tissue resulting from damage to a vessel wall without laceration of the tissue. This trauma to the vessel can be a result of which of the following?
   a. Forceps manipulation
   b. Pressure of the presenting part on pelvic structures
   c. Excessive fundal pressure on the uterus
   d. All of the above

Ms. P is a 24-year-old woman who is G1, P1. She was in labor for 28 hours. A cesarean section was performed because of failure to progress. She delivered a 3629-g (8-lb) boy in good health. After delivery, her vital signs were stable, and lochia was slight, red, and contained no clots. A Foley catheter has been inserted to straight drainage. Her dressing is clean and dry. Forty-eight hours after delivery, her temperature is 38° C (100.4° F) and continues to rise.

9. Which type of puerperal infection does she likely have?

a. Breast
b. Bladder
c. Vaginal
d. Uterine

10. What factors have predisposed her to a postpartum infection?
    a. Age
    b. Length of labor
    c. Parity
    d. Type of delivery
        (1) a, d
        (2) b, d
        (3) c, d
        (4) a, b

11. Daily inspection of the perineum may reveal problems with the episiotomy, such as which of the following?
    a. Hematoma
    b. Infection
    c. Edema
    d. All of the above

12. To promote healing of an episiotomy and prevent infection, the nurse should do which of the following?
    a. Teach the mother perineal care.
    b. Teach the mother about how infections are transmitted.
    c. Teach the mother about the importance of rest, nutrition, and fluid intake.
    d. All of the above are correct.

Ms. G is a 27-year-old overweight woman who is a G3, P3 who had delivered a girl weighing 2800 g (6 lb, 3 oz) by cesarean section. She underwent a prolonged labor of 27 hours.

13. What factor predisposes Ms. G to thrombophlebitis?
    a. Obesity
    b. Parity
    c. Length of labor
    d. Weight of infant

14. Ms. G is prescribed warfarin for thrombophlebitis. You advise her to avoid which of the following?

a. Aspirin
b. Massage of extremities
c. Oral contraceptives
d. All of the above

15. Ms. G asks if her children can come see her in the hospital. You respond that:
    a. Her condition is very serious and she needs to rest right now.
    b. Only children over the age of 14 years can visit the unit.
    c. Her children may visit when she wants.
    d. You will call the social worker and the children can be cared for so she does not have to worry about them.

16. As part of your daily assessment for thrombophlebitis, you look for all except which of the following?
    a. Generalized pallor
    b. Dyspnea
    c. Tachycardia
    d. Positive Homans' sign

17. The physiologic changes during pregnancy in the veins of the thighs or pelvis predispose a postpartum woman to which of the following?
    a. Deep-vein thrombophlebitis
    b. Ecchymosis
    c. Inflammation
    d. Edema

18. In taking a history for thrombophlebitis, you assess for which of the following?
    a. Contraceptive use
    b. Obesity
    c. Postpartum pelvic infection
    d. All of the above

Ms. Q is a 21-year-old woman who is G1, P1. At 39 weeks' gestation, she vaginally delivered an infant girl late last night who is in good health. Ms. Q was excited about being pregnant and felt well throughout her pregnancy. She is eager to breastfeed but feels anxious about being a new mother. You enter her room and she is crying because her husband cannot come to visit because he must work overtime.

19. Your nursing diagnosis is risk for impaired adjustment related to "baby blues." Which of the following is correct?
    a. This is a wrong diagnosis because the blues occur later in the postpartum period.
    b. She is suffering from depression based on her pregnancy course.
    c. She is suffering from psychosis because she has phobias.
    d. She is severely depressed based on social and personal history.

20. Puerperal depression appears predominantly in women with labile emotions who are which of the following?
    a. Initially anxious during pregnancy
    b. Worried about caring for their other children
    c. Depressed during the prenatal period
    d. All of the above

21. A controversy in the literature exists about women who severely harm or kill their babies during the postpartum period. This controversy centers on mothers who:
    a. Are usually depressed
    b. Breastfeed and have high levels of prolactin
    c. Have a crisis in their family
    d. All of the above

22. Treatment for postpartum depression includes which of the following?
    a. Active empathic listening
    b. Psychiatric care
    c. Antidepressive agents
    d. All of the above

23. Postpartum psychosis includes the following symptom:
    a. Fear
    b. Tearfulness
    c. Delusions
    d. Elation

24. When taking a history for depression, it is important to assess for:
    a. Low self-esteem
    b. Guilt
    c. Substance use
    d. All of the above

ANSWERS TO STUDY QUESTIONS

1. b	7. d	13. a	19. a
2. d	8. d	14. d	20. d
3. c	9. d	15. c	21. b
4. d	10. 2	16. a	22. d
5. a	11. d	17. a	23. c
6. c	12. d	18. d	24. d

REFERENCES

Austin, M.P., & Mitchell, P.B. (1998). Use of psychotropic medications in breast-feeding women: Acute and prophylactic treatment. *Australian-New Zealand Journal of Psychiatry*, 32(6), 778-784.

Beck, C.T. (2002). Revision of the postpartum depression predictors inventory. *Journal* of Obstetric, Gynecologic, and Neonatal Nursing, 31(4), 394-402.

Beeber, L. (2002). The pinks and the blues: Symptoms of chronic depression in mothers during their children's first year. American Journal of Nursing, 102(11), 91-95.

Beeber, L.S. (1998). Treating depression through the nurse-patient relationship. Nursing Clinics of North America, 33(1), 153-172.

Beeber, L.S. (2002). Hildahood: Taking the interpersonal theory of nursing to the neighborhood. Journal of the American Psychiatric Nurses Association, 6(2), 49-55.

Bozoky, I., & Corwin, E.J. (2002). Fatigue as a predictor of postpartum depression. Journal of Obstetric, Gynecologic, and Neonatal Nursing, 31(4), 436-443.

Brown, G.W., & Moran, P.M. (1997). Single mothers, poverty and depression. Psychological Medicine, 27(1), 21-33.

Cizza, G., Gold, P.W., & Chrousos, G.P. (1997). High-dose transdermal estrogen, corticotrophin-releasing hormone and postnatal depression. Journal of Clinical Endocrinology and Metabolism, 82(2), 704.

Field, T. (1998). Maternal depression effects on infants and early intervention. Preventive Medicine, 27(2), 200-203.

Hiscock, H., & Wake, M. (2002). Randomized controlled trial of behavioural infant sleep intervention to improve infant sleep and maternal mood. British Medical Journal, 324(7345), 1062-1065.

Hixson, M.J., & Collins, J.H. (2001). Postpartum herpes simplex endometritis. A case study. Journal of Reproductive Medicine, 45(9), 849-852.

Humphrey, R., Carlan, S.J., & Greenbaum, L. (2001). Rectus sheath hematoma in pregnancy. Journal of Clinical Ultrasound, 29(5), 306-311.

Kobler, J., Waterman, M., & DuMenil, S. (1997). Alterations in the health status of postpartum mothers. In F. Nichols & E. Zwelling (Eds.), Maternal newborn nursing (pp. 1281-1330). Philadelphia: Saunders.

Kruckman, L. (2000). Rituals as prevention. The case of postpartum depression. In R. Inge Heinze (Ed.), The nature and function of rituals (pp. 227-241). Westport, CT: Greenwood/Praeger Publishing.

Kruckman, L. (2002). An introduction to postpartum illness. Accessed December 14, 2002 at www.postpartum.net/posttrial2.htm.

Kruckman, L. (2003). An introduction to postpartum illness. Accessed January 19, 2003 at www.postpartum.net/intro%20to%20postpartum%20illness.html.

Luckas, M., & Smith, G.D. (1997). Serum cholesterol concentration and postpartum depression. British Medical Journal, 314(7074), 143.

Meyer, M. (2002). Beyond the baby blues. Accessed December 16, 2002 at www.depressionafterdelivery.com.

Murray, S.S., McKinney, E.S., & Gorrie, T.M. (2002). Foundations of maternal-newborn nursing (3rd ed.). Philadelphia: Saunders.

Normand, M.C., & Damato, E.G. (2001) Postcesarean infection. Journal of Obstetric, Gynecologic, and Neonatal Nursing, 30(6), 642-648.

Olds, S., London, M., & Ladewig, P. (2000). Maternal-newborn nursing: A family and community-based approach (6th ed.). Upper Saddle River, NJ: Prentice Hall Health.

Righetti-Veltema, M., Conne-Perreard, E., Bousquet, A., & Manzano, J. (1998). Risk factors and predictive signs of postpartum depression. Journal of Affective Disorders, 49(3), 167-180.

Rona, R.J., Smeetom, N.C., Beech, R., Barnett, A., & Sharland, G. (1998). Anxiety and depression in mothers related to severe malformation of the heart of children and fetus. Acta Paediatrics, 87(2), 201-205.

Scott, J.R., Hamond, C., & Gordon, J.D. (Eds.). (2003). Danforth's obstetrics and gynecology (2nd ed.). Philadelphia: Lippincott Williams & Wilkins.

Scott, L.D., & Hasik, K.J. (2001). The similarities and differences of endometritis and pelvic inflammatory disease. Journal of Obstetric, Gynecologic, and Neonatal Nursing, 30(3), 332-341.

Simpson, K., & Creehan, P.A. (Eds.). (1996). AWHONN perinatal nursing. Philadelphia: Lippincott Williams & Wilkins.

U.S. Department of Health & Human Services, The National Women's Health Information Center, Office of Women's Health. (2003). Postpartum depression. Accessed January 5, 2003 at www.4women.gov/faq/postpartum.htm.

Vieira, T. (2003). When joy becomes grief: Screening tools for postpartum depression. Lifelines, 6(6), 506-513.

Walker, L.O. (1997). Weight and weight-related distress after childbirth: Relationship to stress, social support, and depressive symptoms. *Journal of Holistic Nursing, 15*(4), 389-405.

Warner, R., Appleby, L., Whitton, A., & Faragher, B. (1997). Attitudes towards motherhood in postnatal depression: Development of the maternal attitudes questionnaire. *Journal of Psychosomatic Research, 43*(4), 351-358.

Williams, K.L., & Wheeler, S.B. (1997). Obsessive-compulsive disorder in pregnancy, the puerperium, and the premenstruum. *Journal of Clinical Psychiatry, 45*(12), 1191-1196.

ETHICS AND ISSUES

31 Ethics

SANDRA L. GARDNER

OBJECTIVES

1. Define common terms used in ethical discussions.
2. Identify three theories or approaches to ethical thinking.
3. Discuss the principle of autonomy and the concept of informed consent.
4. Discuss the principles of beneficence and nonmaleficence and the concept of paternalism.
5. Discuss the principle of justice and the concepts of microallocation and macroallocation.
6. Discuss proxy-decision-makers for care of the newborn.
7. Explain the influences of spirituality and culture on ethical decision-making by parents and professionals.
8. Explain the female versus male and nursing versus medical perspectives brought to ethical discussions.
9. Distinguish between autonomy, substituted judgment, and best interests as a basis for ethical decisions.
10. Define the purpose and goals of palliative care and infants for whom this type of care may be chosen by parents.
11. Identify five clinical issues that commonly lead to ethical dilemmas for nurses.
12. Identify two professional issues that commonly lead to ethical dilemmas for nurses.
13. Outline key points of a teaching plan for patients and families regarding ethics and ethical dilemmas.

INTRODUCTION

A. Terminology

1. Morals: from the Latin word *mores*, which means "custom" or "habit"; the moral principles that guide nursing practice are respect, autonomy, beneficence, nonmaleficence, veracity, confidentiality, fidelity, justice, and privacy (American Nurses Association [ANA], 2001)
2. Morality: one's belief about what is right or the best thing to do; general rules of conduct and standards for evaluating behavior; learned through socialization and association with groups such as family, religious, ethnic groups
3. Moral agent: one who has the power to act; one who is making a moral decision
4. Values: standards that are a person's basic beliefs about the self and relationships to others
5. Value system: a learned, organized set of principles and beliefs concerning conduct and behavior that helps a person choose options, make decisions, and resolve conflicts
6. Ethics: from the Greek word *ethos*, meaning "custom" or "character"; established by Socrates, the discipline dealing with what is good or bad and with moral duty and obligation

7. Bioethics: a subdivision of ethics to determine the most morally desirable course of action in health care, when there are conflicting values inherent in varying treatment options (American Hospital Association, 1985)
8. Ethical-moral dilemma: a difficult choice between two alternatives when there is a conflict of values, no clear consensus about what is right and wrong, and all options are morally justifiable and equally defendable
9. Law: set of rules for social behavior; enforced by the police, courts, and prisons
10. Quality of life: total well being, including both physical and psychosocial determinants (Hack, 1999) so that the individual can lead his or her life and function as part of the human family, both individually and collectively (Kirschbaum, 1996; Swaney, English, & Carter, 2002); to ensure that quality of life decisions not be reduced to arbitrary judgments based on personal preference or the perceived social worth of the patient, justified criteria of benefits and burdens must be considered (Beauchamp & Childress, 2001)

B. **Ethical approaches and theories**
   1. Nonnormative ethics: an approach to ethics that denies that universal principles exist to guide behavior
      a. Descriptive ethics: represents the work of sociologists, anthropologists, psychologists, historians, and others who describe or attempt to explain moral behaviors
      b. Metaethics: from the Greek word *meta,* meaning "behind, beyond, higher"; the division of ethics wherein professional ethicists or philosophers attempt to analyze reasons behind the principles
   2. Principle-based ethics: an approach to ethics that identifies and defines fundamental principles to guide behavior and decision-making
      a. Duty and obligation–based approach: *deontology*
         (1) From Greek word *deonteis,* meaning "duty"
         (2) Devises norms or rules from duties human beings owe one another because of commitments made.
         (3) Duty to follow universally accepted rules of what is right and wrong
         (4) Looks at motives behind an action.
         (5) Related principles (and the moral principles guiding nursing practice) (ANA, 2001)
            (a) Autonomy
               (i) From Greek words *auto,* meaning "self," and *nomos,* meaning "law"
               (ii) Respect for the unconditional worth of people; for their thoughts and actions; and for their free choice and personal decisions (Joffe, Manocchia, Weeks, & Cleary, 2003)
               (iii) The right of people to be left alone and to define their own destiny without interference; self-determination
               (iv) In health care, based on the doctrine of informed consent
            (b) Beneficence
               (i) From the Hippocratic oath; a duty to help others; to balance good and harm; to prevent harm, to remove harm, and to not inflict harm
               (ii) An obligation to accomplish good in service to others through acts such as mercy, kindness, and generosity
            (c) Nonmaleficence
               (i) From the Hippocratic oath; an obligation to "first, do no harm" to others; the duty to avoid intending, causing, permitting, or imposing harm or the risk of harm to another person

          (ii) Harm must be ultimately justified to achieve some greater good or to prevent a greater harm.
    (d) Justice
        (i) Rule derived from Aristotle; the obligation to treat individuals equally or comparably; to distribute benefits and burdens equally throughout society
        (ii) Must guard against arbitrary, inconsistent decision-making.
        (iii) Macroallocation: distribution at a societal level; example: which program is funded?
        (iv) Microallocation: distribution at a personal level; example: who receives the transplant?
    (e) Veracity: obligation to tell the truth and to give full, complete, and truthful information to patient and parents for decision-making
    (f) Fidelity: obligation to keep promises or commitments; to remain loyal
    (g) Privacy: right of an individual or group to decide when and to what extent information about themselves can be revealed to others; freedom from intrusion
    (h) Confidentiality: an extension of privacy; right to limit the access of others to private information revealed by a patient to his or her provider
    (i) Respect: reverence for persons and for human dignity
 b. Goal outcome consequences–based approach: *teleology, utilitarianism,* or *consequentialism*
    (1) The rightness or wrongness of an act depends on its utility or usefulness.
    (2) Rights consist of actions that have good consequences, and wrong consists of actions that have bad consequences; acts are judged according to their value.
    (3) Achieving the greatest good or happiness for the greatest number of people by balancing the good that is possible with the harm that might result from performing or not performing an action; the end justifies the means.
    (4) Related principles (Lagana & Duderstadt, 1995)
        (a) Allocation of resources versus cost effectiveness; relates to the distribution of scarce resources.
        (b) Quality of life versus sanctity of life; addresses the question of a good life compared with life at all costs.
        (c) Paternalism versus autonomy; addresses the question of who knows best and who should make the decision for an individual.
        (d) Withholding of care versus starting care; relates to the delivery of care to individuals and society; questions when care should be initiated, withheld, or withdrawn.
 c. Virtue character–based approach
    (1) Traced to Aristotle; decisions about actions are based on what a virtuous person would do.
    (2) Ethics is not about following rules, but about character and virtues (e.g., respect, fidelity, honesty, benevolence); rules and principles come later.
 d. Case-based approach (casuistry)
    (1) The claims or grounds of a particular case are compared with similar cases.
    (2) Casuistry is about how a general moral principle should be understood in a similar set of circumstances.

e. Story-based approach (narrative)
  (1) The narrative story is a method of ethical reasoning.
  (2) Specific *narratives* for each case, such as the person or people involved, the subjective experience, the illness and caring, are the focus of consideration.
f. Care-based approach (feminist)
  (1) Related to virtue theory; not based on fixed rules, principles, or theories, but on regard for the person; in health care, is relationship-based and stresses the context of a situation: a person has a life before and after the illness, and caregivers should ensure continuity and connectedness to that life.
  (2) Nurses have looked at this model carefully as a basis for their practice because it stresses holism, connectedness, hearing the patient's story, and the ethics of care.
g. Social ethics (Swaney, English, & Carter, 2002)
  (1) Concern for the individual and for the common good of all; moral judgments affect the larger social community of which the individual and institutions are a part; example: society may bear the financial, physical, educational, and social costs of severely disabled infants.
  (2) How individual moral behavior and the range of moral responsibility and accountability are influenced by social context, social structures, and public policy issues
h. Protection of human subjects in research (Swaney, English, & Carter, 2002)
  (1) Introduction of interventions or treatments without appropriate research into safety, efficacy, and long-term outcomes
  (2) Professional responsibility to evaluate the quality of evidence regarding the use and benefit of both traditional and newer clinical practices; evidence-based practice (Orleans, Tappero, Glicken, & Merenstein, 2002)
  (3) Importance of empirical studies to contribute to the ethical aspects of clinical practice and the impact of ethical decision-making (McHaffie, Laing, Parker, & McMillan, 2001)
C. Related principles and concepts
  1. Informed consent: based on principle of autonomy or the right to make decisions without coercion (Joffe, Manocchia, Weeks, & Cleary, 2003)
   a. The fundamental right of a person to determine what happens to his or her own body; to decide what is harmful or beneficial in treatment and care; should be interfered with only to prevent harm to others.
   b. Supported by considerable court decisions in the United States; stresses patient rights; to accomplish informed consent, the *reasonable person standard* may be applied: "What would the reasonable person want in this circumstance?"
   c. Requires that professionals have a positive attitude about autonomy.
   d. Rests on an assumption of competence and capacity.
    (1) Competence
      (a) A legal status; decided by the courts, usually based on age of majority; definition of *adult*
      (b) All adults are competent unless a court decides otherwise.
    (2) Capacity
      (a) A clinical judgment; decided by caregivers based on patient's ability to understand alternatives and consequences of treatment and no treatment, to weigh options, to think about life goals and

values, to choose the best option for self, and to communicate the decision
   (b) Levels of capacity
      (i) Decisional capacity: ability to make decisions
      (ii) Executional capacity: ability to carry out decisions
   (c) Nuances to capacity
      (i) Capacity may come and go, depending on such factors as time of day, effects of medication and anesthesia, environment, stress, and pain.
      (ii) Must use caution when determining capacity; should not manipulate or control patient's capacity; should not judge quickly; should not assume anyone who disagrees does not have capacity; be careful about words used, time of day, condition of patient.
      (iii) Consider ways to restore capacity so patient can make own decision (e.g., hold medications temporarily to restore capacity).
      (iv) Determine whether the decision can be delayed while patient regains capacity.
e. The process of informed consent
   (1) Process is important; paper is often used as evidence that process occurred.
   (2) The right to consent also includes the right to refuse.
   (3) Components of informed consent are defined by each state, but usually include:
      (a) A health care professional's recommendation for treatment
      (b) Determination of competence and capacity
      (c) Truthful and honest disclosure of information such as medical condition, nature and purpose of procedure, consequences, risks, alternatives, and name and qualifications of person performing treatment
      (d) Patient understanding of information
      (e) Voluntary consent or refusal, with a lack of coercion
      (f) Documentation of process
   (4) Responsibility for obtaining consent remains with the person performing procedure or care.
   (5) Types of consent
      (a) Blanket consent: signed on admission to a hospital
      (b) Battery consent: signed for a procedure such as surgery
      (c) Detailed consent: signed for such things as a research drug or treatment
   (6) Who gives consent
      (a) Competent adult: age of majority; determined by state law
      (b) Incompetent adult: court-appointed guardian; person close to adult who knows wishes if no court-appointed guardian is available
      (c) Minors: parent or guardian
      (d) Emancipated minor: when no longer subject to parental control (e.g., after marriage)
      (e) Mature minor: age limits and scope determined by state law; usually applies to consent for situations such as pregnancy care, sexually transmitted diseases care, and substance abuse treatment
   (7) Research consent requires detailed information and a lengthy, special process.

2. Concept of paternalism-maternalism-parentalism
   a. A competent, capable adult being treated as if he or she were a child by a person or people acting as if they had the authority and concern of a parent (Cahill, 2001)
      (1) Paternalism or patriarchal health care system: fathering behaviors (Woodward, 1998)
      (2) Maternalism: mothering behaviors
      (3) Parentalism: nonsexist term; parenting behaviors
   b. Person or people claim they are acting on behalf of the patient; they know what is best and good for the patient (Cahill, 2001).
   c. Is based on the assumption that a patient's lack of technical or medical expertise justifies the provider in making the decision for the patient (Cahill, 2001).
   d. A way to induce, coerce, or direct others to do what one wants them to do (Cahill, 2001)
   e. May include a variety of behaviors such as nonverbal pretenses, withholding of relevant information, lying, and coercion, with the goal being that the patient complies with what the provider wants to do.
   f. Anyone can be parental: spouse, family, friends, clergy, provider, or administrator.
3. Proxy decision-makers
   a. Newborns are incompetent and unable to make their own decisions.
   b. Parents have primary authority (*parental autonomy*) to act as proxy or surrogate decision-makers for their infants.
   c. Legally, through court rulings, society has designated parents as primary decision-makers because: they love the infant and are concerned for the infant's well being; they have the best interests of their infant in mind; they know the values of the family culture and environment in which the infant will be raised; and generally parents are interested in the welfare of their children; as a general matter of law, except in cases of abuse and neglect, courts have ruled that parents have the right to make medical decisions about their children (Rushton & Hogue, 1993; Annas, 1994).
   d. Some professional guidelines state that *parental autonomy* should not be absolute and that the decisions made by parents of premature infants should not be considered absolute (American Academy of Pediatrics [AAP], & American College of Obstetricians and Gynecologists [ACOG], 1995; ACOG, 1989) and that "physicians should not be forced to undertreat or overtreat an infant if, in their best medical knowledge, the treatment is not in compliance with the standard of care for that infant" (AAP, 1995); in protecting the rights of nonautonomous patients, guidelines to facilitate decision-making, establish a standard of care and support health care professionals in making the decision to remove life-sustaining support have been published (AAP, Committee on Bioethics, 1994).
   e. Double effect: principle that asserts that an action is considered *good* if the intent has positive value, even if secondary effects of the action might be considered harmful if undertaken as a primary goal (e.g., using narcotics for a dying newborn [the positive goal is relief of suffering, even at the expense of shortening life]) (Swaney, English, & Carter, 2002).
   f. Problem of uncertainty (Swaney, English, & Carter, 2002)
      (1) Medical uncertainty about the long-term prognosis or quality of life of a newborn infant complicates decision-making about what is in the best interests of the child and family (Stutts & Schloemann, 2002a).

(2) Parental question: "Will my infant be OK when he [she] grows up?" Professional responses: a statistical approach gives probabilities about similar babies, but not about the parent's individual infant; "I don't know" about their individual infant's outcome may be the most honest answer.

(3) How prognostic uncertainty is (or is not) communicated to parents before delivery will influence decision-making when the prognosis or quality of life becomes more certain over time.

g. Treatment versus nontreatment

(1) Treatment goals should be established by parents *(parental autonomy)* with input or participation from health care professionals so that both are working towards the same goals (Culver, Fallon, Londner, Montalvo, Vila, Ramsey, et al., 2000; Glassford, 2003; Harrison, 1993; McHaffie, Laing, Parker, & McMillan, 2001; Swaney, English, & Carter, 2002).

(2) For parents to be decision-makers, they must be fully informed to consent to or refuse treatment for their newborn infant or infants (Culver, Fallon, Londner, Montalvo, Vila, Ramsey, et al., 2000; Harrison, 1993).

(a) Professionals have an ethical and legal obligation (AAP, 1995, Clark, 1996; Doroshow, Hodgman, Pomerance, Ross, Michel, Luckett et al., 2000; Tyson, 1995) to inform parents with facts about the neonate's condition, illnesses, outcomes, and risks and benefits of various interventions or noninterventions so they are able to give informed consent or refusal (Culver, Fallon, Londner, Montalvo, Vila, Ramsey, et al., 2000; Harrison, 1993; Siegel, Gardner, & Merenstein, 2002).

(b) Professional attitudes or intuition that interfere with open, honest communication of information to parents include (Harrison, 1993; McHaffie, Laing, Parker, & McMillan, 2001):

(i) Assuming that parents are too emotional to assimilate information or make a rational decision

(ii) Assuming that information about poor outcomes or complications may disrupt parental attachment to the infant

(iii) Assuming that parental guilt or psychologic harm will result from decision-making and that the final decision is too much for the parents to bear

(iv) Health care providers' efforts to persuade parents: a difficult question between a respect for parental autonomy or an attempt to overcome it; professionals must be careful not to usurp parental authority.

(c) Use of an evidence-based table of the likely outcomes (i.e., mortality, ventilator or oxygen use, brain scan results, long-term neurodevelopmental outcomes) may be useful for parental decision-making (Koh, Harrison, & Morley, 1999; Koh, Casey, & Harrison, 2000).

(d) In several studies, prenatal consultation with a neonatologist for the woman has been found to be useful (Paul et al., 1999; Neufeld, Woodrum, & Tarczy-Hornoch, 2000).

(e) Research (McHaffie, Laing, Parker, & McMillan, 2001) has indicated that parents believe:

(i) They can or should accept responsibility for making difficult decisions; the majority state that the ultimate decision should be theirs.

        (ii) They are able to understand medical issues or information and to assess consequences for their own child.

        (iii) They can make a decision and do so without guilt, doubt, or adverse consequences and believe that the right decision was made.

    (f) Decisions are often based on the infant's medical condition and less by the parent's wishes (Partridge, Freeman, Weiss, & Martinez, 2001); parental choices can be limited by:

        (i) A lack of information on options for limited resuscitation

        (ii) Differing resuscitation thresholds and an unwillingness by physicians to accept parental requests not to resuscitate above these thresholds

(3) In addition to what kind of treatment is in the best interests of the infant, the appropriateness of any treatment must be considered.

    (a) A nontreatment decision is withholding or withdrawing of treatment.

    (b) A nontreatment decision should not be referred to as withholding or a withdrawing care.

    (c) Care, whether curative (with treatment) or palliative (with comfort care), is always provided.

    (d) Nonbeneficial: treatment considered not to benefit the patient may be withheld or withdrawn.

        (i) No ethical obligation exists to provide nonbeneficial treatment, but a standard definition of *nonbeneficial* is lacking.

        (ii) A medical effect may be obtained without a medical benefit as determined by family goals for the newborn or child; may include physiologic, psychologic, social, and religious reasons (Lantos, Singer, Walker, Gramelspacher, Shapiro, Sanchez-Gonzalez, et al., 1989).

4. Creating an ethical environment: one that promotes ethical practice and preserves integrity (Rushton & Scanlon, 1995)

    a. When faced with a moral or ethical dilemma, four elements necessary to ensure an integrity-preserving compromise (Winslow & Winslow, 1991):

        (1) Sharing a common moral language

        (2) Developing a mutual respect

        (3) Understanding and acknowledging moral complexity

        (4) Defining the compromise's limits

    b. Legal versus ethical perspective

        (1) Legal means something fulfills the terms of the law.

            (a) Types of laws:

                (i) Constitutional law: source of the law is the federal or state constitution; it guarantees individuals certain rights or freedom (e.g., right to free speech).

                (ii) Statutory law: source of the law is the federal or state legislature; law is made by men and women in legislature (e.g., a living will, Health Insurance Portability and Accountability Act [HIPPA] regulations) (Chesney, 2001; Gotlieb, 2002; Welch, 2001).

                (iii) Common law, judicial law, decisional law, and case law: source is the decision handed down by courts on a particular case and the opinion that is written to accompany the decision; helps shape conduct in future cases of same type; for example, the

       Cruzan decision: surrogate decision-makers' expression of an incompetent patient's wishes should be respected.

    (iv) Administrative law (agency rules and regulations): source is the federal or state legislature; rules and regulations are made by men and women in legislature (e.g., board of nursing rules and regulations).

  (b) Case law's importance to ethics: increasing recognition in court decisions of importance of individual autonomy with regard to treatment decisions, even if treatments are life saving and the patient is not suffering from a terminal illness (Nelson, 1989)

(2) Ethical means something fulfills the terms of ethics and is higher than the law.

  (a) Actions are in one of four categories:

    (i) Ethical and legal

    (ii) Ethical and illegal

    (iii) Legal and unethical

    (iv) Illegal and unethical

  (b) In ethical discussions, the individual focuses on what is ethical, not on what is legal.

  (c) If an individual chooses an option that is ethical and illegal, he or she must be aware of the impact and have a plan to deal with it.

  (d) Courts do not decide questions of ethics; courts decide questions of law.

  (e) Attempts should be made to keep ethical dilemmas out of the courts.

  (f) Ethical codes

    (i) Religious codes

    (ii) Professional codes developed by professional organizations

      ■ The International Council of Nurses Code for Nurses (1973)

      ■ American Nurses Association Code for Nurses (1950, 1976, 1985, 2001)

    (iii) Medical codes

c. Cultural and spiritual influences

(1) Culture: beliefs and values that impart a sense of identity, security, and belonging; a guide for emotional expression, behavior, and experiencing of life events (Kagawa-Singer, 1998; Stutts & Schloemann, 2002a)

(2) Spirituality: the dynamic, interpretive relationship between one's self and a higher power that is an integral part of human life (De Marco 2000); also defined as a belief system that transmits meaning to life's events by focusing on intangible elements expressed through religious or ritual practices and inner piety (Daaleman & VandeCreek, 2000; Maugans, 1996; Stutts & Schloemann, 2002a)

(3) Every culture and religious tradition has its own ways of defining, celebrating, ritualizing, and acknowledging:

  (a) The two major life passages of birth and death

  (b) The meaning of health, illness, and disability (Stutts & Schloemann, 2002a, 2002b; Ott, Al-Khadhuri, & Al-Junaibi, 2003; National Perinatal Association, 2001)

(4) The belief systems of all participants in decision-making and providing care for a patient should be considered.

  (a) Pastoral care services may be needed by both parents and the health care team.

    (b) *Spiritual distress* can be a commonly unrecognized consequence for professionals (Catlin et al., 2001).

  (5) Parental cultural differences can influence their:

    (a) Emotional response to and perceptions of illness, disability, and death

    (b) Use of community and professional services

    (c) Interactions with health care providers (Stutts & Schloemann, 2002b; Ott, Al-Khadhuri, & Al-Junaibi, 2003; National Perinatal Association, 2001)

  (6) Innovative strategies to offer culturally or spiritually sensitive care include (Catlin & Carter, 2002; Stutts & Schloemann, 2002b):

    (a) Assess the needs of parents and health care professionals.

    (b) Educate professionals about their own culture and the culture of others.

    (c) Provide translation services for verbal encounters and written culturally sensitive materials in primary language.

    (d) Encourage parent-to-parent support from parents of familiar religious, cultural, language, and customs backgrounds.

    (e) Identify and link the family with community services (e.g., outpatient health care provider who speaks family's own language).

    (f) Using culturally sensitive practices to facilitate grief and loss: viewing or touching dead body as desired, appropriate use of eye contact and touch, autopsy, grief counseling, establishing trust among different cultures.

d. Female versus male perspective; according to Gilligan's (1982) viewpoint:

  (1) Men and women have different approaches to ethical questions, so there is a need to appreciate and understand both perspectives.

  (2) Men tend to focus on the concept of justice and also tend to:

    (a) See the world as separate individuals in competition for everything.

    (b) Believe the goal is to equalize the playing field and give everyone an equal opportunity.

    (c) Emphasize the application of universal *rules* to ensure fairness and justice.

  (3) Women, in general, tend to focus on relationships and also tend to:

    (a) See relationships as more desirable than competition.

    (b) Strive to establish and preserve relationships.

    (c) Allow individuals to be different.

    (d) Bend the rules and try to find a way to accommodate differences among people.

    (e) Focus on feelings and interactions of the people involved.

    (f) Look for resolution in the details of the problem.

  (4) Female physicians, according to Gilligan, tend to be:

    (a) Guided by their feelings of responsibility and concern for others.

    (b) Less paternalistic and somewhat less directive than male physicians (Gilligan, 1982).

e. Nursing versus medical perspective

  (1) The foundation of medical practice is curing; medical intervention treats disease in a patient.

  (2) The foundation of nursing practice is caring; nursing interventions protect and restore health and prevent disease in a patient.

    f. Standard of best interest
- (1) Best interest standard, advocated by the President's Commission (1983) and others (Weil, 1984; Weir, 1984), obliges decision-makers for newborns "to try to evaluate benefits and burdens from the infant's own perspective" (President's Commission, 1983).
- (2) Preservation of life without the benefit of the human capabilities to think, be self-aware, and relate to others is controversial and challenged in quality-of-life decisions (Arras, 1984; Duff & Campbell, 1973; Kuhse & Singer, 1985; Lorber, 1971; Weir, 1984).
- (3) Two models of determining best interest have been proposed (Leuthner, 2001).
  - (a) Expertise model: the best outcome data are presented to the parents and used in a directive counseling approach based on the best medical judgment; limited moral weight is given to the views of the parents when they are the opposite of the views of the responsible physician.
  - (b) Negotiated model: maximizes parental input, recognizes physicians as moral agents, and incorporates the moral values of both the parents and the physician into the decision.

    g. Ethics and infant bioethics committees (AAP, 2001a; Swaney, English, & Carter, 2002; Stutts & Schloemann, 2002b)
- (1) Promotes quality decisions regarding difficult ethical issues by being a resource for consultation and advice; may or may not be a decision-making committee.
- (2) Confirms the plan of care when the parents and professionals agree.
- (3) Clarifies ethical principles, values, and various treatment options that are consistent with ethical and legal standards.
- (4) Educates families and professionals; provides a venue for expressing views and feelings; may be a mediator or liaison between the health care providers and the family.
- (5) Develops policy statements for the institution.
- (6) Retrospectively reviews case management.
- (7) Has a multidisciplinary membership (nurses, physicians, administrators, lawyers, parents and families, clergy, ethicists, consumer or community representatives); any interested party, including parents or families, may request a consultation from the committee.

5. Ethical decision-making
    a. The decision-makers need to be determined and need to comprehend (Swaney, English, & Carter, 2002):
- (1) Their philosophy of relationship to the patient and to each other
- (2) Their interpretation of ethical principles and values
- (3) The theoretical basis of ethics (utilitarian, feminist, deontologic, and so forth) used in the decision-making process
- (4) The source from which morality is derived

    b. Steps in ethical decision-making (Swaney, English, & Carter, 2002)
- (1) Consider all people who are involved in making and implementing the decision.
- (2) Decide who makes the final decision and whether a referral to an ethics committee is indicated.
- (3) Consider and clarify all medical facts in the case: all indications, alternatives, and consequences of every action and inaction.

    (4) Understand significant human factors and values for all participants in the process, as well as the patient.

    (5) Identify the moral or ethical conflict or dilemma.

    (6) Decide: list options as problem solutions; weigh and prioritize values and then make a decision.

    (7) Reevaluate for moral and rational defensibility.

CLINICAL PRACTICE

Nurses are closer to patients and families than any other health provider, they spend more time with the patient and family, and they are usually the first to identify an ethical dilemma. Once a dilemma is identified, assessment begins.

A. Assessment

  1. Assess the situation for time constraints.

    a. Is an immediate decision needed?

    b. How much time is available for discussion?

  2. Assess the possible treatment options.

    a. Do everything.

    b. Do some thing or things selectively.

    c. Do nothing but comfort.

    d. Withdraw and comfort.

  3. Assess the basis for decision-making and who will be the decision-maker.

    a. Autonomy (based on competence and capacity)

      (1) The competent, capable person makes the decision about his or her own care, including refusing or discontinuing treatment; permission is needed to treat; verbal refusal can occur at any time for any aspect of care.

      (2) The person continues to exercise autonomy even after capacity is lost through the written document called *a living will.*

        (a) Legal document

        (b) Providers are obligated to follow it.

        (c) Goes into effect only after the patient is no longer competent, capable, or both.

      (3) Parental autonomy in decision-making for the newborn

    b. Substituted judgment (based on former competence and capacity)

      (1) A surrogate stands in the place of the patient and states what the patient would want to say if the patient had capacity.

      (2) The durable power of attorney for health care decisions allows patients to name a surrogate to make decisions for them after they lose capacity.

      (3) If a surrogate has not been established, search for someone who had discussion with the patient, knows the values, lifestyle, and choices of the patient, and can likely speak for patient.

      (4) Parents are the proxy decision-makers for their newborns or infants.

    c. Best interests (based on no competence, no capacity, or no surrogate available)

      (1) Decision is made in the context of what is best for the patient in current circumstances through an analysis of benefits and burdens.

      (2) Question: what would a reasonable person in these circumstances do?

      (3) Examples of situations

        (a) Patient is never able to communicate preferences (e.g., a retarded adult).

        (b) Patient has not yet developed a value system or ability to communicate (e.g., a newborn).

(c) Patient was competent and capable but is no longer, and no one is available who knows the patient or can speak for the patient (e.g., a homeless person who is now in a vegetative state).
  4. Assess patient and family's ethnic, cultural, and spiritual background, and understand how these influence communication and collaboration, decision-making, and ethical dilemmas (Leininger, 1991, 1997; National Perinatal Association, 2001; Ott, Al-Khadhuri, & Al-Junaibi, 2003).
B. **Nursing Diagnoses** (can be psychosocial, psychologic, or both)
  1. Spiritual distress related to ethical dilemma
  2. Anticipatory grieving related to ethical dilemma
  3. Powerlessness related to ethical dilemma
  4. Hopelessness related to ethical dilemma
  5. Fear related to ethical dilemma
  6. Ineffective individual or family coping related to ethical dilemma
  7. Alteration in parenting or family processes related to ethical dilemma
  8. Knowledge deficit related to ethical dilemma
  9. Sleep pattern disturbance related to ethical dilemma
  10. Alteration in nutrition related to ethical dilemma
C. **Interventions**
  1. Interventions for each of the nursing diagnoses mentioned involve the following:
    a. Select and follow a recognized process.
    b. Focus the discussion with participants according to the selected process.
    c. Do a complete data collection according to selected process.
    d. Maintain objectivity and depersonalize issues according to selected process.
  2. Use an ethics committee as an available resource to assist in providing interventions for patients, families, and providers.
    a. Determine whether an ethics committee exists in the agency or institution.
    b. Determine how to access the ethics committee.
  3. Provide culturally sensitive patient and family support during the decision-making and while the plan is being implemented.
  4. Perform the roles of advocate, communicator, facilitator, coordinator, and planner.
    a. Prepare the family for what will happen and how it will appear.
    b. Work with key players, other professionals, and family to develop a plan for implementing the decision—what, when, how, by whom, and so forth—in a culturally sensitive manner.
    c. Encourage all participants to follow the plan.
    d. Assist the patient and family to identify and cope with "unfinished business."
    e. Assess coping abilities, and make referrals as needed.
    f. Identify a primary contact person who will communicate and coordinate the decision-making.
  5. Provide palliative or comfort care as needed.
    a. A family-centered, interdisciplinary, holistic, comprehensive approach to the care of patients with life-threatening or life-limiting conditions and their families is best (Catlin & Carter, 2001, 2002; Swaney, English, & Carter, 2002).
    b. A shift from rescue or cure mode to comfort care should occur at the earliest recognition of life-threatening or life-limiting conditions—futile technologic support is withheld or withdrawn (Catlin & Carter, 2002; Glicken & Merenstein, 2002); may be combined with efforts to prolong life (Beltrin & Coluzzi, 1997; Levetown, 2001; Swaney, English, & Carter, 2002).

    c. Newborn infants with the following conditions may be candidates (Catlin & Carter, 2002; Glassford, 2003; Glicken & Merenstein, 2002):

      (1) Those at the threshold of viability (very low birth weight under 500 g and under 24 weeks' gestation; under 750 g and under 27 weeks' gestation may initially do well but may develop life-limiting complications)

      (2) Those with complex or multiple congenital anomalies that are incompatible with any substantial length of life (e.g., trisomy 13, 15, 18; thanatophoric dwarfism; anencephaly, encephalocele; hypoplastic left heart syndrome) (Zeigler, 2003)

    d. Palliative care may be provided in the community hospital, in a community hospice, at home, or in the neonatal intensive care unit (NICU) where the family has social, familial, and spiritual support (Catlin & Carter, 2001, 2002; Glassford, 2003; Glicken & Merenstein, 2002).

D. Outcomes: the patient, family, or significant others will:

    1. Identify and discuss their beliefs or values that affect decision-making.

    2. Verbalize knowledge of the situation and what is causing the dilemma.

    3. Express feelings and emotions appropriately and freely.

    4. Participate or collaborate in decision-making and problem-solving.

    5. Visit regularly and participate in care.

    6. Demonstrate ability to relate to one another and support one another in coping.

    7. Express some sense of control over the outcome.

    8. Adjust lifestyle by initiating changes that help them deal with the crisis.

    9. Identify their needs; identify support systems available; use outside resources as needed.

    10. Acknowledge that the infant's life is limited and provide for a pain-free, dignified death (Glicken & Merenstein, 2002).

    11. Integrate psychologic, spiritual, cultural, and physiologic aspects of care into their decision-making (Catlin & Carter, 2001, 2002; Glicken & Merenstein, 2002; Swaney, English, & Carter, 2002).

    12. If needed, receive aggressive management of pain, discomfort, and any other distressing symptoms (Catlin & Carter, 2001, 2002; Glicken & Merenstein, 2002; Swaney, English, & Carter, 2002).

    13. Receive social, emotional, physical, spiritual, and cultural support during illness or in the event of death (Catlin & Carter, 2001, 2002; Glicken & Merenstein, 2002; Swaney, English, & Carter, 2002).

Health Education

A. Inform patients and families about the Patient Self Determination Act and the need to prepare for important decisions before a crisis occurs.

    1. Explain the purpose of written documents, what is included, and how to complete them (e.g., living will or durable power of attorney for health decisions).

    2. Encourage patients and families to discuss their wishes and decisions with family members and to give copies of written documents to appropriate persons.

B. Discuss the importance of being involved in decision-making regarding their health care: how to be involved, what questions to ask, and how to ask them.

C. Explain other important patient rights.

    1. The right to change providers to find one who will honor their values, beliefs, or decisions

2. The right to information about their diagnosis, treatment, other options, and anticipated outcomes
3. The right to say *no* to anything or anyone at any time

D. **If an ethics committee exists, explain the purpose and how to access it, if needed.**

DILEMMAS COMMON IN MATERNAL-NEWBORN NURSING PRACTICE

A. **Clinical issues**
   1. Reproductive choice or freedom
      a. Contraception or sterilization: voluntary or involuntary
      b. Abortion: first trimester or second trimester (Garel, Gosme-Seguret, Kaminiski, & Cuttini, 2002)
      c. Lesbian motherhood (Chan, Fox, McCormick, & Murphy, 1993)
   2. Assisted reproductive technology
      a. Artificial insemination
      b. Surrogate motherhood
      c. Cytoplasmic transfer
      d. In vitro fertilization
         (1) Frozen embryos
         (2) Orphaned embryos
      e. Gamete intrafallopian transfer
      f. "Made-to-order babies": preimplantation genetic diagnosis
      g. Cloning
   3. Prenatal screening, testing, and diagnosis: the option to consent or decline (AAP, 2001b; Anderson, 1999; Fioravanti, 2002; Zechmeister, 2001)
      a. Maternal alpha-fetoprotein
      b. Amniocentesis
      c. Chorionic villus sampling
      d. Ultrasound
      e. Genetic counseling, testing, and therapy
      f. Drug screening
      g. Human immunodeficiency virus (HIV) screening
   4. Human fetal tissue research or transplant donation
   5. High-risk pregnancy
      a. Intrauterine fetal treatment or surgery
      b. Substance abuse
      c. Treatments for preterm labor
      d. Pregnancy (selective) reduction
   6. Court-ordered obstetrical treatment: cesarean section and other therapies (Cahill, 1999)
   7. Neonatal intensive care issues (Raeside, 1997; Swaney, English, & Carter, 2002)
      a. Resuscitation of infants at the threshold of viability (low birth weight, very low birth weight)
      b. Rights of infants as individuals
      c. Parents as decision-makers; parental autonomy; proxy decision-makers
      d. Application of experimental or invasive technologies (Zeigler, 2003)
      e. Neonates as research subjects
      f. Pain management in neonates
      g. Palliative or comfort care
         (1) Withholding or withdrawing of resuscitation or life support
         (2) Nutrition, hydration, and pain relief

        (3) Supportive care
        (4) Futility
    h. Organ transplant and donating organs

B. General professional nursing issues

1. A majority of surveyed nurses confront ethical issues daily or weekly, yet they reported that they did not receive sufficient ethics content in their education (Scanlon, 1994a).
2. Resources for nurses with ethical problems were identified as literature or journals (44%), ethics committees (42%), and continuing education (39%); 11% were unable to identify any available resources (Scanlon, 1994a).
3. The most frequently occurring (over 50%) ethics and human rights issues were cost containment, end-of-life decisions, and confidentiality (Scanlon, 1994b); other important issues were pain management, use of advance directives, informed consent, access to health care, care of patients with human immunodeficiency virus or acquired immunodeficiency syndrome, and futile care (Scanlon, 1994b).
4. Code of Ethics (ANA, 2001; can be viewed at *www.ana.org/ethics.htm*):
   a. Practices with compassion and respect for the dignity, worth, and uniqueness of every individual.
   b. Has a primary commitment or responsibility to patient: an individual, family, group, or community.
   c. Promotes, advocates, and protects the health, safety, and rights of the patient.
   d. Is responsible and accountable for individual nursing practice and delegation of tasks to others.
   e. Owes same duties to self as to others: responsibility to preserve integrity, provide safety, maintain competence, and to grow personally and professionally.
   f. Through individual and collective action, nurses establish, maintain, and improve health care environments and conditions of employment necessary to provide quality care and that are consistent with the values of the profession.
   g. Participates in the advancement of the profession by contributions to practice, knowledge development, education, and administration, in accord with national practice standards and guidelines.
   h. Collaborates with other health professionals and members of the community to promote local, national, and international health efforts.
   i. Profession, through associations and members, is responsible for articulating nursing values, maintaining professional and practice integrity, and shaping social policy.

CASE STUDY AND STUDY QUESTIONS

After 4 years of infertility treatments, Mr. and Mrs. S had their first child. Within hours of the infant's birth, complications developed. Over several days, the following diagnosis was made: multiple congenital anomalies involving the cardiac, neurologic, and renal systems. Baby S is in the NICU under the care of a neonatologist. She is on a ventilator with high pressures, has a central line, and is on multiple intravenous medications to maintain the function of her kidneys and heart and to prevent seizures. Decisions about dialysis will need to be made in the next 24 hours. The oximeter reads in the low 70s. She has frequent seizure activity in spite of the medications. She is unresponsive except to painful stimuli. The infant will not live much longer, and no therapy is available to resolve the multiple problems. The physician has been talking with the parents constantly to prepare them for the inevitable and to provide information they will need to make the tough decisions. Until now, the parents have refused to acknowledge the infant's condition and are convinced that a cure must be available. Both parents are educated professionals, they are financially stable, and they are committed to having a family. Grandparents on both sides are supportive and involved. The family has no specific church affiliation.

One of the NICU residents told the parents about an article he read that discussed experimental surgical procedures on babies such as Baby S. The article said only one infant had survived the procedures. An hour ago, Mr. and Mrs. S angrily confronted the neonatologist and demanded that their infant be sent for the experimental surgery immediately.

1. In this situation, the patient:
   a. Has competence and capacity.
   b. Has competence but no capacity.
   c. Has capacity but no competence.
   d. Has neither capacity nor competence.

2. In this dilemma, the conflicting principles are:
   a. Justice and fidelity
   b. Beneficence and nonmaleficence
   c. Veracity and confidentiality
   d. Beneficence and privacy

3. The decision is being made from the perspective of:
   a. Autonomy
   b. Substituted judgment
   c. Best interests

4. The physician has an obligation and duty to:
   a. Do everything the parents demand.
   b. Offer all experimental procedures available.
   c. Do good for the infant.
   d. Follow the legal advice of the hospital attorney.

5. The best way to handle this conflict between physician and parents is to:
   a. Let the court decide.
   b. Petition the court to appoint a guardian.
   c. Ask for an ethics committee consultation.
   d. Not allow the residents to talk with families.

6. The nurse can assist and support the family by:
   a. Testifying at the court hearing.
   b. Encouraging them to get another physician.
   c. Giving them time with the infant and making sure they understand the issues and information.
   d. Restricting visiting hours.

7. The family acknowledges the terminal condition of the infant, and a decision is made not to pursue experimental surgery. What is the immediate next step?
   a. Develop a plan of what will happen, when it will happen, how it will happen, and who will be involved.
   b. Tell the NICU residents to stop talking with the families about experimental procedures.
   c. Discontinue the ventilator and all intravenous medications.
   d. Move the infant to an isolation room to discontinue care.

8. The decision not to offer experimental surgery is:
   a. Illegal and unethical
   b. Legal and unethical
   c. Ethical and illegal
   d. Ethical and legal

9. Which type of law would offer the most support for this decision?
   a. Administrative rules and regulations
   b. Case law
   c. Statutory law
   d. Constitutional law

ANSWERS TO STUDY QUESTIONS

1. d	4. c	7. a
2. b	5. c	8. d
3. c	6. c	9. b

REFERENCES

American Academy of Pediatrics. (1995). The initiation or withdrawal of treatment for high-risk newborns. *Pediatrics, 96*(2, Pt 1), 362-363.

American Academy of Pediatrics, Committee on Bioethics. (1994). Guidelines on foregoing life-sustaining medical treatment, *Pediatrics, 93*(3), 532-536.

American Academy of Pediatrics, Committee on Bioethics. (2001a). Institutional ethics committees. *Pediatrics, 107*(1), 205-209.

American Academy of Pediatrics, Committee on Bioethics. (2001b). Ethical issues with genetic testing in pediatrics. *Pediatrics, 107*(6), 1451-1455.

American Academy of Pediatrics and American College of Obstetricians and Gynecologists. (1995). Perinatal care at the threshold of viability, *Pediatrics, 96*(5), 974-976.

American Academy of Pediatrics and American College of Obstetricians and Gynecologists. (2002). *Guidelines for perinatal care* (5th ed.). Washington, DC: AAP and ACOG.

American College of Obstetricians and Gynecologists. (1989, Nov). Ethical decision-making in obstetrics and gynecology, *ACOG Technical Bulletin, 136*, 1-7.

American Hospital Association. (1985). *Report of the Special Committee on Biomedical Ethics: Values in conflict: Resolving ethical issues in hospital care.* Chicago: American Hospital Publishing.

American Nurses Association. (1985). *Nursing: A social policy statement* (brochure). Kansas City, MO: American Nurses Association.

American Nurses Association. (2001). *Code for nurses with interpretative statements* (brochure). Washington, DC: American Nurses Association.

Anderson, G. (1999). Nondirectiveness in prenatal genetics: Patients read in between the lines. *Nursing Ethics, 6*(2), 215-218.

Annas, G. (1993). *Standard of care: The law of American bioethics.* New York: Oxford University Press.

Annas, G. (1994). Asking the courts to set the standard of emergency care. *New England Journal of Medicine, 330*(21), 1542-1545.

Arras, J. (1984). Toward an ethic of ambiguity, *Hastings Center Report, 14*(2), 25-33.

Bandman, E., & Bandman, B. (1990). *Nursing ethics through the life span* (2nd ed.). Norwalk, CT: Appleton & Lange.

Beauchamp, T., & Childress, J. (2001). *Principles of biomedical ethics* (5th ed.). New York: Oxford University Press.

Beltrin, J., & Coluzzi, P. (1997, Spring/Summer). A model for comprehensive palliative care. *Talbot Journal of Health Care.*

Benjamin, M., & Curtis, J. (1992). *Ethics in nursing* (3rd ed.). New York: Oxford University Press.

Cahill, H. (1999). An Orwellian scenario: Court-ordered caesarean section and women's autonomy. *Nursing Ethics, 6*(6), 494-505.

Cahill, H. (2001). Male appropriation and medicalization of childbirth: An historical analysis. *Journal of Advanced Nursing, 33*(3), 334-342.

Canadian Nurses Association. (1980). *CNA code of ethics: An ethical basis for nursing in Canada* (brochure). Ottawa: Canadian Nurses Association.

Carper, B. (1979). The ethics of caring. *Advances in Nursing Science, 1*(3), 11-19.

Catalano, J. (1995). *Ethical and legal aspects of nursing* (2nd ed.). Springhouse, PA: Springhouse.

Catlin, A., & Carter, B. (2001). Creation of a neonatal end of life protocol. *Journal of Clinical Ethics, 12*(3), 316-318.

Catlin, A., & Carter, B. (2002). Creation of a neonatal end of life protocol. *Journal of Perinatology, 22*(3), 184-195 and reprinted in *Neonatal Network, 21*(4), 37-49.

Catlin, E.A., Guillemin, J.H., Thiel, M.M, Hammond, S., Wang, M.L., & O'Donnell, J. (2001). Spiritual and religious components of patient care in the neonatal intensive care unit: Sacred themes in a secular setting, *Journal of Perinatology, 21*(7), 426-430.

Chan, C., Fox, J., McCormick, R., & Murphy, T. (1993). Lesbian motherhood and genetic choices. *Ethics Behavior, 3*(2), 211-222.

Chesney, R. (2001). Privacy and its regulation: Too much too soon, or too little too late? *Pediatrics, 107*(6), 1423-1424.

Clark, F. (1996). Making sense of *State v Messenger. Pediatrics, 97*(4), 579-583.

Colorado Collective for Medical Health Care Decisions. (lll). *You are not alone* (film). Denver: Nickel's Worth Publications. E-mail address: *nickel-wrth@ aol.com.*

Culver, G., Fallon, K., Londner, R.B., Montalvo, N., Vila, B., Ramsey, B.J., et al. (2000). Informed decisions for extremely low birth weight infants. *Journal of the American Medical Association, 283*(24), 3201-3202.

Curtin, L., & Flaherty, J. (1982). *Nursing ethics: Theories and pragmatics.* Bowie, MD: Prentice-Hall.

Daaleman, T., & VandeCreek, L. (2000). Placing religion and spirituality in end-of-life care. *Journal of the American Medical Association, 284*(19), 2514-2517.

Davis, A., & Aroskar, M. (1991). *Ethical dilemmas and nursing practice* (3rd ed.). Norwalk, CT: Appleton & Lange.

De Marco, D.G. (2000). Medicine and spirituality. *Annals of Internal Medicine, 133*(11), 920-921.

Doroshow, R.W., Hodgman, J.E., Pomerance, J.J., Ross, J.W., Michel, V.J., Luckett, P.M., et al. (2000). Treatment decisions for newborns at the threshold of viability: An ethical dilemma, *Journal of Perinatology, 20*(6), 379-383.

Dubler, N., & Marcus, L. (1994). *Mediating bioethical disputes.* New York: United Hospital Fund of New York.

Duff, R.S., & Campbell, A.G. (1973). Moral and ethical dilemmas in the special care nursery. *New England Journal of Medicine, 289*(17), 890-894.

Fioravanti, J. (2002). Issues related to prenatal diagnosis of congestive heart disease. *Neonatal Network, 21*(6), 23-29.

Fowler, M., & Levine-Ariff, J. (1987). *Ethics at the bedside: A source book for the critical care nurse.* Philadelphia: Lippincott.

Garel, M., Gosme-Seguret, S., Kaminiski, M., & Cuttini, M. (2002). Ethical decision-making in prenatal diagnosis and termination of pregnancy: Qualitative survey among physicians and midwives. *Prenatal Diagnosis, 22*(9), 811-817.

Gilligan, C. (1982). *In a different voice: Psychological theory and women's development.* Cambridge, MA: Harvard University Press.

Glassford, B. (2003). A case study in caring: Trisomy 18 syndrome, *American Journal of Nursing, 103*(7), 81-83.

Glicken, A., & Merenstein, G. (2002). A neonatal end-of-life protocol—An evolving new standard of care? *Neonatal Network, 21*(4), 35-36.

Gotlieb, E. (2002). Privacy rights, HIPPA, and the AAP: About right, about time. *Pediatrics, 109*(1), 146-149.

Hack, M. (1999). Consideration of the use of health status, functional outcome, and quality-of-life to monitor neonatal intensive care practice. *Pediatrics, 103*(1, suppl E), 319-323.

Harrison, H. (1993). The principles of family-centered neonatal care, *Pediatrics, 92*(5), 643-650.

Hastings Center. (1987). *Guidelines on the termination of life-sustaining treatment and the care of the dying.* Indianapolis: Indiana University Press.

Holmes, H., & Prudy, L. (Eds.). (1992). *Feminist perspectives in medical ethics.* Indianapolis: Indiana University Press.

Hunt, G. (Ed.). (1994). *Ethical issues in nursing.* London: Routledge.

Husted, G., & Husted, J. (1995). *Ethical decision-making in nursing* (2nd ed.). St. Louis: Mosby.

International Council of Nurses. (1973). *ICN code for nurses—Ethical concepts applied to nursing* (brochure). Geneva, Switzerland: International Council of Nurses.

Jameton, A. (1984). *Nursing practice: The ethical issues.* Englewood Cliffs, NJ: Prentice-Hall.

Joffe, S., Manocchia, M., Weeks, J., & Cleary, P. (2003). What do patients value in their hospital care? An empirical perspective on autonomy centered bioethics. *Journal of Medical Ethics, 29*(2), 103-108.

Kagawa-Singer, M. (1998). The cultural context of death rituals and mourning practices. *Oncology Nursing Forum, 25*(10), 1752-1756.

Kirschbaum, M. (1996). Life support decisions for children: What do parents value? *Advances in Nursing Science, 19*(1), 51-71.

Koh, T.H., Harrison, H., & Morley, C. (1999). Gestation versus outcome table for parents of extremely premature infants, *Journal of Perinatology, 19*(6, Pt 1), 452-453.

Koh, T.H., Casey, A., & Harrison, H. (2000). Use of an outcome by gestation table for extremely premature babies: A cross-sectional survey of the views of parents, neonatal nurses and perinatologists, *Journal of Perinatology, 20*(8, Pt 1), 504-508.

Kuhse, H., & Singer, P. (1985). *Should the baby live?* New York: Oxford University Press.

Lagana, K., & Duderstadt, K. (1995). Ethical decision making for perinatal nurses. White Plains, NY: March of Dimes Birth Defects Foundation.

Lantos, J.D., Singer, P.A., Walker, R.M., Gramelspacher, G.P., Shapiro, G.R., Sanchez-Gonzalez, M.A., et al. (1989). The illusion of futility in clinical practice, *American Journal of Medicine, 87*(1), 81-84.

Leininger, M. (1991). *Culture care diversity and universality: A theory of nursing.* New York: National League for Nursing Press.

Leininger, M. (1997). Future directions in transcultural nursing in the 21st century. *International Nursing Review, 44*(1), 19-23.

Leuthner, S.R. (2001). Decisions regarding resuscitation of the extremely premature infant and models of best interest. *Journal of Perinatology, 21*(3), 193-198.

Levetown, M. (2001). Pediatric care: The inpatient/ICU perspective. In Ferrell, G., & Coyle, N. (Eds.), *Textbook of palliative nursing.* New York: Oxford University Press.

Lorber, J. (1971). Results of treatment of myelomeningocele: An analysis of 524 unselected cases, with special reference to possible selection for treatment. *Developmental Medicine and Child Neurology, 13*(3), 279-303.

Lynn, J. (Ed.). (1989). *By no extraordinary means.* Indianapolis: Indiana University Press.

Maugans, T. (1996). The spiritual history. *Archives in Family Medicine, 5*(1), 11-16.

McHaffie, H.E., Laing, I.A., Parker, M., & McMillan, J. (2001). Deciding for imperiled newborns: Medical authority or parental autonomy? *Journal of Medical Ethics, 27*(2), 104-109.

National Association for Home Care. (1990). *Home care bill of rights* (pamphlet). Washington, DC: National Association for Home Care.

National Perinatal Association. (2001). *Transcultural aspects of perinatal care: A resource manual: Part I.* Tampa, FL: National Perinatal Association.

Nelson, L.J. (1989). Bioethics in the courts: Summaries of selected judicial decisions. *Clinical Ethics Report, 3*,1-16.

Neufeld, M., Woodrum, D., & Tarczy-Hornoch, P. (2000). Prenatal and postnatal counseling for parents of infants at the limits of viability, *Pediatric Research, 47*, 420A.

Nurses handbook of law and ethics. (1992). Springhouse, PA: Springhouse.

Omnibus Reconciliation Act of 1990, Sections 4206 and 4751. (The Patient Self Determination Act, 1990).

Orleans, M., Tappero, E., Glicken, A., & Merenstein, G. (2002). Evidence-based clinical practice decisions. In Merenstein, G.B., & Gardner, S.L. (Eds.), *Handbook of neonatal intensive care* (5th ed., pp. 1-8). St. Louis: Mosby.

Ott, B., Al-Khadhuri, J., & Al-Junaibi, S. (2003). Preventing ethical dilemmas: Understanding Islamic health care practices. *Pediatric Nursing, 29*(3), 227-230.

Partridge, J.C., Freeman, H., Weiss, E., & Martinez, A.M. (2001). Delivery room resuscitation decisions for extremely low birth weight infants in California. *Journal of Perinatology, 21*(1), 27-33.

Paul, D.A., Leef, K.H., Epps, S., et al. (1999). Usefulness of the prenatal consult: Mothers' response. *Pediatric Research, 45*, 218A.

Paul, D.A., Epps, S., Leef, K.H., & Stefano, J.L. (2001). Prenatal consultation with neonatologist prior to preterm delivery. *Journal of Perinatology, 21*(7), 431-437.

President's Commission for the Study of Ethical Problems in Medicine and Biomedical and Behavioral Research. (1983). *Deciding to forego life-sustaining treatment.* Washington, DC: Public Health Service, U.S. Department of Health and Human Services.

Raeside, L. (1997). Ethical decision-making in neonatal intensive care. *Professional Nurse, 13*(3), 157-159.

Rushton, C., & Hogue, E. (1993). When parents demand everything. *Pediatric Nursing, 19*(2), 180-183.

Rushton, C., & Scanlon, C. (1995). When values conflict with obligations: Safeguards for nurses. *Pediatric Nursing, 21*(3), 260-261, 268.

Scanlon, C. (1994a). Survey yields significant results. *American Nurses Association Center for Ethics and Human Rights Communique, 3*(3), 1-3.

Scanlon, C. (1994b). Ethics survey looks at nurses' experiences. *American Nurse, 26*(10), 22.

Siegel, R., Gardner, S., & Merenstein, G. (2002). Families in crisis: Theoretic and practical considerations. In Merenstein, G.B. & Gardner, S.L. (Eds.), *Handbook of neonatal intensive care* (5th ed., pp. 725-753). St. Louis: Mosby.

Stutts, A., & Schloemann, J. (2002a). Life-sustaining support: Ethical, cultural, and spiritual conflicts. Part I: Family support—a neonatal case study. *Neonatal Network, 21*(3), 23-29.

Stutts, A., & Schloemann, J. (2002b). Life-sustaining support: Ethical, cultural, and spiritual conflicts. Part II: Staff support—A neonatal case study. *Neonatal Network, 21*(4), 27-34.

Swaney, J., English, N., & Carter, B. (2002). Ethics in neonatal intensive care. In Merenstein, G.B., & Gardner, S.L. (Eds.), *Handbook of neonatal intensive care* (5th ed., pp. 801-821). St. Louis: Mosby.

Thompson, J., & Thompson, H. (1981). *Ethics in nursing.* New York: Macmillan.

Tyson, J. (1995). Evidence-based ethics and the care of premature infants, *Future of Children, 5*(1), 197-213.

U.S. Department of Health and Human Services (USDHHS). (1991). *Federal policy for the protection of human subjects: Notice and rules* (45 C.F.R. 11 [a]). Washington, DC: USDHHS.

Weil, W.B. (1984). Issues associated with treatment and non-treatment decisions: Special reference to newborns with handicaps. *American Journal of Diseases of Children, 138*(6), 519-522.

Weir, R. (1984). *Selective nontreatment of handicapped newborns.* New York: Oxford University Press.

Welch, C.A. (2001). Sacred secrets: The privacy of medical records. *New England Journal of Medicine, 345*(5), 371-372.

White, G. (1992). *Ethical dilemmas in contemporary nursing practice.* Washington, DC: American Nurses.

Winslow, B., & Winslow, G. (1991). Integrity and compromise in nursing ethics. *Journal of Medicine and Philosophy, 16*(3), 307-323.

Woodward, V. (1998). Caring, patient autonomy and the stigma of paternalism. *Journal of Advanced Nursing, 28*(5), 1046-1052.

Yarling, R.R., & McElmurry, B.J. (1986). The moral foundation of nursing. *Advances in Nursing Science, 8*(2), 63-73.

Zeichmeister, I. (2001). Fetal images: The power of visual technology in antenatal care and the implications for women's reproductive freedom. *Health Care Analysis, 9*(4), 387-400.

Zeigler, V. (2003). Ethical principles and parental choice: Treatment options for neonates with hypoplastic left heart syndrome. *Pediatric Nursing, 29*(1), 65-69.

Index

P. *See* American Academy of
    Pediatrics.
andonment, feelings of as
    reaction to labor, 257
breviations for charting electronic
    fetal monitoring, 337b
CD assessment in maternal
    traumatic injury, 710-712
domen
etal, circumference of, in
        gestational age
        determination, 168t
naternal
    changes to during pregnancy,
        101
    trauma to, 639, 704, 713
eonatal, assessment of, 439
dominal examination
holecystectomy and, 735
ollowing maternal traumatic
    injury, 713
uring latent phase of labor, 276
dominal pain
n appendicitis, 737, 738f
lue to gastrointestinal disease, 810
elated to abruptio placentae,
    643-644
dominal wall defects, 450-451
Gs. *See* Arterial blood gases.
ortion
lilemmas regarding, 887
pontaneous
    anticipatory grieving related
        to, 193
    grief and loss associated with,
        132
    impaired adjustment related
        to, 137-138
    risk for compromised family
        coping related to, 191-192
ruptio placentae, 638-644, 652
hypertensive disorder-related, 583
sent variability of fetal heart
    rate, 315, 316f, 317, 318f
nterventions for, 330
stinence for contraception, 412t
periodic, 414t
stinence syndrome, neonatal, 752
use
ntimate partner, 537-553
    assessment of, 544-546
    case study and study questions
        associated with, 551-552
    characteristics of abusers in,
        542-543, 543f

Abuse (*Continued*)
    characteristics of women in
        battering relationships,
        543-544
    cultural and socioeconomic
        factors in, 541-542
    cycle of violence in, 538-540,
        539f
    health education regarding, 550
    incidence of, 537-538
    interventions/outcomes for,
        546-548, 549f
    nursing diagnoses in, 546
    resources for professionals
        regarding, 550
    types of injuries in, 540
substance, 70, 750-770
    of alcohol, 762-767, 769
    anxiety related to, 757
    assessment of, 753-755
    case studies and study
        questions for, 768-769
    of cocaine, 751-752
    deficient knowledge related to,
        755, 756b
    effects of on fetus, 751
    health education regarding, 767
    of heroin, 752-753
    impaired parenting due to,
        758-759
    ineffective health maintenance
        associated with, 758
    interrupted family processes
        related to, 757
    as major public health issue, 750
    of marijuana, 753
    of methadone hydrochloride,
        753
    noncompliance associated
        with, 757
    nursing diagnoses and
        interventions/outcomes
        regarding, 755-759, 756b,
        759f
    nutritional aspects in, 756-757
    outcomes associated with,
        750-751
    risk for injury related to, 758,
        759f
    situational low self-esteem
        associated with, 754
    statistics regarding, 750
    of tobacco, 760-762, 768-769
Abusers
    characteristics of, 542-543, 543f
    childhood of, 542

Accelerations of fetal heart rate
    fetal hypoxia and, 165
    nonperiodic, 344f, 344-345
    periodic, 332-333, 333f
Acceptance
    of child, 127
    of pregnancy, 127
Accutane. *See* Isotretinoin.
Acidosis, metabolic
    fetal, 163-164
        oxygen saturation in, 353
    neonatal
        meconium aspiration
            syndrome and, 514
        respiratory distress syndrome
            and, 504
ACOG. *See* American College of
    Obstetricians and
    Gynecologists.
Acoustic stimulation test, 187-188
Acquired immunodeficiency
    syndrome, 599-609
    assessment of, 605-607
    case study and study questions
        for, 625-626
    counseling and early diagnosis
        of, 603
    first recognition of, 599
    health education regarding,
        623-624
    human immunodeficiency virus
        infection in, 599-603
    nursing diagnoses and
        interventions/outcomes for,
        607-609
    treatment of, 604-605
    women and, 603-604, 604f, 604t
Acrocyanosis, 438
Acrosin, 42
ACT. *See* Activated clotting time.
ACTH. *See* Adrenocorticotropic
    hormone.
Activated clotting time in
    disseminated intravascular
    coagulation, 645
Active phase of labor, 276-277
    emotions of, 256
Active sleep, 440
Active transport in placental
    transfer, 54, 55t
Activities of daily living, altered due
    to thrombophlebitis, 860-861
Activity intolerance
    associated with gastrointestinal
        disease, 810
    related to cardiac disease, 778

Page numbers followed by *b*, *t*, or *f* indicate boxes, tables, or figures, respectively.

Activity intolerance (*Continued*)
  related to fatigue caused by the
    physiologic changes of
    pregnancy, 118
Activity restriction, ethnocultural
    factors in, 80, 91t, 93t
Acute renal failure, 782, 783
Addison's disease, 688-690, 698
Adjustment, impaired, related to
    mood disorder, eating disorder,
    or loss, 137-138
Admission history, latent phase of
    labor and, 274-275
Adolescent pregnancy, 147-152, 156
  case studies and study questions
    associated with, 157-159
  risks associated with, 109
Adoption, 132
Adrenal gland
  changes to during pregnancy, 101
  disorders of, 685-690, 698
Adrenal insufficiency, 688-690, 698
Adrenocorticotropic hormone,
    adrenal insufficiency and, 688
Advanced maternal age, 152-156,
    157-159
AFP. *See* Alpha-fetoprotein.
African-American culture, 91t-95t
  AIDS in, 603, 604t
  intimate partner violence and,
    541
Afterpains, 371
AGA. *See* Appropriate to
    gestational age.
Age
  gestational, 465-496
    assessment of, 441, 442t-443t,
      444b-445b, 445f, 446f
    case studies and study
      questions associated with,
      492-494
    health education regarding,
      490-491
    large for, 482-486
    postterm, 486-490
    preterm, 472-482
    small for, 465-471
  as risk factor for gestational
    hypertension, 556
Age-related concerns, 109, 147-160
  adolescent, 147-152
  in advanced maternal age,
    152-156
  case studies and study questions
    associated with, 157-159
  health education regarding, 156
  during labor and delivery, 253
Aggression in abuser, 542-543, 543f.
    See Also Intimate partner
    violence.
AIDS. *See* Acquired
    immunodeficiency syndrome.
AIDS Hotline, 623
Air leak syndrome, 500
  in meconium aspiration
    syndrome, 511, 512
Air-filled intrauterine pressure
    catheter monitoring of
    contractions, 307

Airway clearance, ineffective
  maternal
    related to respiratory disease,
      790-791, 791t
    related to trauma in pregnancy,
      717, 718f
  neonatal, related to inability to
    adequately clear secretions
    from airway, 429
Airway obstruction, maternal, due
    to traumatic injury, 711
Airway secretion clearance in
    newborn, 429
  in respiratory distress syndrome,
    506
Alanine aminotransferase in
    gestational hypertension and
    HELLP syndrome, 573t
Albumin in gestational
    hypertension and HELLP
    syndrome, 573t
Alcohol related birth defects,
    764-765
Alcohol related
    neurodevelopmental disorder,
    764
Alcohol use, 762-767
  breastfeeding and, 404
Aldomet. *See* Methyldopa.
Alert inactivity, 440
Alkaline phosphatase in gestational
    hypertension and HELLP
    syndrome, 573t
Allele, defined, 23
Allocation, ethics and, 875
Aloneness, feelings of as reaction to
    labor, 257
Alpha-fetoprotein
  in fetal and placental assessment,
    67
  in genetic assessment, 32-33
  maternal serum screening of,
    183-185
  in triple marker test, 185-186
Alprazolam as environmental
    hazard, 213
ALT. *See* Alanine aminotransferase.
Altered consciousness associated
    with disseminated
    intravascular coagulation, 647
Altered functioning related to
    deviation from normal
    anatomical or physiologic status
    of reproductive system, 18
Altered metabolism
  in diabetes mellitus
    gestational, 674
    pregestational, 668-669
  in hyperthyroidism, 681
Altered self-concept
  related to gestational diabetes, 675
  related to inability to provide
    adequate milk supply, 402-403
Alzapam. *See* Lorazepam.
Ambivalence about pregnancy, 126
Amenorrhea, 11-12
American Academy of Pediatrics
  on high risk conditions of
    pregnancy, 161-162

American College of Obstetricians
    and Gynecologists
  classification of hypertensive
    disorders of pregnancy by,
    555
  on high risk conditions of
    pregnancy, 161-162
American Family Physician's
    Management of Newborns
    exposed to Maternal HIV, 623
American Indian culture
  AIDS and, 604t
  attitudes of toward menstruation,
    15
American Liver Foundation, 623
American Social Health
    Association, 623
Aminopterin as environmental
    hazard, 214
Amniocentesis, 174-178, 176f
  in fetal and placental assessment,
    67
  in maternal diabetes mellitus, 665
  risk for deficient fluid volume
    related to, 192
Amnionitis, 177
Amniotic bands, 61-63, 63t
Amniotic fluid, 65f, 65-66
  assessment of during latent
    phase of labor, 275-276
  embolism, 839-841, 846-847
  function of, explained to patient,
    827
  volume of
    in biophysical profile, 172, 173t
    in fetal maturity scoring, 168t
    ultrasonographic assessment
      of, 170-171
Amniotic membranes rupture
  abruptio placentae and, 640
  premature, 827-831, 845-846
  as premonitory sign of childbirth,
    273
  risk for infection related to, 273
  risk for infection related to
    vaginal examination
    following, 281
Amniotomy, 291
  in abruptio placentae, 642
Amobarbital as environmental
    hazard, 216
Amoxicillin for acute
    pyelonephritis, 613
Amphetamines as environmental
    hazard, 210-211
Ampicillin for acute pyelonephritis,
    613
Ampulla, 8
Amytal. *See* Amobarbital.
Analgesics
  as environmental hazard, 211
  for first stage of labor, 277-279
  intrauterine fetal demise and, 837
  for pain management in surgery
    in pregnancy, 734
Anamid. *See* Kanamycin.
Anatomy of female reproductive
    system, 3-13
  external, 3-5, 4f

Anatomy of female reproductive system (*Continued*)
  hypothalamic-pituitary-ovarian axis and, 12-13
  internal, 5f, 5-8, 7f
  menstruation and, 11-12
  support for organs of, 8-10, 9f, 10f
Android pelvis, 235
Anemia
  fetal, impaired fetal gas exchange related to, 192
  maternal, 17, 799-801, 802, 803, 803t, 804
  neonatal, respiratory distress syndrome and, 504
Anencephaly, 49, 252
  fetal surgery for, 743
  maternal serum alpha-fetoprotein screening in, 185
Anesthesia, 728-734
  anesthetic choices in, 732-733
  for cesarean birth, 297
  for delivery, 282-283
  effects of on fetus, 239
  epidural, upright postures for labor and delivery and, 239
  for first stage of labor, 277-279
  intrauterine fetal demise and, 837
  laparotomy *versus* laparoscopic approach, 731-732
  maternal preoperative assessment as, 730-731
  nursing diagnoses and interventions/outcomes for, 733-734
  planning and management of, 728-730
  in uterine rupture, 843
Aneuploidies, 41
Angel kiss, term, 438
Angiotensin II
  altered pressor response to, in preeclampsia, 557
  fetal heart rate and, 309
Ankle dorsiflexion in neonatal neurologic assessment, 444b
Announcement phase of pregnancy, 128
Anorexia due to gastrointestinal disease, 809-810
Anorexia nervosa, 130-132
Anovulatory menstrual cycle, 12
Antabuse. *See* Disulfiram.
Antepartum fetal assessment, 161-200
  biochemical, 174-186
    amniocentesis in, 174-178, 176f
    chorionic villus sampling in, 181f, 181-183
    cordocentesis and percutaneous umbilical blood sampling in, 178-181, 180f
    estriol assays in, 185
    fetal DNA in maternal circulation in, 186
    maternal serum alpha-fetoprotein screening in, 183-185

Antepartum fetal assessment (*Continued*)
    triple marker test in, 185-186
  biophysical, 167-174, 175f
    biophysical profile in, 172-174, 173t
    Doppler ultrasound blood flow assessment in, 174, 175f
    ultrasound for, 167-171, 168t, 169f
  case studies and sample questions regarding, 194-195
  comparison of surveillance tests in, 165
  electronic, 186-190
    contraction stress test in, 188-190
    nonstress test in, 187-188
  fetal movement assessment by client in, 165-166
  health education in, 193
  interventions/outcomes in, 190-193
  nursing diagnoses in, 190
  role of nurse in, 162-165
Antepartum period. *See* Pregnancy.
Anthropoid pelvis, 236
Antialcohol agents as environmental hazard, 211
Antiarrhythmic agents, 779t
Antibiotics
  for acute pyelonephritis, 613
  as environmental hazard, 211-212
Anticipatory grieving
  in acquired immunodeficiency syndrome, 608
  in actual or potential loss of fetus following traumatic injury, 720
  in loss of normal pregnancy or fetus, 193
  in preterm labor, 823
  related to ill or preterm newborn, 138
Anticoagulants
  as environmental hazard, 212
  for maternal cardiovascular disease, 778, 780t
  for postpartum thrombophlebitis, 860
Anticonvulsants as environmental hazard, 212-213
Antidepressants as environmental hazard, 213
Antiemetics as environmental hazard, 213
Antihyperlipidemics as environmental hazard, 213
Antihypertensives
  as environmental hazard, 213
  for hypertensive disorders of pregnancy, 577t-578t
Antimigraine agents as environmental hazard, 213-214
Antineoplastics as environmental hazard, 214
Antiphospholipid antibody syndrome, 793-799

Antithyroid drugs, 678, 682, 697
  as environmental hazard, 214
  risk for injury to fetus associated with, 682-683
Antituberculosis drugs, 790t
Antiulcer agents as environmental hazard, 214
Antiviral agents as environmental hazard, 214
Anxiety
  in abnormal progress of labor, 295
  about breastfeeding related to unexpected childbearing experience, 399-403
    cesarean birth and, 399
    of fussy or irritable infant, 400
    for multiple births, 402
    physiologic jaundice and, 400-401
    of preterm or hospitalized infant, 401-402, 402f
    of sleepy or reluctant infant, 399-400
    for special needs infant, 402-403
  in abruptio placentae, 643
  in adrenal insufficiency, 690
  in advanced maternal age pregnancy, 155
  alcohol use and, 766
  in carcinoma secondary to trophoblastic disease, 651
  in chorioamnionitis, 622
  in complicated pregnancy, 771-772
  in diabetes mellitus
    gestational, 674-675
    pregestational, 669-670
  in disseminated intravascular coagulation, 647
  due to disruption of normal routines and support systems, 259
  ethnocultural factors in, 84-85
  in fear of pain and unknown outcome, 191
  in fear of the unknown, 136
  in fetal heart rate problems, 314, 322, 332, 336-337, 341-343, 349
  in fetal pulse oximetry, 355
  in fetal scalp sampling, 352-353
  in hyperadrenocorticism, 687
  in hypertensive disorders of pregnancy, 583-584
  in hyperthyroidism, 680-681
  in induction or augmentation of uterine contractions, 292
  during labor and delivery, 256-257, 259, 279
  in lack of support during stressful circumstances, 191
  in phenylketonuria, 694
  in placenta previa, 638
  in poor outcome from disease process, 191
  in possible chromosomal abnormality, 155
  in possible fetal conditions that are hindering labor, 259
  related to drug use, 757

Anxiety (*Continued*)
related to hazardous effects of pharmaceuticals, 217
related to initial feeding secondary to experience, 396-397
related to occupational hazard, 208
related to strange environment, 259
related to well being of newborn, 287-288
in sexually transmitted diseases, 611
in situational crisis of labor, 259
in surgery in pregnancy, 734
in surgical delivery, 297
in thrombophlebitis, 860-861
in TORCH disease, 599
in umbilical cord sampling, 357
in uncertainty about onset of labor and ability to cope, 272-273
in urinary tract infection and pyelonephritis, 614
Aorta, coarctation of, 456-457, 457f
Apgar scoring, 426, 426t
fetal scalp pH in, 352
in large-for-gestational-age infant, 483
in meconium aspiration syndrome, 513
Apnea in newborn, 429
premature, 477
Appearance of dead infant, 839
Appendectomy, 737-739, 738f
Appendix, relative position of during progression of pregnancy, 738f
Appropriate to gestational age, 441
Apresoline. *See* Hydralazine hydrochloride.
APS. *See* Antiphospholipid antibody syndrome.
Aquatag. *See* Benzthiazide.
Arab culture, 91t-95t
Arachidonic acid, 229
ARBD. *See* Alcohol related birth defects.
Areola
changes to during pregnancy, 98
of premature infant, 476
ARF. *See* Acute renal failure.
Arm recoil in neonatal neurologic assessment, 444b
ARND. *See* Alcohol related neurodevelopmental disorder.
Arnold-Chiari type malformation, fetal surgery for, 743
Arrhythmias, fetal, 319-321, 321f, 329-332. *See Also* Dysrhythmias.
Arsenic exposure, 204
Arterial blood gases, 582t
maternal in asthma, 787
in persistent pulmonary hypertension of newborn, 516
in transient tachypnea of newborn, 509, 510
umbilical cord, 355-356, 356t

Arterial blood pressure, changes to during pregnancy, 98
Arteries that supply reproductive organs, 8
Arteriolar vasospasm in HELLP syndrome, 561
ASD. *See* Atrial septal defect.
Asherman syndrome, 14
Asian culture, 91t-95t
Aspartate aminotransferase in gestational hypertension and HELLP syndrome, 560, 573t
Asphyxia
biophysical profile in assessment of, 172-174, 173t
due to breech presentation, 243
due to maternal diabetes mellitus, 666
fetal response to, 164
in postterm infant, 487
related to malpresentation, 252
related to meconium aspiration syndrome, 511
in small-for-gestational-age infant, 468-470
surgery and anesthesia and, 729
Aspiration
meconium, 510-515, 511f
in large-for-gestational-age infants, 485-486
in postterm infant, 487, 489
transient tachypnea of newborn associated with, 508
Aspirin
as environmental hazard, 211
persistent pulmonary hypertension of newborn and, 515
Assault, 708, 709
Assessment
antepartum fetal, 161-200
biochemical, 174-186
biophysical, 167-174, 175f
case studies and sample questions regarding, 194-195
comparison of surveillance tests in, 165
electronic, 186-190
fetal movement assessment by client in, 165-166
health education in, 193
interventions/outcomes in, 190-193
nursing diagnoses in, 190
role of nurse in, 162-165
ethnocultural, 78-82
at first prenatal visit, 107-111, 109f
diagnostic procedures in, 114-115, 116f
history in, 107-110, 109f
physical examination in, 111-116
of intimate partner violence, 544-546
intrapartum fetal, 303-368
of newborn, 438-441, 440b, 442t-443t, 444b-445b, 445f, 446f

Assessment (*Continued*)
in delivery room, 425-426, 426t
postpartum, 376-378
preoperative, 730-731
Assignment of fetal position, 246f
Assisted hatching, 153
Assistive reproductive technology, dilemmas regarding, 887
AST. *See* Aspartate aminotransferase.
Asthma, 787-788, 792, 792b
Asynclitism, 246, 247f
Ativan. *See* Lorazepam.
Atony, uterine, postpartum hemorrhage due to, 850, 851
Atresia, esophageal, embryonic development of, 50
Atrial fibrillation, fetal, 325
Atrial flutter, fetal, 325, 325f, 331
Atrial septal defect, fetal, 454-455, 455f
Atrioventricular heart block, 328-329, 329f, 331-332
Attachment, postpartum, 375-376, 379-380
beginning process of, 289
cultural factors in, 82
failure to achieve, 381
impaired related to postpartum infection, 858
Attendant, labor, cultural factors regarding, 254-255
Attention-focusing activity during contractions, 258
Attitude, fetal, 242
Augmentation
of breast, breastfeeding and, 390
of uterine contractions, 290-293, 291t
Auscultation, cardiac
changes during pregnancy, 98
fetal, assessment of, 304-305
Autoimmune disease
antiphospholipid antibody syndrome as, 794
systemic lupus erythematosus as, 793-799
Autonomic nervous system, fetal heart rate and, 308, 315
Autonomy
ethics and, 874, 884
parental, 878-879, 884
Autosomal dominant inheritance, 28, 28f
Autosomal recessive inheritance, 29f, 29-30
Aventyl. *See* Nortriptyline hydrochloride.
AVPU assessment, 712

B
Babinski reflex, 440b
Baby blues, 376, 379, 861-864, 865
breastfeeding and, 404-405
Back
fetal, assessment of in Leopold's maneuvers, 251
neonatal, assessment of, 440

Bacterial vaginosis, 602t
    prematurity and, 472
Bacteriuria in urinary tract
    infection, 613, 614
Bag and mask ventilation for
    newborn, 426, 429
Ballistic wound, 710
Bandl's ring, 294-295, 295f
Barbased. *See* Butabarbital.
Barbiturates
    for analgesia during childbirth,
        278
    as environmental hazard, 216
Baroreceptors, fetal heart rate and,
        308
    variable decelerations and, 334
Bartholin's glands, anatomy of, 4
Basal metabolic rate, increased
        during pregnancy, 101
Base deficit, 356t
Base excess, 356t
Baseline fetal heart rate, 309-315,
        310f, 311f
Bathing of infant, ethnocultural
        factors in, 81
Battering. *See* Intimate partner
        violence.
Battery consent, 877
Battle sign, 713
Battledore placenta, 287f, 286286
Beautification, ritual, 82
Bed rest, preeclampsia and, 580, 580f
Behavior
    ethnocultural factors in, 79
    exhibited during anxiety, 256
    labor and delivery and, 25, 258
    neonatal
        assessment of, 440
        health education regarding, 461
        related to intrauterine fetal
            demise, 836
Beneficence, ethics and, 874
Benzene, 206
Benzphetamine hydrochloride as
        environmental hazard, 211
Benzthiazide as environmental
        hazard, 213
Best interest standard, 883, 884-885
Beta-adrenergic agonist in preterm
        labor, 821-822
Beta-blocking agents for maternal
        cardiovascular disease, 779t
Betadine. *See* Povidone-iodine.
Bicarbonate, 164, 356t, 582t
Bicornuate uterus, labor passage
        and, 234
Bigeminy
    premature atrial contractions
        with, 322f, 322-323, 323
    premature ventricle contractions
        with, 327, 327f
Bilateral cleft lip and palate, 449f
Bilateral tubal ligation, 412t
Bilirubin
    maternal
        in cholecystectomy, 736
        in gestational hypertension
            and HELLP syndrome,
            573t

Bilirubin (*Continued*)
    neonatal
        in hyperbilirubinemia, 518
        impaired skin integrity related
            to excretions of, 527
        normal levels of, 518
        production and conjugation of,
            518-520, 519f
Binding-in, term, 127
Biochemical fetal assessment,
        174-186
    amniocentesis in, 174-178, 176f
    chorionic villus sampling in, 181f,
        181-183
    cordocentesis and percutaneous
        umbilical blood sampling in,
        178-181, 180f, 355-357, 356t
    estriol assays in, 185
    fetal DNA in maternal circulation
        in, 186
    maternal serum alpha-fetoprotein
        screening in, 183-185
    triple marker test in, 185-186
Bioethics, 874, 883
Biophysical assessment, fetal,
        167-174, 175f
    biophysical profile in, 172-174, 173t
    Doppler ultrasound blood flow
        assessment in, 174, 175f
    ultrasound for, 167-171, 168t, 169f
Biophysical profile, 172-174, 173t
Biopsy, endometrial, 17
Biparietal diameter for estimation
        of gestational age, 162, 168
Birth control, 383, 409-418
    breastfeeding plans and, 410
    case study and study questions
        for, 416-418
    contraceptive history and, 409
    contraceptive knowledge and, 410
    contraceptives for, 411, 412t-415t
    obstetric and gynecological
        history and, 409-410
    postpartum fertility and, 410-411
    psychosocial responses
        regarding, 410
Birth defects, 61, 62f, 68-69, 441-460
    alcohol-related, 762, 764-765
    associated with maternal
        diabetes mellitus, 666
    cardiovascular, 453-460
        atrial septal defect, 454-455,
            455f
        coarctation of aorta, 456-457,
            457f
        embryonic development of, 49
        hypoplastic left heart
            syndrome, 459-460
        patent ductus arteriosus,
            453-454, 454f
        tetralogy of Fallot, 457-458, 458f
        transposition of great arteries,
            458-459, 459f
        ventricular septal defect,
            455-456, 456f
    cleft lip and cleft palate as,
        448-450, 449f
    congenital diaphragmatic hernia,
        451-453

Birth defects (*Continued*)
    drug abuse-related, 752
    fear of in advanced maternal age
        pregnancy, 155
    hydrocephalus as, 441-447
    intrauterine fetal surgery for,
        741-744
    related to exposure to teratogens,
        68
    in small-for-gestational-age
        infants, 467
    spina bifida as, 447-448, 448f
    ultrasonographic assessment of,
        171
Birth trauma
    macrosomia-associated, 248
    maternal diabetes mellitus and,
        666
    related to malpresentation, 252
Birth weight
    case studies and study questions
        associated with, 492-494
    cigarette smoking and, 761
    health education regarding,
        490-491
    large-for-gestational-age, 482-486
    in macrosomia, 246
    maternal diabetes mellitus and,
        666
    small-for-gestational-age, 465-471
    transient tachypnea of newborn
        and, 508
Bishop score, 290-291, 291t
Bituberous diameter, 236
Black American culture, 91t-95t
    AIDS in, 603, 604t
    intimate partner violence and, 541
Bladder
    changes to during pregnancy, 100
    postpartum assessment of, 376
    spasm of, 785-786
Blanket consent, 877
Blastocyst, 42-43, 44
Bleeding
    gastrointestinal, endoscopic
        procedures for, 740
    periventricular intraventricular,
        474
    postpartum, 634, 850-854, 864
    related to altered clotting factors
        secondary to heparin
        therapy or
        thrombocytopenia, 806
    related to hypertensive disorders
        of pregnancy, 567, 579-582,
        580f
    scleral, 438
    ultrasonographic assessment of,
        171
    vaginal in advanced maternal
        age pregnancy, 154
Bleeding disorders, 630-659
    abruptio placentae, 638-644, 652
    case studies and study questions
        regarding, 653-656
    disseminated intravascular
        coagulation, 644-647, 652-653
    gestational trophoblastic disease,
        647-651, 653

Bleeding disorders (*Continued*)
  health education regarding, 651-653
  placenta previa, 631-638, 651
    diagnostic procedures in, 635-636
    history in assessment of, 631-632
    ineffective fetal perfusion and oxygenation due to, 637-638
    ineffective maternal tissue perfusion related to, 636-637
    maternal anxiety related to, 638
    nursing diagnoses and interventions/outcomes for, 636-638
    physical findings in, 633-635
    physiologic response to blood loss due to, 632-633
    psychosocial findings in, 635
Bleeding time in gestational hypertension and HELLP syndrome, 573t
Blood
  fetal, percutaneous umbilical sampling of, 178-181, 180f, 192, 355-357, 356t
  maternal
    changes to during pregnancy, 99
    diagnostic procedures during first prenatal visit, 114
    disease of, 799-806
    preeclampsia and, 568
    surgery and, 729
    systemic lupus erythematosus-related symptoms in, 795
    trauma and, 706
  neonatal, disorders of
    related to maternal diabetes mellitus, 667
    respiratory distress due to, 498
  volume of
    postpartum changes in, 373
    during pregnancy, 98, 99
    surgery and, 729
Blood flow
  fetal, 53f, 53-55, 55t
    Doppler ultrasound in assessment of, 174, 175f
  maternal, fetal DNA in, testing of, 186
  placental, 53, 54f
    periodic fetal heart rate patterns and, 338, 340
    placental transfer in, 54-55, 55t
    disorders of, 55-56
Blood glucose
  in diabetes mellitus
    gestational, 675-676
    pregestational, 671
  neonatal, 427
    in large-for-gestational-age infant, 485
    monitoring of in infants of diabetic mothers, 667
  in preterm infant, 475

Blood glucose (*Continued*)
  in respiratory distress syndrome, 502, 507
  in small-for-gestational-age infant, 470
  values of in pregnancy, 661t
Blood loss
  in abruptio placentae, 640
  associated with uterine rupture, 842-843
  cesarean birth-related, 298
  in hemorrhagic disorders, 630, 633-634
  during menstruation, 11
  in placenta previa, 630-638
  during placental expulsion, 288
  in postpartum hemorrhage, 853
Blood pressure
  maternal
    assessment of at first prenatal visit, 111
    changes to during pregnancy, 98
    in chronic hypertension, 559
    during first stage of labor, 274
    in gestational hypertension, 555, 558, 559, 570-571
    postpartum assessment of, 288, 376
    postpartum changes in, 374
    prehypertension, 559
  neonatal, assessment of in respiratory distress syndrome, 503
Blood supply, female reproductive, 8
Blood transfusion
  in abruptio placentae, 642-643
  for anemia associated with respiratory distress syndrome, 504
  intrauterine, 179
  of platelets in HELLP syndrome, 561
Blood type, maternal, hyperbilirubinemia and, 523
Blood urea nitrogen, increased in preeclampsia, 564, 573t
Blood vessels
  damage to in disseminated intravascular coagulation, 645
  embryonic development of, 48-49, 49f
Bloody show, 272, 275
Blunt trauma, 703-704, 709
  abdominal, abruptio placentae due to, 639
BMI. *See* Body mass index.
BMR. *See* Basal metabolic rate.
BMV. *See* Bag and mask ventilation for newborn.
Body mass index, 103
Body temperature
  elevated. *See* Fever.
  maternal
    assessment of at first prenatal visit, 111
    in chorioamnionitis, 621
    dangerous postpartum, 382

Body temperature (*Continued*)
  postpartum changes in, 374
  in urinary tract infection, 612
  neonatal, 422, 438
    in premature infant, 478
    in small-for-gestational-age infant, 470
  regulation of. *See* Thermoregulation.
Bone growth, adolescent pregnancy and, 149-150
Bony pelvis. *See Also* Pelvis.
  anatomy and physiology of, 9f, 9-10, 10f
  examination of
    at first prenatal visit, 111
    in reproductive assessment, 16
Borrelia burgdorferi, 619t
Bottle-feeding, 423, 424-425
Bowel
  inflammatory disease of, 807-811
  postpartum assessment of, 376
Bowel sounds, neonatal, 439
BPD. *See* Bronchopulmonary dysplasia.
BPP. *See* Biophysical profile.
Brachial plexus injury in large-for-gestational-age infant, 484
Bradley technique, 133
Bradycardia, fetal, 311-314, 312f
  sinus, 320
Brain, fetal development of, 56, 57, 58, 59, 60. *See Also* Central nervous system.
Braxton Hicks contractions, 97, 271-272
Breast
  assessment of for breastfeeding, 390
  changes to
    postpartum, 373
    during pregnancy, 97-98
  neonatal
    assessment of, 439, 443t
    prematurity and, 476
  pain in secondary to breastfeeding, 397-399
  postpartum assessment of, 376
  postpartum infection of, 856
Breast milk
  inability of mother to provide adequate supply of, 402-403
  jaundice associated with, 518, 524
  production and ejection of, 388f, 388-389
Breastfeeding, 387-408, 423-424
  assessment regarding, 389-391
  caloric needs in, 423
  case study and study questions for, 406-407
  ethnocultural factors in, 81, 94t, 425
  family planning and, 410
  health education associated with, 405-406
  interventions/outcomes regarding, 391-405
    following cesarean section, 399
    for fussy or irritable infant, 400

Breastfeeding (*Continued*)
for incorrect latching on, 394-396
for infant positioning, 391f, 391-394, 392f, 393f, 394f, 395f
maternal anxiety and, 396-397
for maternal low self-esteem related to inability to supply adequate milk, 402-403
for multiple births, 402
for nipple or breast pain, 397-399
nutrition and, 404-405
physiologic jaundice and, 400-401
for preterm or hospitalized infant, 401-402, 402f
sexual identity and, 405
for sleepy or reluctant infant, 399-400
for special needs infant, 402-403
jaundice associated with, 518, 524
nursing diagnoses associated with, 391
phenylketonuria and, 691, 693
physiology of, 387-389, 388f
pregestational diabetes mellitus and, 695-696
return of ovulation and menstrual cycle and, 372
tuberculosis and, 789
Breath sounds, neonatal, 439
Breathing, periodic, in newborn, 429
premature, 477
Breathing pattern, ineffective
related to shallow or periodic breathing and apnea, 429
related to trauma in pregnancy, 717-719
Breathing strategies in childbirth education, 132-133
Breech presentation, 242-244, 244f
ultrasonographic assessment of, 170
Bronchopulmonary dysplasia, 500
Brow presentation, 242
Brown fat, prematurity and, 474
B-scan, ultrasonographic, 167
Bulimia nervosa, 131-132
Bulk flow in placental transfer, 55, 55t
BUN. *See* Blood urea nitrogen.
Burns, 708-709, 710
Burr red blood cell, 560
Butabarbital as environmental hazard, 216
Butagesic. *See* Phenylbutazone.
Butatran. *See* Butabarbital.
Butazolidin. *See* Phenylbutazone.
Butorphanol for analgesia during childbirth, 278

C
Cadmium, 204
Caffeine, breastfeeding and, 404

Calcium
monitoring of in respiratory distress syndrome, 507
requirements of during pregnancy, 106
gestational hypertension and, 569
Calcium channel blockers
for maternal cardiovascular disease, 780t
in preterm labor therapy, 822
Calculi, renal, 782, 785-786
Caldwell-Moloy classification of pelvis, 235f
Caloric intake
maternal
in adolescent pregnancy, 148
excessive, 107, 117
in gestational diabetes mellitus, 675
inadequate, 107
during lactation, 404
requirements of, 70, 104, 105
in type 1 and type 2 diabetes, 663-664
newborn, 423
in persistent pulmonary hypertension of newborn, 517
in respiratory distress syndrome, 506, 507
small-for-gestational-age, 470
Cancer. *See* Carcinoma.
Cannabis sativa, 753
Capacity, informed consent and, 876-878
Capillary hemangioma, 438
Caput succedaneum, 248-249, 438
on large-for-gestational-age infant, 483
Carbohydrates
altered metabolism of
in gestational diabetes mellitus, 674
in pregestational diabetes mellitus, 668-669
metabolism of in pregnancy, 662
required intake during pregnancy, 70
Carbon dioxide, partial pressure of, 582t
maternal
asthma and, 787
surgery and, 729
traumatic injury and, 706
neonatal in transient tachypnea of newborn, 510
umbilical cord, 356t
Carbon monoxide
in cigarettes, 760
intoxication, 708
Carcinogen, 203
Carcinoma
colorectal, 741
gastric, 741
secondary to trophoblastic disease, 651

Cardiac output
cardiac disease and, 777-778, 779t-780t
changes to during pregnancy, 98
surgery and, 728-729
newborn, decreased, 429-432
normal values in pregnancy, 574t
postpartum changes in, 373
Cardiff method of fetal movement assessment, 166
Cardinal movements, fetal, 249
risk for situational low self-esteem related to impairment of, 252-253
Cardiomyopathy in infants of diabetic mothers, 667
Cardiovascular system
embryonic development of, 48-49, 49f
fetal
development of, 56, 59
maternal drug use and, 752
maternal
changes to during first stage of labor, 273-274
changes to during pregnancy, 98-99
disease of, 773-781, 774b, 775t, 776t, 779t-780t
in nutritional status assessment, 112t
postpartum changes to, 373-374
preeclampsia-related disturbances of, 563, 581-582
surgery and, 728-729
systemic lupus erythematosus-related disease of, 795
trauma and, 705, 711-712
neonatal
assessment of, 439
congenital malformations of, 453-460
in preterm infant, 473
respiratory distress related to disease of, 498
transition of fetal to, 422
Care of newborn
ethnocultural factors in, 77, 81-82, 94t
health education regarding, 383
thrombophlebitis and, 860-861
Care-based approach to ethics, 876
Career, advanced maternal age and, 153-154
Carrier, gestational, 153
Case law, 881
Case-based ethics, 875
Casuistry-based approach to ethics, 875
Catecholamines
cocaine and, 752
fetal heart rate and, 308-309
Catheterization
Foley in abruptio placentae, 642
for intrauterine pressure monitoring during labor, 232
risk of infection related to, 233
Swan-Ganz

Catheterization (*Continued*)
  in abruptio placentae, 642
  in gestational hypertension, 574
  normal values of, 574t
Caudal anesthesia, 278
Cavity planes, pelvic, 236, 237f
CBC. *See* Complete blood count
  with differential.
CDH. *See* Congenital diaphragmatic
  hernia.
Cefixime for gonorrhea, 601t
Ceftriaxone for gonorrhea, 601t
Cell division, 24f, 24-25, 25f
Centers for Disease Control and
  Prevention, 623
Centers on Addiction and
  Substance Abuse, 767
Central nervous system
  fetal
    development of, 56, 57, 58, 59, 60
    fetal heart rate and, 308
    response of to diminished
      oxygen supply, 164
  maternal, preeclampsia's effect
    on, 565-567, 579-581, 580f
  neonatal
    fetal alcohol syndrome and, 763
    respiratory distress related to
      disease of, 499
Central venous pressure
  in abruptio placentae, 642
  normal values in pregnancy, 574t
Cephalic presentation, 242, 243f
Cephalic prominence assessment in
  Leopold's maneuvers, 251
Cephalohematoma, 438
  on large-for-gestational-age
    infant, 483
Cephalosporin for acute
  pyelonephritis, 613
Cerclage, cervical, 739-740
Cerebral edema associated with
  hypertensive disorders of
  pregnancy, 579-581, 580f
Cerebral hemorrhage associated
  with hypertensive disorders of
  pregnancy, 567, 579-581, 580f
Cervical smear, 115
Cervical spine stabilization in
  maternal traumatic injury, 711,
  718f
Cervix
  anatomy and physiology of, 6
  cerclage of, 739-740
  changes to
    postpartum, 372
    during pregnancy, 97
  dilatation of, 240f, 240-241, 273-281
    active phase of, 276-277
    analgesia or anesthesia for,
      277-279
    assessment of, 240f, 240-241
    Bishop score for, 291t
    interventions/outcomes in,
      279-281
    latent phase of, 274-276
    nursing diagnoses related to,
      279
    pain resulting from, 280-281

Cervix (*Continued*)
    physiologic changes during,
      273-274
    during second stage of labor, 281
    transition phase of labor, 277
  effacement of, 240
    during active phase of labor, 276
    Bishop score for, 291t
    for infant expulsion, 281
    during latent phase of labor, 272
    during transition phase of
      labor, 277
  effects of trauma or injury to on
    labor and delivery, 234
  examination of, 16
  incompetent due to repetitive
    dilatation and curettage, 14
  injury to related to
    malpresentation, 252
  postpartum infection of, 855
  premonitory signs of childbirth
    involving, 272
Cesarean birth, 296-299
  in abruptio placentae, 642
  in advanced maternal age
    pregnancy, 154
  breastfeeding following, 399
  incision site for
    pain related to, 376
    postpartum examination of, 376
  in multiple gestation, 833
  platelet transfusions for HELLP
    syndrome and, 561
  postpartum infection from, 856
  respiratory distress syndrome
    and, 501
  in uterine rupture, 843
  vaginal birth after, 296
Chadwick's sign, 97
Character-based ethics, 875
Chemoreceptors, fetal heart rate
    and, 308
  variable decelerations and, 334
Chemstrip, 427
Chenodeoxycholic acid as
    environmental hazard, 215
Chenodiol as environmental
    hazard, 215
Chest
  flail, 718-719
  maternal assessment following
    traumatic injury, 713
  neonatal
    assessment of, 439
    circumference of, 438
    compressions of, 425, 432
Chest radiography
  in meconium aspiration
    syndrome, 513
  in persistent pulmonary
    hypertension of newborn,
    516
  in respiratory distress syndrome
    assessment, 502
  in transient tachypnea of
    newborn, 509
Chest wall of premature infant, 473
CHF. *See* Congestive heart failure.
Chickenpox, maternal, 615t

Childbearing family, 125
Childbirth, 225-368
  assessment in, 228-232, 241-252
  cardinal movements and, 249
  case studies and study questions
    for, 264-268, 299-301
  cervical changes during, 240f,
    240-241
  complications of, 818-849
    amniotic fluid embolism,
      839-841
    case studies and study
      questions for, 844-848
    intrauterine fetal demise,
      835-839
    multiple gestation, 831-835
    postterm pregnancy, 825-827
    premature rupture of
      membrane, 827-831
    preterm labor, 818-825
    uterine rupture, 841-844
  contractions in
    frequency of, 232
    onset of, 228-229
    physiology of, 229f, 229-231
    strength of, 232-233
  diagnostic studies and
    techniques during, 232,
    249-252, 250f, 251f
  dilatation as first stage of,
    273-281
    analgesia or anesthesia for,
      277-279
    interventions/outcomes in,
      279-281
    latent phase of, 274-276
    nursing diagnoses related to,
      279
    physiologic changes during,
      273-274
    transition phase of labor, 277
  dysfunctional grieving related to
    loss of desired, 138
  effects of maternal
    musculoskeletal deformities
    and disease on, 234
  ethnocultural factors in, 76-78,
    77f, 79-80, 92t
  false labor in, 231
  fathers at, 128-129
  fetal assessment during
    arrhythmias and dysrhythmias
      and, 319-329
    baseline fetal heart rate and,
      309-315, 310f, 311f
    case studies and study
      questions related to,
      357-364, 358f, 359f, 360f,
      361f, 362f, 363f, 364f
    electronic methods of, 305-308
    fetal scalp sampling for, 351-353
    health education regarding, 357
    nonelectronic methods of,
      304-305
    nonperiodic fetal heart rate
      patterns and, 344-349
    periodic fetal heart rate
      patterns and, 332-344
    pulse oximetry in, 353-355

Childbirth (*Continued*)
umbilical cord blood sampling
in, 355-357, 356t
uterine activity and, 350f,
350-351, 351f
variability of fetal heart rate
and, 314-329, 316f, 317f,
318f, 319f
fetal attitude and, 242
fetal lie and, 242
fetal position and, 245, 246f
fetal presentation and, 242-245,
243f, 244f, 245f
fetal size assessment in, 246-248
fetal skull and, 248-249
fetal station and, 245-246, 247f
"4 Ps" of, 228
health education regarding,
262-263, 263f, 299
immediate postpartum period as
fourth stage of, 288-290
infant expulsion as second stage
of, 281-286
interventions/outcomes in, 233-
234, 241, 252-253, 272-273
nursing diagnoses during, 233,
241, 252, 272
optimizing power during, 262-263,
263f
pain of, fear related to, 261
pelvis and, 234-240
dimension of, 236f, 236-240, 237f
manual determination of
capacity of, 241
shape of, 234-236, 235f
physical examination in, 231-232,
234-240, 242-249
placental expulsion as third stage
of, 286-288, 287f
premonitory signs of, 271-273
preparation education for, 132-133
previous pregnancies and, 241-242
psychosocial factors in, 253-258,
253-262
behaviors, 258
current pregnancy experience,
253
emotions of labor, 255-256
expectations for birth
experience, 254
interventions/outcomes
related to, 259-262
nursing diagnoses related to,
258-259
personality styles, 257-258
preparation for birth, 254
previous birth experiences, 253
psychologic reactions to labor,
256-257
support system, 254-255
variables influencing, 290-299
cesarean birth, 296-299
dysfunctional labor, 293-296,
294f, 295f
induction or augmentation of
uterine contractions,
290-293, 291t
Children who witness parental
violence, 542

Chlamydia, 601t
Chloasma, pregnancy-induced, 101
Chlordiazepoxide hydrochloride as
environmental hazard, 213
Chloride monitoring in respiratory
distress syndrome, 507
Chloroprene, 204
Cholecystectomy, 735-736
Choledocholithiasis, 740
Cholelithiasis, 740
Chorioadenoma destruens, 648,
649-650
Chorioamnionitis, 620-622, 625
Chorioangioma, 650
Choriocarcinoma, 648-650
Chorionic villi, 45, 45f
Chorionic villus sampling, 181f,
181-183
Chromosomes, 26-28, 27f
Chronic hypertension, 559, 574-575,
576t-578t
with superimposed preeclampsia
or eclampsia, 560
Cigarette smoking, 70, 760-762,
768-769
abruptio placentae and, 639
breastfeeding and, 404
hemorrhagic disorders and, 632
passive, 217-218, 219, 221
prematurity and, 472
Circulation
of amniotic fluid, 65f
female reproductive, 8
fetal, 53f, 53-55, 55t
Doppler ultrasound in
assessment of, 174, 175f
transition from to neonatal, 422
maternal
fetal DNA in, testing of, 186
placental, 53, 54f
trauma and, 711-712
placental transfer in, 54-55, 55t
disorders of, 55-56
Circumcision, ethnocultural factors
in, 81
Circumvallate placenta, 286
Clavicular fracture in large-for-
gestational-age infant, 484, 486
Clean catch urine specimen, 571
Cleft lip and palate, 448-450, 449f
Clitoris, 4
Clothing for newborn,
ethnocultural factors in, 94t
Clotting factors
altered, due to heparin therapy
or thrombocytopenia, 806
in disseminated intravascular
coagulation *versus* HELLP
syndrome, 563t
increased due to pregnancy, 99
Clotting time in disseminated
intravascular coagulation, 645
CMV. *See* Cytomegalovirus.
Coach, expectant father as, 128
Coagulation, disseminated
intravascular, 644-647, 652-653,
838
as cause of postpartum
hemorrhage, 851, 852

Coagulation (*Continued*)
HELLP syndrome *versus,* 561,
563t
related to intrauterine fetal
demise, 836
Coagulation factors
altered, due to heparin therapy
or thrombocytopenia, 806
in disseminated intravascular
coagulation *versus* HELLP
syndrome, 563t
increased due to pregnancy, 99
Coarctation of aorta, 456-457, 457f
Cocaine Hotline, 767
Cocaine use, 751-752, 754f
Code of Ethics, 888
Codes, ethical, 881
Coelom, 48
Cold, therapeutic, ethnocultural
considerations in, 81
Cold stress in premature infant, 474
Colic, renal, 785-786
Colitis, ulcerative, 807-811
Colloid osmotic pressure,
preeclampsia and, 563, 564-565,
565t
Colonoscopy, 741
Colorants, 203
Colorectal cancer, 741
Colostrum
ethnocultural factors regarding,
81
production of during pregnancy,
98, 389
Columnar epithelium, cervical, 6
Combined variability of fetal heart
rate, 317
Comfort, impaired
abruptio placentae-associated,
643-644
in gastrointestinal disease, 810
immobility-related, 314
incorrect latching and, 394-396
in invasive procedures, 193
in maternal immobility for fetal
heart rate problems, 314
in nipple or breast pain
associated with
breastfeeding, 397-399
renal disease-related, 785-786
in sexually transmitted disease,
611
systemic lupus erythematosus-
associated, 797
Committee, ethics, 885
Common law, 880-881
Communication
impaired due to language barrier,
83
social isolation related to
changing patterns of, 262
Community resources
associated with environmental
hazard, 218, 218b
for newborn care, 434, 461
related to substance abuse, 767
Competence
cultural and linguistic, 76
informed consent and, 876

Complete blood count with differential
  in appendectomy, 739
  in cholecystectomy, 736
  in hyperbilirubinemia, 526
  in urinary tract infection, 613
Complete breech presentation, 243
Complete heart block, 328
Complex genetic disorders, 31-32
Complications of childbearing, 535-893
  assessment of at first prenatal visit, 107-108
  cardiac, 773-781
  endocrine and metabolic disorders, 660-702
  gastrointestinal, 806-811
  hematologic, 799-806
  hemorrhagic disorders, 630-659
  hepatic, 811-814, 812t
  hypertensive disorders, 554-591
  intimate partner violence, 537-553
  during labor and delivery, 818-849
    amniotic fluid embolism, 839-841
    intrauterine fetal demise, 835-839
    multiple gestation, 831-835
    postterm pregnancy, 825-827
    premature rupture of membrane, 827-831
    preterm labor, 818-825
    uterine rupture, 841-844
  maternal infections, 592-629
  obesity and, 113
  postpartum, 850-870
    case study and study questions regarding, 865-868
    depression, 861-864
    health education for, 864-865
    hemorrhage, 85-854
    infection, 854-858
    thrombophlebitis, 858-861
  renal, 781-787
  respiratory, 787-793
  substance abuse, 750-770
  surgery, 727-749
  systemic lupus erythematosus and antiphospholipid antibody syndrome, 793-799
  traumatic injury, 703-726
Compound fetal presentation, 245
Compromised family coping
  related to fear of fetal loss, 191-192
  related to significant other excluded from testing sessions, 191-192
Computed tomography in trauma in pregnancy, 715
Conception, 41-42, 42f
  counseling before
    in inflammatory bowel disease, 810-811
    in renal disease, 786
    in systemic lupus erythematosus, 799
  maternal body changes following, 96
  problems with

Conception (Continued)
  in advanced maternal age, 152-153
  psyche during labor and delivery and, 253
Condom, 414t
  female, 414t
  spermicide with, 413t
Conduction heat loss, neonatal, 423
Condyloma acuminatum, 600t-601t
Confidentiality, ethics and, 875
Congenital anomalies, 61, 62f, 68-69, 441-460
  alcohol-related, 762, 764-765
  associated with maternal diabetes mellitus, 666
  cardiovascular, 453-460
    atrial septal defect, 454-455, 455f
    coarctation of aorta, 456-457, 457f
    embryonic development of, 49
    hypoplastic left heart syndrome, 459-460
    patent ductus arteriosus, 453-454, 454f
    tetralogy of Fallot, 457-458, 458f
    transposition of great arteries, 458-459, 459f
    ventricular septal defect, 455-456, 456f
  cleft lip and cleft palate, 448-450, 449f
  congenital diaphragmatic hernia, 451-453
  drug abuse-related, 752
  fear of in advanced maternal age pregnancy, 155
  hydrocephalus, 441-447
  intrauterine fetal surgery for, 741-744
  related to exposure to teratogens, 68
  in small-for-gestational-age infants, 467
  spina bifida, 447-448, 448f
  ultrasonographic assessment of, 171
Congenital diaphragmatic hernia, 451-453
  fetal surgery for, 742
Congestive heart failure, 776, 777-778, 779t-780t
Conjugated bilirubin, 518, 519f, 519-520
Consciousness, altered, associated with disseminated intravascular coagulation, 647
Consent, informed, 876-877
Consequences-based approach to ethics, 875
Consequentialism-based approach to ethics, 875
Constipation, 117, 377-378
Constitutional law, 880
Consumption coagulopathy. See Disseminated intravascular coagulation.
Continuous positive airway pressure, 503

Contraception
  contraceptives for, 411, 412t-415t
    history of use, family planning and, 409
    knowledge concerning, 410
    use of by adolescents, 148
    dilemmas regarding, 887
Contraction stress test, 188-190
Contractions, 350f, 350-351, 351f
  assessment of, 306-307
    during active phase of labor, 275
    for infant expulsion, 282
    during latent phase of labor, 275
    during transition phase of labor, 277
  behaviors during, 258
  Braxton Hicks, 97, 271-272
  frequency of, 232
  induction or augmentation of, 290-293, 291t
  manual palpation of, 232
    by patient, 824
  monitoring of, 232
    following traumatic injury, 716
    risk of infection related to internal, 233
  onset of, 228-229
  pain resulting from, 280-281, 292
  periodic fetal heart rate patterns associated with, 332-344
    accelerations, 332-333, 333f
    combined decelerations, 343f, 343-344
    early decelerations, 342f, 342-343
    late decelerations, 337-342, 338f, 339f, 341b
    variable decelerations, 333-337, 334f, 335f, 337b
  physiology of, 229f, 229-231
  risk for situational low self-esteem related to ineffective pattern of, 233-234
  strength of, 232-233
Controlling personality, 258
Convection heat loss, neonatal, 422
COP. See Colloid osmotic pressure.
Coping
  family
    compromised
      related to fear of fetal loss, 191-192
      related to significant other excluded from testing sessions, 191-192
    ineffective related to physical and/or mental handicap of family member, 35
    related to opportunity for growth/mastery, 136-137
  ineffective
    associated with smoking, 762
    during labor and delivery, 258, 260-261
    related to conflict between personal and cultural expectations, 260-261
    related to health care system's practices, 260-261

Coping (*Continued*)
related to inadequate support systems or absence of a support person, 260-261
related to postpartum mood alteration, 381
systemic lupus erythematosus-associated, 797-798
Copper intrauterine device, 413t
Cord, 63-64
compression of
ineffective tissue perfusion related to, 826-827, 830
in postterm pregnancy, 826-827
embryonic development of, 43
ethnocultural factors regarding, 80, 81-82
hyperbilirubinemia associated with delayed clamping of, 524
inadequate perfusion of, risk for impaired fetal gas exchange related to, 335-336, 337b
velamentous insertion of, 64, 286, 287f, 635
Cord blood sampling, 178-181, 180f, 355-357, 356t
risk for deficient fluid volume related to, 192
Cordocentesis, 178-181, 180f
Corneal injury related to phototherapy, 527
Corona radiata, 41, 42f
Corpus, uterine, 6
Corpus luteum
cysts of, 736
pregnancy and, 97
role in menstruation, 11
Corticosteroids for systemic lupus erythematosus, risk for infection due to, 796-797
Corticotropin-releasing hormone, adrenal insufficiency and, 688
Cortisol in onset of labor, 229
Coumarin as environmental hazard, 212
Counseling
acquired immunodeficiency syndrome, 603
phenylketonuria and, 698-699
preconceptual
in inflammatory bowel disease, 810
in renal disease, 786
in systemic lupus erythematosus, 799
during testing sessions, 193
Court-ordered obstetrical treatment, 887
Couvelaire uterus, 641-642
CPAP. *See* Continuous positive airway pressure.
Cradle-hold position for breastfeeding, 391f, 391-392, 392f
Cranial bones, labor and delivery and, 248
Creatinine, increased in preeclampsia, 564, 573t

CRH. *See* Corticotropin-releasing hormone, adrenal insufficiency and.
Crib, open, 423
CRL. *See* Crown rump length.
Crohn's disease, 807-811
Cross cradle-hold position for breastfeeding, 392-393, 393f, 394f
Crown rump length, 162, 168t
Crying, assessment of, 440-441
Cryopreservation of embryo, 153
CST. *See* Contraction stress test.
CT. *See* Computed tomography.
Cultural considerations. *See* Ethnocultural considerations.
Culture-specific, term, 75
Culture-universal, term, 75
Cushing's syndrome, 685-688, 698
Cutis marmorata, 438
CVP. *See* Central venous pressure.
CVS. *See* Chorionic villus sampling.
Cyanocobalamin for megaloblastic anemia, 800
Cyanosis
in respiratory distress syndrome, 501-502
in tetralogy of Fallot, 458
Cycle of violence, 538-540, 539f
Cyclopia, 49
Cystectomy, ovarian, 736-737
Cystitis, postpartum, 855
Cystocele, 15
Cytomegalovirus in TORCH, 592-599, 593t-597t
Cytotrophoblast, 43, 44

D

Daily fetal movement recording, 166
Danger Assessment tool, 547, 548f
Data collection, cultural, 76
Dating, gestational, assessment of, 111, 825
using ultrasound, 167-168, 168t, 825
Death
maternal
AIDS-associated, 599, 603
cardiac-related, 774
due to diabetes mellitus, 666
pregnancy-induced hypertension as cause of, 555
related to obstetric hemorrhage, 630
related to postpartum hemorrhage, 850
traumatic, 703
perinatal, 835-839, 846
maternal traumatic injury and, 703
ultrasonographic confirmation of, 170
Decelerations of fetal heart rate
fetal hypoxia and, 165
nonperiodic
prolonged, 347-349, 348f
variable, 345-347, 346f

Decelerations of fetal heart rate (*Continued*)
periodic
combined, 343f, 343-344
early, 342f, 342-343
late, 337-342, 338f, 339f, 341b
variable, 333-337, 334f, 335f, 337b
Decidua, 44, 44f, 97
Decisional conflict related to adverse test outcome, 192-193
Decision-making
ethical, 883-884
interventions to help adolescents with, 150, 151
by proxy, 878-880
Decongestants as environmental hazard, 214
Decreased variability of fetal heart rate, 315, 316f
Deep tendon reflexes, assessment of in magnesium sulfate therapy, 821
Deep venous thrombosis, 801-802, 803, 804-805, 858-861
Defibrination syndrome. *See* Disseminated intravascular coagulation.
Deficient fluid volume
maternal
in amniocentesis and PUBS, 192
due to fluid shift in early postpartum period, 289-290
in evacuation of hydatidiform mole, 650
in inflammatory bowel disease, 808-809
in kidney disease, 784-785
in postpartum hemorrhage, 852-853
related to blood loss, 288
related to decreased intake or abnormal loss, 281
in surgical procedure and blood loss, 298
in traumatic injury, 719-720, 720f
neonatal, associated with phototherapy light exposure, 526
Deficient knowledge
acquired immunodeficiency syndrome and, 607-608
adrenal insufficiency and, 690
alcohol use and its effects on pregnancy and, 766
birthing process related to inadequate preparation or unanticipated circumstances and, 261
cesarean birth and, 297-298
chorioamnionitis and, 622
contraceptives and, 411
diabetes mellitus and
gestational, 675-676
pregestational, 670
disease complicating pregnancy and, 773
dysfunctional labor and, 295
genetic assessment and, 34-35

Deficient knowledge (*Continued*)
hazardous effects of
pharmaceuticals and, 216-217
hyperadrenocorticism and, 687-688
hyperthyroidism and, 681-682
inexperience with newborn care
and lack of parenting skills
and, 432
maternal experience in
positioning infant for
breastfeeding and, 391f,
391-394, 392f, 393f, 394f, 395f
maternal phenylketonuria and, 694
normal anatomy and physiology
of female reproductive
system and, 17-18
normal menstrual cycle and, 18
normal physiologic response to
pregnancy and, 116-117
occupational hazards and, 207-208
second hand smoke exposure
and, 218
sexually transmitted diseases
and, 611
smoking during pregnancy and,
761
specific high-risk pregnancy
condition and treatment
options and, 191
substance abuse and, 755, 756b
temperature extremes and, 209-210
TORCH disease and, 598-599
urinary tract infection and
pyelonephritis and, 613
Deficient skill related to maternal
experience in positioning
infant for breastfeeding, 391f,
391-394, 392f, 393f, 394f, 395f
Dehiscence, cesarean, postpartum
infection following, 856, 857
Dehydroepiandrosterone sulfate, 17
Delivery. *See* Labor and delivery.
Delivery date, expected
in advanced maternal age
pregnancy, 154
assessment of, 111
using ultrasound, 167-168, 168t
Delivery room
assessment of newborn in,
425-426, 426t, 433
neonatal resuscitation in, 428f,
430t-431t
congenital diaphragmatic
hernia, 452
Demerol. *See* Meperidine.
Deontologic approach to ethics,
874-875
Deoxyribonucleic acid, 26
fetal in maternal circulation,
testing of, 186
in human immunodeficiency
virus, 599
Depakene. *See* Valproic acid.
Dependent phase of mother, 375
Dependent-independent phase of
mother, 375
Depo-Provera, 415t
Depression, postpartum, 376, 379,
861-864, 865
breastfeeding and, 404-405

DES. *See* Diethylstilbestrol.
Descent of fetus, 249
Descriptive ethics, 874
Desires during pregnancy, 125-126
Detailed consent, 877
Developmental assessment in
adolescent pregnancy, 149
Developmental crisis, pregnancy as,
126
Developmental tasks of pregnancy
maternal, 126, 138, 139
in adolescent pregnancy, 149
paternal, 128, 138, 139
Dexedrine. *See*
Dextroamphetamine.
Dextroamphetamine as
environmental hazard, 210
Dextrostix, 427
DFMR. *See* Daily fetal movement
recording.
DHEAS. *See*
Dehydroepiandrosterone
sulfate.
Diabetes mellitus, 660-676
in advanced maternal age, 154
classification of, 661t, 661-661
ethnic factors in, 95t
gestational, 661, 671-676, 696, 696t
hyperbilirubinemia and, 523
maternal metabolism and
pathophysiology of
pregnancy and, 662
pregestational, 663-671
altered metabolism in, 668-669
anxiety related to, 669-670
deficient knowledge regarding,
670
definition and prognosis for, 663
diagnostic procedures in, 668
history in, 663-665
incidence of, 663, 664t
interrupted family processes
related to, 671
nursing diagnoses and
interventions/outcomes
for, 668-671
physical findings in, 665-667
powerlessness related to, 670
psychosocial considerations in,
668
risk for fetal injury in, 671
primary goals of treatment of, 662
symptoms of, 660
Diabetic ketoacidosis, 663
Diagnostic peritoneal lavage, 716-717
Diagnostic procedures, 161-200
in abruptio placentae, 641
in adrenal insufficiency, 689
in AIDS, 606-607
in amniotic fluid embolism,
839-840
in appendectomy, 739
in assessment of reproductive
anatomy, physiology, and
menstrual cycle, 16-17
associated with alcohol use, 765
biochemical, 174-186
amniocentesis in, 174-178, 176f
chorionic villus sampling in,
181f, 181-183

Diagnostic procedures (*Continued*)
cordocentesis and
percutaneous umbilical
blood sampling in,
178-181, 180f, 355-357, 356t
estriol assays in, 185
fetal DNA in maternal
circulation in, 186
maternal serum alpha-
fetoprotein screening in,
183-185
triple marker test in, 185-186
biophysical, 167-174, 175f
biophysical profile in, 172-174,
173t
Doppler ultrasound blood flow
assessment in, 174, 175f
ultrasound for, 167-171, 168t,
169f
in cholecystectomy, 736
comparison of surveillance tests
in, 165
in comprehensive general health
examination at first prenatal
visit, 114-115
in diabetes mellitus
gestational, 672-673
pregestational, 668
in disseminated intravascular
coagulation, 646
electronic, 186-190
contraction stress test in,
188-190
nonstress test in, 187-188
in endoscopic gastrointestinal
procedures, 741
during expulsion of infant,
283-284
in fetal and placental assessment,
67
fetal movement assessment by
client in, 165-166
following trauma in pregnancy,
714-717
in gestational hypertension, 573t,
573-574
in hematologic complications, 803,
803t
in hepatitis, 813
in hyperthyroidism, 680
in hypothyroidism, 684
interventions/outcomes in,
190-193
in intrauterine fetal demise, 836
during labor and delivery, 232,
249-252, 250f, 251f
in multiple gestation pregnancy,
832-833
nursing diagnoses in, 190
in ovaries cystectomy or
oophorectomy, 737
during periodic prenatal revisits,
115-116, 116f
in placenta previa, 635-636
postpartum, 377
in hemorrhage, 852
in infection, 856
in premature infant, 478
in premature rupture of
membrane, 829

Diagnostic procedures (*Continued*)
for preterm infant, 478
in preterm labor, 820
in renal disease, 783-784
for respiratory distress
    syndrome, 502
role of nurse in, 162-165
in small-for-gestational-age
    infant, 469
in systemic lupus erythematosus,
    796
in thrombophlebitis, 859
Diagnostic studies
in fetal and placental assessment,
    67
in genetic assessment, 32-34
in substance abuse, 755
Diaphragm, pelvic, 8, 9f
Diaphragm with spermicide, 413t
Diaphragmatic hernia, congenital,
    451-453
fetal surgery for, 742
Diarrhea
associated with
    hyperbilirubinemia, 527
due to gastrointestinal disease,
    809-810
inflammatory bowel disease-
    associated, 808-809
Diastolic blood pressure
changes to during pregnancy, 98
in chronic hypertension, 559
in gestational hypertension, 555,
    558, 559
Diazepam as environmental
    hazard, 212, 213
DIC. *See* Disseminated
    intravascular coagulation.
Dicumarol as environmental
    hazard, 212
Didrex. *See* Benzphetamine
    hydrochloride.
Diet. *See Also* Nutrition.
in adolescent pregnancy, 148
ethnocultural factors in, 79, 80-81,
    83-84, 91t, 92t, 93t
for phenylketonuria, 691, 692,
    694-695
type 1 and type 2 diabetes and,
    663-664
vegetarian, 104, 105f, 113
Diethylstilbestrol as environmental
    hazard, 215
Diffusion in placental transfer, 55, 55t
Dilantin. *See* Phenytoin.
Dilatation, 273-281
active phase of, 276-277
analgesia or anesthesia for,
    277-279
assessment of, 240f, 240-241
Bishop score for, 291t
interventions/outcomes in,
    279-281
latent phase of, 274-276
nursing diagnoses related to, 279
pain resulting from, 280-281
physiologic changes during,
    273-274
during second stage of labor, 281
transition phase of labor, 277

Dilatation and curettage, repetitive,
    14
Dilemma, ethical, 874, 887-888
Diploid, 26
Discharge
mucoid, ophthalmologic, 438
vaginal, assessment of during
    latent phase of labor, 275-276
Discharge planning
following surgery in pregnancy,
    745
hyperbilirubinemia and, 527
respiratory distress and, 529
Disseminated intravascular
    coagulation, 644-647, 652-653
as cause of postpartum
    hemorrhage, 851, 852
HELLP syndrome *versus*, 561, 838
related to intrauterine fetal
    demise, 836
Distress, spiritual, 882
Disturbed body, related to eating
    disorders, 133
Disturbed sensory perception
    related to multiple
    environmental distracters,
    261-262
Disulfiram as environmental
    hazard, 211
Diulo. *See* Metolazone.
Diuresis, postpartum, 374
Diuretics for maternal
    cardiovascular disease, 779t
DKA. *See* Diabetic ketoacidosis.
DM. *See* Diabetes mellitus.
DNA. *See* Deoxyribonucleic acid.
Documentation
of electronic fetal monitoring, 336,
    337b
of fetal cardiac auscultation, 305
of intimate partner violence, 548
of nonperiodic fetal heart rate
    patterns, 349
of periodic fetal heart rate
    patterns, 340, 341b
of uterine contractions, 351
Domestic violence. *See* Intimate
    partner violence.
Dominant inheritance, 28, 28f
sex-linked, 30
Donation
of embryo, 153
of oocytes, 153
Dopamine for neonatal
    resuscitation, 431t
Doppler studies
in fetal blood flow assessment,
    174, 175f
in fetal heart rate assessment,
    305-306
gestational hypertension and, 569
in patent ductus arteriosus, 454
in placenta previa, 635
in type 1 and type 2 diabetes
    mellitus, 665
Doptone, 304
Dorsal position for labor and
    delivery, 238
Dorsiflexion, ankle, in neonatal
    neurologic assessment, 444b

Doula, 254
Down syndrome
genetics of, 27
nuchal lucency screening in, 171
triple marker test in, 186
DPL. *See* Diagnostic peritoneal
    lavage.
Drowsy behavioral estate, 440
Drugs
for analgesia or anesthesia for
    labor, 278
breastfeeding and, 404
as environmental hazards,
    210-217
amphetamines, 210-211
analgesics, 211-212
antibiotics, 211-212
anticoagulants, 212
anticonvulsants, 212-213
antidepressants and
    psychotropics, 213
antiemetics, 213
antihyperlipidemics and
    hypocholesterolemic
    agents, 213
antihypertensives, 213
antimigraine agents, 213-214
antineoplastics, 214
antithyroid drugs, 214
antiulcer agents, 214
antiviral agents, 214
case studies and study
    questions for, 220
decongestants, 214
diethylstilbestrol, 215
gallstone-solubilizing agents,
    215
gonadotropic hormones, 215
health education regarding, 219
nicotine polarcrilex, 215
nicotine transdermal patch, 215
retinoids, 215
sedatives and hypnotics,
    215-216
Drug abuse, 70, 750-770
anxiety related to, 757
assessment of, 753-755
of cocaine, 751-752
deficient knowledge related to,
    755, 756b
effects of on fetus, 751
health education regarding, 767
of heroin, 752-753
impaired parenting due to,
    758-759
ineffective health maintenance
    associated with, 758
interrupted family processes
    related to, 757
as major public health issue,
    750
of marijuana, 753
of methadone hydrochloride, 753
noncompliance associated with,
    757
nursing diagnoses and
    interventions/outcomes
    regarding, 755-759, 756b,
    759f
nutritional aspects in, 756-757

Drug abuse (*Continued*)
  outcomes associated with, 750-751
  risk for injury related to, 758, 759f
  situational low self-esteem
    associated with, 754
  statistics regarding, 750
Duct, plugged, breastfeeding and,
  390, 398-399
Duncan's mechanism for placental
  delivery, 286
Durable power of attorney, 884
Duration of contractions, 232, 350
Duty and obligation-based
  approach to ethics, 874-875
Duvall's stages of family
  development, 125
DVT. *See* Deep venous thrombosis.
Dwarfism, maternal, labor passage
  and, 234
Dysmaturity syndrome, 825
Dysplasia, bronchopulmonary, 500
Dysrhythmias, fetal, 319-329
  atrial fibrillation, 325
  atrial flutter, 325, 325f
  history in, 319-320
  interventions for, 331-332
  interventions/outcomes in,
    329-332
  nursing diagnoses in, 329
  premature atrial contractions,
    321-323, 322f, 323f, 324f
  premature ventricular
    contractions, 326f, 326-328,
    327f, 328f
  second-degree heart block, 328
  supraventricular tachycardia,
    323-325, 324f
  third-degree heart block, 328

E
Early decelerations of fetal heart
  rate, 342f, 342-343
Ears
  embryonic development of, 49
  fetal development of, 57, 58, 59, 60
  neonatal
    assessment of, 438-439, 443t
    in premature infant, 476
Eating disorders, 130-132
  impaired adjustment related to,
    137-138
ECD. *See* Expected confinement
  date.
Echocardiography
  neonatal in patent ductus
    arteriosus, 454
  in persistent pulmonary
    hypertension of newborn, 516
Eclampsia, 556, 559, 566-567, 576t
  superimposed, chronic
    hypertension with, 560
Ectoderm, 43, 46
Ectopia cordis, 49
Ectopic pacemakers in physiology
  of contractions, 231
Ectromelia, 49
EDC. *See* Estimated date of
  confinement.

EDD. *See* Expected delivery date.
Edema
  associated with gestational
    hypertension, 558, 571
  cerebral, associated with
    hypertensive disorders of
    pregnancy, 579-581, 580f
  neonatal, 442t
  pulmonary
    decreased cardiac output due
      to, 777-778, 779t-780t
    preeclampsia-associated, 565,
      572, 582, 582t
EDRF. *See* Endothelium-derived
  relaxing factor.
Education, childbirth, 132-133
Effacement, cervical, 240
  during active phase of labor, 276
  Bishop score for, 291t
  for infant expulsion, 281
  during latent phase of labor, 272
  during transition phase of labor,
    277
Effective coping during labor and
  delivery, 258
EFM. *See* Electronic fetal
  monitoring.
EGA. *See* Estimation of gestational
  age.
EIA. *See* Enzyme immunoassay.
Eighth week of fetal development,
  51f, 53
Ejaculation, 41
Electrocardiography
  of atrial fibrillation, 325
  of atrial flutter, 325
  of atrial septal defect, 455
  of patent ductus arteriosus, 454
  of supraventricular tachycardia,
    324
Electrolytes
  altered metabolism of
    in gestational diabetes
      mellitus, 674
    in pregestational diabetes
      mellitus, 668-669
  imbalance of in gastrointestinal
    disease, 807-808, 810
  monitoring of
    in cholecystectomy, 736
    in respiratory distress
      syndrome, 507
Electronic fetal monitoring and
  assessment, 186-190
  during active phase of labor, 276
  contraction stress test in, 188-190
  documentation of, 340, 341b
  following trauma in pregnancy,
    716
  intrapartum, 305-308
  nonstress test in, 187-188
Electronic fetal monitoring tracings,
  358f-364f
  of premature atrial contractions
    with bigeminy, 276
    nonconducted, 323
    with trigeminy, 323
ELISA. *See* Enzyme-linked
  immunosorbent assay.

Elkins procedure, 244
Embolism, amniotic fluid, 839-841,
  846-847
Embryo
  cryopreservation of, 153
  donation of, 153
Embryonic disc, 46f, 46-47, 47f
Embryonic stage of fetal
  development, 46-53
  during eighth week, 51f, 53
  during fifth week, 51f, 51-52
  during fourth week, 49-50, 50f, 51f
  during seventh week, 51f, 52
  during sixth week, 51f, 52
  during third week, 46f, 46-49, 47f,
    48f, 49f
Emetine hydrochloride as
  environmental hazard, 212
Emotional history in
  comprehensive general health
  examination at first prenatal
  visit, 110
Emotions
  ethnocultural variations
    regarding, 91t
  of labor, 255-256
  preparation for, 263
Endocrine system
  fetal development of, 57, 58, 59
  maternal
    changes to during pregnancy,
      101-102
    disorders of. *See* Endocrine
      system disorders.
    postpartum changes to, 373
Endocrine system disorders, 660-702
  adrenal insufficiency, 688-690, 698
  case study and study questions
    for, 699-701
  Cushing's syndrome, 685-688, 698
  diabetes mellitus, 660-676
    classification of, 661t, 661-661
    gestational, 671-676, 696, 696t
    maternal metabolism and
      pathophysiology of
      pregnancy and, 662
    pregestational, 663-671, 695-696
    symptoms of, 660
    treatment of, 662
  health education regarding,
    695-699, 696t
  health history and, 13
  hyperthyroidism, 677t, 677-683,
    697
  hypothyroidism, 683-685, 697-698
  maternal phenylketonuria,
    691-695, 698-699
Endoderm, 43, 46
Endometriosis, 13
Endometritis, postpartum, 854,
  855
Endometrium
  anatomy of, 7
  biopsy of, 17
  menstruation and, 11
  pregnancy-induced changes to,
    97
Endoscopic gastrointestinal
  procedures, 740-741

Endothelial cell damage in development of preeclampsia, 557-558, 563-568
Endothelium-derived relaxing factor, 557, 563
Endotracheal intubation in respiratory distress syndrome, 503
Energy intake
  requirements during pregnancy, 104
  requirements for newborn, 423
Engagement, 245-246, 249
Engorgement, 390, 398
Enterocolitis, necrotizing, 474
Environmental factors
  in anxiety related to labor and delivery, 259
  in congenital disorders, 30-31, 61
  in disturbed sensory perception during labor and delivery, 261-262
  in ethics, 880-883
Environmental hazards, 201-224
  case studies and study questions for, 219-221
  health education regarding, 218b, 218-219
  occupational, 203-208, 205t
  pharmaceuticals, 210-217
    amphetamines, 210-211
    analgesics, 211
    antibiotics, 211-212
    anticoagulants, 212
    anticonvulsants, 212-213
    antidepressants and psychotropics, 213
    antiemetics, 213
    antihyperlipidemics and hypocholesterolemic agents, 213
    antihypertensives, 213
    antimigraine agents, 213-214
    antineoplastics, 214
    antithyroid drugs, 214
    antiulcer agents, 214
    antiviral agents, 214
    decongestants, 214
    diethylstilbestrol, 215
    gallstone-solubilizing agents, 215
    gonadotropic hormones, 215
    nicotine polacrilex, 215
    nicotine transdermal patch, 215
    retinoids, 215
    sedatives and hypnotics, 215-216
  scope of problem, 201, 202b
  second hand smoke as, 217-218
  stages of susceptibility to exposure to, 202
  temperature extremes, 208-210
  terms used in, 202-203
Environmental health history tool, 201, 202b
Enzyme immunoassay in acquired immunodeficiency syndrome, 606
Enzyme-linked immunosorbent assay for pregnancy testing, 114

Enzymes
  hepatic, elevated in HELLP syndrome, 560
  released by sperm, 42
Epidural anesthesia, 278
  for cesarean birth, 297
  for surgery in pregnancy, 732
  upright postures for labor and delivery and, 239
Epinephrine
  fetal heart rate and, 309
  for neonatal resuscitation, 426, 430t
Episiotomy, 283, 373
  impaired tissue integrity related to, 377
  pain related to, 378
  postpartum assessment of, 288
Epithelium, cervical, 6
Equanil. See Meprobamate.
Equipment, ultrasonographic, 167
Erb's palsy, 484
Ergomar. See Ergotamine tartrate.
Ergonomics, 203
Ergostat. See Ergotamine tartrate.
Ergotamine tartrate as environmental hazard, 214
Erythema toxicum, 438
Erythrocyte. See Red blood cell.
Escherichia coli, 782
Esophageal atresia, embryonic development of, 50
Estazolam as environmental hazard, 216
Estimated date of confinement, 162
Estimation of gestational age, 162-163
Estriol assays, 185
  in triple marker test, 186
Estrogen
  changes in pregnancy due to, 102
    uterine, 96
  injections of for contraception, with progesterone, 415t
  postpartum changes in, 373
  role of in conception, 41
Ethambutol, 788, 790t
Ethical-moral dilemma, 874
Ethics, 873-893
  case study and study questions regarding, 888-890
  creating and environment that promotes and preserves, 880-883
  in decision-making, 883-884
  defined, 873
  dilemmas involving, 887-888
    assessment of, 884-885
  health education regarding, 886-887
  informed consent and, 876-877
  nonnormative, 874
  nursing diagnoses and interventions/ outcomes related to, 885-886
  paternalism-maternalism-parentalism concept in, 878
  of prenatal diagnosis of genetic disorders, 34

Ethics (Continued)
  principle-based, 874-876
  proxy decision-makers and, 878-880
  terminology used in, 873-874
Ethics committee, 885
Ethionamide as environmental hazard, 211
Ethnocultural considerations, 75-95
  case studies and study questions for, 85-88
  clinical practice associated with, 78-85
    assessment in, 78-82
    interventions/outcomes in, 83-85
    nursing diagnoses in, 82-83
  in contraception, 410
  cultural and linguistic competence in, 76
  in ethics, 881-882
  in feeding of newborn, 425
  health education regarding, 85
  in health history, 15
  in hyperbilirubinemia, 523-524
  in intimate partner violence, 541-542
  during labor and delivery, 253-254
    ineffective coping related to, 260-261
  nutrition and, 109
  in prematurity, 472
  in psychology of pregnancy, 85
  quick reference guide to, 91t-95t
  transcultural nursing and, 75-76
Ethylene oxide, 203
ETT. See Endotracheal intubation.
Evacuation of hydatidiform mole, 650
Evaporation, neonatal, 423
Examination. See Physical examination.
Excessive fluid volume
  in kidney disease, 784-785
  related to use of oxytocin, 292
Excretion
  bilirubin, 519-520
  placenta's role in, 56
Exercise during pregnancy, 119
  labor and delivery and, 262-263, 263f
Exertion as environmental hazard, 206
Exhaustion, heat, 209
Exogenous surfactant
  in meconium aspiration syndrome, 514
  in respiratory distress syndrome, 504
Expectant family, 125
Expectant fathers
  health history of in comprehensive general health examination at first prenatal visit, 110
  psychological findings during pregnancy, 127-129
Expectant grandparents, 129
Expectant siblings, 129

Expected confinement date,
    assessment of, 111
Expected delivery date
    in advanced maternal age
        pregnancy, 154
    assessment of, 111
    using ultrasound, 167-168, 168t
Expiratory grunting in respiratory
    distress syndrome, 501
Expulsion
    cardinal movements and, 249
    of infant, 281-286
    of placenta, 286-288, 287f
    strength of contractions and,
        231-232
Extension, fetal, 242, 249
External genitalia
    anatomy of, 3-5, 4f
    maternal, examination of, 15
    neonatal
        assessment of, 439, 443t
        prematurity and, 476
External monitoring of
    contractions, 232
External rotation, fetal, 249
Extrachorial placenta, 61
Extraembryonic membranes, 46, 46f
Extrauterine life, adaptation of,
    421-425
Extremities
    maternal
        examination of following
            traumatic injury, 713-714
        in nutritional status
            assessment, 112t
        postpartum assessment of, 377
    neonatal, assessment of, 439-440
Eye shields for phototherapy, 527
Eyes
    fetal development of, 57, 58, 59,
        60
    maternal
        hyperthyroidism and, 679
        in nutritional status
            assessment, 112t
    neonatal
        assessment of, 438
        prophylactic treatment of, 426

F
Face
    fetal
        development of, 57
        presentation of, 242
    maternal
        examination of in traumatic
            injury, 713
        in nutritional status
            assessment, 112t
    neonatal
        malformations of due to fetal
            alcohol syndrome, 763,
            764f
        nerve damage in large-for-
            gestational-age infant,
            483
Facilitated diffusion in placental
    transfer, 55, 55t

Fallopian tubes
    anatomy of, 7-8
    changes to during pregnancy, 97
    postpartum infection of, 855
Falls, 708, 709
False labor, 231
False pelvis, 10, 10f
Family
    Duvall's stages in development
        of, 125
    psychosocial reactions to
        pregnancy and childbirth by,
        129
Family coping
    compromised
        related to fear of fetal loss,
            191-192
        related to significant other
            excluded from testing
            sessions, 191-192
    ineffective related to physical
        and/or mental handicap of
        family member, 35
    readiness for enhanced related to
        opportunity for
        growth/mastery, 136-137
Family history
    in comprehensive general health
        examination at first prenatal
        visit, 109-110
    in genetic assessment, 32, 33f
Family planning, 383, 409-418
    breastfeeding plans and, 410
    case study and study questions
        for, 416-418
    contraceptive history and, 409
    contraceptive knowledge and,
        410
    contraceptives for, 411, 412t-415t
    obstetric and gynecological
        history and, 409-410
    postpartum fertility and, 410-411
    psychosocial responses
        regarding, 410
Family process, interrupted
    acquired immunodeficiency
        syndrome and, 608-609
    alcohol use and, 766
    complicated pregnancy-
        associated, 772-773
    development stressors of
        pregnancy or loss and,
        135-136
    following diagnosis of genetic
        disorder in fetus or
        newborn, 35
    related to acceptance of newborn,
        289
    related to demands of care for
        diabetes mellitus
        gestational, 675
        pregestational, 671
    related to value differences
        between woman and her
        partner about contraceptive
        choices, 411-416
    substance abuse and, 757
FAS. *See* Fetal alcohol syndrome.
Fast spin-echo imaging, 306

Fasting glucose, impaired, 661-662
Fat
    brown, prematurity and, 474
    metabolism of in pregnancy, 662
Fatalistic personality, 258
Fathers
    health history of in
        comprehensive general
        health examination at first
        prenatal visit, 110
    psychological findings during
        pregnancy, 127-129
Fatigue
    activity intolerance related to,
        caused by physiologic
        changes of pregnancy, 118
    anemia-related, 804
    due to postpartum hemorrhage,
        853
    during labor and delivery, 257
    prolonged, 280
    systemic lupus erythematosus-
        associated, 797
Fats
    altered metabolism of
        in gestational diabetes
            mellitus, 674
        in pregestational diabetes
            mellitus, 668-669
    required intake during
        pregnancy, 70
FBM. *See* Fetal breathing
    movements.
Fear
    acquired immunodeficiency
        syndrome and, 608
    advanced maternal age
        pregnancy and, 155
    in amniotic fluid embolism, 841
    anticipation of pain during labor
        and, 261
    complicated pregnancy and,
        771-772
    discomfort of labor and, 280
    ethnocultural factors in, 84
    in hypertensive disorders of
        pregnancy, 583-584
    in multiple gestation pregnancy,
        833-834
    of pain related to impending
        labor, 273
    possible chromosomal
        abnormality and, 155
    postpartum hemorrhage and,
        853-854
    postterm pregnancy and, 826
    premature rupture of membrane
        and, 830
    preterm labor and, 823
    as reaction to labor, 257
    sexually transmitted diseases
        and, 611
    threat of potential harm to self or
        fetus and, 261
    TORCH disease and, 599
    unknown of labor and, 261
    urinary tract infection and
        pyelonephritis and, 614
    uterine rupture and, 843-844

Feedback loop, hypothalamic-pituitary-ovarian axis, 13
Feeding of infant, 423-424
  ethnocultural factors in, 81
  in persistent pulmonary hypertension of newborn, 517
  premature, 479-480
  with respiratory distress syndrome, 506-507
  small-for-gestational-age, 470-471
  in transient tachypnea of newborn, 510
Female condom, 414t
Female perspective regarding ethics, 882
Female reproductive system, 3-22
  case studies and study questions related to, 19-22
  changes to
    postpartum, 371-373
    during pregnancy, 96-98
  clinical practice associated with, 13-18
    assessment in, 13-17
    interventions/outcomes in, 17-18
    nursing diagnoses in, 17
  external, 3-5, 4f
    neonatal, assessment of, 439, 443f, 476
  health education related to, 18-19
  hypothalamic-pituitary-ovarian axis and, 12-13
  internal, 5f, 5-8, 7f
  menstruation and, 11-12
  support for organs in, 8-10, 9f, 10f
Feminist approach to ethics, 876
Femur length in gestational age determination, 168t
Fentanyl for analgesia during childbirth, 278
Ferritin, serum, 803t
Fertility
  anorexia nervosa's effect on, 131
  postpartum, 410-411
Fertilization, 41-42, 42f
  in vitro, 153
Fetal alcohol syndrome, 762-767, 763, 763b, 764f
Fetal assessment
  antepartum, 161-200
    biochemical, 174-186
    biophysical, 167-174, 175f
    case studies and sample questions regarding, 194-195
    comparison of surveillance tests in, 165
    electronic, 186-190
    fetal movement assessment by client in, 165-166
    health education in, 193
    interventions/outcomes in, 190-193
    nursing diagnoses in, 190
    role of nurse in, 162-165
    following traumatic injury in pregnancy, 714, 716

Fetal assessment (*Continued*)
  intrapartum, 303-368
    arrhythmias and dysrhythmias and, 319-329
    baseline fetal heart rate and, 309-315, 310f, 311f
    case studies and study questions associated for, 357-364, 358f, 359f, 360f, 361f, 362f, 363f, 364f
    electronic methods of, 276, 305-308
    fetal scalp sampling for, 351-353
    health education regarding, 357
    nonelectronic methods of, 304-305
    nonperiodic fetal heart rate patterns and, 344-349
    periodic fetal heart rate patterns and, 332-344
    pulse oximetry in, 353-355
    umbilical cord blood sampling in, 355-357, 356t
    uterine activity and, 350f, 350-351, 351f
    variability of fetal heart rate and, 314-329, 316f, 317f, 318f, 319f
Fetal breathing movements in biophysical profile, 173, 173t
Fetal development, 41-72
  amniotic fluid in, 65f, 65-66
  clinical practice associated with, 66-69
  conception in, 41-42, 42f
  congenital malformations in, 61, 62f
  embryonic stage of, 46-53
  fetal stage of, 53-61
    at 9 to 12 weeks, 56-57
    between 13 and 16 weeks, 57-58
    at 17 to 20 weeks, 58
    at 21 to 24 weeks, 58-59
    at 25 to 29 weeks, 59
    at 30 to 34 weeks, 60
    at 35 to 38 weeks, 60
    at 39 to 40 weeks, 60-61
    congenital malformation and, 61, 62f
    placental growth and function in, 53-54, 54f, 56
    placental transfer in, 54-56, 55t
  health education related to, 70
  placental abnormalities in, 61-63, 63t
  pre-embryonic stage of, 42-45, 43f, 44f, 45f
  pregenesis in, 41
  role of nurse in assessment of, 162-163
  study questions related to, 70-71
  umbilical cord in, 63-64
Fetal heart rate, intrapartum
  arrhythmias and dysrhythmias and, 319-329
    atrial fibrillation, 325
    atrial flutter, 325, 325f
    history in, 319-320

Fetal heart rate (*Continued*)
    interventions/outcomes in, 329-332
    nursing diagnoses in, 329
    physical findings in, 320
    premature atrial contractions, 321-323, 322f, 323f, 324f
    premature ventricular contractions, 326f, 326-328, 327f, 328f
    second-degree heart block, 328
    sinus node variants, 321f, 321-321
    supraventricular tachycardia, 323-325, 324f
    third-degree heart block, 328-329, 329f
  assessment of in preterm labor, 820
  baseline, 309-315, 310f, 311f
  electronic methods for assessment of, 305-308
  fetal factors influencing, 308-309
  maternal bleeding or shock and, 634, 641
  monitoring during surgery in pregnancy, 732-733
  nonelectronic methods for assessment of, 304-305
  nonstress testing of, 187-188
  normal, 309, 310f
  periodic, 332-344
    accelerations, 332-333, 333f
    combined decelerations, 343f, 343-344
    early decelerations, 342f, 342-343
    late decelerations, 228f, 337-342, 339f, 341b
    variable decelerations, 333-337, 334f, 335f, 337b
  postterm infant and, 488
  variability of, 314-329, 316f, 317f, 318f, 319f
Fetal movement assessment, 165-166
  in nonstress test, 187
Fetal scalp sampling, 164, 351-353
Fetal spiral electrode, 317
Fetoscopy, 404
  in procedures for congenital diaphragmatic hernia, 742
Fetus
  adaptation of to diminished oxygen supply, 163-165
  assessment of. *See* Fetal assessment.
  attitude of, 242
  cardinal movements of, 249
    risk for situational low self-esteem related to impairment of, 252-253
  danger to related to hypertensive disorders of pregnancy, 583
  descent of, pain related to, 285
  development of. *See* Fetal development.
  effects of anesthesia on, 729-730
  effects of maternal hyperthyroidism on, 680
  effects of substance abuse on, 751, 758, 759f

Fetus (*Continued*)
   intrauterine demise of, 835-839, 846
      ultrasonographic confirmation
         of, 170
   lie of, 242
   life-threatening complications to
         associated with hypertensive
         disorders, 554-555
   loss of
      anticipatory grieving related
         to, 720
      compromised family coping
         related to, 191-192
   maternal nutrition for optimal
         health of, 107
   movement of, assessment of by
         client, 165-166
   positioning of, 245, 246f
   presentation of, 242-245, 243f,
         244f, 245f
      placenta previa and, 635
      risk for injury related to, 252
      ultrasonographic assessment
         of, 170
   size of, 246-248
   skull of, 248-249
   station of, 245-246, 247f
   surgery and
      effects of on, 729-730
      intrauterine fetal, 741-744
      maternal, 733-734
   transition of to neonate, 421-425
   viability of, 163
      ultrasonographic assessment
         of, 170
FEV₁. *See* Forced expiratory volume
      in 1 second.
Fever
   in chorioamnionitis, 621
   due to postpartum infection, 854,
         855, 856, 857
   in postpartum thrombophlebitis,
         859
   in urinary tract infection, 612
FHR. *See* Fetal heart rate.
Fibrillation, atrial, 325
   interventions for, 331
Fibrin split products in gestational
         hypertension and HELLP
         syndrome, 573t
   disseminated intravascular
         coagulation *versus*, 563t
Fibrinogen
   in disseminated intravascular
         coagulation, 563t, 573t, 645
   in gestational hypertension and
         HELLP syndrome, 573t
Fibrocystic breast, breastfeeding
      and, 390
Fibroids, uterine, 13
   in advanced maternal age, 154
Fifth disease, 618t
Fifth week of fetal development, 51f,
      51-52
First trimester
   estimation of gestational age
         during, 162
   health education regarding
         physiology of pregnancy
         during, 118-119, 138

First trimester (*Continued*)
   tasks of pregnancy during
      maternal, 127
      paternal, 128
Fistula, tracheoesophageal,
      embryonic development of,
      50
Flagyl. *See* Metronidazole.
Flail chest, 718-719
Flat nipples, 390
   incorrect latching on related to,
      394-396
Flexion, fetal, 242, 249
Floating fetal station, 246
Fluid intake
   in gestational hypertension, 569
   for postpartum constipation,
      377
Fluid therapy
   in abruptio placentae, 642
   in amniotic fluid embolism, 840
   in disseminated intravascular
      coagulation, 646
   in maternal traumatic injury,
      719-720
   in placenta previa, 636
   in postpartum thrombophlebitis,
      860
   for prevention of preterm labor,
      820
   in surgery during pregnancy,
      733
Fluid volume
   deficient
      maternal
         in amniocentesis and PUBS,
            192
         due to fluid shift in early
            postpartum period,
            289-290
         in evacuation of
            hydatidiform mole, 650
         in inflammatory bowel
            disease, 808-809
         in kidney disease, 784-785
         in postpartum hemorrhage,
            852-853
         related to blood loss, 288
         related to decreased intake
            or abnormal loss, 281
         in surgical procedure and
            blood loss, 298
         in traumatic injury, 719-720,
            720f
      neonatal, associated with
         phototherapy light
         exposure, 526
   excessive
      in kidney disease, 784-785
      related to use of oxytocin,
         292
Fluid-filled intrauterine pressure
      catheter monitoring of
      contractions, 307
Fluorescence polarization test,
      177
Flutter, atrial, 325, 325f
   interventions for, 331
Fluvastatin sodium as
      environmental hazard, 213

FM. *See* Fetal movement
      assessment.
Foam stability index, 177, 502
Focusing phase of pregnancy, 128
Foley catheterization in abruptio
      placentae, 642
Folic acid
   deficiencies of, effect on fetus, 107
   for megaloblastic anemia, 800
   requirements of during
      pregnancy, 105-106
      in adolescent, 150
Follicle-stimulating hormone, 13
   anovulation during pregnancy
      due to suppression of, 97
   assessment of, 17
   postpartum changes in, 373
Follicular phase of menstruation, 11
Fontanelles, labor and delivery and,
      248
Food and Drug Administration,
      210
Food guide pyramid, 110f
   vegetarian, 105f
Football-hold position for
      breastfeeding, 393, 394f, 395f
Footling breech presentation, 243
Forced expiratory volume in 1
      second in tuberculosis, 789
Forceps delivery, 284
Foremilk, 389
Formula-feeding, 423, 424-425
Foundation for Children with
      AIDS, 623
Fourchette, 5
Fourth week of fetal development,
      49-50, 50f, 51f
Fracture
   clavicular, in large-for-gestational-
      age infant, 484, 486
   humeral, in large-for-gestational-
      age infant, 484
Frank breech presentation, 243
Fraternal twins, 835
FRC. *See* Functional residual
      capacity.
Free thyroxine, 677t
Free thyroxine index, 677t
Frequency of contractions, 232, 350
Friedman curve, altered, 294, 294f
Frontum presentation, 242
Fruit intake during pregnancy, 105
Frustration, feeling of, during
      pregnancy, 126
FSH. *See* Follicle-stimulating
      hormone.
Functional residual capacity
   in gestational hypertension and
      HELLP syndrome, 573t
   surgery and, 729
Functioning, altered, related to
      deviation from normal status
      of reproductive system, 18
Fundal height
   in advanced maternal age
      pregnancy, 154
   assessment of at periodic
      prenatal visits, 115, 116f
   in estimation of gestational age,
      162

Fundal height (*Continued*)
  postpartum, 371
    hemorrhage and, 853
  in postterm pregnancy, 825
Fundus, uterine, 6
  examination of in Leopold's
    maneuvers, 250
  postpartum assessment of, 288
Furosemide for hypertensive
  disorders of pregnancy, 578t
Fussy infant, 440
  breastfeeding of, 400

G
G-6-PD. *See* Glucose-6-phosphate
  dehydrogenase deficiency.
Gait of pregnancy, 101
Gallbladder, changes to during
  pregnancy, 100
Gallstone-solubilizing agents as
  environmental hazard, 215
Gamete intrafallopian transfer,
  153
Gametogenesis, 24-25, 25f
Gas, waste anesthetic, 207
Gas exchange, impaired
  fetal
    anemia and, 192
    in decelerations of fetal heart
      rate, 335-336, 337b, 340,
      341b
    in decreased placental
      perfusion, 192
    fetal pulse oximetry and,
      354-355
    fetal scalp sampling and, 352
    in impaired placental
      transport, 69
    in nonperiodic fetal heart rate
      patterns, 348-349
    in periodic fetal heart rate
      patterns, 340, 340b
    in tachycardias and
      bradycardias, 313-314
    in variability of fetal heart rate,
      329-332
  maternal, related to respiratory
    disease, 790-791, 791t
  neonatal
    in congenital diaphragmatic
      hernia, 192, 452
    in preterm infant, 481
    related to poor respiratory
      effort and retained lung
      fluid, 429
    related to umbilical cord
      sampling, 356-357
Gastric cancer, 741
Gastrointestinal system
  embryonic development of, 52, 53
  fetal
    development of, 57, 58
    maternal drug use and, 751
  maternal
    changes to during first stage of
      labor, 274
    changes to during pregnancy,
      100
    constipation and, 117

Gastrointestinal system (*Continued*)
  disease of, 806-811
  endoscopic procedures
    involving, 740-741
  in nutritional status
    assessment, 112t
  postpartum changes in, 374
  premonitory signs of childbirth
    involving, 272
  systemic lupus erythematosus-
    related symptoms in, 795
  trauma and, 706
  neonatal
    congenital anomalies of,
      448-451, 449f
    transition of fetal to, 422
Gastroschisis, 451
Gastrulation, embryonic, 46
GDM. *See* Gestational diabetes
  mellitus.
Gender roles, intimate partner
  violence, 542
Gene, 26
  defined, 23
General anesthesia
  for cesarean birth, 297
  for surgery in pregnancy, 732
General appearance in maternal
  nutritional assessment, 111t
General survey
  maternal, 15-16, 16f
  neonatal, 438
Genetic disorders, 31-32
Genetics, 23-40
  case studies and study questions
    related to, 36-39
  clinical practice associated with,
    32-36, 33f
  complex disorders of, 31-32
  definitions in, 23
  health education associated with,
    36
  inheritance and
    foundations of, 24f, 24-28, 25f,
      27f
    modes of, 28f, 28-30, 29f, 31f
  National Human Genome Project
    and, 23
  polygenic or multifactorial
    disorders of, 30-31
  testing of in advanced maternal
    age, 154
Genitalia
  anatomy of, 3-5, 4f
  maternal
    examination of, 15
    traumatic injury to, 713
  neonatal
    assessment of, 439, 443t
    prematurity and, 476
Genitourinary system
  embryonic development of, 52
  fetal development of, 57-58, 59,
    60
  maternal, trauma and, 706
Genogram, 32, 33f
Genome, defined, 23
Genotype, defined, 23
German measles in TORCH,
  592-599, 593t-597t

Gestation, multiple, 831-835, 846
  in advanced maternal age, 154
  breastfeeding interventions for,
    402
  case study and study questions
    regarding, 265-266
  ultrasonographic assessment of,
    170
Gestational age, 465-496
  assessment of, 441, 442t-443t,
    444b-445b, 445f, 446f
  case studies and study questions
    associated with, 492-494
  estimation of, 162-163
  health education regarding,
    490-491
  large for, 482-486
  posterm infants, 486-490
  preterm infant, 472-482
    assessment of, 475-478
    cardiovascular system of, 473
    diagnostic procedures for, 478
    diminished sucking processes
      in, 479-480
    hypocalcemia in, 474
    hypoglycemia in, 474-475
    immune system of, 473-474
    impaired skin integrity in,
      480-481
    impaired urinary elimination
      and retention in, 481
    liver of, 474
    necrotizing enterocolitis in, 474
    nursing diagnoses and
      interventions/outcomes
      for, 478-482
    organ maturity and, 472
    periventricular intraventricular
      hemorrhage in, 474
    physical findings in, 476-478
    renal system of, 474, 481
    respiratory distress syndrome
      in, 502-506
    respiratory system of, 472-473,
      481-482
    risk factors for, 472
    thermoregulation in, 474, 478-479
  small for, 465-471
  uterine size and location
    indicating, 707f
Gestational carrier, 153
Gestational dating assessment,
  111
  using ultrasound, 167-168, 168t
Gestational diabetes mellitus, 661,
  671-676, 696, 696t
Gestational hypertension, 558-559,
  568-574
  in adolescent, 150
  in advanced maternal age, 154
  transient, 560
Gestational trophoblastic disease,
  647-651, 653
GFR. *See* Glomerular filtration rate.
GIFT. *See* Gamete intrafallopian
  transfer.
Glasgow Coma Scale, 715t
Glomerular filtration rate
  in preeclampsia, 564
  in premature infant, 474

Glucocorticoids for
thrombocytopenia, 801
Glucose, blood
in diabetes mellitus
gestational, 675-676
pregestational, 671
neonatal, 427
in large-for-gestational-age
infant, 485
monitoring of in infants of
diabetic mothers, 667
in preterm infant, 475
in respiratory distress
syndrome, 502, 507
in small-for-gestational-age
infant, 470
values of in pregnancy, 661t
Glucose-6-phosphate
dehydrogenase deficiency,
hyperbilirubinemia-associated,
525
Glucosuria due to pregnancy, 100
Glycol, 206
Goal outcome consequences-based
approach to ethics, 875
Gonadotropic hormones as
environmental hazard, 215
Gonads, female, 8
Gonorrhea, 601t-602t
Goodell's sign, 97, 103
Graafian follicle, 11
anovulatory cycles and, 12
Grandparents
cultural factors in labor and
delivery regarding, 254
psychologic findings in, 129
Grasp reflex, 440b
Graves' disease, 677, 678. See Also
Hyperthyroidism.
Grieving, 132
anticipatory
in acquired immunodeficiency
syndrome, 608
related to ill or preterm
newborn, 138
related to loss of fetus
following traumatic injury,
720
related to loss of normal
pregnancy or fetus, 193
related to preterm labor, 823
dysfunctional, related to
stillbirth, ill, or preterm
newborn, loss of perfect
child, loss of pregnancy, or
loss of desired labor or birth
experience, 138
following diagnosis of genetic
disorder in fetus or
newborn, 36
related to fetal demise, 837-838
Group B streptococcus, 617t-618t
Growth and development
adolescent, pregnancy and,
149-150
fetal, 41-72
at 9 to 12 weeks, 56-57
between 13 and 16 weeks, 57-58
at 17 to 20 weeks, 58
at 21 to 24 weeks, 58-59

Growth and development
adolescent (*Continued*)
at 25 to 29 weeks, 59
at 30 to 34 weeks, 60
at 35 to 38 weeks, 60
at 39 to 40 weeks, 60-61
amniotic fluid in, 65f, 65-66
conception in, 41-42, 42f
congenital malformation and,
61, 62f
delayed, due to inadequate
maternal nutrition, 68
embryonic stage of, 46-53
fetal stage of, 53-61
health education related to, 70
maternal diabetes mellitus and,
666
placental abnormalities in,
61-63, 63t
placental growth and function
in, 53-54, 54f, 56
placental transfer in, 54-56, 55t
pre-embryonic stage of, 42-45,
43f, 44f, 45f
pregenesis in, 41
restricted in adolescent
pregnancy, 150
role of nurse in assessment of,
162-163
small-for-gestational-age and,
465-471
study questions related to,
70-71
umbilical cord in, 63-64
intrauterine, restricted
due to heroin abuse, 752
due to maternal diabetes
mellitus, 666
of newborn, health education
associated with, 460-461
Growth charts, human intrauterine,
163
Growth parameters, neonatal, 438
Grunting, expiratory, in respiratory
distress syndrome, 501
Gums, changes to during
pregnancy, 100
Gunshot wound, 709, 710
Gynecoid pelvis, 235
Gynecologic history
in comprehensive general health
examination at first prenatal
visit, 108
family planning and, 409-410

H
Hair
changes to during pregnancy, 101
fetal development of, 57, 58, 59,
60
in nutritional status assessment,
112t
of premature infant, 476
Halcion. See Triazolam.
Haldol. See Haloperidol.
Halogenated gases, 207
Halogenated hydrocarbons, 204
Haloperidol as environmental
hazard, 213

Hand placement
for cradle hold, 392f
for cross-cradle hold, 394f
for football hold, 395f
Haploid, 26
Hashimoto's thyroiditis, 683
Hatching, assisted, 153
Hazards, environmental, 201-224
assessment of, 201-202
case studies and study questions
for, 219-221
health education regarding, 218b,
218-219
occupational, 203-208, 205t
pharmaceuticals, 210-217
scope of problem, 201, 202b
second hand smoke as, 217-218
stages of susceptibility to
exposure to, 202
temperature extremes, 208-210
terms used in, 202-203
hCG. *See* Human chorionic
gonadotropin.
HCS. *See* Human chorionic
somatomammotropin.
Head
embryonic development of, 49-50,
50f
maternal assessment of following
traumatic injury, 713
neonatal
assessment of, 438
premature, 476
Head lag in neonatal neurologic
assessment, 444b
Health care system, ineffective
coping related to practices of
during labor and delivery,
260-261
Health history, 13
Health interview in assessment of
reproductive anatomy,
physiology, and menstrual
cycle, 13-15
Health maintenance, ineffective
associated with insufficient
knowledge to prevent
preterm labor, 823-824
associated with substance abuse,
758
in multiple gestation pregnancy,
833
in trophoblastic disease, 650-651
Health Resource Center on
Domestic Violence, 550
Hearing, neonatal, 441
Heart
embryonic development of, 49,
49f
fetal
development of, 56, 59
maternal drug use and, 752
transition of to neonatal, 422
maternal
changes to during first stage of
labor, 273-274
changes to during pregnancy,
98-99
disease of, 773-781, 774b, 775t,
776t, 779t-780t

Heart (*Continued*)
  in nutritional status
    assessment, 112t
  postpartum changes to,
    373-374
  systemic lupus erythematosus-
    related, 795
  valvular disease of,
    thromboembolism
    secondary to, 778-781
  neonatal
    assessment of, 439
    in preterm infant, 473
Heart block, 328-329, 329f
  interventions for, 331-332
Heart defects, 453-460
  atrial septal defect, 454-455, 455f
  coarctation of aorta, 456-457,
    457f
  hypoplastic left heart syndrome,
    459-460
  patent ductus arteriosus, 453-454,
    454f
  tetralogy of Fallot, 457-458, 458f
  transposition of great arteries,
    458-459, 459f
  ventricular septal defect, 455-456,
    456f
Heart failure, congestive, 776,
  777-778, 779t-780t
Heart murmur, neonatal, 439
Heart rate
  fetal. *See* Fetal heart rate.
  maternal
    changes to during pregnancy,
      98
    in hyperthyroidism, 679
    postpartum changes in, 374
  neonatal, 438
    in Apgar scoring, 426t
    in respiratory distress
      syndrome, 502, 505
Heartburn development during
  pregnancy, 100
Heat, therapeutic, ethnocultural
  considerations in, 81
Heat exhaustion, 209
Heat loss, neonatal, 422-423
  in preterm infant, 474, 479
Heat stroke, 209
Heavy metals, environmental
  exposure to, 204
Hegar's sign, 103
Height, fundal
  in advanced maternal age
    pregnancy, 154
  assessment of at periodic
    prenatal visits, 115, 116f
  in estimation of gestational age,
    162
  postpartum, 371
    hemorrhage and, 853
  in postterm pregnancy, 825
HELLP syndrome, 560-561, 562f,
  563t
Helplessness, feelings of as reaction
  to labor, 257
Hemangioma, 650
  capillary, 438

Hematocrit
  maternal
    assessment of at first prenatal
      visit, 114
    decreased levels of due to
      pregnancy, 99
    in gestational hypertension and
      HELLP syndrome, 573t
    in hemorrhagic disorders, 630
    indices of for iron homeostasis,
      803t
    postpartum changes in values
      of, 373
    in reproductive assessment, 17
  neonatal, in small-for-gestational-
    age infant, 471
Hematologic system
  maternal
    changes to due to trauma in
      pregnancy, 706
    changes to during pregnancy, 99
    disease of, 799-806
    preeclampsia and, 568
    surgery and, 729
    systemic lupus erythematosus-
      related symptoms in, 795
    trauma and, 706
  neonatal
    disturbances of related to
      maternal diabetes
      mellitus, 667
    respiratory distress related to
      disease of, 498
Hematoma as cause of postpartum
  hemorrhage, 851, 852
Hematuria in preeclampsia, 564
Hemoconcentration, preeclampsia-
  associated, 568
Hemodynamic monitoring in
  gestational hypertension, 574
Hemodynamics, maternal, changes
  to during pregnancy, 98
Hemoglobin
  bilirubin from destruction of, 518
  fetal, cordocentesis and
    percutaneous umbilical
    blood sampling for, 180-181
  maternal
    abnormal, ethnic factors in,
      95t
    appendectomy and, 739
    assessment of at first prenatal
      visit, 114
    decreased levels of due to
      pregnancy, 99
    in gestational diabetes and
      preeclampsia, 573t
    indices of for iron homeostasis,
      803t
    postpartum changes in values
      of, 374
    testing of in reproductive
      assessment, 17
  neonatal
    anemia and, 504
    in small-for-gestational-age
      infant, 471
Hemolysis in HELLP syndrome,
  560

Hemorrhage
  gastrointestinal, endoscopic
    procedures for, 740
  periventricular intraventricular,
    474
  postpartum, 634, 850-854, 864
  related to altered clotting factors
    secondary to heparin
    therapy or
    thrombocytopenia, 806
  related to hypertensive disorders
    of pregnancy, 567, 579-582,
    580f
  scleral, 438
  ultrasonographic assessment of,
    171
  vaginal in advanced maternal
    age pregnancy, 154
Hemorrhagic disorders, 630-659
  abruptio placentae, 638-644, 652
  case studies and study questions
    regarding, 653-656
  disseminated intravascular
    coagulation, 644-647, 652-653
  gestational trophoblastic disease,
    647-651, 653
  health education regarding,
    651-653
  placenta previa, 631-638, 651
    diagnostic procedures in,
      635-636
    history in assessment of,
      631-632
    ineffective fetal perfusion and
      oxygenation due to,
      637-638
    ineffective maternal tissue
      perfusion related to,
      636-637
    maternal anxiety related to, 638
    nursing diagnoses and
      interventions/outcomes
      for, 636-638
    physical findings in, 633-635
    physiologic response to blood
      loss due to, 632-633
    psychosocial findings in, 635
Hemorrhoids
  development of during
    pregnancy, 100
  postpartum, pain related to, 378
Hemothorax, traumatic, 718
Heparin, 806
  in disseminated intravascular
    coagulation therapy, 646
  for postpartum thrombophlebitis,
    860
Hepatic enzymes, elevated in
  HELLP syndrome, 560
Hepatic system
  maternal
    changes to during pregnancy,
      100
    disease of, 811-814, 812t
    preeclampsia-related injury to,
      582
    systemic lupus erythematosus-
      related symptoms in, 795
  neonatal

Hepatic system (*Continued*)
assessment of, 439
hyperbilirubinemia due to
dysfunction of, 520
in preterm infant, 474
Hepatitis, 592-599, 593t-597t,
811-814, 812t
Hepatitis Foundation International,
623624
Hepatosplenomegaly,
hyperbilirubinemia-associated,
525
Herbicides, 204
Hernia, congenital diaphragmatic,
451-453
fetal surgery for, 742
Heroin abuse, 752-753
Herpes simplex virus, 592-599,
593t-597t
Hindmilk, 389
Hispanic culture, 91t-95t
AIDS in, 603, 604t
intimate partner violence and, 541
History
in abruptio placentae, 639-640
in advanced maternal age
assessment, 152-154
in breastfeeding assessment, 389
in comprehensive general health
examination at first prenatal
visit, 107-110, 109f
in disseminated intravascular
coagulation, 644-645
in fetal and placental assessment,
66-67
in fetal arrhythmias and
dysrhythmias, 319-320
in fetal heart rate variability,
315-319, 316f, 317f, 318f,
319f
in gestational hypertension,
568-569
in intimate partner violence
assessment, 545
in placenta previa, 631-632
in pregestational diabetes
mellitus, 663-665
in preterm labor, 819
in psychological factors in
pregnancy assessment,
124-125
in reproductive anatomy,
physiology, and menstrual
cycle assessment, 13-15
in traumatic injury, 712
Histrelin acetate as environmental
hazard, 215
HIV. *See* Human immunodeficiency
virus.
HMD. *See* Hyaline membrane
disease.
Homan's sign, 859
Home care management of
placenta previa, 638
Home pregnancy test, 114
Honeymoon stage of intimate
partner violence, 539f, 540
Horizontal postures for labor and
delivery, 238

Hormones
fetal heart rate and, 308-309
maternal
associated with breastfeeding,
387-389, 388f
changes to during pregnancy,
101-102
postpartum changes to, 373
postpartum depression and, 862
placental, 56
Hospitalized infant, breastfeeding
of, 401-402, 402f
Hot or cold theory of health and
diet, 79, 80, 83, 93t
Hot tub exposure, 209
HPL. *See* Human placental
lactogen.
HPV. *See* Human papilloma virus.
HSV. *See* Herpes simplex virus.
Human chorionic gonadotropin
as environmental hazard, 215
in genetic assessment, 32-33
in gestational trophoblastic
disease, 649
postpartum changes in, 373
for pregnancy test, 114
in triple marker test, 186
Human chorionic
somatomammotropin,
postpartum changes in, 373
Human immunodeficiency virus,
599-609
case study and study questions
for, 625-626
counseling and early diagnosis
of, 603
first recognition of, 599
health education regarding,
623-624
nursing diagnoses and
interventions/outcomes for,
607-609
treatment of, 604-605
women and, 603-604, 604f, 604t
Human papilloma virus, 600t-601t
Human placental lactogen,
postpartum changes in, 373
Humeral fracture in large-for-
gestational-age infant, 484
Hyaline membrane disease, 477,
500-508
Hyaluronidase, 42
Hydatidiform mole, 647
assessment of, 648
evacuation of, risk for deficient
fluid volume related to, 650
Hydralazine hydrochloride for
hypertensive disorders of
pregnancy, 577t
Hydramnios, 66
ultrasonographic assessment of,
171
Hydration of infant with
respiratory distress syndrome,
507
Hydrex. *See* Benzthiazide.
Hydrocarbons, halogenated, 204
Hydrocephalus, 441-447
fetal surgery for, 743

Hydrocephaly, 252
Hydroxyzine for analgesia during
childbirth, 278
Hymen, 4
Hyperadrenocorticism, 685-688, 698
Hyperbilirubinemia, 517-528
assessment of, 523-526
causes of, 517-521, 519f
discharge planning in, 529
due to maternal diabetes
mellitus, 667
interventions/outcomes for,
526-528
long-term follow-up in, 529
nursing diagnoses in, 526
in preterm infant, 474
treatment of, 521-523, 523f
Hypercarbia, risk for impaired fetal
gas exchange related to,
335-336, 337b
Hypercoagulability, 778-781
Hyperemesis gravidarum, 806-811
Hyperglycemia, maternal, 661, 661t,
665
Hyperinsulinemia, fetal, 662
Hyperphenylalaninemia, 691-695
Hyperpigmentation, pregnancy-
induced, 101
Hyperplasia, uterine, due to
pregnancy, 96
Hypertension
abruptio placentae and, 639
in advanced maternal age, 154
chronic, 559, 574-575, 576t-578t
with superimposed
preeclampsia or
eclampsia, 560
gestational, 558-559, 568-574
in adolescent, 150
in advanced maternal age, 154
pulmonary
maternal, 782
persistent, 515-517
related to congenital
diaphragmatic hernia, 453
secondary, 575-579
transient, 560, 579
Hypertensive disorders of
pregnancy, 554-591
assessment of, 568-579
cardiovascular system
disturbances associated
with, 581-582
case studies and study questions
for, 585-587
central nervous system injury
resulting from, 579-581,
580f
chronic hypertension as, 559
with superimposed
preeclampsia or
eclampsia, 560
complications of, 554-555, 563-565
generalized vasospasm and
endothelial cell damage in,
563-568
gestational hypertension as,
558-559, 568-574
health education for, 584-585

Hypertensive disorders of pregnancy (*Continued*)
HELLP syndrome as, 560-561, 562f, 563t
hepatic injury associated with, 581-582
impaired fetal well being related to, 583
maternal anxiety and fear associated with, 583-584
nursing diagnoses and interventions/outcomes for, 579-584
renal system disturbances associated with, 581
risk factors for, 556-557
terminology describing, 555-556
transient hypertension as, 560
Hyperthermia, 208-210
Hyperthyroidism, 677t, 677-683, 697
thyroid function tests in, 17
Hypertonia, uterine, 294
Hypertrophy, uterine, due to pregnancy, 96
Hyperventilation for treatment of persistent pulmonary hypertension of newborn, 516
Hypnotics as environmental hazard, 215-216
Hypoadrenocorticism, 688-690, 698
Hypocalcemia
due to maternal diabetes mellitus, 667
in large-for-gestational-age infant, 484
in preterm infant, 474
Hypocholesterolemic agents as environmental hazard, 213
Hypoglycemia
maternal, 662, 665, 669
neonatal
in large-for-gestational-age infant, 485
in postterm infant, 489-490
in preterm infant, 474-475, 477
related to maternal diabetes mellitus, 667
in respiratory distress syndrome, 502, 504
Hypoperfusion in development of preeclampsia, 557-558
Hypoplastic left heart syndrome, 459-460
Hypotension
maternal
late decelerations of fetal heart rate and, 338
supine, due to pregnancy, 98
neonatal
associated with respiratory distress syndrome, 504
in meconium aspiration syndrome, 514
Hypothalamic-pituitary-ovarian axis, 12-13
Hypothermia, newborn, 427-429
respiratory distress syndrome and, 504

Hypothermia, newborn (*Continued*)
in small-for-gestational-age infant, 470, 471
transient tachypnea of newborn and, 509
Hypothyroidism, 683-685, 688-690, 697-698, 698
thyroid function tests in, 17
Hypotonia, uterine, 294
Hypoxia
fetal
due to dysrhythmias, 332
due to early decelerations of fetal heart rate, 343
due to variable decelerations of fetal heart rate, 335-336, 337b
persistent pulmonary hypertension of newborn and, 515
response to, 163-165
maternal, due to respiratory disease, 791
Hysterotomy, 734
for congenital diaphragmatic hernia, 742

I

IBD. *See* Inflammatory bowel disease.
Ibuprofen as environmental hazard, 211
ICSI. *See* Intracytoplasmic sperm injection.
Identical twins, 835
IDMs. *See* Infants of diabetic mothers.
IFG. *See* Impaired fasting glucose.
Ilium, 9, 9f
Ill newborn, 497-534
anticipatory grieving related to, 138
case studies and study questions associated with, 530-532
dysfunctional grieving related to, 138
health education regarding, 490-491, 528-529
hyperbilirubinemia in, 517-528
meconium aspiration syndrome in, 510-515, 511f
persistent pulmonary hypertension of newborn in, 515-517
respiratory distress in, 498-499
respiratory distress syndrome in, 500-508
transient tachypnea in, 508-509
Imbalanced body temperature due to postpartum infection, 857
Imbalanced nutrition: less than body requirements
maternal
in acquired immunodeficiency syndrome, 609
in gastrointestinal disease, 809-810

Imbalanced nutrition (*Continued*)
in lactation and/or depression, 404-405
in phenylketonuria, 694-695
related to alcohol use, 766
related to inadequate information about nutritional needs during pregnancy, 118
related to smoking during pregnancy, 761
in substance abuse, 756-757
neonatal
associated with cleft lip and palate, 432
in large-for-gestational-age infants, 485
in persistent pulmonary hypertension, 517
in postterm infant, 489-490
in preterm infant, 479-480
related to inability to suck and swallow with cleft lip and palate, 450
in small-for-gestational-age infants, 470-471
in transient tachypnea, 510
Imbalanced nutrition: more than body requirements
related to blood glucose management in diabetes mellitus, 675
related to excessive intake of calories, 117
Immobility, maternal, impaired comfort related to, 314
Immune system
changes to during pregnancy, 102
fetal development of, 57, 58, 59
postpartum changes in, 375
preeclampsia and, 557
in preterm infant, 473-474
of small-for-gestational-age infant, 467
Immune thrombocytopenic purpura, 801
Immunoglobulin G
deficiency of in premature infant, 474
pregnancy-induced changes in levels of, 102
Immunoglobulins
intravenous for thrombocytopenia, 801
pregnancy-induced changes in levels of, 102
Impaired adjustment related to mood disorder, eating disorder, or loss, 137-138
Impaired comfort
in abruptio placentae, 643-644
in gastrointestinal disease, 810
immobility and, 314
incorrect latching on and, 394-396
invasive procedures and, 193
in maternal immobility for fetal heart rate problems, 314

Impaired comfort (*Continued*)
in nipple or breast pain
associated with
breastfeeding, 397-399
renal disease-associated, 785-786
in sexually transmitted disease,
611
systemic lupus erythematosus-
associated, 797
Impaired fasting glucose, 661-662
Impaired gas exchange
fetal
in decelerations of fetal heart
rate, 335-336, 337b, 340,
341b
in decreased placental
perfusion, 192
in fetal anemia, 192
in fetal pulse oximetry,
354-355
in fetal scalp sampling, 352
in impaired placental
transport, 69
in nonperiodic fetal heart rate
patterns, 348-349
in periodic fetal heart rate
patterns, 340, 340b
in tachycardias and
bradycardias, 313-314
in variability of fetal heart rate,
329-332
maternal, related to respiratory
disease, 790-791, 791t
neonatal
in congenital diaphragmatic
hernia, 192, 452
in poor respiratory effort and
retained lung fluid, 429
in preterm infant, 481
umbilical cord sampling and,
356-357
Impaired infant attachment, related
to postpartum infection, 858
Impaired oxygenation
in persistent pulmonary
hypertension of newborn,
516-517
in transient tachypnea of
newborn, 509-510
Impaired parenting
drug abuse and, 758-759
following diagnosis of genetic
disorder in fetus or newborn,
35-36
inadequate bonding secondary to
infant with cleft lip and
palate and, 450
lack of knowledge and skills and,
137
late childbearing and, 155-156
multiple births and, 834-835
parent-infant separation
secondary to phototherapy
treatments and, 527-528
postpartum depression and,
863
postpartum infection and, 858
taking on role of mother and,
380-381

Impaired skin integrity
maternal, related to delivery
process, 285
neonatal
associated with
hyperbilirubinemia, 527
in preterm infant, 480-481
Impaired social interaction, due to
extended hospital stay for
postpartum infection, 857-858
Impaired tissue integrity, related to
episiotomy or laceration, 377-378
Impaired urinary elimination
maternal
related to pressure of
presenting part, 284-285
related to process of labor and
delivery, 289
related to progression of labor,
279
in preterm infant, 481
Impaired ventilation and/or
oxygenation
in persistent pulmonary
hypertension of newborn,
516-517
related to meconium aspiration
syndrome, 513-515
Implantation, 42, 43f
In vitro fertilization, 153
Incision
for cesarean birth
examination of, 376
pain related to, 378
for uterine rupture repair, 842, 844
Incubator, 423
Individual coping, ineffective
related to acquired
immunodeficiency
syndrome, 609
related to chorioamnionitis, 622
related to progression of labor,
280
during second stage of labor, 285
Indomethacin
persistent pulmonary
hypertension of newborn
and, 515
in preterm labor therapy, 822
Induction of uterine contractions,
290-293, 291t
Ineffective airway clearance
maternal
related to respiratory disease,
790-791, 791t
related to trauma in pregnancy,
717, 718f
neonatal, related to inability to
adequately clear secretions
from airway, 429
Ineffective breathing pattern
related to shallow or periodic
breathing and apnea, 429
related to trauma in pregnancy,
717-719
Ineffective coping
acquired immunodeficiency
syndrome and, 609
associated with smoking, 762

Ineffective coping (*Continued*)
chorioamnionitis and, 622
health care system's practices
and, 260-261
inadequate support systems or
absence of a support person
and, 260-261
during labor and delivery, 258,
260-261
physical and/or mental handicap
of family member and, 35
postpartum mood alteration and,
381
progression of labor and, 280
related to conflict between
personal and cultural
expectations, 260-261
during second stage of labor, 285
systemic lupus erythematosus-
associated, 797-798
Ineffective health maintenance
associated with insufficient
knowledge to prevent
preterm labor, 823-824
associated with substance abuse,
758
in multiple gestation pregnancy,
833
in trophoblastic disease, 650-651
Ineffective role performance related
to taking on new roles, 133
Ineffective sexuality patterns
related to changes in libido
during pregnancy, 134-135
Ineffective thermoregulation
in preterm infant, 478-479
related to phototherapy, 526-527
Ineffective tissue perfusion
fetal
in abruptio placentae, 643
in disseminated intravascular
coagulation, 647
due to umbilical cord
compression, 826-827, 830
following traumatic injury in
pregnancy, 721
related to maternal blood loss
from placenta previa,
637-638
maternal
in abruptio placentae, 642-643
in amniotic fluid embolism,
840-841
deep venous thrombosis and,
804-805
in disseminated intravascular
coagulation, 646-647
due to thrombophlebitis,
804-805, 859-860
expulsive efforts and, 285
placenta previa and, 636-637
position in labor and, 279
preeclampsia and, 563-568,
581
neonatal
congenital diaphragmatic
hernia-associated
pulmonary hypertension
and, 453

Ineffective tissue perfusion
(*Continued*)
decreased cardiac output and,
429-432
polycythemia and
hypothermia in small-for-
gestational-age infant and,
471
in preterm infant, 481
Infants of diabetic mothers, 666-667
Infection
maternal, 592-629
acquired immunodeficiency
syndrome, 599-609, 623-624
of breast, 390, 399, 855
cardiac disease and, 778
chorioamnionitis, 620-622, 625
due to invasive procedures, 192
due to premature rupture of
membranes, 828, 829-830
due to spontaneous rupture of
membranes, 273
group B streptococcus, 617t-618t
influenza, 616t
intrauterine pressure catheter-
related, 233
labor and delivery-associated,
290
listeriosis, 619t
Lyme disease, 619t
measles, 616t
mumps, 616t
parvovirus B19, 618t
postpartum, 854-858, 865
prematurity and, 472, 475
prolonged second stage of
labor and, 285-286
related to corticosteroid
therapy, 796-797
renal, 784
resistance to during pregnancy,
102
as a result of cesarean birth, 298
resulting from prolonged labor,
296
sexually transmitted diseases,
599-611, 600t-602t, 624
small-for-gestational-age
infants exposed to, 467
TORCH, 592-599, 593t-597t,
622-623
tuberculosis, 617t, 791-792
urinary tract infection and
pyelonephritis, 611-614,
624, 783
vaginal examination after
ROM and, 281
varicella zoster, 615t
neonatal, 432
maternal transmission of
hepatitis, 814
prematurity and, 477-478
related to infant's poor
physiologic response to
pathogens, 432
in small-for-gestational-age
infant, 471
Inferior vena cava, compression of,
705

Inflammatory bowel disease, 807-811
Influenza, maternal, 616t
Informed consent, 876-877
Infundibulum, 8
Inhalation injury, 708-709
Inheritance
foundation of, 24f, 24-28, 25f, 27f.
See Also Genetics.
modes of, 28f, 28-30, 29f, 31f
Injury
birth
macrosomia-associated, 248
related to malpresentation, 252
cervical, effects of on delivery,
234
fetal
related to alcohol use, 767
related to antithyroid drugs,
682-683
related to drug abuse, 758, 759f
related to gestational diabetes
mellitus, 675
related to hazardous effects of
pharmaceuticals, 216
related to
hyperadrenocorticism, 688
related to malpresentation, 252
related to maternal
phenylketonuria, 693-694
related to maternal steroid
replacement therapy, 690
related to occupational
hazards, 207
related to pregestational
diabetes mellitus, 671
related to second hand smoke
exposure, 218
related to smoking during
pregnancy, 761
related to temperature
extremes, 209
related to test complications,
190-191
related uterine rupture, 843
from intimate partner violence, 540
maternal
pelvic, effects of on delivery,
234
perineal, 377
psychologic, related to failure
to achieve parent-infant
attachment, 381
related to alcohol use, 767
related to drug abuse, 758, 759f
related to induction of uterine
contractions, 292-293
related to malpresentation, 252
related to smoking during
pregnancy, 761
related to test complications,
190-191
related to TORCH disease, 599
related to uterine rupture,
842-843
neonatal
corneal, related to
phototherapy, 527
in large-for-gestational-age
infants during birth, 486

Injury (*Continued*)
related to birth asphyxia in
small-for-gestational-age
infant, 469-470
related to maternal
pyelonephritis, 613-614
in pregnancy, 703-726
abdominal, abruptio placentae
and, 639
assessment of, 709-714, 715t
case studies and study
questions for, 723-725
cause or mechanism of injury
in, 708-709
complications of, 709
concepts for, 704
diagnostic procedures for,
714-717
gastrointestinal changes in, 706
genitourinary changes in, 706,
707f
health education regarding,
721-722, 722f
hematologic changes in, 706
incidence and epidemiology of,
703-704
ineffective airway clearance
related to, 717, 718f
nursing diagnoses and
interventions/outcomes
for, 717-721, 718f, 720f
pelvic changes in, 707
physiologic considerations for,
704-705, 705f
respiratory changes in, 706
types of, 707
Inlet, obstetric conjugate of, 236,
236f
Innervation, female reproductive, 10
Inotropic agents for maternal
cardiovascular disease, 779t
Insensible water loss in premature
infant, 480, 481
Insulin, increased production of
during pregnancy, 101
Insulin therapy, 664-665, 668
Insulin-dependent diabetes
mellitus. *See* Type 1 diabetes.
Integumentary system
fetal development of, 57, 58, 59,
60
maternal
changes to during pregnancy,
101
impaired integrity of related to
delivery process, 285
in nutritional status
assessment, 112t
postpartum changes to, 375
neonatal
assessment of, 438, 442t
color of in Apgar scoring, 426
hyperbilirubinemia and, 527
in postterm infant, 487-488
in premature infant, 476
preterm infant and, 480-481
Intensity of contractions, 230, 350
Intensive care unit, neonatal,
dilemmas regarding, 887-888

Interdependent phase of mother, 375
Internal female genitalia
anatomy of, 5f, 5-8, 7f
examination of, 15-16
Internal monitoring of contractions, 232
Internal os, 6
Internal rotation, fetal, 249
Interpreter, 83
Interrupted family process
acceptance of newborn and, 289
acquired immunodeficiency syndrome and, 608-609
alcohol use-related, 766
complicated pregnancy and, 772-773
development stressors of pregnancy or loss and, 135-136
following diagnosis of genetic disorder in fetus or newborn, 35
related to demands of care for diabetes mellitus
gestational, 675
pregestational, 671
related to value differences between woman and her partner about contraceptive choices, 411-416
substance abuse and, 757
Interview, health, in assessment of reproductive anatomy, physiology, and menstrual cycle, 13-15
Intimate partner violence, 537-553, 704
assessment of, 544-546
case study and study questions associated with, 551-552
characteristics of abusers in, 542-543, 543f
characteristics of women in battering relationships, 543-544
cultural and socioeconomic factors in, 541-542
cycle of violence in, 538-540, 539f
health education regarding, 550
incidence of, 537-538
interventions/outcomes for, 546-548, 549f
nursing diagnoses in, 546
during pregnancy, 538, 544
resources for professionals regarding, 550
traumatic injury due to, 708, 709
types of injuries in, 540
Intracytoplasmic sperm injection, 153
Intraembryonic coelom, 48
Intrapartum period, 225-368
assessment in, 228-232, 241-252
cardinal movements and, 249
case studies and study questions related to, 264-268, 299-301
cervical changes in, 240f, 240-241
contractions in

Intrapartum period (Continued)
frequency of, 232
onset of, 228-229
physiology of, 229f, 229-231
strength of, 232-233
diagnostic studies and techniques during, 232, 249-252, 250f, 251f
dilatation as first stage of labor in, 273-281
analgesia or anesthesia for, 277-279
interventions/outcomes in, 279-281
latent phase of, 274-276
nursing diagnoses related to, 279
physiologic changes during, 273-274
transition phase of labor, 277
ethnocultural factors in, 76-78, 77f, 79-80, 92t
expectant fathers during, 128-129
false labor in, 231
fetal assessment during, 303-368
arrhythmias and dysrhythmias and, 319-329
baseline fetal heart rate and, 309-315, 310f, 311f
case studies and study questions associated with, 357-364, 358f, 359f, 360f, 361f, 362f, 363f, 364f
electronic methods of, 305-308
fetal scalp sampling for, 351-353
health education regarding, 357
nonelectronic methods of, 304-305
nonperiodic fetal heart rate patterns and, 344-349
periodic fetal heart rate patterns and, 332-344
pulse oximetry in, 353-355
umbilical cord blood sampling in, 355-357, 356f
uterine activity and, 350f, 350-351, 351f
variability of fetal heart rate and, 314-329, 316f, 317f, 318f, 319f
fetal attitude and, 242
fetal lie and, 242
fetal position and, 245, 246f
fetal presentation and, 242-245, 243f, 244f, 245f
fetal size and, 246-248
fetal skull and, 248-249
fetal station and, 245-246, 247f
"4 Ps" of, 228
health education regarding, 262-263, 263f, 299
immediate postpartum period as fourth stage of, 288-290
infant expulsion as second stage of, 281-286
interventions/outcomes in, 233-234, 241, 252-253, 272-273

Intrapartum period (Continued)
maternal musculoskeletal deformities and disease, effects of on delivery, 234
nursing diagnoses during, 233, 241, 252, 272
pelvis and, 234-240
dimension of, 236f, 236-240, 237f
manual assessment of capacity of, 241
shape of, 234-236, 235f
physical examination in, 231-232, 234-240, 242-249
placental expulsion as third stage of, 286-288, 287f
premonitory signs of, 271-273
previous pregnancies and, 241-242
psychosocial factors in, 253-258, 253-262
behaviors, 258
current pregnancy experience, 253
emotions of labor, 255-256
expectations for birth experience, 254
interventions/outcomes related to, 259-262
nursing diagnoses related to, 258-259
personality styles, 257-258
preparation for birth, 254
previous birth experiences, 253
psychologic reactions to labor, 256-257
support system, 254-255
variables influencing, 290-299
cesarean birth, 296-299
dysfunctional labor, 293-296, 294f, 295f
induction or augmentation of uterine contractions, 290-293, 291t
Intrathecal narcotic, 278
Intrauterine device
copper, 413t
high-dose progesterone-only, 415t
Intrauterine fetal demise, 835-839, 846
ultrasonographic confirmation of, 170
Intrauterine fetal surgery, 741-744
Intrauterine growth restriction, 465
due to heroin abuse, 752
due to maternal diabetes mellitus, 666
Intrauterine pressure catheter monitoring of contractions, 232, 307-308
risk for infection related to, 233
Intrauterine system, levonorgestrel, 414t
Intrauterine transfusion, 179
Intravascular coagulation, disseminated
as cause of postpartum hemorrhage, 851, 852
related to intrauterine fetal demise, 836

Intubation
  indications of for neonate, 426
  for respiratory distress
    syndrome, 503
Inverted nipples, 390
  incorrect latching on related to,
    394-396
Involution, uterine, 371-372
  pain related to, 289
Iodine
  radioactive as environmental
    hazard, 214
  requirements of during
    pregnancy, 107
Ionizing radiation exposure, 204-205
IPV. See Intimate partner violence.
Iris, neonatal, 438
Iron
  changes to levels in blood during
    pregnancy, 99
  deficiencies of, effect on fetus, 107
  requirements of during
    pregnancy, 106
  supplementations for, 104
Iron-deficiency anemia, 800, 802,
  803, 803t
Irritability during pregnancy, 126
Irritable infant, breastfeeding of, 400
Ischium, 9f, 10
Isoimmunization
  red blood cell, 180-181
  Rh, 54
    amniocentesis for evaluation
      of, 177-178
Isolation, feelings of as reaction to
  labor, 257
Isoniazid for tuberculosis, 788,
  790t
Isotretinoin as environmental
  hazard, 215
Isthmus, uterine, 6, 8
ITP. See Immune thrombocytopenic
  purpura.
IUD. See Intrauterine device.
IUGR. See Intrauterine growth
  restriction.
IUPC. See Intrauterine pressure
  catheter monitoring of
  contractions.
IVF. See In vitro fertilization.
IWL. See Insensible water loss in
  premature infant.

J
Jacuzzi exposure, 209
Jaundice, 517-528
  assessment of, 523-526
  breastfeeding and, 400-401
  causes of, 517-521, 519f
  discharge planning in, 529
  interventions/outcomes for,
    526-528
  in large-for-gestational-age
    infant, 486
  long-term follow-up in, 529
  nursing diagnoses in, 526
  in preterm infant, 474
  treatment of, 521-523, 523f

Johns Hopkins AIDS Service
  Guidelines, 623-624
Judgment, substituted, 884
Justice, ethics and, 875

K
Kanamycin as environmental
  hazard, 211
Kangaroo care, 423
Kantrex. See Kanamycin.
KB. See Kleihauer-Betke test.
Kegel exercise, 263
Kernicterus, 521
Ketoacidosis, diabetic, 663, 668
Ketones
  testing of at first prenatal visit, 115
  testing of in diabetes mellitus,
    665, 668-669
Kidney
  maternal
    changes to during first stage of
      labor, 274
    changes to during pregnancy,
      99-100, 781
    disease of, 781-787
    postpartum changes in, 374
    preeclampsia and, 563-564
    systemic lupus erythematosus-
      related symptoms in, 795
  neonatal
    assessment of, 439
    in preterm infant, 474, 481
Kidney stones, 782, 785-786
Kilocalorie intake during
  pregnancy, 105
Klebcil. See Kanamycin.
Kleihauer-Betke test, 67, 715
Klumpe's palsy, 484
Kneeling breech presentation,
  243
Kneeling postures for labor and
  delivery, 240
Knowledge, deficient
  acquired immunodeficiency
    syndrome and, 607-608
  adrenal insufficiency and, 690
  alcohol use and its effects on
    pregnancy and, 766
  birthing process related to
    inadequate preparation or
    unanticipated circumstances
    and, 261
  cesarean birth and, 297-298
  chorioamnionitis and, 622
  diabetes mellitus and
    gestational, 675-676
    pregestational, 670
  disease complicating pregnancy
    and, 773
  dysfunctional labor and, 295
  effective use of contraceptive
    method of choice and, 411
  genetic assessment and, 34-35
  hazardous effects of
    pharmaceuticals and, 216-217
  hyperadrenocorticism and,
    687-688
  hyperthyroidism and, 681-682

Knowledge (Continued)
  inexperience with newborn care
    and lack of parenting skills
    and, 432
  maternal phenylketonuria and, 694
  normal anatomy and physiology
    of female reproductive
    system and, 17-18
  normal menstrual cycle and, 18
  normal physiologic response to
    pregnancy and, 116-117
  occupational hazards and, 207-208
  related to maternal experience in
    positioning infant for
    breastfeeding, 391f, 391-394,
    392f, 393f, 394f, 395f
  second hand smoke exposure
    and, 218
  sexually transmitted diseases
    and, 611
  smoking during pregnancy and,
    761
  specific high-risk pregnancy
    condition and treatment
    options and, 191
  substance abuse and, 755, 756b
  temperature extremes and,
    209-210
  TORCH disease and, 598-599
  urinary tract infection and
    pyelonephritis and, 613
Kyphoscoliosis, labor passage and,
  234

L
Labetalol hydrochloride for
  hypertensive disorders of
  pregnancy, 577t
Labia majora, 3
Labia minora, 3
Labor and delivery, 225-368
  assessment in, 228-232, 241-252
  cardinal movements and, 249
  case studies and study questions
    for, 264-268, 299-301
  cervical changes during, 240f,
    240-241
  complications of, 818-849
    amniotic fluid embolism, 839-841
    case studies and study
      questions for, 844-848
    intrauterine fetal demise,
      835-839
    multiple gestation, 831-835
    postterm pregnancy, 825-827
    premature rupture of
      membrane, 827-831
    preterm labor as, 818-825. See
      Also Preterm labor.
    uterine rupture, 841-844
  contractions in
    frequency of, 232
    onset of, 228-229
    physiology of, 229f, 229-231
    strength of, 232-233
  diagnostic studies and
    techniques during, 232,
    249-252, 250f, 251f

Labor and delivery (*Continued*)
  dilatation as first stage of, 273-281
    analgesia or anesthesia for,
      277-279
    interventions/outcomes in,
      279-281
    latent phase of, 274-276
    nursing diagnoses related to,
      279
    physiologic changes during,
      273-274
    transition phase of labor, 277
  dysfunctional grieving related to
    loss of desired, 138
  effects of maternal
    musculoskeletal deformities
    and disease on, 234
  ethnocultural factors in, 76-78,
    77f, 79-80, 92t
  false labor and, 231
  fathers at, 128-129
  fetal assessment during
    arrhythmias and dysrhythmias
      and, 319-329
    baseline fetal heart rate and,
      309-315, 310f, 311f
    case studies and study
      questions associated for,
      357-364, 358f, 359f, 360f,
      361f, 362f, 363f, 364f
    electronic methods of, 305-308
    fetal scalp sampling for, 351-353
    health education regarding, 357
    nonelectronic methods of,
      304-305
    nonperiodic fetal heart rate
      patterns and, 344-349
    periodic fetal heart rate
      patterns and, 332-344
    pulse oximetry in, 353-355
    umbilical cord blood sampling
      in, 355-357, 356t
    uterine activity and, 350f,
      350-351, 351f
    variability of fetal heart rate
      and, 314-329, 316f, 317f,
      318f, 319f
  fetal attitude and, 242
  fetal lie and, 242
  fetal position and, 245, 246f
  fetal presentation and, 242-245,
    243f, 244f, 245f
  fetal size assessment, 246-248
  fetal skull and, 248-249
  fetal station and, 245-246, 247f
  "4 Ps" of, 228
  health education regarding,
    262-263, 263f, 299
  immediate postpartum period as
    fourth stage of, 288-290
  infant expulsion as second stage
    of, 281-286
  interventions/outcomes in,
    233-234, 241, 252-253, 272-273
  in intrauterine fetal demise, 837
  nursing diagnoses during, 233,
    241, 252, 272
  optimizing power during,
    262-263, 263f

Labor and delivery (*Continued*)
  pain of, fear related to, 261
  pelvis and, 234-240
    dimension of, 236f, 236-240, 237f
    manual determination of
      capacity of, 241
    shape of, 234-236, 235f
  physical examination in, 231-232,
    234-240, 242-249
  placental expulsion as third stage
    of, 286-288, 287f
  premonitory signs of, 271-273
  preparation education for, 132-133
  previous pregnancies and, 241-242
  psychosocial factors in, 253-258,
    253-262
    behaviors, 258
    current pregnancy experience,
      253
    emotions of labor, 255-256
    expectations for birth
      experience, 254
    interventions/outcomes
      related to, 259-262
    nursing diagnoses related to,
      258-259
    personality styles, 257-258
    preparation for birth, 254
    previous birth experiences, 253
    psychologic reactions to labor,
      256-257
    support system, 254-255
  variables influencing, 290-299
    cesarean birth, 296-299
    dysfunctional labor, 293-296,
      294f, 295f
    induction or augmentation of
      uterine contractions,
      290-293, 291t
Laboratory testing
  in cholecystectomy, 736
  in endoscopic gastrointestinal
    procedures, 741
  following trauma in pregnancy,
    714-715
  in gestational hypertension and
    HELLP syndrome, 573t,
    573-574
  in hematologic complications,
    803, 803t
  in hepatitis, 813
  in renal disease, 783-784
  in systemic lupus erythematosus,
    796
Laboring down, 282
Laceration resulting from
    childbirth, 283, 373
  impaired tissue integrity related
    to, 377
  postpartum hemorrhage due to,
    852
Lactate dehydrogenase, in
    gestational hypertension and
    HELLP syndrome, 560, 573t
Lactation. *See* Breastfeeding.
Lactic acid buildup, fetal, 163-164
Lactic dehydrogenase, elevated in
    HELLP syndrome, 560
Lacto vegetarian diet, 113

Lactose intolerance, maternal, 114
Lamaze technique, 133
Lamellar body count, 177
Language barrier, 83
Lanugo, 442t
  prematurity and, 476
Laparoscopic approach
  for cholecystectomy, 735
  versus laparotomy, 731-732
Laparotomy *versus* laparoscopic
    approach, 731-732
Large-for-gestational-age infants,
    441, 482-486, 491
Lasix. *See* Furosemide.
Last menstrual period, estimated
    date of confinement and, 162
Latching on, 394-396
Late decelerations of fetal heart rate,
    165, 228f, 337-342, 339f, 341b
Latent phase of labor, 274-276
  emotions of, 255
Lateral position for labor and
    delivery, 238
Lavage, diagnostic peritoneal,
    716-717
LBC. *See* Lamellar body count.
LDH. *See* Lactate dehydrogenase.
Lead exposure, 204
Learning need
  related to hazardous effects of
    pharmaceuticals, 216-217
  related to occupational hazards,
    207-208
  related to second hand smoke
    exposure, 218
  related to temperature extremes,
    209-210
Lecithin, fetal viability and, 163
Lecithin/sphingomyelin ratio, 177
  in maternal diabetes mellitus, 665
  in respiratory distress syndrome
    assessment, 502
Leg recoil in neonatal neurologic
    assessment, 444b
Legal implications of prenatal
    diagnosis of genetic disorders,
    34
Legal *versus* ethical perspective,
    880-881
Length, neonatal, 438
Leopold's maneuvers, 249-251,
    250f, 842
Let-down reflex, term, 389
"Letting-go" phase of mother, 375
Leukorrhea, 97
Levator ani muscles, 8, 9f
Levonorgestrel intrauterine system,
    414t
LGA. *See* Large-for-gestational-age
    infants.
LH. *See* Luteinizing hormone.
Libido, decreased, during
    pregnancy, 134-135
Librium. *See* Chlordiazepoxide
    hydrochloride.
Lie, fetal, 242
Life-threatening complications
    related to hypertensive
    disorders, 554-555

Ligaments, uterine, 7
Ligation, bilateral tubal, 412t
Lightening, 249, 271, 272
Linguistic competence, 76
Lip, cleft, 448-450, 449f
Listeriosis, 619t
Lithium as environmental hazard, 213
Liver
  maternal
    changes to during pregnancy, 100
    preeclampsia-related injury to, 582
    systemic lupus erythematosus-related symptoms in, 795
  neonatal
    assessment of, 439
    hyperbilirubinemia due to dysfunction of, 520
    in preterm infant, 474
Liver enzymes, maternal, elevated in HELLP syndrome, 560
Liver function tests in cholecystectomy, 736
LMP. See Last menstrual period.
LNG-IUS. See Levonorgestrel intrauterine system.
Lochia, 371
  assessment of, 288, 376
Longitudinal fetal lie, 242
Long-term variability of fetal heart rate, 315-316, 316f, 317f
  interventions for, 329-330
Lorazepam as environmental hazard, 213
Lordosis, pregnancy-induced, 101
Loss, 132
  anticipatory grieving related to, 193
  impaired adjustment related to, 137-138
Loss of control as reaction to labor, 257
Lovastatin as environmental hazard, 213
Low spinal anesthesia, 282
L/S ratio. See Lecithin/sphingomyelin ratio.
LTV. See Long-term variability of fetal heart rate.
Luchal lucency screening for congenital anomalies, 171
Lungs
  fetal
    amniocentesis for assessment of maturity of, 177
    development of, 57, 58, 59, 60
    maternal drug use and, 751
  maternal
    amniotic fluid embolism of, 839-841
    changes in during first stage of labor, 274
    changes to during pregnancy, 99
    disease of, 787-793
    preeclampsia and, 564-565, 565t

Lungs (Continued)
    surgery and, 729
    systemic lupus erythematosus-related symptoms in, 795
    trauma and, 706, 711
  neonatal
    assessment of, 439
    fluid in expelled during delivery, 421
    in preterm infant, 472-473
    retained fluid in, 429, 508-510, 516-517
    transition of fetal to, 421-422
Lupus, 793-799
Luteal phase of menstruation, 11
  inadequate, 12
Luteinizing hormone, 13
  anovulation during pregnancy due to suppression of, 97
  assessment of, 17
Lyme disease, 619t
Lymphatic drainage, 8

M
Macroallocation, ethics and, 875
Macrosomia
  associated with gestational diabetes mellitus, 675
  in infants of diabetic mothers, 666
  labor and delivery and, 246-248
Magnesium sulfate
  for eclamptic seizure, 567, 576t
  for hypertensive disorders of pregnancy, 576t
  for preterm labor intervention, 820-821
Magnetic resonance imaging
  following trauma in pregnancy, 716
  in placenta previa, 635
Malattachment, 380
Male external genitalia, assessment of, 439, 443t
  in premature infant, 476
Male perspective regarding ethics, 882
Male sterilization, 412t
Manual palpation of contractions, 232
MAP. See Mean arterial pressure.
Marazide. See Benzthiazide.
March of Dimes Foundation, 767
Marijuana use, 753
Marked sinus arrhythmia, fetal, 321, 321f
Married couple beginning a family, 125
MAS. See Meconium aspiration syndrome.
Mask of pregnancy, term, 101
MAST suit application during pregnancy, 720, 720f
Mastectomy, breastfeeding and, 390
Mastitis, 399, 855
Maternal age, advanced, 152-156
  case studies and study questions associated with, 157-159

Maternal assessment of fetal movement, 165-166
Maternal infections, 592-629
  acquired immunodeficiency syndrome, 599-609
    assessment of, 605-607
    counseling and early diagnosis of, 603
    first recognition of, 599
    health education regarding, 623-624
    nursing diagnoses and interventions/outcomes for, 607-609
    treatment of, 604-605
    women and, 603-604, 604f, 604t
  case studies and study questions for, 625-627
  chorioamnionitis, 620-622, 625
  group B streptococcus, 617t-618t
  health education related to, 622-625
  influenza, 616t
  listeriosis, 619t
  Lyme disease, 619t
  measles, 616t
  mumps, 616t
  parvovirus B19, 618t
  sexually transmitted diseases, 599-611, 600t-602t, 624
  TORCH, 592-599, 593t-597t, 622-623
  tuberculosis, 617t
  urinary tract infection and pyelonephritis, 611-614, 624
  varicella zoster, 615t
Maternal placental circulation, 53-55, 54f, 55t
Maternal risk factors for preterm infants, 475-476
Maternal role, postpartum, 375, 378-379
Maternal serum alpha-fetoprotein screening, 183-185
  in triple marker test, 185-186
Maternal system changes
  postpartum, 371-375
    in breasts, 373
    in cardiovascular system, 373-374
    in endocrine system, 373
    in gastrointestinal system, 374
    in immune system, 375
    in integumentary system, 375
    in musculoskeletal system, 375
    in reproductive system, 371-373
    in respiratory system, 374
    in urinary system, 374
  during pregnancy, 96-102
    in cardiovascular system, 98-99
    in endocrine system, 101
    in gastrointestinal system, 100
    in immunologic system, 102
    in integumentary system, 101
    in musculoskeletal system, 101
    in reproductive system, 96-98
    in respiratory system, 99
    in urinary system, 99-100

Maturational crisis, pregnancy as, 126
Mature milk, 389
McDonald's suture, 739
Mean arterial pressure
maternal, in gestational hypertension, 555, 571
neonatal, assessment of in respiratory distress syndrome, 503
Mean corpuscular hemoglobin concentration, 803t
Mean corpuscular volume, 803t
Measles, 616t
German, 592-599, 593t-597t
Meconium, hyperbilirubinemia due to delayed passage of, 520
Meconium aspiration syndrome, 510-515, 511f
in large-for-gestational-age infants, 485-486
in postterm infant, 487, 489
Medical history, 108, 109-110
Medical perspective regarding ethics, 882-883
Medications. See Drugs.
MedlinePlus AIDS and Pregnancy, 624
Megaloblastic anemia, 800, 803
Meiosis, 24-25, 25f
Melasma, pregnancy-induced, 101
Membranes, rupture of
abruptio placentae and, 640
premature, 827-831, 845-846
risk for infection related to vaginal examination following, 281
spontaneous
as premonitory sign of childbirth, 273
risk for infection related to, 273
Menarche, 11, 12
age at onset of, 148
Mendelian law, 28f, 28-30, 29f, 31f
Meningocele, 447
Meningomyelocele, 50
maternal serum alpha-fetoprotein screening in, 185
Menopause, 11
Menotropins as environmental hazard, 215
Menstruation
anatomy and physiology of, 11-12
case studies and study questions related to, 19-22
clinical practice associated with, 13-18
deficient knowledge regarding, 18
health education related to, 18-19
history regarding
in first prenatal visit assessment, 107
in reproductive assessment, 107
postpartum resumption of, 372
sociocultural attitudes towards, 15

Meperidine for analgesia during childbirth, 278
Meprobamate as environmental hazard, 213
Mercury exposure, 204
Mersilene suture, 739
Mesoderm, 46
Metabolic acidosis
fetal, 163-164
oxygen saturation in, 353
neonatal
meconium aspiration syndrome and, 514
respiratory distress syndrome and, 504
Metabolic disorders, 660-702
adrenal insufficiency, 688-690, 698
case study and study questions for, 699-701
Cushing's syndrome, 685-688, 698
diabetes mellitus, 660-676
classification of, 661t, 661-661
gestational, 671-676, 696, 696t
maternal metabolism and pathophysiology of pregnancy and, 662
pregestational, 663-671, 695-696
symptoms of, 660
treatment of, 662
health education regarding, 695-699, 696t
hyperthyroidism, 677t, 677-683, 697
hypothyroidism, 683-685, 697-698
maternal phenylketonuria, 691-695, 698-699
neonatal
due to maternal diabetes mellitus, 667
respiratory distress related to, 498
Metabolic function
in diabetes mellitus, 662
gestational, 674
pregestational, 668-669
in hyperthyroidism, 681
in small-for-gestational-age infants, feedings and, 470-471
Metaethics, 874
Methadone hydrochloride abuse, 753
Methamphetamine as environmental hazard, 211
Methimazole
as environmental hazard, 214
for hyperthyroidism, 678
Methotrexate as environmental hazard, 214
Methyldopa for hypertensive disorders of pregnancy, 578t
Metolazone as environmental hazard, 213
Metritis, postpartum, 855
Metronidazole for trichomonas, 602t
Microallocation, ethics and, 875
Microcephaly, 252

Microsomia, labor and delivery and, 248
Microviscosimetry, 177
Midforceps delivery, 284
Military attitude, 242
Milk
breast
inability of mother to provide adequate supply of, 402-403
production and ejection of, 388f, 388-389
intake during pregnancy, 105
Milontin. See Phensuximide.
Miltown. See Meprobamate.
Minerals, required intake during pregnancy, 70, 105-107
Minimal variability of fetal heart rate, 315, 316f
Miscarriage
anticipatory grieving related to, 193
grief and loss associated with, 132
impaired adjustment related to, 137-138
risk for compromised family coping related to, 191-192
Misoprostol as environmental hazard, 214
Mitosis, 24, 24f
MN. See Myelomeningocele.
Mobitz type II heart block, 328, 331
Modified biophysical profile, 172-174, 173t
Modified Elkins procedure, 244
Molar pregnancy, 647-651
Molding, fetal, 248, 438
Molimina symptoms, 14
Mongolian spots, 438
Monosomy, 26
Mons pubis, 3
Montevideo units of uterine contractions, 232, 350
Mood disorders, postpartum, 130, 376, 379, 861-864, 865
impaired adjustment related to, 137-138
risk for ineffective coping related to, 381
Mood swings during pregnancy, 126
Moral agent, ethics and, 873
Morality, ethics and, 873
Morals, ethics and, 873
Moratorium phase of pregnancy, 128
Moro reflex, 440b
Morphine for analgesia during childbirth, 278
Morula, 42
Motor nerves of reproductive system, 10
Motor-vehicle crashes, 708, 709
Mouth
embryonic development of, 50
maternal, changes to during pregnancy, 100
neonatal, assessment of, 439
Movement, fetal, assessment of by client, 165-166

MRI. *See* Magnetic resonance imaging.
Mucocutaneous system, systemic lupus erythematosus symptoms in, 795
Mucoid discharge, ophthalmologic, 438
Mucus, cervical, 6, 11
Mucus plug, formation of, 97
Multifactorial genetic disorders, 30-31
Multigravida
interventions for anxiety for, 136
parenting skills intervention in, 137
Multiple gestation, 831-835, 846
in advanced maternal age, 154
breastfeeding interventions for, 402
case study and study questions regarding, 265-266
ultrasonographic assessment of, 170
Mumps, 616t
Murmur, neonatal, 439
Muscles, maternal
in nutritional status assessment, 111t
pelvic, 8, 9f
Muscles tone
maternal, uterine, postpartum hemorrhage and, 850, 851
neonatal
in Apgar scoring, 426t
assessment of, 440
Musculoskeletal system
embryonic development of, 52, 53
fetal development of, 57, 58, 59, 60
maternal
changes to during pregnancy, 101
effects of deformities and disease on labor and delivery, 234
in nutritional status assessment, 112t
postpartum changes in, 375
systemic lupus erythematosus symptoms in, 795
Mutagen, 202
Mutation, defined, 23
MVCs. *See* Motor-vehicle crashes.
MVUs. *See* Montevideo units of uterine contractions.
Mycobacterium tuberculosis, 788
Myelomeningocele, 447, 448f
fetal surgery for, 743
Myeloschisis, 447
Myocardial dysfunction, fetal, 332
Myometrium
anatomy of, 7
in physiology of contractions, 229, 231
Mysoline. *See* Primidone.

N
Nafarelin acetate as environmental hazard, 215
Nägele's rule, 111, 825

Nalbuphine for analgesia during childbirth, 278
Naloxone hydrochloride for neonatal resuscitation, 431t
Narcotics
for analgesia during childbirth, 278
intrathecal, 278
Narrative approach to ethics, 876
Nasal flaring in respiratory distress syndrome, 501
National Clearinghouse for Alcohol and Drug Information, 767
National Coalition for Health Professional Education in Genetics, 32
National Digestive Diseases Information Clearinghouse, 624
National Directory of Shelters, 550
National Herpes Hotline, 624
National Human Genome Project, 23
National Institute of Child Health and Human Development, 767
National Institute on Drug Abuse, 767
National Institutes of Health and Human Development, 304
National Self-Help Clearinghouse, 624
Native American culture, 91t-95t
intimate partner violence and, 541-542
Natural family planning, 414t
Nausea due to gastrointestinal disease, 809-810
NCHPEG. *See* National Coalition for Health Professional Education in Genetics.
Nebcin. *See* Tobramycin sulfate.
NEC. *See* Necrotizing enterocolitis.
Neck
maternal
examination of in traumatic injury, 713
in nutritional status assessment, 112t
neonatal, assessment of, 439
Necrotizing enterocolitis, 474
Neisseria gonorrhoeae, 601t-602t
Neonatal abstinence syndrome, 752
Neonatal intensive care unit, dilemmas regarding, 887-888
Neonatal lupus erythematosus, 794
Neonate. *See* Newborn.
Neoplasm
chorioadenoma destruens, 648, 650
choriocarcinoma, 648-650
ovarian, surgery for, 736-737
uterine, labor passage and, 234
Nephrolithiasis, 782, 785-786
Nephrotic syndrome, 782
Netilmicin sulfate as environmental hazard, 212
Netromycin. *See* Netilmicin sulfate.
Neural crest, 47, 47f
Neural plate, 47, 47f

Neural tube, 47
Neural tube defects, 441-448, 448f
alpha-fetoprotein levels in, 32
diagnostic testing in pregnancy at risk for, 34
fetal surgery for, 743
maternal serum alpha-fetoprotein screening in, 183-185
Neuraminidase, 42
Neurodevelopmental disorder
alcohol related, 764
heroin related, 753
Neurologic system
female reproductive, 10
fetal development of, 56, 57, 58, 59, 60
fetal heart rate and, 308, 315
maternal
acute renal failure and, 783
assessment of in traumatic injury, 712
in nutritional status assessment, 112t
systemic lupus erythematosus-related symptoms in, 796
neonatal
assessment of, 444b-445b, 446f
premature, 476
Neuromuscular assessment
maternal in preeclampsia, 572
neonatal, 445f
Neurulation, 47, 47f
Neutral thermal environment, 469
New York Heart Association Cardiac Disease Classification, 774, 775t
Newborn, 419-534
acceptance of, risk for interrupted family processes related to, 289
adaptation of to extrauterine life, 421-425
admission of to nursery, 426-427
assessment of, 438-441, 440b, 442t-443t, 444b-445b, 445f, 446f
in delivery-room, 425-426, 426t
breastfeeding of. *See Also* Breastfeeding.
case study and study questions for, 406-407
for fussy or irritable, 400
health education associated with, 405-406
maternal low self-esteem related to inability to supply adequate milk, 403-404
maternal nutrition and, 404-405
for multiple births, 402
physiologic jaundice and, 400-401
positioning for, 390, 391f, 391-394, 392f, 393f, 394f, 395f
for preterm or hospitalized infant, 401-402, 402f
for sleepy or reluctant infant, 399-400

Newborn (*Continued*)
for special needs infant, 402-403
care of, 432-433
ethnocultural factors in, 77,
81-82, 94t
health education regarding,
383, 433-434
thrombophlebitis and, 860-861
clearing of airway secretions in,
429
congenital abnormalities in,
441-460
cardiovascular, 453-460
cleft lip and cleft palate as,
448-450, 449f
congenital diaphragmatic
hernia, 451-453
hydrocephalus as, 441-447
spina bifida as, 447-448, 448f
decreased cardiac output in,
429-432
effects of maternal
hyperthyroidism on, 680
effects of maternal substance
abuse on, 756b
expulsion of, 281-286. *See Also*
Childbirth.
gestational age of, 465-496
assessment of, 441, 442t-443t,
444b-445b, 445f, 446f
case studies and study
questions associated with,
492-494
health education regarding,
490-491
large for, 482-486
postterm infant, 486-490
preterm infant, 472-482
small for, 465-471
health education regarding,
460-461
hypothermic, 427-429
infection in, 432
nursing diagnoses related to,
427-433, 428f, 430t-431t
poor nutrition in related to poor
suck-and-swallow
coordination, 432
poor respiratory effort and
retained lung fluid in, 429
in transient tachypnea, 509-510
preterm. *See* Preterm infant.
at risk, identification of, 425-426,
426t
shallow or periodic breathing
and apnea in, 429
sick, 497-534
anticipatory grieving related
to, 138
case studies and study
questions associated with,
530-532
dysfunctional grieving related
to, 138
health education regarding,
490-491, 528-529
hyperbilirubinemia in, 517-528
meconium aspiration
syndrome in, 510-515, 511f

Newborn (*Continued*)
persistent pulmonary
hypertension of newborn
in, 515-517
respiratory distress in, 498-499
respiratory distress syndrome
in, 500-508
transient tachypnea in, 508-509
suckling, assessment of, 391
transition of fetus to, 421-425
Niacin, requirements of during
pregnancy, 106
NICHD. *See* National Institutes of
Health and Human
Development.
Nicotine, 760
fetal heart rate and, 310
Nicotine polarcrilex as
environmental hazard, 215
Nicotine resin complex, 215
Nicotine transdermal patch as
environmental hazard, 215
Nifedipine
for hypertensive disorders of
pregnancy, 577t
in preterm labor therapy, 822
Nipple
maternal
assessment of for
breastfeeding, 390
changes to during pregnancy,
98
incorrect latching onto, 394-396
pain in secondary to
breastfeeding, 397-399
postpartum changes to, 373
stimulation of for contraction
stress test, 189
neonatal, 443t
prematurity and, 476
Nipple confusion, 394-396
Nitrofurantoin for acute
pyelonephritis, 613
NLE. *See* Neonatal lupus
erythematosus.
Noise as environmental hazard,
205, 205t
Noncompliance
in adolescent, 153
associated with drug abuse, 757
related to alcohol use, 767
Nonconducted premature atrial
contractions, 323, 324f
Non-insulin–dependent diabetes
mellitus. *See* Type 2 diabetes
mellitus.
Nonionizing radiation exposure,
205
Nonmaleficence, ethics and,
874-875
Nonnormative ethics, 874
Nonperiodic fetal heart rate
patterns, 344-349
decelerations
prolonged, 347-349, 348f
variable, 345-347, 346f
Nonstress test, 187-188
Norepinephrine, fetal heart rate
and, 309

Normodyne. *See* Labetalol
hydrochloride.
Norplant, 415t
Nortriptyline hydrochloride as
environmental hazard, 213
Nose, neonatal, assessment of, 439
Notochordal process, 46-47
NST. *See* Nonstress test.
NTE. *See* Neutral thermal
environment.
Nubain. *See* Nalbuphine.
Nuchal cord, 64
Nucleoside analogs for human
immunodeficiency virus-
associated infection, 604
Nurse
role of in antepartum fetal
assessment, 162-165
as trained labor attendant, 255
Nursery, admission of newborn to,
426-427
ill, 490
Nursing, transcultural, 75-76. *See
Also* Ethnocultural
considerations.
Nursing perspective regarding
ethics, 882-883
Nutrient requirements during
pregnancy, 104, 105f
Nutrition
fetal, placenta's role in, 56
maternal, 103-107, 105f
adolescent, 148, 150, 151-152
breastfeeding and, 404-405
delayed fetal growth and
development related to
inadequate, 68
gastrointestinal disease and, 810
gestational hypertension and,
569
history in assessment of,
108-109, 110f
imbalanced: less than body
requirements, 118
imbalanced: more than body
requirements, 117
inflammatory bowel disease
and, 808
physical examination in
assessment of, 111t-112t,
111-114
substance abuse and, 756-757
type 1 and type 2 diabetes and,
663-664
neonatal, 423-424, 434
in premature infant, 477
in respiratory distress
syndrome, 506-507
in small-for-gestational-age,
470-471
for phenylketonuria, 691, 692,
694-695
Nutrition: less than body
requirements
maternal
in acquired immunodeficiency
syndrome, 609
in lactation and/or depression,
404-405

Nutrition(*Continued*)
  related to alcohol use, 766
  related to gastrointestinal disease, 809-810
  related to inadequate information about nutritional needs during pregnancy, 118
  related to maternal phenylketonuria, 694-695
  related to smoking during pregnancy, 761
  in substance abuse, 756-757
  neonatal
    associated with cleft lip and palate, 432
    in large-for-gestational-age infants, 485
    in persistent pulmonary hypertension, 517
    in postterm infant, 489-490
    in preterm infant, 479-480
    related to inability to suck and swallow with cleft lip and palate, 450
    in small-for-gestational-age infants, 470-471
    in transient tachypnea, 510
Nutrition: more than body requirements
  related to blood glucose management in diabetes mellitus, 675
  related to excessive intake of calories, 117

O

Obese patient
  body mass index values for, 103
  childbearing complications due to, 113
  weight gain during pregnancy in, 103-104
Obligation-based approach to ethics, 874-875
Oblique fetal lie, 242
Obstetric conjugate of inlet, 236, 236f
Obstetric history
  in comprehensive general health examination at first prenatal visit, 108
  family planning and, 409-410
Obstruction, airway, maternal, due to traumatic injury, 711
Obstructive uropathy, fetal surgery for, 744
Occupational environmental hazards, 203-208, 205t, 219-220
Occupational factors in advanced maternal age, 153-154
OCT. *See* Oxytocin challenge test.
OGTT. *See* Oral glucose tolerance test.
Oligohydramnios, 66
  due to fetal surgery, 742
  ultrasonographic assessment of, 170-171

Oliguria in preeclampsia, 559, 564, 571
Omphalocele, 450-451
Oocytes, donor, 153
Oogenesis, 25
Oophorectomy, 736-737
Oophoritis, postpartum, 855
Open crib, 423
Open pneumothorax, 718
Open-glottis method of pushing, 282
Operculum, 97
Opportunistic infection in human immunodeficiency virus infection, 604-605, 606
Opthalmia, prophylactic treatment of in newborn, 426
Optimistic personality, 258
Oral cavity in nutritional status assessment, 112t
Oral contraceptives, 412t
Oral glucose tolerance test, 673
Organ maturity in preterm infants, 472
Organic solvents, 206
Orthodox Judaism population, attitudes of toward menstruation, 15
Ostium primum, 455
Ostium secundum, 454
Otic placodes, 49
Ovaries
  anatomy of, 8
  changes to during pregnancy, 97, 102
  cystectomy or oophorectomy for tumors of, 736-737
  feedback loop functioning for, 13
  postpartum infection of, 855
Overweight patient
  body mass index values for, 103
  weight gain during pregnancy in, 103
Oviducts, 7-8
Ovolacto vegetarian diet, 113
Ovulation
  anatomy and physiology of, 11
  return of during breastfeeding, 372
Ovum, fertilization and, 41-42, 42f
Oxygen
  increased requirements of during pregnancy, 99
  partial pressure of. *See* Partial pressure of oxygen.
  risk for impaired fetal gas exchange related to intrapartum events that reduce levels of, 313-314, 329-332
Oxygen consumption in gestational hypertension and HELLP syndrome, 573t
Oxygen saturation
  fetal, normal, 353
  in premature infant, 478
Oxygen therapy
  in amniotic fluid embolism, 840
  in meconium aspiration syndrome, 514

Oxygen therapy (*Continued*)
  in persistent pulmonary hypertension of newborn, 516
  in placenta previa, 636
  for respiratory distress syndrome, 503
  in transient tachypnea of newborn, 510
Oxygenation
  fetal
    in abruptio placentae, 643
    adaptation of fetus to decreased, 164
    adequate, 163
    biophysical profile for assessment of, 172-174, 173t
    placenta previa and, 633, 637-638
  maternal in preeclampsia, 563-568
  neonatal
    in meconium aspiration syndrome, 513-515
    in persistent pulmonary hypertension of newborn, 516-517
    related to meconium aspiration syndrome, 513-515
    in transient tachypnea of newborn, 509-510
Oxytocin
  for induction or augmentation of labor, 291
  in intrauterine fetal demise, 837
  in initiation of milk ejection, 389
  in onset of contractions, 228
  risk for excess fluid volume related to use of, 292
Oxytocin challenge test, 189

P

PAC. *See* Premature atrial contractions.
Pacemaker in physiology of contractions, 230
Pacifiers, 424
Pain
  abdominal
    in appendicitis, 737, 738f
    due to gastrointestinal disease, 810
    related to abruptio placentae, 643-644
  of childbirth, 277-278
    fear related to, 261, 273
  due to thrombophlebitis, 860
  due to uterine rupture, 843
  ethnocultural variations regarding, 92t, 254
  related to abnormal labor pattern, 296
  related to descent of fetus and perineal stretching, 285
  related to early uterine involution, 289
  related to episiotomy, hemorrhoids, or cesarean section incision, 378

Pain (*Continued*)
  related to postpartum infection, 856-857
  related to surgery in pregnancy, 734
  related to surgical intervention for cesarean birth, 298
  resulting from uterine contractions and cervical dilatation, 280-281, 292
  systemic lupus erythematosus-associated, 797
Pain management
  for first stage of labor, 277-279
  intrauterine fetal demise and, 837
  in surgery in pregnancy, 734
  in uterine rupture, 843
Palate
  cleft, 448-450, 449f
  neonatal assessment of, 439
Palmar grasp reflex, 440b
Palpation of contractions, 232
  by patient, 824
Palsy in large-for-gestational-age infant, 484, 486
Pancreas, changes to during pregnancy, 101-102
PAP. *See* Pulmonary artery pressure.
Paracervical block, 278
Paradione. *See* Paramethadione.
Paramethadione as environmental hazard, 213
Parametritis, postpartum, 855
Parasympathetic nervous system
  female reproductive, 10
  fetal heart rate and, 308, 315
Parathyroid gland, changes to during pregnancy, 101
Parental autonomy, 878-879
Parent-child attachment, 375-376, 379-380
  beginning process of, 289
  cultural factors in, 82
  failure to achieve, 381
  impaired related to postpartum infection, 858
Parenting, impaired
  associated with parent-infant separation secondary to phototherapy treatments, 527-528
  due to drug abuse, 758-759
  due to multiple births, 834-835
  following diagnosis of genetic disorder in fetus or newborn, 35-36
  related to inadequate bonding secondary to infant with cleft lip and palate, 450
  related to lack of knowledge and skills, 137
  related to late childbearing, 155-156
  related to postpartum depression, 863
  related to postpartum infection, 858

Parenting (*Continued*)
  related to taking on role of mother, 380-381
Parity, nutrition and, 108-109
Partial pressure of carbon dioxide, 582t
  maternal
    asthma and, 787
    surgery and, 729
    traumatic injury and, 706
  neonatal in transient tachypnea of newborn, 510
  umbilical cord, 356t
Partial pressure of oxygen, 582t
  maternal, asthma and, 787
  neonatal in transient tachypnea of newborn, 510
  in premature infant, 478
  umbilical cord, 356t
Partial thromboplastin time
  in disseminated intravascular coagulation, 645
  in gestational hypertension and HELLP syndrome, 573t
  disseminated intravascular coagulation *versus*, 563t
Parvovirus B19, 618t
Passage, labor, 234-241
  maximization of, 263
Passive smoking, 217-218, 219, 221
Patent ductus arteriosus, 453-454, 454f, 477
Paternalism-maternalism-parentalism concept in ethics, 878
Patient Self Determination Act, 886
Patient self-care
  for asthma, 792b
  postpartum, 382
  regarding blood glucose management in mother's with diabetes mellitus, 670, 675-676
PCBs. *See* Polychlorinated biphenyls.
PCWP. *See* Pulmonary capillary wedge pressure.
PDA. *See* Patent ductus arteriosus.
Peak expiratory flow rate in tuberculosis, 789
Pediatric health maintenance and follow-up, 434
PEFR. *See* Peak expiratory flow rate.
Pelvic floor as support for organs of reproduction, 8, 9f
Pelvic tilt, 263, 263f
Pelvis
  anatomy and physiology of, 9f, 9-10, 10f
  blood supply to, 8
  changes to due to trauma in pregnancy, 707
  contracted, labor passage and, 234
  dimension of, effects on delivery, 236f, 236-240, 237f
  examination of
    at first prenatal visit, 111

Pelvis (*Continued*)
    following traumatic injury, 713
    in reproductive assessment, 15-16
  infections of, health history and, 13
  manual assessment of, 241
  postpartum infection of, 855
  risk for situational low self-esteem related to possible reduced capacity of, 241
  shape of, effects on delivery, 234-236, 235f
  trauma and, 707
    effects of on delivery, 234
Penetrating trauma, 704, 709-710
  uterine, 709
Pentobarbital as environmental hazard, 216
Percutaneous umbilical blood sampling, 178-181, 180f, 355-357, 356t
  risk for deficient fluid volume related to, 192
Perineum
  anatomy of, 5, 8
  delivery-related trauma to
    impaired tissue integrity related to, 377
    risk for urinary retention related to, 377
  pain related to stretching of, 285
  postpartum assessment of, 288, 376-377
  postpartum changes to, 373
  postpartum infection of, 855
  as support for organs of reproduction, 8, 9f
Periodic breathing in newborn, 429
  premature, 477
Periodic fetal heart rate patterns, 332-344
  accelerations, 332-333, 333f
  decelerations
    combined, 343f, 343-344
    early, 342f, 342-343
    late, 228f, 337-342, 339f, 341b
    variable, 333-337, 334f, 335f, 337b
Peripheral blood smear in HELLP syndrome, 560
Peristalsis
  postpartum, 377-378
  during pregnancy, 100
Peritoneal lavage, diagnostic, 716-717
Peritonitis, preterm labor and, 738
Periventricular intraventricular hemorrhage, 474
Persistent pulmonary hypertension of newborn, 515-517
Personality styles, labor and delivery and, 257-258
Pesticides, 206
Pet abuse, 545
Petechiae, hyperbilirubinemia-associated, 525
pH
  of amniotic fluid, 65
  of blood

pH (*Continued*)
  fetal, 164, 352, 355, 356t
  maternal, asthma and, 787
  neonatal in transient tachypnea
    of newborn, 510
  of leukorrhea during pregnancy,
    97
Pharmaceuticals
  for analgesia or anesthesia for
    labor, 278
  breastfeeding and, 404
  as environmental hazards, 210-217
    amphetamines, 210-211
    analgesics, 211-212
    antibiotics, 211-212
    anticoagulants, 212
    anticonvulsants, 212-213
    antidepressants and
      psychotropics, 213
    antiemetics, 213
    antihyperlipidemics and
      hypocholesterolemic
      agents, 213
    antihypertensives, 213
    antimigraine agents, 213-214
    antineoplastics, 214
    antithyroid drugs, 214
    antiulcer agents, 214
    antiviral agents, 214
    case studies and study
      questions for, 220
    decongestants, 214
    diethylstilbestrol, 215
    gallstone-solubilizing agents,
      215
    gonadotropic hormones, 215
    health education regarding, 219
    nicotine polarcrilex, 215
    nicotine transdermal patch, 215
    retinoids, 215
    sedatives and hypnotics, 215-216
Phenacemide as environmental
  hazard, 213
Phenergan. *See* Promethazine.
Phenobarbital
  for analgesia during childbirth,
    278
  as environmental hazards, 216
Phenotype, defined, 23
Phensuximide as environmental
  hazard, 213
Phenurone. *See* Phenacemide.
Phenylbutazone as environmental
  hazard, 211
Phenylketonuria, 691-695, 698-699
Phenylpropanolamine as
  environmental hazard, 214
Phenytoin as environmental
  hazard, 212
Phosphatidylglycerol, 502
Phospholipids, fetal viability and, 163
Phosphorus, calcium requirements
  during pregnancy and, 106
Phototherapy
  for hyperbilirubinemia, 521-522
  impaired skin integrity related to,
    527
  risk for deficient neonatal fluid
    volume in, 526

Physical abuse, intimate partner,
  537-553
  assessment of, 544-546
  case study and study questions
    associated with, 551-552
  characteristics of abusers in,
    542-543, 543f
  characteristics of women in
    battering relationships,
    543-544
  cultural and socioeconomic
    factors in, 541-542
  cycle of violence in, 538-540, 539f
  health education regarding, 550
  incidence of, 537-538
  interventions/outcomes for,
    546-548, 549f
  nursing diagnoses in, 546
  during pregnancy, 538, 544
  resources for professionals
    regarding, 550
  types of injuries in, 540
Physical energy demands as
  environmental hazard, 206
Physical examination
  abdominal
    cholecystectomy and, 735
    following maternal traumatic
      injury, 713
    during latent phase of labor, 276
  in adolescent pregnancy
    assessment, 149-150
  in advanced maternal age
    assessment, 154
  in assessment of reproductive
    anatomy, physiology, and
    menstrual cycle, 15-16, 16f
  in comprehensive general health
    examination at first prenatal
    visit, 111t-112t, 111-116, 116f
  following traumatic injury, 710f,
    710-714
  during labor and delivery,
    231-232, 234-240, 242-249
    cardinal movements and, 249
    for fetal attitude assessment, 242
    for fetal lie assessment, 242
    for fetal position assessment,
      245, 246f
    for fetal presentation
      assessment, 242-245, 243f,
      244f, 245f
    for fetal size assessment,
      246-248
    fetal skull and, 248-249
    for fetal station assessment,
      245-246, 247f
    for pelvic capacity
      determination, 234-240,
      235f, 236f, 237f
    for uterine contraction
      assessment, 231-232
  neonatal, 438-440, 440b
  pelvic, 15-16
  postpartum, 376-377
  preoperative, 730-731
  vaginal, 15
    during active phase of labor,
      276

Physical examination (*Continued*)
  in cholecystectomy, 736
  for effacement and dilatation
    assessment, 241
  in intrauterine fetal demise, 836
  during labor and delivery, 251,
    251f, 281
  during latent phase of labor, 275
  in postterm pregnancy, 825
  risk of infection related to,
    after ROM, 281
Physiologic jaundice, 517-528
  assessment of, 523-526
  breastfeeding and, 400-401
  causes of, 517-521, 519f
  discharge planning in, 529
  interventions/outcomes for,
    526-528
  in large-for-gestational-age
    infant, 486
  long-term follow-up in, 529
  nursing diagnoses in, 526
  in preterm infant, 474
  treatment of, 521-523, 523f
Pica, 79, 106, 113-114
Pinocytosis in placental transfer, 55,
  55t
Pitocin, hyperbilirubinemia and, 524
Pituitary gland, maternal
  changes to during pregnancy, 101
  postpartum changes in, 373
PIVH. *See* Periventricular
  intraventricular hemorrhage.
PKU. *See* Phenylketonuria.
Placenta
  abnormalities of, 61-63, 63t,
    286-287, 287f
    postterm infant and, 487
    small-for-gestational-age-
      related to, 466, 469
  decreased function of in postterm
    pregnancy, 826-827
  ethnocultural factors in
    disposition of after delivery,
    80
  expulsion of as third stage of
    labor, 286-288, 287f
  in fetal circulation, 53-56, 54f, 55t
  function of, explained to patient,
    827
  impaired transport by, 69-70
  inadequate blood supply to
    related to late decelerations
    of fetal heart rate, 340,
    341b
  posterm infant and, 487
  preeclampsia and, 567-568
  pre-embryonic development of,
    44-45, 45f
  retained fragments of,
    postpartum hemorrhage due
    to, 852
  study questions related to,
    70-71
  trophoblastic tumors of, 648,
    649-650
  ultrasonographic assessment of,
    168-169, 169f
Placenta accreta, 634

Placenta previa, 631-638
    diagnostic procedures in, 635-636
    health education regarding,
        651-652
    history in assessment of, 631-632
    ineffective fetal perfusion and
        oxygenation due to maternal
        blood loss, 637-638
    ineffective tissue perfusion
        related to blood loss of,
        636-637
    maternal anxiety related to, 638
    nursing diagnoses and
        interventions/outcomes for,
        636-638
    physical findings in, 633-635
    physiologic response to blood
        loss due to, 632-633
    psychosocial findings in, 635
    ultrasonographic assessment of,
        169
Placental barrier, 44
Placental site, postpartum infection
    of, 855
Plantar creases, 442t
    in premature infant, 476
Plantar grasp reflex, 440b
Platelets
    disseminated intravascular
        coagulation and, 563t, 573t,
        645
    hypertensive disorders of
        pregnancy and, 557-558, 561,
        568
Platypelloid pelvis, 236
Plugged duct, breastfeeding and,
    390, 398-399
PMI. See Point of maximal impulse.
Pneumatic antishock garment, 720,
    720f
Pneumonia in meconium aspiration
    syndrome, 510
Pneumonitis in meconium
    aspiration syndrome, 510
Pneumothorax, traumatic, 718
Point of maximal impulse, 439
Polychlorinated biphenyls, 206
Polychromasia in HELLP
    syndrome, 560
Polycythemia
    related to maternal diabetes
        mellitus, 667
    in small-for-gestational-age
        infant, 471
Polygenic disorders, 30-31
Polyhydramnios, ultrasonographic
    assessment of, 170
Polymorphism, defined, 23
Polythiazide as environmental
    hazard, 213
Popliteal angle in neonatal
    neurologic assessment, 444b
Positioning
    arterial blood pressure during
        pregnancy and, 98
    fetal, 245, 246f
        occiput posterior, 295
        vaginal examination for
            determination of, 251
    for labor and delivery

Positioning (Continued)
    ethnocultural factors in, 80, 92t
    pelvic size and contours and,
        237-240
    newborn
        for breastfeeding, 390, 391f,
            391-394, 392f, 393f, 394f,
            395f
        thermoregulation and, 423
    uterine, 7, 7f
Posterior sagittal diameter of
    pelvis, 237, 237f
Postpartum mood disorders, 130,
    376, 379, 861-864, 865
    impaired adjustment related to,
        137-138
    risk for ineffective coping related
        to, 381
Postpartum period, 369-418
    breastfeeding in, 387-408. See Also
        Breastfeeding.
    assessment for, 389-391
    case study and study questions
        for, 406-407
    health education associated
        with, 405-406
    interventions/outcomes for,
        391-405
    nursing diagnoses regarding, 391
    physiology of, 387-389, 388f
    case studies and study questions
        for, 383-385
    complications in, 850-870
        case study and study questions
            regarding, 865-868
        depression, 861-864
        health education for, 864-865
        hemorrhage, 85-854
        infection, 854-858
        thrombophlebitis, 858-861
    emotions during immediate, 256
    ethnocultural factors in, 77, 80-81,
        93t
    family planning in, 409-418
        breastfeeding plans and, 410
        case study and study questions
            for, 416-418
        contraceptive history and, 409
        contraceptive knowledge and,
            410
        contraceptives for, 411, 412t-415t
        obstetric and gynecological
            history and, 409-410
        postpartum fertility and, 410-411
        psychosocial responses
            regarding, 410
    health education regarding,
        382-383
    hemorrhage during, 634
    immediate as fourth stage of
        labor, 288-290
    interventions/outcomes in,
        377-378
    maternal system changes during,
        371-375
    nursing diagnoses in, 377
    physical examination during,
        376-377
    psychologic changes during, 375-
        376, 378-381

Postterm infant, 486-490, 491
Postterm pregnancy, 825-827, 845
Posture
    maternal
        effect of on pelvic size and
            contours, 237-238
        nutritional assessment, 111t
    neonatal assessment, 440, 444b
Potassium iodide as environmental
    hazard, 214
Potassium monitoring in
    respiratory distress syndrome,
        507
Povidone-iodine as environmental
    hazard, 211
Power of labor, 228-234, 229f
    optimization of, 262-263, 263f
Powerlessness related to
    pregestational diabetes
        mellitus, 670
PPHN. See Persistent pulmonary
    hypertension of newborn.
Praise of infant, ethnocultural
    factors in, 94t
Pravastatin sodium as
    environmental hazard, 213
Precipitate labor, 294
Pre-colostrum, 98
Preconceptual counseling
    regarding inflammatory bowel
        disease, 810-811
    in renal disease, 786
    in systemic lupus erythematosus,
        799
Preeclampsia, 556. See Also
    Hypertensive disorders of
        pregnancy.
    complications of, 555, 563-565
    diagnostic procedures in, 573t,
        573-574
    generalized vasospasm and
        endothelial cell damage in,
        563-568
    pathophysiology of, 557-558
    prevention of, 584-585
    in previous pregnancy, 557
    risk factors for, 556-557
    superimposed, chronic
        hypertension with, 560
Pre-embryonic stage of fetal
    development, 42-45, 43f, 44f,
        45f
Pregenesis, 41
Pregestational diabetes mellitus,
    663-671
    altered metabolism in, 668-669
    anxiety related to, 669-670
    deficient knowledge regarding,
        670
    definition and prognosis for, 663
    diagnostic procedures in, 668
    health education regarding,
        695-696
    history in, 663-665
    incidence of, 663, 664t
    interrupted family processes
        related to, 671
    nursing diagnoses and
        interventions/ outcomes for,
        668-671

Pregestational diabetes mellitus
    (*Continued*)
    physical findings in, 665-667
    powerlessness related to, 670
    psychosocial considerations in, 668
    risk for fetal injury in, 671
Pregnancy, 73-143
    case studies and study questions
        associated with normal,
        121-122
    clinical practice, 107-118
        diagnostic procedures in,
            114-116, 116f
        history in, 107-110, 109f
        interventions/outcomes in,
            116-118
        nursing diagnoses in, 116
        physical examination in,
            111t-112t, 111-116, 116f
    ethnocultural considerations
        regarding, 75-95
        case studies and study
            questions for, 85-88
        clinical practice in, 78-85
        cultural and linguistic
            competence in, 76
        health education in, 85
        quick reference guide to,
            91t-95t
        transcultural nursing and,
            75-76
    fetal assessment during, 161-200
        biochemical, 174-186
        biophysical, 167-174, 175f
        case studies and sample
            questions regarding,
            194-195
        comparison of surveillance
            tests in, 165
        electronic, 186-190
        fetal movement assessment by
            client in, 165-166
        health education in, 193
        interventions/outcomes in,
            190-193
        nursing diagnoses in, 190
        role of nurse in, 162-165
    fetal development during, 41-72
        amniotic fluid in, 65f, 65-66
        clinical practice associated
            with, 66-69
        conception in, 41-42, 42f
        congenital malformations in,
            61, 62f
        embryonic stage of, 46-53
        fetal stage of, 53-61
        health education related to, 70
        placental abnormalities in,
            61-63, 63t
        pre-embryonic stage of, 42-45,
            43f, 44f, 45f
        pregenesis in, 41
        study questions related to,
            70-71
        umbilical cord in, 63-64
    health education regarding
        physiology of, 118-200
    history of, 14-15
    hypertensive disorders in, 554-591
        assessment of, 568-579

Pregnancy (*Continued*)
    cardiovascular system
        disturbances associated
        with, 581-582
    case studies and study
        questions for, 585-587
    central nervous system injury
        resulting from, 579-581,
        580f
    chronic hypertension, 559
    chronic hypertension with
        superimposed
        preeclampsia or
        eclampsia, 560
    generalized vasospasm and
        endothelial cell damage in,
        563-568
    gestational hypertension,
        558-559, 568-574
    health education for, 584-585
    HELLP syndrome, 560-561,
        562f, 563t
    hepatic injury associated with,
        581-582
    impaired fetal well being
        related to, 583
    life-threatening complications
        to mother and fetus
        related to, 554-555
    maternal anxiety and fear
        associated with, 583-584
    pathophysiology of
        preeclampsia and, 557-558
    renal system disturbances
        associated with, 581
    risk factors for preeclampsia
        and, 556-557
    secondary hypertension,
        575-579
    terminology describing,
        555-556
    transient hypertension, 560
    intimate partner violence during,
        538, 544
    loss of. *See* Miscarriage.
    maternal system changes during,
        96-102
        in cardiovascular system, 98-99
        in endocrine system, 101-102
        in gastrointestinal system, 100
        in immunologic system, 102
        in integumentary system, 101
        in musculoskeletal system, 101
        in reproductive system, 96-98
        in respiratory system, 99
        in urinary system, 99-100
    molar, 647-651
    multiple, 170, 831-835, 846
        in advanced maternal age,
            154
        breastfeeding interventions for,
            402
        case study and study questions
            regarding, 265-266
        ultrasonographic assessment
            of, 170
    nutritional considerations
        during, 103-107, 105f
    planned *versus* unplanned, 253
    postterm, 825-827, 845

Pregnancy (*Continued*)
    previous, labor and delivery and,
        241-242
    psychology of, 124-143
        assessment of, 124-133
        case study and study questions
            regarding, 139-141
        health education regarding,
            138-139
        interventions/outcomes in,
            134-138
        nursing diagnoses in, 133
    signs and symptoms of, 102-103
    surgery in, 727-749
        anesthetic considerations for,
            728-734
        appendectomy, 737-739, 738f
        case studies and study
            questions for, 745-748
        cervical cerclage, 739-740
        cholecystectomy, 735-736
        endoscopic gastrointestinal
            procedures, 740-741
        health education regarding, 745
        intrauterine fetal, 741-744
        ovarian cystectomy or
            oophorectomy, 736-737
    trauma in, 703-726
        assessment of, 709-714, 715t
        case studies and study
            questions for, 723-725
        cause or mechanism of injury
            in, 708-709
        complications of, 709
        concepts for, 704
        diagnostic procedures for,
            714-717
        gastrointestinal changes in,
            706
        genitourinary changes in, 706,
            707f
        health education regarding,
            721-722, 722f
        hematologic changes in, 706
        incidence and epidemiology of,
            703-704
        ineffective airway clearance
            related to, 717, 718f
        nursing diagnoses and
            interventions/outcomes
            for, 717-721, 718f, 720f
        pelvic changes in, 707
        physiologic considerations for,
            704-705, 705f
        respiratory changes in, 706
        types of, 707
    unintended related to
        inappropriate selection of
        contraceptive, 411
Pregnancy test, 114
Pregnancy-induced hypertension.
    See Gestational hypertension.
Premature atrial contractions,
    321-323, 322f, 323f, 324f
Premature contractions
    atrial, 321-323, 322f, 323f, 324f
    ventricular, 326f, 326-328, 327f,
        328f
Premature infant. *See* Preterm
    infant.

Premature rupture of membranes, 827-831, 845-846
Premature ventricular contractions, 326f, 326-328, 327f, 328f
Premonitory signs of childbirth, 271-273
Prenatal history, latent phase of labor and, 274-275
Prenatal visits
  in adolescent pregnancy, 148-149
  comprehensive general health examination at first, 107-111, 109f
Preoperative assessment, maternal, 730-731
Prepuce of clitoris, 4
Prescriptive cultural customs and beliefs, 76
Presentation, fetal, 242-245, 243f, 244f, 245f
  assessment of in Leopold's maneuvers, 251
  impaired urinary elimination related to pressure of, 284-285
  placenta previa and, 635
  risk for fetal injury related to, 252
  ultrasonographic assessment of, 170
  vaginal examination for determination of, 251
Pressure catheter monitoring of contractions, intrauterine, 232, 307-308
  risk for infection related to, 233
Preterm infant, 472-482
  accelerations of fetal heart rate in, 332
  anticipatory grieving related to, 138
  assessment of, 475-478
  associated with maternal diabetes mellitus, 667
  breastfeeding of, 401-402, 402f
  cardiovascular system of, 473
  diagnostic procedures for, 478
  diminished sucking processes in, 479-480
  dysfunctional grieving related to, 138
  health education regarding, 491
  hypocalcemia in, 474
  hypoglycemia in, 474-475
  immune system of, 473-474
  impaired skin integrity in, 480-481
  ineffective tissue perfusion related to impaired gas exchange in, 481
  liver of, 474
  necrotizing enterocolitis in, 474
  nursing diagnoses interventions/ outcomes for, 478-482
  organ maturity and, 472
  periventricular intraventricular hemorrhage in, 474
  physical findings in, 476-478
  related to maternal pyelonephritis, 613-614
  renal system of, 474

Preterm infant (Continued)
  impaired urinary elimination and retention related to, 481
  respiratory distress syndrome in, 502-506
  respiratory system of, 472-473, 481-482
  retinopathy in, 500
  risk factors for, 472
  thermoregulation in, 474
  interventions/outcomes for, 478-479
Preterm labor, 818-825, 820-824
  diagnostic procedures in, 820
  history in, 819
  induced by premature rupture of membrane, 830
  in multiple gestation, 833
  nursing diagnoses and interventions/outcomes for, 820-824
  peritonitis and, 738
  physical findings in, 819
  prevention of in surgery during pregnancy, 733
  psychosocial findings in, 819-820
Primidone as environmental hazard, 213
Primigravida
  case study and study questions regarding, 264-266
  interventions for anxiety for, 136
  interventions for lack of parenting skills, 137
  nutrition and, 109
  as risk factor for gestational hypertension, 556
Principle-based ethics, 874-876
Privacy, ethics and, 875
Problem-solving skills, interventions to help adolescents with, 151
Procardia. See Nifedipine.
Professional codes, 881
Progesterone
  changes in pregnancy due to, 102
  uterine, 96
  for contraception, 415t
  diagnostic testing of, 17
  postpartum changes in, 373
  withdrawal of in onset of contractions, 228
Prolactin, 17
  in initiation of milk production, 389
  postpartum changes in, 373
Prolapse, uterine, 15
Prolonged decelerations of fetal heart rate, 347-349, 348f
PROM. See Premature rupture of membrane.
Promethazine for analgesia during childbirth, 278
Propene, 206
Propylthiouracil
  as environmental hazards, 214
  for hyperthyroidism, 678
Prostacyclin/thromboxane ratio in preeclampsia, 557, 563

Prostaglandin synthetase inhibitors in preterm labor therapy, 822
Prostaglandins
  for induction or augmentation of labor, 291
  in intrauterine fetal demise, 837
  in onset of contractions, 229
Protease inhibitor for human immunodeficiency virus- associated infection, 604
Proteins
  intake requirements during pregnancy, 70, 105
  metabolism of in pregnancy, 662
    in gestational diabetes mellitus, 674
    in pregestational diabetes mellitus, 668-669
Proteinuria
  development of during first stage of labor, 274
  due to pregnancy, 100
  due to renal disease, 782
  in hypertensive disorders of pregnancy, 558, 559, 564, 579
Prothrombin time
  in disseminated intravascular coagulation, 645
  in gestational hypertension and HELLP syndrome, 573t
  disseminated intravascular coagulation versus, 563t
Protracted nipples, 390
Proxy decision-makers, ethics and, 878-880
Pseudoephedrine as environmental hazard, 214
Pseudosinusoidal undulating patterns in fetal heart rate, 317-318, 319f
  interventions for, 330-331
PSI. See Foam stability index.
Psychologic battering, 539-540
Psychosis, postpartum, 861-862
Psychosocial factors and responses, 124-143
  in abruptio placentae, 641
  during active phase of labor, 277
  affecting perinatal adaptation and outcomes, 130-132
  affecting single mothers, 129-130
  in AIDS, 606
  case study and study questions regarding, 139-141
  childbirth preparation education and, 132-133
  developmental tasks of pregnancy and, 126
  in diabetes mellitus
    gestational, 672
    pregestational, 668
  in disseminated intravascular coagulation, 646
  Duvall's stages of family development and, 125
  ethnocultural considerations in, 82, 130
  of expectant fathers, 127-129

Psychosocial factors and responses (*Continued*)
in expulsion of infant, 283
in family members' reaction to pregnancy and childbirth, 129
in family planning, 410
findings in, 125-126
in gestational hypertension, 572-573
health education regarding, 138-139
history in assessment of, 124-125
in intrauterine fetal demise, 836, 837-838
in labor and delivery, 253-262
behaviors, 258
cultural considerations, 253-254
current pregnancy experience, 253
emotions of labor, 255-256
expectations for birth experience, 254
interventions/outcomes related to, 259-262
nursing diagnoses related to, 258-259
personality styles, 257-258
preparation for birth, 254
previous birth experiences, 253
psychologic reactions to labor, 256-257
support system, 254-255
during latent phase of labor, 276
to multiple gestation pregnancy, 832
in placenta previa, 635
postpartum, 288-289, 375-376, 378-381, 861-864
attachment and, 375-376, 379-380
baby blues and, 376, 379
health education associated with, 382
interventions/outcomes associated with, 380-381
nursing diagnoses related to, 380
role change and, 375, 378-379
in postpartum hemorrhage, 852
in postpartum infection, 856
in potential responses to reproductive assessment, 17
in pregnancy as a developmental crisis, 126
in premature rupture of membrane, 828-829
in preterm labor, 819-820
Rubin's tasks of pregnancy and, 126-127
in substance abuse, 754-755
in thrombophlebitis, 859
during transition phase of labor, 277
in uterine rupture, 842
Psychotropics as environmental hazard, 213
PT. *See* Prothrombin time.
PTT. *See* Partial thromboplastin time.

PTU. *See* Propylthiouracil.
Puberty, 14
Pubic bone, 9f, 10
Public health issue
alcohol use as, 762
substance abuse as, 750
PUBS. *See* Percutaneous umbilical blood sampling.
Pudendal anesthesia, 282
Puerperium. *See* Postpartum period.
Pulmonary artery pressure in abruptio placentae, 642
Pulmonary capillary wedge pressure, normal values in pregnancy, 574t
Pulmonary edema
decreased cardiac output due to, 777-778, 779t-780t
preeclampsia-associated, 565, 572, 582, 582t
Pulmonary function tests in tuberculosis, 789
Pulmonary hypertension
maternal, 782
in newborn
persistent, 515-517
related to congenital diaphragmatic hernia, 453
Pulmonary system
changes to during pregnancy, 99
fetal
amniocentesis for assessment of maturity of, 177
development of, 57, 58, 59, 60
maternal drug use and, 751
transition of to neonatal, 421-422
maternal
amniotic fluid embolism of, 839-841
changes in during first stage of labor, 274
disease of, 787-793
preeclampsia and, 564-565, 565t
surgery and, 729
systemic lupus erythematosus-related symptoms in, 795
trauma and, 706, 711
neonatal
assessment of, 439
in preterm infant, 472-473
Pulmonary vascular resistance, 574t
Pulmonary wedge pressure, 642
Pulse oximetry, fetal, 353-355
Pupils
maternal, examination of in traumatic injury, 713
neonatal, 438
Purification, ritual, 93t
Pushing to facilitate fetal descent, 282
PVC. *See* Premature ventricular contractions.
PVR. *See* Pulmonary vascular resistance.
Pyelonephritis, 611-614, 624, 626-627, 782, 783
Pyrazinamide for tuberculosis, 790t

Pyridoxine
deficiencies of, effect on fetus, 107
requirements of during pregnancy, 106
Pyrimethamine for toxoplasmosis, 593t

Q
Quality of life, ethics and, 874
Quazepam as environmental hazard, 216
Quiet sleep, 440
Quinine sulfate as environmental hazard, 211

R
Racial factors. *See* Ethnocultural considerations.
Radiant warmer, 423
Radiation exposure
ionizing, 204-205
nonionizing, 205
Radiation heat loss, neonatal, 423
Radioactive iodine as environmental hazard, 214
Radiography
following trauma in pregnancy, 715
in meconium aspiration syndrome, 513
in persistent pulmonary hypertension of newborn, 516
in respiratory distress syndrome assessment, 502
in transient tachypnea of newborn, 509
Radioimmunoassay for pregnancy testing, 114
Rales in respiratory distress syndrome, 501
RBC. *See* Red blood cell.
RDA. *See* Recommended dietary allowances.
RDS. *See* Respiratory distress syndrome.
Readiness for enhanced family coping related to opportunity for growth/mastery, 136-137
Recessive inheritance, 29f, 29-30
sex-linked, 30
Recommended dietary allowances during pregnancy, 104, 105-107
of calcium in gestational hypertension, 569
Rectocele, 15
Red blood cell
bilirubin from destruction of, 518
damage to in disseminated intravascular coagulation, 645
fetal, isoimmunization, 180-181
maternal
changes to during pregnancy, 99
destruction of in HELLP syndrome, 560

Reduction surgery of breast, breastfeeding and, 390
Reflex irritability in Apgar scoring, 426t
Reflexes
  deep tendon, assessment of in magnesium sulfate therapy, 821
  neonatal, 440b
Regional anesthesia, 278
  for surgery in pregnancy, 732
Relaxation strategies
  analgesic effects of during childbirth, 279
  in childbirth education, 132-133
Relaxin, 102
Religious views on contraception, 410
Renal colic, 785-786
Renal failure, acute, 782, 783
Renal insufficiency, 784-785
Renal system
  maternal
    changes in during first stage of labor, 274
    changes in during pregnancy, 99-100, 781
    disease of, 781-787
    postpartum changes in, 374
    preeclampsia and, 563-564, 571, 581
    systemic lupus erythematosus-related symptoms in, 795
  neonatal
    assessment of, 439
    in preterm infant, 474, 481
Renese. See Polythiazide.
Renin-angiotensin system, fetal heart rate and, 309
Reproductive history, 14
Reproductive risk, environmental, 202
Reproductive system, female. See Female reproductive system.
Research consent, 877-878
Reserpine as environmental hazard, 213
Resin triiodothyronine uptake, 677t
Resources
  AIDS, 623-624
  associated with environmental hazards, 218, 218b
  for newborn care, 434, 461
  for professionals regarding intimate partner violence, 550
  related to substance abuse, 767
Respect, ethics and, 875
Respiratory distress, 498-499
  in amniotic fluid embolism, 839
  complications of resulting from respiratory distress syndrome, 506-508
  discharge planning in, 529
  in large-for-gestational-age infant, 484-485
  long-term follow-up in, 529

Respiratory distress (Continued)
  in meconium aspiration syndrome, 513
  in persistent pulmonary hypertension of newborn, 517
Respiratory distress syndrome, 500-508
  complications of, 500, 506-508
  diagnostic procedures for, 502
  discharge planning in, 529
  due to prematurity, 472
  nursing diagnoses and interventions/outcomes in, 502-506
  pathophysiology of, 500
  physical findings in, 501-502
  related to maternal diabetes mellitus, 667
  respiratory complications resulting from prematurity in, 502-506
  risk factors for, 500-501
Respiratory effort
  in Apgar scoring, 426t
  poor, 429
    in large-for-gestational-age infant, 484
    in persistent pulmonary hypertension of newborn, 516-517
    related to meconium aspiration syndrome, 513-515
    related to transient tachypnea, 509-510
Respiratory rate
  in respiratory distress syndrome, 505
  in transient tachypnea of newborn, 509
Respiratory system
  fetal
    development of, 57, 58, 59, 60
    maternal drug use and, 751
    transition of to neonatal, 421-422
  maternal
    changes in during first stage of labor, 274
    changes in during pregnancy, 99
    disease of, 787-793
    in disseminated intravascular coagulation, 647
    postpartum changes to, 374
    preeclampsia and, 564-565, 565t
    related to respiratory disease, 790-791, 791t
    surgery and, 729
    systemic lupus erythematosus-related symptoms in, 795
    trauma and, 706, 711
  neonatal
    assessment of, 439
    in preterm infant, 472-473, 481-482
    respiratory distress due to, 499
Resting tone, uterine, 350
Restitution, fetal, 249
Restrictive cultural customs and beliefs, 76

Resuscitation of newborn, 428f, 430t-431t
  with congenital diaphragmatic hernia, 452
  ethical dilemmas regarding, 887
  in small-for-gestational-age infant, 469
Retained lung fluid, 508-509
  in persistent pulmonary hypertension of newborn, 516-517
Retained placental fragments, postpartum hemorrhage due to, 852
Retina, preeclampsia and, 565
Retinoids as environmental hazard, 215
Retinopathy of prematurity, 500
Retraction
  in physiology of contractions, 230
  pulmonary
    in large-for-gestational-age infant, 484
    in respiratory distress syndrome, 501
Retraction ring, pathological, 294-295, 295f
Retrovir, 605
Retrovirus, human immunodeficiency virus, 599
Review of systems in comprehensive general health examination at first prenatal visit, 110
Rh sensitization, 54
  amniocentesis for evaluation of, 177-178
RIA. See Radioimmunoassay.
Ribavirin as environmental hazard, 211, 214
Riboflavin
  deficiencies of, effect on fetus, 107
  requirements of during pregnancy, 106
Ribonucleic acid in human immunodeficiency virus, 599
Rifampin for tuberculosis, 788, 790t
Right arterial pressure, normal values in pregnancy, 574t
Risk assessment in first prenatal visit assessment, 107-108
Risk for altered consciousness associated with disseminated intravascular coagulation, 647
Risk for compromised family coping
  related to fear of fetal loss, 191-192
  related to significant other excluded from testing sessions, 191-192
Risk for constipation, maternal, 377-378
Risk for decreased cardiac output related to maternal cardiac disease, 777-778, 779t-780t
Risk for deficient fluid volume
  maternal
    in amniocentesis and PUBS, 192

Risk for deficient fluid volume (*Continued*)
  due to fluid shift in early postpartum period, 289-290
  in evacuation of hydatidiform mole, 650
  in inflammatory bowel disease, 808-809
  in kidney disease, 784-785
  in postpartum hemorrhage, 852-853
  related to blood loss, 288
  related to decreased intake or abnormal loss, 281
  in surgical procedure and blood loss, 298
  in traumatic injury, 719-720, 720f
  neonatal, associated with phototherapy light exposure, 526
Risk for disturbed body, related to eating disorders, 133
Risk for excessive fluid volume
  in kidney disease, 784-785
  related to use of oxytocin, 292
Risk for hypothermia in small-for-gestational-age infant, 470
Risk for imbalanced body temperature due to postpartum infection, 857
Risk for imbalanced nutrition: less than body requirements
  maternal, in lactation and/or depression, 404-405
  neonatal
    associated with cleft lip and palate, 432
    in large-for-gestational-age infants, 485
    in postterm infant, 489-490
    in preterm infant, 479-480
    in small-for-gestational-age infants, 470-471
Risk for impaired gas exchange
  fetal
    due to impaired placental transport, 69
    related to decelerations of fetal heart rate, 335-336, 337b, 340, 341b
    related to fetal pulse oximetry, 354-355
    related to fetal scalp sampling, 352
    related to nonperiodic fetal heart rate patterns, 348-349
    related to periodic fetal heart rate patterns, 340, 340b
    related to tachycardias and bradycardias, 313-314
    related to variability of fetal heart rate, 329-332
  neonatal
    related to poor respiratory effort and retained lung fluid, 429
    related to umbilical cord sampling, 356-357

Risk for impaired infant attachment related to postpartum infection, 858
Risk for impaired maternal comfort related to incorrect latching on, 394-396
Risk for impaired parenting
  associated with parent-infant separation secondary to phototherapy treatments, 527-528
  due to drug abuse, 758-759
  following diagnosis of genetic disorder in fetus or newborn, 35-36
  related to inadequate bonding secondary to infant with cleft lip and palate, 450
  related to lack of knowledge and skills, 137
  related to late childbearing, 155-156
  related to postpartum infection, 858
  related to taking on role of mother, 380-381
Risk for ineffective coping
  related to physical and/or mental handicap of family member, 35
  related to postpartum mood alteration, 381
Risk for ineffective health maintenance in trophoblastic disease, 650-651
Risk for ineffective tissue perfusion
  fetal, related to hypoxic myocardial dysfunction or anomaly, 332
  maternal, related to position in labor, 279
  neonatal
    in preterm infant, 481
    related to decreased cardiac output, 429-432
    related to polycythemia and hypothermia in small-for-gestational-age infant, 471
Risk for infection
  maternal
    cardiac disease and, 778
    due to invasive procedures, 192
    due to premature rupture of membrane, 829-830
    related to airborne transmission of tuberculosis, 791-792
    related to corticosteroid therapy, 796-797
    related to labor and delivery, 290
    related to prolonged second stage of labor, 285-286
    related to spontaneous ruptures of membranes, 273
    related to use of intrauterine pressure catheter, 233
    related to vaginal examination after ROM, 281

Risk for infection (*Continued*)
    renal, 784
    as a result of cesarean birth, 298
    resulting from prolonged labor, 296
  neonatal
    maternal transmission of hepatitis, 814
    related to infant's poor physiologic response to pathogens, 432
    in small-for-gestational-age infant, 471
Risk for injury
  fetal
    related to alcohol use, 767
    related to antithyroid drugs, 682-683
    related to drug abuse, 758, 759f
    related to gestational diabetes mellitus, 675
    related to hazardous effects of pharmaceuticals, 216
    related to hyperadrenocorticism, 688
    related to malpresentation, 252
    related to maternal phenylketonuria, 693-694
    related to maternal steroid replacement therapy, 690
    related to occupational hazards, 207
    related to pregestational diabetes mellitus, 671
    related to second hand smoke exposure, 218
    related to smoking during pregnancy, 761
    related to temperature extremes, 209
    related to test complications, 190-191
    related to uterine rupture, 843
  maternal
    psychologic, related to failure to achieve parent-infant attachment, 381
    related to alcohol use, 767
    related to drug abuse, 758, 759f
    related to induction of uterine contractions, 292-293
    related to malpresentation, 252
    related to smoking during pregnancy, 761
    related to test complications, 190-191
    related to TORCH disease, 599
    related to uterine rupture, 842-843
  neonatal
    corneal, related to phototherapy, 527
    in large-for-gestational-age infants during birth, 486
    related to birth asphyxia in small-for-gestational-age infant, 469-470
    related to maternal pyelonephritis, 613-614

Risk for interrupted family
  processes
  following diagnosis of genetic
    disorder in fetus or
    newborn, 35
  related to acceptance of newborn,
    289
  related to complicated pregnancy,
    772-773
  related to value differences
    between woman and her
    partner about contraceptive
    choices, 411-416
Risk for situational low self-esteem
  related to impairment of cardinal
    movements, 252-253
  related to inability to provide
    adequate milk supply,
    402-403
  related to ineffective uterine
    contraction pattern, 233-234
  related to possible reduced pelvic
    capacity, 241
  related to pregnancy
    complications, 133
Risk for social isolation associated
  with genetic disorder in
  newborn, 36
Risk for urinary retention related to
  perineal trauma, 377
Ritual beautification, 82
Ritual behaviors during
  contractions, 258
RLF. See Retained lung fluid.
RNA. See Ribonucleic acid.
Role
  changes in related to pregnancy,
    133
  of fathers during childbirth, 128
  ineffective performance related to
    taking on new, 133
  maternal, postpartum, 375,
    378-379
    conflicted, 379
    failure to take on, 380-381
  of nurse in antepartum fetal
    assessment, 162-165
  preparation of in expectant
    family, 125
Rollover test, 571
Rooting reflex, 440b
ROP. See Retinopathy of
  prematurity.
Rotation, fetal, 249
Rubella in TORCH, 592-599, 593t-
  597t
Rubeola, 616t
Rubin's tasks of pregnancy, 126-127
Rupture
  of membranes
    abruptio placentae and, 640
    premature, 827-831, 845-846
    as premonitory sign of
      childbirth, 273
    risk for infection related to, 273
    risk for infection related to
      vaginal examination
      following, 281
  uterine, 841-844, 847

S
Sacrococcygeal teratoma, fetal
  surgery for, 743-744
Sacrum, curve and length of, 237
Saddle block, 282
Safe passage, 127
Safety
  amniocentesis, 175
  chorionic villus sampling, 182
  cordocentesis and percutaneous
    umbilical blood sampling, 179
  newborn, 433
  ultrasonographic, 167
Saliva, changes to during
  pregnancy, 100
Salpingitis, postpartum, 855
Scalp
  fetal sampling, 164, 351-353
  stimulation of
    for bradycardia, 313-314
    for tachycardia, 313
Scar, uterine, hemorrhagic
  disorders and, 632
Scarf sign in neonatal neurologic
  assessment, 444b
Schistocytes, 560
Schultz's mechanism for placental
  delivery, 286
Scleral hemorrhage, 438
Seat belt use, 708, 721-722, 722f
Secobarbital for analgesia during
  childbirth, 278
Seconal. See Secobarbital.
Second hand smoke, 217-218, 219, 221
Second trimester
  estimation of gestational age
    during, 162-163
  health education in
    regarding physiology of
      pregnancy during,
      119-120, 139
    regarding placenta previa,
      651-652
  tasks of pregnancy during
    maternal, 127
    paternal, 128
Secondary hypertension, 575-579
Secondary sex characteristics,
  assessment of, 15, 16f
Second-degree heart block, 328
Secretions, airway, clearance of in
  newborn, 429
  in respiratory distress syndrome,
    506, 507
Sedation of neonate with
  respiratory distress syndrome,
  505, 506
Sedatives as environmental hazard,
  215-216
Sedimentation rate in
  hyperbilirubinemia, 526
Seizure, eclamptic, 566-567, 576t
Self-care
  for asthma, 792b
  postpartum, 382
  regarding blood glucose
    management in mother's
    with diabetes mellitus, 670,
    675-676

Self-concept, altered
  related to gestational diabetes, 675
  related to inability to provide
    adequate milk supply,
    402-403
Sensory function, neonatal,
  assessment of, 441
Sensory nerves of reproductive
  system, 10
Sensory perception related to
  multiple environmental
  distracters, disturbed, 261-262
Septal defect
  atrial, 454-455, 455f
  ventricular, 455-456, 456f
Serum alpha-fetoprotein
  in fetal and placental assessment,
    67
  in genetic assessment, 32-33
  in triple marker test, 185-186
Serum calcium monitoring in
  respiratory distress syndrome,
  507
Serum chloride monitoring in
  respiratory distress syndrome,
  507
Serum cortisol in assessment of
  adrenal insufficiency, 689
Serum creatinine, increased in
  preeclampsia, 564, 573t
Serum ferritin, 803t
Serum glutamic oxaloacetic
  transaminase. See Aspartate
  aminotransferase.
Serum iron, 803t
Serum potassium monitoring in
  respiratory distress syndrome,
  507
Serum sodium monitoring in
  respiratory distress syndrome,
  507
Serum thyroxine, 17
Serum triiodothyronine, 17
Seventh week of fetal development,
  51f, 52
Sex-linked dominant inheritance, 30
Sex-linked recessive inheritance, 30
Sexual history assessment at first
  prenatal visit, 108
Sexual identity of lactating woman,
  405
Sexual intercourse
  contraindications to during
    pregnancy, 135
  postpartum resumption of, 383,
    410
Sexual partners, adolescent
  pregnancy and, 148
Sexuality patterns, ineffective,
  related to changes in libido
  during pregnancy, 134-135
Sexually transmitted diseases,
  600t-602t, 609-611
  acquired immunodeficiency
    syndrome, 599-609
  assessment of, 605-607
  counseling and early diagnosis
    of, 603
  first recognition of, 599

Sexually transmitted diseases (*Continued*)
human immunodeficiency virus infection in, 599-603
nursing diagnoses and interventions/outcomes for, 607-609
treatment of, 604-605
women and, 603-604, 604f, 604t
case study and study questions for, 626
health education regarding, 624
SGA. See Small-for-gestational-age.
Shake test in respiratory distress syndrome assessment, 502
Shields, eye, for phototherapy, 527
Shingles, 615t
Shirodkar procedure, 739
Shock
in disseminated intravascular coagulation, 645
due to traumatic injury, 705
due to uterine rupture, 842-843
hemorrhagic disorder-associated, 632, 634
Short-term variability of fetal heart rate, 316-317, 318f
interventions for, 330
Shoulder presentation, 242, 244-245
Show, 272, 275
Siblings, expectant, 129
Sick newborn, 497-534
anticipatory grieving related to, 138
case studies and study questions associated with, 530-532
dysfunctional grieving related to, 138
health education regarding, 490-491, 528-529
hyperbilirubinemia in, 517-528
assessment of, 523-526
causes of, 517-521, 519f
interventions/outcomes for, 526-528
nursing diagnoses in, 526
treatment of, 521-523, 523f
meconium aspiration syndrome in, 510-515, 511f
persistent pulmonary hypertension of newborn in, 515-517
respiratory distress in, 498-499
respiratory distress syndrome in, 500-508
complications of, 500, 506-508
diagnostic procedures for, 502
nursing diagnoses and interventions/outcomes in, 502-506
pathophysiology of, 500
physical findings in, 501-502
respiratory complications resulting from prematurity in, 502-506
risk factors for, 500-501
transient tachypnea in, 508-509
Sickle cell anemia, 800-801, 802, 803
ethnic factors in, 95t
sickling crisis in, 805-806

Side-lying position for breastfeeding, 393-394, 395f
Sigmoidoscopy, 741
Signal display, ultrasonographic, 167
Silicon nipple shield, 396
Simvastatin as environmental hazard, 213
Single mother, psychosocial needs of, 129-130
Single ventricle, 459-460
Sinus bradycardia, fetal, 320
Sinus node variants, fetal, 320-321, 321f
Sinus tachycardia, fetal, 320-321
Sinusoidal undulating patterns in fetal heart rate, 318-319, 319f
interventions for, 330-331
Sirenomelia, 63
Sitting for labor and delivery, 239
Situational low self-esteem
related to adverse test outcome, 193
related to change in birth plan, 298-299
related to drug abuse, 754
related to impairment of cardinal movements, 252-253
related to inability to provide adequate milk supply, 402-403
related to ineffective uterine contraction pattern, 233-234
related to possible reduced pelvic capacity, 241
related to pregnancy complications, 133
Sixth week of fetal development, 51f, 52
Size, fetal, 246-248
Skeletal system. See Musculoskeletal system.
Skene's glands, 4
Skill, deficient, related to maternal experience in positioning infant for breastfeeding, 391f, 391-394, 392f, 393f, 394f, 395f
Skin
fetal development of, 57, 58, 59, 60
impaired integrity of
associated with hyperbilirubinemia, 527
in preterm infant, 480-481
related to delivery process, 285
maternal
changes to during pregnancy, 101
in nutritional status assessment, 112t
postpartum changes to, 375
neonatal
assessment of, 438, 442t
color if in Apgar scoring, 426
in premature infant, 476
Skull, fetal, 248-249
SLE. See Systemic lupus erythematosus.

Sleep
maternal disturbances of as premonitory signs of childbirth, 272
neonatal, 441
assessment of, 440
ethnocultural factors in, 81
Small-for-gestational-age infant, 441, 465-471, 491
Smear, cervical, 115
Smell, neonatal, 441
Smoking, 70, 760-762, 768-769
abruptio placentae and, 639
breastfeeding and, 404
hemorrhagic disorders and, 632
passive, 217-218, 219, 221
prematurity and, 472
Social ethics, 876
Social history, 110
Social interaction, impaired, due to extended hospital stay for postpartum infection, 857-858
Social isolation
associated with genetic disorder in newborn, 36
related to changing patterns of communication, 262
related to inadequate support system, 262
related to unfamiliar environment, 262
Socioeconomic factors
in health history, 15
in intimate partner violence, 541-542
in maternal role, 378
in nutritional assessment, 109
in prematurity, 472
in small-for-gestational-age infant, 468
Sodium
impaired excretion of in preeclampsia, 564
monitoring of in respiratory distress syndrome, 507
requirements of during pregnancy, 106
Sodium bicarbonate for neonatal resuscitation, 430t
Sodium nitroprusside for hypertensive disorders of pregnancy, 578t
Soft palate cleft, 449f
Somite development, 47-48, 48f
Sore nipple secondary to breastfeeding, 397-398
Spasm of bladder, 785-786
Special needs infant, breastfeeding of, 402-403
Specific gravity
changes in during first stage of labor, 274
preeclampsia and, 564
Sperm
fertilization and, 41-42, 42f
intracytoplasmic injection of, 153
Spermatogenesis, 25

Spermicide, 414t
  with condom, 413t
  diaphragm with, 413t
Spina bifida, 447-448, 448f
  fetal surgery for, 743
  maternal serum alpha-fetoprotein
    screening in, 185
Spinal anesthesia
  for cesarean birth, 297
  low, 282
  for surgery in pregnancy, 732
Spine stabilization in maternal
    traumatic injury, 711, 718f
Spinnbarkeit, 11
Spiral artery erosion, preeclampsia
    and, 558, 567
Spiritual considerations in ethics,
    881-882
Spiritual distress, 882
Spontaneous abortion
  grief and loss associated with,
    132, 193
  impaired adjustment related to,
    137-138
  risk for compromised family
    coping related to, 191-192
Spontaneous rupture of membranes
  as premonitory sign of childbirth,
    273
  risk for infection related to, 273
Squamocolumnar junction, uterine,
    6
Squamous epithelium, cervical, 6
Square window in neonatal
    neurologic assessment, 444b
Squatting for labor and delivery,
    239
SROM. See Spontaneous rupture of
    membranes.
Stab wound, 709-710
Stabilization, cervical spine, 711, 718f
Stadol. See Butorphanol.
Standing for labor and delivery, 239
Startle reflex, 440b
Station, fetal, 245-246, 247f, 276,
    277, 281
  Bishop score for, 291t
  vaginal examination for
    determination of, 251
Statutory law, 880
STD. See Sexually transmitted
    disease.
Sterilization, 412t
Steroid replacement therapy, risk
    for fetal injury related to, 690
Stillbirth
  dysfunctional grieving related to,
    138
  related to maternal diabetes
    mellitus, 666
Stimulation, minimal, in respiratory
    distress syndrome, 505-506
Stork bite, term, 438
Story-based approach to ethics, 876
Strength of contractions, 231-232
Streptococcus, group B, 617t-618t
Streptomycin
  as environmental hazard, 211
  for tuberculosis, 790t

Stress test, 188-190
Striae gravidarum, 101
Stroke, heat, 209
Stroke volume, changes to during
    pregnancy, 98
STV. See Short-term variability.
Sublimaze. See Fentanyl.
Subpubic angle, 236
Substance abuse, 70, 750-770
  of alcohol, 762-767, 769
  anxiety related to, 757
  assessment of, 753-755
  case studies and study questions
    for, 768-769
  of cocaine, 751-752
  deficient knowledge related to,
    755, 756b
  effects of on fetus, 751
  health education regarding, 767
  of heroin, 752-753
  impaired parenting due to, 758-759
  ineffective health maintenance
    associated with, 758
  interrupted family processes
    related to, 757
  as major public health issue, 750
  of marijuana, 753
  of methadone hydrochloride, 753
  noncompliance associated with,
    757
  nursing diagnoses and
    interventions/outcomes
    regarding, 755-759, 756b, 759f
  nutritional aspects in, 756-757
  outcomes associated with, 750-751
  risk for injury related to, 758, 759f
  situational low self-esteem
    associated with, 754
  statistics regarding, 750
  of tobacco, 760-762, 768-769
Substance Abuse and Mental
    Health Services
    Administration, 767
Substituted judgment, 884
Succenturiate placenta, 286, 287f, 635
Suck-and-swallow technique, 423
  poor coordination of, 432
  preterm infant and, 479-480
Sucking reflex, 440b
Suckling infant, assessment of, 391
Suctioning, airway, in respiratory
    distress syndrome, 506, 507
Sufentanil for analgesia during
    childbirth, 278
Sulfonamide for acute
    pyelonephritis, 613
Supine hypotensive syndrome, 98
Supine position for labor and
    delivery, 238
Supplemental Nursing System, 402f
Supplements, nutritional, 104
Support system during labor and
    delivery, 254-255
  anxiety related to disruption of,
    259
  ineffective coping related to
    inadequate, 260-261
  social isolation related to
    inadequate, 262

Supraventricular dysrhythmias,
    321-325, 322f, 323f, 324f, 325f
  interventions for, 331
Supraventricular tachycardia, fetal,
    323-325, 324f
Surfactant, 163, 422
  administration of
    in meconium aspiration
      syndrome, 514
    in respiratory distress
      syndrome, 504
  deficiency of in respiratory
    distress syndrome, 500
Surfactant/albumin ratio for fetal
    lung maturity assessment, 177
Surgery
  breast, breastfeeding assessment
    and, 390
  cesarean birth, 296-299
    in advanced maternal age
      pregnancy, 154
    breastfeeding following, 399
    pain related to incision site for,
      376
    postpartum examination of
      incision site for, 376
    postpartum infection from, 856
    vaginal birth after, 296
Surgery in pregnancy, 727-749
  anesthetic considerations for,
    728-734
    anesthetic choices as, 732-733
    laparotomy *versus* laparoscopic
      approach as, 731-732
    maternal preoperative
      assessment as, 730-731
    nursing diagnoses and
      interventions/outcomes
      for, 733-734
    planning and management as,
      728-730
  appendectomy, 737-739, 738f
  case studies and study questions
    for, 745-748
  cervical cerclage, 739-740
  cholecystectomy, 735-736
  endoscopic gastrointestinal
    procedures, 740-741
  health education regarding, 745
  intrauterine fetal, 741-744
  ovarian cystectomy or
    oophorectomy, 736-737
Surgical delivery, 296-299
Surgical history, 14
Sutures
  for cervical cerclage, 739
  cranial, labor and delivery and, 248
SVR. See Systemic vascular
    resistance.
SVT. See Supraventricular
    tachycardia.
Swallow reflex, 440b
Swan-Ganz catheterization
  in abruptio placentae, 642
  in gestational hypertension, 574
  normal values of, 574t
Sympathetic nervous system
  fetal heart rate and, 308, 315
  of reproductive system, 10

Symphysis-fundal height
measurement, 115
Synclitism, 246, 247f
Syncytiotrophoblast, 43, 44
Syphilis, 602t
Systemic lupus erythematosus,
793-799
Systemic vascular resistance
normal values in pregnancy, 574t
renal disease and, 783
Systolic blood pressure
maternal
changes to during pregnancy, 98
in chronic hypertension, 559
in gestational hypertension,
555, 558, 559
neonatal, assessment of in
respiratory distress
syndrome, 503

T

T$_3$. *See* Triiodothyronine.
T$_4$. *See* Thyroxine.
Taboo, 76
Tachycardia
fetal, 309-311, 311f
interventions for, 313, 331
sinus, 320-321
supraventricular, 323-325, 324f,
331
neonatal in respiratory distress
syndrome, 502
Tachypnea
in respiratory distress syndrome,
501
transient of newborn, 508-509
Tactile stimulation, minimal, in
respiratory distress syndrome,
505-506
"Taking in" phase of mother, 375
"Taking-hold" phase of mother, 375
Tanner Stages of Development, 15,
16f
Tapazole. *See* Methimazole.
Tasks of pregnancy
developmental, 126
Rubin's, 126-127
Taste, neonatal, 441
TB. *See* Tuberculosis.
TDx test, 177
Teammate, expectant father as, 128
Technology
assistive reproductive, dilemmas
regarding, 887
ethnocultural views of, 130
Teeth, changes to during
pregnancy, 100
Teleologic approach to ethics, 875
Temperature
body. *See* Body temperature.
extremes as environmental
hazard, 208-210, 219, 220-221
TENS. *See* Transcutaneous electrical
nerve stimulation.
Tension pneumothorax, 718
Tentative pregnancy, term, 130
Teratogenicity, 68, 202-203
due to surgery in pregnancy, 730

Teratoma, sacrococcygeal, fetal
surgery for, 743-744
Terbutaline therapy
in preterm labor, 821-822
test complications and, 190
Testosterone, diagnostic testing of,
17
Tetrachloroethylene, 204
Tetracycline as environmental
hazard, 211
Tetralogy of Fallot, 457-458, 458f
TGA. *See* Transposition of great
arteries.
Thalassemia, 801, 802, 803
Thalidomide as environmental
hazard, 216
Therapeutic heat and cold,
ethnocultural considerations
in, 81
Thermoregulation
adaptation of to extrauterine life,
422-423
hypothermic newborn and,
427-429
in preterm infant, 474, 476-477,
478-479
interventions/outcomes for,
478-479
related to phototherapy, 526-527
Thiamin requirements during
pregnancy, 106
Thiethylperazine maleate as
environmental hazard, 213
Thioamides for hyperthyroidism,
678
Third trimester
health education in
regarding physiology of
pregnancy during, 120, 139
regarding placenta previa, 652
tasks of pregnancy during
maternal, 127
paternal, 128
Third week of fetal development,
46f, 46-49, 47f, 48f, 49f
Third-degree heart block, 328
Thoughts during pregnancy, 125-126
Three-point seat belt, 721, 721f
Thrombocytopenia, 801, 802-803,
806
in HELLP syndrome, 561
preeclampsia-associated, 568
Thromboembolism, 778-781,
801-802
Thrombophlebitis, 858-861
assessment of, 377
ineffective tissue perfusion
related to, 804-805
Thrombosis, deep venous, 801-802,
803, 804-805, 858-861
Thromboxane, preeclampsia and,
557
Thyroid function tests, 17, 677,
677t
Thyroid gland
changes to during pregnancy, 101
hyperthyroidism and, 677t,
677-683
Thyroid storm, 678-680

Thyroid-stimulating hormone
changes in normal pregnancy
and thyroid disease, 677t
normal nonpregnant values of, 17
Thyroxine
changes in normal pregnancy
and thyroid disease, 677t
normal nonpregnant values of, 17
Tissue perfusion, impaired
fetal
in abruptio placentae, 643
in disseminated intravascular
coagulation, 647
due to umbilical cord
compression, 826-827, 830
following traumatic injury in
pregnancy, 721
related to hypoxic myocardial
dysfunction or anomaly,
332
related to maternal blood loss
from placenta previa,
637-638
maternal
in abruptio placentae, 642-643
in amniotic fluid embolism,
840-841
in disseminated intravascular
coagulation, 646-647
due to thrombophlebitis,
804-805, 859-860
related preeclampsia, 563-568,
581
related to deep venous
thrombosis, 804-805
related to expulsive efforts, 285
related to placenta previa,
636-637
related to position in labor, 279
neonatal
in preterm infant, 481
related to congenital
diaphragmatic hernia-
associated pulmonary
hypertension, 453
related to decreased cardiac
output, 429-432
related to polycythemia and
hypothermia in small-for-
gestational-age infant, 471
placental, impaired fetal gas
exchange related to, 192
Tobacco use, 760-762, 768-769
abruptio placentae and, 639
breastfeeding and, 404
hemorrhagic disorders and, 632
prematurity and, 472
Tobramycin sulfate as
environmental hazard, 211
Tobrex. *See* Tobramycin sulfate.
Tocolytic therapy, 739, 820-821
Tocotransducer monitoring of
contractions, 232, 306-307
TOF. *See* Tetralogy of Fallot.
Tonic neck reflex, 439
Tonus in physiology of
contractions, 230
TORCH, 592-599, 593t-597t,
622-623, 625

Torecan. *See* Thiethylperazine maleate.
Total parenteral nutrition for premature infant, 480
Total thyroxine, 677t
Total triiodothyronine, 677t
Touch
 analgesic effects of during childbirth, 279
 cultural factors in, 254
 sense of, neonatal, 441
Toxoplasmosis, 592-599, 593t-597t
TPN. *See* Total parenteral nutrition.
Tracheoesophageal fistula, embryonic development of, 50
Trandate. *See* Labetalol hydrochloride.
Tranquilizers for analgesia during childbirth, 278
Transcultural nursing, 75-76. *See Also* Ethnocultural considerations.
Transcutaneous electrical nerve stimulation, 278
Transdermal patch
 contraceptive, 413t
 nicotine, 215
Transducer, ultrasonographic, 167
Transfer, placental, 54-55, 55t
 disorders of, 55-56
Transferrin saturation, 803t
Transformation zone, cervical, 6
Transfusion
 in abruptio placentae, 642-643
 for anemia associated with respiratory distress syndrome, 504
 intrauterine, 179
 of platelets in HELLP syndrome, 561
Transient hypertension. *See* Gestational hypertension.
Transient tachypnea of newborn, 508-509
Transition phase of labor, 277
 emotions of, 256
Transitional milk, 389
Translocation of chromosomes, 27, 27f
Transport
 of bilirubin, 519
 placental, 54, 55t
 impaired, 69-70
Transposition of great arteries, 458-459, 459f
Transverse fetal presentation, 242, 244-245, 245f
Trauma, 703-726. *See Also* Injury.
 abdominal, abruptio placentae and, 639
 assessment of, 709-714, 715t
 birth
 macrosomia-associated, 248
 maternal diabetes mellitus and, 666
 related to malpresentation, 252
 case studies and study questions for, 723-725

Trauma (*Continued*)
 cause or mechanism of injury in, 708-709
 complications of, 709
 concepts for, 704
 diagnostic procedures for, 714-717
 gastrointestinal changes in, 706
 genitourinary changes in, 706, 707f
 health education regarding, 721-722, 722f
 hematologic changes in, 706
 incidence and epidemiology of, 703-704
 ineffective airway clearance related to, 717, 718f
 nursing diagnoses and interventions/outcomes for, 717-721, 718f, 720f
 pelvic changes in, 707
 physiologic considerations for, 704-705, 705f
 respiratory changes in, 706
 types of, 707
Traumatized nipples, 390
Trecator-SC. *See* Ethionamide.
Treponema pallidum, 602t
Triazolam as environmental hazard, 216
Tribavirin as environmental hazard, 211
2,4,5,-Trichlorophenoxyaceticacid, 204
Trichomonas, 602t
Trigeminy
 premature atrial contractions with, 323, 323f
 premature ventricle contractions with, 327f, 327-328
Triiodothyronine
 changes in normal pregnancy and thyroid disease, 677t
 normal nonpregnant values of, 17
Trimethadione as environmental hazard, 212
Triple marker test, 185-186
Trisomy, 26
Trisomy 18, triple marker test in, 186
Trophoblast, 42-43
Trophoblastic disease, gestational, 647-651, 653
True labor, assessment of, 231
Trunk incurvation reflex, 440
TSH. *See* Thyroid-stimulating hormone.
TTN. *See* Transient tachypnea of newborn.
Tubal ligation, bilateral, 412t
Tuberculosis, 617t, 788-789, 791-792, 793
 ethnic factors in, 95t
Tumor
 chorioadenoma destruens, 648, 650
 choriocarcinoma, 648-650
 ovarian, surgery for, 736-737
 uterine, labor passage and, 234
24-hour urine collection, 571
Twins. *See* Multiple gestation.

Twin-twin transfusion syndrome, fetal surgery for, 743
Type 1 diabetes mellitus, 661, 663-671
 altered metabolism in, 668-669
 anxiety related to, 669-670
 deficient knowledge regarding, 670
 definition and prognosis for, 663
 diagnostic procedures in, 668
 health education regarding, 695-696
 history in, 663-665
 hyperbilirubinemia and, 523
 incidence of, 663, 664t
 interrupted family processes related to, 671
 nursing diagnoses and interventions/outcomes for, 668-671
 physical findings in, 665-667
 powerlessness related to, 670
 psychosocial considerations in, 668
 risk for fetal injury in, 671
Type 2 diabetes mellitus, 661, 663-671
 altered metabolism in, 668-669
 anxiety related to, 669-670
 deficient knowledge regarding, 670
 definition and prognosis for, 663
 diagnostic procedures in, 668
 health education regarding, 695-696
 history in, 663-665
 incidence of, 663, 664t
 interrupted family processes related to, 671
 nursing diagnoses and interventions/outcomes for, 668-671
 physical findings in, 665-667
 powerlessness related to, 670
 psychosocial considerations in, 668
 risk for fetal injury in, 671
T-zone, cervical, 6

U
Ulcerative colitis, 807-811
Ultrasound
 in abruptio placentae, 641
 in antepartum fetal assessment, 167-171, 168t, 169f
 for calculation of due date, 111
 Doppler
 in fetal blood flow assessment, 174, 175f
 in fetal heart rate assessment, 305-306
 in estimation of gestational age, 162-163
 in fetal and placental assessment, 67
 following trauma in pregnancy, 716
 in formation of fetal death, 170, 836

Ultrasound (*Continued*)
gestational hypertension and, 569
for intrapartum assessment, 252
in multiple gestation, 832-833
in placenta previa, 635
in type 1 and type 2 diabetes mellitus, 665
use of at periodic prenatal visits, 115
Umbilical cord, 63-64
compression of
ineffective tissue perfusion related to, 826-827, 830
in postterm pregnancy, 826-827
embryonic development of, 43
ethnocultural factors regarding, 80, 81-82
hyperbilirubinemia associated with delayed clamping of, 524
inadequate perfusion of, risk for impaired fetal gas exchange related to, 335-336, 337b
velamentous insertion of, 64, 286, 287f, 635
Umbilical cord blood sampling, 178-181, 180f, 355-357, 356t
risk for deficient fluid volume related to, 192
Unconjugated bilirubin, 518
Underweight patient
body mass index values for, 103
weight gain during pregnancy for, 104
Undulating patterns in fetal heart rate, 317-319, 319f
interventions for, 330
Unilateral cleft lip and palate, 449f
Unknown
anxiety related to, 191
fear of, 136, 261
Unsaturated iron-binding capacity, 803t
Upright postures for labor and delivery, 238-239
Ureters, changes to during pregnancy, 99
Urethral meatus, 4
Urge-to-push method to facilitate fetal descent, 282
Uric acid, increased in preeclampsia, 564, 573t
Urinalysis
at first prenatal visit, 115
in renal disease, 783
Urinary elimination, impaired maternal
related to pressure of presenting part, 284-285
related to process of labor and delivery, 289
related to progression of labor, 279
in preterm infant, 481
Urinary retention, related to perineal trauma, 377
Urinary system
changes to during first stage of labor, 274
changes to during pregnancy, 99-100

Urinary system (*Continued*)
embryonic development of, 52
fetal development of, 57-58, 59, 60
postpartum assessment of, 376
postpartum changes in, 374
in preterm infant, 474, 481
trauma and, 706, 707f
Urinary tract infections, 611-614, 624, 626-627, 783, 855
Urine output
increased during pregnancy, 100
monitoring of in infant with respiratory distress syndrome, 507
postpartum assessment of, 376
Urine specific gravity
changes in during first stage of labor, 274
preeclampsia and, 564
Urofollitropin as environmental hazard, 215
Uropathy, obstructive, fetal surgery for, 744
Uterine contractions, 350f, 350-351, 351f
assessment of, 306-307
during active phase of labor, 275
for infant expulsion, 282
during latent phase of labor, 275
during transition phase of labor, 277
behaviors during, 258
Braxton Hicks, 97, 271-272
frequency of, 232
induction or augmentation of, 290-293, 291t
manual palpation of, 232
by patient, 824
monitoring of, 232
following traumatic injury, 716
risk of infection related to internal, 233
onset of, 228-229
pain resulting from, 280-281, 292
periodic fetal heart rate patterns associated with, 332-344
accelerations, 332-333, 333f
combined decelerations, 343f, 343-344
early decelerations, 342f, 342-343
late decelerations, 337-342, 338f, 339f, 341b
variable decelerations, 333-337, 334f, 335f, 337b
physiology of, 229f, 229-231
risk for situational low self-esteem related to ineffective pattern of, 233-234
strength of, 232-233
Uterus
anatomy of, 5-7, 7f
atony of, postpartum hemorrhage due to, 850
bicornuate, labor passage and, 234
changes to

Uterus (*Continued*)
postpartum, 371-372
during pregnancy, 96-97
Couvelaire, 641-642
examination of, 16
fibroids of, 13
in advanced maternal age, 154
injury to related to malpresentation, 252
involution of, 371-372
pain related to, 289
neoplasm of, labor passage and, 234
palpation for assessment of activity of, 305
penetrating trauma to, 709
postpartum assessment of, 376
postpartum infection of, 855
prolapse of, 15
rupture of, 841-844, 847
scarring of, hemorrhagic disorders and, 632
size and location of reflecting gestational age, 707f
small-for-gestational-age-infant and, 466
tocodynamometer for assessment of, 306-307
Utilitarianism-based approach to ethics, 875
UTIs. *See* Urinary tract infection.

V
Vacuum delivery, 284
Vagina
anatomy of, 5
changes to
postpartum, 372
during pregnancy, 97
examination of, 15
during active phase of labor, 276
cholecystectomy and, 736
for effacement and dilatation assessment, 240-241
in intrauterine fetal demise, 836
during labor and delivery, 251, 251f, 281
during latent phase of labor, 275
in postterm pregnancy, 825
risk of infection related to, after ROM, 281
postpartum infection of, 855
Vaginal birth after cesarean, 296
Vaginal bleeding
in advanced maternal age pregnancy, 154
due to placenta previa, 630-638
Vaginal discharge assessment during latent phase of labor, 275-276
Vaginal ring, 413t
Vaginosis, bacterial, 602t
prematurity and, 472
Valium. *See* Diazepam.
Valproic acid as environmental hazard, 213
Value system, ethics and, 873
Values, ethics and, 873

Valvular heart disease, 778-781
Variability of fetal heart rate,
        314-319, 316f, 317f, 318f, 319f
    fetal hypoxia and, 165
    interventions for, 329-331
Variable decelerations of fetal heart
        rate
    nonperiodic, 345-347, 346f
    periodic, 333-337, 334f, 335f, 337b
Varicella zoster, 615t
VAS. See Vibroacoustic stimulation.
Vasa previa, 64, 286-287, 635
Vascular resistance
    normal values in pregnancy, 574t
    renal disease and, 783
Vasectomy, 412t
Vasodilation, pregnancy and, 98
Vasodilators for maternal
        cardiovascular disease, 779t
Vasopressin, fetal heart rate and,
        309
Vasospasm
    arteriolar, in HELLP syndrome,
        561
    in development of preeclampsia,
        557-558, 563-568
VATERS syndrome, 64
VBAC. See Vaginal birth after
        cesarean.
Vegan vegetarian diet, 113
Vegetable intake during pregnancy,
        105
Vegetarian diet, 104, 105f, 113
Velamentous insertion of cord, 64,
        286, 287f, 635
Venous pressure, changes to during
        pregnancy, 98
Venous return, decreased, 778-781
Ventilation
    assisted
        bag and mask for newborn,
            425, 429
        in persistent pulmonary
            hypertension of newborn,
            516
    impaired
        in meconium aspiration
            syndrome, 513-515
        in persistent pulmonary
            hypertension of newborn,
            516-517
Ventral suspension in neonatal
        neurologic assessment,
        444b-445b
Ventricle, single, 459-460
Ventricular contractions, premature,
        326f, 326-328, 327f, 328f
Ventricular septal defect, 455-456,
        456f
Ventricular tachycardia, 331
Veracity, ethics and, 875
Verbal aggression, 542
Vertex presentation, 242, 283-284
Vestibule, 4
Viability of fetus, 163
    ultrasonographic assessment of,
        170
Vibroacoustic stimulation, 187-188
Vinyl chloride, 204

Violence
    intimate partner, 537-553
        assessment of, 544-546
        case study and study questions
            associated with, 551-552
        characteristics of abusers in,
            542-543, 543f
        characteristics of women in
            battering relationships,
            543-544
        cultural and socioeconomic
            factors in, 541-542
        cycle of violence in, 538-540,
            539f
        estimates of during pregnancy,
            538
        health education regarding, 550
        incidence of, 537-538
        resources for professionals
            regarding, 550
        types of injuries in, 540
    other-directed, postpartum, 864
Viral hepatitis, 811-814, 812t
Viramid. See Ribavirin.
Virtue character-based ethics, 875
Vision
    altered in preeclampsia, 565
    neonatal, 441
Vistaril. See Hydroxyzine.
Vital signs
    maternal
        assessment of during latent
            phase of labor, 275
        assessment of following
            traumatic injury, 712
        postpartum assessment of, 288,
            376
        postpartum changes in, 374
        surgery in pregnancy and, 733
    neonatal, 438
Vitamin A, requirements of during
        pregnancy, 106
Vitamin A analogues as
        environmental hazard, 215
Vitamin B
    deficiencies of, effect on fetus, 107
    requirements of during
        pregnancy, 106
Vitamin C, requirements of during
        pregnancy, 106
Vitamin D, calcium requirements
        during pregnancy and, 106
Vitamin E, requirements of during
        pregnancy, 107
Vitamin intake in pregnancy, 70,
        105-107
Vitamin K
    administration of in newborn, 426
    requirements of during
        pregnancy, 106
Volume expanders for neonatal
        resuscitation, 430t
Vomiting
    due to gastrointestinal disease,
        809-810
    hyperbilirubinemia-associated,
        525
    inflammatory bowel disease-
        associated, 808-809

VSD. See Ventricular septal defect.
Vulnerability, feeling of, during
        pregnancy, 126
Vulva
    anatomy of, 3-5, 4f
    changes to during pregnancy, 97
    postpartum infection of, 855

W
Waddle gait of pregnancy, 101
Warfarin
    as environmental hazard, 212
    for postpartum thrombophlebitis,
        860
Warmer, radiant, 423
Waste anesthetic gas, 207
Water
    intake of in gestational
        hypertension, 569
    loss of, insensible, in premature
        infant, 480, 481
WBCs. See White blood cell count.
WBCT. See Whole blood clotting
        time.
Weariness during labor and
        delivery, 257
Weight
    birth
        case studies and study
            questions associated with,
            492-494
        cigarette smoking and, 761
        health education regarding,
            490-491
        large-for-gestational-age,
            482-486
        in macrosomia, 246
        maternal diabetes mellitus and,
            666
        small-for-gestational-age,
            465-471
        transient tachypnea of
            newborn and, 508
    maternal
        in nutritional assessment,
            111t
        nutritional considerations
            during pregnancy and,
            103-104
    neonatal
        normal, 438
        tube size for intubation and,
            503
Weight gain
    neonatal, 460
        in persistent pulmonary
            hypertension of newborn,
            517
        in small-for-gestational-age
            infant, 471
    during pregnancy, 103-104, 119
        in adolescent, 148
        associated with gestational
            hypertension, 571
        diabetes mellitus and, 676
Weight loss, postpartum, 374, 382
Wet lung syndrome, 508-509
Wharton jelly, 64

White blood cell count
  appendectomy and, 739
  changes to during pregnancy, 99
    surgery and, 729
  in chorioamnionitis, 621
  during first stage of labor, 274
  in hyperbilirubinemia, 526
  postpartum, 374
  in premature rupture of
    membrane, 829
  preterm labor and, 820
  in TORCH, 598
White's classification of diabetes in
  pregnancy, modified, 663, 663t

Whole blood clotting time, 645
Withdrawal for contraception,
  414t
Witness, expectant father as, 128
Wound dehiscence, cesarean,
  postpartum infection following,
  856, 857
Wound infection, postpartum,
  855

X
Xanax. *See* Alprazolam.
X-linked inheritance, 30, 31f, 34

Z
Zaroxolyn. *See* Metolazone.
Zidovudine, 605
ZIFT. *See* Zygote intrafallopian
  transfer.
Zinc, requirements of during
  pregnancy, 107
Zona pellucida, 41, 43
Zygote intrafallopian transfer, 153